Respiratory Care
Patient Assessment & Care Plan Development

David C. Shelledy, PhD, RRT, RPFT, FAARC, FASAHP

Professor and Dean
School of Health Professions
The University of Texas Health Science Center
San Antonio, Texas

and

Dean Emeritus and Professor, Departments of Respiratory Care, Clinical
Sciences, and Health Systems Management
College of Health Sciences
Rush University
Rush University Medical Center
Chicago, Illinois

Jay I. Peters, MD

Professor and Chief, Division of Pulmonary and Critical Care Medicine
School of Medicine
The University of Texas Health Science Center
San Antonio, Texas

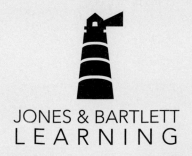

JONES & BARTLETT
LEARNING

World Headquarters
Jones & Bartlett Learning
5 Wall Street
Burlington, MA 01803
978-443-5000
info@jblearning.com
www.jblearning.com

Jones & Bartlett Learning books and products are available through most bookstores and online booksellers. To contact Jones & Bartlett Learning directly, call 800-832-0034, fax 978-443-8000, or visit our website, www.jblearning.com.

Substantial discounts on bulk quantities of Jones & Bartlett Learning publications are available to corporations, professional associations, and other qualified organizations. For details and specific discount information, contact the special sales department at Jones & Bartlett Learning via the above contact information or send an email to specialsales@jblearning.com.

7205-8

Production Credits

Chief Executive Officer: Ty Field
President: James Homer
Chief Product Officer: Eduardo Moura
VP, Executive Publisher: David Cella
Publisher: Cathy L. Esperti
Executive Editor: Rhonda Dearborn
Associate Editor: Kayla Dos Santos
Associate Editor: Sean Fabery
Associate Director of Production: Julie C. Bolduc
Production Manager: Tina Chen

Marketing Manager: Grace Richards
Art Development Editor: Joanna Lundeen
Art Development Assistant: Shannon Sheehan
VP, Manufacturing and Inventory Control: Therese Connell
Composition: Cenveo Publisher Services
Cover Design: Michael O'Donnell
Rights and Photo Research Coordinator: Ashley Dos Santos
Cover Image: © VikaSuh/ShutterStock, Inc.
Manufactured in the United States by RR Donnelley

Library of Congress Cataloging-in-Publication Data
Respiratory care (Shelledy)
  Respiratory care : patient assessment and care plan development / edited by David C. Shelledy, Jay I. Peters.
    p. ; cm.
  Includes bibliographical references and index.
  ISBN 978-1-4496-7244-7
  I. Shelledy, David C., editor.   II. Peters, Jay I., editor.   III. Title.
  [DNLM: 1. Respiratory Therapy—methods.   2. Diagnostic Techniques, Cardiovascular.   3. Diagnostic Techniques, Respiratory System.
4. Patient Care Planning.   5. Physical Examination—methods. WF 145]
  RC735.I5
  615.8'36—dc23
                          2014031648

6048

Printed in the United States of America
18 17 16 15   10 9 8 7 6 5 4 3

Dedication

To my wife, Maga, the light of my life, whose love and support makes this possible, and my daughter, Jennifer. I am very proud of you both.

—DCS

Dedicated to my wife, Jean, and my daughter, Emilee, who are my inspiration, and the support of my Pulmonary/Critical Care Medicine Division, who are truly my second family.

—JIP

Brief Contents

Contents

Preface

This book was created to provide students and clinicians concerned with the assessment and care of patients with cardiopulmonary disorders a comprehensive guide to patient evaluation and implementation of appropriate, evidence-based respiratory care plans.

The book has a natural flow. It begins by describing the purpose of patient assessment (Chapter 1) and methods associated with evidence-based practice. Critical diagnostic thinking is reviewed and then applied to the development and implementation of respiratory care plans (Chapter 2). The book then guides the reader through the review of existing data in the medical record (Chapter 3), the patient interview (Chapter 4), the physical assessment of the patient (Chapter 5), and the ordering and evaluation of the diagnostic studies needed.

Chapters 6 through 8 focus on the assessment of oxygenation, ventilation, and arterial blood gas sampling and interpretation. Chapter 9 reviews laboratory studies related to hematology, clinical chemistry, microbiology,

assessment of sputum, urinalysis, skin testing, histology and cytology, and molecular diagnostics. In Chapter 10, ECG monitoring and interpretation are discussed to include findings with specific cardiac disorders. Chapter 11 focuses on imaging techniques to include the chest radiograph, CT scan, MRI, and other imaging studies used in the evaluation of the respiratory care patient and includes the evaluation of imaging findings associated with specific pulmonary diseases. Pulmonary function testing is described in Chapter 12 to include the evaluation of patients with obstructive and restrictive disease. Chapter 13 details diagnostic bronchoscopy and other diagnostic studies. Acute and critical care monitoring, with a focus on the patient receiving mechanical ventilatory support, is covered in Chapter 14. Chapter 15 addresses the use of sleep studies in the evaluation of the cardiopulmonary patient. Last, but not least, Chapter 16 covers maternal and perinatal/neonatal patient assessment.

How to Use This Book

- **Clinical Focus:** The Clinical Focus exercises are designed to help the reader refine his or her critical-thinking and problem-solving skills. These serve as short case studies with problems for the reader to solve. They can be used for individual study, as course assignments, or as part of a robust class discussion.

CLINICAL FOCUS 14-1

Hypercapnic Respiratory Failure Secondary to Drug Overdose

A 21-year-old male found unresponsive at a public transportation bus stop v arrival, his vitals were heart rate 123 bpm, blood pressure 142/80 mm Hg, re Urine toxicology was performed and found positive for both cocaine and op room air showed pH of 7.15, $Paco_2$ 72 mm Hg, Pao_2 87 mm Hg, HCO_3^- 23.2

Clinical Assessment Questions

1. What is your initial impression of this clinical scenario?
   This patient was in acute ventilatory failure (hypercapnic respiratory f overdose.
2. What are the clinical, laboratory, or radiologic features associated with
   Blood gases typically show elevated $Paco_2$ and normal serum bicarbor with uncompensated respiratory acidosis (i.e., acute ventilatory failure 0.08 for every 10 mm Hg rise in $Paco_2$. For this patient, the $Paco_2$ has with a pH decrease of 0.24 (7.40 – 7.16 = 0.24), which correlates with 10 mm Hg rise in $Paco_2$. The hypercapnia and respiratory acidosis pre

---

- **RC Insights:** Interspersed throughout the text, RC Insights provide the clinician with useful tips on patient assessment and management.

RC Insights

Rule of 4 and 5

To estimate the effect of an increase in $Paco_2$ on Pao_2 in a patient breathing room air, use the Rule of 4 and 5. According to the Rule of 4 and 5, for each increase in $Paco_2$ of 4 mm Hg, the Pao_2 will decrease about 5 mm Hg (when breathing room air).

For example, in a patient breathing room air with a Pao_2 of 60 mm Hg, what would happen to the Pao_2 if the $Paco_2$ increased to 48 mm Hg?

- If the arterial $Paco_2$ increases from 40 to 48 mm Hg:
  - This is an increase of +8 mm Hg = 2 × 4 mm Hg
- Expect the Pao_2 to decrease to 2 × 5 mm Hg = 10 mm Hg:
  - Pao_2 = 60 – 10 = 50 mm Hg
  - The Pao_2 will decrease from 60 to 50 mm Hg.

- **Key Points:** Listed at the conclusion of each chapter, the Key Points provide a summary of the important facts and concepts that students should learn. It can be a helpful study tool.

Key Points

- ▶ Respiratory care patient assessment includes the history, physical examination, and diagnostic testing (laboratory tests and imaging studies).
- ▶ Patient assessment is needed to ensure that patients' problems are properly identified, prioritized, evaluated, and treated.
- ▶ Health may be defined as a person's overall mental, physical, and social well-being.
- ▶ The primary factors that determine health are individual genetic makeup; access to medical care; environmental factors (housing, work, school); and personal health-related behaviors, such as smoking, physical exercise, nutrition, and the use of drugs and alcohol.

- **NBRC 2015:** Integration of the content that will be needed to successfully pass the National Board for Respiratory Care entry level and advanced respiratory care examinations is included throughout (see also Appendix A). As such, this book will also be of great value to individuals preparing for the examinations administered by the National Board for Respiratory Care.
- A brief note on the use of abbreviations:

- *aka* is used in place of "also known as."
- *e.g.* is the abbreviation for the Latin phrase, exemplī grātia, which means "for example."
- *i.e.* comes from the Latin phrase *id est*, which means "that is" or "in other words."

Note from the Authors

Respiratory care may be defined as the healthcare discipline that specializes in the promotion of optimum cardiopulmonary function and health. It is specifically focused on the assessment, diagnostic evaluation, treatment, and care of patients with deficiencies and abnormalities of the cardiopulmonary system. Respiratory care clinicians must also attend to the prevention of cardiopulmonary disease and the management of patients with chronic disease. Thus, the scope of respiratory care extends to the patient, the patient's family, and public education. Respiratory care patient assessment and care plan development may be provided by physicians, advanced practice nurses, physician assistants, and respiratory therapists. Respiratory therapists apply scientific principles to prevent, identify, and treat acute or chronic dysfunction of the cardiopulmonary system. Although this book is primarily aimed at providing the advanced practice respiratory therapist with the knowledge and skills needed to perform patient assessment and develop appropriate respiratory care plans, we believe that the information contained will be of great value to those who prescribe respiratory care and for all healthcare practitioners interested in optimizing outcomes for patients with heart and lung disease. Throughout the text we use the term *respiratory care clinician* to refer to the healthcare practitioners who, as part of the interprofessional team, provide assessment, treatment, and care of patients suffering from heart and lung disorders.

It is our hope that this book will allow the reader to bridge the gap between patient assessment and treatment. Evidence-based practice and critical diagnostic thinking are applied to specific patient situations. The reader will learn how to apply assessment skills to the development, implementation, and evaluation of respiratory care plans. The text should also be of great value to individuals preparing for the examinations administered by the National Board for Respiratory Care.

David C. Shelledy, PhD, RRT, RPFT, FAARC, FASAHP
Jay I. Peters, MD

Acknowledgments

There are a number of people to thank for their contributions to the success of this project. We would like to thank all of the chapter authors whose hard work is demonstrated within these pages. We would also like thank everyone at Jones & Bartlett Learning who patiently assisted us in the process of developing an outstanding book. We would also offer our sincere thanks to the faculty and staff at Rush University, Rush University Medical Center, and the University of Texas Health Science Center. Without their support, this book would not have been possible. And last, but not least, we need to thank Caitlin Coffey for her help in preparing the manuscript.

Reviewers

Kira M. Anderson, MSA, RRT
Assistant Professor, Respiratory Therapy
Baptist College of Health Sciences
Memphis, Tennessee

Janie Castro-Rios, BS, RRT
Director of Clinical Care—Respiratory Care
Arkansas State University
Mountain Home, Arkansas

M. Marcia Fuller, MAE, RRT
Professor and Program Director of Respiratory Care
Bowling Green Technical College
Bowling Green, Kentucky

Rebecca A. Higdon, MS, RRT
Director of Clinical Education
Elizabethtown Community & Technical College
Elizabethtown, Kentucky

Denise I. Kruckenberg, RRT, MS
Program Director of Respiratory Care
College of DuPage
Glen Ellyn, Illinois

Cynthia McKinley, BAAS, RRT
Assistant Professor, Director of Clinical Education
Lamar Institute of Technology
Beaumont, Texas

Gwen Walden, RRT, NPS, CPFT
Program Director of Respiratory Care
Lamar Institute of Technology
Beaumont, Texas

Contributing Authors

Anisha Arora, MD
Pulmonary & Critical Care Medicine Fellow
University of Texas Health Science Center
San Antonio, Texas

Demetra Castillo, MAdEd, MLS (ASCP)
Assistant Professor, Department of Medical Laboratory
    Sciences
Rush University, Rush University Medical Center
Chicago, Illinois

Karla Diaz, MD
Pulmonary Fellow
University of Texas Health Science Center
San Antonio, Texas

Maribeth L. Flaws, PhD, SM (ASCP), SI
Acting Chairman and Associate Professor
Department of Medical Laboratory Science
Rush University, Rush University Medical Center
Chicago, Illinois

Keith R. Hirst, MS RRT-ACCS, NPS
Assistant Professor, Department of Respiratory Care
Rush University, Rush University Medical Center
Chicago, Illinois

Angela C. Hospenthal, MD
Faculty at Pulmonary/Sleep Medicine
University of Texas Health Science Center
Employed at South Texas Veterans Health Care System
San Antonio, Texas

Paul Ingmundson, PhD, FAASM
Clinical Professor, Department of Neurology
University of Texas Health Science Center
San Antonio, Texas

Kyle Jendral, MS-RC, RRT-ACCS
Department of Respiratory Care
Rush University, Rush University Medical Center
Chicago, Illinois

Ramandeep Kaur, MS, RRT
Department of Respiratory Care
Rush University, Rush University Medical Center
Chicago, Illinois

Maureen Koops, MD, FACP
Section Chief Endocrinology
Administration
South Texas Veterans Health Care
San Antonio, Texas

Adriel Malavé, MD
Assistant Professor
Pulmonary & Critical Care Medicine
University of Texas Health Science Center
San Antonio, Texas

Meggan McCarthy, PA-C
Northshore University Health System
Chicago, Illinois

Toni M. Podgorak, MS, RRT, NRP
Clinical Research Associate
Pharmaceutical Product Development
Charlotte, NC

Joan Radtke, MS, MLS (ASCP), SC
Assistant Professor, Department of Medical Laboratory
    Sciences
Rush University, Rush University Medical Center
Chicago, Illinois

J. Brady Scott, MS, RRT-ACCS
Assistant Professor, Department of Respiratory Care
Rush University, Rush University Medical Center
Chicago, Illinois

Viva Jo Siddall, MS, MS, RRT-ACCS
Medical Educator II Research Coordinator
Stritch School of Medicine
Loyola University
Chicago, Illinois

Lisa Tyler, MS, RRT-NPS, CPFT
Manager, Department of Respiratory Care
The Children's Hospital of Philadelphia
Philadelphia, Pennsylvania

**Laura P. Vasquez, MS, RVT (ARDMS),
    RT (R), MR, ARRT**
Associate Chair and Program Director
Department of Medical Physics and Advanced Imaging
Rush University, Rush University Medical Center
Chicago, Illinois

David L. Vines, MHS, RRT, FAARC
Chair and Program Director
Department of Respiratory Care
Rush University, Rush University Medical Center
Chicago, Illinois

Brian K. Walsh, MS, RRT-NPS, FAARC
Clinical Research Coordinator
Department of Anesthesia
Division of Critical Care Medicine
Boston Children's Hospital
Boston, Massachusetts

Joshua Wilson, MS, RRT
Department of Respiratory Care
Rush University, Rush University Medical Center
Chicago, Illinois

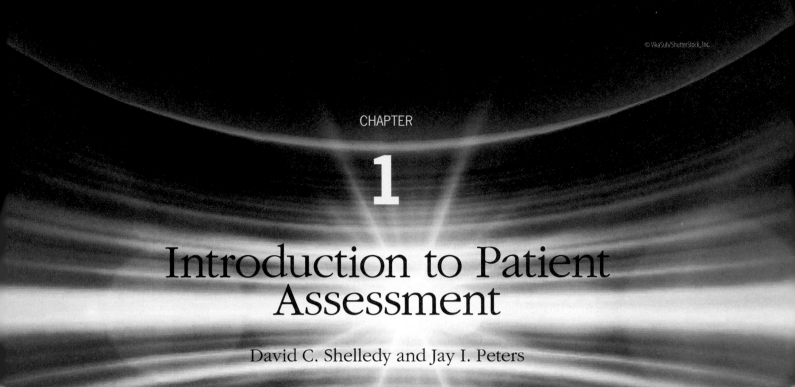

CHAPTER

1

Introduction to Patient Assessment

David C. Shelledy and Jay I. Peters

CHAPTER OUTLINE

Introduction to Patient Assessment
Rationale for Patient Assessment
Evidence-Based Practice
Critical Diagnostic Thinking in Respiratory Care
Typical Presentations of Common Respiratory Problems

CHAPTER OBJECTIVES

1. Explain the rationale for patient assessment.
2. Describe each of the components of a complete patient assessment (history, physical, laboratory tests, imaging studies, and other diagnostic tests).
3. Explain specific factors that affect health.
4. Describe each of the main drivers of the healthcare system (quality, access, and cost).
5. Describe the impact of misallocated care.
6. Describe evidence-based practice.
7. Evaluate sources of evidence.
8. Describe an approach to critical diagnostic thinking.
9. Describe the presentation of common respiratory disorders.

KEY TERMS

activities of daily living (ADL)
acute lung injury (ALI)
acute respiratory distress syndrome (ARDS)
arterial blood gases
asthma
case control
chronic bronchitis
cohort studies
chronic obstructive pulmonary disease (COPD)
critical thinking
emphysema

evidence-based practice (EBP)
health
health-related quality of life (HRQOL)
history
meta-analysis
misallocation
obstructive lung disease
patient outcomes
physical examination
pneumonia
pulmonary function testing (PFT)

randomized controlled trial (RCT)
restrictive lung disease

signs
symptoms

Overview

This chapter reviews the rationale for respiratory care patient assessment, provides an overview of health issues in the United States, describes evidence-based practice, and introduces the skills needed for critical diagnostic thinking and respiratory care plan development. Techniques for hypothesis formulation and evaluation to include identifying and gathering needed information and evaluation of patient problems are introduced. Typical presentations of common respiratory problems are reviewed.

Introduction to Patient Assessment

Physicians, nurses, and respiratory therapists are intimately involved in the diagnosis, treatment, care, and follow-up evaluation of patients with heart and lung problems. Modern healthcare demands that patients receive the right care at the right time and that unnecessary or inappropriate care be reduced or eliminated. In addition, care should promote patients' health and well-being and prevent, when possible, the development of acute and chronic disease. All of these goals demand excellent patient assessment skills.

Respiratory care patient assessment can be divided into three key areas: history, physical examination, and diagnostic testing (laboratory tests and imaging studies). Following initial assessment, hypotheses are formulated and evaluated regarding the patient's

1

problem(s) and the respiratory care plan is developed and implemented.

We begin the assessment process with the patient interview, or **history**. This is where we determine the patient's perceptions of his or her health problem(s), as well as what the patient is experiencing (i.e., **symptoms**). Special emphasis should be placed on noting the difference between the patient's baseline symptoms and current symptoms. We review the patient's past medical history, as well as factors that may affect health, such as smoking, drug and/or alcohol use, nutrition, weight, fitness, occupation, environmental exposures, and family health problems. The patient interview is the first and most important step in identifying the problem. The physical assessment follows and includes observation of the patient (inspection) and his or her level of comfort or distress, auscultation (listening), palpation (touching), and percussion (thumping). Vital signs (i.e., pulse, respirations, blood pressure, and temperature) are measured, and pulse oximetry may be used to assess arterial blood oxygen saturation (SpO_2). During the physical assessment, we look for the presence (or absence) of **signs** associated with specific disease states or conditions. The **physical examination** helps us clarify the patient's problem and guides us in gathering additional information.

Next, we consider diagnostic testing, including laboratory and imaging studies, to gather additional information and further clarify the patient's problem. Laboratory studies may include **arterial blood gases**, pulmonary function tests, blood chemistry, hematology, lipids, blood sugar, microbiology, and cardiac enzymes. Imaging studies may range from the standard chest radiograph to computed tomography (CT), magnetic resonance imaging (MRI), and diagnostic medical sonography (ultrasound).

Last, we begin to formulate and test hypotheses and develop a patient care plan. What do the history and physical suggest? Do the laboratory and imaging studies confirm or refute this hypothesis? What additional information is needed? What are our conclusions at this point? And how should we now treat the problems that have been identified?

Rationale for Patient Assessment

Health is not concerned merely with the absence of disease, but rather the person's overall mental, physical, and social well-being.[1] Modern healthcare should aim not only to treat acute and chronic disease, but to maximize patients' **health-related quality of life (HRQOL)**. Effective assessment skills are essential to ensure that patient problems are properly identified, prioritized, evaluated, and treated. Health promotion, disease prevention, and management of patients with chronic conditions also require strong assessment skills. Patient assessment is essential for evidence-based practice

and care plan development, and patient assessment is required to monitor and evaluate care delivery.

Factors That Affect Health

The factors that determine health include individual genetic makeup, access to medical care, environmental factors (housing, work, and school), and personal health-related behaviors (**Table 1-1**). Although genetics, the environment, and access to healthcare play important roles, much of the cost of healthcare in the

---

TABLE 1-1
Factors That Determine Individual Health

- **Genetic makeup**
- **Natural physical environment** (climate, housing, neighborhood, work, school)
  - ○ Housing factors that may affect health
    - Lead exposures
    - Mold, mites, and other allergens
    - Temperature extremes
    - Indoor air pollution
    - Injuries
    - Residential crowding
  - ○ Neighborhood conditions that may affect health
    - Physical conditions
    - Substandard housing
    - Poor air/water quality, exposure to hazardous substances
    - Crime and safety, safe places to exercise
    - Employment opportunities
    - Access to full-service grocery stores (presence of food deserts)
    - Schools, transportation and other municipal services
    - Social networks and social support
  - ○ Work
    - Exposure to hazardous materials
    - Physical activity
    - Pay, promotions, social support, job satisfaction, stress
    - Access to medical care
  - ○ School
    - Physical activity and nutrition
    - Environment
    - Access to medical care
  - ○ Environmental stress (work, home, other) impacts other health factors, such as
    - Alcohol and drug abuse
    - Mental health
    - Eating habits and obesity
    - Blood pressure and immune response
- **Healthcare services**
  - ○ Quality, access, and cost
  - ○ Acute care
  - ○ Preventative care
  - ○ Rehabilitation
  - ○ Chronic disease management
- **Health-related behaviors**
  - ○ Nutrition
  - ○ Smoking
  - ○ Drugs and alcohol
  - ○ Physical exercise

Adapted with permission from Center on Social Disparities in Health, University of California, San Francisco.

United States is associated with preventable illness due to smoking, obesity, lack of physical exercise, poor nutrition, and the use of drugs and alcohol. Projections place levels of obesity in the United States at 41% by 2015, with consequences for diabetes, heart disease, hypertension, cancer, **asthma**, and osteoarthritis.[2] Cigarette smoking is an important modifiable risk factor for adverse health outcomes, including cancer, **chronic obstructive pulmonary disease (COPD)**, heart disease, and stroke. Cigarette smoking prevalence among adults has decreased 42% since 1965, but declines in current smoking prevalence have slowed during the past 5 years.[3] Cigarette smoking among adults was slightly less than 20% in 2010 and has remained relatively constant. Cigarette use was highest among those with less than a high school education (28%), those with no health insurance (29%), those living below the federal poverty level (28%), and those aged 18 to 24 years (24%).[3] It is interesting to note that the top five leading causes of death in the United States (**Box 1-1**) are heart disease, cancer, chronic lower respiratory diseases (i.e., COPD), cerebrovascular disease (stroke), and accidents, all of which are impacted by personal health-related behaviors.[4]

Environmental factors that may directly affect health include housing, neighborhood of residence, work environment, and access to services near home (Table 1-1). Factors of special concern with respect to respiratory disease include exposure to air pollution, secondhand smoke, occupational dust and fumes, chemicals, pollen, mold, dust mite and cockroach allergens, animal dander, and other allergens and irritants. A complete patient assessment must include review of environmental factors and health-related behaviors that impact patients' health.

Cost, Access, and Quality

The three main drivers of the healthcare system are cost, access, and quality.

Cost

In 2010, the United States spent $2.6 trillion, or about 17% of its gross domestic product (GDP), on healthcare, and this amount is expected to nearly double by 2020.[5] The United States spends twice the European average for healthcare.[6] However, in spite of these expenditures, the United States does poorly in comparison to other industrialized nations (**Table 1-2**), ranking 42nd in life expectancy and 56th in infant mortality.[1]

It is interesting to note that half of the U.S. population spends little or nothing on healthcare, while 5% of the population spends almost half of the total amount.[6] A small number of conditions accounted for most of the growth in total healthcare spending between 1987 and 2000, with heart disease, pulmonary disorders, cancer, mental disorders, and trauma accounting for 31% of the cost.[6]

The U.S. population is aging, and older patients are responsible for higher healthcare costs. The elderly (age ≥ 65) made up around 13% of the U.S. population in 2002, but they accounted for 36% of personal healthcare expenses.[9] By 2020, one in five Americans (20%) will be older than 65 years of age.[7] Over half of the patients over age 65 in the United States have three or more chronic conditions, and patients with multiple chronic conditions cost up to seven times as much as patients with only one chronic condition.[7,8]

Patients with chronic disease have been estimated to account for 75% of overall healthcare spending.[2] Chronic cardiopulmonary conditions include asthma, **emphysema**, **chronic bronchitis**, COPD, combined asthma/COPD, bronchiectasis, cystic fibrosis, interstitial lung disease, chronic hypertension, coronary artery disease (CAD), and congestive heart failure (CHF). Approximately 34 million people were diagnosed with asthma in the United States in 2007, and over 13 million adults were diagnosed with COPD in 2008.[9,10] COPD is currently the third leading cause of death in the United States, and the actual number of COPD patients is probably over 24 million due to underdiagnosis.[4,10]

Inpatient hospital costs represent the largest portion of healthcare expenditures in the United States and average over $2,000 per patient day.[11,12] In 2005,

---

BOX 1-1

The 15 Leading Causes of Death in the United States

1. Diseases of the heart (myocardial infarcts or heart failure)
2. Malignant neoplasms (cancer)
3. Chronic lower respiratory diseases (COPD)
4. Cerebrovascular diseases (including stroke)
5. Accidents (unintentional injuries)
6. Alzheimer disease
7. Diabetes mellitus
8. Influenza and pneumonia
9. Nephritis, nephrotic syndrome, and nephrosis
10. Intentional self-harm (suicide)
11. Septicemia
12. Chronic liver disease and cirrhosis
13. Essential hypertension and hypertensive renal disease
14. Parkinson disease
15. Assault (homicide)

Reproduced from: Kochanek KD, Xu J, Murphy SL, Miniño AM, Kung HC. Deaths: preliminary data for 2009. *Natl Vital Stat Rep.* 2011;59(4).

TABLE 1-2
Health Outcomes by Country for Life Expectancy and Infant Mortality

Life Expectancy at Birth (years)	Infant Mortality (deaths/1000 live births)
1. Monaco (89.57)	1. Monaco (1.81)
2. Macau (84.48)	2. Japan (2.13)
3. Japan (84.46)	3. Bermuda (2.48)
4. Singapore (84.38)	4. Norway (2.48)
5. San Marino (83.18)	5. Singapore (2.53)
6. Hong Kong (82.78)	6. Sweden (2.60)
7. Andorra (82.65)	7. Czech Republic (2.63)
8. Switzerland (82.39)	8. Hong Kong (2.73)
9. Guernsey (82.39)	9. Macau (3.13)
10. Australia (82.07)	10. Iceland (3.15)
11. Italy (82.03)	11. France (3.31)
12. Sweden (81.89)	12. Italy (3.31)
13. Liechtenstein (81.68)	13. Spain (3.33)
14. Canada (81.67)	14. Finland (3.36)
15. France (81.66)	15. Anguilla (3.40)
16. Jersey (81.66)	16. Germany (3.46)
17. Norway (81.60)	17. Guernsey (3.47)
18. Spain (81.47)	18. Malta (3.59)
19. Israel (81.28)	19. Belarus (3.64)
20. Iceland (81.22)	20. Netherlands (3.66)
21. Anguilla (81.20)	21. Andorra (3.69)
22. Netherlands (81.12)	22. Switzerland (3.73)
23. Bermuda (81.04)	23. Ireland (3.74)
24. Cayman Islands (81.02)	24. Jersey (3.86)
25. Isle of Man (80.98)	25. Korea, South (3.93)
26. New Zealand (80.93)	26. Israel (3.98)
27. Ireland (80.56)	27. Slovenia (4.04)
28. Germany (80.44)	28. Denmark (4.10)
29. United Kingdom (80.42)	29. Austria (4.16)
30. Greece (80.30)	30. Isle of Man (4.17)
31. Saint Pierre & Miquelon (80.26)	31. Belgium (4.18)
32. Austria (80.17)	32. Luxembourg (4.28)
33. Malta (80.11)	33. Liechtenstein (4.33)

TABLE 1-2
Health Outcomes by Country for Life Expectancy and Infant Mortality (*continued*)

Life Expectancy at Birth (years)	Infant Mortality (deaths/1000 live births)
34. Faroe Islands (80.11)	34. European Union (4.43)
35. Luxembourg (80.01)	35. Australia (4.43)
36. Belgium (79.92)	36. United Kingdom (4.44)
37. European Union (79.86)	37. Portugal (4.48)
38. Taiwan (79.84)	38. Wallis and Futuna (4.49)
39. Korea, South (79.80)	39. Taiwan (4.49)
40. Virgin Islands (79.75)	40. San Marino (4.52)
41. Finland (79.69)	41. New Zealand (4.59)
42. **United States (79.56)**	42. Cuba (4.70)
43. Turks & Caicos Islands (79.55)	43. Canada (4.71)
44. Wallis & Futuna (79.42)	44. Greece (4.78)
45. Saint Helena, Ascension, & Tristan da Cunha (79.21)	45. French Polynesia (4.78)
46. Gibraltar (79.13)	46. Hungary (5.09)
47. Puerto Rico (79.09)	47. Slovakia (5.35)
48. Denmark (79.09)	48. New Caledonia (5.46)
49. Portugal (79.01)	49. Northern Mariana Islands (5.50)
50. Guam (78.82)	50. Guam (5.51)
51. Bahrain (78.58)	51. Faroe Islands (5.71)
52. Chile (78.44)	52. Bosnia and Herzegovina (5.84)
53. Qatar (78.38)	53. Croatia (5.87)
54. Cyprus (78.34)	54. Lithuania (6.00)
55. Czech Republic (78.31)	55. Serbia (6.16)
56. Panama (78.30)	56. **United States (6.17)**

Data from: Central Intelligence Agency. *The World Factbook*. May 2014 (2014 estimate). Available at: https://www.cia.gov/library/publications/the-world-factbook/rankorder/rankorderguide.html. Accessed May 7, 2014; United Nations Development Programme. *Human Development Reports*. Top 10 most highly developed countries based on the Human Development Index (HDI). Available at: http://hdr.undp.org/en/countries.

coronary artery bypass surgery to treat narrowed or obstructed arteries cost over $20,670 per patient in the United States, and a single hospital stay for **pneumonia** cost up to $15,829.[13,14]

A great deal of respiratory care is provided in the hospital setting, often in the intensive care unit (ICU). Mean ICU cost per patient in 2005 was about $32,000 for patients requiring mechanical ventilation and about $13,000 for those not requiring mechanical ventilation.[15] Interventions that reduce ICU length of stay and/or duration of mechanical ventilation could lead to substantial reductions in total inpatient costs.

Access

All of us want the best care possible for our patients. Unfortunately, not everyone has access to high-quality healthcare, and many people have little or no access to basic or preventative care. Healthcare disparities are of concern for patients with respiratory conditions. For example, African American men have the highest death rate and shortest survival of any racial or ethnic group in the United States for most cancers, including lung cancer.[16] Although health outcomes and life expectancy improve significantly with education and income, racial

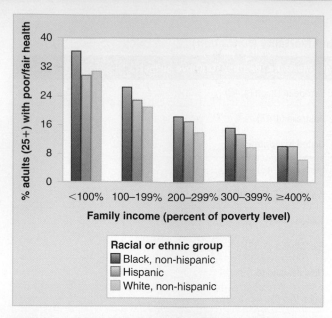

FIGURE 1-1 Racial and ethnic disparities at every income level.

Reproduced from: National Health Interview Survey (NHIS) 2001–2005. Age adjusted. Centers for Disease Control and Prevention.

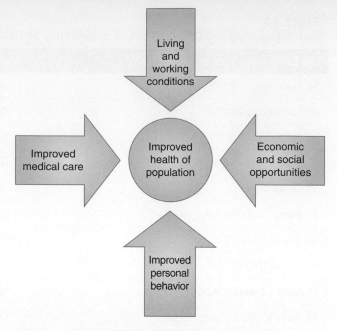

FIGURE 1-2 Conceptual framework for addressing healthcare disparities.

disparities persist at every income level (**Figure 1-1**).[17] The Agency for Healthcare Research and Quality (AHRQ) describes differences in health outcomes based on race/ethnicity, socioeconomic status (SES), insurance status, sex, sexual orientation, health literacy, and language.[18] Cardiopulmonary disease states or conditions that AHRQ has targeted as priorities for reduction in healthcare disparities include asthma, cystic fibrosis, CHF, CAD (ischemic heart disease, myocardial infarction), and hypertension.[18]

Figure 1-2 presents a conceptual framework for addressing healthcare disparities. It is thought that by improving economic and social opportunities, living and working conditions, medical care, and personal behaviors, healthcare disparities will be reduced, leading to improved population health.

Quality

It is clear that high healthcare expenditures may not result in better **patient outcomes**. Although the United States spends more on healthcare than any other industrialized country, measures of health and mortality are worse. In addition, studies point to major differences in healthcare expenses by geographic area within the United States, with no important differences in patient outcomes. One study found that patients in the higher spending areas received 60% more care, and that the increased care could not be attributed to levels of illness or socioeconomic status.[19] A major factor associated with increased cost was higher concentration of medical specialists in high-cost regions.[19]

In the presence of finite resources, should every patient receive all the care he or she prefers to receive, regardless of circumstances? This question gives rise to a number of ethical, moral, and practical dilemmas regarding the cost, quality, and accessibility of care. However, the need for strong assessment skills to help ensure that patients receive appropriate care in a cost-effective and efficient manner is evident.

Misallocation of Respiratory Care

It has been estimated that about 25% of all Medicare expenditures can be attributed to unnecessary variations in care.[2] Only 55% of adults receive recommended levels of general preventive care, and adults with a chronic illness receive only 56% of the care recommended by clinical practice guidelines.[20] **Misallocation** of care increases costs and may result in less than optimal health outcomes.

Respiratory care is not immune to misallocation. In a study of respiratory care in the acute care setting, we found that 25% of ordered basic respiratory care procedures were not indicated. In addition, as much as 32% of ordered aerosolized medications were not indicated, whereas about 12% of the patients assessed were not receiving respiratory care that was indicated. Others have estimated that the frequency of unnecessary respiratory care ranges from 20% to 60%.[21]

There are many reasons for the misallocation of care. Fear of lawsuits is sometimes suggested; however, it is likely that some care is provided simply because healthcare professionals believe it might help, probably won't hurt, and, as such, is low-risk. Medical students and physicians-in-training generally learn very little about respiratory care, and much of what doctors learn about how to care for respiratory patients is not evidence based.

Optimizing Patient Outcomes

In order to ensure that patients receive appropriate, cost-effective care, the respiratory clinician must be able to correctly identify and treat the patient's problem. Patient education, follow-up care, and rehabilitation, if needed, should be provided. Patients should be provided information regarding health promotion and disease prevention, in addition to smoking cessation interventions for smokers.

All of this requires excellent patient assessment skills to ensure that patients receive the right care at the right time and that unnecessary care is reduced or eliminated. Careful assessment of the patient's history, physical, and laboratory and imaging studies is required. The assessment is then followed by the development, implementation, and monitoring of an evidence-based respiratory care plan. The development and implementation of respiratory care plans using evidence-based clinical practice guidelines can reduce unnecessary care, optimize care delivered, and may reduce costs and improve outcomes. Chapter 2 describes the development, implementation, and evaluation of the respiratory care plan.

Evidence-Based Practice

Evidence-based practice (EBP) integrates research findings with clinical expertise and patient values to provide a structured approach to clinical decision making. By integrating the best available scientific evidence into the decision-making process, EBP has the potential to improve patient outcomes and reduce costs.[2] EBP can help tell us if a diagnostic test is accurate, how well the test differentiates between patients with and without a specific disease, and whether the test is appropriate to specific situations. EBP can be useful in predicting a patient's prognosis and is the preferred method for selecting treatment.

Sources of Evidence

EBP requires valid, research-based information about the causes, diagnosis, treatment, prognosis, and prevention of specific conditions. Clinical decisions should not be based solely on preferences or practice patterns. Textbooks may be out-of-date, inaccurate, or based on opinion rather than scientific evidence. EBP requires familiarity with the best evidence and knowledge of how to find it. Sources for EBP include published research reports in peer-reviewed journals, evidence-based systematic reviews (e.g., Cochrane systematic reviews), expert panel recommendations, and clinical practice guidelines. In order to become proficient at EBP, one must become familiar with various Internet-based tools, such as PubMed, Medline, Google Scholar, and the Cumulative Index to Nursing and Allied Health Literature (CINAHL). Evidence-Based Medical Reviews (EBMR) and the Cochrane Library provide additional evidence-based services (**Box 1-2**).

Types of Evidence

The best single source of evidence is the multicenter **randomized controlled trial (RCT)** in which a clear clinical benefit is demonstrated that outweighs the potential risks of the therapy or procedure. Multiple independent RCTs are sometimes combined using a statistical method called **meta-analysis**, and the resulting meta-analyses can provide strong evidence of the value of a particular treatment or technique. In the absence of multicenter RCTs or multiple independent RCTs, evidence from a single-center RCT may be used with caution. Other types of evidence, from best to least preferable, include results from nonrandomized, concurrent **cohort studies**, historic cohort studies, **case-control studies**, case series, case reports, editorials, and animal studies. The best-evidence pyramid is shown in **Figure 1-3**.

Grades of Recommendations for Therapy

In order to perform EBP, the practitioner begins with a series of questions related to diagnosis, treatment, prevention, or prognosis, which are outlined in **Box 1-3**. These questions are designed to help clarify the patient problem and the intervention or treatment being considered. Next, the treatment or comparison options (if any) and the outcomes sought are identified. Once the EPB questions have been answered, an EBP literature search is conducted, using search terms related to the problem, treatment (or technique), comparison, and desired outcomes. The literature search is normally conducted using an electronic database such as Medline or PubMed. The publications located are then evaluated, and the best available evidence is used to guide clinical decisions.

As we have noted, the strongest evidence sources are well-designed RCTs (sometimes combined via meta-analysis) in which the benefits are clear and outweigh the risks. Factors in evaluating the evidence include the study design, size of the treatment effect, patient selection and type of sample, and important outcomes. RCTs that have unclear or inconsistent results or flaws in methodology can sometimes still provide evidence of moderate quality. Other types of studies (e.g., cohort and case control designs, case series), as well as expert panel recommendations and systematic reviews, can also help guide clinical decision making. **Table 1-3** provides one method for rating evidence for grades of recommendations for therapy.

BOX 1-2

Online Resources for Evidence-Based Practice

- **PubMed.** PubMed is a comprehensive online database of peer-reviewed biomedical research papers, reviews, and journal articles (http://www.ncbi.nlm.nih.gov/pubmed/).
- **Medline.** Similar to PubMed, Medline is a comprehensive online database of peer-reviewed biomedical research papers, reviews, and journal articles. It is available through college and university library services via OVIDSP.
- **CINAHL (Cumulative Index to Nursing and Allied Health Literature).** CINAHL is a comprehensive online database of nursing and allied health journal publications. It may include articles not listed in other databases. CINAHL is available through college and university library services via EBSCO Publishing (http://www.ebscohost.com/cinahl/).
- **Google Scholar.** Google Scholar provides an effective search engine which includes an "Advanced Scholar Search" option. When used properly, recall and precision of Google Scholar is similar to PubMed. (http://scholar.google.com)
- **Cochrane Database of Systematic Reviews.** The Cochrane Collaboration (http://www.cochrane.org) and the Cochrane Library (http://www.thecochranelibrary.com/view/0/index.html) provide systematic reviews of the literature for use in evidence-based practice.
- **MD Consult.** This comprehensive medical information service for evidence-based practice is available through college and university library subscription services (http://www.mdconsult.com).
- **UpToDate.** This comprehensive medical information service for evidence-based practice is available through college and university library subscription services (http://www.uptodate.com/index).
- **Centers for Disease Control and Prevention (CDC).** The CDC offers a wealth of tools and resources on its website (http://cdc.gov).
- **National Institutes of Health (NIH).** The NIH is a valuable source of information on evidence-based medicine (http://www.nih.gov).

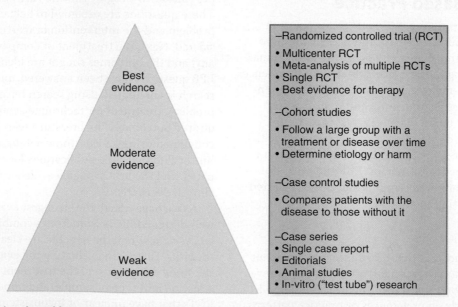

FIGURE 1-3 **Evaluating the evidence (critical appraisal) → best evidence pyramid.**

BOX 1-3

Use of Questions in Evidence-Based Practice

1. Patient problem or population
   - *What patient or problem is being considered?*
     - What is the patient's chief complaint or primary problem? Respiratory examples may include a patient's symptoms or primary disease state or condition:
       - Symptoms: Cough, sputum production, shortness of breath, wheezing, chest tightness, chest pain, other?
       - Disease states or conditions: Asthma "attack," COPD exacerbation, acute respiratory failure, chest trauma, other?
     - What is the larger patient population under consideration?
       - Asthma, COPD, pneumonia, acute lung injury, respiratory failure, ARDS, congestive heart failure (CHF), other?
2. Intervention
   - *What diagnostic method, treatment, medication, procedure or other intervention is being considered?*
     - The intervention is what you plan to do for the patient. Examples might include:
       - Diagnostic procedures (blood gases, pulmonary function testing, laboratory studies, imaging studies, other)
       - Drugs or medications (antimicrobial agents, bronchodilators, anti-inflammatory agents, cardiac drugs, other)
       - Respiratory care procedures (oxygen therapy, directed cough, lung-expansion therapy, bronchial hygiene techniques, other)
       - Mechanical ventilatory support (invasive or noninvasive)
3. Comparison
   - *What alternative treatments or interventions are being considered?*
     - Examples of comparisons for respiratory care might include:
       - Pulmonary rehabilitation versus home care in COPD
       - Peak flow versus symptom monitoring in moderate to severe asthma
       - Volume-control versus pressure-control modes of mechanical ventilation in ARDS
       - Rapid drug-susceptibility tests versus conventional culture-based methods for detection of multi-drug-resistant tuberculosis
     - In some cases, there may not be an alternative treatment or therapy under consideration.
4. Outcome
   - *What outcomes are sought?*
     - Diagnosing a condition
     - Relieving or eliminating specific symptoms
     - Stopping or reversing a pathologic process
     - Improving or maintaining function
     - Prevention
5. Searching the literature
   - *The next step is to define the search terms and perform a literature review:*
     - Search terms should include the problem, intervention, and comparison (if there is to be a comparison).
     - Examples might include:
       - Noninvasive ventilation and COPD
       - Drug treatment and ARDS
       - Medications and acute asthma exacerbation
       - Antibiotics and ventilator-acquired pneumonia
       - Weaning method(s) and mechanical ventilation in ARDS patients

- ◦ The examples of preferred sources for the literature search are:
  - Medline
  - PubMed
  - Established clinical practice guidelines and expert panel reviews
  - Google Scholar
6. Evaluating the evidence (critical appraisal)
   - Following the literature search, the respiratory clinician must evaluate the evidence located. The best evidence sources are well-designed, multicenter RCTs or multiple independent RCTs (sometimes combined via meta-analysis) in which the benefits are clear and outweigh the risks. Factors in evaluating the evidence include the study design, size of the treatment effect, patient selection and type of sample, the importance of the outcomes, cost, and patient values and preferences. RCTs that have unclear or inconsistent results or flaws in methodology can sometimes still provide evidence of moderate quality. Other types of studies (cohort and case-control designs, case series), as well as expert-panel recommendations, can also help guide clinical decision making.
7. Applying the evidence to patient care
   - The clinician must make decisions regarding diagnosis, treatment, prevention, and/or prognosis based on the evidence. Clinical decision should balance potential benefit and harm, cost, as well as patient preferences and values.

TABLE 1-3
Rating the Evidence for Recommendations of Therapy

A number of rating systems have been developed to assess the strength of the evidence for evidence-based practice. The following system evaluates the strength of the recommendation and the quality of the evidence:

Strength of the Recommendation

Level	Strength	Description
1	Stronger	Benefits clearly outweigh the risks and burdens (or vice versa) for nearly all patients.
2	Weaker	Risks and benefits are more closely balanced or are more uncertain.

Quality of the Evidence

Grade	Quality	Description
A	High	Well-performed randomized controlled trials or overwhelming evidence of some other sort. Further research is very unlikely to change our confidence in the estimate of the effect.
B	Moderate	Randomized controlled trials that are less consistent, have flaws, or are indirect in some way to the issue being graded, or very strong evidence of some other sort. Further research is likely to have an important impact on our confidence in the estimate of effect and may change the estimate.
C	Low	Low observational evidence (from observational studies, case series, or clinical experience), or evidence from controlled trials with serious flaws. Further research is very likely to have an important impact on our confidence in the estimate of effect and is likely to change the estimate.
D	Very Low	Any estimate of effect is uncertain.

Reproduced from: Restrepo, RD. AARC Clinical Practice Guideline: From "reference-based" to "evidence-based." *Respir Care.* 2010;55(6):787–789.

Following review of the evidence, the clinician must make decisions regarding diagnosis, treatment, prevention, and/or prognosis. Clinical decisions should balance potential benefit and harm and costs, as well as patient preferences and values.

Critical Diagnostic Thinking in Respiratory Care

Critical-thinking skills needed by respiratory clinicians include the ability to interpret, analyze, and evaluate data; make clinical inferences; and provide explanations.[22] Respiratory clinicians need to be able to prioritize, anticipate, troubleshoot, communicate, negotiate, make decisions, and reflect on experiences.[22] **Critical thinking** is used in establishing the patient's diagnosis and requires the integration of many different pieces of assessment information derived from the medical record, patient history, physical examination, laboratory tests, and imaging studies and from familiarity with the presentation of various disease states and conditions.

Approach to Hypothesis Formulation and Evaluation

Critical thinking to establish the patient's diagnosis should include the key elements of the scientific method.[23] These key elements or steps are:

1. Identify the problem.
2. Gather additional information to clarify the problem.
3. Formulate possible explanations (hypothesis formulation).
4. Test possible explanations (hypothesis testing).
5. Formulate and implement solutions.
6. Monitor and reevaluate.

Identify the Problem

The first step in making a diagnosis is to identify the patient's problem or chief complaint. The classic question, "Why are you here?" is often a good way to identify the problem from the patient's perspective. For respiratory patients, common complaints include acute or chronic cough, sputum production, shortness of breath (acute or chronic), wheezing, whistling, chest tightness, chest pain or discomfort, and hemoptysis (expectorating blood tinged or bloody sputum). Hoarseness, fever, and night sweats are also not uncommon. The time course of symptoms—acute (hours to days), subacute (days to a couple of weeks), or chronic (several weeks to months)—is often helpful in establishing a diagnosis. **Clinical Focus 1-1** lists common problems seen in respiratory care patients.

Gather Additional Information to Clarify the Problem

Following a review of the existing medical record, the respiratory clinician should complete a detailed patient history and perform a thorough physical examination to further identify and clarify the patient's problem(s). The existing medical record review should include patient demographics, previous physician's orders, results of previous history and physical examinations, laboratory and/or imaging reports, and progress notes and reports of procedures. The review of existing medical records is described in Chapter 3.

The patient interview should include the history of the present illness, past medical history, family history, current medications, smoking history, environmental data, and occupational history. The patient should be questioned in more detail regarding specific symptoms associated with pulmonary disease to include cough, sputum production, hemoptysis, dyspnea, and chest pain. The taking of a detailed patient history is discussed in Chapter 4.

The physical examination should include assessment of the patient's general appearance; mental state (anxiety, restlessness, distress) and level of consciousness (alert and awake, sleepy, somnolent); vital signs (pulse, respirations, blood pressure, temperature); skin color, mucosa characteristics, and nail beds (cyanosis); perfusion and capillary refill; and presence of pursed-lip breathing. The chest examination should include inspection, palpation, auscultation, and percussion. Inspection of the chest should include respiratory rate, depth, and pattern; retractions, accessory muscle use, or paradoxical motion of the chest and abdomen; AP (anteroposterior) diameter; and presence of deformity. Palpation should assess for tracheal deviation, chest expansion, vocal fremitus, chest wall tenderness, and subcutaneous emphysema. Percussion should note resonance, hyperresonance, or dullness. Auscultation should include assessment for normal and adventitious (abnormal) breath sounds, including crackles, gurgles, wheezes, rubs, stridor, and bronchial breath sounds over the periphery.

Knowledge of the patient's problem or chief complaint can help guide the physical examination in order to provide evidence to support, reject, or revise specific hypotheses as to the cause of the problem. The physical examination may also identify additional problems such as changes in vital signs, increased work of breathing, abnormal breath sounds, or alterations in mental status. The physical examination is described in Chapter 5.

CLINICAL FOCUS 1-1

Common Respiratory Care–Related History and Physical Findings

Symptoms

Acute or chronic cough
Acute or chronic sputum production
Anxiety, nervousness, excitement, or restlessness
Blurred vision
Chest pain (substernal, pleuritic, musculoskeletal)
  or discomfort
Dizziness, fainting
Fever, chills
Headache
Hemoptysis (expectorating blood tinged or bloody
  sputum)

Hoarseness, sore throat
Night sweats
Palpitations
Sinus pain, runny nose, sneezing, postnasal drip
Shortness of breath (acute or chronic dyspnea,
  orthopnea)
Sleep disturbances
Tremors
Tingling (extremities)
Weight loss, loss of appetite

Signs

Abnormal mental state (confusion, disorientation,
  hallucinations, loss of consciousness, lethargy,
  somnolence, coma)
Blood pressure (hypertension, hypotension)
Abnormal breaths sounds (diminished, crackles,
  gurgles, wheeze, rubs, bronchial breath sounds,
  stridor, egophony)

Heart rate abnormalities (tachycardia, bradycardia)
Skin (pale, cold, clammy, sweating, cyanosis, rash,
  redness)
Seizures, convulsions
Ventilatory disorders (tachypnea; hyperventilation;
  slowed, irregular respirations)

Formulate Possible Explanations (Hypothesis Formulation)

Following identification and clarification of the patient's problem, the next step is formulating possible explanations or hypotheses as to the cause of the problem. Each symptom and sign identified during the history and physical examination is listed, along with more common and less common possible explanations or causes for this sign or symptom. Based on the review of the existing medical records and history and physical examination, a leading, or differential, diagnosis is proposed. Table 1-4 describes the more common and less common causes of typical respiratory care assessment findings.[23] The possible causes or explanations for each sign or symptom identified by the patient assessment provide the hypotheses that then need to be tested.

Test Possible Explanations (Hypothesis Testing)

Following a review of the patient's problems and the more common and less common causes for each, a primary or leading hypothesis as to the cause of the problem is developed. This hypothesis, also known as the leading or differential diagnosis, is then tested via

additional laboratory and imaging studies. These studies may include oximetry, arterial blood gas analysis, **pulmonary function testing (PFT)**, sputum analysis, blood tests to include hematology and blood chemistry, other microbiologic studies, skin tests, and various stains, swabs, and molecular medicine techniques. An electrocardiogram (ECG) may be performed to assess cardiac function, and ECG monitoring is often done in the ICU setting. Imaging studies may include a chest radiograph, CT scan, MRI, and/or ultrasound imaging. Diagnostic bronchoscopy and other diagnostic procedures (e.g., thoracentesis, open lung biopsy) may be also be required. Sleep studies may be needed to evaluate sleep-disordered breathing, and exercise stress testing may be used to evaluate pulmonary and cardiac disease.

Chapters 6 and 7 will discuss assessment of oxygenation and ventilation. Chapter 8 will describe arterial blood gas analysis and acid–base balance. Chapter 9 will describe laboratory studies, including hematology, clinical chemistry, microbiology, sputum examination, urine analysis, skin testing, histology and cytology, and molecular diagnostics. Chapter 10 will discuss the ECG. Chapter 11 will review imaging studies. Chapter 12 will review pulmonary function testing. Chapter 13

TABLE 1-4
Common and Less-Common Causes of Respiratory Care Assessment Findings

Problem	Common Causes	Less-Common Causes
Acute cough	Viral upper respiratory infection (pharyngitis, rhinitis, tracheobronchitis, serous otitis) Bacterial infection (tracheobronchitis, acute bronchitis, mycoplasma, pneumonia, ear infection, sinusitis, abscess) Asthma Sinusitis Gastroesophageal reflux Congestive heart failure, pulmonary edema Inhalation of irritants (smog, smoke fumes, dusts, cold air) Bronchiolitis (RSV)	Tumor, neoplasm Pulmonary emboli Aspiration (foreign body, liquid) Laryngitis ACE inhibitor medication Pleural disease Diaphragm irritation Mediastinal disease Extrabronchial lesions Fungal lung disease Ornithosis
Chronic cough	Postnasal drip (sinusitis, allergic rhinitis) Smoking Asthma Chronic bronchitis Gastroesophageal reflux Congestive heart failure ACE inhibitor medication (20%) HIV Bronchiectasis Neoplasms, bronchogenic carcinoma Lung abscess Recurrent aspiration Aspiration (foreign body, liquid) Mycoplasma pneumonia Pulmonary tuberculosis Pulmonary fibrosis Cystic fibrosis	Chronic pulmonary edema Mitral stenosis Laryngeal inflammation or tumor Fungal pneumonia External or middle ear disease Bronchogenic cyst Mediastinal mass Zenker's diverticulum Aortic aneurysm Vagal irritation Pacemaker wires Pleural disease Pericardial, mediastinal, or diaphragm irritation Psychogenic cough
Acute dyspnea	Acute asthma (intermittent dyspnea) COPD exacerbation (chronic bronchitis, emphysema) Tracheobronchitis Pneumonia or other parenchymal inflammation Left-side CHF Pulmonary edema (acute) Acute pulmonary emboli Myocardial ischemia (coronary artery disease, acute or chronic) Pneumothorax Hyperventilation (anxiety, metabolic acidosis) Hypoxemia Large pleural effusion Upper airway obstruction (stridor, croup, epiglottis, laryngitis, laryngeal edema, foreign body aspiration) Noncardiogenic pulmonary edema Aspiration (gastric liquid, foreign body) Atelectasis Chest trauma (pulmonary contusions, rib fractures, flail chest) Acutely increased work of breathing (decreased compliance and/or increased resistance) Shock Neuromuscular disease	Pulmonary hypertension Fever Anemia Pericardial tamponade Lung cancer Diaphragmatic paralysis Inhalation of noxious fumes or gases Space-occupying lesions of the thorax Anaphylaxis Botulism Increased intracranial pressure
Chronic dyspnea (intermittent or persistent)	COPD (chronic bronchitis, emphysema, cystic fibrosis) CHF Asthma Interstitial fibrosis Hypoxemia Pulmonary hypertension Neuromuscular disease	Pulmonary alveolar proteinosis Alveolar microlithiasis Lipoid pneumonia Lung resection Recurrent pulmonary emboli Lung cancer Persistent large pleural effusion

(continues)

TABLE 1-4
Common and Less-Common Causes of Respiratory Care Assessment Findings (*continued*)

Problem	Common Causes	Less-Common Causes
	Poor physical conditioning with obesity Anemia Ascites Metabolic acidosis Aortic or mitral valve stenosis Arterial hypertension Chronically increased work of breathing (decreased compliance and/or increased resistance) Neuromuscular disease Bronchiectasis	Kyphoscoliosis Tracheal stenosis Mitral stenosis Abdominal mass Pregnancy Congenital heart disease Abnormal hemoglobin Thyroid disease Idiopathic pulmonary hemosiderosis Aortic or mitral valve stenosis or regurgitation
Acute sputum production	Viral infection (tracheobronchitis, bronchiolitis, pneumonia) Bacterial infection (tracheobronchitis, pneumonia) Mycoplasma pneumonia Lung abscess Asthma Inhalation of irritants (smoke, smog, dusts, fumes)	Tuberculosis Lung abscess Neoplasms, lung tumor Foreign body aspiration
Chronic sputum production	COPD (chronic bronchitis, cystic fibrosis) Cigarette smoking Asthma Chronic sinusitis with drainage	Bronchiectasis Tuberculosis Lung abscess Bronchopleural fistula with empyema Recurrent aspiration
Hemoptysis	Bronchitis (acute and chronic) Bronchiectasis Lung abscess Tuberculosis Pneumonia (includes necrotizing pneumonias) Neoplasms, bronchogenic carcinoma Pulmonary embolism, pulmonary infarction Cystic fibrosis Congestive heart failure	Trauma Fungal lung disease (includes allergic bronchopulmonary aspergillosis) Empyema Aspiration (foreign body) Inhalation of toxic gases Arteriovenous fistula Broncholithiasis Goodpasture syndrome Idiopathic pulmonary hemosiderosis Mycetoma Parasitic infection Wegener's granulomatosis Bronchogenic cyst Pulmonary endometriosis (catamenial hemoptysis) Anticoagulation
Pleuritic or chest wall pain	Pleuritis (viral/collagen vascular disease) Pneumonia Pulmonary embolism Empyema Tuberculosis Trauma Rib fracture Pneumothorax Hemothorax	Pulmonary infarction Irritation of intercostal nerves (herpes zoster, spinal nerve root disease) Costochondritis Irritation of the diaphragm
Visceral chest pain	Tumor, neoplasm of major bronchi, mediastinum Abnormalities of the heart, aorta, pericardium Esophageal pain (reflux, tumor) Acute bronchitis	Peptic ulcer Cocaine use Cholecystitis
Substernal pain	Myocardial ischemia, angina pectoris Myocardial infarction Esophagitis, esophageal pain Arrthymias Myocarditis Pericarditis	Dissecting aortic aneurysm Congenital cardiovascular anomalies Aortic stenosis Mitral regurgitation Mitral valve prolapse Psychogenic chest pain

This article was published in Stoller JK, Bakow ED, Longworth DL, eds. *Critical Diagnostic Thinking in Respiratory Care: A Case-Based Approach*; Shelledy D, Stoller JK. An introduction to critical diagnostic thinking, Pages 3–38, Copyright WB Saunders 2002.

will review diagnostic bronchoscopy, thoracentesis, and open lung biopsy. Chapter 14 will describe acute and critical care monitoring and assessment. Chapter 15 will review sleep studies.

It is important to consider all available information from the patient history, physical examination, and laboratory and imaging studies before coming to a final conclusion about the patient's problem or diagnosis. Review of the available medical records can be enormously helpful, and additional laboratory and imaging studies should be limited to those needed to refine the diagnosis and optimize the patient's care. Confirmation or rejection of the primary hypothesis is then dependent on the results of additional diagnostic tests and laboratory studies.

Formulate and Implement Solutions

Based on the findings from the patient history, physical, laboratory and imaging studies, and medical records, the patient's diagnosis is confirmed and the respiratory care plan is designed and implemented. The respiratory care plan may include oxygen and/or humidity therapy, aerosol medication administration, lung expansion therapy, chest physiotherapy, and other techniques for secretion management, airway care, and/or mechanical ventilatory support. Medical treatment may include administration of anti-infective agents, anti-inflammatory agents, diuretics, cardiovascular medications, and other pharmacologic agents. Procedures may include physical therapy and rehabilitation techniques such as diet and exercise and, in some cases, surgical interventions. The development and implementation of the respiratory care plan is discussed in Chapter 2.

Monitor and Reevaluate

Following the establishment of the patient's diagnosis and development and implementation of the respiratory care plan, the patient is monitored and reevaluated. The respiratory clinician assesses the patient for improvement (or deterioration) in his or her condition and the possible development of new problems that may require further evaluation and treatment. Significant changes in vital signs are especially important and should always lead to reevaluation.

Response to therapy is an important aspect of patient assessment. For example, reversible bronchospasm, as demonstrated by a reduction in wheezing and improvement in PFT expiratory flow rates (PEFR, FEV_1) following bronchodilator therapy, provides additional evidence for a diagnosis of reversible airways disease (asthma and some patients with COPD). Improvement in oxygenation in hypoxemic patients following administration of low to moderate concentrations of oxygen therapy (24% to 40%) is associated with pulmonary

disorders with low lung ventilation to perfusion ratios (low $\dot{V}/\dot{Q}$). Examples of conditions in which hypoxemia may be caused by low $\dot{V}/\dot{Q}$ include asthma, chronic bronchitis, emphysema, bronchiectasis, cystic fibrosis, and CHF. Conditions that may require high concentrations of oxygen in order to reverse hypoxemia are associated with intrapulmonary shunting and include atelectasis, severe pneumonia, **acute lung injury (ALI)**, and **acute respiratory distress syndrome (ARDS)**. Thus, response to oxygen therapy can help support (or refute) a specific patient diagnosis.

Common mistakes in clinical problem solving include failure to consider possible causes that should be considered, consideration of only exotic or uncommon diseases, failure to consider that two or more problems may coexist, and inadequate information gathering and processing. Sometimes a diagnosis has been assigned to a patient without adequately considering alternative explanations. For example, a known COPD patient may suffer from a myocardial infarction (MI) and come to the emergency department. By mislabeling the patient as suffering from acute exacerbation of COPD, a potentially catastrophic outcome could result. Any diagnosis should be considered as provisional until confirmed by all of the evidence, including appropriate response to therapy. **Clinical Focus 1-2** provides an example of clinical problem solving.

Typical Presentations of Common Respiratory Disorders

Common respiratory disorders include **restrictive lung disease**, **obstructive lung disease**, and problems of oxygenation and ventilation. Obstructive disorders are associated with a decrease in PFT expiratory flow rates (FEV_1, $FEV_{25-75\%}$, PEF) and include asthma, chronic bronchitis, emphysema, combined/COPD, bronchiectasis, and cystic fibrosis. Because patients have trouble getting air out of the lungs, the FEV_1/FVC ratio is reduced. Restrictive disorders are associated with a decreased ability to take a deep breath in, as indicated by a reduced inspiratory capacity (IC), vital capacity (VC), and total lung capacity (TLC) as assessed by PFT. Acute restrictive problems include pneumonia, atelectasis, ALI, ARDS, pleural effusion, pneumothorax, and pulmonary edema associated with CHF. Chronic restrictive disorders include pulmonary fibrosis, lung cancer, thoracic deformity, neuromuscular weakness, and obesity. Both restrictive and obstructive disorders can lead to problems with oxygenation and ventilation. Other common respiratory care–related problems often seen in the acute care setting that may affect oxygenation and or ventilation are listed in **Clinical Focus 1-3**. Typical presentations of common respiratory disease states and conditions are described in **Table 1-5**.

CLINICAL FOCUS 1-2

Clinical Problem Solving

Identify the Problem

Mr. Smith, a 56-year-old male patient, presents to the emergency department (ED) with complaints of increasing shortness of breath *(dyspnea)*, difficulty breathing in the supine (flat) position *(orthopnea)*, and a history of *chronic cough* with *increasing sputum production.*

Gather Additional Information to Clarify the Problem

Upon *interview,* Mr. Smith indicates he has had a recent change in the color, consistency, and volume of sputum production and worsening ability to perform **activities of daily living (ADL)** due to increasing shortness of breath. Mr. Smith has an extensive smoking history (two packs a day for 20 years, or 40 pack-years) as well as chronic cough with over a tablespoon per day of generally clear sputum produced. The cough with sputum production has been present most days for over 2 consecutive years. Sputum production has increased over the last several days and is now purulent (containing pus). Current medications include use of an albuterol (a bronchodilator) inhaler at home.

On *physical examination*, Mr. Smith has an increased AP diameter of the chest, accessory muscle use on inspiration, and diminished breath sounds with a prolonged expiratory phase, along with crackles and bronchial breath sounds. Vital signs include an increased heart rate (pulse = 115, tachycardia), increased respiratory rate (f = 26, tachypnea), and elevated temperature. Pulse oximetry indicates a reduced arterial oxygen saturation (Spo_2 = 82%) while breathing room air. Together, the symptoms and signs identified on history and physical exam make up the patient's problem list.

Formulate Possible Explanations (Hypothesis Formulation)

Mr. Smith's findings so far can be summarized as follows:
- History findings are associated with a chronic respiratory problem:
  - Chronic cough with sputum production
  - Decreased ability to perform ADLs
  - Smoking history of 40 pack years
  - Home use of inhaled medications (albuterol inhaler)
- Physical examination findings are associated with acute distress:
  - Tachypnea, accessory muscle, and tachycardia.
  - Increasing dyspnea, orthopnea.
  - Diminished breath sounds indicate decreased air movement and a prolonged expiratory phase is associated with air trapping.
  - Crackles upon auscultation are associated with alveolar fluid or, in some cases, fibrosis.
  - Bronchial breath sounds heard over the periphery of the chest are associated with consolidation.
  - Increased chest diameter is associated with overinflation of the lungs.
  - Reduced Spo_2 on room air indicates hypoxemia.

Common causes for these findings include *chronic bronchitis, bronchiectasis,* and *acute exacerbation of COPD.* Acute exacerbation of COPD can be precipitated by increased air pollution, upper respiratory tract infection, flu virus, bacterial infection, or pneumonia.

Test Possible Explanations (Hypothesis Testing)

Mr. Smith presents with increasing dyspnea, tachypnea, tachycardia, reduced Spo_2, accessory muscle use, and chronic cough with recently increased purulent sputum production. These findings, along with a significant smoking history, increased AP chest diameter, abnormal breath sounds, and prolonged expiratory phase suggest that Mr. Smith is likely suffering from an *acute exacerbation of COPD*; however, other acute and chronic pulmonary problems will need to be ruled out.

Common causes of acute exacerbation of COPD include viruses, bacteria, and possibly air pollution. Rhinovirus (common cold virus), respiratory syncytial virus (RSV), influenza, parainfluenza, adenovirus, and bacterial infection have all been associated with COPD exacerbation. Consequently, an upper respiratory tract infection, the common cold or flu, and possible development of pneumonia will need to be considered. Laboratory and imaging studies that should be considered include *arterial blood gas analysis, complete blood count (CBC), blood chemistry,* and *chest radiograph* to test our hypothesis that the patient is suffering from an acute exacerbation of COPD. *Pulmonary function testing* should also be performed when the patient has recovered in order to document the presence and severity of COPD.

Formulate and Implement Solutions

Mr. Smith's history, physical examination, and vital signs are consistent with acute exacerbation of COPD. Arterial blood gases while breathing room air show chronic ventilatory failure with moderate to severe hypoxemia (pH = 7.35; Pao_2 = 47 torr; $Paco_2$ = 55 torr; Sao_2 = 82%). CBC indicates slightly elevated hemoglobin and an increased white blood cell count. Blood chemistry indicates electrolytes in the normal range, except for potassium, which is slightly reduced. The chest radiograph indicates hyperinflation and what appear to be new infiltrates. *These findings are consistent with acute exacerbation of COPD associated with a superimposed pneumonia.*

Treatment of acute exacerbation of COPD should include *oxygen therapy* and *aerosolized bronchodilators* (β_2-agonists and/or anticholinergic agents). A short course of *steroids* may be considered and *antibiotics* to treat pneumonia as well as the exacerbation of COPD. *Noninvasive positive pressure ventilation* (NIPPV) should be considered in the presence of elevated $Paco_2$ with acidosis and continuing ventilatory distress. If NIPPV fails, invasive mechanical ventilation may be required in the presence of worsening hypoventilation with acidosis. Potassium replacement may be needed in the presence of low potassium, and diuretics may be given to treat peripheral edema and fluid overload.

Monitor and Reevaluate

The respiratory care plan for Mr. Smith includes oxygen therapy at 2 L/min via nasal cannula to maintain his Spo_2 in the range of 88% to 90% and avoid further (oxygen-induced) hypercapnea (due to his preexisting chronic CO_2 retention). Bronchodilator therapy, steroids, and antibiotics are ordered. Mr. Smith should now be monitored for adequate oxygenation, ventilation, and acid-base balance. Once the acute COPD exacerbation/pneumonia has been reversed, a smoking cessation program should begin and pulmonary function testing completed. Inhaled bronchodilators, in combination with inhaled steroids, may be useful to reduce future hospitalizations. Triple therapy, which may combine tiotropium (an anticholengeric bronchodilator), salmeterol (a long-acting β_2 bronchodilator [LABA]), and an inhaled steroid may be useful to reduce future hospitalizations. A formal pulmonary rehabilitation program should also be considered.

CLINICAL FOCUS 1-3

Common Disease States and Conditions Seen in Respiratory Care

Acute Restrictive Disease

Acute bronchitis	Lung cancer
Acute lung injury (ALI)*	Pleural effusion/pleural disease
Acute respiratory failure	Pneumonia
Acute respiratory distress syndrome (ARDS)	Pneumothorax
Atelectasis	Pulmonary edema

*Recently, the Berlin Definition of ARDS has incorporated variables and related criteria for mild ARDS that were previously described as ALI.

Chronic Restrictive Disease

Interstitial lung disease (pulmonary fibrosis/other)	Sarcoidosis (restrictive/obstructive)
Lung cancer	Obesity
Thoracic deformity	Pneumoconiosis

Obstructive Disease

Asthma
Bronchiectasis
Chronic bronchitis
COPD

Cystic fibrosis
Emphysema
Sarcoidosis (restrictive/obstructive)
Upper airway obstruction

Cardiac and Circulatory Problems

Abdominal aortic aneurysm
Abnormal cardiac stress test
Cardiac arrhythmias
Chronic hypertension
Acute myocardial ischemia
Aortic valve disease
Heart murmur
Congestive heart failure (CHF)
Coronary artery disease (CAD)
Hyperlipidemia

Mitral valve prolapse
Myocardial infarction (MI)
Chronic, stable angina
Congenital heart disease
Peripheral artery disease (claudication)
Peripheral edema
Pulmonary vascular disease (pulmonary embolus, pulmonary hypertension)
Syncope

Other Problems Affecting the Cardiopulmonary System

Alcohol and drug abuse
Anemia
Burns and smoke inhalation
Chest trauma
Diabetes
Drug overdose
Fluid and electrolyte disturbances
Fungal lung disease
Hypersensitivity pneumonitis
Malnutrition
Neurologic problems affecting ventilatory drive
Neuromuscular disease affecting respiration

Obesity
Postoperative care
Preoperative care
Renal failure
Sepsis
Shock (cardiogenic, hypovolemic, septic, anaphylactic)
Sleep-disordered breathing
Tobacco addiction/dependence
Trauma
Upper respiratory tract infection

TABLE 1-5
Typical Presentation of Common Respiratory Disease States and Conditions

Disease State or Condition	History	Physical Examination	Laboratory Tests
Viral upper respiratory infection	Nasal congestion, runny nose, scratchy sore throat, laryngitis, cough, sputum production	Mucopurulent nasal discharge; fever; pharynx pale, boggy, swollen Breath sounds may show gurgles or coarse rhonchi	Chest radiograph may be clear, throat culture to rule out streptococcal infection
Sinusitis	Postnasal drip, cough, sneezing, nasal congestion, facial pain, pressure or fullness	Headache pain worsened by touch	Sinus CT scan
Mycoplasma bronchitis or pneumonia	Dry hacking cough progressing to cough with purulent sputum	Fever, crackles, signs of pneumonia	Chest radiograph shows signs of pneumonia, Gram stain negative except for neutrophils, bedside cold agglutinins positive, ESR elevated

TABLE 1-5
Typical Presentation of Common Respiratory Disease States and Conditions (*continued*)

Disease State or Condition	History	Physical Examination	Laboratory Tests
Pneumonia	Cough, purulent or rusty sputum, fever, chills, dyspnea, pleuritic chest pain **(in elderly patients: sometimes only confusion, fatigue, with minimal or no pulmonary complaints)**	Sudden onset, spiking fever with rigors, mental status changes associated with hypoxemia, tachycardia, tachypnea, cyanosis, crackles, bronchial breath sounds, egophony, vocal fremitus, diminished breath sounds, dull percussion note	New or progressive infiltrate on chest radiograph, sputum analysis (color, amount, consistency, odor, Gram stain, direct fluorescent antibody stain, fungal stains, acid-fast stains, culture and sensitivity), WBC with differential
Atelectasis	History of recent abdominal or thoracic surgery, immobilization, chest wall pain, muscular weakness, thoracic or abdominal limitation to diaphragmatic excursion (ascites, obesity, peritonitis, thoracic deformity, etc.), weakness, neuromuscular disease, pneumonia or other acute restrictive disease, other chronic restrictive pulmonary disease, sedatives or narcotics	Decreased chest wall movement over affected side, absent or diminished breath sounds, dull percussion node, crackles	Findings associated with atelectasis on chest radiograph, decreased inspiratory capacity, vital capacity
COPD exacerbation (chronic bronchitis, emphysema)	Chronic cough with sputum production (chronic bronchitis), increased dyspnea, orthopnea, decreased mobility	Diffuse wheezing, cyanosis (chronic bronchitis), dependent edema, clinical manifestations of hypoxemia, increased AP diameter, accessory muscle use, pursed lip breathing, diminished breath sounds, prolonged expiration, wheezing, crackles, rhonchi	Decreased FEV_1/FVC; hyperinflation on chest radiograph, possible new infiltrates
Pleural effusion	Dyspnea, pleuritic chest pain, cough	Chest wall movement reduced over affected side, dull percussion note, absent or diminished breath sounds over effusion, egophony and/or bronchial breath sounds above effusion, pleural rub may be present	Chest x-ray consistent with pleural effusion, thoracentesis, pleural fluid analysis (appearance, WBC and differential, Gram stain, culture, glucose, amylase)
Pneumothorax	Chest pain, dyspnea	Tachycardia, tachypnea, respiratory distress, tracheal deviation to opposite side with tension, decreased chest wall movement on affected side, resonant or hyperresonant percussion note, absent or decreased breath sounds	Chest x-ray consistent with pneumothorax, arterial blood gases, oximetry may show hypoxemia with or without hypercapnea

ESR, erythrocyte sedimentation rate; WBC, white blood cell count.

This article was published in Stoller JK, Bakow ED, Longworth DL, eds. *Critical Diagnostic Thinking in Respiratory Care: A Case-Based Approach*; Shelledy D, Stoller JK. An introduction to critical diagnostic thinking, Pages 3–38, Copyright WB Saunders 2002.

Key Points

▶ Respiratory care patient assessment includes the history, physical examination, and diagnostic testing (laboratory tests and imaging studies).

▶ Patient assessment is needed to ensure that patients' problems are properly identified, prioritized, evaluated, and treated.

▶ Health may be defined as a person's overall mental, physical, and social well-being.

▶ The primary factors that determine health are individual genetic makeup; access to medical care; environmental factors (housing, work, school); and personal health-related behaviors, such as smoking, physical exercise, nutrition, and the use of drugs and alcohol.

▶ The top five leading causes of death in the United States are heart disease, cancer, COPD, stroke, and accidents.

▶ The major drivers of the modern healthcare system are quality, access, and cost.

▶ Patients with chronic disease, such as asthma, COPD, heart disease, and diabetes, account for about 75% of overall healthcare spending.

▶ In spite of spending more on healthcare, the United States ranks below many other nations in measures of overall health.

▶ Careful patient assessment may reduce misallocation of care, decrease costs, and save valuable resources.

▶ A major goal of patient assessment is to ensure that patients receive the right care at the right time and that unnecessary care is reduced or eliminated.

▶ Evidence-based practice uses research findings to aid in clinical decision making.

▶ The best sources of evidence for clinical decision making include the results of well-designed randomized controlled trails (RCTs), systematic reviews, expert panel recommendations, and national/international clinical practice guidelines and standards.

▶ Critical thinking to establish a patient's diagnosis includes identifying the problem, gathering additional information, formulating hypotheses, hypothesis testing, formulating and implementing solutions, and monitoring and reevaluating the patient.

▶ Common respiratory problems include cough, dyspnea, sputum production, hemoptysis, and chest pain.

▶ Common respiratory disease states or conditions requiring patient assessment include upper respiratory tract infection, pneumonia, atelectasis, asthma, emphysema, COPD, acute or chronic bronchitis, acute respiratory failure, ALI, ARDS, pulmonary edema, chest trauma, interstitial lung disease, and lung cancer.

References

1. World Health Organization. Frequently asked questions: what is the WHO definition of health? http://ww.who.int/suggestions/faq/en/index.html. Accessed January 10, 2012.
2. Yong PL, Saunders RS, Olsen L. *The Healthcare Imperative: Lowering Costs and Improving Outcomes—Workshop Series Summary.* Washington, DC: National Academies Press; 2010.
3. Centers for Disease Control and Prevention. Clusters of acute respiratory illness associated with human enterovirus 68—Asia, Europe, and United States, 2008–2010. *MMWR.* 2011;60(38):1301–1336.
4. Kochanek KD, Xu J, Murphy SL, Miniño AM, Kung HC. Deaths: preliminary data for 2009. *Natl Vital Stat Rep.* 2011;59(4).
5. Kocher R, Sahni NR. Rethinking health care labor. *N Engl J Med.* 2011;365(15):1370–1372.
6. Stanton MW, Rutherford MK. The high concentration of U.S. health care expenditures. *Research in Action Series,* Issue 19. Rockville, MD: Agency for Healthcare Research and Quality; 2006: 1–11.
7. Keehan SP, Lazenby HC, Zezza MA, Catlin AC. Age estimates in the national health accounts. *Health Care Financ Rev* (Web Exclusive). 2004;1(1):1–16.
8. Wolff JL, Starfield B, Anderson G. Prevalence, expenditures, and complications of multiple chronic conditions in the elderly. *Arch Intern Med.* 2002;162:2269–2276.
9. Centers for Disease Control and Prevention, National Asthma Control Program. Asthma fast facts. http://www.cdc.gov/asthma/pdfs/asthma_fast_facts_statistics.pdf. Accessed January 3, 2012.
10. American Lung Association. Chronic obstructive pulmonary disease (COPD) fact sheet 2011. http://www.lungusa.org/lung-disease/copd/resources/facts-figures/COPD-Fact-Sheet.html. Accessed January 3, 2010.
11. Stranges E, Kowlessar N, Elixhauser A. Components of growth in inpatient hospital costs, 1997–2009. *HCUP Statistical Brief.* No. 123. Rockville, MD: Agency for Healthcare Research and Quality; 2011. http://www.hcup-us.ahrq.gov/reports/statbriefs/sb123.pdf. Accessed January 3, 2012.
12. Chen LM, Jha AK, Guterman S, Ridgway AB, Orav EJ, Epstein AM. Hospital cost of care, quality of care, and readmission rates: penny-wise and pound-foolish? *Arch Int Med.* 2010;170(4):340–346.
13. Costs of coronary artery bypass graft surgery in U.S. more than Canada. *Medical News Today.* July 19, 2005. http://www.medicalnewstoday.com/printerfriendlynews.php?newsid=27589. Accessed January 3, 2011.
14. Thorpe KE, Florence CS, Joski P. Which medical conditions account for the rise in health care spending? *Health Affairs* (Web Exclusive) 2004: W4-437-45. http://content.healthaffairs.org/content/early/2004/08/25/hlthaff.w4.437.short. Accessed April 24, 2014.
15. Dasta JF, McLaughlin TP, Mody SH, Piech CT. Daily cost of an intensive care unit day: the contribution of mechanical ventilation. *Crit Care Med.* 2005;33(6):1266–1271.

16. American Cancer Society. Cancer facts and figures for African Americans 2011–2012. http://www.cancer.org/acs/groups /content/@epidemiologysurveilance/ documents/document /acspc-027765.pdf. Accessed January 3, 2012.

17. Center on Social Disparities in Health, University of California–San Francisco. http://www.familymedicine.medschool.ucsf.edu /csdh. Accessed December 29, 2011.

18. Quality improvement interventions to address health disparities: evidence-based practice center systematic review protocol. *Closing the Quality Gap: Revisiting the State of the Science Series.* Rockville, MD: Agency for Healthcare Research and Quality; 2011. http://www.ahrq.gov/clinic/tp/gapdisptp.htm. Accessed December 28, 2011.

19. Fisher ES, Wennberg DE, Stukel TA, Gottlieb DJ, Lucas FL, Pinder EL. The implications of regional variations in Medicare spending. Part 1: The content, quality, and accessibility of care. *Ann Int Med.* 2003;138(4):273–287.

20. Elhauge E. Why we should care about health care fragmentation and how to fix it. In: E. Elhauge, ed. *The Fragmentation of U.S. Health Care Causes and Solutions.* New York: Oxford University Press; 2010: 1–16.

21. Shelledy DC, LeGrand TS, Peters JI. An assessment of the appropriateness of respiratory care delivered at a 450-bed acute care Veterans affairs hospital. *Respir Care.* 2004;49(8):907–916.

22. Mishoe SC. Critical thinking in respiratory care. In: Mishoe SC, Welch MA, eds. *Critical Thinking in Respiratory Care: A Problem-Based Approach.* New York: McGraw-Hill; 2002: 33–64.

23. Shelledy DC, Stoller, JK. *An Introduction to Critical Diagnostic Thinking.* In: Stoller, JK, Bakow, ED, Longworth, DL, eds. *Critical Diagnostic Thinking in Respiratory Care: A Case-Based Approach.* Philadelphia: W.B. Saunders; 2002: 3–38.

CHAPTER

2

Development and Implementation of Respiratory Care Plans

David C. Shelledy and Jay I. Peters

CHAPTER OUTLINE

Introduction to Respiratory Care Plans
Common Conditions Requiring Care Plan Development
Respiratory Care Plan Development
Maintain Adequate Tissue Oxygenation
Treat and/or Prevent Bronchospasm and Mucosal Edema
Mobilize and Remove Secretions
Provide Lung Expansion Therapy
Critical Care and Mechanical Ventilation
Diagnostic Testing
Respiratory Care Plan Format

CHAPTER OBJECTIVES

1. Describe the purpose of a respiratory care plan.
2. Identify the key elements of a respiratory care plan.
3. Describe common conditions that may require development of a respiratory care plan.
4. Define *respiratory failure*, and give examples of several types of respiratory failure.
5. Define *ventilatory failure*, and contrast acute ventilatory failure and chronic ventilatory failure.
6. Give examples of appropriate outcome measures for a respiratory care plan.
7. Outline the key steps in the development and implementation of a respiratory care plan.
8. Develop a respiratory care plan to maintain adequate tissue oxygenation.
9. Create a respiratory care plan for the treatment and/or prevention of bronchospasm and mucosal edema.
10. Describe the care of patients with asthma and COPD.
11. Design a respiratory care plan to mobilize secretions.
12. Propose a respiratory care plan for the treatment and/or prevention of atelectasis and pneumonia.
13. Give examples of types of respiratory care plans used in the intensive care unit.
14. Explain the role of diagnostic testing in the development of a respiratory care plan.

KEY TERMS

acute lung injury (ALI)
acute respiratory distress syndrome (ARDS)
acute respiratory failure
acute ventilatory failure (AVF)
anti-inflammatory agents
antiasthmatic medications
asthma
atelectasis
bronchial hygiene
bronchiectasis
bronchodilator therapy
bronchospasm
chest physiotherapy (CPT)
chronic bronchitis
chronic ventilatory failure (CVF)
chronic obstructive pulmonary disease (COPD)

history
hypoxemia
incentive spirometry (IS)
intermittent positive pressure breathing (IPPB)
lung expansion therapy
mechanical ventilation
mucosal edema
oxygen therapy
physical
pneumonia
positive airway pressure (PAP)
protocol
pulmonary edema
respiratory care plan
retained secretions
SOAP notes
treatment menu

Overview

This chapter provides a guide to the development, implementation, and evaluation of respiratory care plans. In order to develop an appropriate respiratory care plan, the clinician must first perform a thorough patient assessment, including a review of the patient's existing medical record, a patient interview, and a physical assessment. The bedside measurement of clinical parameters related to oxygenation, ventilation, and pulmonary function may be performed. Pulse oximetry (Spo_2) is often used to assess oxygenation status. Arterial blood gases should be obtained if there is concern regarding the patient's ventilatory status, acid–base balance, or the reliability of Spo_2 values. Laboratory, imaging, and other diagnostic studies may be needed to further define and clarify the patient's problem and diagnosis. Following establishment and clarification of the patient's diagnosis and/or problem list (see Chapter 1), a respiratory care plan is developed, implemented, and evaluated.

Introduction to Respiratory Care Plans

The **respiratory care plan** provides a written description of the care the patient is to receive. The plan is based on a careful patient interview and physical assessment, review of diagnostic test results, and consideration of the treatment modalities available, sometimes known as the **treatment menu**. The respiratory care plan may take the form of physician's orders, a detailed progress note in the medical record, an established **protocol**, completion of a standardized respiratory care consultation and treatment plan, or the use of problem-oriented medical records (e.g., SOAP notes). The respiratory care plan can be viewed as an individualized protocol for the patient.

A basic respiratory care plan often includes the following elements:

- Goals of therapy
- Device or procedure to be used or medications to be given
- Method or appliance to be used
- Gas source or oxygen concentration
- Device pressure, volume, and/or flow
- Frequency of administration and duration of therapy

SOAP notes are sometimes used to document patient care plans:

S (Subjective): Refers to what the patient says or subjective information obtained from chart.
O (Objective): Refers to what the clinician observes or objective test results.
A (Assessment): Refers to the clinician's assessment.
P (Plan): Refers to the plan of care.

The respiratory care plan may also include a statement of how the intensity and/or duration of therapy will be adjusted and when the therapy will be discontinued. Assessment of the outcomes of therapy may also be included, as well as measurable objectives of the care delivered.

In summary, the respiratory care plan provides the written plan of treatment that the patient will receive. The plan may include goals, rationale, significance, and a description of how care will be assessed. Following a careful patient assessment, the respiratory care plan is

---

TABLE 2-1
Types of Care Provided in the Respiratory Care Plan

Basic Respiratory Care
- Oxygen therapy
- Secretion management
- Sputum induction
- Management of bronchospasm and mucosal edema
- Lung expansion therapy

Critical Respiratory Care
- Invasive mechanical ventilatory support
- Noninvasive mechanical ventilatory support
- Physiologic monitoring
- Cardiac and hemodynamic monitoring
- Suctioning and airway care
- Airway intubation
- Advanced cardiovascular life support
- Metabolic studies
- Extracorporeal membrane oxygenation
- Mechanical circulatory assistance
- Basic care in the intensive care setting

Diagnostic Testing
- Oximetry
- Arterial blood gases
- Pulmonary function testing
- Cardiac testing (e.g., ECG, invasive cardiology, cardiac catheterization laboratory)
- Ultrasound (echocardiography, other)
- Sleep studies
- Exercise testing

Special Procedures
- Transport
- Patient education
- Smoking cessation
- Disease management
- Pulmonary rehabilitation
- Cardiac rehabilitation

---

developed, implemented, and evaluated. A summary of the types of care often included in the respiratory care plan is provided in **Table 2-1**.

Common Conditions Requiring Respiratory Care Plan Development

Problems that affect oxygenation and/or ventilation often require the development of a respiratory care plan. Other common respiratory problems include **bronchospasm** and **mucosal edema**, **retained secretions**, airway plugging, infection, consolidation, inadequate lung expansion, **atelectasis**, and **pulmonary edema**. Common disease states or conditions encountered in the physician's office, clinic, or acute care setting that may require respiratory care include upper respiratory tract infection, **pneumonia**, acute bronchitis, **asthma**, **chronic obstructive pulmonary disease** (COPD; including emphysema and **chronic bronchitis**), pulmonary hypertension, congestive heart failure (CHF), lung cancer, pulmonary fibrosis, pulmonary emboli, postoperative pulmonary complications, and acute respiratory failure (see Chapter 1).

Respiratory Failure

Respiration refers to the exchange of oxygen (O_2) and carbon dioxide (CO_2) across the lung and pulmonary capillaries (external respiration) and at the tissue level (internal respiration). Respiratory failure, broadly defined, is an inability of the heart and lungs to provide adequate tissue oxygenation and/or carbon dioxide removal.[1,2] **Acute respiratory failure** may be defined as a sudden decrease in arterial blood oxygen levels with or without carbon dioxide retention.[1,2] **Acute lung injury (ALI)** and **acute respiratory distress syndrome (ARDS)** are two special cases of respiratory failure that are characterized by oxygenation problems that generally do not respond well to basic **oxygen therapy**. The term *hypoxemic respiratory failure* (aka "lung failure") is sometimes used when the primary problem is oxygenation.[3] Chapter 6 describes the assessment of a patient's oxygenation status. **Box 2-1** summarizes the various types of respiratory failure.

The most common reason for initiation of mechanical ventilatory support is *hypercapnic respiratory failure* (aka "ventilatory failure" or "pump failure").[3,4] **Acute ventilatory failure (AVF)** can be defined as a sudden rise in arterial CO_2 levels (as assessed by $Paco_2$) with a corresponding decrease in pH.[5] Respiratory muscle fatigue and an increased work of breathing may lead to acute ventilatory failure. Decreased ventilatory drive due to narcotic or sedative drug overdose, head trauma, or stroke can also result in AVF. Common disease states or conditions associated with the development of AVF include severe pneumonia, ALI, ARDS, massive or submassive pulmonary emboli, CHF, and pulmonary edema. Shock, trauma, smoke or chemical inhalation, aspiration, and near drowning may also cause AVF. Acute exacerbation of COPD, acute severe asthma, severe burns, upper airway obstruction, obesity, and thoracic deformity all predispose patients to the development of AVF. Neuromuscular disease such as Guillain-Barré syndrome, myasthenia gravis, and spinal cord injury may also precipitate AVF.

Chronic ventilatory failure (CVF) (aka "chronic hypercapnea") may be defined as a chronically elevated $Paco_2$ with a normal (compensated) or near-normal pH.[5] The most common cause is severe COPD, although not all COPD patients develop chronic ventilatory failure. Ventilatory failure usually suggests that less than 25% of alveoli are functioning. Acute pneumonia in COPD patients often will result in AVF that resolves as the pneumonia improves and inflammatory cells are cleared from the airway. Other chronic lung diseases, such as late-stage cystic fibrosis, severe interstitial lung disease, and obesity-hypoventilation syndrome, are associated with the development of CVF. Evaluation of ventilation is described in Chapter 7.

Respiratory failure requires careful patient assessment and then the development and implementation of the respiratory care plan. Common causes of respiratory failure are listed in **Box 2-2. Clinical Focus 2-1** provides an example of a specific type of respiratory failure.

Respiratory Care Plan Development

The process for respiratory care plan development generally includes the receipt of an order for a specific type of respiratory care or for a respiratory care consult. The process for developing a respiratory care plan may begin when a patient enters the healthcare setting with a problem or complaint. Sometimes the need for respiratory care is not immediately apparent and, in the acute care setting, patients often require respiratory care at some point following admission to the hospital.

Following initial assessment and verification of the patient's problem or diagnosis by the physician, nurse practitioner, or physician assistant, an order for respiratory care may be written. Upon receipt of an order, the respiratory care clinician performs a medical records review, patient interview, and physical assessment. Bedside measurement of Spo_2 and basic pulmonary function parameters may be performed. Following this assessment, the respiratory care clinician may then select the appropriate care based on the patient's condition. The goal is to optimize the match between the care needed and the care "menu," or treatment options that are available. Basic respiratory care options include techniques to improve oxygenation and manage secretions, treatment for bronchospasm and mucosal edema, and **lung expansion therapy**.

A typical basic respiratory care treatment menu is provided in **Table 2-2**. Following selection of a respiratory care treatment regimen, the patient's physician should be notified and given the opportunity to review and/or modify the care plan. The care is then delivered. The patient is monitored, and the care plan is reevaluated based on the patient's response to therapy. **Figure 2-1** summarizes the steps in respiratory care plan development and implementation.

Goals of Respiratory Care Plans

Respiratory care plans may be developed for basic and critical respiratory care, diagnostic testing, and specialized procedures (Table 2-1). Goals of the respiratory care plan may include maintaining or improving oxygenation and ventilation, managing secretions, treating or preventing bronchospasm and mucosal edema, and treating and/or preventing atelectasis and pneumonia. Basic respiratory care plans may include oxygen

BOX 2-1

Types of Respiratory Failure

Respiratory Failure

Respiratory failure is a general term that indicates the inability of the heart and lungs to provide adequate tissue oxygenation and/or carbon dioxide removal.

Acute Respiratory Failure

Acute respiratory failure may be defined as a sudden decrease in arterial blood oxygen levels (arterial partial pressure of oxygen [Pao_2] < 50 to 60 mm Hg; arterial oxygen saturation [Sao_2] < 88% to 90%), with or without carbon dioxide retention (arterial partial pressure of carbon dioxide [$Paco_2$] > 45 mm Hg):
- *Hypoxemic respiratory failure* (lung failure) refers to a primary problem with oxygenation.
- *Hypercapnic respiratory failure* (pump failure) refers to a primary problem with ventilation. Hypercapnic respiratory failure is also known as *ventilatory failure*.

Ventilatory Failure

Ventilatory failure may be defined as an elevated $Paco_2$ (> 45 to 50 mm Hg). An increased $Paco_2$ may also be called hypoventilation or hypercapnea:
- *Acute ventilatory failure* is defined as a sudden increase in arterial $Paco_2$ with a corresponding decrease in pH.
- *Chronic ventilatory failure* is defined as a chronically elevated $Paco_2$ with a normal or near-normal pH owing to metabolic compensation.
- *Acute on chronic ventilatory failure* is defined as a chronically elevated Pco_2 followed by an acute increase in the Pco_2 and a corresponding fall in pH.

Acute Lung Injury and Acute Respiratory Distress Syndrome

Acute lung injury (ALI) and *acute respiratory distress syndrome* (ARDS) are forms of noncardiogenic hypoxemic respiratory failure as defined by the Pao_2/Fio_2 ratio. The characteristics of ALI/ARDS are:
- Bilateral pulmonary infiltrates on chest x-ray
- Pulmonary capillary wedge pressure < 18 mm Hg
- Pao_2/Fio_2 < 300 = ALI. This is equivalent to a Pao_2 of less than 63 torr while breathing room air (Fio_2 = 0.21).
- Pao_2/Fio_2 < 200 = ARDS. This is equivalent to a Pao_2 of less than 42 torr while breathing room air (Fio_2 = 0.21)

More recently, the Berlin definition of ARDS was proposed based on symptom timing, chest imaging, and Pao_2/Fio_2 ratio while receiving at least 5 cm H_2O of PEEP or CPAP. This revised definition combines aspects of ALI and ARDS and requires (1) identification of respiratory symptoms within 1 week of new or worsening symptoms or a known clinical insult; (2) bilateral opacities upon chest imaging (chest x-ray or CT scan); (3) opacities that cannot due to lobar collapse, lung collapse, pulmonary effusion, or pulmonary nodules; (4) pulmonary edema that cannot be due to cardiac failure or fluid overload as assessed by echocardiography or other measures to exclude hydrostatic edema (e.g. PCWP < 18 mm Hg); and (5) Pao_2/Fio_2 ≤ 300 mm Hg with PEEP or CPAP ≥ 5 cm H_2O where:
- Pao_2/Fio_2 ≤ 300 mm Hg—mild
- Pao_2/Fio_2 ≤ 200 mm Hg—moderate
- Pao_2/Fio_2 ≤ 100 mm Hg—severe

CPAP, continuous positive airway pressure; Fio_2, fraction of inspired oxygen; $Paco_2$, partial pressure of arterial carbon dioxide; Pao_2, partial pressure of arterial oxygen; PEEP, positive end-expiratory pressure. If altitude is higher than 1000 m, then correction factor should be calculated as follow: [Pao_2/Fio_2 × (barometric pressure/760)].
Data from: ARDS Definition Task Force, Ranieri VM, Rubenfeld GD, Thompson BT, et al. Acute respiratory distress syndrome: the Berlin Definition. *JAMA*. 2012;307(23):2526-2533. doi: 10.1001/jama.2012.5669.

BOX 2-2

Common Causes of Respiratory Failure

Oxygenation Problems

Low ventilation/perfusion ratio (low $\dot{V}/\dot{Q}$)
- Underventilation with respect to pulmonary perfusion
- Examples: Asthma, emphysema, COPD, cystic fibrosis, bronchiectasis

Pulmonary shunt
- No ventilation with respect to pulmonary perfusion
- Examples: ALI/ARDS, atelectasis, pneumonia, rarely pulmonary edema

Diffusion problems
- Impaired diffusion due to increased diffusion distance, block
- Example: Early pulmonary fibrosis

Hypoventilation
- Increases in Pa_{CO_2} result in a corresponding decrease in Pa_{O_2}

Low blood oxygen content
- Low Pa_{O_2}, Sa_{O_2}, or hemoglobin
- Examples:
  - Low Pa_{O_2} may be due to low $\dot{V}/\dot{Q}$, shunt, diffusion problems, or hypoventilation
  - Low hemoglobin (anemia), abnormal hemoglobin (carbon monoxide poisoning)

Increased pulmonary dead space
- Examples: Pulmonary embolus, obliteration of the pulmonary capillaries (as in severe emphysema)

Ventilation Problems

Acute ventilatory failure (AVF)
- A sudden increase in Pa_{CO_2} with a corresponding decrease in pH
- Examples of conditions associated with AVF:
  - ALI/ARDS, severe pneumonia.
  - Shock, chest trauma, pneumothorax, head trauma, stroke, spinal cord injury, smoke or chemical inhalation, aspiration, near drowning.
  - Sedative or narcotic drug overdose, paralytic drugs, deep anesthesia.
  - Respiratory muscle fatigue and increased work of breathing due to acute exacerbation of COPD, acute severe asthma, severe obesity, thoracic deformity.
  - Neuromuscular disease associated with respiratory failure, such as Guillain-Barré, amyotrophic lateral sclerosis (ALS), myasthenia gravis, polio, critical illness/steroid myopathy, botulism, tetanus.
  - Patients recovering from abdominal or thoracic surgery may need mechanical ventilatory support.

Chronic ventilatory failure
- A chronically elevated Pa_{CO_2} with normal or near-normal pH
- Examples: Chronic bronchitis, severe COPD, obesity-hypoventilation syndrome

Data from: West JB. Acute respiratory failure. In: West JB, ed. *Pulmonary Physiology and Pathophysiology: An Integrated, Case-Based Approach*, 2nd ed. Philadelphia: Lippincott, Williams & Wilkins; 2007: 116–133.

therapy, secretion management, treatment of bronchospasm and mucosal edema, and lung expansion therapy.

Diagnostic respiratory care procedures include techniques to assess oxygenation, ventilation, acid–base balance, and pulmonary function and to obtain sputum samples (e.g., sputum induction) for Gram stain, cultures, and cytologic examination. Critical respiratory care may include mechanical ventilatory support, airway care, physiologic monitoring, cardiovascular stabilization, mechanical circulatory assistance, and extracorporeal membrane oxygenation (ECMO). We will now turn to the development of specific respiratory care plans based on an assessment of the patient's needs and the related goals of therapy.

CLINICAL FOCUS 2-1

Respiratory Failure

A 30-year-old male was admitted to the hospital following a motor vehicle accident with chest trauma. The patient's increasing respiratory distress, tachypnea, and hypoxemia while breathing room air led to intubation and the initiation of mechanical ventilation. The chest x-ray shows bilateral pulmonary infiltrates; however, there is no evidence of cardiogenic pulmonary edema. Current arterial blood gases while being supported in the assist-control mode of ventilation with an F_{IO_2} of 0.60 are:

pH: 7.36
Pa_{CO_2}: 36 mm Hg
Pa_{O_2}: 62 mm Hg
Sa_{O_2}: 90%
HCO_3: 20 mEq/L
B.D.: −5 mEq/L

How would you describe the patient's respiratory condition? (Hint: Before describing the patient's condition, review the definitions and descriptions of respiratory failure found in Box 2-1).

The patient is in acute respiratory failure. The patient has bilateral pulmonary infiltrates, no evidence of cardiogenic pulmonary edema, and a Pa_{O_2}/F_{IO_2} ratio of 103, which is consistent with a diagnosis of ARDS.

The definition of ARDS was clarified by a 1992 American-European Consensus Conference. Rubenfeld GD, Herridge MS. Epidemiology and outcomes of acute lung injury. *Chest.* 2007;131(2):554–562.

TABLE 2-2
Respiratory Care Treatment Menu

Oxygenation • Nasal cannula • Oxygen masks (simple/partial/nonrebreather) • High-flow systems ("Venturi" masks, large-volume air-entrainment nebulizers) • CPAP by mask • PEEP (may require invasive mechanical ventilation)	**Bronchospasm/Mucosal Edema** • Bronchodilator therapy (small-volume nebulizer, MDI, DPI) • Anti-inflammatory agents (steroids) • Antiasthmatic aerosol agents (cromolyn, etc.)
Ventilation • Noninvasive mechanical ventilation (includes BiPAP) • Invasive mechanical ventilation	**Lung Expansion Therapy** • Cough and deep-breathing techniques • Suctioning • Incentive spirometry • IPPB
Secretion Management • Directed cough and deep-breathing instruction • Suctioning (NT, ET, tracheostomy suctioning) • Chest physiotherapy (postural drainage, percussion, vibration) • High-volume bland aerosol therapy (ultrasonic nebulizer, heated large-volume nebulizer) • Mucus-controlling agents (mucolytics)	**Frequency of Treatment Options** • Continuous • Every 1 to 2 hours • Every 4 hours • Every 6 hours • Four times a day • Three times a day • Two times a day • Daily • As needed
Sputum Induction/Obtain Specimen • Directed cough • Hypertonic saline aerosol • Suctioning (NT, ET, tracheostomy suctioning)	

CPAP, continuous positive airway pressure; PEEP, positive end expiratory pressure; BiPAP, bilevel positive airway pressure; NT, nasotracheal; ET, endotracheal; MDI, metered dose inhaler; DPI, dry powder inhaler; IPPB, intermittent positive pressure ventilation.

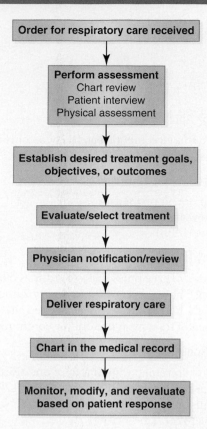

Order for respiratory care received

↓

Perform assessment
Chart review
Patient interview
Physical assessment

↓

Establish desired treatment goals,
objectives, or outcomes

↓

Evaluate/select treatment

↓

Physician notification/review

↓

Deliver respiratory care

↓

Chart in the medical record

↓

Monitor, modify, and reevaluate
based on patient response

FIGURE 2-1 **Steps in the development and implementation of the respiratory care plan.**

Key Elements of a Respiratory Care Plan

The key elements of a basic respiratory care plan are listed in **Box 2-3** and include the goals of therapy, devices, medications, methods, gas source, and frequency of administration. Assessment of basic respiratory care should note improvement in oxygenation and ventilation, work of breathing, breath sounds, and, in some cases, pulmonary function and blood gases. **Box 2-4** lists the key elements of a respiratory care plan for mechanical ventilatory support.

Maintain Adequate Tissue Oxygenation

Oxygen therapy is indicated for documented or suspected **hypoxemia**, severe trauma, acute myocardial infarction (MI), and immediate postoperative recovery.[6] It also may be indicated to support the patient with chronic lung disease during exercise and to prevent or treat right-side CHF (cor pulmonale) due to chronic pulmonary hypertension.[6] A $Pa_{O_2} < 60$ and/or a $Sp_{O_2} < 90\%$ to 92% are considered clear indications for oxygen therapy in most patients.[6] Exceptions to this rule include patients with chronic carbon dioxide retention and the premature neonate. A critical value in the COPD patient may be a Pa_{O_2} of ≤ 55 torr with a Sp_{O_2} of ≤ 88% while breathing room air or a Pa_{O_2} of 56 to

59 and a $Sa_{O_2} < 89\%$ in the presence of cor pulmonale, pulmonary hypertension, CHF, or erythrocythemia with a hematocrit > 56.[7] A critical Pa_{O_2} for the newborn may be a $Pa_{O_2} < 50$ torr and/or a $Sp_{O_2} < 88\%$ or a capillary $P_{O_2} < 40$ torr.[8]

Hypoxemia should be suspected whenever the patient is exhibiting the signs and symptoms of hypoxia. Initial signs of hypoxia include tachycardia, increased blood pressure, tachypnea, hyperventilation, dyspnea, and use of accessory muscles. Other early manifestations of hypoxia include restlessness, disorientation, dizziness, excitement, headache, blurred vision, impaired judgment, and confusion. Clinical manifestations of severe hypoxia may include slow, irregular respirations; bradycardia; hypotension; dysrhythmias; loss of consciousness; somnolence; convulsions; and coma. These later findings are more common when hypoxia and hypercapnea coexist. Severe hypoxia may lead to respiratory and/or cardiac arrest. The respiratory care clinician should obtain a Sp_{O_2} or arterial blood gas study in order to confirm the presence of hypoxemia. The indications for oxygen therapy in the acute care setting are summarized in **Box 2-5**.

Once it is established that oxygen therapy is required, the respiratory care clinician must decide on the appropriate equipment, the correct oxygen flow (F_{IO_2}), and how the therapy will be assessed. In general, the lowest F_{IO_2} needed to ensure adequate tissue oxygenation should be chosen. Generally, this means a target Pa_{O_2} of 60 to 100 with a Sp_{O_2} of 92% to 98% for most patients, with the exception of the COPD patient and the premature infant.

One should also avoid high oxygen levels (> 50% to 60%) for extended periods of time because of the threat of oxygen toxicity, absorption atelectasis, and depression of ciliary and/or leukocytic function.[6] If high levels of oxygen are needed for more than a brief period of time, alternative methods to improve oxygenation should be considered.

Excessive oxygen levels in patients who are chronic CO_2 retainers may lead to ventilatory depression and increased $\dot{V}/\dot{Q}$ mismatch when the Pa_{O_2} exceeds 60 torr.[6] Oxygen therapy for the COPD patient with chronically elevated Pa_{CO_2} levels should be targeted at maintaining a Pa_{O_2} of 50 to 59 torr with a Sa_{O_2} of 88% to 90% in order to avoid oxygen-induced hypercapnea. The Global Initiative for Chronic Obstructive Lung Disease (GOLD) guide suggests that oxygen therapy in the treatment of COPD exacerbations be titrated to achieve a Sp_{O_2} of 88% to 92%.[9] However, a $Sp_{O_2} > 90\%$ may result in a $Pa_{O_2} > 60$, and consequently should probably be avoided in patients with documented or suspected CO_2 retention. Therefore, titration to a goal of 90% may be ideal.

Providing high oxygen levels to premature infants has been associated with retinopathy of prematurity, a disorder caused by high arterial oxygen concentrations

BOX 2-3

Key Elements of a Basic Respiratory Care Plan

Goals of Therapy

Maintain adequate tissue oxygenation and/or
alveolar ventilation.
Treat/prevent bronchospasm and/or mucosal
edema.
Deliver anti-inflammatory or antiasthmatic
agents.
Manage secretions.
Induce sputum.
Prevent or treat atelectasis.

Device or Procedure

Oxygen therapy (nasal cannula, air-entrainment
mask, other masks)
Aerosol medication via small-volume nebulizer
MDI via holding chamber
Incentive spirometry
IPPB
Chest physiotherapy (postural drainage and chest
percussion)
High-volume bland aerosol with or without sup-
plemental oxygen
Directed cough
Suctioning
Mechanical ventilators (invasive and noninvasive
ventilation; see also Box 2-4)

Medications

Bronchodilators
Mucolytics (Mucomyst, Pulmonzyme)
Anti-inflammatory agents and decongestants
(steroids, racemic epinephrine, others)
Antiasthmatic agents (cromolyn, Tilade)
Bland aerosol (normal saline, one-half normal
saline, sterile distilled water)

Method or Appliance

Mask, mouthpiece, mouthseal, tracheostomy mask,
nose clips, aerochamber, etc.

Gas Source, Flow, and/or Pressure

Oxygen or compressed air
Liter flow and/or FIO_2
Pressure (IPPB)

Frequency and Duration of Therapy

Twice daily, three times daily, four times daily,
every 6 hours, every 4 hours, every 2 hours,
every 1 hour, continuous, as needed, etc.
Duration of therapy in minutes or continuous

Volume Goals

Incentive spirometry minimum of one-third of
predicted IC (1/3 × IBW in kg × 50 mL/kg)
IPPB minimum of one-third predicted IC (or at
least 10 mL/kg)

Assessment

Improvement and/or reversal of clinical signs and
symptoms of respiratory failure
Reversal of the manifestations of hypoxia and/or
hypoventilation
Decreased work of breathing
Decreased cardiac work
Improved breath sounds (air movement, wheez-
ing, rhonchi, crackles)
Pulse oximetry and arterial blood gases
Bedside pulmonary function (rate, volumes, inspi-
ratory force, PEF, IC, FVC, FEV_1)
Chest x-ray or other imaging techniques

MDI, metered dose inhaler; IPPB, intermittent positive pressure breathing; IC, inspiratory capacity; IBW, ideal body weight; PEF,
peak expiratory flow rate; FVC, forced vital capacity; FEV_1, forced expiratory volume in 1 second.
Data from West JB. Acute respiratory failure. In: West JB. Pulmonary Physiology and Pathophysiology: An Integrated, Case-
based Approach, 2nd ed. Philadelphia: Lippincott, Williams & Wilkins; 2007: 116–133.

in the newborn that may result in blindness. In the
past, maintenance of a Pao_2 in the range of 50 to 70 was
thought to be safe; however, current guidelines suggest
a $Pao_2 \leq 80$ torr be maintained in preterm infants of
less than 37 weeks gestation.[10]

Other techniques that may improve the patient's
oxygenation status include positive end-expiratory

pressure (PEEP) or continuous positive airway pressure (CPAP), **bronchial hygiene** techniques to mobilize
secretions, and **bronchodilator therapy**. Prone positioning has been shown to improve oxygenation in patients
with ARDS; however, prone positioning has not been
shown to improve survival.[11–13] Rotational therapy
(turning the patient) may reduce the occurrence of

BOX 2-4

Key Elements of a Respiratory Care Plan for Mechanical Ventilatory Support

Goals of Therapy

Maintain adequate tissue oxygenation.

Maintain adequate ventilation and CO_2 removal.

Maintain adequate acid-base balance.

Maintain adequate circulation, blood pressure, and cardiac output.

Treat bronchospasm/mucosal edema/excess secretions.

Maintain lung volumes/prevent or treat atelectasis.

Device or Procedure

Volume ventilators

Pressure ventilators (includes BiPAP devices)

Humidifiers

Nebulizers

MDI and holding chamber

Positive pressure masks (nasal/oral)

Artificial airways (endotracheal tracheostomy tubes)

Suctioning equipment

Medications

Bronchodilators, anti-inflammatory agents, decongestants, antiasthmatic drugs

Drugs to treat infection

Drugs to support circulation, cardiac function, blood pressure

Sedatives, tranquilizers, pain medications, paralytic agents

Method or Appliance

Mask (oral/nasal)

Endotracheal tube

Tracheostomy tube

Mode of Ventilation

Invasive or noninvasive

Volume limited (volume ventilation) or pressure limited (pressure control and pressure support ventilation)

Assist/control, SIMV, SIMV with pressure support, other

Breath initiation (time or patient trigger)

Inspiratory termination (volume, time, pressure, or flow)

Gas Source, Flow, and/or Pressure

Oxygen concentration

Patient trigger (pressure or flow trigger)

Inspiratory flow or time

Termination of inspiration (pressure, volume, or flow)

Frequency and Duration of Therapy

Continuous mechanical ventilatory support

Intermittent support (ventilator weaning, night only, or for acute distress)

Volume and Pressure

Volume-limited ventilation (mL/kg IBW or mL)

Inspiratory pressure or pressure limit

Baseline pressure (PEEP or CPAP)

Pressure support for "spontaneous" breaths

Assessment

Improvement and/or reversal of clinical signs and symptoms

Reversal of the manifestations of hypoxia and/or hypoventilation

Cardiovascular/hemodynamics (pulse, blood pressure, cardiac output, CVP, other)

Work of breathing

Improved breath sounds (air movement, wheezing, rhonchi, crackles)

Pulse oximetry and arterial blood gases

Bedside pulmonary function (spontaneous respiratory rate, volumes, RSBI, inspiratory force, IC, VC)

Chest x-ray or other imaging techniques

BiPAP, bilevel positive airway pressure; MDI, metered dose inhaler; SIMV, synchronized intermittent mandatory ventilation; IBW, ideal body weight; PEEP, positive end-expiratory pressure; CPAP, continuous positive airway pressure; CVP, central venous pressure; RSBI, rapid shallow breathing index; IC, inspiratory capacity; VC, vital capacity.

BOX 2-5

Indications for Oxygen Therapy

Documented hypoxemia (SpO_2 or arterial blood gases):

- Adults and children: $PaO_2 < 60$ and/or $SpO_2 < 90$
- Neonates (< 28 days): $PaO_2 < 50$ and/or $SpO_2 < 88\%$ or a capillary $PO_2 < 40$ torr

Suspected hypoxemia based on patient condition and/or clinical manifestations of hypoxia (follow with SpO_2 or arterial blood gas measurement)*

- Clinical manifestations of hypoxia include:
  - Tachycardia, increased blood pressure, dysrhythmias
  - Dyspnea, tachypnea, hyperventilation, use of accessory muscles
  - Restlessness, disorientation, dizziness, excitement, headache, blurred vision, impaired judgment, and confusion
- Clinical manifestations of severe hypoxia may include:
  - Slowed, irregular respirations
  - Bradycardia, hypotension
  - Loss of consciousness, somnolence, convulsions, or coma

Severe trauma

Acute myocardial infarction

Postoperative recovery

Treat or prevent pulmonary hypertension secondary to chronic hypoxia:

- $PaO_2 \leq 55$ and/or SpO_2 of $\leq 88\%$ while breathing room air with COPD

OR

- COPD patients with cor pulmonale or hematocrit > 56, PaO_2 of 56 to 59, $SaO_2 < 89\%$, and preexisting pulmonary hypertension

*Hypoxemia should be suspected in the presence of the clinical manifestations of hypoxia.

---

atelectasis and ventilator-associated pneumonia (VAP), and thus improve oxygenation; however, improvements in length of stay have not been shown.[14]

Attention to maintaining cardiac output and blood pressure is required to ensure adequate oxygen delivery to the tissues in patients with cardiovascular instability. Replacement of blood in patients with severe anemia may also be helpful.

The selection of an oxygen delivery method should be based on the desired FIO_2, as well as patient-specific factors such as disease state or condition, ventilatory pattern, patient comfort, and patient acceptance of the oxygen appliance. Generally, hypoxemia due to low $\dot{V}/\dot{Q}$ or hypoventilation responds well to low to moderate concentrations of oxygen. This includes patients with asthma, emphysema, chronic bronchitis, **bronchiectasis**, and cystic fibrosis. Oftentimes, patients with CHF without acute pulmonary edema and patients with coronary artery disease (CAD) also respond well to low to moderate concentrations of oxygen.

The device of choice for most patients requiring low to moderate concentrations of oxygen is the nasal cannula. Setting the nasal cannula oxygen flow at 0.5 to 6.0 L/min will deliver approximately 22% to 40% oxygen.[6] The nasal cannula is well tolerated, easy to use, and effective for most patients and does not require humidification at flows ≤ 4 L/min. The only major problem associated with the cannula is that the delivered FIO_2 will vary with the patient's ventilatory pattern and tidal volume (amount of air moved with each breath). An air-entrainment mask should be considered in patients with a variable ventilatory pattern or those with rapid, shallow breathing. Air-entrainment ("Venturi") masks will deliver a stable FIO_2 for most patients and are available to deliver percentages of 24%, 28%, 30%, 35%, and 40% oxygen.[6] A sample respiratory care plan for providing oxygen therapy by nasal cannula using the SOAP note format is provided in **Clinical Focus 2-2. Figure 2-2** presents a simple oxygen therapy protocol.

Patients with hypoxemia due to pulmonary shunting (ARDS or severe pneumonia) and patients suffering from cardiogenic shock (severe acute MI) or trauma may require moderate to high concentrations of oxygen

CLINICAL FOCUS 2-2

Oxygen Therapy Respiratory Care Plan

A 65-year-old man with a history of COPD has come to the emergency department with worsening shortness of breath, increased sputum production, and production of thick, yellow sputum. The patient has a 50-pack-year history of smoking; however, he quit smoking 3 years ago. The patient has been admitted to the hospital several times over the past 3 years, most recently 8 months ago due to acute exacerbation of COPD with documented CO_2 retention. On physical assessment, the patient displays accessory muscle use and tachypnea with an increased pulse and blood pressure. Oximetry on room air reveals a SpO_2 of 85%. On his previous admission, blood gas analysis demonstrated chronic ventilatory failure.

Respiratory Care Plan

S (Subjective): "I'm feeling really bad and can barely get my breath. I am having trouble walking, and I have been coughing up some awful-looking stuff."

O (Objective):
- Vital signs: Respiratory rate, 28; pulse, 116; BP, 142/92 mm Hg; temperature, 99.6 °F
- SpO_2 = 85% while breathing room air
- Physical assessment: Accessory muscle use, diminished breath sounds bilaterally, cough with purulent sputum production

A (Assessment): Acute respiratory failure due to exacerbation of COPD

P (Plan):
- Begin oxygen via nasal cannula at 1 to 2 L/min and titrate by oximetry.
- Titrate oxygen flow based on oximetry to maintain an SpO_2 of 88% to 90% and a PaO_2 of 50 to 59 due to the patient's documented history of CO_2 retention (chronic ventilatory failure).
- Obtain arterial blood gases on oxygen to access ventilatory status.
- Begin albuterol and ipratropium bromide (Atrovent) bronchodilator administration per protocol to relieve airflow obstruction.
- Consider administration of systemic corticosteroids to improve outcomes and decrease length of stay
- Consider antibiotics for pulmonary infection.
- Consider labs (CBC, electrolytes) and chest radiograph
- Continue to monitor patient (level of consciousness, dyspnea, vital signs, SpO_2, blood gases) and be alert to possible comorbidities (pneumonia, cardiovascular disease, lung cancer, diabetes, etc.)

therapy. Short-term oxygen therapy for patients who need moderate to high concentrations of oxygen can be provided using a simple mask (35% to 50% O_2 at 5 to 10 L/min), a partial rebreathing mask (40% to 70% O_2 at 5 to 10 L/min), or a non-rebreathing mask (60% to 80% O_2 at 6 to 10 L/min). Air-entrainment nebulizers via aerosol mask, tracheostomy mask, or "T" piece can be very useful in providing a stable oxygen concentration from 28% to 50%. Above 50% oxygen, most air-entrainment nebulizers do not have an adequate total gas flow to deliver a dependable FIO_2. The Misty Ox high-flow, high-FIO_2 nebulizer, however, will deliver 60% to 96% oxygen with total gas flows of 42 to 80 L/min. The Thera-Mist air-entrainment nebulizer is designed to provide 36% to 96% oxygen at flows of 47 to 74 L/min.[15]

Patients with conditions that are unresponsive to basic oxygen therapy may require the use of PEEP or CPAP. PEEP and CPAP may be applied through the use of specialized face masks. Often, however, administration of PEEP or CPAP will require intubation and the use of mechanical ventilatory support.

To summarize, if the patient requires a low to moderate concentration of oxygen, the nasal cannula is the device of choice for oxygen delivery. In patients with unstable ventilatory patterns or rapid shallow breathing, an air-entrainment ("Venturi") mask may be considered. For moderate to high concentrations of oxygen therapy for short-term use, consider a simple, partial-rebreathing or non-rebreathing mask. For stable oxygen concentration via aerosol mask, tracheostomy mask, or "T" piece, consider a standard air-entrainment nebulizer for an FIO_2 of 0.28 to 0.50 and a high-flow, high-FIO_2 entrainment nebulizer for 60% to 96% oxygen. In patients who do not respond to basic oxygen therapy, the use of PEEP or CPAP should be considered.

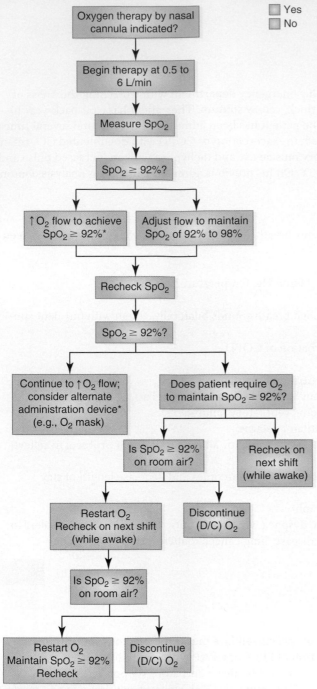

*If flow is > 6 L/min and Spo₂ < 92% consider alternative device to deliver moderate to high F$_{IO_2}$

FIGURE 2-2 Protocol for oxygen therapy by nasal cannula.

Treat and/or Prevent Bronchospasm and Mucosal Edema

Bronchodilator Therapy

The primary indication for bronchodilator therapy is to treat or prevent bronchospasm. Bronchodilator therapy is indicated in the treatment of acute asthma, COPD (to include chronic bronchitis and cystic fibrosis), and whenever wheezing is due to reversible bronchoconstriction. A documented response to bronchodilator therapy may be demonstrated by an improvement in peak expiratory flow rate (PEF), forced expiratory volume in 1 second (FEV_1), or forced vital capacity (FVC) following therapy.[16] An improvement in clinical findings such as decreased wheezing or improved aeration or a subjective improvement in the respiratory status of the patient are also important indicators of bronchodilator effectiveness.[16] In mechanically ventilated patients, bronchodilator therapy may be helpful with increased airway resistance. An improvement in peak inspiratory pressures or expiratory gas flow curves may be useful in documenting the effectiveness of the therapy in these patients. **Box 2-6** summarizes the indications for bronchodilator therapy.

Once the respiratory care clinician has determined that bronchodilator therapy is indicated, the specific medication, method of delivery, and frequency of administration must be determined. Bronchodilators are most commonly administered by inhalation via a metered-dose inhaler (MDI), a small-volume nebulizer (SVN), or a dry powder inhaler (DPI). Bronchodilators may be classified as β_2-agonists or anticholinergics and as short acting or long acting. Short-acting β_2-agonists include albuterol, levalbuterol, and pirbuterol. All have a rapid onset and a duration of effect of 5 to 8 hours. Anticholinergic bronchodilators include ipratropium bromide (short-acting) and tiotropium bromide (long-acting). Asthma and COPD represent two conditions that often require bronchodilator therapy.

Respiratory Care Plans for Asthma

Excellent clinical practice guidelines for the management of asthma have been developed by the National Institutes of Health.[17] Inhaled asthma medications include quick-relief bronchodilators and long-term control agents, usually inhaled corticosteroids. Patients with persistent asthma usually require both types of medications. Most patients with persistent asthma can maintain good control of their asthma with proper patient education (including symptom monitoring and a written asthma action plan), avoidance of asthma triggers, and an appropriate regimen of both bronchodilators (rescue medications) and **anti-inflammatory agents** (controller medications).

With poorly controlled asthma, acute asthma exacerbations often result in visits to the emergency department (ED). Initial ED treatment of acute asthma exacerbation in the adult often includes administration of 2.5 to 5.0 mg (per dose) of aerosolized albuterol via SVN every 20 minutes for a total of three doses. Following the initial bronchodilator administration of three doses, 2.5 to 10 mg of albuterol is then administered by SVN every 1 to 4 hours as needed (or 10 to 15 mg/hour nebulized continuously). Ipratropium may be added, initially beginning with 0.5 mg every 20 minutes

BOX 2-6

Indications for Bronchodilator Therapy

Asthma
COPD (emphysema/chronic bronchitis)
Cystic fibrosis
Wheezing
Documented response to a bronchodilator:
- Increase in FEV_1 > 12% following therapy and at least 200 mL

OR

- Increase in FVC > 12% following therapy and at least 200 mL

OR

- Increase in PEF*:
  - PEF to> 80% of predicted or > 80% personal best = good response
  - PEF to 50% to 79% of predicted or 60% to 80% of personal best = not well controlled.
- Increased airway resistance in patients receiving mechanical ventilation

*PEF monitoring is recommended for patients with moderate to severe chronic asthma. A peak flow > 80% of predicted or > 80% personal best suggests that asthma is in good control; 50% to 79% of predicted or 50% to 79% of personal best suggests that asthma is not well controlled; < 50% suggests asthma is poorly controlled and represents a medical alert that requires immediate treatment and contact with the patient's physician.

FEV_1, forced expiratory volume in 1 second; FVC, forced vital capacity; PEF, peak expiratory flow rate

for three rounds, and then every 2 to 4 hours as needed. Newer guidelines suggest ipratropium may only be beneficial during the initial treatment of acute asthma. These medications may be given via MDI and holding chamber with equal effectiveness, if the patient is able to coordinate the use of the MDI. The frequency of administration is then reduced based on the patient's response and measurement of PEF or FEV_1. **Table 2-3** lists the medication dosages for treatment of asthma exacerbations. An outline of a protocol for management of acute asthma exacerbation is provided in **Figure 2-3**.

Respiratory Care Plans for COPD

Inhaled bronchodilator therapy is central to the management of COPD, as described in the GOLD standards.[18] Bronchodilators are prescribed on an as-needed basis to prevent or reduce symptoms, improve exercise capacity, and reduce airflow limitation. Some evidence suggests that long-acting bronchodilators, such as tiotropium, may improve health status, reduce exacerbations, decrease the number of hospitalizations, and improve the efficacy of pulmonary rehabilitation.[18] Combination of a β_2-agonist and anticholinergic bronchodilator (combination therapy) may result in greater bronchodilation than either drug when used alone. Inhaled triple therapy, which combines a β_2-agonist, anticholinergic agent, and inhaled corticosteroid, has

been advocated for use with severe COPD. **Table 2-4** lists common COPD medications and dosages. **Box 2-7** outlines the management of patients with stable COPD.

Generally, low-risk COPD patients with intermittent symptoms are treated with two puffs of an inhaled short-acting anticholinergic bronchodilator or a short-acting β_2-agonist via MDI, as needed. Low-risk patients with regular or daily symptoms may be treated with a long-acting inhaled anticholinergic bronchodilator or a long-acting inhaled β_2-agonist. High-risk patients with severe to very severe airflow limitation (FEV_1/FVC < 0.70 and FEV_1 < 50% predicted) require the addition of an inhaled corticosteroid to a long-acting bronchodilator. A severe exacerbation of COPD may require a short-acting β_2-bronchodilator via MDI or SVN every one-half to 2 hours and/or increasing the dose of ipratropium. Hospitalized patients with acute exacerbation of COPD are also treated with oral corticosteroids and antibiotics. **Figure 2-4** outlines the pharmacologic management of stable COPD; **Figure 2-5** describes the treatment of COPD exacerbation.

Bronchodilator Therapy for Other Conditions

For other disease states or conditions where bronchospasm is suspected, the frequency of administration of a short-acting bronchodilator generally ranges from

TABLE 2-3
Medication Dosages for Treatment of Asthma Exacerbation

Medication	Child Dose (≤ 12 years)	Adult Dose	Comments
Inhaled Short-Acting Selective β₂-Agonists (SABA)			
Albuterol			
Nebulizer solution (0.63 mg/3 mL, 1.25 mg/3 mL, 2.5 mg/3 mL, 5.0 mg/mL)	0.15 mg/kg (minimum dose 2.5 mg) every 20 minutes for three doses then 0.15–0.3 mg/kg up to 10 mg every 1–4 hours as needed, or 0.5 mg/kg/hour by continuous nebulization.	2.5–5 mg every 20 minutes for three doses, then 2.5–10 mg every 1–4 hours as needed or 10–15 mg/hour continuously.	Dilute aerosols to minimum of 3 mL at gas flow of 6–8 L/min. Use large-volume nebulizers for continuous administration. May mix with ipratropium nebulizer solution.
MDI (90 mcg/puff)	4–8 puffs every 20 minutes for three doses, then every 1–4 hours inhalation maneuver as needed. Use VHC; add mask in children < 4 years.	4–8 puffs every 20 minutes up to 4 hours, then every 1–4 hours as needed.	In mild to moderate exacerbations, MDI plus HC is as effective as nebulized therapy with appropriate administration technique and coaching by trained personnel.
Bitolterol			
Nebulizer solution (2 mg/mL)	See albuterol dose; thought to be half as potent as albuterol on per mg basis.	See albuterol dose.	Not studied in severe asthma exacerbations. Do not mix with other drugs.
MDI (370 mcg/puff)	See albuterol MDI dose.	See albuterol MDI dose.	Not studied in severe asthma exacerbations.
Levalbuterol (R-albuterol)			
Nebulizer solution (0.63 mg/3 mL, 1.25 mg/0.5 mL, 1.25 mg/3 mL)	0.075 mg/kg (minimum dose 1.25 mg) every 20 minutes for three doses, then 0.075–0.15 mg/kg up to 5 mg every 1–4 hours as needed.	1.25–2.5 mg every 20 minutes for three doses, then 1.25–5 mg every 1–4 hours as needed.	Levalbuterol administered in one-half the mg dose of albuterol provides comparable efficacy and safety. Has not been evaluated by continuous nebulization.
MDI (45 mcg/puff)	See albuterol MDI dose.	See albuterol MDI dose.	
Pirbuterol			
MDI (200 mcg/puff)	See albuterol MDI dose; thought to be half as potent as albuterol on a per mg basis.	See albuterol MDI dose.	Has not been studied in severe asthma exacerbations.
Systemic (Injected) β₂-Agonists			
Epinephrine			
1:1,000 (1 mg/mL)	0.01 mg/kg up to 0.3–0.5 mg SQ every 20 minutes for three doses.	0.3–0.5 mg SQ every 20 minutes for three doses.	No proven advantage of systemic therapy over aerosol.
Terbutaline			
(1 mg/mL)	0.01 mg/kg SQ every 20 minutes for three doses then every 2–6 hours as needed.	0.25 mg SQ every 20 minutes for three doses.	No proven advantage of systemic therapy over aerosol.
Anticholinergics			
Ipratropium bromide			
Nebulizer solution (0.25 mg/mL)	0.25–0.5 mg every 20 minutes for three doses, then as needed.	0.5 mg every 20 minutes for three doses, then as needed.	May mix in nebulizer with albuterol. Should not be used as first-line therapy; add to SABA therapy for severe exacerbations. The addition of ipratropium not shown to provide further benefit once the patient is hospitalized.

TABLE 2-3
Medication Dosages for Treatment of Asthma Exacerbation (*continued*)

Medication	Child Dose (≤ 12 years)	Adult Dose	Comments
MDI (18 mcg/puff)	4–8 puffs every 20 minutes as needed up to 3 hours.	8 puffs every 20 minutes as needed up to 3 hours.	Use with HC and face mask for children < 4 years.
Ipratropium with albuterol			
Nebulizer solution (each 3 mL vial contains 0.5 mg ipratropium bromide and 2.5 mg albuterol)	1.5–3 mL every 20 minutes for three doses, then as needed.	3 mL every 20 minutes for three doses, then as needed.	Used for up to 3 hours in initial management of severe exacerbations. Addition of ipratropium to albuterol not shown to provide further benefit once the patient is hospitalized.
MDI (each puff contains 18 mcg ipratropium bromide and 90 mcg of albuterol)	4–8 puffs every 20 minutes as needed up to 3 hours.	8 puffs every 20 minutes as needed up to 3 hours.	Use with HC and face mask for children < 4 years.
Systemic Corticosteroids			
		(Applies to all three corticosteroids)	
Prednisone Methylprednisolone Prednisolone	1–2 mg/kg in two divided doses (maximum = 60 mg/day) until PEF is 70% of predicted or personal best.	40–80 mg/day in one or two divided doses until PEF reaches 70% of predicted or personal best.	Outpatient "burst": use 40–60 mg in one or two divided doses for total of 5–10 days in adults (children: 1–2 mg/kg/day maximum 60 mg/day for 3–10 days).

- There is no advantage for intravenous administration over oral therapy provided gastrointestinal transit time or absorption is not impaired.
- Course of systemic corticosteroids for asthma exacerbation requiring ED visit or hospitalization may be 3–10 days. For less than 1 week, no need to taper dose. For courses up to 10 days, tapering may not be necessary, especially if patients are concurrently taking inhaled corticosteroids.
- Inhaled corticosteroids can be started at any point in the treatment of an asthma exacerbation.

MDI, metered-dose inhaler; HC, holding chamber; PEF, peak expiratory flow; ED, emergency department; SQ, subcutaneous.

Reproduced from: National Institutes of Health, National Heart, Lung, and Blood Institute Guidelines for the Diagnosis and Management of Asthma: Expert Panel 3 Report. (NIH publication). Bethesda, MD: US Department of Health and Human Services; 2007.

every 4 hours to four times a day, depending on the patient's response and the duration of effect of the medication. For example, the recommended dosage of albuterol by SVN is 2.5 mg three or four times per day, with the onset of action occurring in about 15 minutes, a peak effect in 30 to 60 minutes, and a duration of action of 5 to 8 hours.[19] Salmeterol, a long-acting β_2-agonist, has an onset within 20 minutes, a peak effect in 180 to 300 minutes, and a duration of action of 12 hours. The normal dose for salmeterol via DPI is one inhalation every 12 hours.[19] Formoterol also has a duration of 12 hours but an onset of action similar to albuterol. The usual dose for formoterol via MDI is two puffs every 12 hours.

Anti-inflammatory Agents and Antiasthmatic Medications

Anti-inflammatory aerosol agents and **antiasthmatic medications** include inhaled corticosteroids; cromolyn sodium (a mast cell stabilizer); and antileukotrienes, such as zafirlukast (Accolate), montelukast (Singulair), and zileuton (Zyflo), the latter three medications being administered in tablet form. The indications for anti-inflammatory aerosol agents and antiasthmatic agents are listed in **Box 2-8**.

Corticosteroids are the strongest and most effective anti-inflammatory agents currently available and are more effective in asthma control than any other single long-term medication.[17] The appropriate use of corticosteroids in the treatment of asthma is well described in the NIH Guidelines.[17] Inhaled corticosteroids are taken daily on a long-term basis to control persistent asthma; and short courses of oral corticosteroids are often used to gain rapid control during asthma exacerbations.

Cromolyn sodium, administered by inhalation, stabilizes the mast cells in the lungs and may prevent or reduce the inflammatory response in asthma. As a prophylactic agent, cromolyn sodium may be added to the care regimen as an alternative in the long-term

Patient Assessment

- **Review of the patient record and patient interview :** Assess for severity of exacerbation and risk factors associated with death from asthma:
  - **Asthma history**
    - Level of dyspnea (mild, moderate, or severe?)
    - Previous history of exacerbation?
    - Previous emergency department visits ($\geq$3 in the past year?)
    - Previous hospitalizations ($\geq$2 in the past year?)
    - ICU admission and/or intubation for asthma?
    - Use of MDI β_2-adrenergic agonist canisters (>2 per month?)
    - Difficulty perceiving asthma symptoms or severity of exacerbations?
    - Written action plan (in place and followed)?
    - Sensitivity to *Alternaria* (a fungus associated with hay fever and allergic asthma)?
  - **Social history**
    - Low socioeconomic status or inner-city resident?
    - Illicit drug use?
    - Major psychological problems?
  - **Comorbidities**
    - Cardiovascular disease?
    - Other chronic lung disease?
    - Chronic psychiatric disease?

- **Physical assessment:** Observe for:
  - Breathlessness at rest?
  - Ability to talk in sentences, phrases, or only words due to dyspnea?
  - Alertness (agitated, drowsy, confused)?
  - Increased respiratory rate (>30 is severe)?
  - Tachycardia (>120 is severe)? Pulsus paradoxus?
  - Accessory muscle use?
  - Wheezing? (Absence of wheeze may signal an imminent respiratory arrest.)

- **Pulmonary function:** PEF percent predicted or percent personal best (for asthma):
  - Mild severity: $\geq$70%
  - Moderate severity: 40% to 60%
  - Severe: <40%

- **Oximetry and arterial blood gases breathing room air:**
  - Normal: SpO_2 > 95% and/or PaO_2 80 to 100 on room air
  - Moderate severity: SpO_2 90% to 95% and/or PaO_2 $\geq$ 60 but <80
  - Severe: SpO_2 < 90% and/or PaO_2 < 60 – severe
  - Mild or normal: $PaCO_2$ < 42 mm Hg; $\geq$42 mm Hg may progress to ventilatory failure requiring mechanical ventilation

- **Treatment**
  - Supply oxygen therapy to relieve hypoxemia and maintain SaO_2 $\geq$ 90%.
  - Administer inhaled short-acting β_2-agonist to relieve airflow obstruction, with addition of inhaled ipratropium bromide in severe exacerbations.
  - Administer systemic corticosteroids to decrease airway inflammation in moderate or severe exacerbations or for patients who fail to respond promptly and completely to a short-acting β_2-agonist/
  - Monitor vital signs, SaO_2.
  - Consider adjunct therapy in severe exacerbations unresponsive to the initial treatment:
        Intravenous magnesium sulfate
        Heliox
  - Monitor response with serial measurements of lung function (FEV_1 or PEF).
  - Prevent recurrence:
    - Refer to follow-up asthma care within 1 to 4 weeks of discharge.
    - Provide asthma care plan with instructions for medications prescribed at discharge and for increasing medications or seeking medical care if asthma worsens.
    - Review/teach inhaler use/techniques.
    - Consider initiating inhaled corticosteroids.

FIGURE 2-3 Management of acute asthma exacerbation.

Data from: National Institutes of Health, National Heart, Lung, and Blood Institute Guidelines for the Diagnosis and Management of Asthma: Expert Panel 3 Report. NIH publication. Bethesda, MD: U.S. Department of Health and Human Services; 2007.

TABLE 2-4
COPD Medications

Drug	Trade Names	Inhaler (mcg)	DPI/MDI Dose	Solution for Nebulizer	Nebulizer Dose	Duration of Action (hours)
β₂-agonists						
Short Acting						
Albuterol	Proventil HFA; Ventolin HFA; ProAir HFA; AccuNeb; VoSpire ER	90 mcg/puff (MDI)	2 puffs three to four times per day	0.5% solution—0.5 mL (2.5 mg), or 0.63 mg, 1.25 mg, and 2.5 mg unit dose	2.5 mg in 3 mL normal saline three to four times per day	5–8
Levalbuterol	Xopenex; Xopenex HFA	45 mcg/puff (MDI)	2 puffs every 4–6 hours	0.31 mg, 0.63 mg, 1.25 mg in 3 mL solution	3 mL three times per day	5–8
Pirbuterol	Maxair Autohaler	200 mcg/puff (MDI)	2 puffs every 4–6 hours	NA	NA	5–8
Long Acting						
Arformoterol	Brovana	NA	NA	15 mcg/2 mL unit dose vial	2 mL every 12 hours	12
Formoterol	Perforomist, Foradil	12 mcg/inhalation (DPI)	1 inhalation every 12 hours	20 mcg/2 mL unit dose vial	2 mL every 12 hours	12
Indacaterol	Arcapta Neohaler	75 mcg/inhalation (DPI)	1 inhalation every day	NA	NA	24
Salmeterol	Serevent Diskus	50 mcg/inhalation (DPI)	1 inhalation every 12 hours	NA	NA	12
Anticholinergics						
Short Acting						
Ipratropium bromide	Atrovent HFA	17 mcg/puff (MDI)	2 puffs four times daily	0.2 mg/mL (0.02% solution) in a 2.5 mL unit dose	2.5 mL unit dose/500 mcg three to four times daily	4–6
Oxitropium bromide (available outside United States)	Oxivent, Tersigan, Tersigat, Ventilat, Ventox	100 mcg (MDI)	2 puffs two to three times daily	NA	NA	7–9
Long Acting						
Tiotropium	Spiriva	18 mcg/inhalation (DPI)	1 inhalation every day	NA	NA	24
Combination Short-Acting β₂-Agonists Plus Anticholinergic						
Albuterol/ Ipratropium	Combivent DuoNeb	Albuterol: 90 mcg Ipratropium: 18 mcg/puff	2 puffs four times a day of 18 mcg/puff ipratropiumand 90 mcg/puff albuterol	Albuterol: 2.5 mg Iprotropium: 0.5 mg in 3 mL	3 mL four times a day	4–6

(continues)

TABLE 2-4
COPD Medications (*continued*)

Drug	Trade Names	Inhaler (mcg)	DPI/MDI Dose	Solution for Nebulizer	Nebulizer Dose	Duration of Action (hours)
Fenoterol/ Ipratropium (available in Canada)	Duovent UDV	NA	NA	Fenoterol: 1.25 mg Ipratropium: 0.5 mg in 4 mL	4 mL every 6 hours	6–8
Methylxanthines						
Aminophylline	Phyllocontin; Truphylline (Canada)	• IV 5.7 mg/kg loading dose in patients not currently receiving • IV maintenance dose in adults 16–60 years: 0.51 mg/kg/hr; maximum 400 mg/day to achieve a serum theophylline level of 5–10 mcg/mL • IV maintenance dose in adults > 60 years: 0.38 mg/kg/hr; maximum 400 mg/day • Dose should be adjusted for shock, sepsis, cardiac decompensation, cor pulmonale, or liver dysfunction to 0.25 mg/kg/hr; maximum 400 mg/day				Variable, up to 24
Theophylline	Theochron, Elixophyllin, Theo-24	• Initial dose (oral): 300–400 mg once daily • Maintenance: 400–600 mg once daily (maximum 600 mg/day)				Variable, up to 24
Phosphodiesterase-4 inhibitors						
Roflumilast	Dalisresp	500 mcg oral tablet once daily				24
Inhaled Corticosteroids						
Beclomethasone diprorionate HFA	Qvar	40 mcg/puff and 80 mcg/puff (MDI)	40–80 mcg twice daily or 40–160 mcg twice daily*	NA	NA	NA
Budesonide	Pulmicort, Pulmicort Respules	90 mcg/actuation and 180 mcg/actuation (DPI)	180–360 mcg twice daily or 360–720 mcg twice daily**	NA	NA	NA
Fluticasone propionate	Flovent HFA, Flovent Diskus	44 mcg/puff, 110 mcg/puff, and 220 mcg/puff (MDI)	88 mcg twice daily***	NA	NA	NA
Combination Long-Acting β_2-Agonists Plus Corticosteroids						
Formoterol/ Budesonide	Symbicort	160 mcg budesonide/4.5 mcg formoterol per puff (MDI)	2 puffs twice daily	NA	NA	NA
Salmeterol/ Fluticasone	Advair Diskus, Advair HFA	100, 250, or 500 mcg fluticasone/50 mcg salmeterol (DPI) 45, 115, or 230 mcg fluticasone/21 mcg salmeterol (MDI)	1 inhalation every 12 hours (DPI) 2 puffs every 12 hours (MDI)	NA	NA	12

TABLE 2-4
COPD Medications (*continued*)

Drug	Trade Names	Inhaler (mcg)	DPI/MDI Dose	Solution for Nebulizer	Nebulizer Dose	Duration of Action (hours)
Systemic Corticosteroids May Improve Outcomes When Used in the Treatment of Acute Exacerbation of COPD						
Methyl-prednisolone	Medrol; Meprolone	Methylprednisolone suggested dosage for COPD exacerbation with impending respiratory failure is 60 mg IV, one to two times daily.				
Prednisone	Prednisone Intensol™	Oral prednisone dose of 30–60 mg/day for 7–10 days has been suggested.				

MDI, metered dose inhaler; DPI, dry powder inhaler; SMI, smart mist inhaler; NA = not applicable.
*Beclomethasone recommended starting dose if previously taking inhaled corticosteroids.
**Budesonide starting dose if only taking bronchodilators and/or inhaled corticosteroids previously. Starting dose should be higher (360 to 720 mcg twice daily) if previously taking oral corticosteroids.
***Fluticasone starting dose if only taking bronchodilators previously. Starting dose should be 88 to 220 mcg twice daily if previously taking inhaled corticosteroids and 880 mcg twice daily if previously taking oral corticosteroids.
Data from: Gardenhire D. *Rau's Respiratory Care Pharmacology*, 8th ed. St. Louis: Elsevier Health; 2012: 98–108; Global Initiative for Chronic Obstructive Lung Disease. *Pocket Guide to COPD Diagnosis, Management, and Prevention: A Guide for Health Care Professionals*. 2011. Available at: http://www.goldcopd.org /uploads/users/files/GOLD_PocketGuide_2011_Jan18.pdf.

BOX 2-7

Management of Stable COPD

Smoking cessation
Pharmacological therapy
- Short-acting β_2-agonists (albuterol)
- Short-acting anticholinergic bronchodilator (ipratropium)
- Combined short-acting β_2-agonists and short-acting anticholinergic bronchodilators
- Long-acting inhaled β_2-agonists (salmeterol, formoterol)
- Long-acting anticholinergic bronchodilator (tiotropium)
- Combined long-acting β_2-agonists and long-acting anticholinergic bronchodilators
- Phosphodiesterase-4 inhibitor (roflumilast)*
- Inhaled corticosteroids (beclomethasone, budesonide, triamcinolone, fluticasone, flunisolide)
- Combining long-acting inhaled β-agonists and inhaled corticosteroids in one inhaler
- Mucolytics/antioxidant therapy (oral *N*-acetylcysteine)
- α-Trypsin augmentation therapy (identified α_1-antitrypsin deficiency)
Vaccination (influenza, pneumococcal disease)
Oxygen therapy
Long-term oxygen therapy
Pulmonary rehabilitation
Nutrition
Surgery in or for COPD
Sleep (assess for sleep issues and/or sleep disorders)
Air travel considerations (evaluate the need for oxygen)

*For chronic bronchitis with frequent exacerbations
Data from the American Thoracic Society–European Respiratory Society Standards for the Diagnosis and Management of Patients with COPD. http://www.thoracic.org/clinical/copd-guidelines/resources/copddoc.pdf.

LESS RISK, LESS SYMPTOMS

Patients with low risk, less symptoms, and mild to moderate airflow limitation ($FEV_1/FVC < 0.70$ and $FEV_{1.0} > 50\%$ predicted) and one or fewer exacerbations per year.

First Choice

Short-acting anticholinergic bronchodilator PRN OR
Short acting β_2-agonist PRN

Second Choice

Long-acting anticholinergic bronchodilator OR
Long-acting β_2-agonist OR
Long-acting anticholinergic and long-acting β_2-agonist

LESS RISK, MORE SYMPTOMS

Patients with low risk, more symptoms, and mild to moderate airflow limitation ($FEV_1/FVC < 0.70$ and $FEV_1 > 50\%$ predicted) and one or fewer exacerbations per year.

First Choice

Long-acting anticholinergic bronchodilator OR
Long-acting β_2-agonist

Second Choice

Long-acting anticholinergic bronchodilator and long-acting β_2-agonist

HIGH RISK, LESS SYMPTOMS, BUT SEVERE AIRFLOW LIMITATION

Patients with high risk, less symptoms, but severe to very severe airflow limitation and two or more exacerbations per year ($FEV_1/FVC < 0.70$ and $FEV_1 < 50\%$ predicted [severe] or $FEV_1 < 30\%$ predicted [very severe]).

First Choice

Inhaled corticosteroids AND
Long-acting β_2 agonist OR long-acting anticholinergic

Second Choice

Long-acting antichololinergic and long-acting β_2-agonist

HIGH RISK, MORE SYMPTOMS, AND SEVERE AIRFLOW LIMITATION

Patients with high risk, more symptoms, and severe to very severe airflow limitation and two or more exacerbations per year.

First Choice

Inhaled corticosteroids AND
Long-acting β_2-agonist OR long-acting anticholinergic

Second Choice

Inhaled corticosteroids and long-acting anticholinergic OR
Inhaled corticosteroids and long-acting β_2-agonist and long-acting anticholinergic OR
Inhaled corticosteroids and long-acting β_2-agonist and phosphodiesterase-4 inhibitor OR
Long-acting anticholinergic and long-acting β_2-agonist OR
Long-acting anticholinergic and phosphodiesterase-4 inhibitor

FIGURE 2-4 Pharmacologic treatment for the stable COPD.

Data from: Global Initiative for Chronic Obstructive Lung Disease. *Pocket Guide to COPD Diagnosis, Management, and Prevention 2011.* Available at: http://www.goldcopd
.org/guidelines-pocket-guide-to-copd-diagnosis.html.

Patient Assessment

- **Interview:** Question patient regarding increased dyspnea, orthopnea, cough, sputum production, sputum purulence, decreased ability to conduct activities of daily living (ADLs).

- **Physical assessment:** Observe for increased respiratory rate, tachycardia, color (cyanosis, pale, skin flushed/red), accessory muscle use, pursed-lip breathing, chest configuration (overinflation; barrel chest), level of consciousness (oriented, anxiety, sleepy, lethargic, somnolent), breath sounds (diminished, crackles, gurgles, wheezing), cough, purulent sputum.

- **Oximetry and arterial blood gases**
  - $SpO_2 < 88\%$ to 90% is consistent with a $PaO_2 < 55$ to 58 ($SpO_2 < 85\%$ is consistent with a $PaO_2 < 50$).
  - $PaO_2 < 60$ on $FIO_2 = 0.21$ (with or without CO_2 elevation) indicates respiratory failure.

- **Chest radiograph:** Review for infiltrates, pneumonia, exclude alternative diagnoses.

- **Laboratory studies**
  - Complete blood count (polycythemia, anemia, elevated WBC)
  - Electrolytes
  - Renal function

Treatment

- **Oxygen therapy**
  - Low-flow cannula (0.5 to 4 L/min) to achieve SpO_2 of 90% to 92% and PaO_2 of 60 to 70 mm Hg.
  - High-flow air-entrainment mask (24% to 28%) may be considered in the presence of an irregular ventilatory pattern or rapid shallow breathing.

- **Bronchodilators:** Short-acting β_2-agonist with or without short-acting anticholinergics for treatment of an exacerbation.

- **Systemic corticosteroids**
  - Corticosteroids may improve patient outcomes and reduce length of stay.
  - IV or oral prednisone 30 to 60 mg, once daily for 7 to 10 days (dose may be tapered for another 7 days; however, tapering is not necessary for therapy of less than 3 weeks).
  - Prednisolone dose suggested by the GOLD standards is 30 to 40 mg/day for 10 to 14 days (oral route preferred).

- **Antibiotics:** Antibiotics should be considered in the presence of:
  - Increased dyspnea, increased sputum volume and increased sputum purulence OR
  - Increased sputum purulence AND
  - Increased sputum volume OR increased dyspnea OR
  - Ventilatory failure requiring mechanical ventilatory support.

- **Other therapy:** Attention should be paid to:
  - Fluid balance (consider diuretics for fluid overload)
  - Nutrition
  - Treatment of comorbidities such as pneumonia, cardiovascular disease (ischemic heart disease, CHF, hypertension, atrial fibrillation), lung cancer, renal failure, liver failure, osteoporosis, diabetes, anxiety and depression.

FIGURE 2-5 Outline of the management of COPD exacerbation.

Data from: Global Initiative for Chronic Obstructive Lung Disease. *Pocket Guide to COPD Diagnosis, Management, and Prevention—2011.* Available at: http://www.goldcopd .org/guidelines-pocket-guide-to-copd-diagnosis.html; Jong YP, Vil SM, Grotjohan HP, Postma DS, Kerstjens H, Vanden Berg J. Oral or IV prednisolone in the treatment of COPD exacerbations: a randomized controlled, double-blind study. *Chest.* 2007;132(6):1741–1747.

management of asthma and as a preventive measure prior to exercise or exposure to known allergens.[17]

Leukotriene modifiers that reduce or block inflammation include montelukast (Singulair), zafirlukast (Accolate), and zileuton (Zyflo). Montelukast and zafirlukast are leukotriene receptor antagonists (LTRAs) and may be useful as alternatives in the treatment of mild to moderate asthma.[17] LTRAs may be used in combination with inhaled corticosteroids, although in adults the addition of long-acting bronchodilators should be considered first.[17] Zileuton is a 5-lipoxygenase pathway inhibitor that may also be considered for asthma prophylaxis. Zileuton requires assessment of liver enzymes prior to initiation and ongoing liver function monitoring.[19]

Treatment of Upper Airway Inflammation

A cool, bland aerosol is indicated in the treatment of upper airway edema, including laryngotracheobronchitis and subglottic edema, and for postoperative management of the upper airway.[20] Upper airway edema is common following extubation, and the use of a cool, bland aerosol with supplemental oxygen is recommended. Nebulized racemic epinephrine (0.5 mL of 2.25% in 3 mL of diluent) or dexamethasone (1 mg in 4 mL of diluent) by nebulizer have also been suggested for the treatment of postextubation laryngeal edema; however, the evidence to support this recommendation is weak. Helium–oxygen mixtures (60% He and 40% O_2) by nonrebreathing mask may be helpful in decreasing the severity of stridor and reducing the need for reintubation. Helium–oxygen therapy (60% to 80% helium) may also be of value in treatment of acute severe asthma exacerbation and has been used in an attempt to reduce the need for intubation and **mechanical ventilation** in these patients.

For pediatric patients suffering from croup (laryngotracheobronchitis), treatment typically consists of cool mist therapy.[20] Aerosolized racemic epinephrine (0.05 mL/kg of a 2.25% solution not to exceed 0.5 mL per dose diluted to 3 mL) may provide rapid improvement in upper airway obstruction in moderate to severe croup. Aerosolized dexamethasone or budesonide may also be effective in reducing severity of symptoms in patients suffering from croup, although dexamethasone is most commonly administered intravenously (IV), intramuscularly (IM), or orally.

Mobilize and Remove Secretions

Disease states or conditions in which mucus clearance may be a problem include chronic bronchitis, bronchiectasis, and cystic fibrosis. Mucus hypersecretion, inflammation, and bronchospasm are sometimes seen in asthma, acute bronchitis, and acute pulmonary infections. Mucus plugging can cause atelectasis, and copious secretions are sometimes seen with atelectasis and pneumonia.

Techniques to Mobilize Secretions

Techniques to mobilize or remove secretions include directed cough, suctioning, use of high-volume aerosol therapy, and bronchial hygiene. Bronchial hygiene techniques include **chest physiotherapy (CPT)** (postural drainage, percussion, and vibration), kinetic therapy (turning), and directed cough. Indications for bronchial hygiene therapy include difficulty with secretion clearance, evidence of retained secretions, the presence of copious secretions (generally expectorated sputum production > 25 to 30 mL/day in the adult), atelectasis associated with mucus plugging, and the presence of a foreign body in the airway.[20–25] Bronchial hygiene therapy is probably not helpful in acute exacerbation of COPD, pneumonia without excess secretion production, and acute asthma exacerbation. A complete list of bronchial hygiene techniques are listed in **Box 2-9**. Specific indications for therapy to mobilize secretions are listed in **Box 2-10**.

Directed Cough

Directed cough to clear secretions may be employed in patients with an inadequate spontaneous cough and should be included as an integral part of other bronchial hygiene therapies to mobilize and remove secretions.[25] The indications for a directed cough include retained secretions, atelectasis, and lung disease with excess secretions (chronic bronchitis, bronchiectasis, cystic fibrosis, and necrotizing pulmonary infection).[25] Directed cough is also indicated in patients at risk of developing postoperative complications and to obtain sputum specimens for diagnostic analysis, and it has been suggested for patients with spinal cord injury.[25] A mechanically provided artificial cough, using an insufflation–exsufflation device (also known as cough-assist device) may be especially helpful in patients with spinal cord injury or neuromuscular disease.[26]

High-Volume Bland Aerosol Therapy

High-volume heated, bland aerosols (normal saline, half normal saline, and sterile, distilled water) may minimize or eliminate humidity deficits in patients with artificial airways and thus help maintain mucociliary clearance. Heated bland aerosols are used routinely to

BOX 2-9

Bronchial Hygiene Techniques

Directed cough: A cough technique taught and supervised by a healthcare professional.

Postural drainage: The use of gravity and position to mobilize secretions.

Chest percussion (aka clapping or cupping) and vibration: Manual or mechanical percussion and vibration of the chest wall in order to mobilize secretions.

Kinetic therapy (turning): Rotation of the body to improve lung expansion, oxygenation, and secretion mobilization.

High-frequency chest wall oscillation (HFCWO): A technique that uses a mechanical device attached to an inflatable vest worn by the patient. Air is pulsed into the vest at a high frequency to vibrate the chest and lungs and thus improve mucus clearance.

Positive airway pressure (PAP): Adjunct techniques for secretion mobilization that incorporates the use of a mechanical device to generate continuous positive airway pressure (CPAP), positive expiratory pressure (PEP), or expiratory positive airway pressure (EPAP).

Flutter valve: A mechanical device that combines EPAP and high-frequency airway oscillations at the airway as the patient exhales through the device.

Intrapulmonary percussive ventilation (IPV): An IPV device is used to produce high-frequency oscillation of the inspired gas in combination with PAP.

Forced expiratory technique (FET): A modified version of the directed cough, also known as a "huff" cough.

Active cycle breathing (ACB): A breathing exercise cycle that incorporates the FET.

Autogenic drainage: A modification of the directed cough that incorporates diaphragmatic breathing at varied lung volumes.

Mechanical insufflation–exsufflation: The use of a mechanical device that uses positive pressure on inspiration to produce a deep breath followed by negative pressure on exhalation to simulate a cough.

BOX 2-10

Indications for Therapy to Mobilize Secretions

Directed Cough

Retained secretions

Atelectasis

At risk for postoperative pulmonary complications

Cystic fibrosis, bronchiectasis, chronic bronchitis, necrotizing pulmonary infection, or spinal cord injury

During/following other bronchial hygiene therapies

To obtain sputum specimens

Suctioning

Presence of endotracheal or tracheostomy tube

Inability to clear secretions in spite of best cough effort (secretions audible in large/central airways)

Need to remove accumulated pulmonary secretions in presence of an artificial airway

Coarse or noisy breath sounds (rhonchi, gurgles)

Increased PIP during mechanical ventilation or decreased V_T during pressure-controlled ventilation

Ineffective spontaneous cough

Visible secretions in airway

(continues)

Suspected aspiration

Increased work of breathing

Deterioration of arterial blood gases

Chest radiograph changes consistent with retained secretions

To obtain sputum specimen

To maintain artificial airway patency

To stimulate cough

Presence of atelectasis or consolidation presumed to be associated with secretion retention

Chest Physiotherapy (Postural Drainage and Percussion)

Suggestion/evidence of problems with secretion clearance

Difficulty clearing secretions with volume > 25 to 30 mL/day (adult)

Retained secretions in presence of an artificial airway

Atelectasis caused/suspected to be due to mucus plugging

Cystic fibrosis, bronchiectasis, cavitating lung disease

Presence of a foreign body in airway

Mucolytic Therapy

Evidence of viscous/retained secretions that are not easily removed via other therapy

Chronic bronchitis, cystic fibrosis, bronchiectasis

High-Volume Bland Aerosol

Cool Large-Volume Nebulizer with Bland Solution

Following extubation

Delivery of precise F_{IO_2} via aerosol mask and humidity

Upper airway edema:

- Laryngotracheobronchitis (croup)
- Subglottic edema

Heated Large-Volume Nebulizer with Bland Solution

Evidence/potential for secretion clearance problem

Deliver precise F_{IO_2} via aerosol mask and high humidity

Mobilization of secretions

Hypertonic Saline Administration

Need to induce sputum specimens

PIP, peak inspiratory pressure; V_T, tidal volume.

provide humidification in patients with artificial airways for which there is evidence or potential for secretion problems. High-volume bland aerosols may be useful for mobilization of secretions and induction of sputum specimens; however, the efficacy of using bland aerosols to reduce mucus has not been established.[20] Most pneumatic cool-mist aerosol generators do not deliver a substantial amount of water to the airway and have little potential for mobilizing secretions. Heated pneumatic nebulizers and ultrasonic nebulizers may deliver sufficient volumes of water to the airway to assist in mobilizing secretions; however, the physical properties of mucus are only minimally affected by the use of bland aerosols.[20,21] Heated aerosols and ultrasonic nebulizers are used to administer either sterile distilled water or a hypertonic saline solution (3% to 7% NaCl) for sputum induction.

Mucolytic Therapy

Mucolytic agents may promote secretion clearance by reducing mucus viscosity. Aerosolized dornase alfa (Pulmozyme) is indicated for clearance of purulent secretions in cystic fibrosis.[18,19] Acetylcysteine (Mucomyst) thins mucus by breaking down mucoprotein disulfide bonds. Acetylcysteine may be given orally, by inhaled aerosol, or directly installed into the airway. Aerosolized acetylcysteine should always be accompanied by a bronchodilator to avoid inducing bronchospasm. There is little evidence to support the use of aerosolized acetylcysteine in patients.

Oral acetylcysteine may be helpful in COPD patients with viscid secretions, but oral acetylcysteine is not approved for use in the United States.[18]

The least expensive and effective method for mobilization of secretions should be selected. For example, a well-hydrated patient with chronic bronchitis who is able to easily expectorate secretions using a directed cough probably has no need for chest physiotherapy or use of an oral mucolytic. A cystic fibrosis patient with abundant secretions that are not easily cleared by directed cough might require vigorous chest physiotherapy or use of alternative techniques for secretion management, such as administration of aerosolized dornase alfa.

Frequency of therapy will vary with the respiratory care modality selected and the patient's condition. For example, aerosolized dornase alfa is indicated specifically in the management of cystic fibrosis using 2.5 mg in a 2.5 mL solution administered once daily.

Directed cough should follow any therapy used to mobilize secretions and may be useful in obtaining a sputum specimen. Suctioning should be applied to patients with artificial airways on an as-needed basis. Routine suction schedules (every 2 hours, every 4 hours, etc.) should be avoided.

Chest Physiotherapy

Chest physiotherapy may include postural drainage, percussion, and vibration accompanied by directed cough. Postural drainage positions are generally applied for 3 to 15 minutes per position for a total treatment time of 30 to 40 minutes, as tolerated by the patient.[22,23] Chest percussion or vibration may be applied for each postural drainage position for 3 to 5 minutes per position.[22] Frequency of performance of chest physiotherapy should be based on the patient's ability to tolerate the procedure and the effectiveness of the procedure in mobilizing secretions. Generally, postural drainage and chest percussion in the acute care setting are applied every 4 to 6 hours.

Other techniques sometimes used as an aid to mobilizing secretions include the use of the huff cough (forced expiratory technique, or FET), active-cycle breathing, autogenic drainage, mechanical insufflation–exsufflation, positive expiratory pressure (PEP), and high-frequency compression/oscillation (high-frequency chest wall compression, flutter valve, and intrapulmonary percussive ventilation).[22,24]

An example of a respiratory care plan designed to assist in mobilizing secretions in a patient with bronchiectasis is found in **Clinical Focus 2-3**.

CLINICAL FOCUS 2-3

Respiratory Care Plan to Mobilize Secretions in a Hospitalized Patient with Bronchiectasis

A 68-year-old man with a history of bronchiectasis is admitted to the hospital for acute exacerbation. The patient has a been coughing up more than approximately 25 mL/day of thick, dark yellow muco-purulent sputum and has some difficulty clearing secretions. The patient is short of breath, has some pleuritic chest pain, and is receiving oxygen by nasal cannula at 2 L/min with a resultant Spo_2 of 92%.

Treatment of acute exacerbation of bronchiectasis is aimed at treating infection, providing supportive care, and delivering bronchial hygiene therapy. The following is the care plan for this patient:

- The goals of therapy are to treat infection, provide bronchial hygiene, manage secretions, maintain oxygenation, and treat/prevent bronchospasm associated with inflammation.
- Obtain a sputum sample for culture and sensitivity followed by antibiotics to treat acute infection.
- Ensure adequate patient hydration via oral liquids.
- Provide 2.5 mg of albuterol in 3 mL of 0.9% NaCl by small-volume nebulizer every 4 hours while awake and as needed at night powered by compressed air (keep cannula in use during therapy; see below).
- Follow aerosol therapy with postural drainage and chest percussion to right lower lobe and left lower lobe and anterior, posterior, and lateral segments.
- Directed cough following aerosol therapy and chest physiotherapy.
- Continue nasal cannula at 1 to 4 L/m to maintain Spo_2 > 90% to 92% with a Pao_2 of 60 to 70. Monitor Spo_2 during chest physiotherapy.
- Assessment includes monitoring breath sounds, cough, sputum production (color, volume consistency), shortness of breath, Spo_2, and vital signs. Review results of sputum culture and sensitivity to tailor antibiotic therapy.

Note that inhaled corticosteroids may improve lung function and dyspnea and reduce cough in bronchiectasis and may be added. Bronchiectasis may be accompanied by gastroesophageal reflux, requiring medication to suppress gastric acid.

Nasotracheal Suctioning

Nasotracheal (NT) suctioning is indicated in cases where the patient's spontaneous or directed cough is ineffective. Specifically, NT suctioning may be required to maintain a patent airway in the presence of excess pulmonary secretions, blood, saliva, vomitus, or foreign material in the trachea or central airways.[27] NT suctioning may also be useful to stimulate a cough or to obtain a sputum sample for microbiologic or cytologic analysis.[27] NT suctioning is contraindicated with nasal bleeding, epiglottitis, croup, laryngospasm, bronchospasm, or an irritable airway. It also is contraindicated in the presence of coagulopathy or bleeding disorders; acute head, facial, or neck injury; gastric surgery with high anastomosis; and myocardial infarction.[27]

Provide Lung Expansion Therapy

The primary indications for lung expansion therapy are in the treatment and/or prevention of atelectasis and the prevention of the development of respiratory failure, particularly in postoperative patients.[26,28,29] Patients who are bedridden, immobilized, or prone to shallow breathing with a weak cough may also be candidates for lung expansion therapy. The two primary techniques for applying lung expansion therapy are **incentive spirometry (IS)** and **intermittent positive pressure breathing (IPPB)**. In addition, **positive airway pressure (PAP)** is sometimes used to mobilize secretions and treat atelectasis.[24]

Incentive spirometry should be considered in patients who are able to perform the maneuver every 1 to 2 hours while awake and are able to achieve an inspired volume of at least one-third of the predicted inspiratory capacity (IC).[25] Inspiratory capacity may be estimated by multiplying the patient's calculated ideal body weight (IBW) in kilograms by 50 mL (i.e., IBW kg × 50 mL/kg). **Clinical Focus 2-4** provides an example of the application of incentive spirometry. Recommended frequency and duration of an incentive spirometry session should be every hour while awake for 10 to 15 breaths of at least one-third predicted IC each (or > 10 mL/kg). Also see the RC Insight.

RC Insights

Inspiratory capacity (IC) in adults can be estimated as follows:

$$IC = 50 \text{ mL/kg of ideal body weight (IBW)}$$
where IBW in kg is:
$$IBW \text{ men} = [106 + 6(H - 60)] / 2.2$$
$$IBW \text{ women} = [105 + 5(H - 60)] / 2.2$$

CLINICAL FOCUS 2-4

Application of Incentive Spirometry

A preoperative 54-year-old coronary artery bypass graft (CABG) patient is seen by the respiratory care clinician for assessment and patient education. The patient is alert, awake, and cooperative, and has no history of pulmonary disease. Vitals signs, breaths sounds, and oximetry are normal, and the patient is in no distress. The patient's spontaneous inspiratory capacity prior to surgery is 3000 mL. The patient is 5'11" and weighs 200 pounds.

In order to prevent postoperative atelectasis and related respiratory problems, a respiratory care plan for this patient should include lung expansion therapy:

- Goal of therapy is to prevent postoperative atelectasis and respiratory failure.
- Device or procedure is incentive spirometry every hour while awake for 10 to 15 breaths followed by directed cough.
- Calculated ideal body weight (IBW) for this patient 172 pounds, or 78 kg:

$$IBW \text{ (lbs.)} = 106 + 6(H - 60) = 106 + 6(71 - 70) = 172 \text{ lbs.}$$
$$kg = lbs/2.2 = 172/2.2 = 78 \text{ kg}$$

- Predicted inspiratory capacity (IC) for this patient is approximately 3900 mL:

$$\text{Predicted IC} = 50 \text{ mL/IBW (kg)} = 50 \times 78 = 3900 \text{ mL}$$

- Volume goal should be at least one-third predicted IC, or about 1200 mL per breath:

$$1/3 \times 3900 \text{ mL} = 1287 \text{ mL}$$

- Assessment includes monitoring volumes and compliance with IS and watching patient for development of the signs and symptoms of atelectasis and postoperative respiratory failure:

$$\text{Minimum volume for incentive spirometry} = IBW \times 50 \text{ mL/kg} \times 1/3$$

IPPB should generally be reserved for patients who have clinically important atelectasis in which other therapy has been unsuccessful.[26] When used as a form of lung expansion therapy, minimum delivered tidal volumes during IPPB therapy should probably be at least one-third of predicted IC, or about 1200 mL in a typical adult.[26] IPPB may also be considered for patients at risk for developing atelectasis who cannot or will not take a deep breath on their own. IPPB may also be useful in a few patients for delivery of bronchodilators or other medications where patient coordination and the ability to take a deep breath is compromised. IPPB as a form of lung expansion therapy usually includes the administration of an aerosolized bronchodilator, and therapy is usually given three times a day, four times a day, or every 2 to 4 hours for approximately 10 to 20

minutes. The indications for lung expansion therapy are listed in **Box 2-11**. A sample protocol for delivery of lung expansion therapy is found in **Figure 2-6**.

Critical Care and Mechanical Ventilation

Respiratory care plans for patients in the intensive care unit (ICU) may include therapy to improve oxygenation and/or ventilation, provide secretion management and airway care, treat bronchospasm and mucosal edema, or deliver lung expansion therapy to treat or prevent atelectasis. The goals of invasive and noninvasive ventilatory support in the ICU include maintaining adequate tissue oxygenation, ventilation, carbon dioxide removal, and acid–base balance. Respiratory care in the ICU is

BOX 2-11

Indications for Lung Expansion Therapy

Incentive Spirometry

Patient is able to achieve an inspired volume of at least one-third of predicted IC (or VC ≥ 10 mL/kg).

AND

Patient is able to perform the maneuver every 1 to 2 hours while awake.

AND ONE OR MORE OF THE FOLLOWING:

- Patient is predisposed to development of atelectasis: upper/lower abdominal, cardiac, or thoracic surgery; surgery in COPD; patient debilitated/bedridden; acute chest syndrome in patients; sickle cell disease.
- Preoperative screening/instruction for surgical patients to obtain baseline volume or flow
- Presence of atelectasis
- Quadriplegic and/or dysfunctional diaphragm
- Lack of pain control
- Thoracic or abdominal binders
- Restrictive lung defect with a dysfunctional diaphragm or involving the respiratory musculature
- IC < 2.5 L
- Neuromuscular disease or spinal cord injury

Intermittent Positive Pressure Breathing (IPPB)

Other therapy has been unsuccessful (incentive spirometry, chest physical therapy, deep breathing exercises, positive airway pressure).

AND AT LEAST ONE OF THE FOLLOWING:

- Clinically important atelectasis
- At risk for postoperative pulmonary complications (e.g. atelectasis, pneumonia, respiratory failure)
- Inability to spontaneously deep breath with inadequate cough and/or secretion clearance (inspired volumes less than one-third predicted IC or VC < 10 mL/kg)
- To deliver aerosol medication in patients unable to adequately deep breath and/or unable to coordinate the use of other aerosol devices
- For short-term ventilatory support in an attempt to avoid intubation and continuous mechanical ventilation, a noninvasive positive pressure (NPPV) device should be considered

IC, inspiratory capacity; VC, vital capacity.

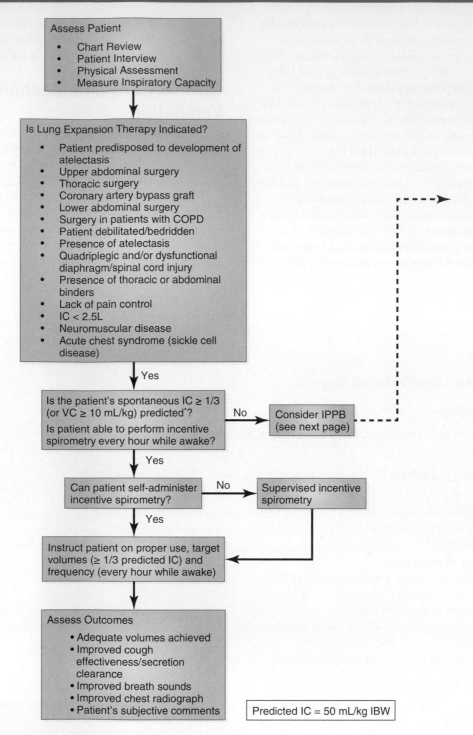

FIGURE 2-6 Protocol for lung expansion therapy.

Modified from: the American Association for Respiratory Care. Clinical Practice Guideline: Intermittent positive pressure breathing—2003 revision and update. *Respir Care*.2003; 48(5):540–546.

Diagnostic Testing

also concerned with maintaining adequate circulation, blood pressure, and cardiac output and monitoring ventilatory and hemodynamic function. Chapters 6 and 7 describe assessment of oxygenation and ventilation; Chapter 8 reviews arterial blood gases and acid–base balance. The focus of Chapter 14 is acute and critical care monitoring and assessment.

Patient assessment and care plan development may require measurement of clinical parameters related to oxygenation, ventilation, and cardiopulmonary function. Chapters 6 and 7 describe assessment of oxygenation and ventilation; Chapter 8 reviews arterial blood gases and acid-base balance. Laboratory, imaging, and

Is IPPB indicated?

- Presence of clinical significant atelectasis when other therapy (incentive spirometry, chest physiotherapy, deep breath exercises, positive airway pressure) has been unsuccessful.
- Inability to spontaneously deep breath (inspired volumes less than 1/3 predicted IC or VC < 10 mL/kg) in patients with inadequate cough and/or secretion clearance and other therapy has been unsuccessful.
- Patient at risk for postoperative pulmonary complications (e.g., atelectasis, pneumonia, respiratory failure) AND other lung-expansion therapy has been unsuccessful.
- To deliver aerosol medication in patients who are unable to adequately deep breathe and/or coordinate the use of other aerosol devices and therapy (metered-dose inhaler [MDI], small-volume nebulizer) has been unsuccessful.
- Patients with ventilatory muscle fatigue, neuromuscular disease, kyphoscoliosis, spinal injury or chronic conditions requiring intermittent ventilatory support may also benefit from IPPB to deliver aerosol therapy.
- Provide short-term ventilatory support as an alternative to tracheal intubation and continuous mechanical ventilation. Devices specifically for noninvasive positive pressure ventilation (NPPV) should be considered.
- Decrease dyspnea and discomfort during nebulized therapy in patients with severe hyperinflation.

Yes →

Is IPPB contraindicated?

Absolute contraindication: untreated tension pneumothorax

Relative contraindications:

- Intracranial pressure (ICP) > 15 mm Hg
- Hemodynamic instability
- Recent facial, oral, or skull surgery
- Tracheoesophageal fistula
- Recent esophageal surgery
- Active hemoptysis
- Nausea
- Air swallowing
- Active untreated tuberculosis
- Radiographic evidence of bleb
- Singulation (hiccups)

 No

Determine volume goals, medications, and frequency of administration

- ≥ 1/3 predicted IC or ≥ 10 mL/kg or ≥ 1200 mL in most adults
- Frequency for critical care: every 1–6 hours
- Frequency for acute care or home care: two to four times daily
- Bronchodilators are normally administered with IPPB

Apply Therapy

Reassess Patient

- Adequate volumes achieved?
- Improved cough effectiveness?
- Secretion clearance/sputum production?
- Chest radiograph improved?
- Breath sounds improved?
- Patient's subjective comments?
- Improved FEV$_1$ or peak flow following bronchodilator administration?

FIGURE 2-6 (*continued*)

other diagnostic studies may be needed to further define and clarify the patient's problem and diagnosis. Chapter 9 reviews laboratory studies, Chapter 10 describes the use of the electrocardiogram (ECG), and Chapter 11 describes medical imaging. Chapter 13 reviews pulmonary function testing. Following establishment the patient's diagnosis, a respiratory care plan is developed, implemented, and evaluated.

Respiratory Care Plan Format

Many institutions have developed various forms and formats for use in writing and organizing the respiratory care plan. One common format uses problem-oriented charting, including the use of a SOAP note for the respiratory care plan, as described earlier. **Figure 2-7** contains a suggested format for organizing a respiratory care plan using the SOAP technique. Another format may include problems or complaints, possible sources of problems or complaints, actions taken to relieve problems or complaints, short- and long-term goals, and evaluation and documentation.

A third possible format for the respiratory care plan is found in **Figure 2-8**. This format includes patient demographic data, indications for specific respiratory care, and a care plan oriented towards maintaining oxygenation, treating and preventing bronchospasm and/or mucosal edema, delivering anti-inflammatory and antiasthmatic medications, initiating therapy to mobilize and remove secretions, and providing lung expansion therapy.

S: The patient's **subjective** expression of the symptoms that have brought him or her before the clinician.
- The chief complaint is the leading statement reported by the patient.
- The history of present illness and past medical history are also subjective.

O: The **objective** signs that are exhibited by the patient.
- Includes physical assessment, vital signs, inspection, palpation, percussion, and auscultation.
- Diagnostic data such as the results of arterial blood gas analysis, chest radiography, pulmonary function, and other laboratory tests may also be recorded.

A: The clinician's **assessment** of the findings noted in the S & O sections of the clinical note.
- Commonly an assessment of the clinical signs and symptoms followed by the disease or disorder that is suggested by the findings.
- For example, the symptoms, physical findings, and diagnostic data noted during examination of the asthmatic patient present a very characteristic disease pattern.

P: Describes the care **plan** that has been formulated based on the assessment findings.
- The plan should address the treatment and/or monitoring of the patient's disease state, conditions, or compliant.

SOAP Note Format

Patient Name: _____   Age: _____
Physician(s): _____   Height: _____
Hospital ID No.: _____   Weight: _____
   Sex: _____

Admitting Diagnosis: _____

Problems or Complaints:
1. _____   4. _____
2. _____   5. _____
3. _____   6. _____

Subjective Findings: _____
_____
_____

Objective Findings: _____
_____
_____

Assessment: _____
_____

Plan: _____
_____
_____
_____

FIGURE 2-7 SOAP format for organizing a respiratory care plan. The problem-oriented medical record (POMR) may be used to collect and document data, assess the patient, and develop an appropriate treatment plan. The most common POMR technique is the SOAP note. The SOAP note allows the clinician to report a patient assessment and treatment plan. The four letters of the acronym are described in the figure.

CHART REVIEW

Patient Name: _____   Age: _____
Physician(s): _____   Height: _____
Hospital ID No.: _____   Weight: _____
Floor/Unit: _____   Sex: _____
Admitting Diagnosis: _____

Other Problems from Problem List or Patient History and Physical:
1. _____   4. _____
2. _____   5. _____
3. _____   6. _____
Current Physician Orders for Respiratory Care: _____
_____

Most Recent ABGs and/or SpO_2: _____
_____

Most Recent Chest X-ray Reports: _____
_____

Most Recent Pulmonary Function Testing: _____

PATIENT INTERVIEW

Cough: _____   Sputum Production: _____
Hemoptysis: _____   Wheezing, Whistling or Chest Tightness: _____
Breathlessness: _____
Chest Illness: _____
Smoking: _____
Occupational History: _____
Hobby and Leisure History: _____
Medicines or Respiratory Care Used: _____
Response to Current Respiratory Care: _____

PHYSICAL ASSESSMENT

General Appearance: _____
Pulse: _____   Respirations: _____   Blood Pressure: _____
Level of Consciousness: _____
Chest Inspection: _____
Auscultation: _____
Percussion: _____
Palpation: _____
Bedside Spirometry: IC: _____   PEFR: _____   VC: _____ FEV_1: _____

ASSESSMENT FOR THERAPY

Evaluate whether each specific therapy listed is indicated and/or appropriate for this patient based on your chart review, patient interview, and physical assessment data. NOTE: Check all indications present REGARDLESS of whether the patient is currently receiving a particular therapy or not.

Assessment for Oxygen Therapy (check all indications present for oxygen therapy; see Box 2-5)

Yes   No
☐   ☐   documented hypoxemia
☐   ☐   corrected hypoxemia
☐   ☐   suspected hypoxemia
☐   ☐   severe trauma
☐   ☐   acute M.I.
☐   ☐   immediate post-op recovery (recovery room or ICU)

Assessment for Bronchodilator Therapy (check all indications present for bronchodilator therapy; see Box 2-6)

Yes   No
☐   ☐   asthma
☐   ☐   COPD
☐   ☐   wheezing
☐   ☐   documented response to a bronchodilator

FIGURE 2-8 Detailed respiratory care plan format. Format includes patient demographic data, indications for specific respiratory care, and a care plan oriented towards maintenance of oxygenation, treatment and prevention of bronchospasm and/or mucosal edema, delivery of anti-inflammatory and antiasthmatic medications, therapy to mobilize and remove secretions, and lung expansion therapy.

Assessment for Anti-inflammatory Aerosol Agents (inhaled steroids) (check all of the indications present; see Box 2-8)

Yes   No
- ☐   ☐ asthma
- ☐   ☐ COPD
- ☐   ☐ upper airway edema

Assessment for Antiasthmatic Aerosol Agents (cromolyn, etc.) (check all of the indications present; see Box 2-8)

Yes   No
- ☐   ☐ asthma

Assessment for Directed Cough (check all of the indications present for this patient; see Box 2-10)

Yes   No
- ☐   ☐ retained secretions, excess secretion production
- ☐   ☐ following bronchial hygiene therapy
- ☐   ☐ at risk for atelectasis/post-op pulmonary complications
- ☐   ☐ to obtain sputum specimen

Assessment for Suctioning (check all of the indications present for this patient; see Box 2-10)

Yes   No
- ☐   ☐ inability to clear secretions with cough
- ☐   ☐ need to remove secretions with artificial airway
- ☐   ☐ need to stimulate cough
- ☐   ☐ to obtain sputum specimen

Assessment for Mucolytic Therapy (check the indications present for this patient; see Box 2-10)

Yes   No
- ☐   ☐ evidence of viscous/retained secretions which are not easily removed via other therapy
- ☐   ☐ chronic bronchitis, cystic fibrosis, bronchiectasis

Assessment for Chest Physiotherapy (check all of the indications present for this patient; see Box 2-10)

<u>Postural Drainage and Percussion</u>

Yes   No
- ☐   ☐ suggestion/evidence of problems with secretion clearance
- ☐   ☐ difficulty clearing secretions with volume >25–30 mL/day (adult)
- ☐   ☐ retained secretions in presence of an artificial airway
- ☐   ☐ atelectasis caused/suspected to be due to mucus plugging
- ☐   ☐ cystic fibrosis, bronchiectasis, cavitating lung disease
- ☐   ☐ presence of a foreign body in airway

Assessment for High Volume Bland Aerosol (see Box 2-10)

<u>Cool Mist Bland Solution</u>

Yes   No
- ☐   ☐ post extubation
- ☐   ☐ deliver precise FIO_2 via air-entrainment nebulizer
- ☐   ☐ upper airway edema
- ☐   ☐ to obtain sputum specimen

<u>Heated Large-Volume Nebulizer</u>

Yes   No
- ☐   ☐ evidence/potential for secretion clearance problem
- ☐   ☐ deliver precise FIO_2 with high humidity
- ☐   ☐ mobilize secretions

<u>Hypertonic Saline Administration</u>

Yes   No
- ☐   ☐ induce sputum

FIGURE 2-8 *(continued)*

Assessment for Lung Expansion Therapy (see Box 2-11)

Incentive Spirometry (check all of the indications present for this patient)

Yes	No	
☐	☐	Patient is able to perform the maneuver q1–2 hours while awake and is able to achieve adequate inspired volume.

AND:
Check as many as apply:

Yes	No	
☐	☐	Patient is predisposed to development of atelectasis (surgery, debilitated, bedridden, ventilatory impairment/restrictive/ neuromuscular defect).
☐	☐	Presence of atelectasis.
☐	☐	Preoperative screening/education of patients at risk.
☐	☐	Patient has reduced inspiratory capacity (<2.5 L).

IPPB (check all the indications present for this patient)

Yes	No	
☐	☐	Presence of clinically important atelectasis AND other therapy has been unsuccessful.
☐	☐	Patient cannot or will not spontaneously deep breathe and is at risk for atelectasis.
☐	☐	To deliver aerosol medication with coordination or cooperation issues.
☐	☐	NPPV to provide short-term ventilatory support in an attempt to avoid intubation and continuous mechanical ventilation.

IS, incentive spirometry; CPT, chest physiotherapy.

FIGURE 2-8 (*continued*)

Summary

The respiratory care plan is simply a written explanation of the respiratory care that the patient is to receive. The respiratory care plan may take the form of physician's orders, a detailed progress note in the medical record, an established protocol, completion of a standardized respiratory care plan form, or the use of problem-oriented medical records using SOAP notes. In the clinical setting, respiratory care plan development requires an initial physician's order, a well-designed protocol or policy, and careful patient assessment. The physician's order may be specific, or it may simply state "respiratory care per protocol."

Developing and implementing the respiratory care plan requires a careful patient assessment. Following the patient assessment, the respiratory care clinician selects the appropriate care based on the patient's condition and the indications for each type of therapy. The respiratory care plan may include the goals of therapy, the device or procedure that will be used, medications given, method or appliance used, gas source and/or flow, volume goals, frequency of therapy, and duration of therapy. The care plan may also include a statement of how the intensity and/or duration of therapy will be adjusted and when the therapy will be discontinued. Assessment of the outcomes of therapy may also be included. These may include evidence of clinical improvement, measurement of bedside pulmonary function data such as PEF or FEV_1, improvement in oxygenation or SpO_2, improved quality of life, patient subjective improvement, and the absence of adverse side effects.

In summary, the respiratory care plan is the written plan of treatment that the patient will receive. The respiratory care plan may include goals, rationale, and significance and a description of how care will be assessed.

Key Points

▸ The respiratory care plan provides a written description of the care the patient is to receive.

▸ Respiratory care plans include the goals of therapy, the device or procedure to be used, medications to be given, frequency of administration, and duration of therapy.

▸ SOAP refers to **S**ubjective, **O**bjective, **A**ssessment, and **P**lan.

▸ Acute respiratory failure (ARF) is defined as a sudden decrease in arterial oxygen levels with or without carbon dioxide retention.

▸ Acute ventilatory failure (AVF) is defined as a sudden rise $Paco_2$ with a corresponding decrease in pH.

▸ Chronic ventilatory failure is defined as a chronically elevated $Paco_2$ with a normal (compensated) or near-normal pH.

▶ Respiratory care plans may be developed for basic and critical respiratory care, diagnostic testing, or specialized procedures.

▶ Oxygen therapy is indicated for documented or suspected hypoxemia, severe trauma, acute myocardial infarction (MI), and immediate postoperative recovery.

▶ For delivery of low to moderate concentration of oxygen, the nasal cannula is the device of choice.

▶ With unstable ventilatory patterns or rapid, shallow breathing, an air-entrainment mask may be considered.

▶ For moderate to high concentrations of oxygen therapy for short-term use, consider a simple partial-rebreathing or nonrebreathing mask.

▶ The primary indication for bronchodilator therapy is to treat or prevent bronchospasm.

▶ Bronchodilator therapy is indicated in acute asthma, COPD, and whenever wheezing is due to reversible bronchoconstriction.

▶ Anti-inflammatory aerosol agents and antiasthmatic drugs include inhaled corticosteroids, cromolyn sodium, and antileukotrienes.

▶ Techniques to mobilize or remove secretions include directed cough, suctioning, use of high-volume aerosol therapy, and bronchial hygiene.

▶ Directed cough should be included as an integral part of bronchial hygiene therapy.

▶ Forced expiratory technique (FET), also known as a "huff" cough, is a modified version of the directed cough.

▶ A cool bland aerosol is indicated in the treatment of upper airway edema and for postoperative management of the upper airway.

▶ Bronchial hygiene techniques include chest physiotherapy, kinetic therapy, high-frequency chest wall oscillation (HFCWO), positive airway pressure (PAP), the flutter valve, intrapulmonary percussive ventilation (IPV), and mechanical insufflation–exsufflation.

▶ Nasotracheal (NT) suctioning is indicated in cases where the patient's spontaneous or directed cough is ineffective.

▶ The primary indications for lung expansion therapy are in the treatment and/or prevention of atelectasis.

▶ Lung expansion therapy may be used to prevent the development of respiratory failure, particularly in postoperative patients.

▶ The two primary techniques for applying lung expansion therapy are incentive spirometry and intermittent positive pressure breathing (IPPB).

▶ Incentive spirometry should be considered in patients who are able to perform the maneuver every 1 to 2 hours while awake and are able to achieve an adequate inspired volume.

▶ IPPB should generally be reserved for patients who have clinically important atelectasis in which other therapy has been unsuccessful.

▶ PAP is sometimes used to mobilize secretions and treat atelectasis.

▶ The goals of ventilatory support in the ICU include maintaining adequate tissue oxygenation, ventilation, and acid–base balance.

▶ Patient assessment and care plan development may require measurement of clinical parameters related to oxygenation, ventilation, and cardiopulmonary function.

References

1. Aboussouan L. Respiratory failure and the need for ventilatory support. In: Wilkins RL, Stoller JK, Kacmarek RM, eds. *Egan's Fundamentals of Respiratory Care*, 9th ed. St. Louis, MO: Mosby; 2009: 949–964.

2. West JB. Acute respiratory failure. In: West JB, ed. *Pulmonary Physiology and Pathophysiology: An Integrated, Case-Based Approach*, 2nd ed. Philadelphia: Lippincott, Williams & Wilkins; 2007: 116–133.

3. Weinberger SE, Cockrill B, Manel J. *Principles of Pulmonary Medicine*, 3rd ed. Philadelphia: W.B. Saunders; 1998.

4. Esteban A, Anzueto A, Alia I, et al. How is mechanical ventilation employed in the intensive care unit? An international utilization review. *Am J Respir Crit Care Med.* 2000;161(5):1450–1458.

5. Shapiro BA, Peruzzi WT, Kozelowski-Templin R. *Clinical Application of Blood Gases*, 5th ed. St. Louis, MO: Mosby; 1994.

6. American Association for Respiratory Care Clinical Practice Guideline: oxygen therapy in the acute care hospital—2002 revision and update. *Respir Care.* 2002;47(6):717–720.

7. American Association for Respiratory Care Clinical Practice Guideline: oxygen therapy in the home or alternate site health care—2007 revision and update. *Respir Care.* 2007;52(1):1063–1068.

8. Boatright J, Ward JJ. Therapeutic gases: management and administration. In: Hess DR, MacIntyre NR, Mishoe SC, Galvin WF, Adams AB, eds. *Respiratory Care Principles and Practice*, 2nd ed. Sudbury, MA: Jones & Bartlett Learning; 2012: 271–302.

9. Global Initiative for Chronic Obstructive Lung Disease. Pocket guide to COPD diagnosis, management, and prevention 2011. http://www.goldcopd.org/guidelines-pocket-guide-to-copd-diagnosis.html.

10. American Association for Respiratory Care Clinical Practice Guideline: selection of an oxygen delivery device for neonatal and pediatric patients—2002 Revision & Update. *Respir Care.* 2002;47(6):707–716.

11. Curley MA. Prone positioning in patients with acute respiratory distress syndrome: a systematic review. *Am J Crit Care.* 1999;8(6):397–405.

12. Gattinoni L, Tognoni G, Pesenti A, Taccone P, Mascheroni D, Labarta V. Effect of prone positioning on the survival of patients with acute respiratory failure. *N Engl J Med.* 2001;345:568–573.

13. Guerin C, Gaillard S, Lemasson S, et al. Effects of systematic prone positioning in hypoxic acute respiratory failure: a randomized controlled trial. *JAMA.* 2004;292(19):2379–2387.

14. Ahrens T, Kollef M, Stewart J, Shannon W. Effect of kinetic therapy on pulmonary complications. *Am J Crit Care.* 2004;13:376–383.

15. Gardner DD, Vines DL, Wettstein RB, Garcia J, Peters JI. The effectiveness of the Misty-Ox high fraction of inspired oxygen (F_{IO_2})–high-flow nebulizer and the Theramist air entrainment nebulizer in delivering high oxygen concentrations. *Chest.* 2005;128(4):305S.

16. American Association for Respiratory Care Clinical Practice Guideline. Assessing response to bronchodilator therapy at point of care. *Respir Care*. 1995;40(12):1300–1307.

17. National Institutes of Health, National Heart, Lung, and Blood Institute Guidelines for the Diagnosis and Management of Asthma: Expert Panel 3 Report. Bethesda, MD: U.S. Department of Health and Human Services; 2007.

18. Global Strategy for Diagnosis, Management, and Prevention of COPD Global Strategy for Diagnosis, Management, and Prevention of COPD. Revised 2011. http://www.goldcopd.org /guidelines-global-strategy-for-diagnosis-management.html.

19. Gardenhire D. *Rau's Respiratory Care Pharmacology*, 8th ed. St. Louis, MO: Elsevier Health; 2012.

20. American Association for Respiratory Care Clinical Practice Guideline: bland aerosol administration—2003 revision and update. *Respir Care*. 2003;48(5):529–533.

21. Hess, DR. Humidity and aerosol therapy. In: Hess DR, MacIntyre NR, Mishoe SC, Galcin B, Adams AB, eds. *Respiratory Care Principles and Practice*, 2nd ed. Sudbury, MA: Jones & Bartlett Learning; 2012: 303–341.

22. Myslinski MJ, Scanlan CL. Bronchial hygiene therapy. In: Wilkins RL, Stoller JK, Kacmarek, RM, eds. *Egan's Fundamentals of Respiratory Care*, 9th ed. St. Louis, MO: Mosby; 2009: 921–946.

23. American Association for Respiratory Care Clinical Practice Guideline: postural drainage therapy. *Respir Care*. 1991;36(12): 1418–1426.

24. American Association for Respiratory Care Clinical Practice Guideline: use of positive airway pressure adjuncts to bronchial hygiene therapy. *Respir Care*. 1993;38(5):516–521.

25. American Association for Respiratory Care Clinical Practice Guideline: directed cough. *Respir Care*. 1993;38(5):495–499.

26. American Association for Respiratory Care Clinical Practice Guideline: intermittent positive pressure breathing—2003 revision and update. *Respir Care*. 2003;48(5):540–546.

27. American Association for Respiratory Care Clinical Practice Guideline: nasotracheal suctioning—2004 revision and update. *Respir Care*. 2004;49(9):1080–1084.

28. American Association for Respiratory Care Clinical Practice Guideline: incentive spirometry. *Respir Care*. 2011;56(10): 1600–1604.

29. Hess, DR. Sputum collection, airway clearance, and lung expansion therapy. In: Hess DR, MacIntyre NR, Mishoe SC, Galcin B, Adams AB, eds. *Respiratory Care Principles and Practice*, 2nd ed. Sudbury, MA: Jones & Bartlett Learning; 2012: 342–375.

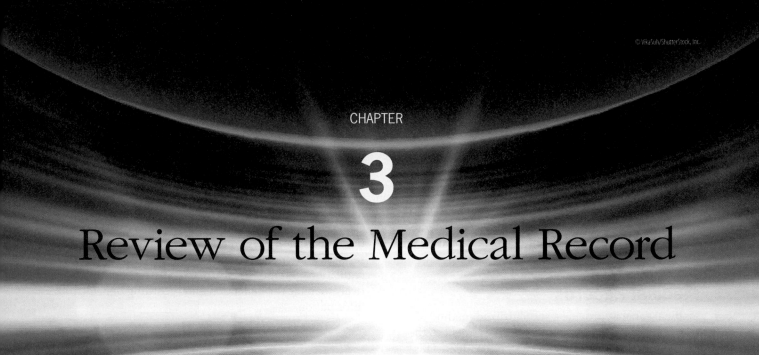

CHAPTER

3

Review of the Medical Record

Toni M. Podgorak and David C. Shelledy

CHAPTER OUTLINE

Medical Records
Review of the Medical Record
Charting

CHAPTER OBJECTIVES

1. Define the term *medical record*.
2. Explain the four functions of a chart.
3. Compare the electronic medical record (EMR) with the electronic health record (EHR).
4. Contrast the advantages and disadvantages of EMRs, EHRs, and paper-based medical records.
5. Explain the term *problem-oriented medical record* (POMR).
6. Provide examples of objective and subjective comments that may be included in a SOAP note.
7. Write an appropriate SOAP note given information about a patient requiring respiratory care assessment.
8. Categorize the types of information that may be found in each of the major sections of the patient medical record.
9. Distinguish the major admitting diagnoses seen in the acute care setting.
10. Summarize the important pulmonary and critical care diagnoses seen in the hospital.
11. Describe the types of physician's orders that are important to review as a part of a respiratory care consult.
12. Write an appropriate order for a basic respiratory care treatment or procedure.
13. Provide examples of medications that may be prescribed for cardiopulmonary patients and explain the significance of each.
14. Describe the types of respiratory care orders found in the patient chart and explain the significance of each.
15. Explain the significance of do not resuscitate (DNR) orders in the patient chart.
16. List the components of a typical history and physical examination report found in the patient chart and explain the significance of each.
17. Give examples of other information to be reviewed in the patient chart, including vital signs, progress notes, and results of laboratory and imaging studies.
18. Interpret common symbols and abbreviations sometimes encountered in the patient medical record.
19. Utilize the rules for charting when recording information in the medical record.
20. Formulate an appropriate medical record entry for a basic respiratory care procedure.

KEY TERMS

admitting diagnosis
Centers for Medicare and
  Medicaid Services (CMS)
charting
critical care monitoring
electronic health record
  (EHR)
electronic medical record
  (EMR)
history and physical
  examination

imaging studies
laboratory studies
medical record
physician's orders
problem-oriented medical
  record (POMR)
SOAPIER
The Joint Commission (TJC)

Overview

Medical records have evolved from simple documentation of care provided to a patient by a physician or other healthcare provider to an interdisciplinary/interprofessional tool used to track, monitor, and evaluate patient care. They can also be used to identify trends in the health of a population. Because the medical record allows the clinician to document, organize, and review patient data directly related to the development of the respiratory care plan, it plays a central role in patient management. One must also always remember that the medical record is a legal document and that any information in the medical record may be used in court or other legal proceedings. The medical record is also used to determine healthcare reimbursement by insurance companies, Medicare, Medicaid, and other third-party payers. Consequently, it is essential that the information recorded in the medical record be timely, accurate, legible, and written in understandable and clear language.

This chapter will explore components of the medical record while differentiating between the various types of records currently used in healthcare. We will then review existing data in the patient's medical record and highlight the major sections of the medical record that should be reviewed. A brief overview of **charting** as it relates to the hospitalized patient follows in order to provide the respiratory care clinician a foundation for solid clinical documentation skills.

Medical Records

Medical records provide a standardized method of recording and collating information pertinent to the care and treatment of the hospitalized patient. This information is then shared in paper (written) or electronic form. Chart organization can vary from one hospital to the next; however, the functions of the medical record will always include: (1) serving as a database clinicians can access for data collection and review; (2) providing a legal record of all care and services provided; (3) establishing clear documentation of diagnosis and care provided for reimbursement; and (4) offering a central location for interdisciplinary communication and documentation to monitor and improve patient outcomes. Review of the existing medical record ("chart review") is the first step in developing a comprehensive respiratory care plan. With the exception of medical emergencies, the patient medical record should also be reviewed prior to initiation of any ordered respiratory care. **Box 3-1** lists the major sections found in the typical hospitalized patient medical record or chart.

BOX 3-1

Components of the Medical Record

Patient information/admissions sheet
Physician's orders
Reports of history and physical examination(s)
Consultation reports
Laboratory study results
Imaging reports
Cardiac testing reports
Progress notes
Nurses notes
Respiratory therapy notes
Medication records
Reports of procedures and operations
Patient education (previous)

Certain content in the medical record is required in order to meet federal and state law and regulations as well as standards of accrediting agencies. In addition, health records must meet the standards set forth by the **Centers for Medicare and Medicaid Services (CMS)** of the U.S. Department of Health and Human Services. **The Joint Commission (TJC)** accredits and certifies hospitals, healthcare organizations, and related programs in the United States (see www.jointcommission .org). TJC is authorized by CMS to review patient medical records to ensure that clinicians provide detailed, timely, confidential, and accurate depictions of the services and/or care provided. Together, CMS and TJC regulations attempt to ensure that institutions effectively manage the collection and recording of health information.

RC Insights

Always check the patient's chart or medical record before providing care. The only exception is for providing emergency care or immediate life support.

Reimbursements for healthcare are dependent on accurate diagnosis and appropriate treatment. In addition, both must be documented; in the eyes of the law, if something is not recorded in the medical record, it did not happen. The respiratory care clinician could be accused of negligence if failure to properly record information results in harm to the patient. Respiratory therapists (RTs) tend to be named as plaintiffs in lawsuits less frequently than physicians or registered nurses (RNs). However, RTs are increasingly being included in cases involving airway management, intubation, mechanical ventilation, and cardiopulmonary resuscitation (CPR). The number of medical malpractice cases related to breaches of confidentiality has also increased. In the event that a patient brings legal action against a hospital, four basic criteria must be met for the medical record to be deemed admissible as evidence.[1] The medical record must be:

1. Documented in the normal course of providing care
2. Kept in the regular course of business
3. Made at or near the time of the matter recorded
4. Made by a person within the hospital or healthcare agency with knowledge of the acts, events, conditions, opinions, or diagnoses recorded

---

RC Insights

Clinicians should only view the medical records of patients under their direct care.

Types of Medical Records

The following provides an overview of three types of medical records: paper-based medical records, **electronic medical records (EMRs)**, and **electronic health records (EHRs)**.

EMRs Versus EHRs

In the United States, physicians and hospitals are transitioning from paper medical records to EMRs/EHRs, which allow documentation through the electronic collecting, storing, and organizing of individual patient information. EMR and EHR are not interchangeable terms. In 2008, The National Alliance for Health Information Technology (NAHIT) established the following definitions for EMRs and EHRs[2]:

- *EMR*: "an electronic record of health-related information on an individual that can be created, gathered, managed, and consulted by authorized clinicians and staff within one health care organization."
- *EHR*: "an electronic record of health-related information on an individual that conforms to nationally recognized interoperability standards and that can be created, managed, and consulted by authorized clinicians and staff across more than one health care organization."

The 2009 American Recovery and Reinvestment Act (ARRA) included financial incentives for physician practices and hospitals to adopt EHR systems starting in 2011; disincentives for not adopting these systems start in 2015.[3,4] In 2011, 57% of office-based physicians used an EHR system.[5] Studies indicate that adoption of EHRs can vary greatly based on the hospital's size, teaching status, and location.[6] In 2008, a total of 11% of nonfederal U.S. hospitals had implemented basic EHR systems, and less than 2% had implemented comprehensive systems in at least one clinical unit.[7] Despite the low percentage of total implementations, many hospitals have begun implementation of key EHR functionalities, such as physician's notes or clinical-decision support systems involving practice guidelines.[8]

> **RC Insights**
>
> A breach of confidentiality is disclosure to a third party, without patient consent, of private information related to the health and care of the patient.

Paper Charts

Traditional paper charting is easy for the novice clinician to navigate. Paper charts provide a snapshot of everything that must be documented. Charts are typically two- or three-ring notebooks or charts with papers held within by a clasp. The traditional paper chart is divided into categories such as: Patient Information/Admission Sheet; Physician Orders; History and Physical; Progress Notes; Nurses Notes; Medication Record; Laboratory Results; Radiology/Imaging; Cardiovascular (ECG); Patient Care Flow Sheets (vital signs, fluid-I/O, hemodynamics, ventilation flow sheets, other); Reports of Operations (surgical and anesthesia records); Consultation Reports; Respiratory Therapy Notes; Medications; Discharge; and Other Records. A major drawback to paper documentation is that only one person can access the chart at a time. In addition, paper charts can be time-consuming to locate if they are not returned to the designated area for chart storage. **Figure 3-1** illustrates a paper document used by respiratory therapists to chart respiratory care treatments, procedures, progress notes, assessments, and care plans. **Figure 3-2** provides an example of a paper flow sheet for mechanical ventilation.

Benefits of EHRs/EMRs

The EMR provides a centralized electronic "chart" that can be accessed from multiple workstations, thus enhancing access and clinical efficiency. In today's busy clinical environment, real-time, bedside charting is made possible via stationary bedside computers, computers-on-wheels, handheld tablet PCs, personal digital assistants (PDAs), and smartphones. Clinicians undergo extensive orientation and training on the proper use of the software used at a specific hospital. Unfortunately, there are multiple EMR software system vendors, and no one system has been universally accepted. In fact, it would not be unusual to encounter different EMR systems in different hospitals in the same city or region. This may pose a challenge to healthcare providers who work across different hospital systems as they seek to consolidate important patient information. Cerner Corporation, McKesson, and Meditech have been reported to have greater than 50% of the EMR/EHR market; Epic, Allscripts (Eclipsys), Siemens, CPSI, Healthcare Management Systems, and Healthland are among the top 10 most widely used EHRs.[9] EHRs have the potential to improve patient care and safety. For example, hospital personnel have, on rare occasion, caused severe patient harm, and hospitals have endured public relations disasters, as a result of inappropriate and/or lethal doses of medications being administered by mistake. EHRs have the potential to greatly reduce these errors. **Box 3-2** lists the advantages and disadvantages of EMRs.

Problem-Oriented Medical Records

The **problem-oriented medical record (POMR)** was created in 1968 by Dr. Lawrence Weed. The POMR focuses on problem-solving while providing complex care by encouraging ongoing assessments and care

BAR CODE LABEL				
	Patient Name			
	MR #			
ABC UNIVERSITY MEDICAL CENTER				

Date	Time	Comments		Therapist

FIGURE 3-1 Respiratory care notes.

adjustments by the healthcare team.[10] The format of the POMR varies from institution to institution. Essential components include a database, a problem list, a plan of care, and progress notes.

The POMR begins with compiling a *database*. This is done by using information from interviews with the patient and family, the results of assessments and physical exams, and findings from laboratory and imaging studies. The database helps to generate a differential diagnosis, or *problem list*. Items on a problem list should be verifiable facts that are indexed into active/inactive problems, including the date of onset. An initial *plan of care* is then formulated in which each problem is named and described using a *progress note* format. Shortly after the initial development of

the POMR, the SOAP note was developed to further standardize medical evaluation entries made into the healthcare record.[11] SOAP notes enable respiratory care clinicians to quickly document the plan of care. The four components of the SOAP format are:

S (Subjective): Subjective information is what the patient (or family member) says. Subjective information is obtained from the patient, his or her relatives, or a similar source.

O (Objective): Objective information is what you can see, hear, touch, or smell. Objective information is based on the healthcare professional's direct observations of the patient as well as the results of laboratory or imaging testing.

BAR CODE LABEL		Patient Name		
		MR #		

ABC UNIVERSITY MEDICAL CENTER

DAY OF VENTILATION (number):			AIRWAY INFORMATION		
			Time/Initials		
Date:			Airway Type		
DX:			Airway Size		
Oxygen Equipment:			Secured @ Lip (cm)		
Inubation Date/Time:		Extubation Date/Time:	Cuff Pressure (cm H_2O)		
			Position in mouth		

Time					
Mode			SUCTIONING RECORD		
Set V_T (mL)			Time/Initials		
Set RR			Sputum Volume		
PEEP			Sputum Consistency		
F_{IO_2}			Sputum Color		
Pressure Support					
Tube Comp.					
Insp. Pressure		BREATH SOUNDS			
Heart Rate		Time/Initials			
V_T Spont.		Aeration	Good / Poor /↓ Bases		
V_T Mand.		Aeration Balance	R = L / R > L / R < L		
Total RR		Right Lung			
MV		Rhonchi	RUL / RML / RLL		
Peak Pressure		Crackles	RUL / RML / RLL		
Plateau Pressure		Wheeze	RUL / RML / RLL		
Mean Pressure		Clear	RUL / RML / RLL		
Static Comp.					
Dynamic Comp.		Left Lung			
RAW		Rhonchi	LUL / LLL		
PEEP		Crackles	LUL / LLL		
Spo_2		Wheeze	LUL / LLL		
$ETCO_2$		Clear	LUL / LLL		
I Time					
I:E Ratio					
Flow		COMMENTS			
Rise Time					
Wave Form					
Sensitivity					
Temp/HME					
Initials					
ALARMS					
Time/Initials					
Peak Pressure High/Low					
MV High/Low		SIGNATURE	Initials		
High RR					
V_T High/Low					
$ETCO_2$ High/Low					
D-Sens					

FIGURE 3-2 **Mechanical ventilation flow sheet.**

BOX 3-2

Advantages and Disadvantages of Electronic Medical Records

Advantages	Disadvantages
Facilitate effective quality assurance	Initial high cost
Produce a legible record	Large training investment
Accessible by multiple people at the same time	Power failures
Expedite the transfer of data between facilities	Hardware crashes and breakdowns
Reduce the number of lost records	Software glitches
Speed the retrieval of data and expedite billing	Sabotage of the system by disgruntled employees and hackers
Provide analysis of practice patterns and research activities	Unauthorized access
Allow for a complete set of backup records at little or no cost	Reluctance of physicians to use tightly controlled note format
Easily identify patients due for preventative screenings or vaccinations	
Practice enhancers and a public relations tool	

Data from: Haskins M. Legible charts! Experiences in converting to electronic medical records. *Can Fam Physician.* 2002;48(4):768–771; van Wingerde FJ, Sun Y, Harary O, Mandl KD, Salem-Schatz S, Homer CF, Kohane IS. Linking multiple heterogeneous data sources to practice guidelines. *Proc AMIA Symp.* 1998;391–395; Kapp M. *Our Hands Are Tied: Legal Tensions and Medical Ethics.* Westport, CT: Auburn House; 1998; Evans RS, Pestotnik SL, Classen DC, Horn SD, Bass SB, Burke JP. Preventing adverse drug events in hospitalized patients. *Ann Pharmacother.* 1994;28(4):523–527; Buckner F. The duty to inform, liability to third parties and the duty to warn. *J Med Prac Manage.* (Sept/Oct 1998): 100; Loomis GA, Ries JS, Saywell RM, Thakker NR. If electronic medical records are so great, why aren't family physicians using them? *J Fam Pract.* 2002;51(7):25.

A (Assessment): The assessment section of the SOAP note provides the interpretation or conclusions regarding the objective and subjective information. The patient's problem(s) and/or diagnosis may be listed and described here.

P (Plan): The plan of action to be taken to resolve the problem(s) and/or treat the patient is described. All subsequent plans and modifications should be added to the SOAP note.

Box 3-3 gives examples of respiratory care–related findings that may be recorded under the subjective and objective sections of a SOAP note. Some institutions have modified the SOAP note so that care providers are able to document revisions to the care plan based on a patient's response to therapy. **SOAPIER** is a newer acronym being used, which includes the following additions:

I (Intervention): The specific interventions that have actually been performed by the caregiver.

E (Evaluation): Patient responses to interventions and medical treatments.

R (Revision): Care plan modifications suggested by the evaluation. Changes may target revised outcomes, interventions, or target dates.

Clinical Focus 3-1 provides an example of a SOAPIER note for a respiratory care patient.

Review of the Medical Record

Review of the medical record, better known as "chart review," is the first step in development of a comprehensive respiratory care plan. A careful review of the existing medical record or patient chart should precede the administration of care by the respiratory clinician. The only exception to this rule is cases where immediate or emergency care is essential to supporting the patient or treating a medical emergency. Review of the patient's chart or medical record by the respiratory care clinician should include review of the patient admissions sheet, **admitting diagnosis** and problem list, **physician's orders**, results of **history and physical**

BOX 3-3

Examples of Subjective and Objective Data for Respiratory Care–Related SOAP Notes

Subjective: Symptoms, what the patient (or family member) says or experiences.

- Fever
- Sweating or night sweats
- Fatigue and/or lethargy
- Anxiety
- Problems sleeping
- Cough and sputum production
- Hemoptysis
- Shortness of breath
- Wheezing, whistling, or chest tightness
- Chest pain

- Palpitations
- Headache
- Sinus pain
- Hoarseness
- Ankle swelling
- Heartburn
- Nausea
- Vomiting
- Diarrhea
- Lack of appetite

Objective: Signs and tests, what the clinician observes.

- Heart rate
- Respiratory rate
- Respiratory pattern
- Accessory muscle use
- Temperature
- Breath sounds
- Cough effort
- Sputum volume, consistency, color, and odor
- Physical examination findings

- Pulse oximetry values
- Arterial blood gas results
- ECG results
- Hemodynamic monitoring results
- Pulmonary function test results
- Medical laboratory results (sputum culture and sensitivity, CBC, blood chemistry, etc.)
- Imaging studies (chest x-ray, CT scan, MRI, other)

CBC, complete blood count; CT, computed tomography; MRI, magnetic resonance imagery.

CLINICAL FOCUS 3-1

SOAPIER Note for a Respiratory Care Patient

A 51-year-old obese female is status post coronary artery bypass graft (CABG). The patient was intubated for surgery and extubated 6 hours post operatively and placed on oxygen at 2 L via nasal cannula. Forty-eight hours postop, the respiratory care clinician enters the patient's room to perform a respiratory care assessment, because the patient has recurrent desaturations and is unable to perform incentive spirometry. The patient is found sitting upright in bed; the nasal O_2 therapy has been taken off and is on standby at the bedside. On physical examination, the patient is found to be afebrile (temperature: 98.1°F). Vital signs are respiratory rate (RR) 31/minute and shallow; blood pressure 122/74 mm Hg; pulse (HR) 96/minute; Spo_2 87% on room air. Auscultation reveals faint, slight inspiratory wheeze and late inspiratory crackles bilaterally with dullness to chest percussion. Chest x-ray reveals atelectasis/infiltrate in lower lobes. Room air arterial blood gas results are pH 7.49, Pao_2 64, Pco_2 30, and HCO_3^- 22.

Soapier Note

Problem 1: Atelectasis, 7:15 a.m., 05/16/15

Subjective: "My chest hurts when I take a deep breath."

Objective: Patient sitting upright in bed; pale, dry skin; RR 31/minute, thoracic in nature, shallow; HR 96/minute, regular and faint to palpation; Spo_2 87% on RA; BP 122/74 mm Hg; temp 98.6°F (38.3°C); slight wheeze, late inspiratory crackles bilaterally—lower lobes; chest x-ray suggestive of bibasilar atelectasis. ABG: pH 7.49, Pao_2 64, Pco_2 30, HCO_3^- 22. Ineffective cough. The patient's calculated ideal body weight is 115 lbs (52 kg). Predicted inspiratory capacity is 2600 mL (50 mL/kg × 52 kg).

(continues)

(*continued*)

Assessment: Atelectasis; poor ability to cough, deep breathe, and mobilize secretions; acute respiratory alkalosis with mild hypoxemia.

Plan: Initiate O_2 therapy by nasal cannula to maintain $SpO_2 \geq 92\%$; provide cough instruction and assist with coughing and deep breathing every 1 to 2 hours; initiate incentive spirometry and evaluate patient's inspiratory capacity. Begin bronchodilator therapy via small-volume nebulizer every 4 hours while awake. Ambulate as tolerated. Monitor breath sounds, secretion clearance, and SpO_2 before and after each nebulizer treatment. Provide additional cough and incentive spirometry instruction and assess inspiratory capacity via incentive spirometry after each nebulizer treatment.

Intervention: O_2 therapy initiated at 2 L/min; small-volume nebulizer aerosol therapy given with albuterol solution (2.5 mg in 3 mL of normal saline) × 10 minutes followed by cough and deep breathing instruction. Incentive spirometry begun with target goal of a minimum of 1000 mL × 10 to 15 breaths repeated every hour while awake. Minimum incentive goal is at least one-third of the predicted inspiratory capacity (1/3 × 2600 mL = 860 mL).

Evaluation: SpO_2 improved to 93% following O_2 initiation. Pulse before, during, and after initial nebulizer treatment was 88-86-86. Respiratory rate before during and after initial nebulizer therapy was 22-18-20. Diminished breath sounds noted before nebulizer therapy; aeration improved following therapy. Cough productive of 1 to 2 mL of colorless, mucoidal secretions following nebulizer treatment. Patient able to achieve an incentive spirometry volume of 1000 mL × 10 breaths, which is acceptable.

Revision: 48 hours of therapy completed. Diagnostic: Chest x-ray shows resolution of atelectasis; SpO_2 98% on room air. Patient has been using incentive spirometry every 1 to 2 hours while awake and achieving an inspired volume of at least 1000 mL/breath. Continue ambulation as per physician orders and patient tolerance; discontinue nebulizer and O_2 therapy.

> **RC Insights**
>
> An EHR should meet nationally recognized interoperability standards.

examinations, consultation reports, and diagnostic testing results (laboratory tests, **imaging studies**, blood gases, and pulmonary functions test results). The respiratory care clinician should also review any progress notes, data or monitoring flow sheets, and reports of operations or special procedures. The following items should be reviewed, if available, under each of the major medical record sections:

Patient Admissions Sheet

The patient admissions sheet will include the patient's name, age, sex, admission date and time, attending physician, and other demographic information.

Admitting Diagnosis and/or Problem List

The admitting diagnosis provides a starting point for the respiratory care clinician to assess the patient, evaluate ordered respiratory care, and develop a respiratory care plan. Common general hospital admission diagnoses include:

- Childbirth (see Chapter 16 for maternal and perinatal/neonatal assessment)
- Heart disease (acute myocardial infarction [MI], coronary atherosclerosis [coronary artery disease, CAD], other ischemic heart disease, arrhythmias, and congestive heart failure [CHF])
- Mental health issues (including depression)
- Malignant neoplasms (cancer)
- Pneumonia
- Chronic obstructive pulmonary disease (COPD)
- Asthma
- Acute cerebrovascular disease (stroke)
- Bone fractures
- Osteoarthritis
- Back problems
- Septicemia
- Diabetes mellitus
- Surgical procedures (including cardiac catheterization, endoscopy, and orthopedic, abdominal, and thoracic surgery)

Many of the common diagnoses associated with hospitalization are chronic in nature. Important chronic diseases that sometimes require acute care include CHF, stroke, COPD, cancer, asthma, and diabetes.

Acute pulmonary and critical care diagnoses that are often seen by the respiratory care clinician include respiratory failure, cardiac disease, neuromuscular disease, musculoskeletal disease, shock (anaphylactic, cardiogenic, septic, hypovolemic, and neurogenic), renal failure, and traumatic injury.[12–14] Commonly encountered traumatic injuries include chest trauma (rib fractures, sternal injury, and lung contusions), cervical spine and/or spinal cord injury, long bone fractures, burns, head trauma, and abdominal trauma.[12–14] Acute and critical care–related causes of respiratory failure, acute lung injury (ALI), and acute respiratory distress syndrome (ARDS) include:

- Aspiration
- Atelectasis
- Drug overdose (sedatives, narcotics)
- Hypoventilation syndrome
- Morbid obesity
- Musculoskeletal disease (ICU myopathy, rhabdomyolysis [breakdown of muscle tissue leading to release of myoglobin into the blood], spinal cord injury, other)
- Neuromuscular disease (myasthenia gravis, Guillain-Barré syndrome, other)
- Obstructive lung disease
- Pneumonia
- Postoperative respiratory failure
- Pulmonary contusion
- Pulmonary edema (cardiac, noncardiac)
- Pulmonary embolism
- Restrictive lung disease
- Sleep apnea
- Transfusion-related lung injury
- Upper airway obstruction

Physician's Orders

The respiratory care clinician should carefully review the current physician's orders for medications, respiratory care (to include oxygen therapy, respiratory care procedures, or mechanical ventilatory support), and diagnostic testing (to include laboratory and imaging studies). Review of the current orders provides an excellent overview of the treatment the patient is receiving, diagnostic testing that has been ordered and/or performed, and any planned procedures or operations. Orders may also be written by certain mid-level healthcare providers, such as advanced practice nurses and physician assistants. Examples of current physician orders that should be noted related to assessment of the respiratory care patient are described in the following section.

Medications

Orders for the following types of medications should be noted:

- *Antimicrobials:* These may include antibiotics or antiviral and/or antifungal agents used to treat lung infection.

- *Respiratory care medications:* These may include bronchodilators, inhaled corticosteroids, other antiasthma medications, inhaled antimicrobials, mucus-controlling agents, surfactant agents, nasal decongestants, nasal anti-inflammatory agents, and cough and cold medications. Certain patients with α_1-proteinase inhibitor (α_1-PI) deficiency–associated emphysema may have an α_1-proteinase inhibitor medication (Zemaira) prescribed for intravenous (IV) administration.
- *Cardiac/cardiovascular agents:* These may include vasopressors, inotropic agents, antiarrhythmic agents, antihypertensives, antianginal agents, antithrombotic drugs, and diuretics.
- *Sedatives, hypnotics, narcotics, and pain medications:* Remember that opioids (morphine, meperidine [Demerol], codeine, fentanyl, oxycodone, and hydrocodone) act as sedatives and may depress ventilation.
- *Systemic steroids:* These are sometimes prescribed in the treatment of acute, severe asthma and in exacerbation of COPD. Steroids that may be given systemically include cortisone, hydrocortisone, prednisone, prednisolone, triamcinolone, methylprednisolone, dexamethasone, and betamethasone.
- *Neuromuscular blocking agents:* These may include vecuronium, succinylcholine, and cisatracurium. Neuromuscular blocking agents are sometimes used during surgical procedures to paralyze the patient while providing ventilation via an anesthesia ventilator. Neuromuscular blocking agents are also sometimes used to immobilize/paralyze patients receiving invasive mechanical ventilation. Great care must be taken with the use of neuromuscular blocking agents during mechanical ventilatory support because a ventilator malfunction or disconnect can be catastrophic in the paralyzed patient who is unable to breathe on his or her own.
- *Airway medication instillations:* Medications that may be instilled directly into the airway include epinephrine, lidocaine, and cold saline. On rare occasions, topical thrombin may be directly instilled into the airway during bronchoscopy to stop or help control airway bleeding or hemoptysis.
- *Drugs that may cause methemoglobinemia:* Lidocaine, benzocaine spray, dapsone, chloroquine, nitric oxide, and nitroprusside may cause methemoglobinemia. An elevated level of methemoglobin may interfere with the blood's oxygen-carrying capacity. Methylene blue may be used to treat severe methemoglobinemia.
- *Reversal agents:* A number of agents are used to reverse the effects of another drug. Naloxone is used to reverse the effects of opioid drugs or

narcotics. Flumazenil may be used to reverse the effects of benzodiazepines, a class of tranquilizers also sometimes used to treat insomnia. Neostigmine is a reversal agent that can reverse the effects of nondepolarizing muscle relaxants such as vecuronium and rocuronium. Edrophonium is sometime used in the "tensilon test" to differentiate between a myasthenic versus a cholinergic crisis in myasthenia gravis.

Intravenous Fluid Administration and Parenteral Nutrition

Orders should be noted for IV fluid administration. IV orders should include the solution to be used, the rate of infusion, and any medications or electrolytes that may be included. The respiratory care clinician should also note orders for parenteral nutrition.

Respiratory Care Orders

Respiratory care orders that should be reviewed include orders for oxygen therapy, respiratory care treatments and procedures, diagnostic studies related to respiratory care (e.g., blood gases, pulmonary function testing, sleep studies, exercise testing), and orders related mechanical ventilatory support. Examples of typical physician's orders for respiratory care are found in **Box 3-4**. The following list describes each of these areas:

- *Oxygen therapy.* The clinician should note any oxygen therapy orders to include the device, liter flow, desired F_{IO_2}, and associated orders for oximetry (Sp_{O_2}) and/or blood gases. It should be noted whether the therapy is to be delivered "per protocol," which may allow titration of the oxygen therapy based on assessment of Sp_{O_2} and/or blood gas results. Ideally—though not essential—a pretherapy blood gas on room air will have been ordered and reported in order to establish baseline values for Pa_{O_2}, Sa_{O_2}, and Ca_{O_2}. It should also be noted if oxygen therapy is ordered PRN (as needed) or for continuous use. In the acute care setting, PRN oxygen therapy orders should be avoided because intermittent oxygen therapy can result in severe hypoxemia when the oxygen therapy is removed during meals, visits to the bathroom, or patient transport. Continuous positive airway pressure (CPAP) devices may also be ordered to improve oxygenation.
- *Respiratory therapy.* Respiratory therapy orders, sometimes known as "treatments," may include orders for inhaled aerosol medications (bronchodilators, corticosteroids, nonsteroidal antiasthma medications, anti-infective agents, mucus controlling agents); lung expansion therapy (incentive spirometry, intermittent positive pressure breathing [IPPB]; airway clearance techniques (cough and deep breathing instruction, positive expiratory pressure [PEP] therapy, high-frequency chest wall oscillation); chest physiotherapy (postural drainage, chest percussion, vibration and use of chest percussors and/or vibrators); and other therapies aimed at improving respiratory function. Humidification and/or nebulizer therapy may also be ordered.
- *Respiratory care diagnostic tests and procedures.* Respiratory care consults may be ordered to assess and treat patients using established protocols or to generate a new respiratory care plan. Orders may include diagnostic procedures such as oximetry, blood gas studies, pulmonary function testing, exercise testing, or sleep studies. Airway care and ventilatory and/or hemodynamic monitoring may be prescribed. Therapeutic and/or diagnostic bronchoscopy and insertion of chest tubes to treat pleural effusion and/or pneumothorax may be ordered. Special life-support techniques such as extracorporeal membrane oxygenation (ECMO) and mechanical circulatory assistance may also be ordered.
- *Mechanical ventilatory support.* Orders for invasive or noninvasive mechanical ventilatory support should be reviewed carefully to include whether protocols should be used for ventilator initiation, patient stabilization, F_{IO_2}, and positive end-expiratory pressure (PEEP) titration and/or weaning. The clinician should note orders for the following:
  - Noninvasive ventilation and desired support levels
  - Invasive ventilation to include mode of ventilation
  - Initial ventilator settings (patient trigger; tidal volume; rate; inspiratory pressure, flow and time; F_{IO_2}; PEEP/CPAP)
  - Protocols to manage ventilation (initial settings, patient stabilization, weaning, PEEP titration, other)
  - Special modes (high-frequency ventilation, inverse ratio ventilation, independent lung ventilation, other)
  - Procedures to improve oxygenation to include bronchial hygiene, recruitment maneuvers, and/or prone positioning
  - Inhaled vasodilators (nitric oxide, prostacyclin)
  - Specialty gas orders (e.g., helium–oxygen mixtures)
  - Airway care to include humidification, suctioning, cuff maintenance, tube position monitoring, and tracheostomy care

BOX 3-4

Examples of Typical Physician's Orders for Respiratory Care

Oxygen Therapy

Orders should specify the device and liter flow and/or desired F_{IO_2}. PRN (as needed) orders should be avoided. The following are examples of orders for oxygen therapy:
- "Begin nasal cannula at 2 L/min; titrate to maintain $SpO_2 \geq 92\%$."
- "Venturi mask at 28%."
- "Nonrebreathing mask at 8 to 10 L/min. Follow with ABG in 30 minutes."
- "O_2 by nasal cannula to maintain $SpO_2 \geq 92\%$."
- "Cool aerosol by mask at 40% O_2."
- "$\downarrow F_{IO_2}$ to .30 and get an ABG in 30 minutes. Call office with results."
- "O_2 cannula per protocol."

Treatments
- Bronchodilator via metered dose inhaler (MDI) to treat asthma exacerbation in the emergency department: "MDI albuterol (90 mcg/puff) with holding chamber × 4 to 8 puffs every 20 minutes × 3."
- Bronchodilator via MDI to treat hospitalized adult asthma patient: "MDI albuterol (90 mcg/puff) with holding chamber × 4 to 8 puffs q1–4 hours PRN."
- Bronchodilator via MDI to treat hospitalized COPD patient:
  - "MDI albuterol (90 mcg/puff) via holding chamber × 4 to 8 puffs with spacer qid."
  - "MDI ipratropium bromide (Atrovent) (18 mcg/puff) via holding chamber × qid."
- Bronchodilator via small-volume nebulizer (SVN) for routine use in the hospitalized patient with bronchospasm: "SVN with 2.5 mg albuterol in 3 mL of NS qid and PRN at night."
- Intermittent positive pressure breathing (IPPB) for lung expansion therapy: "IPPB with 2.5 mg albuterol in 3 mL of NS qid to achieve an inspiratory $V_T \geq 1200$ mL."
- Incentive spirometry for postoperative lung expansion therapy: "IS every hour while awake × 10 to 15 breaths. Goal is inspiratory volume ≥ 1200 mL."
- Chest physiotherapy with postural drainage and chest percussion to concentrate over the left lower lobe (LLL): "Postural drainage and chest percussion qid to follow aerosol therapy; concentrate over LLL."

Respiratory Care Procedures
- Tracheostomy care: "Trach care every morning."
- Oximetry: "Oximetry in A.M. Call if $SpO_2 < 90\%$."
- Respiratory therapist consults (basic care):
  - "RT consult for bronchial hygiene therapy."
  - "Respiratory care to evaluate for therapy."
- Mechanical ventilatory support:
  - "Initiate mechanical ventilation in assist/control mode at $V_T = 8$ mL/kg IBW; Rate = 10 to 12 bpm; $F_{IO_2} = .50$; PEEP = 5 cm H_2O. Adjust F_{IO_2} and PEEP to maintain PaO_2 60 to 100; SpO_2 92% to 98% per protocol."
  - "Evaluate patient for weaning in AM."
  - "Wean per protocol."

Orders for Laboratory and Imaging Tests and Procedures

A review of the physician's orders section of the medical record for ordered laboratory tests or imaging studies can provide the respiratory care clinician with an idea of what diagnoses have been considered by the admitting physician, as well as any follow-up tests ordered and any orders from consulting physicians. **Laboratory studies** that may have been ordered include hematology, blood chemistry, microbiology, urinalysis, cytology, histology, and molecular techniques. Orders for imaging studies may include chest x-rays, other radiography studies, computed tomography (CT scans), magnetic resonance imaging (MRI), positron emission testing (PET scans), diagnostic ultrasound studies (abdominal, vascular, echocardiography), and other imaging studies. Cardiac tests may include orders for electrocardiograms (ECGs), cardiac stress testing, or angiography. Skin tests for tuberculosis (TB) or fungal lung disease may also be ordered. By reviewing the physician's orders section of the medical record, the clinician can also anticipate what laboratory and imaging reports to expect to be available in other sections of the medical record.

Do Not Resuscitate (DNR) Orders

Generally, in the acute care setting, if a patient suffers a cardiac or respiratory arrest, the healthcare professional on the scene will "call a code" alerting the hospital code team to come to the site of the arrest as soon as possible and begin cardiopulmonary resuscitation and advanced life support. A "do not resuscitate" (DNR) order, sometimes known as a "no code," is a form of advanced directive in which the patient (or family) indicates in advance that he or she does not wish to receive cardiopulmonary resuscitation (CPR) and advanced life support in the event of a cardiac or respiratory arrest. The respiratory care clinician should review the medical record and physician's orders in order to note any advanced directives in place.

Results of the History and Physical Examination(s)

Reviewing reports of the admitting history and physical (H&P) examination(s) found in the patient chart can be invaluable in preparing for a respiratory care assessment, developing a respiratory care plan, and evaluating ordered respiratory care. An outline of the format of a typical medical history and physical examination report follows (see also Chapters 4 and 5). The typical medical history and physical report generally includes:

- *Date of admission.* The date the patient was admitted to the hospital or other inpatient care facility will be noted.
- *History of the present illness.* For the cardiopulmonary patient, this may include a description of cough and sputum production, shortness of breath (to include dyspnea on exertion), chest pain, fever, night sweats, significant weight changes, and associated symptoms.
- *Past medical history.* This may include such things as previous hospitalizations for cardiac or pulmonary problems, prior heart or lung surgery, or thoracic trauma, along with the relevant dates. Chronic heart disease (such as CHF or prior MI) or lung problems (such as COPD or asthma) and other chronic disease (cancer, diabetes, hypertension, and obesity) should be noted. Home use of oxygen or ventilatory assist devices (such as BiPAP or CPAP) should also be noted. Any testing

performed, such as allergy testing, chest or cardiac imaging studies, and pulmonary function or sleep studies may be reported. Skin testing for TB or fungal disease should also be noted, along with any immunizations for influenza or pneumococcal pneumonia.

- *Medications.* A description of pulmonary medications, cardiac medications, or drugs to control blood pressure taken by the patient on a regular basis should be recorded.
- *Allergies.* Any allergies to foods, insect stings, or medications should be noted.
- *Personal and social history.* This should include employment, home environment, exposure to infectious disease, and hobbies. The personal history should also note the patient's nutritional status, fitness and exercise tolerance, tobacco use, and use of alcohol or recreational drugs.
- *Family history.* The family history should note pulmonary or cardiac disease among family members.
- *Review of symptoms.* The review of symptoms should provide a summary of the symptoms noted during the patient history and may be organized by body system. A review of symptoms organized by body system and with examples related to the cardiopulmonary patient follows:
  - General symptoms (e.g., fever, chills, and fatigue)
  - Symptoms related to the skin (e.g., sweating, rash, cyanosis, cold or clammy skin)
  - Musculoskeletal symptoms (e.g., muscle aches and pain)
  - Head-related symptoms (e.g., headache or dizziness)
  - Eyes (e.g., blurred vision or other vision disturbances)
  - Ears (e.g., pain, hearing loss, or discharge)
  - Nose (e.g., nasal discharge, postnasal drip, sinus pain, sneezing, or nasal obstruction)
  - Throat (e.g., pain, hoarseness, or other symptoms)
  - Endocrine system (e.g., enlarged thyroid, diabetes, or pregnancy)
  - Respiratory system (e.g., cough, sputum production, and dyspnea)
  - Cardiac-related symptoms (e.g., chest pain or palpitations)
  - Blood-related symptoms (e.g., bruising or bleeding)
  - Lymph nodes (e.g., tender, enlarged)
  - Gastrointestinal tract (e.g., appetite, diet, digestion, heartburn, nausea, vomiting, diarrhea)
  - Genitourinary system (e.g., urine output)
  - Neurologic symptoms (e.g., fainting, seizures, convulsions, coma, paralysis, or tremors)
  - Mental status (e.g., anxiety, depression, or confusion)

- *Previous patient education.* This may include asthma education received; smoking cessation instruction; information related to the chronic care and management of COPD, CHF, or diabetes; and weight loss or nutritional education.
- *Physical examination.* The typical report of the physical examination found in the patient medical record or chart will include:
  - General appearance
  - Vital signs
  - Skin
  - HEENT (head, eyes, ears, nose, and throat)
  - Neck
  - Back and spine
  - Heart and blood vessels
  - Chest (inspection, palpation, percussion, auscultation)
  - Abdomen/gastrointestinal (abdominal distension, ileus [bowel obstruction], GI bleeding, feeding-tube placement)
  - Extremities
  - Musculoskeletal
  - Neurologic
  - Mental status
  - Other (skin, hair, nails; lymphatic system; breasts and axillae; genitalia; pelvis; anus, rectum, and prostate)
- *Assessment or impression.* The medical history and physical report will generally conclude with a section entitled "Assessment" or "Impression" in which the physician or other clinician describes what he or she has established as the principle, initial, or working diagnosis or problem list.
- *Plan.* The last section of the history and physical report describes what is to be done to complete the differential diagnosis and to manage the patient's problems. This may include further diagnostic tests to confirm or refute the leading diagnosis as well as the therapy to be provided and any monitoring or patient follow-up that is planned.

RC Insights

The pulmonary history should focus on how the patient feels (to include the level of activity at which the patient becomes dyspneic), cough and sputum production, wheezing, crackles, chest tightness or history of pulmonary problems, smoking history, and, finally, environmental and/or occupational exposure to causative agents such as allergens, chemicals, fumes, and mold.

Vital Signs

The respiratory care clinician should review the patient monitoring flow sheets and related data found in the medical record for vital signs (pulse, blood pressure, respirations, temperature) and oximetry (Sp_{O_2}). Data

may also be available on monitoring flow sheets regarding intake and output (I&O) to monitor fluid balance and results of arterial blood gas studies, ECG studies, and ECG monitoring (see also the sections following).

Progress Notes and Reports of Procedures

Hospitalized patients are often seen by consultants with special expertise in areas such as cardiology, pulmonology, oncology, neurology, or psychiatry, and review of reports of these consultations can be very helpful when developing a respiratory care plan. In addition, the chart should contain nursing, respiratory care, and physician progress notes and reports of special procedures or operations. In summary, the respiratory care clinician should review the following reports in the medical record:

- Pulmonary, cardiology, or other consultation reports
- Progress notes (nurses, physicians, physician assistants, respiratory therapists)
- Reports of operations or special procedures, such as bronchoscopies, thoracentesis, or lung biopsy

Laboratory Reports

An essential part of the medical record or chart contains the reports of laboratory studies (see also Chapter 9). Laboratory testing results found in the chart may include the results of tests for:

- Complete blood count (CBC)
- Blood chemistry (electrolytes, magnesium, calcium, phosphate, lactate levels)
- Coagulation studies (indices, platelet count, risk for deep vein thrombosis)
- Cardiac enzymes
- Troponin associated with heart muscle damage and MI
- Brain natriuretic peptide (BNP; a normal BNP level helps to rule out heart failure)
- Microbiology (sputum Gram stain, culture, and sensitivities)
- Kidney function (blood urea nitrogen [BUN], creatinine)

Imaging Studies

Another essential part of the medical record contains the reports of the various imaging studies that may have been performed (see also Chapter 11). Imaging studies that may be of special interest to the respiratory care clinician include reports of medical radiography such as the chest radiograph and upper airway radiograph. Other imaging studies of special interest include reports of CT scans, MRIs, diagnostic ultrasound studies, PET scans, and $\dot{V}/\dot{Q}$ scans. Results of angiography (coronary, pulmonary, bronchial, gastrointestinal) can also be very helpful in identifying such conditions as coronary artery disease or pulmonary embolus.

Respiratory Care–Related Diagnostic Studies

The respiratory care clinician should review reports of respiratory care–related diagnostic studies found in the medical record relevant to the diagnosis, treatment, and follow-up care of patients with heart and lung problems. Data that are often found in the patient record that are important in the evaluation and care of the cardiopulmonary patient include:

- Oximetry results (Spo_2)
- Arterial blood gas studies (see also Chapter 8)
- ECG studies (see also Chapter 10)
- Pulmonary function test results (see also Chapter 12)
- Sleep study results (see also Chapter 15)

Critical Care Monitoring

Results of tests and studies found in the patient chart and directly related to cardiac, respiratory, and hemodynamic function (see also Chapter 14) includes **critical care monitoring** flow sheets and reports related to:

- Cardiac and hemodynamic monitoring
  - ECG monitoring (heart rate, rhythm, presence of arrhythmias)
  - Blood pressure monitoring
  - Fluid balance (intake and output, I&O)
  - Central venous pressure monitoring (CVP)
  - Pulmonary artery pressure monitoring (PAP and pulmonary capillary wedge pressure [PCWP])
  - Left heart preload (often assessed by estimates of left atrial end-diastolic pressure)
  - Left heart afterload (often assessed by arterial blood pressure)
  - Cardiac output/index

- Respiratory monitoring
  - Pulse oximetry (Spo_2)
  - Respiratory rate, tidal volume, minute volume, I:E ratio, rapid shallow breathing index (RSBI).
  - Peak expiratory flow rate (PEFR)
  - Pulmonary mechanics (maximum inspiratory pressure [MIP], bedside vital capacity [VC)])
  - Compliance, airway resistance, and work of breathing (WOB)
  - Capnography, deadspace (V_D/V_T), CO_2 clearance
  - Transcutaneous O_2/CO_2
  - O_2 delivery, $C_{(a-v)}O_2$ difference, shunt fraction
- Intracranial pressure monitoring (ICP)

Patient Education

Education provided to the patient should be recorded in the medical record. For example, patients with moderate to severe asthma should be provided asthma education and an asthma action plan. Asthma education may include an overview of the disease, instruction regarding recognition of symptoms and how to handle an asthma episode, and information about asthma triggers and medication use. COPD patients may receive education related to the chronic care of their disease, and this may be included as a part of a formal pulmonary rehabilitation program. Other types of patient education include instruction on the use and care of respiratory care equipment, nutrition instruction, smoking cessation programs, diabetes education, and education as a part of a cardiac rehabilitation program.

Respiratory Care Plan Development

Box 3-5 provides a summary of the items the respiratory care clinician should review in the medical record for patient assessment and respiratory care plan development. **Figure 3-3** provides an example of a form that can be used to review the patient's medical record in preparation for developing a respiratory care plan.

BOX 3-5

Items in Medical Record for Review in Respiratory Care Plan Development

Prior to developing and implementing a respiratory care plan, the respiratory care clinician should review each of the following items (if available) in the patient's medical record or chart:

Patient data/demographics (name, age, gender, race/ethnicity)

Admission date and time and admitting diagnosis and/or problem list

Current physician's orders

- General care
- Antibiotic and antimicrobial drugs
- Cardiac drugs (inotropes, antiarrhythmic agents, antianginal medications)
- Antihypertensive agents
- Antithrombotics

(*continued*)

- Medications to treat hypotension (e.g., vasopressors)
- IV therapy
- Diuretics
- Systemic steroids
- Analgesics, sedatives, tranquilizers, hypnotics, neuromuscular blocking agents
- Nutrition, diet, and any restrictions (e.g., nothing by mouth, salt, other)

Respiratory care orders

- Oxygen therapy
- Bronchodilators
- Anti-inflammatory agents (e.g., steroids, antiasthmatic agents)
- Other aerosol therapy (humidity therapy, sputum induction, antibiotics, other)
- Lung expansion therapy (e.g., incentive spirometry, IPPB, other)
- Cough and deep breathing
- Bronchial hygiene therapy (e.g., chest physiotherapy, PEP therapy, high-frequency chest wall oscillation, other)
- Suctioning and airway care
- Ventilatory support (mechanical ventilation, BiPAP, etc.)

Orders for diagnostic testing (laboratory, imaging, pulmonary, cardiac, other)

Orders for procedures or operations

Results of history and physical examination(s)

Reports of consultations

Pulmonary consults

Cardiology consults

Other consult reports (neurologic, renal, cancer, psychiatric, etc.)

Cardiopulmonary laboratory studies

- Arterial blood gas studies and oximetry
- Pulmonary function testing
- Pulmonary stress testing
- Cardiac stress testing
- ECG
- Sleep laboratory

Laboratory study results

- Sputum cultures, cytology
- Blood chemistry (electrolytes, BUN, creatinine, serum enzymes, glucose)
- Hematology (CBC, other)
- Microbiology
- Urinalysis
- Histology and cytology
- Skin testing

Imaging reports

- Chest x-rays
- CT scan
- MRI
- Other advanced imaging studies (echocardiography, PET scanning, nuclear medicine procedures, vascular ultrasound, other)

Progress notes/SOAP notes

Reports of procedures and operations

- Surgeries (heart, lung, abdominal, head, other)
- Bronchoscopy
- Cardiac catheterization laboratory

Flow sheets

- Vital signs
- Cardiac and hemodynamic monitoring
- Ventilator/ventilatory support monitoring flow sheets

Respiratory care notes

Patient education (previous)

IPPB, intermittent positive pressure breathing; PEP, positive expiratory pressure; BiPAP, bi-level positive airway pressure; CBC, complete blood count; CT, computed tomography; MRI, magnetic resonance imaging.

Indicate information based on your review of the patient's chart. If a specific item or information is not available, mark that section N/A.

PATIENT DATA

Patient Name:

Physician:

Hospital I.D. Number:

Date:

Floor/Unit:

Room/Bed Number:

Gender: ☐ Male ☐ Female

Age (please write in):_____ Height:_____ Weight:_____ IBW:_____

ADMISSION INFORMATION

Admission Diagnosis:

Past Medical/Surgical History:

Problem List:

CURRENT PHYSICIAN ORDERS

Medications (antibiotics, respiratory, pain, cardiac, diuretic, hypertension/hypotension, etc.):

Respiratory care orders:

Diagnostic tests ordered:

Procedure orders:

DNR/DNI status:

RESULTS OF HISTORY AND PHYSICAL EXAMINATION(S)

General History and Physical (Impression/Assessment):

Pulmonary (Impression/Assessment):

Other (Impression/Assessment):

DIAGNOSTIC/LABORATORY DATA

Most Recent **ABG:**
Date/Time: _____
F_{IO_2}: _____
O_2 device: _____
Liter flow: _____
Pa_{O_2}: _____
pH: _____
Pa_{CO_2}: _____
HCO_3^-: _____
B.E. _____
Settings for **ABG** if mechanically ventilated:
Mode: _____
F_{IO_2}: _____
Machine rate: _____
Total rate: _____
Machine V_T: _____
PEEP/CPAP: _____
Pressure support: _____
Pressure control: _____

ECG ☐ Yes ☐ No If yes, indicate date and results:

Sputum sample ☐ Yes ☐ No If yes, indicate date(s) and findings:

Serum electrolytes/enzymes ☐ Yes ☐ No If yes, indicate date(s) and findings:

Fluid balance status ☐ Yes ☐ No If yes, summarize:

Chest x-ray reports ☐ Yes ☐ No If yes, indicate date(s) and results:

FIGURE 3-3 Respiratory care assessment medical record review data collection form.

	Yes	No	Date(s):
Atelectasis on CXR	☐	☐	_____
Pneumonia on CXR	☐	☐	_____
Pulmonary edema on CXR	☐	☐	_____
Lung over inflation on CXR	☐	☐	_____
Infiltrate(s)	☐	☐	_____

If yes, to any of the above, indicate description and location(s) (RUL/RML/RLL/LUL/LLL, etc.):

Other imaging findings (please write in):

Sleep Study/Pulmonary Stress Testing/Pulmonary Function Testing (please note):

	Yes	No	
Sleep study testing completed?	☐	☐	If yes, indicate date(s) and results:
Pulmonary stress testing completed?	☐	☐	If yes, indicate date(s) and results:
Pulmonary function testing completed?	☐	☐	If yes, indicate date(s) and results:

PFT Results	Before Bronchodilator			Post Bronchodilator		
	Actual	Predicted	% Predicted	Actual	Predicted	% Predicted
FVC						
FEV_1						
FEV_1/FVC						
$FEF_{25-75\%}$						
TLC						
RV						
FRC						
DLCO						
DLCO/VA						

CURRENT RESPIRATORY SERVICES

OXYGEN THERAPY: ☐ Yes   ☐ No

If yes, check device and indicate device, F_{IO_2}, and flow

☐ Low-flow device _____ % F_{IO_2} and _____ L/M
☐ High-flow device _____ % F_{IO_2} and _____ L/M
☐ Large-volume aerosol nebulizer _____ % F_{IO_2} and _____ L/M
☐ Other _____ % F_{IO_2} _____ L/M
Device Name:_____

AEROSOL /MDI MEDICATION (bronchodilators, steroids and/or mucolytics): ☐ Yes   ☐ No

Frequency (QID, BID, etc):
Medication (Albuterol, etc.):
Dose (0.3 mL in 3 mL NS, 2 puffs, etc.):

	Yes	No
Documented wheezing?	☐	☐
Documented improvement in wheezing following therapy?	☐	☐
Documented patient cough following treatments?	☐	☐
Documented productive cough?	☐	☐

FIGURE 3-3 (*continued*)

If yes, specify sputum appearance and amount:

BRONCHIAL HYGIENE THERAPY: ☐ Yes   ☐ No

COUGH ASSIST   ☐ Yes   ☐ No
POSTURAL DRAINAGE   ☐ Yes   ☐ No
VEST THERAPY   ☐ Yes   ☐ No
CPT (postural drainage and/or chest percussion)   ☐ Yes   ☐ No

LUNG EXPANSION THERAPY: ☐ Yes   ☐ No

INCENTIVE SPIROMETRY: ☐ Yes   ☐ No

      If yes, please indicate volumes achieved and use:

Is patient able to reach prescribed volume?   ☐ Yes   ☐ No

      If no, indicate volume achieved (Example: 1200 mL):
Is patient using device?

      If yes, _____per/hour and _____ breaths per use

Has anyone measured and recorded the patients spontaneous IC, or VC?   ☐ Yes   ☐ No

      If yes, enter values IC:_____ (mL)   VC:_____ (mL)

                                                      ☐ Yes   ☐ No

IPPB or IPV:

    Frequency (TID, Q 4 hrs., etc.):
    Prescribed mode
    Prescribed pressure (20 cm H_2O, etc.):
    Prescribed volume (1200 mL, etc.):
    Measurements for V_T, VC or IC?   ☐ Yes   ☐ No
    If yes, please note: V_T:_____ (mL)   VC:_____mL IC:_____mL
    Cough documented post treatments?   ☐ Yes   ☐ No
    Productive cough?   ☐ Yes   ☐ No
    If yes, specify sputum volume and appearance:

FIGURE 3-3 (*continued*)

Charting

Respiratory care clinicians routinely review a patient's medical record prior to performing patient assessment and providing care. Based on the review of the medical record, the respiratory care clinician should determine the patient's current disease state or condition, what respiratory care has been ordered, and what current therapy the patient is receiving. The clinician should then make a preliminary judgment, based on the information that is in the medical record or chart. Specifically, the clinician should ask:

1. Is the ordered therapy indicated and appropriate?
2. Could another form of therapy be more effective?
3. How should the therapy be assessed?

As reviewed in Chapter 1, misallocation of care increases costs and may result in less than optimal health outcomes. Respiratory care clinicians need to exhibit critical diagnostic thinking and evidence-based decision making to optimize patient outcomes. To accomplish this goal, clinicians must demonstrate good clinical documentation and charting skills. Failure to chart information related to the care of the patient may result in duplicate procedures, interventions, and/or

therapy. In addition, clinicians are obligated to notify the responsible licensed caregiver of any critical results of tests and diagnostic procedures. Values that fall outside of normal range may indicate a life-threatening situation. Accurate and timely documentation of a patient's response to care contribute to improved planning, intervening, evaluating, and revising of the patient's care.

Box 3-6 provides rules for charting that should be followed by the respiratory care clinician. Every effort should be made to chart accurately noting the time, effect, and results of all treatments and procedures. Note any patient complaints or adverse reactions. Use correct spelling, grammar, and approved abbreviations. The respiratory care clinician should avoid terms that may be vague or difficult to interpret. For example, when charting volume of sputum production, terms such as "small amount," "moderate amount," and "large amount" should be avoided because different clinicians may have different concepts of the actual volumes associated with each term. Instead, the clinician should approximate the volume of sputum produced in cubic centimeters (ccs) or other units of measure, such a teaspoonfuls. In a similar fashion, terms such as "tolerated

BOX 3-6

Rules for Charting

General Rules for Charting

1. Chart accurately.
2. Document patient complaints and unusual behavior. Describe type, location, onset, and duration of pain or adverse reactions.
3. Use correct spelling, grammar, and approved abbreviations.
4. Use present tense, never future, to describe care.
5. Avoid criticism.
6. Avoid documenting for others.

Rules for Paper Charting

1. Write legibly.
2. Be exact in noting the time, effect, and results of all treatments and procedures.
3. Only use approved abbreviations.
4. Do not erase unwanted entries. A single line should be drawn through a mistake and the word "error" printed above it and initialed.
5. Do not leave blank lines. Draw a line through empty fields.
6. Verify that client-identifying information is on each page of the written chart.
7. Paper entries should be handwritten and signed using an initial, your last name, and your title (e.g., S. Valdez, Resp Care Student; J. Johnson, RRT). Institutional policies may require student entries to be countersigned by supervisory personnel.

Rules for Electronic Charting

1. Document in real time.
2. Document only services performed.
3. Avoid "charting by exception."
4. Perform closed-loop medication administration. Scan patient band and medication prior to administration.
5. Do not delete unwanted entries without documentation. A comment stating "charted in error" should be made to justify the deletion.

well," "tolerated fairly," or "tolerated poorly" should be avoided and a more specific description provided. For example, when charting the patient response to a respiratory therapy treatment, the terms "patient alert and cooperative" and "no adverse reaction noted" would be more descriptive than the term "tolerated well." The term "the patient was uncooperative and seemed confused" would provide a better description of events than the term "tolerated poorly."

When charting in the patient medical record, medical abbreviations should be used sparingly. Some institutions have a published list of approved abbreviations. However, common abbreviations can often be confused. For example, B.S. has been used by various care providers to indicate "breath sounds," "bowel sounds," and "bedside." Commonly used medical abbreviations related to respiratory care are listed in **Table 3-1**, and **Box 3-7** lists commonly used symbols.

Table 3-2 provides a list of medical abbreviations developed by TJC that should *not* be used when charting in the patient record. This "do not use" list of abbreviations was published in 2010 as a part of National Patient Safety Goal (NPSG) 02.02.01.[15] When in doubt as to whether specific abbreviations are approved, it is best to avoid their use. **Box 3-8** provides a list of items that should be charted following administration of a basic respiratory care treatment or procedure. **Clinical Focus 3-2** provides an example of charting for a patient receiving mechanical ventilation using an EMR.

RC Insights

To avoid miscommunication, use medical abbreviations sparingly.

TABLE 3-1
Commonly Used Medical Abbreviations in Respiratory Care

Abbreviation	Meaning	Abbreviation	Meaning
BID, bid	administered twice a day	DC, dc	discontinue
TID, tid	administered three times a day	DOB	date of birth
QID, qid	administered four times a day	Dx	diagnosis
q4h	administered every 4 hours	ECG, EKG	electrocardiogram
q6h	administered every 6 hours	EEG	electroencephalogram
q8h	administered every 8 hours	e.g.	for example
q12h	administered every 12 hours	ENT	ear, nose and throat
ABG	arterial blood gas	ETOH	ethyl alcohol
A/C	assist-control mode	Fx	fracture
AMI	acute myocardial infarction	GERD	gastroesophageal reflux disease
ARDS	acute respiratory distress syndrome	Hgb	hemoglobin
ALI	acute lung injury	Hct	hematocrit
ASAP	as soon as possible	H_2O	water
BUN	blood urea nitrogen	HS	hour of sleep or bedtime
c/o	complaints of	Ht	height
CABG	coronary artery bypass graft	Hx	history
CAD	coronary artery disease	IPPB	intermittent positive pressure breathing
CBC	complete blood count	I&O	intake and output
CF	cystic fibrosis	IC	inspiratory capacity
CHD	coronary heart disease	ICU	intensive care unit
CHF	congestive heart failure	IS	incentive spirometry
CNS	central nervous system	IM	intramuscular
COPD	chronic obstructive pulmonary disease	IV	intravenous
CO_2	carbon dioxide	LUL	left upper lobe
CPAP	continuous positive airway pressure	LLL	left lower lobe
CPR	cardiopulmonary resuscitation	MDI	metered dose inhaler
CVA	cerebral vascular accident	MI	myocardial infarction
CVP	central venous pressure		

TABLE 3-1
Commonly Used Medical Abbreviations in Respiratory Care (*continued*)

Abbreviation	Meaning	Abbreviation	Meaning
MRI	magnetic resonance imaging	RML	right middle lobe
MRSA	methicillin-resistant *Staphylococcus aureus*	RLL	right
NG, NGT	nasogastric tube	RRT	registered respiratory therapist
NSAID	nonsteroidal anti-inflammatory drug	SOB	short of breath
NS	normal saline solution (0.9% salt)	S/P	status post
MIP	maximum inspiratory pressure	Staph	*Staphylococcus*
1/2 NS	half normal saline solution (0.45% salt)	Stat	immediately
O_2	oxygen	STD	sexually transmitted disease
PA	physician assistant	Subq	subcutaneous
PCWP	pulmonary capillary wedge pressure	SVN	small-volume nebulizer
PEFR	peak expiratory flow rate	Sx	symptom
PEEP	positive end-expiratory pressure	TB	tuberculosis
PIP	peak inspiratory pressure	TIA	transient ischemic attack
PFT	pulmonary function test	T/O	telephone order
Prn	as needed	TPR	temperature, pulse and respirations
PO	by mouth	Tsp	teaspoon measurement
PSV	pressure support ventilation	Tx	treatment
Pt	patient	URI	upper respiratory infection
PVC	premature ventricular contraction	WBC	white blood cell
pH	hydrogen ion concentration	VC	vital capacity
RBC	red blood cell	VO	verbal order
RN	registered nurse	V_T	tidal volume
R/O	rule out	w/o	without
Rx	treatment	wt	weight
RN	registered nurse	y/o	years old
RUL	right upper lobe	yr	year

BOX 3-7

Commonly Used Symbols for Charting

Symbol	Meaning
↑	increase, up
↓	decrease, down
♀	female
♂	male
=	equal
>	greater than
<	less than
≤	less than or equal to
≥	greater than or equal to
#	number
~	approximately
%	percent
@	at

TABLE 3-2
The Joint Commission Official "Do Not Use" Abbreviation List*

Do Not Use	Potential Problem	Use Instead
U, u (unit)	Mistaken for "0" (zero), the number "4" (four), or "cc"	Write "unit"
IU (International Unit)	Mistaken for IV (intravenous) or the number 10 (ten)	Write "International Unit"
Q.D., QD, q.d., qd (daily) Q.O.D., QOD, q.o.d, qod (every other day)	Mistaken for each other Period after the Q mistaken for "I" and the "O" mistaken for "I"	Write "daily" Write "every other day"
Trailing zero (X.0 mg)** Lack of leading zero (.X mg)	Decimal point is missed	Write X mg Write 0.X mg
MS MSO$_4$ and MgSO$_4$	Can mean morphine sulfate or magnesium sulfate Confused for one another	Write "morphine sulfate" Write "magnesium sulfate"

*Applies to all orders and all medication-related documentation that is handwritten (including free-text computer entry) or on preprinted forms.
**Exception: A "trailing zero" may be used only where required to demonstrate the level of precision of the value being reported, such as for laboratory results, imaging studies that report size of lesions, or catheter/tube sizes. It may not be used in medication orders or other medication-related documentation.
© The Joint Commission, 2014. Reprinted with permission.

BOX 3-8

Items to Chart Following Administration of Respiratory Care Treatments and Procedures

Following administration of respiratory therapy, the clinician should record the following information:

Date: Date therapy given.

Time: When the therapy was started.

What was given: Device or procedure. For example:
- "Aerosol therapy given via small-volume nebulizer."
- "MDI 2 puffs given via holding chamber."
- "Postural drainage and chest percussion given."

Medication: The medication, if any, should be listed. For example:
- "0.5 mL of albuterol (0.5%) in 3 mL of normal saline."
- "2.5 mg of albuterol in 3 mL of normal saline."
- "2 puffs of salmetorol via MDI given."

Method or appliance: The method or appliance used for therapy should be listed. This may include use of a mouthpiece, mouth seal, face mask, trach mask, nose clips, or holding chamber or spacer.

Gas source and flow or pressure: The delivered gas (O_2 or compressed air), flow (L/min), and/or pressure used (cm H_2O) should be recorded.

Length of therapy: The duration of the treatment should be listed. For example: "×10 minutes."

Pulse and respiratory rate: For most intermittent procedures (such as bronchodilator therapy administration), pulse and respiratory rate should be recorded before, during, and after the procedure.

Breath sounds: For most respiratory therapy treatments, breath sounds before and after therapy should be recorded. Breaths sounds should also be assessed during therapy to make sure wheezing or aeration is not getting worse.

Cough and sputum production: Patients should be instructed to cough following most therapy, and the nature of the cough and sputum production should be recorded.

Patient comments: Following most therapy, the respiratory care clinician should ask the patient if he or she thinks the treatments are helping and if he or she can "breathe better" following treatment.

Patient cooperation: The respiratory care should note if the patient is cooperative and seems to understand the purpose of the therapy.

Adverse reactions/side effects: Examples include increased shortness of breath, increased wheezing, tachycardia, tachypnea, chest pain, or discomfort.

Physical appearance: Note if the patient appears in distress (or not).

IC/VC/V_T: For lung expansion therapy, record the inspired volume achieved.

Name, signature, and credentials: First initial and last name, followed by credential (e.g., RN, RRT, PA, or MD).

CLINICAL FOCUS 3-2

Routine Charting Using the Electronic Medical Record

The respiratory care clinician should approach the bedside with a clearly formulated plan for documentation. In addition, clinicians must remember that billing for services is required. Reimbursements are made only when charges match documented procedures.

Let's use the example of ventilator initiation. Following a review of the medical record, what are the major components to performing ventilator initiation and assessment?

(continues)

(*continued*)

The steps are as follows:

Step 1   Confirm emergency equipment at the bedside (mask, bag-valve mask, spare oral endotracheal tube or tracheostomy).

Step 2   Perform respiratory patient assessment (see Chapters 3, 4, and 5).

Step 3   Document artificial airway (size, cuff pressure, how/where it is secured).

Step 4   Complete ventilator documentation (see Chapter 14).

Step 5   Create care plan.

Step 6   Charge.

Examples of documentation for each of these steps in the EMR is as follows.

Step 1: Confirm Emergency Equipment

The clinician should approach the bedside and verify that there is suction equipment and supplies and a resuscitation bag with oxygen supply, appropriately fitting mask, and adaptors for connection of the artificial airway (endotracheal tube or tracheostomy tube). If the patient has an artificial airway, additional sizes of oral endotracheal tubes or tracheostomy tubes should be kept at or near the bedside, along with intubation equipment (e.g., laryngoscope, stylets, and colorimetric capnometers). The clinician should then chart in the medical record, as per the pediatric patient example shown here:

							6/1/12								
	0600	0700	0800	0900	1000	1100	1200	1300	1400	1500	1600	1700	1800	1900
Safety															
Hospital Band Applied			ID;Allerg...											
Security ID Number														
Airway Emergency Supplies			Yes											
Emergency Drug Sheet At Bedside			Yes											
Password														
Call Light Accessible			Yes											
Bed Type			Bed											
Isolation Precautions														
Precautions			Fall risk											
Pediatric Visitation															
Primary Visitor Banded 1			Father											
Primary Visitor Banded 2														
Parental Involvement															
Parent Telephone Call to RN														
Parent Visited Child			Parent											
Visit Duration (In Minutes)														
Overnight with Child														
Parental Participation			Verbalize...											
Basic Care															
Bath			No											
Care Assistance			Partial As...											
Oral Care			Mouth Sw...											
Eye Care			Yes											
Catheter Care														
Eating Assistance			Independ...											
Linen Change			No											
Additional Care Needed			No											
Head of Bed			Flat											
Bladder Assessment Method														
Activities															
Bed Rest														
Activity			Up with a...											
Position Change			Assist wit...											

© 2014 Epic Systems Corporation. Used with permission.

Step 2: Perform Respiratory Patient Assessment

Flow sheets record measurements made over time. The following screenshot shows the "Adult Assessment" flow sheet. Additional options can be made based on patient population (e.g., pediatric, infant, neonate assessment).

(*continued*)

The clinician can enter a patient's respiratory status and breath sounds as noted in the adult ICU patient shown here:

	6/1/12						
	0200	0300	0400	0600	0700	0800	0820
Respiratory							
Regular			Yes			Yes	
Respiratory Effort			Ventilated			Ventilated	
🔲 Cough			Yes			Yes	
Cough Effort			Fair			Fair	
🔲 Sputum			Yes			Yes	
Amount			Moderate			Moderate	
Consistency			Thick			Thick	
Color			Yellow;T...			Blood tin...	
🔲 Respiratory Distress			No 🔲🔍			No	
Substernal Retractions							
Clavicular Retractions							
Dyspnea							
Cough/Deep Breathe						Yes	
Incentive Spirometer Volume (L)							
Spirometer Frequency							
Suction			Endotrac...			Endotrac...	
Delivery Device	Ventilator	Ventilator	Ventilator	Ventilator	Ventilator	Ventilator	Manual in...ᵉ
O2 Flow Rate (l/min)							
🔲 Respiratory - Additional Assessment						No	
Breath Sounds							
🔲 Lungs Clear			No			No	
Anterior/Lateral Right Upper			Clear			Rhonchi	
Anterior/Lateral Right Lower			Rhonchi;...			Rhonchi	
Anterior/Lateral Right Middle			Clear			Rhonchi	
Anterior/Lateral Left Upper			Clear			Rhonchi	
Anterior/Lateral Left Lower			Rhonchi;...			Rhonchi	
Lingula						Rhonchi	
Posterior Right Upper							
Posterior Right Lower							
Posterior Right Middle							
Posterior Left Upper							
Posterior Left Lower							

Step 3: Document Artificial Airway (Inpatient Department)

An artificial airway can be entered by inputting data such as airway properties (i.e., type, intubation date and time, intubation performed by), how and where tube is secured, depth of insertion and location, and cuff pressure, as shown in the following screenshot:

⊟ Airway 06/01/12 1730 Oral endotracheal tube	
Airway Properties	Intubation Date/Intubation Time: 06/01/12 1730 Airway Type: Oral endotracheal tube Airway Size: 7.5
Last Filed Value:	
@ Lip (cm)	▢ 🔲 📰 📊
Last Filed Value: 23 cm taken at 06/04/12 0817 by Geda, Meron A	
Lip to Tip (cm)	▢ 🔲 📰 📊
Last Filed Value: "No data filed"	
Cuff Pressure (cm H2O)	▢ 🔲 📰 📊
Last Filed Value: 28 cm H2O taken at 06/04/12 0817 by Geda, Meron A	
Secured With	ETAD Sutured Taped Trach Ties Other (Comment) 📰 📊
Last Filed Value: ETAD *[comment: Checked]* taken at 06/04/12 0817 by Geda, Meron A	
Airway Status	Spontaneous Mechanical ventilation 📰 📊
Last Filed Value: Mechanical ventilation taken at 06/04/12 0817 by Geda, Meron A	
Airway Location	Right Midline Left 📰 📊
Last Filed Value: Left taken at 06/04/12 0817 by Geda, Meron A	

(*continues*)

(*continued*)

Step 4: Complete Ventilator Documentation

When initiating ventilator support, the first day on a ventilator will always count as Day 1. This is true whether mechanical ventilation is initiated at 00:02 or 23:59. It is important to select the proper mode of ventilation prior to beginning documentation, because the fields that populate the documentation sheet are preprogrammed based on the initial mode selected, as shown in the following screenshot:

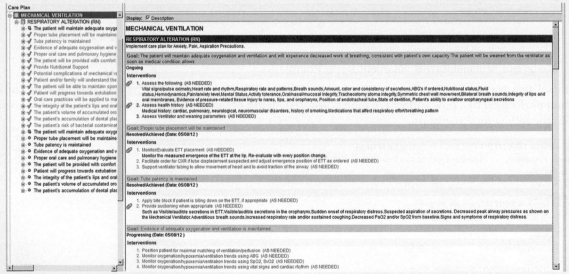

© 2014 Epic Systems Corporation. Used with permission.

Step 5: Create Care Plan

Care plans are a general way for clinicians to update revised care based on interventions and evaluations. In the intensive care environment, patients may need mechanical ventilatory support or other forms of respiratory therapy, such as oxygen therapy; bronchodilator therapy via small-volume nebulizer or metered dose inhaler; or bronchial hygiene therapy. A progress note may be written to detail a specific intervention, such as: "Patient was transported off unit for CT using transport ventilator with no change in ventilator settings. Upon being placed in supine position for scan, patient became asynchronous with the ventilator and required manual bagging and suctioning. Flow on transport ventilator increased from baseline to meet patient inspiratory demand. Scan performed without incident, and patient transported back to ICU and successfully placed on previous ventilator settings." The EMR care plan documentation provides an example:

© 2014 Epic Systems Corporation. Used with permission.

Step 6: Charge

As stated previously, failing to chart gives the impression that care was never given (negligence). Charging without documentation will result in refusal of payment for undocumented services. Charges are often done based on initial or subsequent days. For instance, a clinician may charge a ventilator "first day" on the day the ventilator was

(continued)

initiated; each additional day of support would be billed as "subsequent." The following screenshot shows the new charges.

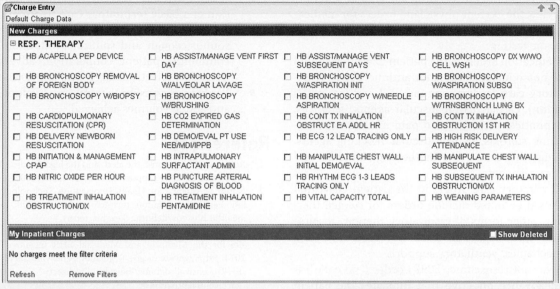

Summary

Review of the patient's medical record is an essential step taken prior to delivering ordered respiratory care, and it is indispensable in the development of an appropriate respiratory care plan. The medical record may be electronic or paper-based; however, it must conform to standards set by governmental, regulatory, and accreditation agencies. Review of the medical record should include review of the patient's admission sheet, diagnosis, physician's orders, results of history and physical examinations, laboratory and imaging test results, and cardiac diagnostic tests. The respiratory care clinician should also review monitoring and related flow sheets for vital signs and respiratory, cardiac, and hemodynamic monitoring reports. Progress notes, reports of consultations, reports of operations, and discharge plans should also be reviewed. Charting must be timely, accurate, and legible. Avoid terms that may be vague or difficult to interpret and use medical abbreviations sparingly. Recording the respiratory care plan in the medical record in a clear, understandable fashion, along with the patient's response to therapy and any needed care plan modifications, is an essential skill for the respiratory care clinician.

Key Points

▶ Medical records are used to record, track, monitor, and evaluate patient care and to identify trends in population health.

▶ Information in the medical record must be timely, accurate, and legible.

▶ The functions of the medical record include serving as a database for clinicians, providing a legal record of care provided, documenting diagnosis and care for reimbursement, and establishing a central location for interprofessional communication.

▶ Types of medical records include paper-based records, electronic medical records (EMRs), electronic health records (EHRs).

▶ The problem-oriented medical record (POMR) focuses on problem-solving while providing complex care by encouraging ongoing assessments and care adjustments by the healthcare team.

▶ The four sections of the POMR SOAP note are subjective, objective, assessment, and plan. The SOAPIER note adds intervention, evaluation, and revision.

▶ Common hospital admitting diagnoses include childbirth, heart disease, mental health issues, cancer, pneumonia, stroke, and surgery.

▶ Important chronic diseases that sometimes require acute care include congestive heart failure (CHF), COPD exacerbation, acute asthma, and diabetes.

▶ Important respiratory and critical care diagnoses to note include respiratory failure, acute lung injury (ALI), acute respiratory distress syndrome (ARDS), pneumonia, postoperative respiratory failure, pulmonary edema, pulmonary embolism, cardiac disease, neuromuscular disease, musculoskeletal disease, drug overdose, shock, renal failure, and traumatic injury.

▶ The respiratory care clinician should carefully review the current physician's orders for medications, respiratory care orders, and orders for diagnostic testing.

▶ Medication orders in the patient chart that should be noted include orders for antimicrobials, respiratory care medications (aerosol and for installation), cardiac/cardiovascular agents, sedatives, hypnotics, narcotics, and pain medications, systemic steroids, neuromuscular blocking agents, drugs that may cause methemoglobinemia, and reversal agents.

▶ Respiratory care orders in the patient chart that should be noted include orders for oxygen therapy, other forms of respiratory therapy, respiratory care diagnostic tests, and procedures and mechanical ventilatory support.

▶ A do not resuscitate (DNR) order ("no code") is an advance directive that indicates the patient does not wish to receive cardiopulmonary resuscitation (CPR).

▶ The history and physical (H&P) report in the patient chart should include date of admission, history of the present illness, past medical history, medication history, allergies, personal and social history, family history, patient education, review of symptoms, and physical examination findings.

▶ The H&P review of symptoms should provide a summary of the symptoms noted during the patient history organized by body system.

▶ The physical examination portion of the H&P report should include findings related to general appearance, vital signs, skin, HEENT, neck, back and spine, heart and blood vessels, chest, abdomen/gastrointestinal, extremities, musculoskeletal, neurologic, and mental status.

▶ The H&P report in the medical record will generally conclude with sections entitled "Assessment" or "Impression" and "Plan."

▶ Other sections of the patient's medical record that should be reviewed by the respiratory care clinician include vital signs, progress notes, laboratory studies, imaging studies, and results of respiratory and critical care monitoring.

▶ Following review of the patient chart regarding orders for respiratory care, the clinician should ask himself or herself if the ordered therapy is indicated and appropriate, if another form of therapy might be more effective, and how the therapy should be assessed.

▶ When charting a basic respiratory care treatment or procedure, record the date and time the therapy was given, what was given, any medications administered, method of administration, appliance used, gas source and flow or pressure, oxygen concentration, and duration of therapy.

▶ Assessment data recorded following administration of a basic respiratory care treatment or procedure may include pulse, respiratory rate, breath sounds, cough and sputum production, patient comments, patient cooperation, adverse reactions/side effects, and physical appearance.

▶ For lung-expansion therapy, chart volume targets and actual volumes achieved.

References

1. Rollins G. The prompt, the alert, and the legal record: documenting clinical decision support systems. *J AHIMA.* 2005;76(2):24–28.
2. National Alliance for Health Information Technology. Defining key health information technology terms. 2008. http://www.healthit.hhs.gov/defining_key_hit_terms.
3. Centers for Medicare and Medicaid Services. The official web site for the Medicare and Medicaid EHR Incentive Programs. 2014. http://www.cms.gov/Regulations-and-Guidance/Legislation/EHRIncentivePrograms/index.html?redirect=/ehrincentiveprograms/.
4. Blumenthal D, Tavenner M. The "meaningful use" regulation for electronic health records. *N Engl J Med.* 2010;363(6):501–504.
5. Hsiao CJ, Hing E, Socey TC, Cai B. Electronic health record systems and intent to apply for meaningful use incentives among office-based physician practices: United States, 2001–2011. NCHS Data Brief, No 79. Hyattsville, MD: National Center for Health Statistics; 2011.
6. Desroches CM, Worzala C, Joshi MS, Kralovec PD, Jha AK. Small, nonteaching, and rural hospitals continue to be slow in adopting electronic health record systems. *Health Aff (Millwood).* 2012;31(5):1092–1099.
7. Jha AK, DesRoches CM, Campbell EG, et al. Use of electronic health records in U.S. hospitals. *N Engl J Med.* 2009;360:1628–1638.
8. Hsiao C-J, Beatty PC, Hing ES, Woodwell DA, Rechtsteiner EA, Sisk JE. Electronic medical record/electronic health record use by office-based physicians: United States, 2008 and preliminary 2009. National Center for Health Statistics, December 2009. http://www.cdc.gov/nchs/data/hestat/emr_ehr/emr_ehr.htm.
9. McBride M. Ranking top 10 hospital EMR vendors by number of installed symptoms. Dark Daily. March 25, 2011. http://www.darkdaily.com/ranking-top-10-hospital-emr-vendors-by-number-of-installed-systems-32511#axzz1w63ZSouo. Accessed May 6, 2012.
10. Jacobs L. Interview with Lawrence Weed, MD—the father of the problem-oriented medical record looks ahead. *Perm J.* 2009;13(3):84–89.
11. Weed LL. *Medical Records, Medical Education, and Patient Care.* Cleveland, OH: Press of the Case Western Reserve University; 1971.
12. National Board for Respiratory Care. Entry level CRT examination detailed content outline. Lenexa, KS: Author; 2007.
13. National Board for Respiratory Care. Therapist written RRT examination detailed content outline. Lenexa, KS: Author; 2007.
14. National Board for Respiratory Care. Adult critical care specialist examination detailed content outline. Lenexa, KS: Author; 2009.
15. The Joint Commission. Critical Access Hospital: 2012 National Patient Safety Goals. 2012. http://www.jointcommission.org/standards_information/npsgs.aspx. Accessed May 20, 2012.

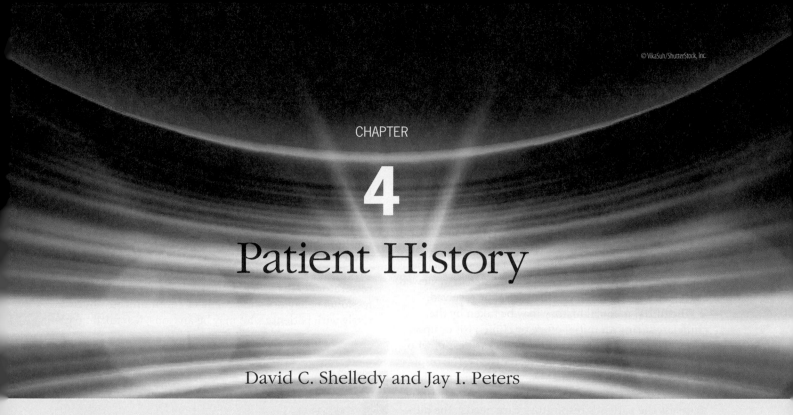

© VikaSuh/ShutterStock, Inc.

CHAPTER

4

Patient History

David C. Shelledy and Jay I. Peters

CHAPTER OUTLINE

Patient Interview Guidelines
Demographic Data and Patient Profile
Chief Complaint
History of the Present Illness
Cough and Sputum Production
Hemoptysis
Whistling, Wheezing, and Chest Tightness
Chest Pain
Dyspnea
Sleep Issues
Past Medical History
Family History
Personal and Social History
Smoking History
Occupational and Environmental History
Current Medications
Current Respiratory Care
Exercise Tolerance
Nutritional Status
Advanced Directives
The Patient's Learning Needs
Health-Related Quality of Life
Review of Symptoms

CHAPTER OBJECTIVES

1. List the components of a successful patient interview and explain each.
2. Discuss the collection and use of demographic data in patient assessment.
3. Define the term *chief complaint* and give examples related to respiratory care.
4. Describe the components of a history of the present illness (HPI) and explain the significance of each.
5. Evaluate the significance of cough and sputum production.

6. Describe types and causes of hemoptysis.
7. Explain the significance of wheezing, whistling, and chest tightness.
8. Describe types and causes of chest pain.
9. Classify levels of dyspnea.
10. Formulate a treatment approach to a patient with dyspnea.
11. Apply interview questions in assessment of sleep issues and disorders.
12. Assess a patient's past medical history.
13. Explain the importance of each of the following in patient assessment: social history, family history, occupational history, and environmental history.
14. Explain the importance of assessing current medication use.
15. Assess a patient's current respiratory care based on the patient interview.
16. Evaluate exercise tolerance.
17. Assess a patient's nutritional status.
18. Explain the application of advanced directives and DNR status.
19. Evaluate a patient's learning needs.
20. Develop a respiratory care plan based on the review of symptoms.

KEY TERMS

angina
Borg scale
chief complaint
DNR status
dyspnea
family history
health-related quality of life (HRQOL)
hemoptysis
history of the present illness (HPI)

musculoskeletal chest pain
myocardial infarction (MI)
pleuritic chest pain
patient profile
smoking history
sputum
substernal chest pain
wheezing

Overview

This chapter reviews the interview and medical history as an integral part of patient assessment and care plan development. Patient interview guidelines, collection and review of pertinent demographic data, and assessment of the patient's chief complaint are discussed. We will then describe how to take a complete history as it relates to the cardiopulmonary patient. The history of the present illness, past medical history, family history, and development of a patient profile are included in a complete medical history. Current medications, smoking, alcohol abuse, and/or illicit drug use, and occupation and environmental factors should also be reviewed, as well as any respiratory care ordered or received.

The initial medical history may be taken by the clinician during an initial office or clinic visit or upon admission to the acute care facility. Regardless of who obtains the patient's initial medical history, the respiratory care clinician should always perform a chart review and, when possible, a patient interview in order to assess the patient's respiratory care needs. The purpose of the patient interview performed by the respiratory care clinician is to determine the appropriateness of ordered care and the goals of therapy and to monitor, evaluate, and modify or discontinue therapy based on the patient's response. A patient interview is essential for respiratory care plan development, implementation, and evaluation.

An overview of the interview and medical history follows, with an emphasis on findings related to the cardiopulmonary patient. Typical findings on history with common respiratory problems are reviewed.

Patient Interview Guidelines

The patient interview is an essential part of the assessment performed by the respiratory care clinician. The purpose of the patient interview is to collect subjective data from the patient and/or his or her family members. During the interview, the clinician asks a series of questions to get a clear idea of the patient's condition, problem(s), and symptoms.

The respiratory care clinician must have competence in effective listening and excellent communication skills in order to conduct a successful patient interview. Factors that may affect the interview include the patient's emotional and mental state, cognitive function, and any perceptual deficits, such as hearing impairment.[1] Fear, stress, anxiety, and pain can all impact the effectiveness of communication.[1] The environment in which the interview takes place can also have an impact, and privacy, noise, and factors such a room temperature, lighting, and general patient comfort may influence the patient–clinician interaction.[1] Interviewing skills can improve with practice and experience and attention to those factors that may impact the interview.

Many additional factors may affect communication between patients and clinicians. Use of jargon should be avoided, and choice of words, explanations, and questions should be such that communication is clear and direct. Voice tone and nonverbal communication cues such as facial expression and body language should project warmth, interest, and professionalism. Language barriers should be addressed by use of a trained medical interpreter. The clinician should also be alert to communication difficulties that may occur due to differences in culture, religion, attitudes, beliefs, and values. **Box 4-1** highlights professional behaviors that should be included in any patient encounter. The respiratory care clinician must display appropriate professional behaviors and be able to communicate effectively with patients who may be anxious, fearful, angry,

---

BOX 4-1

Professional Behaviors Associated with the Patient Encounter

Introduce yourself by name and role (e.g., respiratory therapist, physician, nurse, physician assistant, other).

Explain why you are seeing the patient.

Address the patient by his or her formal name.

Be warm, friendly, and set the patient at ease:
- Face the patient directly.
- Use an open posture.
- Use appropriate eye contact.
- Express genuine concern.
- Maintain professional demeanor; do not be informal or make jokes.

Observe the patient for responses, cooperation, and understanding:
- Make eye contact.
- Watch the patient's body language.
- Listen carefully to the patient's questions and responses.

Respect the patient's social, personal, and intimate space:
- Social space (4 to 12 feet distant from patient) should be used for the initial encounter between the clinician and the patient for introductions.
- Person space (18 inches to 4 feet distant from the patient) should be used for the interview.
- Ask permission before entering the patient's intimate space (0 to 18 inches distant) for the physical assessment (auscultation, vital signs, etc.).

or depressed. The successful patient interview includes the following components:

1. Establish patient rapport so you can obtain the most accurate description of the patient's condition.
2. Gather information about the patient's condition, including a chronology of events and the patient's impressions of his or her health.
3. Obtain feedback from the patient regarding your understanding of the patient's answers to your questions.
4. Involve the family, especially family caregivers, in the patient interview whenever possible.
5. Demonstrate to the patient and the family that you understand the patient's problems and will work with them to obtain the appropriate care.
6. Build on initial rapport to enhance further assessment, evaluations, and treatment plans.
7. Provide additional assessment, evaluation, and a treatment plan for chronic cardiopulmonary conditions to facilitate disease management.

The patient interview should include questions to assess cough; sputum production; hemoptysis; wheezing, whistling, or chest tightness; dyspnea; past history of chest illness; smoking history; occupation; and, where appropriate, hobby and leisure activities. The patient interview should also include questions regarding the patient's current medications, use of oxygen in the home, use of other respiratory care equipment, and history of previous episodes requiring intubation or mechanical ventilatory support. The patient interview should also include questions to assess the benefits of any respiratory care the patient is currently receiving, as well as any adverse effects of respiratory care the patient may have experienced. **Table 4-1** outlines the key elements to assess during the patient interview for respiratory care plan development.

TABLE 4-1
Items to Be Included in the Patient Interview for Respiratory Care Plan Development

Cough
Sputum production
Hemoptysis
Wheezing, whistling, or chest tightness
Breathlessness
History of chest illness
Previous hospitalizations and/or ICU admissions
Smoking
Occupational history
Hobby and leisure history
Medications
History of intubation and/or mechanical ventilation
Response to respiratory care received
Home respiratory care

Demographic Data and Patient Profile

Following review of the medical record (see Chapter 3), the next step in patient assessment and care plan development is to identify and clarify the patient's problem by performing a patient history. The patient history begins with collection of the patient's demographic data, development of a patient profile, and identification of the patient's chief complaint.

Demographic data and the patient profile provide a description or overview of the patient and his or her condition. Demographic data collected should include the patient's name, address, age, gender, race/ethnicity, admitting diagnosis (if available), and any other already-identified medical problems. Other information helpful in describing the patient may include place of birth, education, socioeconomic status, marital status, religion, and languages spoken. The name(s) of the physician(s) caring for the patient, sources of referral for care, and a brief description of why the patient sought medical care should also be included.

As the assessment process proceeds, the clinician should begin to develop an outline or summary of the patient's characteristics and problems, sometimes known as the **patient profile**. The patient profile provides a narrative description, or "snapshot," of the patient; that is, the "who, why, what, when and where" of the patient's current condition.

If there is an available medical record or chart, any previous blood gases, chest x-rays, pulmonary function tests, the results of diagnostic studies, including sputum AFB stains, culture, sensitivity, cytology, and silver stain (for evaluating fungal infections and pneumocystis pneumonia) and other relevant reports should be sought and reviewed. Previously performed history and physical examination reports and consultations found in the patient's medical record can also be extremely helpful to establish the patient's baseline condition from which current findings may differ in ways that provide important diagnostic clues.

Chief Complaint

The **chief complaint** is a concise statement by the patient (or family member) relating his or her reason for seeking medical attention.[1] The simple question "Why are you here?" or "What medical problem brought you to the hospital?" provides a good way to identify the patient's perceived problem. Common chief complaints of patients with respiratory problems include shortness of breath, cough, sputum production, hemoptysis, fever, and chest pain or tightness. The chief complaint is the patient's primary symptom described in his or her own terms.

Breathlessness is perhaps the most common pulmonary complaint.[2] For example, the patient may state

irritants or chemicals) that stimulate the cough receptors, it is abnormal to cough. Cough is considered the "watch dog" of the lung, and a new-onset cough often signals the development of respiratory disease. A cough may be classified as acute (< 3 weeks), subacute (3 to 8 weeks), or chronic (> 8 weeks). The development of a new cough may signal development of a pulmonary problem, and a change in a chronic cough may indicate a change in a chronic lung disease or condition.[2] The respiratory care clinician should ask the patient specific questions about the onset, timing, nature, pattern, and severity of the cough. A cough may be characterized as effective or ineffective, strong or weak, and productive or nonproductive. The nature of the cough may help identify specific respiratory problems. Wheezing with cough is associated with obstruction, such as asthma. A hoarse, brassy, or barking cough is seen with upper airway or laryngeal disorders such as croup. The nature of a cough may progress from being dry to productive, and the volume of sputum produced may also vary over time. The patient should also be asked if he or she smokes or has postnasal drip, two conditions associated with a chronic cough. Cough-related symptoms and efforts to treat the cough should be assessed and sputum production and characteristics reviewed. For example, a harsh, explosive cough can cause other symptoms, such as headache and chest muscle pain.

The most common cause of an acute cough is acute respiratory tract infection. Acute bronchitis is generally caused by a viral infection, although bacterial infection, inhalation of noxious substances, or aspiration may also cause acute bronchitis. Cough in patients with acute bronchitis typically lasts for 5 days or more and may persist for several weeks.[4]

Common causes of subacute and chronic cough are postnasal drip (now referred to as the *upper airway cough syndrome*), chronic bronchitis, asthma, and gastroesophageal reflux disease (GERD).[2] Postnasal drip is a common cause of subacute or chronic cough. Causes of postnasal drip include rhinitis, sinusitis, nasopharyngitis, and the common cold, all of which may cause frequent nasal discharge, throat clearing, and cough. Sinusitis and rhinitis are often seen in asthma as comorbidities. Treatment of sinusitis may include use of saline washes, corticosteroids administered as nasal sprays, antileukotriene agents, nonsedating antihistamines, and antibiotics or antifungal agents for infection.

A chronic morning cough is common with smokers. A cough on most days for as much as 3 months of 2 consecutive years that is productive of a tablespoonful or more of sputum in the absence of other pulmonary disease is the definition chronic bronchitis. Chronic bronchitis is a form of chronic obstructive pulmonary disease (COPD) and is associated with cigarette smoking or chronic exposure to inhaled irritants, such as air pollution, industrial irritants, or chronic exposure to dust or fumes.

Asthma is a leading cause of persistent cough. The typical presentation of acute asthma includes wheezing and shortness of breath; however, in some patients cough may be the only symptom. This is known as *cough-variant asthma*.[2] Pulmonary function testing, including bronchial challenge testing, can help in making the diagnosis of asthma in patients where cough is the primary or only symptom (see Chapter 12). Improvement following treatment for asthma can help confirm asthma as the cause of the cough. A cough associated with plants, pets, dusts, or other allergens may be helped by avoidance of the allergen or irritant or use of a bronchodilator or antiinflammatory medication prior to exposure.

GERD is a very common cause of chronic cough. GERD occurs when the acidic contents of the stomach leak backwards from the stomach into the esophagus.[5] Conditions associated with gastric reflux include hiatal hernia, pregnancy, obesity, alcohol consumption, and certain medications, including sedatives, antidepressants, bronchodilators, and blood pressure medications.[5] GERD is sometimes seen in asthma as a comorbidity. Symptoms of GERD include heartburn and a sour taste in the mouth, which may worsen during the night and in the supine position, although reflux can occur without these symptoms. Treatment includes lifestyle modifications, dietary changes, and use of antacids and histamine-2 (H-2) receptor antagonists.[5] Fatty foods and other foods that cause symptoms should be avoided. Weight loss, smoking cessation, and alcohol restriction may also be helpful. Elevation of the head of the bed and avoidance of meals before bedtime may also help to alleviate symptoms.

Timing of the cough and change in the nature of the cough over time should also be assessed. Cough at night may be associated with asthma, heart failure, or GERD.[2] A cough or shortness of breath that subsides over the weekend and recurs on Monday morning with the return to work may be a sign of an occupationally related disorder. A classic example is byssinosis, which is caused by inhalation of cotton brac. Cotton workers exposed to cotton brac will develop a COPD-like syndrome and complain of shortness of breath, chest tightness, or wheezing on Monday mornings when they return to work after the weekend. A chronic morning "smoker's cough" with sputum production suggests that the patient has airway inflammation.

Cough may also be a complication of angiotensin converting enzyme (ACE) inhibitors used to treat high blood pressure and congestive heart failure (CHF). Other causes of chronic cough include neoplasm, foreign body inhalation, interstitial lung disease, and chronic pulmonary infections (including tuberculosis, fungal infections, and lung abscess). **Box 4-4** lists common causes of acute, subacute, and chronic cough.

BOX 4-4

Common Causes and Classification of Cough as Acute, Subacute, or Chronic

Acute cough: A cough that has been present for < 3 weeks.
- Acute respiratory tract infection
- Acute exacerbation of chronic lung disease
- Pneumonia
- Pulmonary embolus

Subacute cough: Cough has been present for 3 to 8 weeks.
- Postnasal drip
- Postinfectious cough
- Pertussis (whooping cough)

Chronic cough: Cough present > 8 weeks.
- Postnasal drip
- Asthma
- GERD
- ACE inhibitor medications
- Chronic bronchitis
- Bronchiectasis
- Lung cancer/neoplasm
- Foreign body aspiration
- Interstitial lung disease
- Lung abscess
- Nonasthmatic eosinophilic bronchitis
- Pertussis (whooping cough)
- Chronic idiopathic cough

GERD, gastroesophageal reflux disease; ACE, angiotensin converting enzyme.

A change in the nature of the cough may indicate a major change in the patient and should be carefully assessed. Although lung cancer is a less common cause of chronic cough, it should always be considered in current or former smokers with a new cough or change in a chronic cough. Remember, in any case, that a cough is *not* normal and its presence may indicate a problem that should be carefully assessed. Interview questions to assess a patient's cough are listed in **Table 4-2**. Items to include when describing the cough based on interview findings are found in **Table 4-3**.

Sputum Production

The term **sputum** refers to material expelled from the upper or lower airways, whereas the term *phlegm* technically refers to secretions from the lower airways (lungs and tracheobronchial tree). More than occasional sputum production should be considered abnormal.[2] Excessive sputum production is a common symptom of pulmonary disease and is generally associated with acute or chronic infection or inflammation of the respiratory mucosa. Conditions in which excessive sputum production is often seen include asthma, acute and chronic bronchitis, bronchiectasis, emphysema, pneumonia, and tuberculosis. The respiratory care clinician should question the patient regarding sputum volume, consistency, color, odor, and presence or absence of blood.[2] The clinician should also ask the patient when he or she coughs and produces sputum in a typical 24-hour period. For example, patients with chronic bronchitis generally produce the most sputum during the first hour after arising in the morning, though sputum production continues throughout the day.[6]

In additional to questioning the patient about sputum production, whenever possible the respiratory care clinician should directly observe and record the appearance and characteristics of sputum produced (see **Table 4-4**). With respect to gross examination of sputum, the following items are important for assessment.

Sputum Volume

Whenever possible, the actual volume of sputum produced should be estimated using a standard measurement system. Patients may be able to describe the volume of sputum produced in terms of a teaspoon, tablespoon, or portion of a cup (1/4, 1/2, full cup). For example, a diagnostic criterion for chronic bronchitis is the presence of a cough productive of a tablespoon or more of sputum on most days for at least 3 months of the year in at least 2 consecutive years. Vague terms to describe sputum volume, such a "scant," "moderate," and "copious," should be avoided, because these terms may mean different things to different people.

One method of monitoring sputum production is to simply place a clean graduated sample container at the bedside for a 24-hour period. The able and cooperative patient is instructed to deposit all sputum produced into the container. Frequently, the respiratory care clinician only records sputum produced following a specific treatment or procedure. The use of a 24-hour collection system such as just described will give a more complete picture of the patient's sputum production.

Color

Sputum is normally colorless or clear. Sputum color may be characterized as clear, cream, white, green, yellow-green, rust, yellow, red, and brown.[3,7] Cellular debris and white blood cells associated with inflammation or infection can affect sputum color.[3,7] Sputum purulence occurs when inflammatory cells or sloughed mucosal epithelial cells are present.[7] This can occur in the presence of either viral or bacterial infection.[7]

TABLE 4-2
Patient Interview Questions Related to the Cough

The patient should be questioned using clear and direct language. A positive patient response should be followed by specific questions to provide more detail regarding onset, nature of the cough, pattern, frequency, associated symptoms, and related items.

Onset and Nature of the Cough
1. When did your cough start?
2. Was the onset sudden or gradual?
3. Did something seem to trigger your cough?
4. How would you describe your cough?
   a. Dry?
   b. Moist or wet?
   c. Hoarse?
   d. Barking?
   e. Whooping?
   f. Bubbling?
   g. Other?
5. Has the nature of your cough changed over time?
6. Do you cough up phlegm, mucus, sputum, or bloody sputum? (See Table 4-13 for interview questions for tobacco users.)
7. Do you clear your throat a lot?

Pattern and Frequency of the Cough
1. How long have you had this cough?
2. Is the cough occasional or regular?
3. Do you usually cough first thing in the morning?
4. Do you usually cough at other times during the day or night?
5. Does your cough wake you up at night?
6. Does your cough get better or worse in certain locations?
   a. At work?
   b. At home?
   c. Outdoors?
   d. When you are near plants, birds, or pets?
   e. Other?
   If yes to any of the above, please describe.
7. Do you cough on most days as much as 3 months of the year? If so, how many years have you had this cough?
8. Does your cough seem to vary with the time of day?
9. Does your cough seem to get better or worse with certain activities, such as:
   a. Walking?
   b. Exercise?
   c. Talking?
   d. Eating or drinking?
   e. Sleeping?
   f. Lying down?
   g. In certain positions?
   h. When working on a hobby, such as woodworking? If so, please describe.
   i. Other?
10. Does your cough seem to change with changes in the weather?
11. Do you cough more on any particular day of the week? If "Yes," which day?
12. Does your cough get worse (or better) during certain times of the year?

Related Symptoms
1. Do you experience any of the following symptoms or conditions that may be related to your cough?
   a. Chest pain?
   b. Wheezing, whistling, or chest tightness?
   c. Shortness of breath?
   d. Headache?
   e. Cold or flu?
   f. Allergies?
   g. Runny nose?
   h. Fever?
   i. Hoarseness?
   j. Gagging or choking?
2. What have you done to treat your cough?
   a. Prescription cough medications?
   b. Over-the-counter (nonprescription) cough medications?
   c. Use of a vaporizer or nebulizer?

TABLE 4-2
Patient Interview Questions Related to the Cough (*continued*)

    d. Are you receiving any form of respiratory care?
       i. Oxygen therapy?
       ii. Aerosol therapy?
       iii. Chest physical therapy?
       iv. Other?
What, if anything, has helped relieve your cough?

Other Questions Related to Cough
1. Do you smoke (see Table 4-15)?
2. Do you have sinusitis, allergic rhinitis, or nasal allergies?
3. Do you have postnasal drip or a runny nose?
4. Do you have asthma?
5. Do you have COPD?
6. Do you have any other lung disease or condition?
   a. Tuberculosis?
   b. Other?
7. Do you have a heart condition or high blood pressure?
   a. If so, are you taking any medications for your heart or blood pressure, such as ACE inhibitors?
   b. What medications are you taking?
8. Do you have gastric reflux or heartburn?
   a. Do you ever have an acid or bitter taste in our mouth? If so, when?
   b. Do you use antacid medications?
9. Are you under a great deal of stress at home or work? If yes, please describe.

Sputum that is cream colored, white, or clear generally has few bacteria present.[7] Sputum that is green, yellow-green, yellow, or rust in color generally has a much higher concentration of bacteria.[7] Table 4-4 summarizes sputum appearance associated with specific conditions.

Consistency

The viscosity of sputum is partly a function of the sputum's water content. Normal sputum is thin and mucoidal. With excess secretion production, dehydration, inflammation, or infection, sputum may become colored, thick, viscous, and tenacious (sticky). It should be noted whether the sputum is tenacious (associated with dehydration), mucoidal, or purulent. Purulent sputum indicates the presence of white blood cells. The term *mucopurulent sputum* generally refers to mucus that is thicker, white, or yellow in color and sticky. With advanced cases of bronchiectasis, sputum placed in a container may settle out into three layers:

1. Top layer—cloudy
2. Middle layer—clear saliva
3. Bottom layer—cloudy and purulent

TABLE 4-3
Description of Cough and Sputum Production Based on Interview Findings

Cough onset: Sudden, gradual; duration
Nature of cough: Dry, moist, wet, hacking, hoarse, barking, whooping, bubbling, productive, nonproductive
Cough pattern: Occasional, regular, recurrent; persistent; paroxysmal (sudden, convulsive); related to time of day, weather, activities, talking, deep breaths; change over time
Cough severity: Severe enough to tire patient or disrupt sleep or conversation; causes chest pain
Sputum production: Duration, frequency, with activity, at certain times of day
- *Sputum characteristics*: Amount, color (clear, mucoid, purulent, blood tinged, mostly blood), foul odor
- *Frequency of sputum production*: Daily, mornings, days of the week, such as the first workday of the week, or associated with specific activities
- *Sputum amount or volume* (estimate in mL, teaspoons, or tablespoons)
- *Color*: Green, yellow, brown, colorless, red brick, frothy pink
- *Consistency*: Purulent, viscous, tenacious, watery, saliva
- *Other*: Blood tinged, bloody, mucous plugs
Associated symptoms: Shortness of breath, chest pain or tightness with breathing, fever, upper respiratory signs, noisy respirations, hoarseness, gagging, choking, stress
Efforts to treat: Prescription or nonprescription drugs, vaporizers, other

TABLE 4-4
Sputum Appearance

Sputum color may be characterized as clear, cream, white, green, yellow-green, rust, yellow, or red.
Sputum consistency may be thin, thick, viscous (high resistance to flow), or tenacious (sticky).
Normal sputum is colorless (clear) and thin or mucoidal.
Muciodal (clear, thin, sometimes viscid) sputum is seen in emphysema and asthma and chronic bronchitis without infection and neoplasms.
- Sputum purulence occurs when inflammatory cells or sloughed mucosal epithelial cells are present.
  - Causes of purulent sputum are infection and inflammation. Inflammation can occur from inhaled irritants, smoking, or allergy
  - Purulent sputum can occur without bacterial infection.
Green-colored sputum is generally associated with acute infection or inflammation.
- Green sputum is sometimes seen from draining sinuses.
- *Pseudomonas aeruginosa* infection has been traditionally associated with green sputum; however, yellow-green, yellow, and rust have been reported as frequently in the outpatient setting.
- Inflammation from chronic asthma can also produce discolored sputum.
White, pale yellow, or yellow purulent sputum is sometimes seen with infection, such as in pneumonia or bronchitis.
- Gram-negative bacteria are more commonly cultured from yellow sputum in the outpatient setting.
- Gram-positive bacteria are more commonly cultured from white-gray sputum in the outpatient setting
Brown or off-white brownish sputum is associated with a long-standing infection, such as chronic bronchitis.
- Cigarette smokers may produce brownish sputum.
Rust- or red-colored sputum has been associated with specific types of infection.
- A classic "currant jelly" appearance or red brick color is associated with a *Klebsiella* pneumonia infection, although yellow-green sputum may also occur with *Klebsiella*.
- Alcoholics and elderly diabetics are at risk to develop *Klebsiella* pneumonia.
- *Streptococcus* pneumonia traditionally has been associated with rust-colored sputum; however, yellow-green, yellow, or cream sputum may be more common with this bacteria.
Pulmonary edema fluid sometimes contains red blood cells.
- Frothy white or pink sputum may indicate pulmonary edema.
- Some older inhaled medications turn pink.
Blood-streaked sputum may be seen with bronchogenic carcinoma, tuberculosis, chronic bronchitis, abscess, and other conditions.
Colored sputum does not always indicate bacterial infection, contrary to common opinion.
Clear, cream, or white sputum has a lower yield of acceptable Gram stains than yellow, green, or rust-colored sputum specimens in the outpatient setting.

Data from: Johnson AL, Hampson DF, Hampson NB. Sputum color: potential implications for clinical practice. *Respir Care*. 2008;53(4):450–454; and Gardner D, Wilkins R. Cardiopulmonary symptoms. In: Wilkins RL, Dexter JR, Heuer AJ (eds.). *Clinical Assessment in Respiratory Care*, 6th ed. St. Louis, MO: Mosby-Elsevier; 2010: 28–50.

Odor

Foul-smelling (fetid) sputum is associated with long-term infections such as those found with bronchiectasis, lung abscess, cystic fibrosis, or aspiration. *Pseudomonas* has a peculiar "sweet" smell.

Change in Sputum Production

A change in sputum production may mean that the patient is getting better or worse. Increased sputum production may occur with improved airway humidification and effective bronchial hygiene therapy. Sputum production should then decrease gradually with further improvement. A sudden increase in sputum production may be associated with the rupture of an abscess or release of blocked bronchi. A sudden decrease in sputum production could be caused by airway obstruction, bronchospasm, or inadequate humidification of the inspired gases, particularly in the presence of an artificial airway. Interview questions to assess a patient's sputum production are found in **Table 4-5**.

Hemoptysis

Blood-tinged sputum is associated with a large number of pulmonary disorders. If the blood is bright red and in significant amounts, the origin is probably the lower airway and most often secondary to cancer, bronchiectasis, or tuberculosis (see following).

Curschmann's Spirals

Curschmann's spirals are mucus plugs or casts that have been coughed out and are associated with bronchial asthma. In difficult-to-control asthma, brown plugs or bronchial casts in the sputum are associated with bronchopulmonary aspergillosis, a disorder most often caused by hypersensitivity to *Aspergillus fumigatus*.[2]

Sputum Collection

Sputum Gram stain and culture should be performed in patients with hospital-acquired pneumonia and in hospitalized patients with community-acquired

TABLE 4-5
Patient Interview Questions Related to Phlegm, Sputum, or Mucus Production

The patient should be questioned using clear and direct language. A positive patient response should be followed by specific questions to provide more detail regarding onset, nature of the cough, pattern, frequency, associated symptoms, and related items.

1. Do you USUALLY bring up phlegm (sputum, mucus) from your chest first thing in the morning?   ☐ Yes ☐ No
2. Do you USUALLY bring up phlegm (sputum, mucus) from your chest at other times during the day or night?   ☐ Yes ☐ No
3. Do you bring up phlegm (sputum, mucus) from your chest on most days for as much as 3 months of the year?   ☐ Yes ☐ No
4. (If yes to #3) For how many years have you raised phlegm (sputum, mucus) from your chest?
   _____ years
5. What is the USUAL color of the phlegm (sputum, mucus) you bring up from your chest?
   - Clear
   - Cream of off-white
   - White
   - Yellow
   - Green
   - Yellow/green
   - Rust
   - Pink
   - Red
   - Brown
   - Don't know
   - Other (give details):
     _____
6. How much sputum do you raise each day?
   - Less than a teaspoon
   - About a teaspoon full
   - About a tablespoon full
   - More than a tablespoon full
   - Don't know

pneumonia.[8,9] Sputum cultures are probably not useful in otherwise healthy patients with acute bronchitis. Obtaining a satisfactory sputum specimen for Gram stain, culture, and sensitivity or cytology requires special care. Methods for obtaining a sputum specimen include the directed cough and use of ultrasonic nebulizers with sterile distilled water or hypertonic (3% to 8% NaCl) heated aerosols. The latter must be used with caution because hypertonic saline may induce bronchospasm. The high salt content of the inhaled aerosol may literally pull water out of the mucosa (osmolaric transudation) to help provide a sputum specimen. Table 4-4 provides an introduction to the interpretation of sputum production, color, consistency, and other characteristics. Table 1-4 (Chapter 1) describes common and less-common causes of acute and chronic cough and sputum production.

Hemoptysis

The term **hemoptysis** simply means coughing up blood. The most common causes of blood in the sputum are bronchitis (in the United States) and pulmonary tuberculosis (worldwide).[2] Other common causes of hemoptysis include lung cancer, pneumonia, bronchiectasis, lung abscess, pulmonary embolus/infarction, and cystic fibrosis.[10,11] The respiratory care clinician must be careful to distinguish the source of blood as pulmonary or lower respiratory tract. Other possible sources of expectorated blood include the upper airway (nose,

pharynx) and upper gastrointestinal tract (esophagus, stomach). Nasal mucosal bleeding (epistaxis, or nosebleed) and vomiting blood from the upper gastrointestinal tract (hematemesis) must be ruled out. Spitting blood without cough is associated with an upper airway source, and a careful upper airway examination should be done. Vomiting blood is associated with gastrointestinal disease, such as esophageal varices, which can result in life-threatening bleeding from the submucosal veins in the lower part of the esophagus. The development of esophageal varices is associated with portal hypertension and is commonly due to liver cirrhosis. Blood-streaked sputum is sometimes seen with pulmonary infection, such as bacterial pneumonia, chronic bronchitis, and bronchiectasis. Blood-streaked sputum is also seen with lung cancer and pulmonary embolus. Broncholithiasis is a condition in which calcified material (broncholiths) are found in the airways, and small stones or gravel mixed with blood may be found in the sputum. **Box 4-5** lists the most common causes of hemoptysis. **Table 4-6** provides a list of patient interview questions regarding hemoptysis.

Submassive and Massive Hemoptysis

Scant hemoptysis is a term sometimes used for small amounts of blood-streaked sputum (which is usually due to bronchitis). Hemoptysis may also be classified as massive ($\geq$ 500 mL of expectorated blood per 24-hour period or $\geq$ 100 mL per hour) or submassive (< 500 mL

BOX 4-5

Common Causes of Hemoptysis

Bronchitis (acute and chronic)
Bronchiectasis
Lung abscess
Tuberculosis
Pneumonia (includes necrotizing pneumonias)
Neoplasms (bronchogenic carcinoma)
Pulmonary embolism (pulmonary infarction)
Cystic fibrosis

per 24-hour period).[2,3] Submassive hemoptysis generally resolves with treatment of the underlying cause.[2] Though much less common, massive hemoptysis represents a life-threatening emergency that requires prompt action to maintain the airway, ensure adequate cardiopulmonary function, and control the bleeding. Causes of massive hemoptysis are varied and include trauma, infection, cancer, vasculitis, other pulmonary disease, hematological disease, cardiac and cardiovascular problems, certain drugs, and complications of medical or surgical procedures. Evaluation and treatment of massive hemoptysis may include diagnostic imaging (chest CT), endotracheal intubation, bronchoscopy, interventional angiography, and surgery.[2,3] **Box 4-6** lists causes of massive hemoptysis. Table 1-4 (Chapter 1) describes common and less-common causes of hemoptysis.

TABLE 4-6
Patient Interview Questions Related to Hemoptysis

1. Have you coughed up blood from your chest in the past 2 years?   ☐ Yes ☐ No
2. If yes, when, and how many times? _____
   _____

3. Please describe the amount of blood produced (teaspoon, tablespoon, cup, etc.):
   _____

4. Please describe the appearance of the blood and sputum produced: _____

5. Please describe the color of the blood and sputum produced: _____

6. Please describe the odor of the blood and sputum produced: _____
   _____

7. Would you describe your sputum or phlegm as blood-tinged?   ☐ Yes ☐ No
8. Would you describe the blood and sputum as streaky or blood-streaked?   ☐ Yes ☐ No
9. Did you see any blood clots in your sputum?   ☐ Yes ☐ No
10. Where there any associated symptoms, such as chest pain, a sensation of warmth, or a bubbling sensation?   ☐ Yes ☐ No
11. Did you seek and/or receive medical care?   ☐ Yes ☐ No
12. If yes, please describe any treatment received: _____
    _____

13. Did you have a chest x-ray or CT scan?   ☐ Yes ☐ No

BOX 4-6

Causes of Massive Hemoptysis

Trauma: Blunt or penetrating chest injury, ruptured bronchus, fat embolus, tracheal-innominate artery fistula)
Infection: Fungal lung disease, tuberculosis, necrotizing pneumonia, lung abscess, viral or parasitic infection
Cancer: Bronchogenic carcinoma, bronchial adenoma, metastatic cancer
Other pulmonary disease: Bullous emphysema, bronchiectasis, cystic fibrosis, pulmonary embolus
Hematologic disorders: Platelet and clotting disorders, use of anticoagulants
Cardiac/cardiovascular disease: Mitral stenosis, endocarditis, congenital heart disease, pulmonary hypertension, aortic aneurysm, arteriovenous malformation)
Drugs: Aspirin overdose, crack cocaine, others
Procedure related: Bronchoscopy, transtracheal aspiration, lung surgery

This article was published in *Clinics in Chest Medicine* 15(3), Cahill BC, Ingbar DH. Massive hemoptysis: assessment and management, pages 147–67, Copyright Elsevier 1994.

Whistling, Wheezing, and Chest Tightness

Patients with cardiopulmonary disease may describe wheezing, chest pain, and/or chest tightness. **Wheezing** may be described as a high-pitched, whistling sound during breathing. Recurrent wheezing, chest tightness, difficulty in breathing, or a cough that may be worse at night are associated with a diagnosis of asthma.[12,13] Asthma is characterized by airway inflammation, hyperreactive airways, and reversible airway obstruction, all of which may cause wheezing, whistling, and/or chest tightness.[12] Exposure to allergens such as animal dander, dust mites, cockroach debris, cigarette smoke, and air pollution may precipitate an asthma episode.[12] Remember, however, that all that wheezes is *not* asthma, and the many other possible causes of wheezing should be considered.

Patients should be asked about their breathing using open-ended questions. The interviewer should ask direct questions to determine any changes in the frequency, duration, or related circumstances associated with wheezing, chest tightness, shortness of breath, or cough. A change in symptoms and what factors are associated with that change should be noted. For example, exercise-induced asthma is associated with breathing cold air while exercising.[12] Occupational or environmental irritants or allergens may be isolated by a careful patient interview. Materials associated with the development of occupational asthma include red cedar wood dust and chemicals found in spray paints.[12] Some patients may experience acute shortness of breath at night, which is called paroxysmal nocturnal dyspnea (PND). PND is associated with CHF. CHF causes edema of the airways and may lead to wheezing and shortness of breath (also known as cardiac asthma).

Wheezing is a continuous, musical sound heard upon auscultation of the chest, although with severe wheezing the sound can sometimes be heard at a distance without the use of a stethoscope. Wheezing is caused by narrowing of the upper or lower airway due to obstruction, bronchospasm, tumor, or asthma. Wheezing is most commonly heard on expiration, though inspiratory wheezing is not uncommon. The most common cause of wheezing in the outpatient setting is postnasal drip.[14] Wheezing may also be caused by extrathoracic airway obstruction (such as tumor or vocal cord disorders) or intrathoracic upper airway obstruction due to such things as tracheal stenosis, airway tumors, or foreign body aspiration.[14] Stridor is associated with upper airway obstruction and requires prompt attention, because it may progress to complete airway obstruction.[14] Chest tightness is a common complaint in the early stages of an asthma attack and is associated with bronchoconstriction.[15]

Although all that wheezes is *not* asthma, episodic wheezing is a hallmark of that disease, and asthma

TABLE 4-7
Possible Causes of Wheezing

Upper Airway Obstruction: Extrathoracic
- Postnasal drip
- Croup and laryngotracheobronchitis
- Other laryngeal problems
  - Post extubation edema
  - Laryngeal stenosis
  - Vocal cord dysfunction
- Epiglottitis
- Anaphylaxis
- Retropharyngeal abscess
- Tumor

Upper Airway Obstruction: Intrathoracic
- Airway tumors
- Foreign body aspiration
- Tracheal stenosis
- Tracheal malacia

Lower Airway Obstruction
- Asthma
- Other chronic obstructive lung disease
  - COPD
  - Bronchiectasis
  - Cystic fibrosis
- Bronchiolitis
- Aspiration
  - Fluid aspiration, including gastric contents
  - Small foreign body aspiration
- Heart failure (cardiac asthma)
- Noncardiogenic pulmonary edema
- Pulmonary embolus
- Miscellaneous
  - Carcinoid syndrome
  - Lymphangitic carcinomatosis
  - Parasitic infections

should always be considered when wheezing is present. The asthma patient generally responds well to bronchodilator therapy, although improvement following bronchodilator administration can occur with other conditions. In addition to asthma, other possible lower airway causes of obstruction and wheezing include COPD, bronchiectasis, cystic fibrosis, and bronchiolitis. Aspiration (fluid or foreign body), pulmonary edema, and pulmonary embolus may also cause lower airway narrowing with wheezing. Pulmonary function testing (see Chapter 12) can be useful to differentiate between extrathoracic upper airway obstruction, intrathoracic upper airway obstruction, and lower airway obstruction.[14] Causes of wheezing are summarized **Table 4-7**.

Chest Pain

Chest pain is a common symptom in patients with a wide variety of cardiopulmonary problems, ranging from heart disease to pneumonia, pleurisy, rib fracture, pneumothorax, and tumor. Chest pain is typically not life threatening; however, it requires immediate attention because some causes of chest pain may lead to sudden death if not treated promptly. Potentially life-threatening causes of chest pain include myocardial infarction, pulmonary embolus, tension pneumothorax, aortic dissection, and esophageal rupture.[16] The patient with acute chest pain should be questioned as to the location and nature of the pain, timing, and any associated symptoms and/or risk factors. Physical assessment should follow, along with appropriate diagnostic testing such as electrocardiogram (ECG) and imaging studies.

The three basic types of chest pain a patient may describe are substernal, pleuritic, and musculoskeletal.

Substernal Chest Pain

Substernal chest pain may be caused by coronary artery disease and related cardiac ischemia, myocardial infarction, or other heart disease, such as pericarditis or heart valve disease. Substernal chest pain, shortness of breath, and diaphoresis are common cardiovascular effects of cocaine abuse.[16,17] Chest trauma, pleural disease, pulmonary embolus, aortic dissection, pneumothorax, tracheal or large airway problems, hyperventilation, and esophageal disease may also cause chest pain. Emotional problems, stress, and panic disorder are also sometimes associated with substernal chest pain.

Angina Pectoris

Patients with ischemic heart disease may exhibit a form of substernal chest pain known as angina pectoris. **Angina** is caused by reduced blood flow to the myocardium (myocardial ischemia), usually due to coronary artery disease. One type of angina, "variant angina," is caused by coronary vasospasm.

Typical angina is characterized by stable, intermittent substernal chest pain or discomfort that may be brought on by or worsen with exertion. Angina generally increases gradually over a period of several minutes, but only lasts about 5 to 10 minutes. Angina lasting longer may signal acute myocardial infarction (MI, see below). Anginal pain does not change with position or respirations. Patients may describe the sensation associated with angina as chest discomfort, tightness, or pressure. The patient may complain that it feels as if someone is "sitting on my chest." The pain may radiate down the arms or to the shoulder, neck, lower jaw, or teeth.[16] The "Levine sign" is when the patient places his or her fist in the center of the chest to indicate the location of the pain or discomfort. Angina is often accompanied by other symptoms such as shortness of breath, sweating, lightheadedness, dizziness, and fatigue. Some patients confuse angina with heartburn, and indigestion and nausea may be reported. Angina often improves with rest and administration of nitroglycerin, a coronary artery vasodilator.

Myocardial Infarction

Myocardial infarction (MI) is a major cause of death and disability worldwide. MI is defined as myocardial cell death, most commonly caused by prolonged ischemia.[18] New-onset chest pain should be considered a potential medical emergency. Unexplained severe central chest pain in at-risk patients with no known cardiac disease and lasting 2 minutes or longer may indicate a developing MI, and action should be taken accordingly. Current guidelines suggest that patients, caregivers, or family members should activate the emergency medical system (EMS) within 5 minutes of MI symptom development. Patients who may be suffering an acute MI should be given a 325-mg tablet of aspirin to chew. Patients with ongoing symptoms who may be unstable based on history, associated risk factors, and physical examination should be immediately transported via ambulance to a hospital emergency department.[16] A defibrillator should be available and oxygen therapy and venous access established. Pain due to myocardial ischemia may be treated by administration of sublingual nitroglycerin unless contraindicated due to low blood pressure or recent ingestion or administration of a vasodilator (such as Viagra).[16] It should also be recognized that some MIs are "silent," having no clinical symptoms; these occur most often in elderly patients or patients with diabetes.

Acute MI is confirmed by elevated cardiac biomarker laboratory studies indicating myocardial tissue damage (troponin or creatine kinase [CK-MB]) and development of ECG changes associated with MI (Q-wave development and/or ST-segment elevation or depression). Imaging studies may confirm loss of functional heart tissue. Treatment of ST-elevation myocardial infarction includes medical care and rapid transport to a facility where reperfusion therapy via percutaneous coronary intervention (PCI) using coronary artery balloon angiography can be accomplished rapidly and safely.[19] Early use of thrombolytic therapy is the treatment of choice when PCI is not readily available.

Pleuritic Chest Pain

Pleuritic chest pain is often described as a sharp, knifelike localized pain, often at the periphery of the chest. Pleuritic pain changes with breathing motion and coughing. Common causes of pleuritic chest pain include pleurisy, pneumonia, pulmonary embolus, pleuropericarditis, and pneumothorax.

Musculoskeletal Chest Pain

Musculoskeletal chest pain may be caused by rib fractures, chest trauma or bruising, thoracic or cardiac surgery, and sprain or injury to the muscles of the chest. Musculoskeletal pain often varies as the patient breathes and moves about and may persist from a few hours to weeks. Musculoskeletal chest pain may improve with the administration of nonsteroidal anti-inflammatory drugs (NSAIDs). Other causes of chest wall pain include costochondritis, stenoclavicular arthritis, and cervical disc disease. Chest radiographs or CT scan may help separate the cause of pleurtic pain from musculoskeletal chest pain.

Onset, Duration, and Timing of Chest Pain

The onset, duration, and timing of chest pain and whether the pain is associated with trauma, coughing, movement, or lower respiratory infection should be noted. For example, sudden onset of pain is common with pneumothorax, aortic dissection, or acute pulmonary emboli.[16] Cardiac ischemic pain generally begins more gradually.[16] Chest pain associated with exertion is common with ischemic cardiac disease and may improve when activity is stopped.[16] Musculoskeletal pain may have a less-well-defined onset.[16] The patient should also be questioned as to what, if anything, makes the pain better or worse. For example, esophageal pain may worsen with swallowing and improve following ingestion of antacids.[16] Pain that worsens with movement or upon palpation is often musculoskeletal in origin.[16] Pleuritic chest pain also may worsen when breathing and when lying down.[16]

Associated symptoms such as shallow breathing, fever, uneven chest expansion, coughing, anxiety about getting air, or radiation of the pain to the neck or arms should also be noted during the patient interview. Efforts to treat chest pain with heat, splinting, or pain medication should be noted.

Dyspnea

Shortness of breath is often the chief complaint in patients with cardiopulmonary disorders. It affects up to 25% of all patients seen in the ambulatory care setting and up to 50% of all patients seen in the hospital.[15,20] **Dyspnea** may be defined as the conscious sensation (as experienced by the patient) of being short of breath. This subjective experience of breathing discomfort is thought to be derived from the interaction of various physiological, psychological, social, and environmental factors.[15,20] The underlying cause of dyspnea may be pulmonary, cardiac, hematologic, neurologic, psychogenic, metabolic, or mechanical.[15,20]

Patients may describe the experience of dyspnea as an increased work of breathing, chest tightness, or the sensation of not getting enough air ("air hunger"). Patients may say "I feel short of breath," "I'm having difficulty breathing," or "I can't catch my breath."[15,20] Patients with air hunger may complain that they are starved for air, have feelings of suffocation, or that they cannot get a deep enough breath.[15,20] Dyspnea may be described as acute or chronic, intermittent or continuous, and progressive or stable. Dyspnea may be a new symptom for which a cause has not yet been identified, or it may be associated with known respiratory, neuromuscular, or cardiovascular disease.[15,20] In any case, dyspnea is a serious finding, and patients with severe dyspnea are at much greater risk of mortality.[15,20]

The actual physiologic mechanisms involved in the generation of the sensation of dyspnea are complex and may be similar to those experienced when exercising other skeletal muscle groups.[15,20] The causes of dyspnea, however, can be generally described as being due to an increased respiratory drive (increased ventilatory demand) and/or impaired ventilatory mechanics (decreased ventilatory capacity or increased work of breathing).[15,20] Causes of an increased respiratory drive include hypoxemia, hypercapnea, and acidosis. Hypoxemia and hypercapnea may be caused by a wide variety of disorders that may lead to respiratory failure (see Box 2-1, Chapter 2). Disease states or conditions that may decrease oxygen delivery to the tissues may also cause dyspnea. These include cardiac disease, anemia, carbon monoxide poisoning, and disorders of the hemoglobin. Metabolic acidosis may be caused by such things as diabetic ketoacidosis (as seen in a diabetic crisis); acute severe hypoxia leading to lactic acidosis; diarrhea; and renal failure. Acute respiratory acidosis is simply caused by elevations in arterial $Paco_2$ due to hypoventilation and a corresponding drop in arterial pH (see Chapter 8). Respiratory drive may also be elevated by neurologic disease, cardiac disease, metabolic disorders, and psychogenic factors, such as pain and anxiety.

Disease states that may impair ventilatory mechanics (decreased ventilatory capacity) include conditions that affect ventilatory muscle strength and conditions that decrease lung or chest wall compliance. Obstructive lung disease (e.g., asthma and COPD) may impair ventilatory mechanics by increasing the resistive work of breathing (due to bronchospasm or mucosal edema) or increasing the elastic work of breathing (due to lung hyperinflation). The major contributing factors to the dyspnea experienced by COPD patients are the combination of increased ventilatory demand and reduced respiratory muscle function.[15,20] A patient's emotional state and psychological makeup may also impact the perception of dyspnea, and anxiety, panic attacks, and psychogenic hyperventilation may cause dyspnea. In general, reductions in the ability to ventilate or sustain the desired level of ventilation result in increasing dyspnea. **Table 4-8** lists causes of dyspnea grouped by physiologic mechanism.

The most common clinical causes of dyspnea are asthma, COPD, interstitial lung disease, heart disease, and obesity with deconditioning (**Box 4-7**).[20] In assessing the specific cause of dyspnea in an individual patient, the respiratory care clinician should consider the pace with which dyspnea began, the characteristics

TABLE 4-8
Causes of Dyspnea

Causes of dyspnea may be grouped into two broad categories:
1. Increased Ventilatory Workload
   a. Increased drive to breathe
      - Hypoxemia (e.g., $\downarrow \dot{V}/\dot{Q}$, $\uparrow$ shunt, $\downarrow Ca_{O_2}$, $\downarrow D_{O_2}$)
      - Hypercapnia
      - Acidosis (e.g., diabetic ketosis, renal failure)
      - Lung disease (e.g., "J" receptor stimulation, hypoxemia)
      - Heart disease (e.g., decreased cardiac output, congestive heart failure, MI)
      - Neurologic disease (e.g., head trauma, stroke, cerebral vascular accident [CVA], brain tumor)
      - Pain
      - Anxiety
   b. Decreased system compliance
      - Decreased lung compliance
      - Decreased thoracic (chest wall) compliance
   c. Increased resistance
      - Increased airway resistance (e.g. bronchospasm, mucosal edema, secretions)
      - Airway obstruction (e.g., laryngeal edema, foreign body obstruction)
      - Artificial airways (e.g., endotracheal or tracheostomy tube)
   d. Exercise or increased level of activity
      - Normal exertional dyspnea with vigorous exercise
      - Dyspnea with increasing levels of activity in patients with heart disease, lung disease, or poor physical conditioning (e.g., obesity, poor physical fitness)
2. Decreased Ventilatory Capacity
   a. Neuromuscular disease
   b. Ventilatory muscle weakness or fatigue
   c. Spinal cord injury
   d. Diaphragmatic dysfunction
   e. Poor conditioning
   f. Obesity
   g. Pregnancy
   h. Abdominal distension, ascites
   i. Partial or complete airway obstruction

Data from: Parshall MB, Schwartzstein RM, Adams L, et al. An official american thoracic society statement: update on the mechanisms, assessment, and management of dyspnea. *Am J Respir Crit Care Med.* 2012;185(4):435–452. Available at: http://www.thoracic.org/statements/resources/respiratory-disease-adults/update-on-mamd.pdf

BOX 4-7

Common Causes of Dyspnea

Acute asthma
COPD exacerbation (includes chronic bronchitis and emphysema)
Interstitial lung disease
Myocardial dysfunction
Obesity
Deconditioning

or qualities of the dyspnea, the presence of any accompanying symptoms, triggers of the dyspnea, the duration and character of the dyspnea, and any maneuvers that relieve or reduce it. For example, dyspnea may occur only with exertion. In the absence of specific cardiopulmonary disease, this may suggest poor cardiovascular fitness or obesity/deconditioning as the cause. Dyspnea at rest or on simply standing upright is more severe and may indicate a more serious condition. The sudden development of dyspnea in an otherwise healthy patient generally signals an acute problem, whereas chronic dyspnea is seen with chronic lung disease and may progressively worsen over months or years.

The patient's description of the character or nature of his or her dyspnea may be useful in identifying the underlying cause. For example, the sensation of increased breathing effort or work is associated airway obstruction, neuromuscular disease, and reduced lung or chest wall compliance. Air hunger is associated with an increased drive to breathe as may occur with acute severe hypoxia or acidosis. The sensation of inability to get a deep enough breath may be seen in patients with restrictive lung disease, such as pulmonary fibrosis, or in cases of dynamic lung hyperinflation, as seen in COPD or acute asthma. Chest tightness or constriction is associated with bronchospasm or interstitial edema. The sensation of suffocation or smothering is associated with acute pulmonary edema, as well as other conditions.

Dyspnea may be positional, occurring only when the patient is lying down (orthopnea). Orthopnea is common with patients with severe COPD or CHF. PND is sometimes seen in patients with CHF and is associated with sleeping in the recumbent position. Trepopnea refers to dyspnea associated with lying on one side and may be caused by unilateral lung or chest disease, such as unilateral pleural effusion or rib fractures. Platypnea is a less common form of dyspnea in which the patient becomes more short of breath in the upright position (the opposite of orthopnea), but improves when lying down. Platypnea is caused by conditions in which oxygenation gets worse in the upright position and improves when lying down (orthodeoxia). Clinical causes of platypnea include liver disease affecting the pulmonary vasculature and right-to-left cardiac shunting that worsens in the upright position.

By asking the patient questions that focus on the character, pace, duration, triggers, and relievers of dyspnea, the clinician is often able to clarify the likely cause. Physical examination, laboratory studies, and imaging may then help further identify the cause of the patient's shortness of breath. For example, the chest x-ray may identify pulmonary disease, such as pneumonia or interstitial lung disease. Arterial blood gas studies may show hypoxemia, hypercapnea, and/or acidosis. Laboratory testing may identify anemia as the cause of a reduction in oxygen content of the blood.

D-dimer laboratory screening may help rule out pulmonary embolus as the cause of dyspnea. D-dimer is a substance present in blood after blood-clot breakdown. This laboratory study is most useful in the assessment of ambulatory patients in the outpatient setting because many conditions associated with hospitalization will increase D-dimer values. In the acute care setting, B-type natriuretic peptide (BNP) or N-terminal prohormone precursor (NTproBNP) laboratory measurement may help in evaluating the patient with acute dyspnea due to heart failure. BNP is an amino acid associated with overstretch of the heart. Cardiopulmonary exercise testing can be especially useful in separating chronic problems that are primarily pulmonary or cardiac in origin or due to deconditioning.

Quantification of Dyspnea

It is very helpful to quantify the degree of dyspnea a patient suffers. Although dyspnea is a subjective experience that does not necessarily correlate with the patient's physical appearance, one objective way to quantify the dyspnea is to ask the patient about activity and any resulting breathlessness, as described in **Table 4-9**. Shortness of breath only upon extreme exertion would be described as appropriate dyspnea, whereas dyspnea at rest would be classified as very

BOX 4-8

Modified Medical Research Council (MMRC) Dyspnea Scale

The MMRC uses a simple grading scale to assess dyspnea:

Grade	Description of Breathlessness
0	I only get breathless with strenuous exercise.
1	I get short of breath when hurrying on level ground or walking up a slight hill.
2	On level ground, I walk slower than people of the same age because of breathlessness, or have to stop for breath when walking at my own pace.
3	I stop for breath after walking about 100 yards or after a few minutes on level ground.
4	I am too breathless to leave the house or I am breathless when dressing.

Reproduced from British Medical Journal, Fletcher CM, Elmes PC, Fairbairn MB, et al., 2, pp. 257–266, Copyright (c) 1959 with permission from BMJ Publishing Group Ltd.

TABLE 4-9
Severity of Dyspnea *The severity of a patient's dyspnea can be estimated by the associated level of activity at which the patient becomes short of breath. Dyspnea may then be characterized as follows:*

Level	Description
Appropriate	Dyspnea occurs only with severe exertion or heavy exercise (e.g., vigorous aerobic exercise)
Mild	The patient can keep pace with someone of the same age and build on a level surface; however, not on stairs or inclined surfaces, such as hills or ramps
Moderate	The patient can walk a mile at his or her own pace without becoming short of breath; however he or she cannot keep pace with a normal person on a level surface
Severe	The patient becomes short of breath after walking only about 100 yards on a level surface or when climbing only 1 flight of stairs
Very Severe	The patient is short of breath at rest or with minimal activity

Data from: Committee on Rating of Mental and Physical Impairment: guides to the evaluation of permanent impairment—the respiratory system. *JAMA.* 1965;194:919–932.

severe. The Modified Medical Research Council Dyspnea Scale (MMRC; see **Box 4-8**) provides a similar scale to grade the severity of a patient's dyspnea based on a scale of 0 to 4, where 0 is shortness of breath only on extreme exertion and a score of 4 is dyspnea so severe that the patient is unable to leave the house. The MMRC can be used with other measures to calculate the BODE index, where B is body mass index (BMI), O is obstruction (as assessed by FEV_1), D is dyspnea (via the MMRC), and E is exercise (as assessed by the 6-minute walk). The BODE index may be useful in predicting hospitalization and mortality in COPD patients, where a score of 0 is very good and a maximum score of 7 to 10 is associated with an increased risk of hospitalization and death (see **Box 4-9**).[21,22]

The modified **Borg scale** (see **Box 4-10**) provides a more subjective method of rating a patient's dyspnea. To use the Borg scale, the patient is asked to describe his or her sensation of being short of breath using a scale of 0 to 10 where "none" receives a score of 0 and "maximal" is scored a 10. The visual analog scale (VAS) provides a similar subjective method of assessing the severity of dyspnea. With the VAS, dyspnea is reported as the number of millimeters marked by the patient to the right of "no shortness of breath" on the scale provided (see **Figure 4-1**). The scale range is 0 cm (no shortness of breath) to 10 cm (maximum shortness of breath).

BOX 4-9

The BODE Index

The BODE* scale range is from 0 to a maximum of 10 points, where a 10 indicates an increased risk of hospitalization and mortality.

Variable	Points			
	0	1	2	3
FEV_1 (% predicted)	≥ 65	50–64	36–49	≤ 35
6-minute walk test (meters)	≥ 350	250–349	150–249	≤ 149
MMRC dyspnea scale	0–1	2	3	4
BMI	> 21	≤ 21	—	—

*B, body mass index (BMI); O, obstruction as assessed by FEV_1% predicted; D, dyspnea using the MMRC dyspnea scale; E, exercise as assessed by distance walked using the 6-minute walk test.
Data from: Celli BR, Cote CG, Lareau SC, Meek PM. Predictors of survival in COPD: more than just the FEV_1. *Respir Med.* 2008;102(Suppl 1):S27–S35; Celli BR, Cote CG, Marin JM, et al. The body-mass index, airflow obstruction, dyspnea, and exercise capacity index in chronic obstructive pulmonary disease. *N Engl J Med.* 2004;350(10):1005–1012.

BOX 4-10

The Modified Borg Scale for Evaluation of Dyspnea

Patient instructions: Please rate your shortness of breath using a scale of 0 to 10, where 0 means you have no shortness of breath and 10 means your shortness of breath is maximal.

Rating	Sensation of Shortness of Breath
0	Nothing at all
0.5	Very, very slight (just noticeable)
1	Very slight
2	Slight breathlessness
3	Moderate
4	Somewhat severe
5	Severe breathlessness
6	
7	Very severe breathlessness
8	
9	Very, very severe (almost maximum)
10	Maximal

The patient is instructed to indicate how much shortness of breath he or she is experiencing by marking the line. If the patient is experiencing no shortness of breath, he or she is instructed to circle the marker at the left end of the line. The line is constructed 100 mm in length, and the VAS score is recorded as the number of millimeters marked by the patient to the left of "no shortness of breath." The scale range is from 0 mm (no shortness of breath) to 100 mm (extremely breathless).

No shortness   Maximum shortness
  of breath   of breath

FIGURE 4-1 The visual analog scale (VAS).

Data from: Meek PM, Lareau SC. Critical outcomes in pulmonary rehabilitation: assessment and evaluation of dyspnea and fatigue. *J Rehab Res Develop.* 2003;40(5):13–24 and College of Nursing, University of New Mexico, Albuquerque, NM; New Mexico Veterans Affairs Health Care System, Albuquerque, NM.

The University of California, San Diego (UCSD) Shortness of Breath Questionnaire (SOBQ) is a newer system for quantifying dyspnea (**Table 4-10**). The SOBQ questionnaire has the patient rate his or her shortness of breath on 24 different items related to activities of daily living (ADLs) such as walking, eating, dressing, and shopping. The resultant scores are summed, and possible scores range from 0 (no shortness of breath) to 120 (extreme dyspnea). Factors to be considered when evaluating a patient's shortness of breath are summarized in **Box 4-11**.

Treatment of Dyspnea

The treatment of dyspnea should be aimed at the underlying cause. For example, dyspnea caused by asthma-associated bronchospasm and mucosal edema may be relieved by administering inhaled bronchodilators and the use of corticosteroids as anti-inflammatory agents. Dyspnea due to heart failure may improve with the administration of diuretics (to get rid of excess fluid by increasing urine output) and drugs to reduce cardiac afterload.[15,20] Dyspnea due to hypoxemia with increased respiratory demand may benefit from oxygen therapy. Because dyspnea is usually caused by an increase in the work of breathing, support with noninvasive or invasive

TABLE 4-10

The University of California, San Diego (UCSD) Medical Center Pulmonary Rehabilitation Program Shortness-of-Breath Questionnaire (SOBQ)

Instructions: For each activity listed below, please rate your breathlessness on a scale **between zero (0) and five (5), where 0 is not at all breathless and 5 is maximally breathless or too breathless to do the activity**. If the activity is one which you do not perform, please give your best estimate of breathlessness. Your responses should be for an "average" day during the past week. Please respond to all items.

How short of breath do you get?

1. At rest	0	1	2	3	4	5
2. Walking on a level at your own pace	0	1	2	3	4	5
3. Walking on a level with others your age	0	1	2	3	4	5
4. Walking up a hill	0	1	2	3	4	5
5. Walking up stairs	0	1	2	3	4	5
6. While eating	0	1	2	3	4	5
7. Standing up from a chair	0	1	2	3	4	5
8. Brushing teeth	0	1	2	3	4	5
9. Shaving and/or brushing hair	0	1	2	3	4	5
10. Showering/bathing	0	1	2	3	4	5
11. Dressing	0	1	2	3	4	5
12. Picking up and straightening	0	1	2	3	4	5
13. Doing dishes	0	1	2	3	4	5
14. Sweeping/vacuuming	0	1	2	3	4	5
15. Making bed	0	1	2	3	4	5
16. Shopping	0	1	2	3	4	5
17. Doing laundry	0	1	2	3	4	5
18. Washing car	0	1	2	3	4	5
19. Mowing lawn	0	1	2	3	4	5
20. Watering lawn	0	1	2	3	4	5
21. Sexual activities	0	1	2	3	4	5

How much do these limit you in your daily life?

22. Shortness of breath	0	1	2	3	4	5
23. Fear of "hurting myself" by overexerting	0	1	2	3	4	5
24. Fear of shortness of breath	0	1	2	3	4	5

To score the SOBQ, sum the responses for all 24 items. Total score range is from 0 to 120 points.

Modified with permission from the American College of Chest Physicians: G. Eakin, EG, Resnikoff PM, Prewitt LM, Ries AL, Kaplan RM. Validation of a new dyspnea measure: The UCSD Shortness of Breath Questionnaire. *Chest.* 1998;113;619–624.

BOX 4-11

Factors to Be Considered When Taking a Patient History for Evaluating Dyspnea

1. Onset and duration: Sudden or gradual; persistence; gagging or choking event few days before onset
2. Pattern
   a. Position most comfortable, number of pillows used
   b. Related to extent of exercise, certain activities, time of day, eating
   c. Harder to inhale or exhale
3. Severity: Tiring or fatigue with breathing, anxiety about getting air
   a. Level of activity associated with dyspnea (severe exertion, exercise, stairs, walking, at rest)
   b. Extent of activity limitation
4. Associated symptoms: Pain or discomfort (relationship to specific point in respiratory exertion, location), cough, diaphoresis, swelling of ankles

mechanical ventilation may be necessary while the underlying cause is being treated.

Pulmonary rehabilitation and exercise training should be considered for patients with reduced functional capacity and long-standing dyspnea due to chronic lung disease.[15] Pulmonary rehabilitation interventions are aimed at reducing ventilatory demand and/or reducing ventilatory workload. Techniques to reduce ventilatory demand include exercise training, oxygen therapy, nutritional assessment and intervention, and inspiratory muscle training. Ventilatory workload may be reduced by administration of bronchodilators and anti-inflammatory agents. Lung volume-reduction surgery may be helpful to treat lung hyperinflation and air trapping in certain patients with severe emphysema.

Although treatment of the cause of dyspnea is the best approach, it is sometimes not possible to identify the cause, and dyspnea may persist despite optimal treatment. Opioid medications, such as morphine, reduce dyspnea for the short term and should be considered in the palliative care of severe dyspnea that does not respond to other treatment. Opioid drugs may depress ventilation, though this is unlikely with appropriate dosing. Table 1-4 (Chapter 1) lists more common and less common causes of dyspnea to consider in the differential diagnosis of acute and chronic dyspnea.

Sleep Disorders

The most common sleep disorders are insomnia, sleep deprivation, excessive daytime sleepiness, circadian rhythm disorders, restless legs syndrome, and sleep-related breathing disorders (see **Box 4-12**). Difficulty falling asleep (insomnia) or difficulty staying awake in the daytime affects up to 40% of the adult population in the United States.[23] Sleep disorders can cause memory problems, slowed responses, and emotional problems. Drowsiness or falling asleep while driving or operating machinery can be a cause of serious accidents.

BOX 4-12

Common Sleep Disorders

Insomnia: Difficulty getting to sleep, maintaining sleep, or poor quality sleep.

Sleep-related breathing disorders: Abnormal breathing during sleep that includes obstructive sleep apnea (OSA) and central sleep apnea.

Hypersomnias of central origin: CNS-mediated excessive daytime sleepiness.

- *Narcolepsy*: A CNS disorder characterized by excessive sleepiness and frequent daytime sleep "attacks."
- *Idiopathic hypersomnia*: Sleeping too much without an obvious cause.
- *Sleep deprivation*: Leads to excessive sleepiness.

Circadian rhythm sleep disorders: Sleep disturbances caused by misalignment between the subjects' sleep cycle and the environment due to such factors as jet lag due to travel across time zones and rotating shift work.

Parasomnias: Movements, behaviors, or experiences while asleep, including sleep walking, night terrors, sleep paralysis, or sleep-related hallucination.

Sleep-related movement disorders: Movements during sleep such as restless legs syndrome, periodic limb movements, and teeth grinding.

Isolated symptoms and normal variants: These are normal sleep variations and include sleep starts and talking in one's sleep.

Other sleep disorders: Includes sleep disorders due to environmental noise, a restless sleep partner, or other environmental discomfort.

Data from: Iber C, Ancoli-Israel S, Chesson AL, et al. *The AASM Manual for the Scoring of Sleep and Associated Events*. West Chester, IL: American Academy of Sleep Medicine; 2007.

As a part of a complete patient history, patients should be questioned regarding any unusual factors or difficulties related to their sleep. The simple question "Are you getting enough sleep?" is a good way to begin to investigate whether the patient is experiencing sleep-related problems. Patients may also be questioned as to whether they experience excessive daytime sleepiness (drowsiness) or fall asleep during normal daily activities such as reading, watching television, sitting, or driving, or if they struggle to stay awake during the day.

Sleep-related breathing disorders include obstructive sleep apnea, central sleep apnea, and sleep-associated hypoventilation/hypoxemia. Obstructive sleep apnea occurs when there is an absence or near absence of airflow due to airway obstruction accompanied by ventilatory efforts to breathe. Less common is central sleep apnea, which occurs when both airflow and ventilatory efforts are absent. **Box 4-13** describes the various types of sleep-related breathing disorders.

Snoring is caused by the movement of air across a partially obstructed upper airway. Complaints regarding snoring should alert the respiratory care clinician of the possibility of the presence of obstructive sleep apnea. Patients should be asked if they snore, and if so, how often. Snoring that disturbs the patient's bed partner tends to be very loud and correlates with the severity of partial airway obstruction. The patient should also be questioned as to whether anyone has ever noticed that he or she quits breathing during sleep (sleep apnea). Snoring followed by complete airway obstruction with resultant apnea that lasts for more than 10 seconds is a hallmark of obstructive sleep apnea. Similar to apnea, hypopnea occurs when a reduction in airflow causes a corresponding decrease in oxygen saturation. The apnea–hypopnea index (AHI) is the average number of apnea/hypopnea events per hour of sleep. An AHI of five or greater is diagnostic of sleep apnea syndrome in patients with signs or symptoms of disturbed sleep.[24]

Gastroesophageal reflux is a common complaint and is often most troublesome at night, when the patient is in the supine position. "Silent aspiration" occurs during sleep in normal subjects, and this may be exacerbated with stroke, depressed central nervous system (CNS) function, or ingestion of sedatives, narcotics or alcohol.[25] Aspiration during sleep may introduce bacteria or other microorganisms into the respiratory tract and may lead to pneumonia in at-risk patients.

PND may cause sleep problems due to left-sided CHF and the resultant increase in pulmonary vascular fluid and congestion in the recumbent position. Typically with PND, the patient awakens due to discomfort after 1 to 2 hours of sleep, sits up in bed or a chair, and finds some relief in the upright position. PND is caused by the reabsorption of fluid during sleep and can occur from 1 to 6 hours after retiring at night, depending on the amount of edema.

Mukerji,[26] Chapter 15, describes sleep studies to evaluate the various forms of sleep disordered breathing.

Past Medical History

The past medical history should provide an overview of the patient's general state of health, past illnesses (childhood and adult), past accidents or injuries, past surgical procedures and operations (if any), and any previous hospitalizations. Immunizations, allergies, medications, and the results of recent health screening tests should be reviewed. The past medical history should also provide a history of any cardiopulmonary disease (pulmonary disease or cardiac problems), cancer, or other major disease the patient may have experienced. A history of exposure to respiratory infections (e.g., tuberculosis, influenza) or other related environmental exposures (e.g., dust, fumes, spores) should be noted. A childhood history of early-life injury to the airways such as pneumonia, parental smoking, or bronchopulmonary dysplasia (a lung disease associated with premature birth) have all been implicated in the development of asthma.[13] Past cardiopulmonary testing and results, as well as imaging studies and laboratory test results, should be included, if available.

BOX 4-13

Sleep-Related Breathing Disorders

Obstructive sleep apnea: Periods of apnea due to airway obstruction.

Central sleep apnea: Periods of apnea without respiratory efforts and due to

- CNS disorder
- Medical condition
- Drugs or medications
- Infant sleep apnea

Hypoventilation and hypoxemia associated with sleep:

- Alveolar hypoventilation due to an unknown cause (idiopathic alveolar hypoventilation)
- Congenital hypoventilation syndrome
- Hypoventilation and hypoxemia due to heart or lung disease or other medical condition

Data from: Iber C, Ancoli-Israel S, Chesson AL, et al. *The AASM Manual for the Scoring of Sleep and Associated Events*. West Chester, IL: American Academy of Sleep Medicine; 2007.

The extent of the past medical history is determined, in part, by the nature of the illness, the patient's age, and his or her health history. For example, the past medical history for a 70-year-old COPD patient with comorbid diabetes and CHF will greatly exceed that of an otherwise healthy 22-year-old college student with acute bronchitis. Information that should be included in the general past medical history is summarized in **Box 4-14**.

BOX 4-14

Patient History

Items to review in the patient history include:

Chief Complaint (CC)

- Breathlessness
- Cough
- Sputum production

- Hemoptysis
- Wheezing
- Chest tightness

History of the Present Illness (HPI)

- Nature of complaint
- Onset
- Duration
- Frequency

- Severity
- Location
- Progression
- Treatment

Past Medical History (PMH)

- *Childhood respiratory and cardiac disease*
  - Neonatal or infant respiratory disease (e.g., respiratory distress syndrome [RDS] of the neonate, meconium aspiration, bronchopulmonary dysplasia [BPD])
  - Congenital cardiac/cardiovascular disease (e.g., aortic valve stenosis, pulmonary valve stenosis, atrial septal defect, ventricular septal defect, patent ductus arteriosis, tetralogy of Fallot, coarctation of the aorta)
  - Pediatric respiratory disease (e.g., asthma, cystic fibrosis, bronchiolitis, pneumonia, croup, epiglottitis, pertussis ["whooping cough"], respiratory syncytial virus [RSV])
- *Other childhood illnesses* (e.g., polio, infectious disease [measles, mumps, rubella, chickenpox, rheumatic fever, scarlet fever, diphtheria], childhood aspiration
- *Adult respiratory disease* (e.g., pneumonia, tuberculosis, asthma, bronchitis, emphysema, COPD, bronchiectasis, upper respiratory tract infection, influenza, pulmonary embolus)
- *Adult heart disease* (e.g., congestive heart failure [CHF], angina, myocardial infarction [MI], cor pulmonale)
- *Adult infectious disease* (e.g., hepatitis, rheumatic fever, HIV/AIDS)
- *Adult chronic illness* (e.g., diabetes; high blood pressure; neuromuscular disease)
- *Other adult disease* (e.g., cancer, leukemia, stroke, kidney disease, liver disease, anemia, obesity)
- *Immunizations*—polio; diphtheria; pertussis (Td/Tdap); tetanus; influenza; hepatitis A, hepatitis B; measles, mumps, rubella (MMR); varicella, herpes zoster; pneumococcus, meningococcus, human papillomavirus; travel-related immunizations (typhoid, cholera, yellow fever)
- *Allergies*—drugs, medications, foods, other substances
- *Medications*—dose, frequency, duration; home remedies or nonprescription medications
- *Recent health screening tests and results*—cholesterol, glucose, C-reactive protein (CRP), Pap smear, colonoscopy, prostate specific antigen (PSA), mammogram, pulmonary health screens, PPD or other skin tests (tuberculosis, fungal, sensitivity to diphtheria antitoxin)
- *Laboratory testing*—hematology, blood chemistry, microbiology, urinalysis, spinal fluid, pleural fluid, sputum, cardiac enzymes
- *Imaging studies*—chest X-ray, CT, MRI, ultrasound
- *Cardiopulmonary diagnostics*—pulmonary function testing, ECG, stress testing
- *Accidents and injuries*—thoracic trauma, broken bones, head trauma, other
- *Hospitalizations*—dates, hospital, diagnosis, procedures

(*continued*)
- *Operations (surgery)*—dates, hospital, diagnosis, procedure, complications
- *Pregnancy*—to include any complications
- *Respiratory care received*—oxygen, history of intubation, history of mechanical ventilation, use of metered dose inhalers (MDI) or aerosolized medication, other
- *Psychiatric illnesses or mood disorders*—anxiety, depression, other
- *Limitations to function or disabilities*—ability to perform activities of daily living (ADLs)
- *Names of physicians or other healthcare providers*

Social History

- Birthplace
- Place of residence
- Housing
- Education
- Marital status

- Smoking
- Alcohol use
- Sexual activity
- Geographic exposure
- Social support

Family History (FH)

- Relatives and their ages (spouse, parents, children)
- Relatives' causes of death and age at death
- Family diseases (e.g., heart disease, lung disease, cancer, genetic disease)
- Family support

Occupational History (OH)

- Occupation
- Work environment
- Hours worked
- Work history

- Exposure to chemicals, dust, fumes
- Protective devices worn at work
- Military record (dates and location of assignment)

Miscellaneous

- Primary care provider
- Access to care (insurance coverage, ability to pay)
- Transportation needs

Data from: Seidel HM, Ball. JW, Dains, JE, Flynn JA, Solomon BS, Stewart RW. Partnership with patients: building a history. In: *Mosby's Guide to Physical Examination*, 7th ed. St. Louis, MO: Mosby Elsevier; 2011:1–31.

When taking the patient's past medical history, the interviewer should assess the patient's ability to accurately answer specific questions. Family members may provide reliable information if the patient is unconscious, confused, disoriented, or experiencing cognitive deficits. Past medical information on file may also be helpful. Language barriers, hearing impairment, and speech problems can also affect communications. Cultural differences may impact the patient's health history in a variety of ways. For example, beliefs and practices regarding food and nutrition, use of alternative medicines, spiritual practices, and attitudes toward mental illness may be influenced by cultural values. Attitudes and values regarding medical care may be influenced by culture, and disparities in access to healthcare services exist across different racial, ethnic, social, and economic groups. **Figure 4-2** provides a list of interview questions for a general past medical history.

A past history of chest illness can be useful in assessing a patient's current cardiopulmonary status (see **Table 4-11**). The patient should be questioned as to the frequency of chest colds, bronchitis, or pneumonia. The patient should also be asked if he or she has ever been told that he or she has any type of heart or lung disease. In the case of preexisting cardiopulmonary disease, age of onset, diagnosis, and progression over time (better or worse) should be ascertained, as well the effectiveness of treatment and current management of the condition. Respiratory care–related medications that the patient may currently be taking or has taken in the past for breathing should be noted. As noted earlier, exposure to tuberculosis (TB) or influenza should be recorded. Ancillary information regarding the patient's occupation, hobbies, and leisure activities may be helpful in pointing to a specific pulmonary problem.

Careful attention should be given to a history of emergency care or unscheduled treatment or

PATIENT INFORMATION

Name: _____   Home Phone: _____

Address: _____   Daytime Phone: _____

_____

Date of Birth: _____   E-mail Address: _____

Sex: ☐ Male   ☐ Female   Religion: _____

Marital Status: ☐ Single   ☐ Married   ☐ Widowed   ☐ Civil Union   ☐ Domestic Partnership

Spouse's Name: _____

Emergency contact information: _____

_____

Education: ☐ High School/GED   ☐ Some College   ☐ Undergrad   ☐ Post-grad/Doctorate   ☐ Other

Employer: _____

Occupation: _____

Habits (smoking, other tobacco use, alcohol use, coffee/tea; diet, exercise, sleep): _____

_____

Current medications: _____

_____

Allergies:

Are you allergic to:

Penicillin?	☐ Yes	☐ No
Sulfa drugs?	☐ Yes	☐ No
Tetanus antitoxin?	☐ Yes	☐ No
Any other drugs or medications?	☐ Yes	☐ No

If yes, please describe: _____

Immunizations:

Have you been immunized for or received any of the following vaccines?

Hepatitis A?	☐ Yes	☐ No	Meningococcal vaccine?	☐ Yes	☐ No
Hepatitis B?	☐ Yes	☐ No	Pertussis vaccine (Td/Tdap)?	☐ Yes	☐ No
Herpes zoster?	☐ Yes	☐ No	Pneumococcal vaccine?	☐ Yes	☐ No
Human papilloma virus (HPV, male or female)?	☐ Yes	☐ No	Polio?	☐ Yes	☐ No
			Smallpox vaccine?	☐ Yes	☐ No
Influenza vaccine?	☐ Yes	☐ No	Tetanus, diphtheria, Pertussis (Td/Tdap)?	☐ Yes	☐ No
Measles, Mumps, Rubella (MMR)?	☐ Yes	☐ No	Varicella vaccine?	☐ Yes	☐ No

Recent Health Screens:

Have you recent had any of the following health screens or tests?

Blood pressure?	☐ Yes	☐ No	Obesity (height, weight, body mass index [BMI])?	☐ Yes	☐ No
Cholesterol?	☐ Yes	☐ No			
Colorectal cancer?	☐ Yes	☐ No	Prostate (PSA)?	☐ Yes	☐ No
HIV/AIDS?	☐ Yes	☐ No	Pulmonary function screening?	☐ Yes	☐ No

If yes to any of the above, please provide dates and details: _____

_____

FIGURE 4-2 **Form for general past medical history.**

PAST MEDICAL HISTORY

Cardiac/Cardiovascular:

Have you ever had or been told you had:

Abnormal bleeding?	☐ Yes	☐ No	High blood pressure		
Anemia?	☐ Yes	☐ No	(hypertension)?	☐ Yes	☐ No
Angina?	☐ Yes	☐ No	Irregular heart beat?	☐ Yes	☐ No
Blood transfusion?	☐ Yes	☐ No	Low blood pressure?	☐ Yes	☐ No
Congestive heart failure?	☐ Yes	☐ No	Myocardial infarction?	☐ Yes	☐ No
Coronary artery disease?	☐ Yes	☐ No	Other blood disease?	☐ Yes	☐ No
Heart attack?	☐ Yes	☐ No	Other heart disease?	☐ Yes	☐ No
Heart murmur?	☐ Yes	☐ No			

If yes to any of the above, please provide dates and details: _____

Pulmonary:

Have you had or ever been told you had:

Acute bronchitis?	☐ Yes	☐ No	Interstitial lung disease?	☐ Yes	☐ No
Asthma?	☐ Yes	☐ No	Lung cancer?	☐ Yes	☐ No
Chest pain?	☐ Yes	☐ No	Other lung disease?	☐ Yes	☐ No
Chronic bronchitis?	☐ Yes	☐ No	Pleurisy?	☐ Yes	☐ No
COPD?	☐ Yes	☐ No	Pneumonia?	☐ Yes	☐ No
Cough?	☐ Yes	☐ No	Shortness of breath?	☐ Yes	☐ No
Emphysema?	☐ Yes	☐ No	Sinusitis?	☐ Yes	☐ No
Hay fever?	☐ Yes	☐ No	Tuberculosis?	☐ Yes	☐ No

If yes to any of the above, please provide dates and details: _____

Infectious Disease:

Have you ever had:

Bladder infections?	☐ Yes	☐ No	Meningitis?	☐ Yes	☐ No
Diphtheria?	☐ Yes	☐ No	Mumps?	☐ Yes	☐ No
Hepatitis B or C?	☐ Yes	☐ No	Polio?	☐ Yes	☐ No
Herpes?	☐ Yes	☐ No	Rheumatic fever?	☐ Yes	☐ No
HIV/AIDS?	☐ Yes	☐ No	Scarlet fever?	☐ Yes	☐ No
Infectious mononucleosis?	☐ Yes	☐ No	Sexually transmitted disease (STD)?	☐ Yes	☐ No
Malaria?	☐ Yes	☐ No	Shingles?	☐ Yes	☐ No
Measles?	☐ Yes	☐ No			

Whooping cough?   ☐ Yes   ☐ No

If yes to any of the above, please provide dates and details: _____

FIGURE 4-2 (*continued*)

Other Disease:

Have you ever had:

Alcoholism?	☐ Yes	☐ No	Gastroesophageal reflux?	☐ Yes	☐ No
Allergies?	☐ Yes	☐ No	Glaucoma?	☐ Yes	☐ No
Alzheimer's disease?	☐ Yes	☐ No	Gout?	☐ Yes	☐ No
Anaphylaxis?	☐ Yes	☐ No	Hemorrhoids?	☐ Yes	☐ No
Arthritis?	☐ Yes	☐ No	Hives or rash?	☐ Yes	☐ No
Back problems?	☐ Yes	☐ No	Hypoglycemia?	☐ Yes	☐ No
Bruise easily?	☐ Yes	☐ No	Kidney problems?	☐ Yes	☐ No
Cancer?	☐ Yes	☐ No	Leukemia?	☐ Yes	☐ No
Chemotherapy?	☐ Yes	☐ No	Liver disease or yellow jaundice?	☐ Yes	☐ No
Convulsions?	☐ Yes	☐ No	Nose bleeds?	☐ Yes	☐ No
Diabetes?	☐ Yes	☐ No	Psychiatric care?	☐ Yes	☐ No
Drug addiction?	☐ Yes	☐ No	Radiation treatments?	☐ Yes	☐ No
Epilepsy or seizures?	☐ Yes	☐ No	Sickle cell disease?	☐ Yes	☐ No
Fainting or dizziness?	☐ Yes	☐ No	Stomach/intestinal disease?	☐ Yes	☐ No
Frequent diarrhea?	☐ Yes	☐ No	Stroke?	☐ Yes	☐ No
Frequent headaches?	☐ Yes	☐ No	Thyroid disease?	☐ Yes	☐ No
			Ulcer?	☐ Yes	☐ No

If yes to any of the above, please provide dates and details: _____

_____

Surgery or Operations:

Appendix?	☐ Yes	☐ No
Breast?	☐ Yes	☐ No
Cardiac Pacemaker?	☐ Yes	☐ No
Coronary artery bypass surgery?	☐ Yes	☐ No
Coronary angiography?	☐ Yes	☐ No
Gallbladder?	☐ Yes	☐ No
Heart valve replacement?	☐ Yes	☐ No
Hemorrhoids?	☐ Yes	☐ No
Hernia?	☐ Yes	☐ No
Other heart operations?	☐ Yes	☐ No
Prostate?	☐ Yes	☐ No
Stomach?	☐ Yes	☐ No
Thyroid?	☐ Yes	☐ No
Tonsils?	☐ Yes	☐ No
Uterus and/or ovary?	☐ Yes	☐ No
Varicose veins?	☐ Yes	☐ No

If yes to any of the above, please provide dates and details: _____

_____

FIGURE 4-2 (*continued*)

Accidents or Injuries:

Abdomen?	☐ Yes	☐ No
Back?	☐ Yes	☐ No
Broken bones?	☐ Yes	☐ No
Chest?	☐ Yes	☐ No
Head?	☐ Yes	☐ No
Motor vehicle accidents with injuries?	☐ Yes	☐ No
Other accidents or injuries?	☐ Yes	☐ No

If yes to any of the above, please provide dates and details: _____

_____

FIGURE 4-2 (*continued*)

hospitalizations related to cardiopulmonary disease. An account of any respiratory care received (oxygen, aerosol medications, etc.) should be included. Prior intensive care unit (ICU) admissions and any history of intubation or mechanical ventilation are of particular interest. For example, in the asthmatic patient any of the following events as noted in the past medical history place the patient at much greater risk for death from asthma:[13]

- Intubation
- Prior admission to an ICU
- Two or more hospitalizations or three or more emergency department (ED) visits in the past year

TABLE 4-11
History of Chest Illness

The patient should be asked each of the following interview questions:
1. During the past 3 years have you had chest colds, bronchitis, or pneumonia?
   a. None _____ 2 or 3 bouts _____ More than 3 bouts _____
   b. During the past 3 years have any of these kept you off work or in bed for as long as a week?
      Yes _____ No _____
2. Have you ever had or been told that you had:
   a. Asthma?   Yes _____ No _____
   b. Allergies?   Yes _____ No _____
   c. Bronchitis?   Yes _____ No _____
   d. Emphysema?   Yes _____ No _____
   e. Pneumonia?   Yes _____ No _____
   f. Influenza?   Yes _____ No _____
   g. Occupational lung disease?   Yes _____ No _____
   h. Pneumoconiosis?   Yes _____ No _____
   i. Interstitial lung disease (ILD)?   Yes _____ No _____
   j. Pleurisy?   Yes _____ No _____
   k. Tuberculosis (TB)?   Yes _____ No _____
   l. Lung cancer?   Yes _____ No _____
   m. Chest injury such as fractured rib or spine?   Yes _____ No _____
   n. Pneumothorax?   Yes _____ No _____
   o. A chest operation?   Yes _____ No _____
   p. A bronchoscopy?   Yes _____ No _____
   q. A pulmonary function test?   Yes _____ No _____
   r. A heart condition?   Yes _____ No _____
   s. A heart operation?   Yes _____ No _____
   t. An allergy or reaction to food or drugs?   Yes _____ No _____
   u. Chest pain?   Yes _____ No _____
   v. Frequent colds?   Yes _____ No _____
   w. Sinus infections?   Yes _____ No _____

If "YES" to any of the above, please give details to include dates and details:

_____

_____

- Use of more than two canisters per month of short-acting bronchodilators
- Systemic steroid use
- ER visit or hospitalization due to asthma in the last month

A summary of the items that should be included in the medical history for an asthma patient is found in **Table 4-12**.

The impact of a chronic illness on the family, finances, and school or work performance should be explored. School or work days missed due to illness and any limitation in activity should be assessed. Chronic illness may affect the patient's psychological, social, and economic well-being and health-related quality of life.

TABLE 4-12
Medical History for the Patient with Asthma

A detailed medical history of the new patient who is known or thought to have asthma should address:

Symptoms
- Cough
- Wheezing
- Shortness of breath
- Chest tightness
- Sputum production

Pattern of Symptoms
- Perennial, seasonal, or both
- Continual, episodic, or both
- Onset, duration, frequency (number of days or nights, per week or month)
- Diurnal variations, especially nocturnal and on awakening in early morning

Precipitating and/or Aggravating Factors
- Viral respiratory infections
- Environmental allergens, indoor (mold, dust mite, cockroach, animal dander or secretory products) and outdoor (pollen)
- Characteristics of home, including age, location, cooling and heating system, wood-burning stove, humidifier, carpeting over concrete, presence of molds or mildew, characteristics of rooms where patient spends time (bedroom and living room with attention to bedding, floor covering, stuffed furniture)
- Smoking (patient and others in home or daycare)
- Exercise
- Occupational chemicals or allergens
- Environmental change (moving to new home; going on vacation; and/or alteration in workplace, work processes, or materials used)
- Irritants (tobacco smoke, strong odors, air pollutants, occupational chemicals, dusts and particulates, vapors, gases, and aerosols)
- Emotions (fear, anger, frustration, hard crying or laughing)
- Stress
- Drugs (aspirin, nonsteroidal anti-inflammatory drugs; β-blockers, including eye drops; other)
- Food, food additives, and preservatives (sulfites)
- Changes in weather, exposure to cold air
- Endocrine factors (menses, pregnancy, thyroid disease)
- Comorbid conditions (sinusitis, rhinitis, GERD)

Development of Disease and Treatment
- Age of onset and diagnosis
- History of early life injury to airways (bronchopulmonary dysplasia, pneumonia, parental smoking)
- Progression of disease (better or worse)
- Present management and response, including plans for managing exacerbations
- Frequency of using short-acting β-agonists
- Need for oral corticosteroids and frequency of use

Family History
- History of asthma, allergy, sinusitis, rhinitis, eczema, or nasal polyps in close relatives

Social History
- Daycare, workplace, and school characteristics that may interfere with adherence
- Social factors that interfere with adherence, such as substance abuse
- Social support/social networks
- Level of education completed
- Employment

TABLE 4-12
Medical History for the Patient with Asthma (*continued*)

History of Exacerbations

- Usual early signs and symptoms
- Rapidity of onset
- Duration
- Frequency
- Severity (need for urgent care, hospitalization, ICU admission)
- Life-threatening exacerbations (intubation, ICU admission)
- Number and severity of exacerbations in the past year
- Usual patterns and management (what works?)

History of Exacerbations

- Usual early signs and symptoms
- Rapidity of onset
- Duration
- Frequency
- Severity (need for urgent care, hospitalization, ICU admission)
- Life-threatening exacerbations (intubation, ICU admission)
- Number and severity of exacerbations in the past year
- Usual patterns and management (what works?)

Impact of Asthma on Patient and Family

- Episodes of unscheduled care (emergency department, urgent care, hospitalization)
- Number of days missed from school/work
- Limitation of activity, especially sports and strenuous work
- History of nocturnal awakening
- Effect on growth, development, behavior, school or work performance, and lifestyle
- Impact on family routines, activities, or dynamics
- Economic impact

Assessment of Patient's and Family's Perceptions of Disease

- Patient's, parents', and spouse's or partner's knowledge of asthma and belief in the chronic nature of asthma and in the efficacy of treatment
- Patient's perception and beliefs regarding use and long-term effects of medications
- Ability of patient and parents, spouse, or partner to cope with disease
- Level of family support and patient's and parents', spouse's, or partner's capacity to recognize severity of an exacerbation
- Economic resources
- Sociocultural beliefs

Modified from: National Institutes of Health, National Heart, Lung, and Blood Institute Guidelines for the diagnosis and management of asthma: Expert Panel 3 Report. (NIH publication). Bethesda, MD: US Department of Health and Human Services; 2007.

Family History

Obtaining a **family history** is necessary because the health status of relatives, including parents, siblings, and grandparents, often plays an important role in establishing a familial link with hereditary diseases. Two examples of gender-linked genetic disease are color blindness and hemophilia, a blood disorder with impaired blood clot formation and increased risk of bleeding. If a disease seems to run in the family, sometimes a genetic pedigree diagram is developed. The pedigree diagram will cover at least three generations of the family to document the family history of major health problems that may have a genetic component. An example of a pedigree diagram for cystic fibrosis is found in **Figure 4-3**.

Major diseases that should be included in the family history include hypertension, cancer, heart disease, lung disease (including asthma, COPD, pneumonia, and TB), diabetes, stroke, kidney disease, thyroid problems, and Alzheimer disease.[27] The list of cardiopulmonary diseases with a hereditary association is extensive, and the family history should include questions regarding blood relatives who may have had heart or lung problems. Asthma, cystic fibrosis, and panlobular emphysema caused by an alpha-1 antitrypsin deficiency are notable pulmonary diseases with a hereditary disposition. A family history of asthma, allergy, sinusitis, rhinitis, eczema, or nasal polyps in close relatives is common in asthmatics.[13] Less-common genetic lung diseases include primary ciliary dyskinesia (Kartagener syndrome) and Niemann-Pick disease, a fatal metabolic disorder that affects the lungs, liver, spleen, bone marrow, and brain. Cardiovascular diseases that have a genetic component include congenital heart disease, hypertension, coronary artery disease, MI, and CHF.

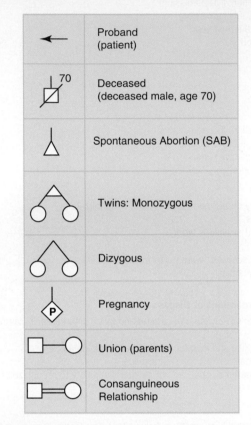

(A)

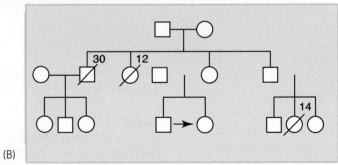

(B)

FIGURE 4-3 Pedigree charts. (A) Pedigree chart symbols. (B) Example of a three-generation pedigree chart for an autosomal recessive genetic condition, such as cystic fibrosis.

Data from: Seidel HM, Ball JW, Dains JE, et al. Recording information. In: *Mosby's Guide to Physical Examination*. St. Louis, MO: Mosby-Elsevier; 2011: 792–813.

Genetically associated neuromuscular diseases that may affect patients' ability to breathe include amyotrophic lateral sclerosis (ALS or Lou Gehrig disease) and Duchenne muscular dystrophy.

For infectious diseases, the nuclear family is typically the focus of the family history. Pneumonia and tuberculosis are infectious diseases that often spread via contact with immediate family members.

Personal and Social History

Items that are included in an in-depth personal and social history are outlined in Box 4-14 and include personal status, habits, self-care, sexual history, home conditions, occupation, environment, military record, religious and cultural preferences, and access to care.[28] Items included in the patient's personal and social history will vary, depending on the possible impact specific items may have on health. In addition to the demographic data already collected, the interviewer may wish to inquire about the patient's cultural and ethnic background, religion, spiritual needs, and any religious prohibitions regarding healthcare.[27] Economic resources, availability of transportation, and type of health insurance coverage may influence the patient's access to care.

The patient's emotional state may serve as a precipitating or aggravating factor with lung disease, such as COPD or asthma. Fear, anger, frustration, or sources of stress should be investigated. In addition, the interviewer may wish to inquire about the home environment (living conditions, number of occupants, pets) and neighborhood of residence (see below). Social and family support may be an important factor in the patient's ability to cope with the problems associated with illness. In patients with asthma, daycare, school, or workplace issues that make medication compliance more difficult should be noted.

Items included in the patient's personal and social history will vary depending on the possible impact specific items may have on health. Nutrition, diet, and eating patterns may also impact overall health. Consumption of tea, coffee, alcohol, and use of tobacco products should be determined. The personal and social history should also incorporate habits such as use of tobacco, alcohol, or illicit drugs. Substance abuse can pose serious health threats as well as interfere with a patient's compliance with a treatment or monitoring regimen. Alcohol dependence and abuse is a major health problem that affects about 17 million people in the United States.[29] Major organs that may be damaged by alcohol included the liver, pancreas, heart, brain, and bone.[29] Cardiovascular complications of alcohol abuse include hypertension, cardiomyopathy, stroke, and arrhythmias.[29] Alcohol abuse markedly increases the risk of accidents, trauma, violence, and suicide. Alcoholics are prone to the development of aspiration pneumonia, as well as many other health problems. Other commonly abused drugs include sedative-hypnotics (tranquilizers, barbiturates), opioid and morphine derivatives (heroin, codeine, oxycodone), stimulants (amphetamine, cocaine), and cannabinoids (marijuana, hashish). Sedative-hypnotic drugs and the opioids are CNS depressants, and an overdose may result in respiratory depression and apnea. Tobacco, marijuana, and cocaine use are discussed in the following sections.

Smoking History

In 1964, the U.S. Surgeon General's report entitled *Smoking and Health: Report of the Advisory Committee to the Surgeon General* held cigarette smoking responsible for a 70% increase in the mortality rate of smokers over nonsmokers.[30] The report described the adverse health consequences of tobacco use and identified smoking as the cause of lung cancer and chronic bronchitis. The report also highlighted the correlation between smoking, emphysema, coronary heart disease, and low-birth-weight babies born to mothers who used tobacco during pregnancy.[30]

Currently, the adverse health effects of cigarette smoking in the United States account for nearly 20% of all deaths (> 443,000 deaths/year due to smoking).[31] For people with COPD, about 90% of deaths are smoking related, and smoking causes 80% of all lung cancer deaths in women and 90% of all lung cancer deaths in men.[31] Smokers have a marked increase in the risk of coronary heart disease and stroke, and smoking causes many other types of cancer, including cancers of the mouth, pharynx, larynx, esophagus, stomach, pancreas, kidney, and bladder. Smokers also are at risk for developing more severe disease in the presence of coal miner's pneumoconiosis (CWP) and asbestosis. Although cigarette smoking is the primary cause of COPD, it should be noted that only about 20% of smokers develop clinically significant COPD.[32] **Box 4-15** summarizes the adverse health effects of smoking.

Tobacco History

Because of the profoundly negative effects of smoking on health and the corresponding benefits of smoking cessation, the **smoking history** is an essential part of the patient interview. The first patient interview question related to smoking history is "Have you ever smoked tobacco?" This should be followed by a series of questions to determine the nature of the patient's tobacco use, amount consumed per day, number of years smoked, and current tobacco use status (see **Table 4-13**). The patient should be questioned about the use of cigarettes, pipes, cigars, and other tobacco products. For cigarettes, the number of years smoked and the number of packs smoked per day are often multiplied to create a measure called "pack years." For example, a pack per day smoked for 1 year is: 1 pack/day × 1 year = 1 pack year. As an alternative to the use of pack years, some interviewers prefer to ask patients how many cigarettes per day they smoke. Any previous attempts to quit smoking should be noted and the method used, such as "cold turkey" or a formal smoking cessation program. The use of any smoking cessation aids such as nicotine patches, nicotine gum, other medications or counseling should be noted. The respiratory care clinician should also ask patients who continue to smoke if they are willing to give quitting a try.

BOX 4-15

The Adverse Health Effects of Tobacco Smoking

Smoking accounts for nearly one of every five deaths each year in the United States.

More deaths are caused by tobacco use than by all deaths from human immunodeficiency virus (HIV), illegal drug use, alcohol use, motor vehicle injuries, suicides, and murders combined.

Smoking causes:

- COPD: 90% of all deaths from COPD are due to smoking
- Cancer:
  - Oral cavity (mouth cancer)
  - Pharynx (throat cancer)
  - Lung cancer:
    - 90% of all lung cancer deaths in men are due to smoking
    - 80% of all lung cancer deaths in women are due to smoking
  - Acute myeloid leukemia
  - Bladder cancer
  - Cancer of the cervix
  - Cancer of the esophagus
  - Kidney cancer
  - Cancer of the larynx (voice box)
  - Pancreatic cancer
  - Stomach cancer
- Coronary heart disease (the leading cause of death in the United States)
- Reduced circulation
- Abdominal aortic aneurysm

Smoking increases the risk of:

- Coronary heart disease by 2 to 4 times
- Stroke by 2 to 4 times
- Men developing lung cancer by 23 times
- Women developing lung cancer by 13 times
- Dying from COPD by 12 to 13 times

Smoking has adverse reproductive and early childhood effects, including increased risk for:

- Infertility
- Preterm birth, still birth, and low birth weight
- Sudden infant death syndrome (SIDS)

Smoking has adverse effects on women's' health:

- Postmenopausal women who smoke have lower bone density
- Women who smoke have an increased risk for hip fracture.

Secondhand smoke has similar effects as smoking itself.

Modified from: Centers for Disease Control and Prevention. Health effects of smoking. http://www.cdc.gov/tobacco/data_statistics/fact_sheets/health_effects/effects_cig_smoking/.

Public health efforts over the past 48 years have been effective in educating the public about the hazards of cigarette smoking. Studies also demonstrate a significant health risk from secondhand smoke and a history of exposure to secondhand smoke should also be obtained. Increased taxation of cigarettes; smoke-free zones, including workplaces, airports, and airplanes; and laws banning smoking in many public places have reduced tobacco consumption and exposure to secondhand smoke. All of these efforts have had an impact on both the perception and practice of tobacco smoking in the United States. Because of embarrassment or the desire to please their healthcare provider, patients may underreport current tobacco use. Inspection of the patient's fingers for nicotine stains may help identify continuing smokers. Measurement of blood carboxyhemoglobin levels via co-oximetry or measurements of urinary cotinine (a longer-lasting

TABLE 4-13
Smoking and Tobacco Use Interview Questions

Please check the correct response or fill in the requested information:

A. Have you ever smoked cigarettes? — Yes _____ No _____
   If "Yes":
   1. How old were you when your first started smoking? _____
   2. How many total years have you smoked? _____
   3. What is the average number of packs of cigarettes you smoked (or continue to smoke) per day? _____
   4. Have you stopped smoking? — Yes _____ No _____
      a. If "Yes," how long has it been since you stopped smoking? _____
      b. If "No," have you ever tried to quit smoking? — Yes _____ No _____
      c. Would you like to try and quit smoking? — Yes _____ No _____
B. Have you ever smoked cigars regularly? — Yes _____ No _____
   If "Yes":
   1. How many years? _____
   2. How many cigars per day? _____
   3. Do you still smoke cigars? — Yes _____ No _____
   4. Do you (did you) inhale? — Yes _____ No _____
   5. Have you stopped smoking cigars? — Yes _____ No _____
   If "Yes," how long has it been since you stopped smoking cigars? _____
C. Have you ever smoked a pipe regularly? — Yes _____ No _____
   If "Yes":
   1. How many years? _____
   2. How many pipefuls a day? _____
   3. Do you still smoke a pipe? — Yes _____ No _____
   4. Do you (did you) inhale? — Yes _____ No _____
   5. Have you stopped smoking a pipe? — Yes _____ No _____
      If "Yes," how long has it been since you stopped smoking a pipe? _____
D. Have you ever used, or do you now use any of the following tobacco products? — Yes _____ No _____
   1. Snuff (such as Skoal or Copenhagen)? — Yes _____ No _____
   2. Chewing tobacco? — Yes _____ No _____
   3. Other tobacco products? — Yes _____ No _____
      If "Yes," please describe: _____
E. Does anyone smoke cigarettes, cigars, or pipes anywhere inside your home? — Yes _____ No _____
   If "Yes," please describe: _____
F. Have you ever smoked marijuana? — Yes _____ No _____
   If "Yes":
   1. How long? _____
   2. How many times per week? _____
   3. Have you stopped smoking marijuana? — Yes _____ No _____
      If "Yes," how long has it been since you stopped smoking marijuana? _____
G. Have you ever smoked any other recreational drugs, such as crack cocaine? — Yes _____ No _____
   If "Yes":
   1. What drug(s)? _____
   2. How long? _____
   3. How many times per week? _____
   4. Have you stopped smoking? — Yes _____ No _____
      If "Yes," how long has it been since you stopped smoking? _____

Data from: National Institutes of Health, National Heart, Lung, and Blood Institute Guidelines for the Diagnosis and Management of Asthma: Expert Panel 3 Report. (NIH publication). Bethesda, MD: US Department of Health and Human Services; 2007.

metabolite of nicotine) may also help identify "hidden" smokers.

Smoking Cessation

Although the rate of cigarette smoking in the United States has declined significantly since the 1964 Surgeon General's report on smoking and health, about 19% of U.S. adults continue to smoke (based on 2010 data), and over a billion people smoke tobacco worldwide.[31] Almost 70% of adult smokers in the United States report that they want to quit.[32] Quitting, however, can be very difficult, and only about 4% to 7% of smokers are successful on any given attempt in quitting without assistance.[33,34] Most cigarette smokers who are able to quit successfully do so without using a formal smoking cessation program.[33,34] The use of evidence-based smoking cessation treatments can increase cessation success rates two- to threefold to a success rate of about 10% to 26%.[33–39] **Box 4-16** summarizes effective, evidence-based smoking cessation techniques.

BOX 4-16

Effective Smoking Cessation Techniques

The majority of cigarette smokers who quit do so without using smoking cessation treatments. However, the following evidence-based treatments are proven effective and may increase success rates substantially.

Advisement, assistance, counseling, and behavioral therapy:

- Brief clinical interventions: Clinician takes < 10 minutes to deliver advice and assistance about quitting.
- Counseling: Individual, group, or telephone counseling.
- Behavioral cessation therapies: Training in problem solving.
- Treatments with more person-to-person contact and intensity: More time with counselors.

Medications:

- Nicotine replacement products
  - Over-the-counter (nicotine patch, gum, lozenge)
  - Prescription (nicotine inhaler, nasal spray)
- Prescription non-nicotine medications:
  - Bupropion SR (Zyban)
  - Varenicline tartrate (Chantix)

The combination of medication and counseling is more effective for smoking cessation than either medication or counseling alone.

Data from: Centers for Disease Control and Prevention. Smoking Cessation and Interventions Fact Sheet. Available at: http://www.cdc.gov/tobacco/data_statistics/fact_sheets/cessation/quitting/index.htm; Tobacco Use and Dependence Guideline Panel. *Treating tobacco use and dependence: 2008 update.* Rockville (MD): US Department of Health and Human Services; 2008 May. http://www.ncbi.nlm.nih.gov/books/NBK63952/

The first step in successful smoking cessation intervention is to identify all current tobacco users.[34,35] Interview questions regarding a patient's smoking history are found in Table 4-13.

The recommended approach to smoking cessation can be summarized as ask, advise, assess, assist, and arrange, which is outlined in **Table 4-14**.[34,35] The respiratory care clinician should *ask* every patient about tobacco use and document tobacco use status at every visit.[34,35] The respiratory care clinician should then *advise* all tobacco users to quit. Next, the clinician should *assess* the willingness of all tobacco users to make a quit attempt.[34,35] The respiratory care clinician should then *assist* willing patients by offering to provide medication and counseling. The clinician should then *arrange* for appropriate follow-up to begin within the first week of the quit date.[34,35]

As noted, the respiratory care clinician should ask every patient about tobacco use and document tobacco use status for every patient at every visit. Patients who continue to smoke should be advised to quit using clear, strong, and personalized language. An assessment should be made as to the patient's willingness to quit. Assistance is then provided to willing patients to include help with the development of a quit plan,

practical counseling to solve problems, and assistance in obtaining family and social support (see Table 4-14).[40] The most successful smoking cessation programs include both counseling and medication. Nicotine is highly addictive, and nicotine replacement therapy in the form of gum, lozenges, nasal sprays, nicotine inhalers, or transdermal skin patches can help ease withdrawal symptoms. Bupropion SR (Zyban) is a non-nicotine atypical antidepressant that reduces the cravings and other withdrawal symptoms associated with smoking cessation. Bupropion for smoking cessation is typically prescribed in a stepwise fashion, starting with a 150 mg sustained-release tablet taken once per day for the first 3 days. The dose is then increased to 300 mg per day taken as two doses of 150 mg each separated by at least 8 hours. Treatment should begin about 1 week before the patient's actual smoking quit date and then continue for 7 to 12 weeks. Generally, if patients have not successfully quite smoking by week 7, the medication should be discontinued, as success is unlikely. Varenicline tartrate (Chantix) is another medication used as therapy for smoking cessation. Varenicline tartrate is a nicotinic receptor partial agonist that reduces nicotine withdrawal symptoms (see **Clinical Focus 4-1**).

TABLE 4-14
The 5 A's for Treating Tobacco Dependence

1. *Ask* about tobacco use.
   - Identify and document tobacco use status for every patient at every visit.
2. *Advise* tobacco users to quit. Be clear, strong, and personalized; urge every tobacco user to quit.
   - Clear: "It is important that you quit smoking (or using other tobacco products) now, and I can help you."
   - Strong: "As your clinician, I need you to know that quitting smoking is the most important thing you can do to protect your health now and in the future. We (staff) will help you."
   - Personalized: Link tobacco use to current symptoms and health concerns. For example, "Continuing to smoke makes your asthma (or COPD) much worse. Quitting may dramatically improve your health."
3. *Assess* willingness to quit. Assess every tobacco user's willing to make a quit attempt at each new patient encounter. Ask the patient "Are you willing to give quitting a try?"
4. *Assist* in quit attempt. If the patient is willing to make a quite attempt, offer medication and provide or refer for counseling or additional treatment to help the patient quit.
   - Help the patient make a quit plan:
     - Set a quit date, usually within 2 weeks.
     - Tell family, friends and coworkers about quitting and request understanding and support.
     - Anticipate challenges to the upcoming quit attempt, especially during the critical first few weeks. These include reviewing nicotine withdrawal symptoms:
       - Symptoms may include irritability, anxiety, depression, difficulty concentrating, weight gain, restlessness, and impatience.
       - Assure the patient that the withdrawal symptoms will subside, though they may last for several weeks.
     - Remove tobacco products from environment.
     - Prior to quitting, avoid smoking in places were a great deal of time is spent such as work, home, or car. Make the home smoke-free.
   - Recommend the use of approved medication (pharmacotherapy), unless contraindicated or insufficient evidence of effectiveness (e.g., pregnant women, smokeless tobacco users, light smokers, adolescents).
   - Provide practical counseling (e.g., problem-solving and skills training).
     - Stress abstinence. No smoking, not even a single puff, after the quit date.
     - Review past quit experience. Identify what helped and what hurt in previous attempts to quit.
     - Anticipate triggers and challenges and discuss how the patient will successfully overcome them.
       - Avoid triggers.
       - Alter routines.
     - Review relationship of alcohol to tobacco use.
       - Limit or abstain from alcohol use while quitting.
     - Point out that having other smokers in the home will increase the difficulty.
       - Encourage housemates to quit with the patient.
   - Provide treatment and social support in the clinical environment.
     - Provide a supportive clinical environment.
     - Inform patient that staff are available to assist him or her.
   - Help obtain extra treatment, social support.
   - Help obtain patient–environment support from family, friends, and coworkers.
   - Provide supplementary materials, including information on quitline telephonic services:
     - Sources: Organizations that promote smoking cessation, including federal, state, and nonprofit organizations.
     - 1-800-QUIT-NOW.
     - Materials should be appropriate for the patient, in relation to culture, race, education, and age.
     - Location: Materials should be readily available at every clinician's workstation.
5. *Arrange* follow-up. Schedule follow-up contacts in person or via telephone.
   - Timing:
     - Follow up within the first week of the quit date.
     - Follow up again within the first month.
     - Schedule further follow-up contacts, as needed.
   - Actions during follow-up:
     - Review.
     - Stress abstinence.
     - Identify problems already encountered and anticipate challenges in the immediate future.
     - Assess medication use and problems.
     - Remind patients of quitline support (1-800-QUIT-NOW).
     - Congratulate abstinent patients on their success.
     - If tobacco use has occurred, review circumstances and elicit recommitment to total abstinence.
       - Remind the patient that a lapse is a learning experience.
       - Consider increased intervention when necessary.

(continues)

TABLE 4-14
The 5 A's for Treating Tobacco Dependence (*continued*)

If patient is not willing to quit, the clinician should ask patient to identify negative consequences of smoking and highlight those most relevant to the patient.

- Emphasize that low-tar, low-nicotine, and other forms of tobacco do not eliminate risk.
- Acute risks:
  - Shortness of breath.
  - Exacerbation of asthma.
  - Harm in pregnancy.
  - Impotence.
  - Infertility.
  - Increased serum carbon monoxide.
- Long-term risks:
  - Heart attack.
  - Stroke.
  - Cancer: Lung, larynx, oral cavity, pharynx, esophagus, pancreas, bladder, cervix.
  - COPD.
  - Long-term disability.
- Environmental risks (secondhand smoke, other):
  - Increased risk of lung cancer and heart disease in spouse.
  - Higher rate of smoking among children of tobacco users.
  - Increased risk of low birth weight, sudden infant death syndrome, asthma, middle ear disease, and respiratory infections in children of smokers.

Modified from: Fiore, MC, Bailey WC, Cohen SJ, et al. Treating tobacco use and dependence. Clinical Practice Guideline. Rockville, MD: U.S. Department of Health and Human Services. Public Health Service. June 2000. Available at http://www.surgeongeneral.gov/tobacco/tobaqrg.htm; and Marlow SP, Stoller JK. Smoking cessation. *Respir Care.* 2003;48(12):1238–1254.

Follow-up care should occur within the first week of the quit date, with follow-up again within the first month.[34,35] At each follow-up session, the respiratory care clinician should review how the patient is doing and offer congratulations for his or her continuing efforts. The clinician should also help the patient identify current and potential problems, stress the need for continued abstinence, and assess pharmacotherapy provided. If a patient has used tobacco, the clinician should review the circumstances, elicit a recommitment to total abstinence, and consider more intensive treatment.[34,35]

CLINICAL FOCUS 4-1

Smoking Cessation

Upon patient interview, the respiratory care clinician finds that the patient has smoked for 30 years, starting smoking at age 16. The patient typically smokes two packs of cigarettes per day and has a chronic cough, with about a tablespoon of sputum or produced per day. The clinician advises the patient that she must quit smoking and informs the patient of the consequences of not quitting. The patient states that she wants to quit smoking, but that she has been unsuccessful in past attempts to quit. What should the clinician now do?

The clinician has completed the first three A's of smoking cessation: *ask, advise* and *assess.* The patient seems ready to stop smoking. The next steps are to *assist* the patient in the quit attempt and to *arrange* for follow-up care. Assistances should include helping the patient to develop a quit plan and providing recommendations of approved medications (see Table 4-15). One medication that may be useful is varenicline tartrate (Chantix). Medication should be started 1 week before the set quit date and continued as follows:

- Starting week: 0.5 mg once daily on days 1 through 3 and 0.5 mg twice daily on days 4 through 7.
- Continuing weeks: 1 mg twice daily for a total of 12 weeks.
- An additional 12 weeks of treatment is recommended for those who are successful to increase likelihood of long-term abstinence.

Dose should be reduced in patients with renal impairment and in patients who cannot tolerate adverse effects. Practical counseling should be provided, as well as treatment and social support in the clinical environment.

Last, the respiratory care clinician should arrange for follow-up care (see Table 4-14).

The Five R's of Cessation Motivation: Relevance, Risks, Rewards, Roadblocks, and Repetition

For patients who are *not* ready to quit smoking, the respiratory care clinician should employ the five R's for motivating patients to quit smoking (**Table 4-15**).[34,35] To begin, the clinician should ask the patient about the importance of quitting in terms that are personally *relevant*. For example, it may be important for patients to live longer, have a better quality of life, save money currently being spent on tobacco products, or to reduce the harmful effects of secondhand smoke on their spouses or children.

Next, the clinician should ask the patient to identify the *risks* (negative consequences) of continued tobacco

---

TABLE 4-15
The 5 R's for Motivation for Smoking Cessation

1. **Relevance**
   - Encourage the patient to indicate why quitting is personally relevant.
   - Be as specific as possible.
   - Motivational information has the greatest impact if it is relevant to a patient's:
     - Disease status or risk.
     - Family or social situation (e.g., having children in the home).
     - Health concerns.
     - Age or gender.
   - Other important consideration (e.g., prior quitting experience, personal barriers to cessation).

2. **Risks**
   - Ask the patient to identify potential negative consequences of tobacco use.
   - Suggest and highlight those that seem most relevant to the patient.
   - Emphasize that smoking low-tar/low-nicotine cigarettes or use of other forms of tobacco (e.g., smokeless tobacco, cigars, and pipes) will not eliminate these risks.
   - Examples of risks include:
     - *Acute risks*: Shortness of breath, exacerbation of asthma, increased risk of respiratory infections, harm to pregnancy, impotence, and infertility.
     - *Long-term risks*: Heart attacks and strokes, lung and other cancers (e.g., larynx, oral cavity, pharynx, esophagus, pancreas, stomach, kidney, bladder, cervix, and acute myelocytic leukemia), COPD (chronic bronchitis and emphysema), osteoporosis, long-term disability, and need for extended care.
     - *Environmental risks*: Increased risk of lung cancer and heart disease in spouses; increased risk for low birth-weight, sudden infant death syndrome (SIDS), asthma, middle ear disease, and respiratory infections in children of smokers.

3. **Rewards**
   - Ask the patient to identify potential benefits of stopping tobacco use.
   - Suggest and highlight those that seem most relevant to the patient such as:
     - Improved health.
     - Food will taste better.
     - Improved sense of smell.
     - Saving money.
     - Feeling better about oneself.
     - Home, car, clothing, breath will smell better.
     - Setting a good example for children and decreasing the likelihood that they will smoke.
     - Having healthier babies and children.
     - Feeling better physically.
     - Performing better in physical activities.
     - Improved appearance, including reduced wrinkling/aging of skin and whiter teeth.

4. **Roadblocks**
   - Ask the patient to identify barriers or impediments to quitting.
   - Provide treatment (problem-solving counseling, medication).
   - Barriers might include:
     - Withdrawal symptoms
     - Fear of failure
     - Weight gain
     - Lack of support
     - Depression
     - Enjoyment of tobacco
     - Being around other tobacco users

5. **Repetition**
   - Motivational intervention should be repeated every time an unmotivated patient visits the clinical setting.
   - Those who have previously failed are told that most people make repeated quit attempts before they are successful.

Modified from: Tobacco Use and Dependence Guideline Panel. Treating tobacco use and dependence: 2008 update. Rockville, MD: U.S. Department of Health and Human Services; 2008. Available at: http://www.ncbi.nlm.nih.gov/books/NBK63952/.

use.[34,35] Examples include increasing shortness of breath, development or worsening of COPD, exacerbation of asthma, loss of lung function, and/or elevated blood levels of carbon monoxide. Other negative consequences of smoking include increased risk of cancer, heart attack, and stroke.[34,35] For women who are pregnant or plan to become pregnant, smoking reduces the weight of newborn babies. Patients should be told that complete abstinence from smoking is required and that low-tar, low-nicotine, and other forms of tobacco do not eliminate risk.[34,35] As noted earlier, cigarette smoking is the primary cause of COPD, and smoking cessation is the most effective means of stopping the progression of the disease. **Figure 4-4** illustrates the loss of lung function (as assessed by FEV_1) over time in susceptible smokers, as well as the benefits of smoking cessation.

Following a review of the negative consequences of smoking, the clinician should then ask the patient to identify the most important *rewards* (positive consequences) he or she associates with quitting.[34,35] These may include improved overall health and physical condition, higher self-esteem, and improved overall appearance. Other benefits may include improved ability to taste food and improved sense of smell; improvement in the smell of the home, car, clothing, and breath; reduced wrinkling and aging of skin; and whiter teeth.[35] Some patients may value setting a good example for their children, reducing the chance their children will smoke or eliminating the negative health effects (and associated worry) of smoking on family and friends.

Roadblocks or barriers to success are then identified and discussed. These may include withdrawal symptoms, fear of failure, fear of weight gain, and depression. Other barriers to success may include the enjoyment of smoking, lack of family and social support, and being exposed to other smokers. Discussion and counseling should include methods to deal with these roadblocks.

The motivational intervention (the five R's) should be respectfully *repeated* at every patient visit. Motivational interviewing strategies may be effective. These generally include expressing empathy with the patient while pointing out discrepancies between the patient's behavior and expressed priorities, goals, ambitions, and fears regarding his or her own health and the impact of continuing to smoke on others. The respiratory care clinician should avoid conflict and maintain a supportive, but firm, approach regarding the need for the patient to quit smoking.

To summarize, tobacco dependence is a chronic disease that often requires repeated intervention and multiple attempts to quit. The respiratory care clinician should ask every patient if he or she uses tobacco, advise patients to quit, and assess the patient's willingness to make a quit attempt. For those patients willing to make a quit attempt, the clinician should assist in the quite attempt and arrange for follow-up. The respiratory care clinician should discuss the risks of continuing to smoke and the benefits of quitting. Successful smoking cessation programs include an individualized patient evaluation, patient-specific counseling and education, medication therapy, follow up and relapse prevention. According to Marlow and Stoller:

> one of the most effective behavioral interventions is advice from a healthcare professional; it seems not to matter whether the advice is from a doctor, respiratory therapist, nurse, or other clinician, so smoking cessation should be encouraged by multiple clinicians. However, since respiratory therapists interact with smokers frequently, we believe it is particularly important for respiratory therapists to show leadership in implementing smoking cessation.[34]

Inhalation of Illicit Drugs

Another widespread smoking problem in terms of lung disease is the use of marijuana. Similar to tobacco smoking, marijuana smoking is associated with the development of chronic cough, sputum production, wheeze, and an increase in pulmonary infections such as acute bronchitis.[41,42] Marijuana smoke contains carcinogens, although the link between marijuana smoking and cancer has not been established.[42] Cardiovascular effects of marijuana include increased heart rate, palpitations, arrhythmia, and an increased risk of heart attack in the first hour after use.[42]

The smoking of crack cocaine has been associated with the development of cough, dyspnea, hemoptysis, airway burns, and other acute respiratory symptoms. Cocaine intoxication may cause irritability, restlessness, anxiety, sweating, and even severe psychosis. Intranasal

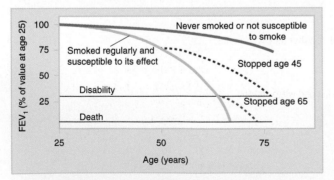

FIGURE 4-4 Decline in FEV₁ in susceptible smokers in comparison with a normal subject who has never smoked or a smoker who is not susceptible to the effects of smoking on lung function. Smoking cessation does not restore lost lung function in the susceptible smoker; however, it does reduce the rate of decline.

Reproduced from: 36 Tobacco Use and Dependence Guideline Panel. Treating Tobacco Use and Dependence: 2008 Update. Rockville (MD): US Department of Health and Human Services; 2008 May. http://www.ncbi.nlm.nih.gov/books /NBK63952/

use may cause problems with swallowing, hoarseness, and nosebleeds.[43] Cardiovascular effects associated with acute cocaine intoxication include tachycardia, elevated blood pressure, cardiac ischemia, substernal chest pain, and the possible development of a myocardial infarction.[43]

Because of the adverse health effects of smoking or inhaling illicit drugs, the respiratory care clinician should ask patients about drug use. If the patient admits using marijuana or cocaine, the clinician should inquire about the amount and frequency of drug use and describe the risks of continued use and the benefits of quitting. For those patients who are willing to try and quit, the clinician should offer assistance and follow-up care.

Occupational and Environmental History

A large number of lung diseases are associated with environmental conditions or specific occupations. Patients should be questioned regarding occupational exposure and environmental factors associated with the development of lung disease.

Environmental History

Geographic location, environmental exposure to contagious diseases, travel, and the home and work environment can all have an impact on the development and course of cardiopulmonary disease. School, work, and home environmental conditions that may affect health include the age, condition, and location of the home; cooling and heating systems; availability of safe places to exercise; and access to transportation, grocery shopping, healthcare, and work. In the context of asthma, questions regarding exposure to dust mites, cockroaches, pollen, pets, or animal danders may help to identify specific asthma triggers. Presence of molds or mildew, use of a wood-burning stove, use of a humidifier in the home, type of bedding used, stuffed furniture, carpeting over concrete, tobacco smoke, strong odors, and other irritants may all contribute as aggravating or precipitating factors for asthma exacerbation. Changes in the weather or exposure to cold air may also be precipitating factors for acute asthma.

Any recent environmental changes should be noted, such as a new job, moving to a new house, or a recent vacation that may expose the patient to things that precipitate or aggravate cardiopulmonary disease.

Travel History

Travel to or residence in undeveloped parts of the world or the tropics may result in exposure to infectious diseases that are less common in the United States. For example, typhoid fever is a serious health threat endemic to certain parts of Asia, Africa, and Latin America. Cases seen in the United States are usually travel-related. Typhoid fever is typically contracted from food or water contaminated with *Salmonella typhi* bacteria, although direct contact with an infected person can transmit the disease.[44] Signs and symptoms of typhoid fever include very high fever, fatigue and weakness, headache, sore throat, abdominal pain, rash, and diarrhea or constipation.[44] The most serious complication of typhoid fever is intestinal bleeding, which can lead to hypotension and shock.[44] The treatment of typhoid fever includes antibiotics and supportive care.[44]

Malaria is another severe and potentially fatal disease seen in many parts of the world, including sub-Saharan Africa, India, and South Asia. Malaria is caused by a protozoal parasite of the genus *Plasmodium* that is carried by the *Anopheles* mosquito and transmitted to people when bitten by an infected insect.[45] Travelers to areas where malaria is common should consider precautions, which may include taking an antimalarial drug as a preventative measure and use of mosquito repellent, protective clothing, and mosquito bed nets or sleeping in an air-conditioned or well-screened room.[45] Clinical manifestations of malaria include high fever and flulike symptoms, including cough, malaise, and shaking chills. Gastrointestinal symptoms may include nausea, vomiting, and diarrhea.[44] Neurologic symptoms may include headache, dizziness, confusion, disorientation, and coma.[44] The diagnosis of malaria can be confirmed by laboratory antigen testing, use of molecular diagnostic techniques, and examination of blood droplet smears for the presence of parasites using the Giemsa stain. Treatment of malaria includes administration of antimalarial medications such as chloroquine, quinine sulfate, hydroxychloroquine, mefloquine, or a combination of atovaquone and proguanil (Malarone). It is of interest to note that carriers for sickle cell disease (one sickle hemoglobin gene and one normal hemoglobin gene) have some resistance to malaria.[45] Because of this advantage, the number of sickle cell carriers in areas where malaria is endemic tends to be higher.[45]

Geographic Location

Some fungal lung diseases are endemic to certain geographic areas. For example, histoplasmosis is endemic to the Ohio and Mississippi River valleys. Histoplasmosis is caused by inhalation of airborne *Histoplasma capsulatum* spores, which are sometimes found where there are large deposits of bat or bird droppings. Most people infected are asymptomatic or develop only mild symptoms, whereas some patients will develop a self-limited pneumonia that generally resolves without treatment. Symptoms of respiratory infection include fever, chest pain, and dry, nonproductive cough.[46] Diagnosis is made based on the clinical picture and confirmed via fungal cultures (blood, sputum, bone marrow, liver, or skin), blood or urine testing for the presence of the antigen, or direct microscopic examination of infected tissue. Antifungal medications (itraconazole or amphotericin B) are used to treat severe cases of histoplasmosis.[46] Past infection can provide partial protection if a person becomes reinfected later in life.[46]

Blastomycosis is a fungal disease caused by *Blastomyces dermatitidis* that affects humans and animals, especially dogs. *Blastomyces dermatitidis* is endemic to the Ohio and Mississippi River valleys, although cases of blastomycosis have been reported in Canada and the Southeastern United States. *Blastomyces dermatitidis* most often causes skin disease, but it may also cause a self-limited pulmonary infection. Treatment is with amphotericin B or itraconazole for immunocompromised patients.[47]

Coccidioidomycosis is a fungal lung disease caused by *Coccidioides immitis*, which is prevalent in the San Joaquin valley of California and parts of New Mexico, Utah, and Texas. Coccidioidomycosis typically results in a self-limited respiratory infection or pneumonia; however it can cause pulmonary nodules, cavities, and overwhelming pneumonia in people more susceptible to this fungus.[47] Treatment of progressive or extrapulmonary coccidioidomycosis includes antifungal medications such as fluconazole, itraconazole, or amphotericin B.[47]

Cryptococcoses is another fungal lung disease caused by inhalation of airborne spores of the genus *Cryptococcus*. *C. neoformans* and *C. gattii* are the two most common causes of cryptococcoses.[48,49] *C. gattii* is found in tropical and subtropical regions of the world and in the U.S. Pacific Northwest, Vancouver Island, and mainland British Columbia.[48] *C. neoformans* is found in soil throughout the world.[49] *C. neoformans* infection typically causes meningitis in HIV and immunosuppressed persons, whereas *C. gattii* infections more often cause pneumonia in persons without immune defects.[47–49] Symptoms of pulmonary infection include shortness of breath, cough, and fever.[47–49] Diagnosis is made via use of the cryptococcal antigen test performed on blood or cerebrospinal fluid and by microscopic examination and culture of tissue or body fluids. Respiratory infection may be self-limited or a chronic pneumonia may occur. Mild or moderate cryptococcosis may be treated with fluconazole or itraconazole. Severe cryptococcal infections may require amphotericin B in combination with flucytosine. Fluconazole is also used for maintenance therapy in HIV patients with cryptococcal meningitis.

Hobbies and Pets

Hobbies and pets may also be associated with the development of certain types of lung disease. For example, bird fanciers, pet shop employees, and veterinarians may develop psittacosis (aka ornithosis or parrot fever), a bacterial infection associated with pet birds and poultry. Psittacosis can result in a severe pneumonia with complications that range from endocarditis to hepatitis and neurologic disease.[50,51] Psittacosis is caused by the *Chlamydophila psittaci* bacterium excreted in the feces and nasal discharges of infected parrots, parakeets, macaws, and cockatiels.[50,51] Other birds, including turkeys, ducks, doves, pigeons, birds of prey, and shore birds, may carry and transmit the bacteria to humans, and outbreaks of psittacosis in poultry processing plants have been reported.[50,51] Human infection typically occurs following inhalation of bacteria that have been aerosolized from dried feces or respiratory tract secretions of infected birds. Handling of infected birds and mouth-to-beak contact may also transmit the disease.[50] Symptoms of respiratory infection include fever, chills, dyspnea, dry cough, chest tightness, headache, muscle aches, and malaise. Chest radiograph may show pneumonia with lobar or interstitial infiltrates, and respiratory failure requiring intensive care may occur.[50] Diagnosis is based on the clinical presentation and confirmed by the presence of antibodies against *C. psittaci* using microimmunofluorescence (MIF) laboratory test methods.[50] The bacteria may also be cultured from sputum, pleural fluid, or blood, although technical and safety issues limit the availability of culture capability. Real-time polymerase chain reaction (rt-PCR) assays have recently been developed for the detection of *C. psittaci* in respiratory specimens.[50] Treatment consists of supportive care and administration of antibiotics (tetracycline or doxycycline).[50]

Pets may also play a significant role in poorly controlled asthma. Although any warm-blooded animal can produce antigens that worsen asthma, cat dander, house dust mite, and cockroach antigen are the three most common allergens that trigger an inflammatory response in asthmatic airways. A careful environmental history is very important in identifying triggers of persistent asthma.

Hobbies that may impact pulmonary disease include gardening, woodworking, and any hobby that involves working around dust or fumes. For example, woodworking and the inhalation of wood dust may be a causative factor in the development of occupational asthma, and asthma exacerbation can be triggered by wood dust inhalation, as well as the inhalation of sprays, paint fumes, or airborne chemicals or dusts from hobby activities.

Interstitial Lung Diseases

The interstitial lung diseases (ILDs) are a large group of lung diseases associated with chronic lung injury, inflammation, and the development of fibrosis (scar tissue in the lung). Many ILDs are associated with specific environmental or occupational exposures. For example, hypersensitivity pneumonitis is a form of ILD characterized by inflammation of the alveoli caused by a number of different organic materials found in the environment, including bird feathers, molds (moldy hay; aka "farmer's lung"), microbial antigens (mycobacteria avian complex; aka "hot tub lung"), proteins within flour (aka "baker's lung"), and numerous other organic antigens. Other occupational ILDs include the pneumoconises (inhalation of inorganic material), such as coal miners pneumoconiosis, silicosis, and asbestos (see occupational history below). Clinical findings with ILDs often include decreased oxygen saturation, especially upon exertion, crackles at the lung bases on auscultation, and a restrictive pattern on pulmonary function testing.

Occupational History

Occupational history should include occupation, current and previous jobs, working conditions, occupational exposure to dust or toxins, and military service.[27,28] Occupational lung disease can be caused by inhalation of inorganic dusts (silicates, carbon, metals), organic dusts (fungi, bacteria, animal proteins), chemicals, gases, fumes, vapors, or aerosols.[52] The patient should be asked if his or her symptoms are better or worse at home or at work or on weekends or work days. Exposure to aluminum, asbestosis, beryllium, sugar cane, cotton brac, barium, coal dust, moldy hay, clay, iron, silica dust, talc, and other substances are all associated with the development of lung disease.[52] The pneumoconioses (inorganic dust-induced lung disease) include coal worker's pneumoconiosis, asbestosis, silica-induced ILD, and berylliosis.[52] The pneumoconioses due to silica or asbestos exposure are less common today, due to various occupational safeguards now in place.[52] The development of occupational asthma has been associated with exposure to many substances, including animal-derived materials, plant and vegetable products, enzymes, chemicals (such as isocyanates used in plastic manufacture), drugs, wood dust, and metals. Granulomatous pneumonitis has been reported in lifeguards due to mold exposure at indoor swimming pools.[52] Diagnosis of occupational lung disease is based on a careful work history, physical examination, and laboratory testing, including pulmonary function testing. A list of occupations associated with specific lung disease is located in **Table 4-16**.

TABLE 4-16
Occupations Associated with Specific Lung Disease*

Lung Disease	Occupation	Lung Disease	Occupation
Aluminum pneumoconiosis	Ammunition maker Fireworks maker	Bagassosis	Sugar cane worker
		Byssinosis	Cotton flax or hemp mill worker
Asbestosis (associated with smoking)	Asbestos weaver Brake manufacturer Clutch manufacturer Filter maker Floor tile maker Insulator Lagger Mill worker Miner or miller Roofer Shipbuilder Steam fitter	Baritosis (barium)	Barite miller and miner Ceramics worker Fluorescent lamp maker Glassmaker Metallurgist Missile worker Neon sign maker Nuclear energy worker Phosphor maker Propellant manufacturer Toxicologist X-ray tube maker
Beryllium disease	Alloy maker Bronze maker Ceramics worker Demolition person Electronic tube maker Extraction worker Fettler Flame cutter Foundryman Grinder Metalworker Metalizer Polisher Scarfer	Coal workers' pneumoconiosis (Black Lung associated with smoking)	Coal miner Motorman Roof bolter Tipple worker Trimmer
		Interstitial lung disease (ILD)	Farm worker (associated with moldy hay)
		Kaolinosis (clay)	Brick maker Ceramics worker China maker Miner Potter

(continues)

TABLE 4-16
Occupations Associated with Specific Lung Disease* (continued)

Lung Disease	Occupation
Occupational asthma	Animal-derived materials
	Laboratory workers (medical labs, veterinarians)
	Breeders (birds, rabbits, other)
	Food processors (poultry, seafood)
	Plants and vegetable products
	Food processors
	Grain handlers
	Textile workers
	Bakers
	Printers
	Laxative manufacturers
	Enzymes, chemicals, and drugs
	Detergent manufacturers
	Food processors
	Pharmaceutical workers
	Printers
	Chemical workers
	Foam manufacturers
	Plastic workers
	Dye workers
	Farmers
	Hairdressers
	Hospital workers
	Food wrappers
	Wood dust
	Carpenters
	Woodworkers
	Aluminum soldering, metal plating, etc.
	Metal workers
Siderosis (iron)	Ship breaker
	Welder

Lung Disease	Occupation
Silicosis	Abrasives worker
	Bentonite mill worker
	Brick maker
	Ceramics worker
	Coal miner
	Diatomite worker
	Enameler
	Fettler
	Filter maker
	Foundryman
	Miner or miller
	Motorman
	Paint maker
	Polisher
	Quarry man
	Sandblaster
	Shotblaster
	Stonecutter
	Stone driller
	Well driller
Talcosis (certain talcs)	Ceramics worker
	Cosmetics worker
	Miner or miller
	Papermaker
	Plastics worker
	Rubber worker

*Most pneumoconiosis (dust-caused disease) results in scar tissue formation in the lung (fibrotic lung disease). Important exceptions are bagassosis, byssinosis, and farmers' lung. The latter disorders are thought to be related to an immune or allergic response to an irritant.
Data from: Shelledy DC, Mikles SP. Patient assessment and respiratory care plan development. In: Mishoe SC and Welch MA, eds. *Critical thinking in respiratory care: a problem based approach.* New York: McGraw-Hill;2002:181–234

Current Medications

All current medications should be recorded as part of a complete history. Use of nasal decongestants, antihistamines, expectorants, and cough and cold medications are important to record. Antibiotics, pulmonary drugs (bronchodilators, steroids; see below), cardiac drugs, antihypertensive medications, and diuretic use should be identified. β-blockers and ACE inhibitors are used to control hypertension and in the treatment of CHF. β-blockers can exacerbate bronchospasm; ACE inhibitors can cause cough. Alpha-1 proteinase inhibitor medications (Prolastin, Bayer, West Haven, Connecticut; and Zemaira, CSL Behring, King of Prussia, Pennsylvania) are used to treat a genetic protein deficiency (alpha-1 antitrypsin deficiency), which is a cause of severe panacinar emphysema. Nicotine replacement therapy (transdermal patch, gum, or nasal spray) and other medications (e.g., bupropion, varenicline tartrate) taken as a part of a smoking cessation program should also be noted. Aspirin, NSAIDs such as ibuprofen, β-blockers (also found in some eye drops), and sulfites used in foods as a preservative all may precipitate or aggravate asthma.[13]

Medications taken for pain, anxiety, or sleep should be noted, especially those that are CNS depressants. Psychotherapeutic agents taken should also be recorded. Vaccination status should be reviewed to include whether the patient has received the pneumococcal vaccine, flu vaccine, and other immunizations (see Figure 4-2). Vitamins and any herbal or other complementary therapy should also be noted.

Current Respiratory Care

Current and previous respiratory care received should be noted. Current or past use of oxygen therapy should be carefully documented, both use in the hospital and in the home or extended care facility. Oxygen concentration, flow, device used, and use pattern (continuous, intermittent, during exercise, etc.) should be noted. The respiratory care clinician should also inquire about the use of bronchodilators, anti-inflammatory agents (e.g., inhaled corticosteroids), and antiasthmatic agents (e.g., cromolyn, nedocromil, zafirlukast, zileuton). In asthma, the frequency of use of short-acting bronchodilators and the need for oral corticosteroids and frequency of use should be determined. Emergency department or hospital admissions should be explored and a history of endotracheal intubation, tracheotomy, and/or receipt of mechanical ventilatory support should be noted. For example, asthmatics with a history of intubation, mechanical ventilation, heavy use of short-acting bronchodilators, or use of systemic steroids are at much greater risk for death from asthma.[13] Other respiratory care received may include mucolytics (e.g., acetylcysteine, dornase alpha, guaifenesin) or aerosolized anti-infective agents (e.g., pentamidine, ribavirin, antibiotics). Home equipment, such as nebulizers, oxygen equipment, CPAP/BiPAP equipment, or any mechanical ventilatory support devices used in the home should also be noted.

Exercise Tolerance

Any deficit in the patient's ability to participate in the normal ADLs should be noted. For example, does the patient have difficulty dressing, bathing, doing household chores, walking, or shopping due to shortness of breath? Can the patient walk on the level, climb stairs, or participate in more vigorous exercise, such as using a treadmill or bicycle ergometer? Is the patient's health status adequate for participation in sports? For children or younger adults, a preparticipation physical evaluation (PPE) may be required that includes evaluation of possible cardiac, respiratory, neurologic, vision-related, orthopedic, or psychosocial problems that may limit participation in certain sports.

Nutritional Status

Good nutrition is essential to optimizing a patient's health. The patient history should include eating habits, usual calorie intake, and types of foods consumed to include fat, protein, and carbohydrates in the diet. Patient access to healthy foods should be assessed to include adequate income to purchase food and the ability to shop, prepare, and store healthy foods. Use of vitamin, mineral, and herbal supplements should be noted, as well as use of any liquid or powder nutrition supplements.

Recent weight loss or gain should be documented and include intentional weight loss through dieting. Unintentional weight loss should be noted to include the total weight lost, time period, whether the loss was sudden or gradual, and any associated symptoms, such as loss of appetite, difficulty in swallowing,

vomiting, diarrhea, or anxiety and stress. Acute illness, such as fever, burns, trauma, or cancer may markedly increase metabolic rate and nutritional requirements. Medications that may affect nutritional status and body weight include laxatives, appetite suppressants, fat-blockers, and chemotherapy. Eating disorders such as anorexia and bulimia may also have a profound effect on nutritional status.

Obesity is a major health problem in the United States, and measurement of the patient's height and weight can be used to calculate the body mass index (BMI). A BMI ≥ 25–29.9 indicates the patient is overweight, and a BMI ≥ 30 indicates obesity. Waist-to-hip circumference ratio is a measure of central body fat distribution. Ratios > 1.0 in men and > 0.85 in women indicate a high level of central fat with associated obesity-related health risks. Overweight and obese people are at increased risk for the development of heart disease, hypertension, stroke, sleep apnea, type 2 diabetes, cancer, liver and gallbladder disease, osteoarthritis, and dyslipidemia (i.e., high total cholesterol, high triglycerides). Patients should be advised of the benefits of good nutrition and the health hazards of being overweight or obese. The U.S. Department of Agriculture provides a website for consumers and health professionals to assist in development of a healthy diet (see http://www.choosemyplate.gov).

Advance Directives

Advance directives provide patients with a mechanism to indicate the types of end-of-life care they would prefer to receive if they are unable to communicate in the presence of a catastrophic illness. *Living wills* are one type of advance directive in which patients indicate whether they wish to be resuscitated in the event of a cardiac or respiratory arrest, as well as their preferences regarding such things as being placed on a ventilator, tube-feedings, dialysis, and/or organ donation. A *durable power of attorney for medical decisions* provides a mechanism for patients to name a spouse, friend, or relative to make healthcare decisions in the event they are unable to do so themselves. Both living wills and durable power of attorney are legal documents in most states in the United States. A *do not resuscitate* (**DNR**) order is another form of advance directive in which the patient (or family) indicates in advance whether the patient should receive cardiopulmonary resuscitation (CPR) and advanced life support in the event of a cardiac or respiratory arrest. DNR orders apply in all U.S. states. The respiratory care clinician often is called to administer CPR and advanced life support in the event of a cardiopulmonary arrest and often is asked to provide mechanical ventilatory support. Consequently, the clinician should inquire about and be aware of any advance directives in place.

The Patient's Learning Needs

Patient education provides patients with the knowledge and skills needed to understand and participate in meeting their healthcare needs. Patients' learning needs may range from knowledge of their medical condition to information on their medications, therapy, equipment, and treatment plans. Other learning needs may include personal care, hygiene, diet and nutrition, exercise, and pain management. Respiratory care learning needs may include use of aerosolized medications, cough and bronchial hygiene techniques, smoking cessation, and/or pulmonary rehabilitation. Asthma patients may need to learn about asthma triggers, use of asthma action plans, and how to measure and monitor symptoms and peak flow. Health maintenance, disease prevention, and chronic disease management may need to be addressed with the patient. The patient may also need assistance with discharge planning, follow-up care, and availability of health resources. Barriers to patient education may include limited education, lack of prior knowledge, poor health literacy, a lack of motivation, poor reading or language skills, cultural factors, cognitive limitations, or emotional issues.

Most patients, particularly those with chronic disease, need to be able to perform some level of self-care to optimize their health. To do this, they need to have a basic understanding of their disease state or condition and why specific treatments, medications, or other interventions are prescribed. They should understand what medications they are taking, how often and when to take the medications, and be able to recognize side effects and know what to do in the event of an adverse reaction to the medication. Other important learning needs include ensuring that patients know what is wrong with them, when to seek help, what things they are allowed to do (and not do), what their treatment is, and when they should begin to feel better. Information provided to patients should be appropriate for their age, education level, cognitive skills, and native language.

Health-Related Quality of Life Questionnaires

Health can be defined as "a state of complete physical, mental, and social well-being and not merely the absence of disease."[53] **Health-related quality of life (HRQOL)** is determined by a number of factors, including physical, social, emotional, and cognitive functioning; pain and discomfort; vitality; and a person's overall sense of well-being (aka the seven domains of health, see **Box 4-17**). In order to quantify HRQOL, a number of general health status questionnaires have been developed. Perhaps the best known are the Medical Outcomes Study (MOS) Short Form (SF) Health Survey family of questionnaires (the SF-36, SF-12, SF-8). The SF-36 is a 36-question survey that asks patients questions related to their health status in all of the major health domains except cognitive function. The SF-36 has excellent validity and reliability, is easy and fast to administer (taking 5 to 10 minutes to complete), and can be used to assess individual patient progress following health interventions, such as a pulmonary rehabilitation program. The SF-36 is also an excellent tool for health outcomes research. The SF-8 is an abbreviated eight-question version of the SF-36 better suited for large population studies. Similar to the SF-36, the SF-8 asks the patient to rate his or her health status using

---

BOX 4-17

Seven Domains of Health

The seven domains of health have a direct impact on health-related quality of life (HRQOL).

1. *Physical functioning*: Range of motion of limbs, feeding and bathing, walking, shopping and cleaning.
2. *Social functioning*: Visits with friends and family, restrictions on working, ability to babysit grandchildren.
3. *Emotional functioning*: Feeling depressed or psychologically distressed, feeling happy.
4. *Cognitive functioning*: Problems remembering important dates or events, awareness of current time and place.
5. *Pain/discomfort*: Feeling bodily pain when getting out of bed, feeling aches when lifting light objects, itching.
6. *Vitality:* Lacking energy, feeling tired, needing to nap frequently.
7. *Overall well-being*: Feeling satisfied with overall health, feeling content in general.

Modified from: Kane RL. *Understanding Health Care Outcomes Research.* Gaithersburg, MD: Aspen; 1997.

the rating scales provided on the following questions (see also http://www.sf-36.org/demos/SF-8.html):

1. Overall, how would you rate your health in the past 4 weeks?
2. How much did physical health problems limit your usual physical activities (such as walking or climbing stairs)?
3. How much difficulty did you have doing your daily work, both at home and away from home, because of your physical health?
4. How much *bodily* pain have you had?
5. How much energy did you have?
6. How much did your physical health or emotional problems limit your usual social activities with family or friends?
7. How much have you been bothered by emotional problems (such as feeling anxious, depressed, or irritable)?
8. How much did personal or emotional problems keep you from doing your usual work, school, or other daily activities?

The SF-36, SF-12, and SF-8 allow for calculation of scores for four physical health domains (physical functioning, role functioning/physical, bodily pain, general health perceptions) and four mental health domains (vitality, social functioning, role functioning/emotional, mental health). The results are then used to calculate a physical component summary score (PCS) and a mental component summary (MCS) score. For more information about the SF surveys, visit the SF website (http://www.SF-36.org). Other general health status surveys include the Sickness Impact Profile (SIP), the Nottingham Health Profile (NHP), the Duke-University of North Carolina Health Profile (DUHP), the Quality of Well-Being Scale (QWB), the Dartmouth COOP Charts, and the Patient Reported Outcomes Measurement Information System (PROMIS).

A number of disease-specific health-status questionnaires are also available. Two of particular interest to the respiratory care clinician are the Chronic Respiratory Disease Questionnaire (CRQ) and the St. George's Respiratory Questionnaire (SGRQ).[54,55] The CRQ includes questions to assess dyspnea, fatigue, emotional function, and mastery (i.e., feeling control over the disease) and allows for calculation of a summary score.[54] Both the CRQ and SGRQ have good validity and reliability and can be used to assess HRQOL in patients with respiratory disease.[54,55] The CRQ may be the instrument of choice for the COPD patient, whereas the SGRQ has been used successfully to assess HRQOL in patients with asthma, COPD, cystic fibrosis, bronchiectasis, kyphoscoliosis, and sarcoidosis.[54,55] Disease-specific quality-of-life questionnaires such as the Asthma Quality of Life Questionnaire (AQoLQ) have been designed and validated for several pulmonary diseases.

Review of Symptoms

After taking a complete patient history, the respiratory care clinician should develop a problem list for the patient based on a review of the symptoms noted during the patient history. A review of the medical history is often organized by body system:

- *General symptoms*: Problems that may be related to pulmonary or cardiac/cardiovascular disease may include fever, chills, malaise, fatigue, lethargy, night sweats, and weight problems (obesity, underweight, and/or weight loss).
- *Skin and nails*: The respiratory care clinician should note the color, temperature, and appearance of the skin and nails. Problems include pale skin and if the skin is cold or clammy; these findings may be associated with low cardiac output, shock, or other circulatory problems. Very warm skin may be associated with fever or overheating. Rash, redness, or itching may indicate an allergic reaction. Excessive sweating may indicate distress. Cyanosis of the skin, lips, or nails is associated with more than 5 g of desaturated hemoglobin and associated hypoxemia.
- *Head, eyes, ears, nose, and throat (HEENT)*: Problems to note include:
  - *Head:* Frequent or unusual headaches, dizziness, fainting, head injury, loss of consciousness, concussion.
  - *Eyes:* Blurred vision, diplopia (double vision), conjunctivitis, eye disease or blindness, use of glasses or contact lenses, pupils (dilated, contracted, or fixed).
  - *Ears:* Pain, hearing loss, pain, vertigo, tinnitus (ringing in the ears).
  - *Nose*: Sinus pain, colds, nasal obstruction or runny nose, sneezing, nasal flaring, postnasal drip, nosebleeds
  - *Throat:* Hoarseness, voice change, sore throat, tooth pain or abscess, throat sores or ulcers, bleeding or swelling of gums, appearance of mucous membranes (color, cyanosis), bad taste in mouth.
- *Endocrine:* The clinician should note problems such as thyroid enlargement or tenderness. Diabetes or pregnancy should also be noted.
- *Respiratory*: The clinician should note any of the following problems:
  - Respiratory symptoms, including cough; sputum production; hemoptysis; dyspnea; orthopnea; wheezing, whistling or chest tightness; chest pain; exposure to infection (TB, etc.); night sweats; or use of accessory muscles.
  - Chest discomfort or pain or other abnormalities such as trauma, surgical scars, rib fractures, or chest deformity.

- Any history of asthma, COPD, pneumonia, or other pulmonary disease.
- *Cardiac/cardiovascular:* The clinician should note any chest pain or discomfort, palpitations, dyspnea, orthopnea, exercise tolerance, and past tests done (ECG, other cardiac tests).
  - *Peripheral vasculature:* Thrombophlebitis may result in pulmonary embolus and should be noted. Peripheral edema (ankle swelling, other) is often seen in patients with CHF and fluid overload.
  - A history or cardiac problems (MI, CHF, other) or high blood pressure should be noted.
- *Hematologic.* Problems may include anemia, bleeding, and blood loss. Bruising may be caused by trauma or problems with clotting. Elevated hemoglobin levels (polycythemia) are associated with chronic hypoxia or living at altitude.
- *Lymph nodes:* The clinician should note if the lymph nodes are tender, swollen, or enlarged.
- *Gastrointestinal (GI):* The clinician should note any problems with diet, appetite, digestion, food problems or restrictions, and any food allergies. Use of caffeine and/or alcohol should be noted. Other problems to note include heartburn, nausea, vomiting, or diarrhea. Additional GI problems include constipation, blood in the stool, stomach ulcers, esophagitis (associated with painful swallowing, heartburn), esophageal varices (dilated veins in the lower esophagus), and cancer.
- *Genitourinary:* The clinician should note any problems with urination or urine output.
- *Musculoskeletal:* Problems to note include joint stiffness or pain, swelling, fractures, or trauma or restrictions to motion.
- *Neurologic and mental status*: Problems that should be noted include headache, disorientation, excitement, fainting, dizziness, confusion, somnolence, loss of consciousness, or coma. Weakness, tremors, seizures, convulsions, or paralysis should be noted. Mental health issues should also be noted, including depression, restlessness, anxiety, mood swings, or sleep disturbances.

Timing of Signs and Symptoms

Triggers that bring on a symptom, things that improve the symptom, and other temporal aspects of a patient's symptoms, such as the rate of onset, may allow the respiratory care clinician to identify or clarify the likely cause. For example, occupational asthma may first become noticeable at the beginning of the work week. Symptoms may steadily worsen over the course of the work week and remit during time off work.[56] Many cardiopulmonary related problems worsen at night, often due to sleeping in a supine position. Problems that sometimes worsen at night include the dyspnea

associated with COPD or CHF and some cases of asthma. Postnasal drip and gastroesophageal reflux may also worsen at night in the supine posture.

The rate of change of signs and symptoms over time can also be helpful diagnostic features. For example, chronic bronchitis is defined by the chronic nature of associated symptoms. Specifically, chronic bronchitis is defined as a chronic cough with phlegm production that occurs daily for at least 3 months of the year in at least 2 consecutive years. Asthma is typically characterized by intermittent symptoms, and the asthmatic patient often has "good days" and "bad days."[56] In contrast, dyspnea that consistently progresses over the course of months to years is more characteristic of a parenchymal lung disease, such as idiopathic pulmonary fibrosis. Pulmonary hypertension also generally progresses over the course of months to years.[56]

Digital clubbing provides another example related to symptom timing. Clubbing may be caused by many conditions, including bronchiectasis, interstitial lung diseases (e.g., pulmonary fibrosis), congenital cyanotic heart disease, chronic liver disease (e.g., cirrhosis), inflammatory bowel disease, and hypothyroidism as a familial trait or as a complication of many malignancies, including lung cancer.[56] Lung cancer is described by cell type and includes adenocarcinoma, squamous cell cancer, non-small cell cancer, and small cell cancer.[56] Clubbing is thought to be rare with small cell cancer. This may be due to the generally aggressive, rapid time course of small cell carcinoma, which would not allow digital clubbing to develop. To summarize, timing of the patient's symptoms may provide valuable diagnostic clues. Following a complete pulmonary history, the respiratory care clinician should be able to describe the patient's symptoms in terms of onset, duration, and timing:

1. At what time of day (week, season, or year) does the symptom occur?
2. Does anything seem to trigger the symptom?
3. How does the symptom change over time?
4. Does the symptom steadily get worse?
5. Does the symptom come and go, with some "good days" and some "bad days"?
6. Does anything seem to relieve the symptom or make it better?

Summary

To summarize, the pulmonary history should gather information regarding the patient's cough and sputum production; wheezing, whistling, and chest tightness; breathlessness; and past chest illness. The respiratory care clinician should note the patient's smoking history, occupational history, and environmental history. Commonly identified respiratory problems include shortness of breath, cough, sputum production, and hemoptysis. Other possible problems might include chest pain, restlessness, nervousness, excitement, tremors, headache, palpitations, disorientation, dizziness, headache, blurred vision, daytime sleepiness, fatigue, or confusion. Each problem should be described in some detail as to the nature, onset, location, and progression over time. After writing the problem list, a list of diseases or conditions that produce these symptoms is developed. This list generates the initial hypotheses that can then guide the subsequent physical examination and laboratory studies.

For example, the symptoms of shortness of breath, cough, sputum production, and fever may generate the hypothesis that these problems are caused by a respiratory tract infection. While performing the physical examination, the respiratory care clinician should specifically look for signs that can help evaluate this hypothesis, such as increased respiratory rate, other signs of hypoxemia, or abnormal findings on chest examination.

Key Points

▶ The patient interview follows the review of the patient medical record and is the next step in identifying and/or clarifying the diagnosis and problem list.

▶ The patient interview is essential for respiratory care plan development, implementation, and evaluation.

▶ The interview should establish rapport, gather information, obtain feedback, involve the family, demonstrate understanding, and provide for assessment.

▶ The interview should assess cough; sputum production; hemoptysis; wheezing, whistling, or chest tightness; dyspnea; past history of chest illness; smoking history; occupation; and, where appropriate, hobby and leisure activities.

▶ Current medications, use of home oxygen or other respiratory care equipment, and history of previous episodes requiring intubation or mechanical ventilatory support should be assessed.

▶ The interview should assess the benefits of care received and any adverse effects or complications.

▶ The chief complaint is a concise statement of the reason for seeking medical attention.

▶ The history of the present illness (HPI) describes the symptoms, chronology of events, and impact on the patient of the current illness or problem.

▶ Cough is one of the most common symptoms for which medical care is sought.

▶ Common causes of cough include infection, postnasal drip, GERD, asthma, and other chronic lung diseases.

▶ Sputum volume, color, consistency, and odor should be assessed.

▶ Causes of hemoptysis include bronchitis, tuberculosis, lung cancer, pneumonia, bronchiectasis, lung abscess, cystic fibrosis, and pulmonary embolus/infarction.

▶ Causes of wheezing include asthma, obstruction, bronchospasm, and tumor.

▶ Types of chest pain include substernal, pleuritic, and musculoskeletal chest pain.

▶ Dyspnea may be quantified using the Borg scale or the VAS, MMRC, or SOBQ assessment tools.

▶ Sleep-related disorders include central and obstructive sleep apnea.

▶ A history of intubation, ICU admission, multiple hospital admissions, elevated bronchodilator use, or use of systemic steroids indicates a higher risk of mortality in asthmatic patients.

▶ The 5 A's of smoking cessation are *ask, advise, assess, assist,* and *arrange.*

▶ Environmental history should assess location, exposure to contagious diseases, travel, and the home, school, and work environments.

▶ Occupational history should include occupation, current and previous jobs, working conditions, occupational exposure to dust or toxins, and military service.

▶ All current medications and current respiratory care should be recorded as part of a complete history.

▶ The patient's exercise tolerance, nutritional status, and learning needs should be assessed.

▶ Advanced directives, including DNR status, should be noted.

▶ HRQOL questionnaires include the SF-36, SGRQ, and CRQ.

▶ Review of symptoms should include general symptoms and symptoms related to each body system: skin and nails, HEENT, endocrine, respiratory/chest, cardiac/cardiovascular, peripheral vasculature, hematologic, lymph nodes, gastrointestinal, genitourinary, musculoskeletal, and neurologic, as well as mental status.

References

1. Wilkins RL. The medical history and the interview. In: Wilkins RL, Dexter JR, Heuer AJ (eds.). *Clinical Assessment in Respiratory Care,* 6th ed. St. Louis, MO: Mosby-Elsevier; 2010: 10–27.
2. Casserly B, Rounds S. General approach to patients with respiratory disorders. In: Andreoli TE, Benjamen IJ, Griggs RC, Wing EJ, Fitz, G (eds.). *Andreoli and Carpenter's Cecil Essentials of Medicine,* 8th ed. Philadelphia: Saunders-Elsevier; 2010: 192–197.
3. Gardner D, Wilkins RL. Cardiopulmonary symptoms. In: Wilkins RL, Dexter JR, Heuer AJ (eds.). *Clinical Assessment in Respiratory Care,* 6th ed. St. Louis, MO: Mosby-Elsevier; 2010: 28–50.
4. Wenzel RP, Fowler AA 3rd. Clinical practice: acute bronchitis. *N Engl J Med.* 2006;355(20):2125–2130.
5. PubMed Health. Gastroesophageal reflux disease. A.D.A.M. Medical Encyclopedia, 2011. http://www.ncbi.nlm.nih.gov/pubmedhealth/PMH0001311/. Accessed May 15, 2012.

6. Ashcroft T. Daily variations in sputum volume in chronic bronchitis. *Br Med J.* 1965;1(5430):288–290.

7. Johnson AL, Hampson DF, Hampson NB. Sputum color: potential implications for clinical practice. *Resp Care.* 2008;53(4):450–454.

8. Mandell LA, Wunderink RG, Anzueto A, et al. Infectious Diseases Society of America/American Thoracic Society consensus guidelines on the management of community-acquired pneumonia in adults. *Clin Infect Dis.* 2007;44(Suppl 2):S27–S72.

9. American Thoracic Society; Infectious Diseases Society of America. Guidelines for the management of adults with hospital-acquired, ventilator-associated, and healthcare-associated pneumonia. *Am J Respir Crit Care Med.* 2005;171(4):388–416.

10. Mukerji V. Dyspnea, orthopnea, and paroxysmal nocturnal dyspnea. In: Walker HK, Hall WD, Hurst JW (eds.). *Clinical Methods: The History, Physical, and Laboratory Examinations*, 3rd ed. Boston: Butterworths; 1990: 78–80.

11. Haponik EF, Fein A, Chin R. Managing life-threatening hemoptysis: has anything really changed? *Chest.* 2000;118(5):1431–1435.

12. Jankowich MD. Obstructive lung diseases. In: Andreoli TE, Benjamen IJ, Griggs RC, Wing EJ, Fitz, G (eds.). *Andreoli and Carpenter's Cecil Essentials of Medicine*, 8th ed. Philadelphia: Saunders-Elsevier; 2010: 213–224.

13. National Institutes of Health, National Heart, Lung, and Blood Institute Guidelines for the Diagnosis and Management of Asthma: Expert Panel 3 Report. (NIH publication). Bethesda, MD: US Department of Health and Human Services; 2007.

14. Irwin RS, Barnes PJ, Hollingsworth H. Diagnosis of wheezing illnesses other than asthma in adults. In: UpToDate, Barnes, PJ (ed.), UpToDate, Waltham, MA, 2012.

15. Parshall MB, Schwartzstein RM, Adams L, et al. An official American Thoracic Society statement: update on the mechanisms, assessment, and management of dyspnea. *Am J Respir Crit Care Med.* 2012;185(4):435–452.

16. Meisel JL. Diagnostic approach to chest pain in adults. In: UpToDate, Aronson MD, Rind DM (eds), UpToDate, Waltham, MA, 2012.

17. McCord J, Jneid H, Hollander JE, et al. Management of cocaine-associated chest pain and myocardial infarction a scientific statement from the American Heart Association Acute Cardiac Care Committee of the Council on Clinical Cardiology. *Circulation.* 2008;117:1897–1907.

18. Thygesen K, Alpert JS, White HD. Universal definition of myocardial infarction. *Circulation.* 2007;116:2634–2653.

19. Faxon, DP. Development of systems of care for ST-elevation myocardial infarction patients. *Circulation.* 2007;116:e29–e32.

20. Schwartzstein RM. Approach to the patient with dyspnea. In: UpToDate, King TE, Holingsworth H (eds.), UpToDate, Waltham, MA, 2012.

21. Celli BR, Cote CG, Lareau SC, Meek PM. Predictors of survival in COPD: more than just the FEV_1. *Respir Med.* 2008;102(Suppl 1):S27–S35.

22. Celli BR, Cote CG, Marin JM, et al. The body-mass index, airflow obstruction, dyspnea, and exercise capacity index in chronic obstructive pulmonary disease. *N Engl J Med.* 2004;350(10):1005–1012.

23. Hossain JL, Shapiro CM. The prevalence, cost implications, and management of sleep disorders: an overview. *Sleep Breath.* 2002;6(2):85–102.

24. Young T, Palta M, Dempsey J, Skatrud J, Weber S, Badr S. The occurrence of sleep-disordered breathing among middle-aged adults. *N Engl J Med.* 1993;328:1230–1235.

25. Gleeson K, Eggli DF, Maxwell SL. Quantitative aspiration during sleep in normal subjects. *Chest.* 1997;111(5):1266–1272.

26. Mukerji V. Dyspnea, orthopnea, and paroxysmal nocturnal dyspnea. In: Walker HK, Hall WD, Hurst JW (eds.). *Clinical Methods: The History, Physical, and Laboratory Examinations*, 3rd ed. Boston: Butterworth; 1990: 78–80.

27. Recording information. In: Seidel HM, Ball JW, Dains JE, Flynn JA, Solomon BS, Stewart RW (eds.). *Mosby's Guide to Physical Examination*, 7th ed. St. Louis, MO: Mosby-Elsevier; 2011: 792–814.

28. Partnership with patients: building a history. In: Seidel HM, Ball JW, Dains JE, Flynn JA, Solomon BS, Stewart RW (eds.). *Mosby's Guide to Physical Examination*, 7th ed. St. Louis, MO: Mosby-Elsevier; 2011: 13.

29. Lang RA, Hillis LD. Alcohol and substance abuse. In: Andreoli TE, Benjamen IJ, Griggs RC, Wing EJ, Fitz, G (eds.). *Andreoli and Carpenter's Cecil Essentials of Medicine*, 8th ed. Philadelphia: Saunders-Elsevier; 2010: 1220–1233.

30. National Institutes of Health, Department of Health & Human Services; U.S. National Library of Medicine. The reports of the surgeon general: the 1964 report on smoking and health. http://profiles.nlm.nih.gov/ps/retrieve/Narrative/NN/p-nid/60. Accessed June 8, 2012.

31. Centers for Disease Control and Prevention. Vital signs: current cigarette smoking among adults aged ≥ 18 Years—United States, 2005–2010. *MMWR Morb Mortal Wkly Rep.* 2011;60(35):1207–1212.

32. Jankowich MD. Obstructive lung diseases. In: Andreoli TE, Benjamen IJ, Griggs RC, Wing EJ, Fitz, G (eds.). *Andreoli and Carpenter's Cecil Essentials of Medicine*, 8th ed. Philadelphia: Saunders-Elsevier; 2010: 213–224.

33. Centers for Disease Control and Prevention; Office on Smoking and Health; National Center for Chronic Disease Prevention and Health Promotion. Smoking cessation and interventions fact sheet. Updated 2011. http://www.cdc.gov/tobacco/data_statistics/fact_sheets/cessation/quitting/index.htm. Accessed July 23, 2012.

34. Marlow SP, Stoller JK. Smoking cessation. *Respir Care.* 2003;48(12):1238–1254.

35. Fiore MC, Jaén CR, Baker TB, et al. Treating tobacco use and dependence: 2008 update. Clinical Practice Guideline. Rockville, MD: U.S. Department of Health and Human Services. Public Health Service. http://www.surgeongeneral.gov/tobacco/treating_tobacco_use08.pdf. Accessed February 16, 2011.

36. Hendrick B. Computer is an ally in quit-smoking fight: study shows web- and computer-based programs help smokers quit. WebMD Health News. http://www.webmd.com/smoking-cessation/news/20090526/computer-is-an-ally-in-quit-smoking-fight. Accessed February 21, 2011.

37. Myung SK, McDonnell DD, Kazinets G, Seo HG, Moskowitz JM. Effects of web- and computer-based smoking cessation programs: meta-analysis of randomized controlled trials. *Arch Intern Med.* 2009;169(10):929–937.

38. Civljak M, Sheikh A, Stead LF, Car J. Internet-based interventions for smoking cessation. *Cochrane Database Syst Rev.* 2010;(9).

39. Hutton HE, Wilson LM, Apelberg BJ, et al. A systematic review of randomized controlled trials: web-based interventions for smoking cessation among adolescents, college students, and adults. *Nicotine Tob Res.* 2011;13(4):227–238.

40. Centers for Disease Control and Prevention. Quitting smoking among adults—United States, 2001–2010. *MMWR Morb Mortal Wkly Rep.* 2011;60(44):1513–1519. http://www.cdc.gov/tobacco/data_statistics/mmwrs/byyear/2011/mm6044a2/intro.htm. Accessed November 10, 2011.

41. Tashkin DP, Coulson AH, Clark VA, et al. Respiratory symptoms and lung function in habitual heavy smokers of marijuana alone, smokers of marijuana and tobacco, smokers of tobacco alone, and nonsmokers. *Am Rev Respir Dis.* 1987;135(1):209–216.

42. National Institutes of Health, National Institute on Drug Abuse. Drug facts: marijuana. Revised November 2010. http://www.drugabuse.gov/publications/drugfacts/marijuana. Accessed July 23, 2012.

43. National Institutes of Health, National Institute on Drug Abuse. Drug facts: cocaine. Revised November 2010. http://www.drugabuse.gov/publications/drugfacts/cocaine. Accessed July 23, 2012.

44. Mayo Clinic. Typhoid fever. April 9, 2010. http://www.mayoclinic.com/health/typhoid-fever/DS00538. Accessed July 23, 2012.

45. Centers for Disease Control and Prevention; Global Health–Division of Parasitic Diseases. About malaria. Updated 2010. http://www.cdc.gov/malaria/about/index.html. Accessed July 23, 2012.

46. Centers for Disease Control and Prevention; National Center for Emerging and Zoonotic Infectious Diseases; Division of Foodborne, Waterborne, and Environmental Diseases. Histoplasmosis. Updated 2012. http://www.cdc.gov/fungal/histoplasmosis/. Accessed July 23, 2012.

47. Rodriguez B, Lederman MM. Organisms that infect humans. In: Andreoli TE, Benjamen IJ, Griggs RC, Wing EJ, Fitz, G (eds.). *Andreoli and Carpenter's Cecil Essentials of Medicine*, 8th ed. Philadelphia: Saunders-Elsevier; 2010: 884–897.

48. Centers for Disease Control and Prevention. Definition of *C. gattii* cryptococcosis. http://www.cdc.gov/fungal/cryptococcosis-gattii/definition.html. Accessed July 23, 2012.

49. Centers for Disease Control and Prevention. *C. neoformans* cryptococcosis. http://www.cdc.gov/fungal/cryptococcosis-neoformans/. Accessed July 23, 2012.

50. Smith KA, Campbell CT, Murphy J, Stobierski MG, Tengelsen LA. Compendium of measures to control *Chlamydophila psittaci* infection among humans (psittacosis) and pet birds (avian chlamydiosis), 2010 National Association of State Public Health Veterinarians (NASPHV). http://www.nasphv.org/Documents/Psittacosis.pdf. Accessed July 23, 2012.

51. Centers for Disease Control and Prevention. Psittacosis. Disease listing. 2009. http://www.cdc.gov/ncidod/dbmd/diseaseinfo/psittacosis_t.htm. Accessed July 23, 2012.

52. Aliotta JM, Jankowich MD. Interstitial lung diseases. In: Andreoli TE, Benjamen IJ, Griggs RC, Wing EJ, Fitz, G (eds.). *Andreoli and Carpenter's Cecil Essentials of Medicine*, 8th ed. Philadelphia: Saunders-Elsevier; 2010: 225–240.

53. Preamble to the Constitution of the World Health Organization as adopted by the International Health Conference, New York, June 19–22, 1946; signed on July 22 1946 by the representatives of 61 States (Official Records of the World Health Organization, no. 2, p. 100) and entered into force on 7 April 1948. World Health Organization (WHO) Definition of Health. www.who.int/about/definition/en/print.html.

54. Chauvin A, Rupley L, Meyers K, Johnson K, Eason J. Outcomes in cardiopulmonary physical therapy: chronic respiratory disease questionnaire (CRQ). *Cardiopulm Phys Ther J*. 2008;19(2):61–67.

55. Jones PW, Forde Y; St. George's University of London. St. George's respiratory questionnaire manual, version 2.3. June 2009. http://www.healthstatus.sgul.ac.uk/SGRQ_download/SGRQ%20Manual%20June%202009.pdf.

56. Shelledy DC, Stoller JK. An introduction to critical diagnostic thinking. In: Stoller JK, Bakow ED, Longworth DL (eds.). *Critical Diagnostic Thinking in Respiratory Care: A Case-Based Approach*. Philadelphia: W.B. Saunders Company; 2002: 3–38.

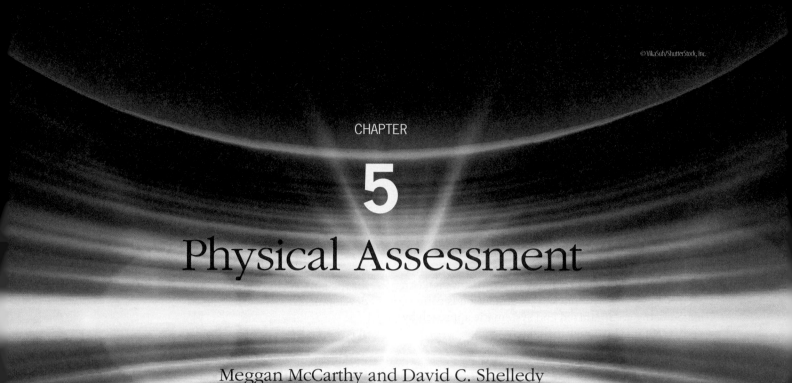

CHAPTER

5

Physical Assessment

Meggan McCarthy and David C. Shelledy

CHAPTER OUTLINE

CHAPTER OBJECTIVES

1. Describe normal vital signs and explain causes of common alterations in vital signs.
2. Explain the causes and significance of alterations in body temperature.
3. Explain methods for assessment of pain.
4. Explain causes of abnormal body weight and the importance of alterations in body weight.
5. Summarize assessment of the patient's general appearance.
6. Explain the assessment of cyanosis.
7. Describe assessment of the patient's mental status and level of consciousness.
8. Overview the main components of the neurologic examination.
9. Summarize the examination of the head, eyes, ears, nose, and throat (HEENT).
10. Describe the examination of the thorax (inspection, auscultation, palpation, percussion) to include the significance of specific alterations.
11. Describe the cardiac exam to include the significance of normal and abnormal heart sounds.
12. Describe examination of the extremities to include important alterations (e.g., clubbing, capillary refill, color, and edema).
13. Summarize the examination of the abdomen.
14. Explain the significance of ancillary equipment in use.
15. Integrate physical assessment findings to formulate a problem list or diagnosis.

KEY TERMS

adventitious breath sounds	hypertension
ascites	hypotension
auscultation	hypothermia
body mass index (BMI)	inspection
bradycardia	obesity
bradypnea	palpation
cachexia	percussion
crackle	pitting edema
cyanosis	pupillary response
diaphoresis	retractions
fever	subcutaneous emphysema
fremitus	tachycardia
heart murmur	tachypnea
heat exhaustion	wheeze

Overview

The physical examination is an important part of the assessment and evaluation of patients with suspected or confirmed cardiopulmonary disease. Taken together, the history and physical guide further assessment and laboratory testing. The history and physical examination also play an important role in maintaining and monitoring a patient's health, as well as in caring for patients with a chronic disease. In addition, the physical assessment provides important information needed to develop, implement, and assess the respiratory care plan. The core physical examination techniques of inspection, palpation, percussion, and auscultation will be described throughout this chapter. This chapter will emphasize key components of the cardiopulmonary physical examination to include the interpretation of the findings.

Introduction to the Physical Examination

The physical examination techniques of inspection, palpation, percussion, and auscultation are essential skills that every respiratory care clinician must acquire and refine. The respiratory care clinician must be able to integrate the results of the patient history, physical examination, and diagnostic tests in confirming the diagnosis and creating an effective treatment plan. An accurate and effective physical examination is completed using an organized and systematic approach by body system, which may include:

- Vital signs
- Skin
- Head, eyes, ears, nose, and throat (HEENT)
- Neck
- Back and spine
- Heart and blood vessels
- Thorax and lungs
- Abdomen/gastrointestinal
- Extremities
- Musculoskeletal
- Neurologic
- Other (skin, hair, nails; lymphatic system)

The respiratory care clinician will often complete a physical examination directed at assessing the cardiopulmonary system. The results of this examination may be used to monitor the patient's condition and evaluate the effects of therapy and to develop, implement, and evaluate the respiratory care plan. This assessment should include review of the patient's general appearance, level of consciousness, and assessment of oxygenation and perfusion. Chest **inspection** should include ventilatory pattern, use of accessory muscles, chest excursion, and observation of the right to left chest wall motion and chest–abdominal synchrony. Assessment of breath sounds should include noting aeration and any adventitious (i.e., abnormal) breath sounds. Palpation techniques may be used to determine the presence of tactile rhonchi or vocal fremitus. Percussion of the chest may be helpful in assessing for hyperinflation or pneumothorax and diminished aeration or pleural fluid.

Bedside measurement of pulse and respirations should be performed and blood pressure should be assessed. Temperature should be taken to assess for the presence of hyperthermia or hypothermia. SpO_2 should be measured in most patients, given that it is a simple and low-cost method of determining oxygenation

status. Inspiratory capacity should be measured in patients at risk for developing atelectasis and in all patients being considered for or receiving lung expansion therapy. Patients receiving bronchodilator therapy should also have before and after measurement of $FEV_{1.0}$ or, at a minimum, peak expiratory flow rate (PEFR) in asthma patients. Arterial blood gases may be obtained to confirm suspected hypoxemia, identify suspected hypoventilation, and assess acid-base balance. Lastly, bedside measurement of vital capacity and maximum inspiratory force may be helpful in assessing ventilatory muscle strength and the ability to cough and deep breathe. **Box 5-1** provides a checklist for the physical examination for respiratory care plan development.

Approach to the Patient

Building trust and rapport with the patient is important in completing the physical examination. Patients and their families may be experiencing a great deal of stress and uncertainty. The respiratory care clinician's initial interaction with the patient can often alleviate some of the patient's anxiety associated with the current illness. Building trust and rapport begins as soon as the clinician enters the room. The clinician should always begin by introducing himself or herself and asking the patient how he or she would like to be addressed. A professional and supportive demeanor should be adopted. The clinician should smile, make eye contact with, and listen to the patient. Small aspects of the clinician–patient interaction, such as these, can help establish a trusting environment for the patient and family. Setting clear and realistic expectations for the encounter is also important. As much as possible, the patient should be allowed to remain in control. The patient should be allowed to ask questions, and the clinician should ensure that the patient has a clear understanding of the clinician's role and the purpose of the encounter.

At the beginning of the patient interaction, the clinician should always wash his or her hands and put on examination gloves, if needed. Next, the examination that will be completed should be outlined. Patients and family members will often be more relaxed and cooperative if the clinician clearly explains what will be done and, most important, the reason for each action. Establishing as much privacy as possible will help reduce the patient's anxiety or discomfort. If there are family members in the patient's room, the clinician should also introduce himself or herself to the family. The clinician should ask the patient and family members what their preferences are in regards to who remains in the room during the physical exam. If the clinician must examine areas of sensitivity such as the breasts or perineum, a chaperone should be present regardless of the patient's gender.[1]

BOX 5-1

Checklist for the Physical Assessment for Respiratory Care Plan Development

General Appearance

☐ Anxious, agitated, restless, or distressed

☐ Other signs of hypoxia

Level of Consciousness

☐ Awake, alert, and oriented to person, place, and time

☐ Confusion, disorientation

☐ Somnolent

☐ Sedated

☐ Unconscious

☐ Coma

☐ Other symptoms of hypoxia

Pulse, Respirations, and Blood Pressure

☐ Tachycardia

☐ Bradycardia

☐ Tachypnea

☐ Bradypnea

☐ Hypertension

☐ Hypotension

Temperature

☐ Fever

☐ Hypothermia

SpO_2

☐ Hypoxemia

Oxygenation and Perfusion

☐ Skin color and characteristics

☐ Nail beds and mucosa

☐ Capillary refill

Chest Inspection

☐ Respiratory pattern

☐ Use of accessory muscles

☐ Chest excursion

☐ Right-to-left chest wall synchrony

☐ Chest-to-abdominal synchrony

☐ Flail, trauma

Inspiratory Capacity (IC) and/or Vital Capacity (VC)

☐ Normal IC is about 50 mL/kg of ideal body weight

☐ Normal VC is about 70 mL/kg of ideal body weight

Peak Expiratory Flow Rate (PEFR) and/or FEV_1

☐ Before and after bronchodilator therapy

Assessment of the Work of Breathing

☐ Respiratory distress, accessory muscle use, sweating

Breath Sounds

☐ Normal

☐ Diminished

☐ Absent

☐ Bronchial breath sounds

☐ Crackles

☐ Gurgles

☐ Wheezing

Palpation

☐ Chest excursion

☐ Right-to-left chest wall synchrony

☐ Trachea position

☐ Tactile fremitus

☐ Vocal fremitus

Percussion

☐ Dullness

☐ Resonance

☐ Hyperresonance

TABLE 5-1
Patient Position for the Physical Examination

Area or Exam	Patient Position	Provider Position
Vital signs, general inspection	Sitting or reclining	Standing before patient or at bedside
Head and neck	Sitting	Standing before patient
Anterior torso	Sitting	Standing before patient initially, later behind the patient
Posterior torso	Sitting	At patient's side
Anterior chest and abdomen	Supine	Before the patient
Gait, station, coordination	Variable positions	Behind the patient

Patient Position

Patient positioning is important to completing certain physical examination procedures. **Table 5-1** outlines the ideal patient position for each component of the physical examination. As outlined in the table, the patient should be sitting, standing, or lying down, depending on the part of the examination being completed. A systematic approach that reduces multiple movement changes is preferred. For example, the clinician should attempt to complete all exams requiring the patient to be standing at the same time. Although it is ideal to have patients in certain positions for each discrete exam, this is not always possible when considering patient comfort, type of illness, and ancillary equipment in use. Many patients who require physical assessment are acutely ill or have little physical reserve. In these cases, minimizing movement may help prevent patient distress.

Clinician ergonomics should be taken into consideration when completing a physical exam. In the case of hospitalized patients, the bed should be raised or lowered to a comfortable height to alleviate clinician back strain.[2] A well-lit examination room is preferred; if overhead lighting is not adequate, a mobile light source, such as a pen light or gooseneck light, should be utilized. Although room temperature is not always under the clinician's control, a warm and comfortable exam room is preferred.

Completing a thorough physical examination requires exposure of the patient's bare skin. The patient should be informed before the exam as to which body parts will be exposed. Drapes should be used, and the patient should not be exposed for prolonged periods without redraping. If the clinician is unexpectedly called out of the exam room, he or she should completely re-cover the patient to maintain comfort and modesty. At the completion of the exam, the clinician should return the room to the pre-examination state. If bed rails were lowered in order to complete the exam, they must be returned to their upright position in order

to prevent patient injury.[3] If the bed was raised or lowered for the examination, it should be returned to its original height. Before leaving the room, the clinician should ask if the patient has any questions or needs any assistance.

Order of the Physical Examination

Completing the physical examination in a systematic manner will ensure that all key components are completed and that the patient's comfort is taken into consideration. **Box 5-2** lists the suggested steps for a complete physical examination. This list may be individualized depending on the patient's presentation and ability to cooperate.

Vital Signs

The vital signs are pulse, respirations, blood pressure, and temperature. Vital signs are routinely monitored in patients who are admitted to the hospital and who are assessed during routine office or clinic visits. Recently, the patient's pain perception has been included as an additional vital sign.[4,5] Pain is often documented using a standardized pain scale. O_2 saturation via pulse oximetry (SpO_2) is also suggested as an added vital sign (see Chapter 8). Measurement of height and weight is routinely performed as a part of the physical examination.

Assessment of the patient's vital signs provides essential information regarding the cardiopulmonary system. Hypoxia and ventilatory failure are often first detected by observing changes in heart rate, respiratory rate, and blood pressure. Fever may be the only sign of infection. Assessment of vital signs before, during, and after delivery of therapy can provide important information regarding the patient's response to therapy or the effect of a procedure. Assessment of vital signs may alert the clinician as to the need for additional evaluation and testing in order to identify the cause of any detected abnormalities. Vital sign values should be critically evaluated in light of the patient's overall condition.

BOX 5-2

Steps in the Physical Examination

1. Introduce yourself.
   a. Address the patient by his/her formal name.
   b. Ask the patient how he/she would like to be addressed.
2. Explain the agenda for the encounter. This will vary depending on the patient's presentation, but a brief explanation of the physical exam process should be given.
3. Wash your hands. Apply personal protective equipment if necessary (gloves, gown, mask, etc.).
4. Ensure the patient's comfort.
   a. Ensure patient privacy by either closing doors or pulling drape.
   b. If necessary, obtain a chaperone for the exam.
   c. Make sure that the patient is in a comfortable and relaxed position.
   d. Properly gown or drape the patient for modesty.
5. Prepare the examination environment.
   a. Adjust the examination table or bed height appropriate for the examiner.
   b. Lower bed rails if necessary.
   c. Arrange light sources if necessary.
   d. Remove distractions if present.
   e. Turn television sets, radios, and other noisy distractions off or at least decrease the volume.
6. Vital signs and general inspection.
   a. Evaluate the radial pulse for heart rate and rhythm.
   b. Obtain blood pressure.
   c. Evaluate the respiratory rate.
   d. Obtain body temperature.
   e. Assess pain, if present (the "fifth" vital sign), utilizing an appropriate pain scale.
   f. Inspect nails, skin, and hair.
   g. Note the general appearance, body habits, hair distribution, muscle mass, movement coordination, odors, and breathing pattern.
7. Head.
   a. *Eyes*: Examine the conjunctiva, sclera, cornea, and iris of each eye. Test pupils for irregularity, accommodation, and reaction. Evaluate visual fields and visual acuity (cranial nerve II). Assess extraocular movements (cranial nerves III, IV, VI). Test the corneal reflex (cranial nerve V).
   b. *Ears*: Examine the pinnae and periauricular tissues. Test auditory acuity. Perform the Weber and Rinne maneuvers (cranial nerve VIII).
   c. *Nose*: Connect the nasal speculum to the otoscope and examine the nares, noting the condition of the mucosa, septum, and turbinates.
   d. *Mouth*: Examine the vermilion border, the oral mucosa, and the tongue. Identify the salivary duct papillae. Assess the dentition for decay and repair and the condition of the bite. View the pharynx. Evaluate the function of cranial nerves IX, X, and XII. If appropriate, evaluate sensory divisions of cranial nerves V and VII.
   e. *Face*: Evaluation of symmetry, smile, frown, and jaw movement will provide information about motor divisions of cranial nerves V and VII.
8. *Neck*: Palpate the neck with emphasis on the salivary glands, lymph nodes, and thyroid. Look for tracheal deviation. Identify the carotid arteries and auscultate for bruits. Note jugular venous distention. Certain parts of evaluation of this area, such as jugular venous filling, may warrant review with the patient reclining. Test shoulder strength of the sternocleidomastoid and trapezius muscles (cranial nerves XI and XII).
9. *Anterior torso:* With the patient sitting, examine the epitrochlear and axillary nodes. Examine the breasts. Define the point of maximal impulse (PMI) and examine the heart, having the patient lean forward if necessary.

(continues)

(*continued*)

10. *Posterior torso:* Observe for spinal curvature or chest deformity. Evaluate the vertebral column and the costovertebral areas. Auscultate the posterior and lateral lung fields.
11. Complete the "sitting" portion of the examination. Evaluate proximal and distal motor strength, deep tendon reflexes, distal pulses and sensation.
12. With the patient supine:
    a. *Thorax:* Reexamine the heart, turning the patient to the left lateral decubitus position if appropriate.
    b. *Lungs:* Auscultate the anterior lung structures.
    c. *Abdomen:* After inspection, auscultate, listening for bowel sounds and bruits. Next inspect, percuss, and palpate the abdomen, taking special notice of hepatic or splenic enlargements.
    d. *Proximal lower extremities:* Examine the inguinal, femoral, and popliteal regions for adenopathy and pulses.
13. With the patient standing, evaluate station and gait.

Monitoring trends in vital signs can indicate if the patient is getting better or worse. Observing changes over time, especially as compared to "baseline" values when the patient is in his or her normal state of health, can be particularly important. For example, a healthy male marathon runner may have a baseline resting heart rate of 50 beats per minute (bpm) due to a well-conditioned heart. In comparison, a heart rate of less than 60 bpm may represent a clinically important bradycardia in a 75-year-old patient with a history of cardiac disease whose "normal" resting heart rate is 88 bpm. It is important to note that many elderly subjects are on medications (β-blockers/calcium channel blockers) that lower heart rate.

As another example of the importance of monitoring trends in vital signs, a patient with a history of chronic hypertension in the intensive care unit (ICU) may have a current blood pressure of 95/70 mm Hg. Although this would be considered in the normal range for most patients, it represents a large deviation from baseline for this patient and could indicate a problem, such as early sepsis. Although single measures of vital signs provide helpful information, trends and changes are very important to note.

Heart Rate

Most commonly, heart rate is assessed by taking the patient's pulse. Heart rate may also be assessed using pulse oximetry or electrocardiographic (ECG) monitoring equipment. Heart rate varies considerably with age, activity, and the patient's baseline health status. A normal adult resting heart rate (HR) is between 60 and 100 beats per minute (bpm).[5,6] Heart rate tends to increase with age in adults. In infants and young children, heart rate declines as the child gets older. For example, a heart rate of 130 bpm in the newborn would be considered normal, whereas a normal heart rate for a 2- to 3-year-old child is about 110 bpm.[5,6] Regardless of age, the pulse should be regular with little variation with the respiratory cycle. **Box 5-3** lists the normal range for adult heart rate. **Box 5-4** lists the normal heart rate in infants and children.

BOX 5-3

Heart Rate in Adults

Classification	Beats per Minute (bpm)	Common Causes
Normal	80 (range 60–100)	—
Tachycardia	> 100	Hypoxia, cardiac disease, fever, exercise, and anxiety.
Bradycardia	< 60	Very severe hypoxia, heart disease, arrhythmia, and vagal stimulation. Well-trained athletes may have a "normal" resting heart rate in the 50s.

BOX 5-4

Heart Rate in Infants and Children

	Normal (beats per minute)	Range (beats per minute)
Infants	135 (approximate)	110–150
Children (age):		
1 year	125	80–140
2 years	110	80–130
3 years	105	80–120
4 years	100	70–115
10 years	80	70–110

Heart rate can be assessed in a variety of ways; however, it is important to consistently use the same technique in the same patient. For a fast assessment, if the pulse is regular, the clinician may palpate the patient's radial pulse and count the heart rate for 15 seconds and then multiply this number by four to calculate the estimated heart rate. A more accurate assessment is obtained by counting the pulse for 30 seconds and then multiplying by two. If the pulse is irregular, the heart rate should be counted for a full minute. When assessing the pulse, the clinician should also note the regularity and quality of the pulse using common terminology for describing pulse quality (see **Box 5-5**). **Box 5-6** describes the steps in assessing the radial pulse.

Tachycardia

In adults, a HR > 100 bpm is defined as **tachycardia**.[6,7] An elevated heart rate is a normal physiologic response to vigorous activity, such as running or walking up multiple flights of stairs. With exercise, the predicted maximum HR in adults can be estimated as:

$$HR\ max = 220 - Age\ in\ years$$

Thus, a 20-year-old would have an expected maximum heart rate of 200 bpm (HR max = 220 − 20 = 200 bpm); this would decline to 140 bpm for an 80-year-old (HR max = 220 − 80 = 140 bpm).

Anxiety and fear may elevate HR as a part of the normal "flight-or-fight" response to a perceived external threat. HR also increases with body temperature; for each 1 degree Fahrenheit increase, HR increases about 10 bpm.[7]

Tachycardia is associated with a many pathologic conditions, including, but not limited to, hypoxia, anemia, blood loss, hypovolemia; hypotension, shock, heart disease, arrhythmia (e.g., sinus tachycardia, supraventricular tachycardia, and ventricular tachycardia), uncontrolled pain, and fever. Certain drugs may elevate HR to the point of tachycardia. Examples include the sympathomimetics (e.g., epinephrine, isoproterenol, and dopamine), anticholinergic drugs (e.g., atropine), xanthenes (e.g., theophylline, caffeine), nicotine, and cocaine. Although an increased heart rate is a normal response to vigorous exercise, a HR > 100 bpm is considered tachycardia, regardless of the cause.

Bradycardia

A HR < 60 bpm is considered **bradycardia**.[5,7] Bradycardia can be caused by severe hypoxia, vagal stimulation, severe acidosis, cardiac disease, arrhythmia (e.g., heart block), and the administration of certain medications, such as β-blockers.

Many athletes have a larger than normal heart and a corresponding larger stroke volume and reduced resting heart rate. Well-trained endurance athletes often maintain resting heart rates in the forties or fifties. Overall, it is important to note the patient's symptoms when experiencing an episode of bradycardia. Asymptomatic bradycardia requires prompt evaluation, whereas symptomatic bradycardia may require emergent intervention either with chronotropic medications or artificial pacing.

BOX 5-5

Characteristics of the Pulse

Rate	Rapid, normal, or slow
Rhythm	Regular or irregular
Strength	Weak vs. strong
Amplitude	4 = Bounding[1] 3 = Full, increased 2 = Normal or expected 1 = Diminished, barely palpable[2] 0 = Absent, not palpable

[1] A full, bounding pulse is associated with exercise or distress.
[2] A weak, thready pulse is associated with diminished cardiac output.

BOX 5-6

Procedure for Assessing the Radial Pulse

1. Wash hands.
2. Identify the patient.
3. Position patient's arm across the lower chest-upper abdomen (in lap), palm down.
4. Place the index, middle, and fourth fingers gently on the skin at the site where the artery passes next to a bony prominence.
5. If pulse is regular, count for 30 seconds and multiply by 2.
   a. If the pulse is very regular or for a quick check, count for 15 seconds and multiply by 4.
   b. If the pulse is irregular, count for a full minute.
6. Record the following:
   a. Rate: Record the number of beats per minute.
   b. Rhythm: Regular, irregular (pulse may be regular, regularly irregular, or irregularly irregular).
   c. Strength: By pressing gently against side of vessel, note the strength of the pulse (weak or thready vs. strong, full, or bounding). Note: You can cut off the pulse if you press too hard.
   d. Amplitude: bounding (4), full (3), expected (2), diminished (1), absent (0).

Key Points

- Radial, brachial, or femoral sites can be used to assess pulse.
- Do not use your thumb (it has a pulse).
- Assess for 30 seconds and multiply by 2. Assessing for 15 seconds and multiplying by 4 provides a quick check. If the pulse is irregular, assess for 1 full minute.

Character of the Pulse

The character of the pulse should be assessed, because it may provide useful information about the patient's condition. The pulse rhythm may be regular or irregular. An irregular pulse is associated with cardiac arrhythmia. The amplitude of the arterial pulse may be described as bounding, full, expected, diminished, or absent (see Box 5-5). A weak, thready pulse is associated with diminished blood flow. The pulse can be diminished for many reasons, including hypovolemia, hypotension, shock, myocardial infarction (MI), congestive heart failure (CHF), or poor or blocked peripheral perfusion (e.g., clots, atherosclerosis). Unequal or delayed pulses may help diagnose specific abnormalities. For example, aortic dissection or stenosis of the left subclavian artery may result in a strong right radial pulse and a weak left radial pulse. "Pulse pressure," the difference between the systolic and diastolic pressure, is also helpful and is increased in sepsis and narrowed in hypovolemia. Abnormal arterial pulses include pulsus alternans, pulsus paradoxus, and pulsus bisferiens (see Box 5-7).

Respiratory Rate

Respiratory rate varies with age and level of activity. A healthy full-term newborn may have a respiratory rate of 40 breaths per minute (range of 35 to 45

per minute).[5,6] A healthy 2- to 3-year-old child might have a respiratory rate of about 28 breaths per minute, whereas a 12-year-old child might have a normal respiratory rate of 18 breath per minute.[5] The normal adult respiratory rate is 12 to 20 breaths per minute.[5,6] Respiratory rate increases with activity and is reduced with relaxation and sleep. **Table 5-2** lists normal values for respiratory rate for infants, children, and adults, as well as terms sometimes used to describe alterations in respiratory rate. **Box 5-8** describes the steps in assessing respiration.

TABLE 5-2
Normal Values of Respiratory Rate

Age Group	Normal Range of Breaths per Minute
Adults	12–20
Infants	30–40
Children	18–30, but varies with age

Terms used to describe rate and depth of breathing:

Eupnea: Normal breathing (rhythm and rate).

Tachypnea: Rapid respiratory rate (remember that tachypnea does not equal hyperventilation)

Bradypnea: Decreased respiratory rate.

Depth (apparent): Normal, shallow, deep.

BOX 5-7

Abnormalities of the Pulse

Pulsus bisferiens: A pulse characterized by two systolic peaks and associated with aortic regurgitation. Hypertropic cardiac myopathy, large patent ductus arteriosis, mitral valve prolapse, and hyperdynamic circulatory states (such a septic shock) have been associated with pulsus bisferiens.

Pulsus parvus: A small, weak pulse that seems to rise and fall slowly in magnitude. Associated with aortic stenosis and increased peripheral vascular resistance.

Pulsus paradoxus: Decrease in force (not rate), almost to the point of disappearance during inspiration (only). Constrictive pericarditis, pericardial effusion, and cardiac tamponade are important causes. Hypvolemic shock, heart failure, increased venous return on inspiration, severe emphysema, and asthma have been associated with pulsus paradoxus. It is significant if inspiratory blood pressure (systolic) falls more than 20 mm Hg on inspiration.

Pulsus alternans: Strong beats alternating with weak beats. Left ventricular failure is the most important cause. Severe hypertension, cardiac tamponade, severe aortic regurgitation, and coronary artery disease have been associated with pulsus alternans.

BOX 5-8

Procedure for Assessing Respirations

Normally pulse and respirations are assessed in the same session. Because patients may change their ventilatory rate or pattern if they think their respirations are being counted, it is suggested that the clinician take the pulse and then continue as if still checking the pulse while counting the respiratory rate.

1. Wash hands and put on gloves (if needed).
2. Make sure chest and abdominal movements are easy to see.
3. Observe a complete inspiration and expiration to make sure you can detect a full breath.
4. Count respirations.
   a. In adults, if the rhythm is regular, then count for 30 seconds and multiply by 2.
   b. In children, infants, or adults with an irregular rhythm, count the rate for a full minute.
5. Observe respirations for:
   a. Rate
   b. Apparent depth
   c. Regularity (rhythm)
   d. Diaphragm–chest wall synchrony
6. Record data.
7. Wash hands.

Tachypnea

In adults, a respiratory rate > 20 breaths per minute is described as **tachypnea**.[5,6] Tachypnea is a normal physiologic response to hypoxemia (see Chapter 6). Causes of hypoxemia include reduced inspired oxygen tension (such as occurs at altitude); obstruction of the conducting airways; mismatch of alveolar gas to pulmonary capillary blood flow (e.g., low $\dot{V}/\dot{Q}$, shunt, or increased deadspace); and problems with diffusion across the lung (e.g., interstitial lung disease often causing only exercise hypoxemia). Pulmonary diseases seen in the acute care setting that may lead to respiratory failure and the development of tachypnea include atelectasis, pneumonia, pulmonary edema (cardiogenic and noncardiogenic), asthma exacerbation, and acute exacerbation of chronic obstructive pulmonary disease (COPD).

Sudden onset dyspnea, tachypnea, and pleuritic chest pain are often seen in patients with acute pulmonary embolus, though these findings are highly variable and nonspecific.[8] Cardiac insufficiency may cause circulatory hypoxia and tachypnea. Tachypnea and hyperventilation are also physiologic responses to metabolic acidosis, including lactic acidosis, diabetic ketoacidosis, and acidosis due to kidney failure. Other causes of tachypnea include anxiety or panic attack and severe pain.

Tachypnea and Alveolar Ventilation

It is important to distinguish between tachypnea, hyperventilation, and hypoventilation. *Hyperventilation* is defined as a level of alveolar ventilation that results in a $Paco_2$ < 35 mm Hg, whereas tachypnea in adults is simply a respiratory rate > 20 breaths per minute. *Hypoventilation*, in contrast, is a level of ventilation that results in a $Paco_2 > 45$ mm Hg. Tachypnea and hyperventilation are two different conditions that may or may not occur together. In fact, many patients with ventilatory failure exhibit tachypnea and alveolar hypoventilation at the same time for reasons that are discussed below. The relationship between $Paco_2$ and alveolar ventilation is discussed more thoroughly in Chapter 7.

Rapid Shallow Breathing and Respiratory Failure

Many patients with acute respiratory failure experience a decline in lung compliance due to pulmonary disease, such as atelectasis, pneumonia, or pulmonary edema. With reductions in compliance, the lung becomes more difficult to inflate, and the work of breathing is increased. This often results in a reduction in inspired tidal volume. A normal adult tidal volume (V_T) is approximately 500 mL (range 400 to 600 mL), and a normal respiratory rate (f) is 12 breaths per minute (range 12 to 20 breaths/min). A normal minute volume (V_E) is respiratory rate (f) multiplied by the tidal volume (V_T):

$$\dot{V}_E = f \times V_T$$

$$\dot{V}_E = 12 \times 500 \text{ mL} = 6000 \text{ mL/min} = 6.0 \text{ L/min}$$

In order to maintain minute volume, patients with reduced tidal volumes will often attempt to increase their respiratory rate. For example, a patient with atelectasis and pneumonia may have a tidal volume of only 200 mL because the lung has low compliance and is difficult to inflate. This patient may try and compensate by increasing his or her respiratory rate to 30 breaths per minute. The resultant minute volume is calculated as follows:

$$\dot{V}_E = f \times V_T$$

$$\dot{V}_E = 30 \times 200 \text{ mL} = 6000 \text{ mL/min} = 6.0 \text{ L/min}$$

By definition, this patient has tachypnea (f = 30 breaths/min). The patient also has a reduced tidal volume (V_T = 200 mL) and thus is exhibiting *rapid shallow breathing*, which is one of the most common findings in acute respiratory failure. With rapid shallow breathing, the increase in respiratory rate can sometimes maintain the patient's minute volume, as was shown in the example. Unfortunately, the small tidal volumes and rapid respiratory rates may be insufficient to maintain adequate alveolar ventilation, causing an increase in $Paco_2$. This is because of the increasing proportion dead space assumes for each breath.

Dead space is the volume of gas in the conducting airways plus any alveoli that are ventilated but not perfused. Normal dead space (V_D) is about 150 mL (about 2.2 mL/kg of ideal body weight). Alveolar ventilation per breath ($\dot{V}_A$) is tidal volume minus dead space (V_T

$- V_D$) and alveolar ventilation per minute ($\dot{V}_A$) is tidal volume minus dead space multiplied by the rate:

$$\dot{V}_A = (V_T - V_D) \times f$$

With a normal V_D and V_T, the alveolar ventilation ($\dot{V}_A$) per breath and per minute would be 350 mL and 4200 mL, respectively:

$$\dot{V}_A \text{ per breath} = V_T - V_D = 500 - 150 = 350 \text{ mL}$$

$$\dot{V}_A \text{ per minute} = (V_T - V_D) \times f = (500 - 150)12 = 4200 \text{ mL/min}$$

However, with reduced V_T, alveolar ventilation can be dramatically reduced. In our previous example, the patient was exhibiting rapid shallow breathing (f = 30; V_T = 200 mL). Assuming a normal dead space of 150 mL, the patient's minute volume and alveolar ventilation would be:

$$\dot{V}_A \text{ per breath} = V_T - V_D = 200 - 150 = 50 \text{ mL}$$

$$\dot{V}_A \text{ per minute} = (V_T - V_D) \times f = (200 - 150)30$$

$$= 1500 \text{ mL/min} = 1.5 \text{ L/min}$$

$$\dot{V}_E = 30 \times 200 \text{ mL} = 6000 \text{ mL/min} = 6.0 \text{ L/min}$$

This example demonstrates that with rapid shallow breathing there is often a significant decrease in alveolar ventilation, even when minute volume is maintained. In the previous example, a $\dot{V}_A$ of 1.5 L/min could result in a $Paco_2$ of over 100 mm Hg*—severe hypoventilation.

RC Insights

A respiratory rate of greater than 30 breaths per minute when combined with a spontaneous tidal volume of ≤ 300 mL is associated with impending ventilatory failure.

Bradypnea

Bradypnea is defined as a respiratory rate of < 12 breaths per minute in adults.[5,6] Bradypnea is often associated with neurologic depression of the medullary center. Common causes of bradypnea include overdose of central nervous system (CNS) depressants (intentional or iatrogenic) and neurologic insult from trauma or disease. CNS depressants that may cause bradypnea include the opiates (e.g., morphine, heroin, hydrocodone), benzodiazepines (e.g., valium, lorazepam), barbiturates, and alcohol. Severe hypoxia can lead to bradypnea, irregular breathing, and respiratory arrest.

---

*$Paco_2 = (0.863 \times \dot{V}CO_2) \div \dot{V}_A$; assuming a normal $\dot{V}CO_2$ of 200 mL/min and a $\dot{V}_A$ of 1.5 L/min, then $Paco_2 = (0.863 \times 200) \div 1.5 = 115$ mm Hg. For more information regarding $Paco_2$ and $\dot{V}_A$, see Chapter 7.

Blood Pressure

Arterial blood pressure is a measure of the pressure within the arteries as the blood moves through the arterial system. Arterial blood pressure is determined by the force of ventricular contraction and cardiac output, blood volume and viscosity, systemic vascular resistance, and the elasticity of the arterial vessel walls. Cardiac output is determined by stroke volume and heart rate. There are several arterial pressure measurements of interest:

- *Systolic arterial pressure*: The peak pressure within the artery during left ventricular contraction (systole).
- *Diastolic pressure*: The lowest pressure within the artery during left ventricular filling (diastole).
- *Pulse pressure*: Systolic pressure minus diastolic pressure.
- *Mean arterial pressure (MAP)*: The mean pressure within the artery. MAP is approximately equal to the diastolic pressure plus one-third of the pulse pressure.

Blood pressure is typically recorded as the systolic pressure (top number) over the diastolic pressure (bottom number) in mm Hg. At the bedside, blood pressure can be measured in a variety of manners; the most accurate is an invasive method that requires cannulation of an artery, commonly the radial artery. Arterial cannulation (arterial line placement) is generally reserved for critically ill patients requiring close monitoring. It should be noted that arterial line measurement of blood pressure tends to overestimate systolic pressure and underestimate diastolic pressure, but accurately reflects MAP. In most patients, a sphygmomanometer is utilized along with a stethoscope or Doppler device. The sphygmomanometer consists of a cuff with an inflatable bladder, an inflating bulb, a controlled exhaust for deflation, and a manometer. When assessing the patient's blood pressure, it is important that the clinician uses the appropriate size blood pressure cuff. Inaccurate sizing can lead to erroneous readings that are either falsely elevated or too low. To ensure appropriate sizing of the blood pressure cuff the clinician should measure the cuff for each patient. According to the American Heart Association the "ideal" cuff should have a bladder length that is 80% of arm circumference and a width that is at least 40% of arm circumference (a length-to-width ratio of 2:1).[9] **Table 5-3** lists suggested pressure cuff sizes based on arm circumference. **Box 5-9** describes the steps to assess blood pressure.

As noted with heart rate and respiratory rate, blood pressure (BP) varies with age. BP values steadily climb from birth and reach the adult mean normal values of 120/80 mm Hg at approximately 18 to 20 years of age.[6,10] Normal and abnormal arterial blood pressures are listed in **Box 5-10**.

TABLE 5-3
Blood Pressure Cuff Size

Patient's Arm Circumference (cm)	Size
22–26	"Small adult," 1222 cm
27–34	"Adult," 1630 cm
35–44	"Large adult," 1636 cm
45–52	"Adult thigh," 1642 cm

Hypertension

Systemic **hypertension** in adults is defined as a sustained systolic pressure of ≥ 140 mm Hg or a sustained diastolic pressure of ≥ 90 mm Hg.[10] The diagnosis of hypertension using ambulatory blood pressure measurement depends on the time span over which it is measured because blood pressures recorded during sleep are normally lower than waking blood pressures.[10] It is interesting to note that a significant number of patients are thought to have "white coat" hypertension in which blood pressure is normal at home or work, but is elevated when measured in the clinic setting.[10]

Box 5-11 lists risk factors associated with the development of hypertension. Factors associated with the development of hypertension include smoking, obesity, race, heredity, and Type A personality. Persistent hypertension can lead to left ventricular hypertrophy and CHF, MI, ischemic stroke, hemorrhagic stroke, and kidney disease. Severe elevations in blood pressure (diastolic pressure > 120 mm Hg) are life threatening.[10]

Most patients with high blood pressure have primary, or essential, hypertension.[10,11] Secondary hypertension is due to a specific underlying disease such as renal disease or an endocrine disorder. About one-third of the adult population in the United States has hypertension, and in many cases it is poorly controlled.[10,11] Patients with chronic hypertension should be counseled and encouraged to make lifestyle changes. These include weight loss if overweight or obese, sodium restriction, smoking cessation and avoidance of secondhand smoke, increased physical activity (at least 30 minutes per day of aerobic exercise), stress management, and moderation of alcohol consumption.[11] Eating habits should be reviewed and patients should be encouraged to consume a diet rich in fruits and vegetables and to use low-fat dairy products and reduce total fat intake.[11]

Antihypertensive medications should generally be prescribed for patients with a persistent elevation in

BOX 5-9

Assessment of Blood Pressure by Auscultation

1. Introduce yourself.
2. Wash hands.
3. Identify the patient.
4. Explain the procedure.
5. Position patient and expose arm.
6. Palpate brachial artery.
7. Place cuff around arm 2 to 3 cm above anticubital fossa with arrows centered over radial artery.
8. Wrap cuff snug.
9. Position pressure gauge where you can see it.
10. Palpate brachial pulse.
11. Rapidly inflate to peak occlusion pressure (the point at which pulse disappears while palpating brachial pulse). Generally, cuff is inflated to 30 mm Hg above systolic pressure.
12. Position bell of scope over brachial artery just below the lower edge of the cuff.
13. Deflate cuff at a rate of 2 to 3 mm Hg per heartbeat.
14. Systolic pressure is where Korotkoff's sound is first heard.
15. Diastolic pressure is where Korotkoff's sound is muffled (disappears in most patients) or dampened. American Heart Association says diastolic pressure in adults is the fifth Korotkoff sound (fourth in children).

Key Points

- Inflate cuff to approximately 30 mm Hg past the point where the brachial pulse disappears upon palpation.
- Deflate cuff at a rate of 2 to 3 mm Hg per heartbeat.
- Systolic pressure is where Korotkoff's sound is first heard.
- Diastolic pressure is where Korotkoff's sound is muffled (i.e., disappears in most patients).
- Diastolic pressure is usually recorded as the fifth Korotkoff sound (silence as the cuff pressure drops below the diastolic blood pressure).

BOX 5-10

Normal and Abnormal Blood Pressure

Normal: 120/80 mm Hg*
- Normal range for systolic is 90–140 mm Hg
- Normal range for diastolic is 60–90 mm Hg

Prehypertension
- Systolic pressure > 120 but < 139 mm Hg
- Diastolic pressure 80–89 mm Hg

Hypertension
- Stage 1
  - Systolic pressure 140–159 mm Hg

    OR

  - Diastolic pressure 90–99 mm Hg
- Stage 2
  - Systolic pressure ≥ 160 mm Hg

    OR

  - Diastolic pressure ≥ 100 mm Hg

Hypotension: Blood pressure < 90/60 mm Hg

Changes in blood pressure:
- Increased systolic pressure implies increased resistance of arterial tree (thickening of arterial walls, elasticity).
- Decreased systolic pressure implies decreased resistance (peripheral vascular collapse, shock, weak left ventricle).
- Increased diastolic pressure implies increased peripheral vascular resistance.
- Decreased diastolic pressure implies decreased peripheral vascular resistance.
- Pulse pressure = Systolic pressure − Diastolic pressure = 120 − 80 = 40 (normal value).

Pulse pressure is affected by:
- Stroke volume of heart. Decreased stroke volume results in decreased pulse pressure and vice versa.
- Compliance of arteries. Decreased compliance results in decreased pulse pressure.

Mean arterial pressure (MAP) $\cong \frac{1}{3}$ (Systolic pressure − Diastolic pressure) + Diastolic pressure = $\frac{1}{3}$ (120 − 80) + 80 = 93 mm Hg (normal value).

*Blood pressure < 140/90 mm Hg but > 120/80 mm Hg may be considered prehypertension.

BOX 5-11

Risk Factors Associated with the Development of Hypertension

Race: Blacks have greater risk than whites.
Heredity: Risk increases if one or both parents have/had hypertension.
Excessive salt (Na⁺) intake
Alcohol abuse
Obesity
Sedentary lifestyle
Hyperlipidemia
Depression or Type A behavior
Vitamin D deficiency

Data from: Kaplan NM, Domino FJ. Overview of hypertension in adults. In: *UpToDate*, Basow, DS (ed.), UpToDate, Waltham, MA, 2012.

systolic ($\geq$ 140 mm Hg) or diastolic pressures ($\geq$ 90 mm Hg) despite lifestyle and diet changes.[11] A variety of antihypertensive medications are available, including the thiazide diuretics, ACE (angiotensin converting enzyme) inhibitors, angiotensin II receptor blockers, calcium channel blockers, and β-blockers.[11] Choice of antihypertensive medications should be based on evidence-based guidelines, such as those provided by the American Heart Association. Though β-blockers are commonly prescribed, they may not offer the same level of protection against stroke as other medications.[11] The goal of therapy is generally to maintain blood pressure < 140/90 mm Hg, although treatment goals may vary depending on the patient's condition. For example, in patients with diabetes or chronic kidney disease, there may be some benefit from a lower goal for blood pressure (e.g., < 130/80 mm Hg).[11] **Figure 5-1** provides an example of an algorithm for the treatment of hypertension.

Malignant hypertension and hypertensive encephalopathy are life-threatening conditions associated with very high arterial blood pressures, usually $\geq$ 180/120 mm Hg.[12] Hypertensive encephalopathy is associated with the development of cerebral edema, whereas malignant hypertension may occur in patients with chronic, poorly controlled hypertension who have discontinued antihypertensive therapy.[12] Renal artery stenosis may also contribute to the development of malignant hypertension.[12] Initial treatment of a hypertensive emergency should include administration of parenteral antihypertensive medications such as nicardipine or nitroprusside.

Hypotension

Hypotension can be defined as a sustained arterial blood pressure of less than 90 mm Hg over 60 mm Hg (systolic over diastolic).[5,6] Hypotension can be caused by decreased cardiac output, peripheral vasodilatation, or low circulating fluid volume (hypovolemia). Common causes of hypotension include dehydration, blood loss, sepsis, heart disease, and shock.[5] Addison's disease is a rare form of chronic adrenal insufficiency in which low blood pressure worsens when standing (orthostatic hypotension) and may be critically low when patients develop stress (e.g., severe infection).

Shock may be defined as inadequate tissue perfusion and oxygenation, usually due to hypotension.[5,13] Clinical findings in patients with shock include low blood pressure; decreased urine output; cool, clammy skin; altered mental status; and metabolic acidosis.[5,13] Types of shock include cardiogenic shock, hypovolemic shock, and distributive shock. Cardiogenic shock is caused by low cardiac output. Hypovolemic shock is caused by inadequate intravascular volume due to blood or fluid loss. Distributive shock (aka redistributive shock) is caused by inappropriate peripheral vasodilatation resulting in decreased systemic vascular resistance (SVR) and low blood pressure. Types of distributive shock include septic shock, neurogenic shock, adrenal insufficiency, and anaphylactic shock. Shock may lead to cell and organ damage and death. Treatment of shock includes aggressive fluid replacement and treatment of the underlying cause. In the case of cardiogenic shock, drugs to improve cardiac function may be administered.

Temperature

Body temperature is an important vital sign that is routinely measured in adult and pediatric patients. Temperature is usually measured orally, rectally, or using an infrared sensor for tympanic (ear) measurement.[14,15] An infrared sensor for axillary temperature measurement is available and correlates well with core body temperature in neonates. For comparison purposes and to monitor trends, the patient's temperature should be taken the same way each time.

Normal adults have variations in core body temperature throughout the day. Temperature is normally highest in late afternoon and lowest early in the morning in daytime workers; in nightshift workers this pattern is reversed.[5] Temperature also varies with activity level and increases during exercise. The body's central regulation of body temperature is located within the anterior hypothalamus, which maintains a set point for temperature. Information is relayed to the brain regarding the temperature of the blood within the pulmonary artery.[14] The average oral temperature in healthy individuals is approximately 37° C or 98.6° F. The normal range for oral temperature is 36.5° C (97° F) to 37.5° C

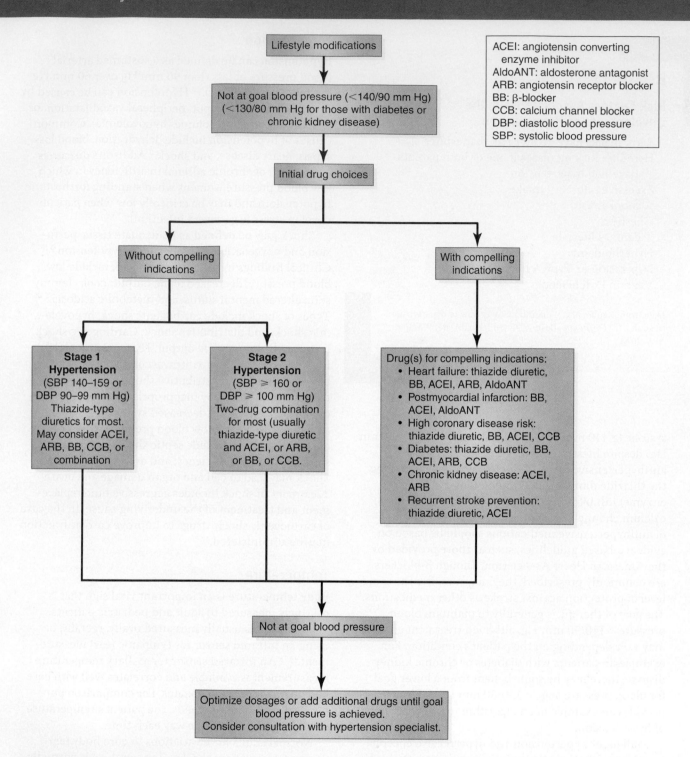

FIGURE 5-1 Algorithm for the treatment of hypertension.

Modified from: The Seventh Report of the Joint Committee on Prevention, Detection, Evaluation, and Treatment of High Blood Pressure. United States Department of Health and Human Services.

(99.5° F). Rectal temperatures are about 1.0° F (or 0.6° C) higher than oral temperatures, whereas axillary temperature in adults is about 1.0° F (0.5° C) less than oral temperature.[5,16] A persistently elevated temperature or low temperature is typically indicative of a pathologic process occurring. Normal temperatures are listed in **Table 5-4. Box 5-12** describes body regulation of temperature and types of fever.

TABLE 5-4
Normal Temperature by Measurement Method

Method	Normal	Accuracy
Oral	97°–99.5° F 36.5°–37.5° C	++
Rectal	98.7°–100.5° F 37.1°–38.1° C	+++
Axillary	96.7°–98.5° F 35.9°–36.9° C	+
Tympanic (ear)	Similar to rectal	Varies, though should be similar to core temperature when done properly

Key Points:
- Rectal > oral > axillary ($\cong 1°$ F < oral).
- Normal temperature fluctuates with daily diurnal cycle.
  - Higher between 4 and 6 pm
  - Lowest at 6 am
- Ranges consistent with life: 24°–45° C (74°–114° F)
- Temperature > 40.6° C or > 105° F is critical and should be considered a medical emergency.

Fever

Elevated body temperature is caused by excessive heat production or inadequate heat dissipation. This can be due to environmental conditions, damage to the normal thermoregulatory response, or elevation in the body's set point for temperature.[5] **Fever** is an abnormally elevated body temperature due to disease that affects the hypothalamic set point. Pyrogens are substances that may be released due to tissue necrosis, infection, inflammation, and certain tumors. Pyrogens cause fever by elevating the body's temperature set point. There has been much debate over what actually defines fever considering the normal variations of body temperature throughout the day. Normal temperature varies throughout the day and night and with activity level. However, in patients with a normal baseline temperature, fever generally corresponds to an oral temperature > 37.5° C (99.5° F) or a rectal temperature > 38.0° C (100.5° F); temperature > 38.3° C (101° F) should be considered fever in most patients.[5,6,16] A fever typically indicates that infection is present in the body, although various autoimmune and inflammatory disorders can cause a persistently elevated temperature.[15] Tachypnea and tachycardia are clinical signs that often occur during a febrile episode due to an increased metabolic rate.

Most fevers are caused by infection, often of viral origin, but bacteria, fungi, and parasites may also cause infection.[16] Common infectious causes of fever include influenza, upper respiratory tract infection, pneumonia, and gastroenteritis. Tuberculosis, Rocky Mountain spotted fever, Lyme disease, malaria, typhoid fever,

and dengue fever provide examples of infectious diseases that may initially present as fever. Causes other than infection are numerous but are less common and may be ruled out during the course of the assessment. These include endocrine disease (e.g., hyperthyroidism); immunologic disease (e.g., systemic lupus erythematosus, and sarcoidosis); tissue destruction (e.g., myocardial infarction, pulmonary infraction, and stroke); reaction to blood products; certain cancers; and metabolic disease, such as gout.[5] Fever with illness of at least 3 weeks duration, temperatures > 38.3° C (100.9° F), and no diagnosis reached following three or more clinic visits or 3 or more days in the hospital is the definition of *fever of unknown origin* (FUO).[5] The most common causes of FUO are noninfectious inflammatory disease, unidentified infection, and malignancies.[5]

The preferred antipyretic medication is acetaminophen, though aspirin or nonsteroidal anti-inflammatory drugs (NSAIDs) such as ibuprofen are often prescribed.[16] Both aspirin and acetaminophen are equally effective in reducing fever; acetaminophen in combination with aspirin has been shown to be more effective than either when used alone.[16] Aspirin and NSAIDs may cause gastrointestinal (GI) irritation, GI tract bleeding, and impair platelet function. Aspirin use in children has been associated with the development of Reye syndrome, a potentially fatal disease that may elevate intracranial pressure and cause liver failure. Allergic reactions are common with NSAIDs, and asthmatics may develop bronchospasm following ingestion of NSAIDs (including aspirin). Because of the potential for precipitating or aggravating an asthma exacerbation, NSAIDs should be avoided in these patients.

It is of interest to note that for each 1 degree increase in temperature above 37° C, there is a 13% increase in oxygen consumption, and this may further impair oxygenation in the presence of cardiac or pulmonary disease.[16] It should also be noted that the ability to develop fever may be impaired in the elderly, and this should be taken into account in the assessment of older patients.[16] Fever may also be reduced or absent with infection in the newborn, patients with chronic renal failure, or those receiving corticosteroids.[16]

Fever may be characterized by the pattern of temperature changes observed over time, and some febrile diseases have characteristic patterns, though the fever pattern may be of little or no value in establishing a diagnosis. Onset of fever may be marked with shivering and chills.[5] Night sweats may occur with chronic infectious disease, inflammatory disease, and certain malignancies.[5] Fever may be continuous and sustained, intermittent, remittent, relapsing, or episodic (see Box 5-12). Fever may also be characterized as mild (37.2° to 38.9° C or 99° to 102° F), moderate (> 38.9° to 40.6° C or > 102° to 105° F) or severe (> 40.6° C or > 105° F), though classification systems vary. The term *hyperpyrexia* is reserved for very high fever, generally > 41.5° C

BOX 5-12

Temperature Regulation and Types of Fever

The body's temperature regulating center is in the hypothalamus. Its main purpose is to regulate body temperature in a changing environment.

Too hot	Sweating, peripheral vasodilatation
Too cold	Shivering, peripheral vasoconstriction
Hypothermia	< 97° F; occurs with prolonged exposure to cold, general anesthesia, damage to hypothalamus
Hyperthermia	> 100° F; occurs in very hot environment, heat stroke, exercise, abnormalities in brain, toxic substances, infection, inflammation, bacterial diseases, brain tumor, dehydration
Pyrogens	Certain fever-producing proteins, breakdown products of proteins (as in disease), or toxins secreted by bacteria leads to increase in set point of hypothalamus, which results in fever and chills.
Treatment of fever	Antipyretics include aspirin/acetaminophen and ibuprofen.
Types of fever	Fever may be continuous, intermittent, remittent, relapsing or episodic.

Continuous fever: Fever remains elevated throughout the day (aka sustained fever) and does not fluctuate more than 0.5° to 1° C in 24 hours.
  - Most common type of fever.
  - Seen with minor infection, lobar pneumonia, urinary tract infection, typhoid fever, and some cases of head injury.

Intermittent fever: Fever spikes with return to normal between spikes.
  - Seen in malaria (*Plasmodium* infection).
  - Variations include quotidian fever (periodicity of 24 hours), tertian fever (periodicity of 48 hours), and quartan fever (periodicity of 72 hours).

Remittent fever: Fever is elevated with marked fluctuations that do not return to normal.
  - Seen in typhoid fever, infective endocarditis.

Relapsing fever: Recurring fever for several days interspersed with periods of normal temperature.

Pel-Epstein fever: Occurs with Hodgkin disease and consists of bouts of several days of continuous or remittent fever.

Episodic fever: Fever that lasts for days or longer followed by at least 2 weeks without fever.
  - May be familial in origin (e.g., congenital familial Mediterranean fever).

Data from: Gardner DD, Wilkins RL. Cardiopulmonary symptoms. In: Wilkins RL, Dexter JR and Heuer AJ, editors. *Clinical Assessment in Respiratory Care*, 6th ed., St. Louis: Mosby Elsevier, 2010: 28–50; Vital signs, anthropometric data and pain. In: LeBlond RF, Brown DD, DeGowin RL, *DeGowin's Diagnostic Examination*, 9th ed. New York: McGraw Hill, 2009: 51–87.

(or > 106.7° F).[16] In addition to the administration of antipyretic medications, cooling blankets should be considered in the treatment of very high fever.[16]

Hyperthermia (as opposed to fever) is an elevated temperature due to excessive heat production or inadequate heat dissipation. Examples of increased heat production include malignant hyperthermia and heavy exertion in a hot, humid environment.[5] Malignant hyperthermia is a rare, inherited condition that may be precipitated by exposure to inhalational anesthetics or succinylcholine.[5]

Heat exhaustion (aka heat prostration) may occur following exertion in a hot, humid environment resulting in fluid loss (due to excessive sweating) and electrolyte disturbances. Symptoms of heat exhaustion include faintness, headache, nausea, vomiting, and cramps.[5] Tachycardia, hypotension, diaphoresis, and dilated pupils may be present. The skin may be moist and cool. Heat exhaustion may lead to *heat stroke*, which occurs when the thermoregulatory system fails and there is a rapid increase in body temperature.[5] The patient may become delirious or lose consciousness. The skin is often hot and dry. Heat stroke can rapidly prove fatal if not treated. Application of cool (not cold) or tepid water applied using a damp sponge to reduce body temperature should be helpful, and intravenous fluid administration to correct dehydration should be considered. Antipyretics are of no use in treating hyperthermia.[16] Causes of inadequate heat dissipation include certain medications and metabolic disease that interferes with thermoregulation.

Hypothermia

Body temperature normally decreases at night, and normal values may be as low as 35.0° C (95.0° F) during sleep.[5] An abnormally low body temperature (**hypothermia**) can occur due to exposure to environmental cold, as may occur during winter or with cold water immersion. An abnormally low body temperature is also sometimes seen in chronic kidney dialysis patients and occasionally in patients with liver cirrhosis and in diabetics in septic shock. Hypothermia reduces the metabolic rate and tissue demand for oxygen. Shivering increases heat production and is a physiologic response to decreased body temperatures. Because of the reduction in metabolic rate, hypothermic patients may exhibit slowed or shallow breathing. The prognosis for cold water near-drowning patients is more favorable when compared to an equal time of submersion for warm water near-drowning patients due to the reduction in oxygen consumption. Intentional body cooling is often used during certain types of surgery, such as cardiac transplant surgery, to prevent or reduce tissue damage.

When hypothermia is observed due to nonenvironmental causes, the clinician should suspect involvement of the hypothalamus. In these cases, low body temperature should alert the clinician to a possibly significant neurologic incident, such as head trauma, stroke, or evolution of a mass.[5] Low body temperature may also occur in patients with severe infections, especially in those with cirrhosis.

Pain

Assessment of pain should be part of the routine physical examination of the cardiopulmonary patient. Pain may be somatic (arising from skin, muscles, soft tissue, bones, ligaments, or tendons), visceral (arising from the viscera in body cavities due to ischemia, inflammation, or injury), or neuropathic (arising from nerve injury).[5] Pain may also be acute or chronic, localized or generalized, and of varying quality and severity. For example, sharp, stabbing, localized pain is often somatic, whereas generalized pain (often described as deep pain, aching, pressing, or squeezing) is more often visceral in origin.[5] Burning or hot pain may be neuropathic.[5]

Patients with cardiopulmonary disease may experience generalized pain and discomfort or localized pain due to specific injury or disease. For example, sinus pain and headache may accompany sinus infection. Hoarseness and sore throat are common complaints following extubation. Chest pain is a common symptom in patients with a wide variety of cardiopulmonary problems ranging from heart disease to pneumonia, pleurisy, rib fracture, pneumothorax, and tumor. Chest pain that responds to nitroglycerin suggests angina, whereas chest discomfort that responds to antacids suggests acid-peptic disease (e.g., gastroesophageal reflux disease; GERD).[5] Although chest pain is not typically life threatening, a number of potentially life-threatening causes of chest pain must be ruled out. These include myocardial infarction, pulmonary embolus, tension pneumothorax, aortic dissection, and esophageal rupture. The three types of chest pain are substernal, pleuritic, and musculoskeletal (see Chapter 4).

Abdominal pain can also be caused by many different disease states and conditions. Examples include gastric or intestinal disease, such as peptic ulcers; gastritis (inflammation of the lining of the stomach or duodenum); GERD; appendicitis; diverticulitis (inflammation of the sacs lining the intestine); colitis (inflammation of the colon); intestinal obstruction; irritable bowel syndrome; and inflammatory bowel disease (e.g., Crohn's disease).[17] Other causes of abdominal pain include pancreatitis (inflammation of the pancreas); cholecystitis (gallbladder inflammation); peritoneal inflammation; abdominal wall disorders (e.g., trauma, hernia); toxins (e.g., lead poisoning); metabolic disorders (e.g., uremia, ketoacidosis), neurologic problems; and referred pain from the heart, lungs, or esophagus.[17] Acute, intense abdominal pain with hemodynamic instability represents a medical emergency requiring immediate attention. Possible causes include dissection of an abdominal aortic aneurysm; obstruction, perforation, or rupture of a hollow organ within the abdomen (hollow viscus rupture); abdominal sepsis; ketoacidosis; and adrenal crisis (inadequate cortisol secretion).[17]

The respiratory care clinician often sees critically ill patients in the ICU or emergency department, where pain management is an important part of patient care. Causes of pain include tissue damage due to specific disease states, injury, trauma, surgery, and medical procedures, such as endotracheal intubation and mechanical ventilatory support.[18] In the ICU, patients may have multiple invasive lines and catheters (e.g., arterial lines, central venous lines, chest tubes, urinary catheters) and are subject to unpleasant or painful procedures, such as suctioning, airway care, arterial and/or venous puncture, and bedside thoracentesis or bronchoscopy. Control of pain and anxiety in the ICU patient is often inadequate, and this may result in hypermetabolism, increased O_2 consumption, and fighting against the ventilator in patients receiving mechanical ventilatory support.[18]

Assessment of pain should be based on what the patient reports. Useful pain scales include numerical ratings, visual analog scales, and questionnaires. A common method is to ask the patient to rate his or her pain on a scale of 0 to 10, where 0 indicates no pain and 10 indicates the worst possible pain.[18] In patients who are semiconscious, unconscious, or unable to otherwise communicate, the presence of the physical signs of pain (including sympathetic nervous system stimulation should) should be noted:[18]

- Grimacing
- Writhing
- Tachycardia
- Hypertension
- Tachypnea
- Diaphoresis
- Piloerection (elevation of the hair follicles of the skin)

The Behavioral Pain Scale (BPS) and Critical Care Pain Observation Tool (CPOT) are valid and reliable instruments developed for use with critically ill patients.[18] The BPS sums subscores for the patient's facial expression, upper limb movements, and compliance with mechanical ventilation; each subscore has a range of 1 to 4 for a total score range of 3 to 12 points (lowest to highest pain). The CPOT uses a similar scoring system based on observation of the patient's facial expression (0 to 2 points), body movements (0 to 2 points), muscle tension (0 to 2 points), and compliance with the ventilator for intubated patients or vocalization for extubated patients (0 to 2 points). Total CPOT scores range from 0 to 8 (absent pain to greatest pain). **Figure 5-2** provides an illustration of CPOT.

Because pain is often underestimated in critically ill patients, when in doubt, the clinician should presume and treat pain.[18] For conscious patients using a rating scale, the goal is a pain rating of ≤ 3 out of 10 or ≤ 2 out of 5 points.[18] Intravenous administration of opiates (e.g., morphine, hydromorphone [Dilaudid], or fentanyl) is generally preferred for analgesia in critically ill patients.[18] Intravenous opiates can be delivered by bolus injection (for moderate pain); continuous infusion (moderate to severe pain that is poorly controlled by bolus injection); or using patient-controlled analgesia (for conscious patients).[18] Morphine and hydromorphone have a longer duration of action than fentanyl and may be preferred for intermittent bolus administration.[18] Fentanyl provides the most rapid

Indicator	Description	Score	
Facial expression	No muscular attention observed	Relaxed, neutral	0
	Presence of frowning, brow lowering, orbit tightening, and levator contraction	Tense	1
	All of the above facial movements plus eyelid tightly closed	Grimacing	2
Body movements	Does not move at all (does not necessarily mean absence of pain)	Absence of movements	0
	Slow, cautious movements, touching or rubbing the pain site, seeking attention through movements	Protection	1
	Pulling tube, attempting to sit up, moving limbs/thrashing, not following commands, striking at staff, trying to climb out of bed	Restlessness	2
Muscle tension Evaluation by passive flexion and extension of upper extremities	No resistance to passive movements	Relaxed	0
	Resistance to passive movements	Tense, rigid	1
	Strong resistance to passive movements, inability to complete them	Very tense or rigid	2
Compliance with the ventilator (intubated patients)	Alarms not activated, easy ventilation	Tolerating ventilator or movement	0
	Alarms stop spontaneously	Coughing but tolerating	1
	Asynchrony: blocking ventilation, alarms frequently activated	Fighting ventilator	2
OR	Talking in a normal tone or no sound	Talking in a normal tone or no sound	0
Vocalization (extubated patients)	Sighing, moaning	Sighing, moaning	1
	Crying out, sobbing	Crying out, sobbing	2
Total, range			0–8

FIGURE 5-2   Critical Care Pain Observation Tool (CPOT).

onset of analgesia and may be preferred in patients with bronchospasm because it causes less histamine release.[18] With renal failure or hemodynamic instability, fentanyl or hydromorphone are recommended in place of morphine.[18] All opioids have similar side effects, which include nausea and vomiting, depressed consciousness, and the potential for causing hallucinations.[18] Cardiopulmonary side effects of the opiates include respiratory drive depression, hypotension (especially in hypovolemic patients), and release of histamine.[18] Histamine release is greatest with morphine and least with fentanyl.[18] Other possible opiate side effects include urinary retention and hypomotility of the GI tract (ileus or bowel obstruction). Opiate withdrawal signs and symptoms (e.g., drug craving, anxiety, sweating, tachycardia, tachypnea, vomiting, fever, and seizures) can occur in patients who have received moderate to high doses of opioids for as little as 1 week.[18] Gradual weaning of opiates has been suggested to avoid withdrawal symptoms. Nonopioid analgesics include acetaminophen and NSAIDs, such as ibuprofen and naproxen. Complications of NSAID use include increased risk of cardiovascular thrombotic events and GI complications (e.g., gastritis, bleeding, ulcers, and perforation).[18]

Height and Weight

Measurement of the patient's height and weight is a routine part of the physical examination. **Obesity** is linked to a variety of adverse health outcomes, and the number of overweight and obese patients in the United States has skyrocketed over the last three decades. Unexplained weight loss, however, could signal the development of acute or chronic disease.

In adult patients, clinicians typically utilize the height and weight measurements to calculate the patient's **body mass index (BMI)**. Calculating the patient's BMI can provide a helpful indicator of body weight adjusted for the patient's height. BMI can be utilized to estimate body fat content, although it is not a direct measure. The BMI is helpful for risk stratification for a variety of chronic and acute disease processes, such as hypertension, coronary heart disease, diabetes, and obstructive sleep apnea.[19] Based on the calculated BMI, patients are placed into four separate categories: underweight, appropriate or normal weight, overweight, and obese (see **Table 5-5**). Overweight or obese patients are at risk for the development of heart disease, high blood pressure, stroke, cancer, osteoarthritis, sleep apnea, diabetes, elevated triglycerides and LDL cholesterol, metabolic syndrome, and other acute and chronic

CLINICAL FOCUS 5-1

Vital Signs

A 72-year-old man is admitted to the hospital from an extended care facility. The patient seems confused and somewhat unresponsive to verbal commands. The respiratory care clinician performs a brief physical assessment and obtains the following information:

    Pulse: 122 bpm
    Respiratory rate: 32 breaths/min
    BP: 90/60 mm Hg
    Temperature: 101°F

What additional nontraditional "vital signs" should be obtained?

Answer: Pulse oximetry for measurement of SpO_2 should be completed. While the patient is somewhat unresponsive to verbal commands, any signs of pain (e.g., grimacing, writhing, tachycardia) should be noted.

A pulse oximeter is used to measure the SpO_2 while breathing room air:

    $SpO_2 = 83\%$

Describe the patient's condition based on the available information.

Answer: The patient is exhibiting tachycardia, tachypnea, and borderline hypotension. The patient is febrile, which may be due to infection. The patient is also somewhat unresponsive and confused, which may be due to hypoxemia (SpO_2 of 83% corresponds to $PaO_2 < 50$ mm Hg).

What steps should the respiratory care clinician now take?

Answer: Oxygen should be started at 4 L/min and oximetry repeated. Oxygen flow should then be adjusted to achieve $SpO_2 \geq 90\%$. Additional assessment should then be completed to include a thorough physical examination and appropriate laboratory studies. Chest imaging may also be required to assess for possible pneumonia.

TABLE 5-5
Body Mass Index (BMI) and Weight Status

BMI	Weight Status
< 18.5	Underweight
18.5–24.9	Normal
25.0–29.9	Overweight
≥ 30.0	Obese

BMI = Weight (kg)/[Height (m)]^2
OR
BMI = Weight (lb)/[Height (in)]^2 × 703

Reproduced from: Centers for Disease Control: About BMI for Adults. Last updated September 2011. Retrieved from: http://www.cdc.gov/healthyweight/assessing/bmi/adult_bmi/index.html)

health problems.[19,20] **Box 5-13** summarizes the health risks associated with overweight and obesity.

In addition to assessing BMI, when patients are admitted to the hospital, especially for cardiovascular disorders, weight can be used to assess the patient's fluid status. Patients with chronic heart failure can be especially sensitive to changes in fluid balance, and daily weights can be helpful to determine whether the patient is fluid-volume overloaded (as indicated by weight gain) or to assess the effectiveness of diuretics to eliminate excess fluid. When considering a patient's weight, a comparison to the patient's baseline and trends are helpful to provide a clear clinical picture. When noting patient's daily weights, it is important that the clinician consider the method used for weight measurement.[21] When patients are hospitalized, there are a variety of ways a patient can be weighed, such as traditional standing scales, wheelchair scales, or bed scales. Measured weight can fluctuate depending on how the weight is obtained. For example, bed weights may vary depending on the contents in the bed (number of blankets on the bed, pillows, etc.). If there is a large fluctuation in weight from one day to the next, it is prudent to assess whether this correlates with other physical exam findings (e.g., breath sounds, edema, or oxygen requirements). Ideally, the patient will be weighed each day with the same scale that has been calibrated to the manufacturer's specifications, wearing the same or similar clothing, and with an empty bladder.[21]

Weight Loss and Cachexia

Significant weight loss in a previously healthy individual can signal serious health problems.[22] Malignant neoplasms (e.g., lung cancer, GI tract cancer, other); chronic infectious disease (e.g., tuberculosis, HIV, other); chronic inflammatory disease (e.g.,

inflammatory bowel disease, other); endocrine and metabolic disorders (e.g., hyperthyroidism, diabetes mellitus, other); and psychiatric disorders (e.g., depression, anxiety, eating disorders, other) may all cause involuntary weight loss.[22] Malnutrition is caused by inadequate caloric intake, impairment of gastrointestinal dietary uptake, excessive energy expenditure, or problems with metabolism.[23] Severe illness, stress from surgery, and chronic cardiac or lung disease are often associated with malnutrition and weight loss.[23] Patients with prolonged illnesses may have severe weight loss and muscle wasting. The clinical term for this is **cachexia**. Common chronic illnesses that are associated with cachexia are CHF; chronic respiratory illnesses, such as COPD; and chronic renal failure.[24] It should be noted if a patient is beginning to experience

---

BOX 5-13

Health Risks of Overweight and Obesity

Overweight or obese patients are at risk for the development of:

- Coronary heart disease
- High blood pressure
- Stroke
- Type 2 diabetes
- Dyslipidemia (abnormal blood fats):
  - Elevated triglycerides
  - Elevated LDL (bad) cholesterol
  - Decreased HDL (good) cholesterol
- Cancer
- Osteoarthritis (e.g., joint problems of the knees, hips, and lower back)
- Obstructive sleep apnea and obesity hypoventilation syndrome
- Menstrual issues and infertility in women
- Gallstones
- Metabolic syndrome:
  - Increases risk of heart disease, diabetes, and stroke
  - Defined by the presence of three or more of the following:
    - Large waistline (abdominal obesity; i.e., "apple shape")
    - Elevated triglycerides
    - Low HDL (good) cholesterol
    - Elevated blood pressure
    - Elevated fasting blood sugar

Modified from: National Institutes of Health, National Heart Lung and Blood Institute. What are the health risks of overweight and obesity? July 13, 2012. http://www.nhlbi.nih.gov/health/health-topics/topics/obe/risks.html. Accessed February 1, 2013.

muscle wasting and weight loss. Regardless of the cause, cachexia is associated with increased morbidity and mortality. Patients with cachexia have less reserve than healthier patients and typically have poorer health outcomes.

General Appearance

When beginning the physical exam, the first step is to observe the patient's general appearance. The goal is to gain a picture of the individual as a whole. Inspection of the patient should begin at the moment the clinician first encounters the patient and continue throughout the assessment. Gender, ethnicity, age, height and weight, and general state of health should be noted. For example, men are more likely to develop hemophilia (a genetic bleeding disorder), whereas sickle cell disease is more common in African Americans and in persons of Middle Eastern, Indian, Mediterranean, and African heritage. Facial expression may provide clues as to the patient's emotional state. For example, the patient may appear to be alert, awake, relaxed, and responsive, or the patient may appear to be anxious, restless, or confused. General appearance can also provide clues as to the patient's nutritional status and whether the patient is underweight, overweight, or obese. Overweight or obese patients are at risk for the development of heart disease, high blood pressure, stroke, cancer, sleep apnea, diabetes, and blood lipid disorders (see Box 5-13). Malnourished patients may be suffering from a number of acute or chronic diseases.[23–26] Important questions to consider regarding the patient's general appearance include:

- Is the patient awake, alert, and responsive?
- Is the patient relaxed and resting quietly?
- Is the patient anxious, restless, or disoriented and/or confused?
- What is the patient's position (lying down, sitting up, other)?
- Are there any signs of respiratory distress?
- What ancillary equipment or supplies are in use (oxygen equipment, monitoring equipment, intravenous lines)?
- What is the patient's general state of health?

The patient's general appearance, overall condition, level of consciousness, respiratory rate and pattern, and signs of respiratory distress (e.g., use of accessory muscles, retractions) should be noted. Positional dyspnea is common in CHF as well as COPD. For example, the patient with severe COPD may have great difficulty breathing while in a supine position. These patients often sit up, with one or more pillows, even while sleeping. The respiratory clinician should note the patient's color and if the patient is sweating excessively (diaphoresis). If pulse oximetry is in use, the patient's SpO_2 should be noted, along with any supplemental O_2 the patient may be receiving. If cardiac monitoring equipment is in use, the clinician should note the cardiac rate and rhythm and observe for gross arrhythmias. The general inspection should include the head and face, neck, hands and fingernails, and skin of the arms and extremities.

When observing the cardiopulmonary patient's general appearance, it is important to be alert for the signs of respiratory failure. Hypoxic patients may exhibit anxiety, excitement, restlessness, impaired judgment, and disorientation or confusion (see Chapter 6). Other signs of respiratory failure include respiratory distress, tachypnea, hyperventilation, and use of the accessory muscles. Cardiovascular signs of respiratory failure include tachycardia, increased blood pressure, and the development of cardiac arrhythmias. With respiratory failure and severe hypoxia, respirations may be slowed and/or irregular, and bradycardia and hypotension may develop. Loss of consciousness, somnolence, convulsions, and coma are findings associated with very severe hypoxia and may portend a respiratory and/or cardiac arrest. Signs of severe respiratory distress include accessory muscle use, retractions, brief fragmented speech, profuse sweating, agitation or altered mental status, and an inability to lie supine.

Skin

Inspecting the patient's skin in order to detect changes in skin color and the presence of edema or diaphoresis provides useful information.[27] Skin color varies with skin pigmentation; however, the nail beds of the fingers and toes and the gums should be pink. Cyanosis is associated with hypoxemia, though it is a variable finding (see below). Capillary refill should be good, and the skin and extremities should be well perfused. A pale appearance, with cold, clammy skin is associated with shock or hypotension. Causes of peripheral edema include fluid overload, CHF, increased capillary permeability (e.g., sepsis), and low plasma albumin (e.g., cirrhosis, nephrotic syndrome, burns). Angioedema is swelling that may appear in the face, tongue, larynx, hands, or feet. Angioedema may be caused by an allergic reaction to a bee sting or insect bite, a drug reaction (e.g., penicillin or other antibiotic), or food allergy (e.g., peanuts, shellfish). Scars may indicate past trauma or surgery, and the past medical history should help clarify the cause of any scars observed.

Diaphoresis

Sweating is a natural mechanism for body temperature regulation and cooling in the face of vigorous exercise or a warm or hot environment.[28] Excessive sweating (**diaphoresis**) can be a sign of acute respiratory distress (e.g., hypercapnea and ventilatory failure) or cardiac disease (e.g., MI, CHF). Sweating can also be caused by fever, infection, certain drugs and medications (e.g., cocaine, morphine, alcohol, and caffeine), anxiety and stress, pain, ingestion of spicy foods, menopause, low blood sugar, and withdrawal from alcohol or narcotic drugs.[28]

Cyanosis

Cyanosis is a bluish discoloration of the skin, nail beds, and mucus membranes caused by an elevated level of desaturated (deoxygenated) hemoglobin (Hb) in the arterial blood.[29] Generally, cyanosis is most readily observed in the lips, gingiva (gums), and nail beds of the fingers and toes. The term *central cyanosis* refers to cyanosis of the oral mucosa or trunk, whereas *peripheral cyanosis* is observed in the hands, fingertips, and nail beds of the hands and feet. Central cyanosis is associated with generalized hypoxemia; peripheral cyanosis may be caused by vascular occlusive disease.

Although central cyanosis is generally considered a sign of hypoxemia, the absence of cyanosis should not be taken to mean that oxygenation is satisfactory. In order to develop cyanosis, the level of unsaturated Hb must exceed 4 to 5 g/dL.[29] A normal Hb level is about 15 g/dL. Thus, a patient with a normal Hb will probably become cyanotic when the oxygen saturation falls to < 67% to 73% (i.e., 4 to 5 g/dL of *desaturated* Hb).

Patients with chronic hypoxemia and polycythemia often present with cyanosis. A patient with an Hb of 20 g/dL (e.g., polycythemia) will probably become cyanotic when the oxygen saturation falls to < 75% to 80%. Patients with anemia or blood loss have a decreased Hb. These patients may not develop cyanosis, even though the blood oxygen content is very low. In a patient with hemoglobin level of only 8 g/dL, the oxygen saturation would have to be less than 50% for cyanosis to appear. Consequently, the presence or absence of cyanosis must be interpreted cautiously, because cyanosis is a variable finding, depending on the oxygen saturation and Hb level. For a further discussion of cyanosis, hemoglobin levels, and hypoxemia, refer to Chapter 7.

Clinicians should also differentiate whether cyanosis is caused by a cardiac or respiratory problem. Respiratory causes of cyanosis include hypoventilation and impaired gas exchange in the lung. Cardiac causes of cyanosis include congenital cardiovascular anomalies in which deoxygenated blood is shunted from the right to left side of the heart and then pumped to the peripheral tissues. Due to improved surgical care, congenital cyanotic heart disorders are typically treated in childhood. There are a variety of congenital heart disorders that can progress to cyanotic heart disease in adulthood, depending on severity, and should be considered in adults who present with cyanosis. A thorough examination of the pulmonary and cardiac systems should be completed in patients who present with cyanosis. Though it is a variable finding, cyanosis can indicate impending or current respiratory failure.

Other Alterations in Skin Color

A pale, cold, clammy appearance may be just as ominous as cyanosis. In particular, a pale, cold, clammy appearance is associated with shock. Other conditions that may affect skin color include skin rash, allergic reactions, carbon monoxide poisoning, methemoglobinemia, cyanide poisoning, and elevated carbon dioxide levels. A skin rash combined with mucosal edema, nasal polyps, and aspirin intolerance are common in allergic asthma and is known as *triad asthma*. Carbon monoxide poisoning may produce a bright cherry red skin color, whereas elevated carbon dioxide levels are sometimes associated with redness of the skin. Cyanide poisoning may also cause the skin to appear red due to increased venous oxygen concentration caused by impaired tissue uptake of O_2. An elevated skin temperature can cause reddening of the skin (erythema) due to vasodilatation, which may occur with a number of different conditions, including scarlet fever, cellulitis, lupus erythematosus, and first-degree burns.[27] Jaundice is a yellowing of the skin associated with liver disease.

Mental Status and Neurologic Examination

Completing an extensive mental status and neurologic examination is not warranted for every cardiopulmonary patient; however, certain components of the mental status and neurologic exam can give valuable insight into the patient's overall health, respiratory status, and the severity of disease. The clinician can often assess aspects of cognitive function and neurologic status during the patient interview. The patient's family and prior medical records can be helpful to assess alterations from baseline. It is important to note alterations in the neurologic examination because these can signal systemic or focal neurologic disorders.

Assessment of Mental Status and Levels of Consciousness

The assessment of a patient's mental status should begin with sensorium (the sensory components of the brain and nervous system), level of consciousness (LOC), and orientation. This assessment begins at the start of the clinician–patient encounter. An astute clinician will observe the patient interacting with his or her environment and other healthcare providers. This often will provide insight to the patient's mental and/or neurologic status. The patient's LOC may be described as alert, lethargic, stuporous, semi-coma, or coma.[30] With semi-coma the patient responds to pain, but nothing else (i.e., eyes open with pain stimulus); with coma there is no response to stimulus (i.e., eyes remain closed). The patient may be oriented to place, person, time, and situation. Questions the clinician should consider when assessing a patient's orientation include:

- Does the patient know who he or she is?
- Does the patient know who others are and their names and role(s)?
- Does the patient know where he or she is (place, city, state, country)?
- Does the patient know the year, season, date, and time?

Appropriate questions to assess the patient's orientation are listed below (see "Mental Status Examination"). The following terms are often used to describe levels of consciousness:

- *Confused*: The patient may have difficulty in understanding directions or be confused regarding person, place, time, or situation.
- *Delirious*: Hallucinations may be present.
- *Lethargic*: Patient is sleepy but can be aroused.
- *Obtunded*: Patient may be difficult to arouse but responds appropriately.
- *Stuporous*: Patient does not completely awaken when attempts are made to arouse.
- *Semi-coma*: Patient responds only to pain.
- *Comatose*: Patient is unconscious, does not respond even to pain.

The difference between an awake, relaxed, and oriented patient versus a confused, anxious, disoriented patient could be the adequacy of oxygenation and/or ventilation. The respiratory care clinician should always be alert to the signs of hypoxia, which may affect cognition, level of consciousness, and neurologic function. Remember, the brain is very sensitive to inadequate oxygen levels. Hypoxia may cause excitement, restlessness, anxiety, overconfidence, impaired judgment, disorientation, or confusion; severe hypoxia may cause somnolence, loss of consciousness, convulsions, and coma.

Level of Consciousness

As noted, patients with neurologic disease and many patients seen in the acute care setting, especially in ICUs, have alterations in their level of consciousness. Trauma, narcotic or sedative drugs, hypoxia, and circulatory disorders (e.g., shock or hypotension) all may affect brain function and consciousness. In addition, patients may be agitated, anxious, restless, or in pain, and drugs are often prescribed to relieve these conditions.

A number of scales and scoring systems have been developed to quantify level of consciousness or levels of sedation. The Glasgow Coma Scale ranges from 3 points (brain death) to 15 points (fully conscious; see Table 5-6). Some have suggested that if scores are "less than 8 then intubate", though this rule of thumb should not be applied indiscriminately. Both the Ramsay Sedation Scale and the Richmond Agitation Sedation

Scale have been developed to rate patients' agitation and level of sedation (see **Tables 5-7** and **5-8**).

Mental Status Examination

The mental status examination begins with the patient encounter. As noted, the clinician should observe the patient's interaction with the environment, healthcare providers, and others (e.g., family members). Reviewing prior medical records, discussing the patient's mental status (or changes in the mental status) with family members, and questioning other providers involved in the patient's care can help in developing a better understanding of the patient's current status and any

TABLE 5-6
Glasgow Coma Scale
The Glasgow Coma Scale ranges from a low score of 3 points (brain death) to a maximum score of 15 points (fully conscious). A patient who spontaneously opens his or her eyes, responds in an oriented manner to verbal stimuli, and obeys motor commands would have a score of 15 points. Points are assigned for eye opening, verbal response, and motor response.

Observation	Score
Eye Opening	
Spontaneous	4
In response to voice	3
In response to pain	2
None	1
Verbal Response	
Oriented response	5
Confused response	4
Inappropriate words	3
Incomprehensible words	2
None	1
Motor Response	
Obeys commands	6
Localizes	5
Withdraws	4
Flexes (decorticate)	3
Extends (decerebrate)	2
None	1

Data from: Center for Disease Control: Glascow Coma Score. Last updated May, 2003. Retrieved from: http://www.bt.cdc.gov/masscasualties/pdf/glasgow-coma-scale.pdf

TABLE 5-7
Ramsey Sedation Scale
The Ramsey Sedation Scale rates the patient's sedation/agitation level from minimal sedation/high agitation (score = 1) to maximum sedation (score = 6). A score of 2 points would be preferred in most patients.

Level	Response
1	Anxious, agitated, restless
2	Cooperative, oriented, tranquil
3	Responding to commands only
4	Asleep, brisk response to stimulus
5	Asleep, sluggish response to stimulus
6	Unarousable

TABLE 5-8
Richmond Agitation Sedation Scale
The Richmond Agitation Sedation Scale (RASS) provides a method to quantify a patient's sedation. The scale range is +4 points (no sedation/combative) to –5 points (unarousable). The preferred score for most patients is 0.

Score	Term	Description
+4	Combative	Overtly combative, violent, immediate danger to staff
+3	Very agitated	Pulls or removes tube(s) or catheter(s), aggressive
+2	Agitated	Frequent nonpurposeful movement, fights ventilator
+1	Restless	Anxious but movements not aggressive or vigorous
0	Alert and calm	
–1	Drowsy	Not fully alert, but has sustained awakening (eye opening/eye contact) to voice (≥ 10 seconds)
–2	Light sedation	Briefly awakens with eye contact to voice (≥ 10 seconds)
–3	Moderate sedation	Movement or eye opening to voice (but no eye contact)
–4	Deep sedation	No response to voice, but movement or eye opening to physical stimulation
–5	Unarousable	No response to voice or physical stimulation

Reprinted with permission of the American Thoracic Society. Copyright © 2014 American Thoracic Society. Sessler CN, Gosnell M, Grap MJ, Brophy GT, O'Neal PV, Keane KA et al. The Richmond Agitation-Sedation Scale: validity and reliability in adult intensive care patients. *Am J Respir Crit Care Med* 2002;166:1338-1344. Official Journal of the American Thoracic Society.

changes. Initially, as the clinician enters the room, the clinician should observe the patient for his or her overall appearance. Is the patient dressed appropriately? Does he or she look disheveled or unkempt? What is the patient's level of consciousness? Does the patient appear to be oriented to person, place, time, and situation? Is the patient able to pay attention and stay on task? Answers to these questions can provide indicators of the patient's overall neurologic and mental status.[30,31] Although not always necessary or feasible, especially in an emergent situation, the components of a complete mental status examination are as follows:

Appearance
The clinician should observe the patient for overall appearance. Questions the clinician should ask himself or herself:

- Does the patient appear older or younger than the stated age?
- Does the patient appear well groomed or unkempt?
- What is the status of the patient's personal hygiene?
- Is the patient's dress appropriate for the season and setting?

Attitude
While interviewing the patient, the clinician should note the patient's general attitude towards the situation and encounter. This can be inferred from the patient's facial expressions and interaction with the clinician. Ideally, the patient will be cooperative, interact in an appropriate fashion, and appear to be interested in the encounter. Table 5-9 provides a variety of different descriptors sometimes used by clinicians to describe patients' attitude or affect. The clinician should be cautious, however, when labeling a patient's affective characteristics, because the possibility of misinterpreting the patient's emotional state is high.

Body Language and Eye Contact
The healthcare provider should observe the patient's body language and use of eye contact. Does the patient make and sustain eye contact? What may be inferred from the patient's body language? For example, does the

TABLE 5-9
Descriptors of Patient Attitude or Affect

Hostile	Apathetic	Open
Secretive	Easily distracted	Defensive
Focused	Suspicious	Vigilant
Tense	Evasive	Argumentative

patient cross his or her arms and look at the floor, or is the patient appropriate, open, and make and sustain good eye contact?

With respect to eye contact, the clinician should take into account the patient's culture, because this can affect the way the patient addresses or looks at the clinician. Generally speaking, it should be noted if the patient makes, avoids, or seems hesitant to make eye contact. This should be documented in the medical record.

Level of Consciousness

The patient's level of consciousness (LOC) should be documented in the patient's medical record. Any changes in LOC should be reported to the healthcare team because it may indicate evolving neurologic, respiratory, or systemic disorders. As noted earlier, LOC may be described as alert, drowsy, lethargic, stuporous, comatose, or confused.

Orientation

As noted earlier, there are four aspects to patient orientation: person, place, time, and situation. The patient's orientation can be assessed by asking the following four questions:

- "What is your full name?"
- "Where are we at (floor, building, city, county, and state)?"
- "What is the full date today (date, month, year, day of the week, and season of the year)?"
- "How would you describe the situation we are in?"

The clinician should note whether the patient is completely oriented or if there is a deficit. This should be recorded in the patient's medical record.

Motor Behavior

The patient's motor behavior can be assessed by observing the patient in the exam room. If possible, have the patient walk to observe the patient's gait. The examiner should note the type and quality of motor behavior. Motor behavior can be described as normal, hyperactive, fidgety, catatonic, dystonia, tremors, dyskinesia, or tics.

Speech and Language

Neurologic and psychiatric disorders can affect the quality and content of the patient's speech. Both should be documented clearly in the medical record. If speech content is abnormal, this should also be documented, providing examples in the medical record. When observing the patient's speech, the clinician should note the rate and flow of speech, intensity of volume, clarity, and quantity. The following are commonly used terms when describing speech:

- *Quantity*: Talkative, spontaneous, expansive, or rambling
- *Rate*: Fast, slow, normal, or pressured

- *Volume* (tone): Loud, soft, monotone, weak, strong, or yelling
- *Fluency and rhythm*: Slurred, articulate or clear, incoherent, hesitant, or aphasic

Mood and Affect

Affect refers to the patient's transient state of emotion, whereas *mood* refers to the patient's sustained feelings. When inquiring about the patient's mood, ask the patient to describe his or her long-term internal emotional state. For example, the clinician may ask how the patient's mood has been over the last 2 weeks.[30] Some questions that may be helpful when assessing the patient's mood are as follows:

- "How are your spirits?"
- "How are you feeling?"
- "Have you been discouraged/depressed/low/blue lately?"
- "Have you been energized/elated/high/out of control lately?"
- "Have you been angry/irritable/edgy lately?"

Affect is observed (and inferred) by the clinician and varies over time. In describing the patient's affect, the clinician should note the emotional range (broad or restricted), intensity (blunted, flat, or normal), and stability of the patient's affect. The four classic affective states are mad, sad, glad, and afraid. Affect may also be described as angry, fearful, worried, or wary.

Thought Process and Content

The patient's thought process can be described as the patient's form and flow of thinking. The rate of thought (extremely rapid thinking is called *flight of ideas*) and flow of thought (whether thought is goal directed or disorganized) should be noted. The patient's thought content describes what the patient is thinking about. Assessment of the patient's thought may include:[30]

- *Content*: Is the patient's thinking appropriate to his or her situation? Does it represent a realistic assessment of what's going on?
- *Sequence*: Do thoughts link in a logical way?
- *Insight*: Is the patient able to look at himself or herself and the current situation with comprehension and understanding?
- *Judgment*: Does the patient make reasonable assessments, choices, and decisions?

Commonly utilized terms to describe thought content are normal, delusional, obsessive, rumination, paranoia depersonalization, suicidality, and homicidality. Questions for assessing the patient include:

- "What's been on your mind lately?"
- "Are you worried/scared/frightened about something?"

- "What do you think about when you are sad or angry?"
- "Do you ever feel detached/removed/changed/different from others around you?"
- "Do you think someone or some group intend to harm you in some way?"

Insight describes the patient's awareness of or ability to understand his or her illness. Judgment describes the patient's ability to identify consequences for his or her actions. Insight and judgment are often assessed concurrently, but they are not exclusive of the other. For example, a patient might have insight into his or her illness but may not have the ability to use appropriate judgment in regards to care and may not understand the consequences for lack of treatment.

Perception

Perception describes how the patient experiences the world through the senses. Perception can be distorted by neurologic or psychiatric disease.[30] Examples of abnormalities of perception include hallucinations, illusions, and problems with structural perception. Hallucinations are visual, auditory, tactile, olfactory, or gustatory patient experiences that are not shared by a competent observer. Visual hallucinations are more common with delirium, such as may be experienced during narcotic drug or alcohol withdrawal. Auditory hallucinations are more common with psychosis.[30] Illusions are incorrect perceptions of objects that both the patient and clinician experience.[30] Structural perception refers to the patient's ability to place objects and shapes in relation to one another.[30]

Personality changes often accompany both acute and chronic cardiopulmonary disease. Patients may become anxious, irritable, or depressed. Denial is another defense mechanism seen with severe disease, in which the patient will not acknowledge the extent of the disease or its limitations. The patient may be uncooperative and noncompliant with treatment. Fear and anger are also common responses. It is important to investigate any feelings of depression or hopelessness. If the patient reports long-term feelings of hopelessness or depression, the clinician should inquire about suicidal ideation. If the patient reports suicidal thoughts, a prompt psychiatric evaluation is warranted. Inform the healthcare team regarding suicidal thoughts reported by the patient to ensure prompt attention and patient safety.

Table 5-10 contains an example of the Mini Mental State Examination (MMSE), which assesses orientation, registry, recall, and language using a simple rating

TABLE 5-10
Mini-Mental State Examination
The Mini-Mental State Examination (MMSE) assesses a patient's orientation to time, place, registration, attention and calculation, recall, language, repetition, and response to complex commands. The MMSE is sometimes used to screen for cognitive impairment and dementia. A score of at least 25 out of 30 points indicates normal cognitive function. Score ranges for impairment are:

Normal: ≥ 25
Mild impairment: 19–24
Moderate impairment: 10–18
Severe impairment: ≤ 9

Category	Possible Points	Questions
Orientation to time	5	What is the time/date/day/month/year? (1 point for each)
Registration	3	Name three objects and ask the patient to repeat them until all three are learned. Record the number of trials.
Orientation to place	5	Where are we (state, county, city, hospital, ward, or floor)? (1 point each)
Attention and calculation	5	Ask the patient to subtract serial 7s for five times. (Up to 5 points)
Recall	3	Ask the patient to recall the three objects named above. (1 point for each)
Language	2	Ask the patient to name a pencil and a watch. (1 point each)
Repetition	1	Ask the patient to speak back a phrase: "No ifs, ands, or buts."
Complex	6	1. Instruct patient to "take paper in your right hand, fold it in half and put it on the floor." (3 points) 2. Have patient read and obey instruction given in writing: "Close your eyes." (1 point) 3. Instruct patient to "write a sentence." (1 point) 4. Ask patient to "Copy this figure." (1 point)

Data from: Crum RM, Anthony JC, Bassett SS, Folstein MF. Population-based norms for the mini-mental state examination by age and educational level. *JAMA*. 1993:269:2386–2391; LeBlond RF, Brown DD, DeGowins RL. The mental status and psychiatric examination evaluation. *DeGowin's Diagnostic Evaluation*. 9th ed. New York; McGraw Hill; 2009: 766–784.

scale. The MMSE is commonly used to screen for cognitive impairment.

Neurologic Examination

The purpose of the neurologic examination is to identify cognitive, sensory, motor, and coordination deficits.[31] The nature and location of specific deficits often points to the site or mechanism of injury or disease process. For example, muscle paralysis that may affect ventilation can be caused by inflammatory/immune system disease (e.g., Guillain-Barré syndrome, myasthenia gravis, multiple sclerosis); infectious disease (e.g., poliomyelitis, postpolio syndrome, West Nile virus); trauma (e.g., spinal cord injury, head trauma); or vascular disease (stroke, subdural or epidural bleeding). A complete neurologic examination includes mental status; the cranial nerves; motor examination (e.g., muscle wasting, muscle tone, strength); examination of reflexes; cerebellar examination (posture, balance, coordination); sensory examination (e.g., pain, touch); peripheral nerves; and movements of specific muscles and nerves.[31] Although a discussion of the complete neurologic examination is beyond the scope of this chapter, the respiratory care clinician should be familiar with the basics of the neurologic exam.

Cranial Nerve Assessment

The 12 cranial nerves include the olfactory nerve (smell), optic nerve (vision), acoustic nerve (hearing), glossopharyngeal nerve (pain, touch, and temperature from the mucosa of the pharynx; gag reflex), and the vagus nerve.[31] The vagus nerve has multiple branches, and vagal stimulation can occur during endotracheal suctioning, resulting in bradycardia. Cranial nerve abnormalities can be indicative of brainstem or neurologic injury. Issues with specific cranial nerves should prompt a thorough neurologic evaluation, because the patient may be at risk for a compromised airway or aspiration.

Common neurologic symptoms sometimes related to cranial nerve problems include visual loss, ringing in the ears (tinnitus), hearing loss, vertigo, double vision (diplopia), difficulty swallowing (dysphagia), difficulty speaking (dysarthria or aphasia), facial pain, asymmetrical smile or facial appearance, hoarseness, and neck or shoulder weakness.[31] Physical signs sometimes caused by cranial nerve problems include visual field loss, abnormal pupils, jaw weakness or spasm, facial weakness or paralysis, balance problems, laryngeal paralysis (coughing or reflux), sternocleidomastoid or trapezius weakness, tongue deviation, and wasting. **Table 5-11** summarizes assessment for the cranial nerves.

Motor Assessment

Assessment of motor function includes inspection of the muscles for the presence of wasting and assessment of muscle tone and strength. Neurologic symptoms sometimes associated with motor problems include weakness, cataplexy (episodic loss of motor control), muscle pain (myalgia), muscle stiffness, twitches and tics, restless legs syndrome, muscle spasm, loss of balance, difficulty walking, vertigo, and tremors.[31] Neurologic signs sometimes seen with motor problems include muscle paralysis or loss of strength, decreased muscle tone (hypotonia), increased muscle tone (hypertonia), spasticity, myoclonus (jerking motion), myotonia (continued muscle contraction), tetany, or twitching.[31] Disease states or condition that may cause motor muscle weakness or paralysis include Guillain-Barré syndrome, myasthenia gravis, multiple sclerosis (MS), poliomyelitis, postpolio syndrome, and spinal cord injury.[31]

Assessment of Reflexes

Pupillary Reflexes

Pupillary reaction (i.e., pupillary reflex) to light is assessed by shining a swinging light onto the retina of the eye and observing **pupillary response**. Normally, both pupils will contract, regardless of the side exposed to the light, and dilate when the light source is removed.[31] Failure to respond normally can be caused by optic nerve damage or oculomotor damage on one side. Fixed, unilateral pupil dilation (mydriasis) may be caused by an elevation in intracranial pressure (ICP). Anticholinergic drugs (e.g., atropine) and some illicit drugs (e.g., LSD) may cause bilateral pupil dilation. Special eye drops containing cyclopentolate or phenylephrine may be used during an eye examination to dilate the pupils for better visualization of the retina. Depressant and opiate drugs may also cause an abnormal pupillary response.[31] In the acute care setting, an abnormal pupillary response (the pupils are dilated and fixed) can be caused by brainstem death.[31]

Muscle Stretch Reflexes

Evaluation of muscle stretch reflexes (also known as *tendon reflexes*) during a neurologic examination can give insight into the patient's spinal reflex arc function.[31] Muscle tendon reflexes are tested by tapping on a tendon with a reflex hammer. Physiologically, the tapping mechanism causes a stretch of the tendon, resulting in contraction of the corresponding muscle. There are two components of the reflex arc that should be noted: the upper motor neurons and lower motor neurons. Damage to either can cause abnormality of the reflex. The upper motor neuron is the component of the reflex arc that is located in the higher brain center. Damage to the higher brain center can cause the reflex arc to become hyperactive because the sensory component of the arc will be uninhibited. In contrast, if the lower motor neuron or peripheral nerve of the reflex arc is damaged, the correlating muscle tendon reflex will be diminished. In a normal muscle tendon reflex,

TABLE 5-11
Cranial Nerve Assessment

Cranial Nerve	Function (what it controls)	Test
(I) Olfactory	Smell (not usually tested)	Patient should close both eyes and occlude one nostril and identify the odor of a common object. Do this for each nostril. Objects frequently used include coffee, cloves, lemon, or soap (avoid ammonia or harsh soaps).
(II) Optic	Visual acuity Visual fields	*Visual acuity*: Snellen eye chart at 14 inches. *Visual fields:* Patient covers one eye and examiner moves fingers of left hand and then right into patient view. Patient identifies when fingers can be seen. Repeat with patient covering the opposite eye.
(III) Oculomotor	Pupillary reactions (pupillary light reflex and accommodation) Eyelid elevation Eye movements up, down, and medially	*Pupillary reactions:* Instruct patient to fix both eyes on an object. Shine the beam of a light directly into each pupil. Note the size, shape, and reaction of the pupils. *Eye movements:* Instruct patient to follow your finger without moving head. Examiner moves finger up, down, left, and right. Note the presence of limited eye movement.
(IV) Trochlear	Eye movement down and in toward nose	Instruct the patient to follow your finger without moving head. Examiner moves finger up, down, left, and right. Note the presence of limited eye movement.
(VI) Abducens	Eye movement laterally toward temporal field	Instruct patient to follow your finger without moving head. Examiner moves finger up, down, left, and right. Note the presence of nystagmus, limited eye movement.
(V) Trigeminal	Sensation of face Corneal reflex Muscles of mastication (jaw movement)	Ask the patient to open mouth as wide as possible Attempt to close mouth by placing one hand under chin and the other on top of head
(VII) Facial	Facial muscles	Have patient wrinkle forehead, smile showing teeth, and wink eyes. Note any asymmetrical movement or facial drooping.
(VIII) Auditory or Acoustic	Hearing and sense of balance	Test using Rinne and Weber tests with tuning fork. Test gross hearing by holding a watch or rubbing fingers together close to ears.
(IX) Glossopharyngeal and (X) Vagus	Cough Gag Swallow Articulation Phonation	Instruct patient to open mouth and say "ahhh." Look for elevation of soft palate and uvula in the midline. Assess gag reflex by stimulating back of pharynx with tongue depressor. Note any difficulties in articulation and/or speech.
(XI) Spinal Accessory	Motor control for the trapezius and sternocleidomastoid muscles Both of these muscles are involved in the movement of shoulder and head, shoulder shrugging	*Trapezius testing:* Ask the patient to raise both shoulders while examiner applies resistance. *Sternocleidomastoid testing:* Ask the patient to turn head to left and then to right while examiner applies resistance.
(XII) Hypoglossal	Tongue movement and strength	Ask the patient to protrude tongue. Normally the tongue should be midline. Note deviation to the right or left.

Data from: Bolek B. (2006). Facing cranial nerve assessment. *Am Nurse Today.* November 2006. http://www.americannursetoday.com/assets/0/434/436/440/5120/5122/5154/5156/904adb93-6d32-4770-83d7-e6f1ad1667d2.pdf.

the rapidity and strength should be equal and symmetrical when comparing one side with the other.

Babinski Sign
The Babinski sign is a descriptor for the plantar reflex. Plantar reflexes are assessed by applying a stimulus (usually using the handle of a reflex hammer) to the bottom of the foot while observing the great toe of the same foot. A normal response is noted when the great toe points downward. When adult patients have upper motor neuron lesions, the great toe will point upward and the other toes will fan. When this occurs, it is

considered a positive Babinski sign and a thorough neurologic evaluation is warranted.[31]

Assessment of Muscle Tendon Reflexes

Reflexes are assessed utilizing a reflex hammer and tapping gently on the tendon associated with the muscle. Reflex responses are graded on a scale of 0 to 4 (sometimes indicated by the number of plus signs [+] assigned) (Table 5-12).[31]

Other Aspects of the Neurologic Examination

The complete neurologic exam should also include assessment of the patient's posture, balance, and coordination. Sensory examination (pain, touch, and pressure) is included in a thorough neurologic examination, and this may incorporate other tests of sensory perception. A number of tests for specific peripheral nerves are available as well as assessment tests of muscle movement.

Common general neurologic symptoms include headache, memory loss, spells (episodic altered perception), and insomnia.[31] Clinical problems sometimes caused by neurologic disease include loss of balance and falls, alteration in consciousness, coma, and seizures.[31] Epidural or subdural hematoma following head trauma, intracerebral hemorrhage, subarchnoid hemorrhage, and bacterial meningitis are forms of neurologic disease often encountered in patients seen in the acute care setting.[31] Stroke may be caused by cerebral venous thrombosis or vessel dissection.[31]

Other neurologic syndromes that may cause muscle weakness and/or atrophy affecting ventilation include multiple sclerosis (weakness, incoordination); amyotrophic lateral sclerosis (ALS; progressive weakness with muscle wasting); poliomyelitis (muscle weakness and atrophy); West Nile virus (muscle weakness and atrophy); postpolio syndrome; and myasthenia gravis.[31] Botulism (*Clostridium botulinum*) and tetanus (*C. tetani*) may lead to ventilatory failure requiring mechanical ventilatory support.[31]

TABLE 5-12
Reflex Response Grading

Score	+	Reflex Response
0	0	No response
1	+	Detectable only with reinforcement
2	++	Normal
3	+++	Brisk with at most a few beats of clonus (clonus is a series of rhythmic, involuntary muscle contractions and relaxations)
4	++++	Sustained clonus

Head, Eyes, Ears, Nose, and Throat Examination

Examination of the head and neck provides a number of clues regarding cardiopulmonary disease.[25,26,32] The patient's facial expression can reveal distress or pain, alertness, mood, and mental status. Nasal flaring suggests an increased work of breathing, especially in infants and children. Cyanosis is often most apparent in the lips, gums, and oral mucosa. Mouth breathing may indicate nasal passage obstruction or respiratory distress, whereas purse-lipped breathing during exhalation is sometimes seen in patients with COPD. Excessive sweating (diaphoresis) is often most apparent upon examination of the head and neck. Jugular vein distension is associated with fluid overload.

Examination of the eyes, pupils, and eyelids can also provide clues regarding the patient's condition.[32] For example, pupillary reflexes may be abnormal with head trauma, CNS disease, brain death, and following administration of certain medications (e.g., catecholamines, atropine). Brain death causes mydriasis in which the pupils are dilated and fixed. Opiate drugs may cause the pinpoint pupils (miosis), whereas atropine tends to dilate the pupils. Droopy eyelids (ptosis) are sometimes seen in patients with neuromuscular disease (e.g., myasthenia gravis).

Inspection of the Head and Neck

Observation of the mouth offers two signs associated with respiratory disease. The presence of central cyanosis indicates that the level of desaturated oxyhemoglobin within the capillaries of the oral mucosa is significantly elevated. The lips and adjacent oral tissue reveal the same bluish hue noted with peripheral cyanosis. Central cyanosis is often associated with severe hypoxemia and warrants immediate intervention.

The patient who appears to be "blowing out candles" upon expiration is exhibiting a pursed-lip breathing pattern. Patients with COPD who are prone to airway collapse upon expiration may intuitively incorporate this technique or, more frequently, are taught this exercise as part of their pulmonary rehabilitation program. The slight expiratory resistance afforded by this maneuver helps to "splint" the airways and prevent their premature collapse and resultant air trapping.

Observation of the neck also offers two distinctive signs associated with COPD. Inspection of the internal and external jugular veins for jugular venous distention (JVD) allows one to assess the degree of right heart failure in patients with pulmonary hypertension due to chronic hypoxemia.[25] JVD is also associated with other clinical disorders, including left heart failure; however, cor pulmonale is the leading cause of this finding.[25] **Figure 5-3** illustrates the technique for jugular venous pressure (JVP) estimation. This evaluation should be

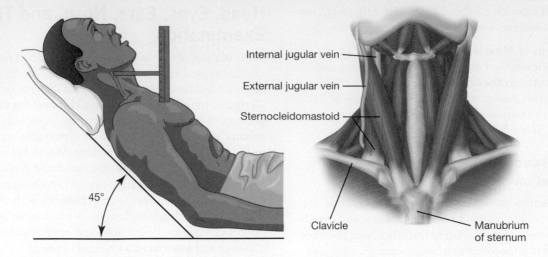

Internal jugular vein

External jugular vein

Sternocleidomastoid

Clavicle

Manubrium of sternum

45°

FIGURE 5-3 Jugular venous distension. To estimate jugular venous pressure (JVP), position the patient supine at 45°. Visualize the internal jugular vein as it ascends the side of the neck between the two heads of the sternocleidomastoid muscle. Measure the height of the distension as a vertical column of blood in relation to the sternal angle. Normal JVP ≤ 3–4 cm above the sternal angle. JVP may increase due to right heart failure (e.g., cor pulmonale), left heart failure, constrictive pericarditis, pleural effusion, obstructed vena cava, and other cardiopulmonary disorders.

done at end-exhalation and is simply graded as normal, increased, or markedly increased.

The head, eyes, ears, neck, and throat (HEENT) examination can be especially useful to identify upper airway problems that may affect oxygenation or ventilation. For example, swelling of the lips, tongue, pharynx, or larynx can occur due to angioedema, which may, in turn, compromise ventilation. Angioedema may be due to allergy or a reaction to certain medications. Food allergies, insect bites, or other allergies may cause anaphylaxis, which may also cause swelling of the upper airway. Upper airway trauma may be caused by smoke inhalation, burns, or blunt or penetrating injuries. Acute epiglottitis, laryngotracheobronchitis (croup), or abscess may also compromise ventilation. Foreign body aspiration may also result in upper airway obstruction.

Use of Accessory Muscles of Inspiration

The accessory muscles of inspiration include the neck muscles (e.g., scalenes, sternocleidomastoids), pectoralis major, and, to a lesser extent, the parasternal intercostals and the external intercostals. Use of the accessory muscles of inspiration often indicates an increased work of breathing (WOB) and difficulty in maintaining adequate ventilation.[25] Accessory muscle use is commonly associated with an increased WOB due to decreases in compliance, obstruction, or increased airway resistance.

Visible contraction of the accessory inspiratory muscles of the neck, notably the sternomastoid and scalenes, is also a common finding in patients with COPD.[25] Hyperinflation of the lungs from gas trapping causes a depression of the diaphragm and thus limits

normal abdominal excursion during inspiration, forcing a more apical adaptation to the breathing pattern and the incorporation of the neck accessory muscles. Patients with advanced obstructive lung disease may develop a "clavicular lift" upon inspiration with intense contraction of the neck accessory muscles.

Thorax

Examination of the thorax includes inspection, palpation, and percussion of the chest; assessment of breath sounds; and auscultation of the heart.[25,26,33,34] **Figure 5-4** provides illustrations of the anatomy of the thorax and underlying lung anatomy.

Inspection of the Chest

For inspection of the chest, the patient should be sitting upright to allow the examiner to adequately observe the anterior, lateral, and posterior aspects of the thorax. The transverse distance across the chest is normally measurably greater than the anteroposterior (AP) distance. This difference decreases with age and is significantly altered with the development of COPD. The term *barrel chest* refers to the dramatic increase in the AP dimension of the chest in some COPD patients. **Figure 5-5** compares a patient with a normal chest to a patient with an increased AP diameter.

The chest should also be inspected for scars, radiation markers, or trauma. For example, cardiac surgery leaves a distinctive sternal scar. Blunt trauma of the chest or rib fractures can often be observed following motor vehicle accidents. Flail chest occurs when there are double fractures of multiple adjacent ribs with

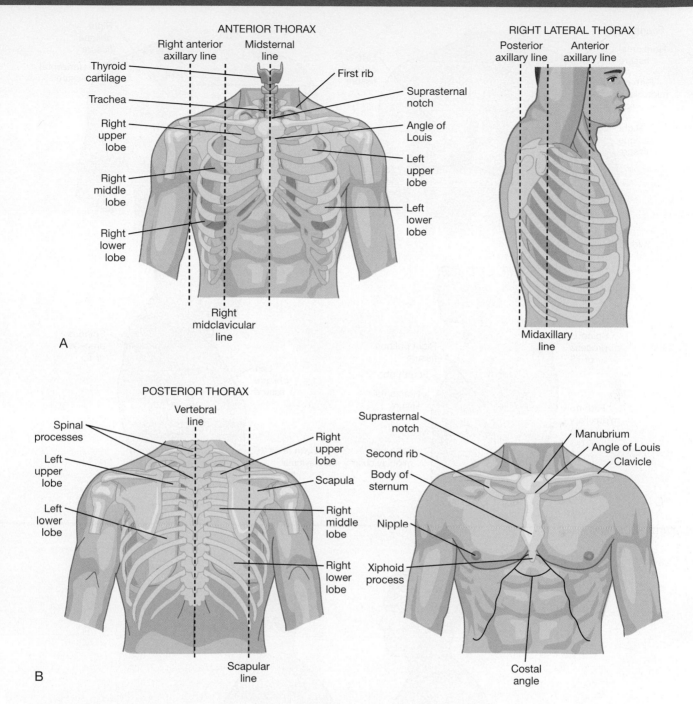

FIGURE 5-4 Anatomy of the thorax. (A) Thoracic landmarks. (B) Topographic landmarks of the chest. (C) Surface anatomy of the thorax.

resulting instability of the chest wall. Flail chest leads to a paradoxical movement of the affected area—in upon inspiration and out upon expiration. Flail chest may be noted following traumatic impact to the chest often incurred in motor vehicle accidents or blunt trauma. Pneumothorax and lung contusions are typical sequelae and warrant immediate medical intervention.

An inward movement of the upper abdomen upon inspiration rather than the normal outward movement characterize abdominal paradox. This phenomenon is associated with paralysis or fatigue of the diaphragm. It is commonly noted in patients with COPD with the development of respiratory failure.

Paralysis of the hemidiaphragm can occur with phrenic nerve damage caused by trauma, mediastinal masses, or surgery. This may result in a lack of chest motion on the affected side of the thorax.

Deformities of the bony thorax should also be assessed, because they are associated with restrictive pulmonary disease. Pectus excavatum is a chest wall

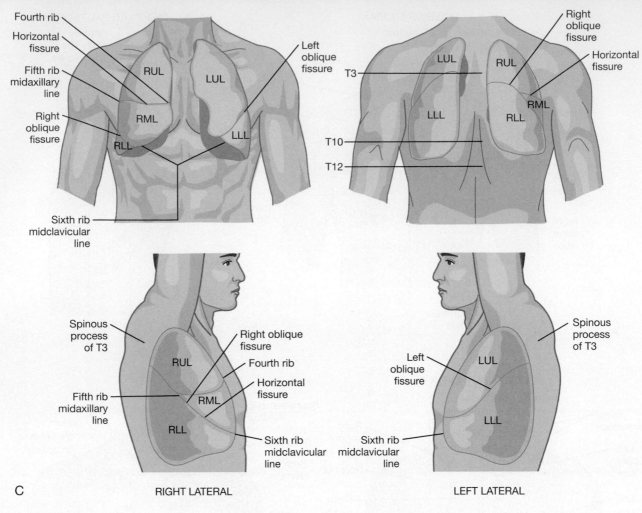

C   RIGHT LATERAL   LEFT LATERAL

FIGURE 5-4 (*continued*)

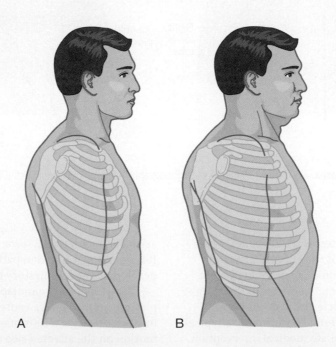

FIGURE 5-5 Increased anterior – posterior (AP) diameter. Normal chest configuration (A) and a patient with increased anteroposterior (AP) diameter (B).

Data from: Wilkins RL. Physical Examination of the Patient with Cardiopulmonary Disease. In: Wilkins R, Krider S, Sheldon R, eds. *Clinical Assessment in Respiratory Care.* 3rd ed. St. Louis: Mosby-Year Book; 1995: 47–77.

deformity in which the chest wall is "sunk in" (see **Figure 5-6**). Scoliosis, a lateral (sideways) spine curvature, is noted upon inspection of the posterior aspect of the chest. **Figure 5-7** provides an example of a patient with scoliosis. Kyphosis, an anteroposterior spine curvature (outward curve of thoracic spine), is noted upon inspection of the lateral aspect of the chest. **Figure 5-8** provides an illustration of a patient with kyphosis. Scoliosis is often congenital in nature, whereas kyphosis is often associated with osteoporosis in the elderly population. Kyphoscoliosis is a combination of the two deformities and causes a more significant restrictive pattern. **Figure 5-9** provides an example of a patient

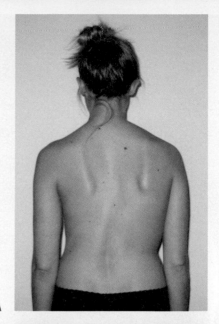

A

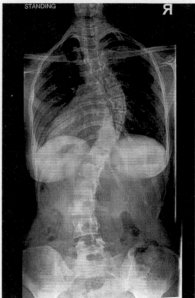

B

FIGURE 5-7 Scoliosis

(A) Courtesy of Darci Manley; (B) Courtesy of Darci Manley

with lordosis (inward curve of lumbar spine). **Box 5-14** provides a summary of important findings upon chest inspection.

Respiratory Rate and Pattern

Respiratory rate and respiratory pattern should be assessed whenever the respiratory clinician interacts with the patient. As described earlier, tachypnea, as well as an uneven respiratory pattern, such as Cheyne-Stokes breathing, should be noted, because their presence may indicate impending ventilatory failure. Bradypnea may be associated with CNS problems, sedatives, hypnotics, or impending respiratory arrest.

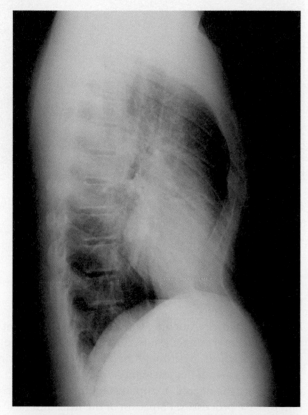

A

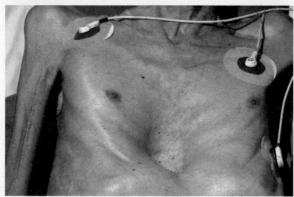

B

FIGURE 5-6 Pectus excavatum.

(A) © Custom Medical Stock Photo; (B) © M. English, MD/Custom Medical Stock Photo.

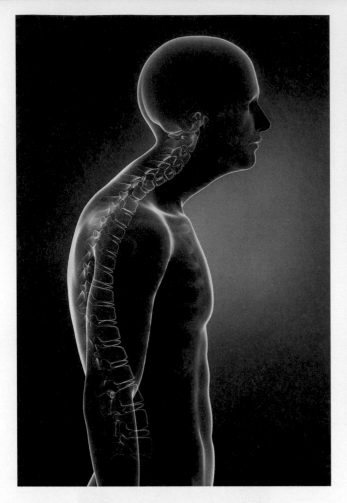

FIGURE 5-8 Kyphosis. An x-ray of a lateral view of a kyphotic spine.

© CLIPAREA I Custom media/ShutterStock, Inc.

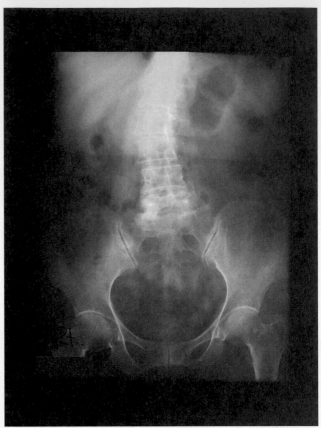

FIGURE 5-9 Lumbar lordosis. A plain film of lumbosacral AP view with demonstrated lumbar lordosis.

© Santibhavank P/ShutterStock, Inc.

Synchronicity of the Chest Wall and Diaphragm

The chest wall and abdomen should rise and fall together as the patient inhales and exhales. Asynchronous and/or spasmodic diaphragmatic contractions are strong indicators of acute ventilatory failure (not including hiccups, of course) and respiratory muscle fatigue. Often this sign is a prelude to respiratory arrest.

Retractions

Retractions between the ribs (intercostal), above the clavicles (supraclavicular), or below the xiphoid process (xiphoid) are noted as the tissue in these areas moves inward with inspiration. They are associated with marked negative pleural pressure on inspiration. Retractions can be caused by upper airway obstruction (supraclavicular), decreased lung compliance (intercostal and/or xiphoid), or inadequate gas flow to the mechanically ventilated patient.

Palpation

Palpation involves touching the chest wall of a patient in order to determine chest expansion and the degree of tactile fremitus.[25] Although palpation is not a routine part of every patient assessment, it may be of help in quantifying the degree of impairment involved in certain disease processes. Palpation of the neck and face can be helpful in identifying **subcutaneous emphysema** (air under the skin), which may occur following pneumothorax or pneumomediastinum. Palpation techniques and findings with common problems are summarized in **Table 5-13**.

Chest Expansion

The degree and symmetry of chest expansion are evaluated as the patient is instructed to take a deep breath from end exhalation. Chest expansion is most easily assessed by positioning the tips of each thumb so that they are touching at approximately the eighth thoracic vertebra along the posterior chest wall. The palmar surface of the hand and fingertips are spread out across the lower chest wall. The tips of the thumbs should move symmetrically away from one another approximately

BOX 5-14

Inspection of the Chest Summary

The following key elements should be noted during chest inspection:

Increased AP diameter: An increase in anteroposterior (AP) diameter of the chest is associated with pulmonary overinflation. This is a common finding with COPD and is sometimes seen with cystic fibrosis and in acute asthma exacerbations.

Unilateral apparent hyperexpansion: A decrease in compliance on one side, a pneumothorax, or bronchial intubation could all result in this appearance. A severe unilateral pneumonia or pneumonectomy are possible causes of decreased or absent chest wall movement on one side. Types of pneumothorax include spontaneous, traumatic, and tension.

Chest wall or spinal deformity: Pectus excavatum, pectus caravatum, kyphosis, kyphoscoliosis, and lordosis may all affect the patient's thoracic compliance.

Flail chest: Flail chest is the instability of the chest wall due to multiple rib fractures (generally two to three consecutive ribs broken in two or more places each). The chest wall sinks in on inspiration with flail chest.

Obesity, pregnancy, or ascites: All of these conditions indirectly reduce compliance (extrapulmonary or thoracic compliance). Obesity is also associated with disorders of ventilatory control and obstructive sleep apnea.

Intercostal retractions. Often caused by upper airway obstruction, increased resistance to air flow, or inadequate gas flows via closed systems such as mechanical ventilators.

Symmetry of respiration: By placing both hands parallel to one another on the chest wall (right and left) and observing chest expansion for symmetry one can sometimes note changes associated with such things as major atelectasis, pneumothorax, or other unilateral disorders of lung or chest wall expansion. Other possible causes of asymmetrical movement of the chest include bronchial intubation, unilateral pneumonia, or pneumonectomy. Trauma and the associated presence of a flail chest may cause paradoxical chest wall movement.

Scars due to trauma or surgery and radiation markers: Surgical scars relating to pneumonectomy, lobectomy, or thoracotomy are of obvious interest, as is sternal scarring from open-heart surgery. Radiation markers are also of obvious interest.

TABLE 5-13
Palpation Techniques and Clinical Implications of Specific Findings

Palpation Technique	Possible Implications
Tactile vocal fremitus: To perform this exam one simply places the lateral edge of one's hand against the patient's chest wall. The patient then repeatedly speaks the number "ninety-nine." The examiner shifts his or her hand from side to side, noting the vibrations felt through the chest wall as the patient speaks.	A marked increase in vibration over a given area is associated with consolidation. Vocal fremitus may be absent or reduced over the affected area with pleural effusion and absent with pneumothorax.
Tactile rhonchi: These are vibrations or a "rumbling" or "gurgling" feeling when the examiner places his or her hands flat (palms down) over portions of the chest wall.	"Rumbling" or tactile rhonchi are associated with secretions in a larger airway. They may clear following a cough or suctioning.
Subcutaneous emphysema: This is air under the skin, usually of the neck and face. Upon palpation, the skin feels "crackly," sort of like the feeling when one balls up a sheet of waxed paper or plastic.	Subcutaneous emphysema is associated with pneumothorax (especially tension pneumothorax) and pneumomediastinum.
Tracheal deviation: This is movement or shift in the trachea away from the midline. One can feel the position of the trachea by placing the index finger in the suprasternal notch.	A shift toward the affected side is caused by massive atelectasis or severe pneumonia on one side. Bronchial intubation, tension pneumothorax, and large pleural effusion may shift the trachea away from the affected site. With spontaneous or traumatic pneumothorax without tension, there tends to be no shift in tracheal position.
Chest wall motion: Chest wall motion can be assessed by placing one hand on the right and left side of the anterior thorax and feeling and observing chest wall motion as the patient breathes.	Chest wall motion may be reduced over the affected side with pleural effusion, consolidation, pneumothorax, or atelectasis. Chest wall motion may be reduced bilaterally with interstitial fibrosis.

3 to 5 cm at the end of an inspiratory vital capacity maneuver. Limitations to chest expansion may be unilateral or bilateral. Bilateral limitation is noted with COPD and neuromuscular disease. Unilateral limitation may be present with unilateral disorders such as lobar atelectasis or lobar pneumonia.

Tactile Fremitus

This technique involves placing the fingertips or ulnar surface of the hand or fist on the anterior and posterior surfaces of the chest wall in a systematic order as the patient repeats a number such as "ninety-nine." The tactile sensation felt by the examiner from the vibrations caused by the patient's phonation is referred to as tactile **fremitus**. Air is a poor transmitter of sound waves and resultant vibration, whereas solid substances tend to enhance said transmission. Conditions that increase the ratio of air to lung tissue such as pneumothorax and emphysema will decrease fremitus. Conditions that decrease the air to lung tissue ratio such as consolidation and atelectasis will increase fremitus.

Percussion

Percussion is also used to assess the ratio of air to lung tissue via the transmission quality of sound waves created by striking the patient's chest wall with one's fingertip. The examiner systematically taps the anterior and posterior aspects of the chest. The resonance that is evoked from percussion over normal lung tissue has been compared the sound heard by tapping on a watermelon.[25] Conditions that increase the air-to-lung tissue ratio, such as pneumothorax and emphysema, will increase resonance (aka hyperresonance). The transmission of sound in the presence of increased resonance can be compared to the sound heard when striking a hollow log. Conditions that decrease the air-to-lung tissue ratio, such as consolidation and atelectasis, will decrease resonance (dullness). Decreased resonance or dullness can be compared to the sound associated with striking a solid log.

There are two basic methods of percussion, mediate and intermediate. With mediate percussion, one thumps directly on the chest wall. With intermediate percussion, one interposes the first and second finger of one hand between the chest wall and the hand used for percussion. **Figure 5-10** illustrates the technique for intermediate percussion of the chest. Diaphragmatic excursion can be determined by percussion along the posterior thorax during a full inspiration and marking the level of the dullness–resonance border. The procedure is then repeated following a full expiration, and the distance traveled represents diaphragmatic excursion (see **Figure 5-11**). **Table 5-14** summarizes chest percussion findings.

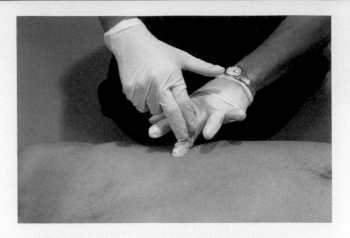

FIGURE 5-10 **Percussion technique (intermediate percussion).**

© Jones & Bartlett Learning. Courtesy of MIEMSS.

TABLE 5-14
Chest Percussion Findings

Percussion Note	Possible Implication(s)
Resonant	Normal lung tissue underlying percussion point
Hyperresonant (tympanic)	Hyperinflation (asthma, emphysema) or pneumothorax
Dull	Pleural effusion, empyema, atelectasis, consolidation or percussion over liver, heart, or kidneys

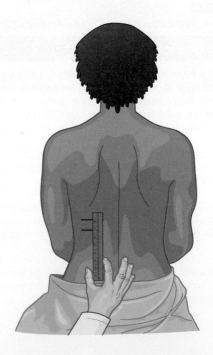

FIGURE 5-11 **Measuring diaphragmatic excursion.**

Auscultation

Auscultation over the chest is performed to identify normal and abnormal heart and lung (breath) sounds using a conventional stethoscope (see **Figure 5-12**). Chest auscultation can provide the examiner with essential information regarding the status of the airways and the lung parenchyma.[25,33] Auscultation is carried out in a systematic manner as the examiner positions the patient in an upright sitting position and proceeds to listen to the patient's breath sounds with his or her stethoscope. Sources differ as to progressing from apices to bases or vice versa, but there is consensus that one should auscultate from side to side over both anterior and posterior aspects of the chest. **Figure 5-13** provides an illustration of the positions on the chest for auscultation of the lung.

Normal Breath Sounds

Tracheal breath sounds are heard over the trachea and are loud and acoustically high in pitch.[25,33] *Bronchial breath sounds* are loud, coarse sounds normally heard over the large central airways. *Bronchovesicular breath sounds* are a combination of bronchial and vesicular sounds and may be heard between the scapulae and around the sternum over the medium-sized airways.[25,33] These sounds are attenuated in intensity and pitch as compared to tracheal breath sounds. *Vesicular breath sounds* are heard over the remaining aspects of the chest and are soft in intensity and low in pitch.[25,33] Bronchial breath sounds have a longer inspiratory phase, whereas vesicular breath sounds have a longer expiratory phase. The differences in these breath sounds is explained by the role that healthy lung tissue plays in "filtering" or actually muffling the harsh sounds produced by turbulent flow in the trachea and large airways.

Adventitious Breath Sounds

Adventitious breath sounds are abnormal and may indicate problems in the lung parenchyma and/or the airways.[25,33] Bronchial breath sounds may be transmitted to the periphery of the chest due to consolidation of the lung parenchyma, which may lead to a loss of the normal alveolar muffling of the tracheal breath sounds from the upper airways. Diminished breath sounds are associated with hypopnea, as noted with neuromuscular disease and drug overdose, or with an increase in the air-to-tissue ratio in the lung, as noted with emphysema and pneumothorax.

Abnormal airway sounds are classified acoustically as continuous or discontinuous. The continuous sound maintains a uniform pattern for at least one-tenth of a second. The discontinuous sound does not hold such a pattern. Wheezes are often continuous during expiration, whereas crackles are often discontinuous and occur during inspiration.

Wheezing and *stridor* are continuous sounds and are associated with narrowing of the airway. Stridor is a sign of upper airway obstruction that can often be heard without the use of a stethoscope, because it

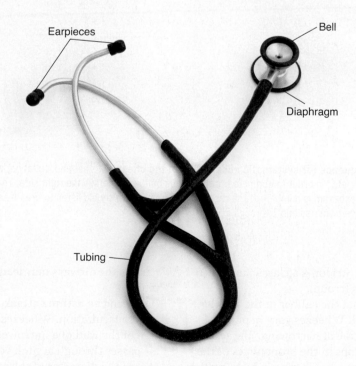

FIGURE 5-12 Stethoscope, illustrating diaphragm and bell.

© Martin Kubát/ShutterStock, Inc.

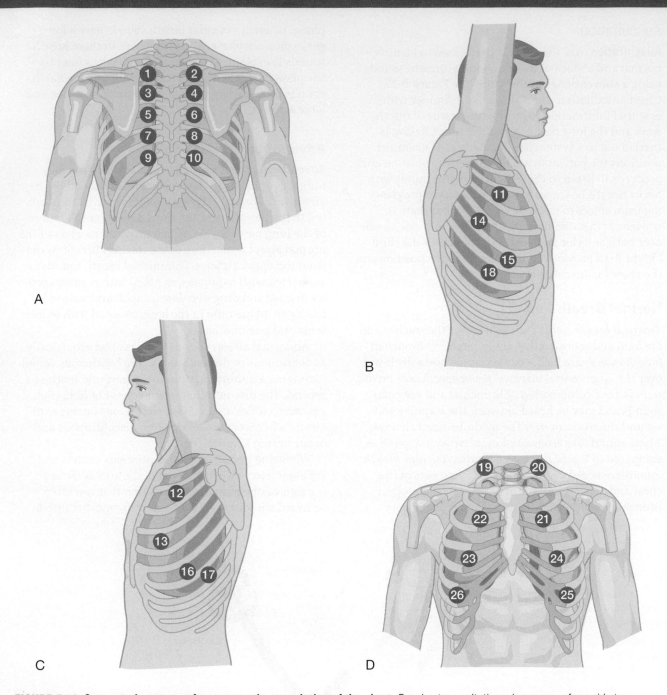

FIGURE 5-13 Suggested sequence for systematic auscultation of the chest. For chest auscultation, always move from side to side (e.g., 1 to 2, 3 to 4, 5 to 6, etc.) in order to compare breath sounds on the left versus the right side. The suggested sequence for auscultation for a complete chest exam is numbered. The respiratory care clinician should listen to breath sounds on inspiration and expiration and move in sequence from position 1 through 25.

is loud and high in pitch. Stridor is a classic finding in laryngotracheobronchitis (croup).

Wheezing indicates that the caliber of the smaller airways has been reduced. Wheezes vary in pitch based on the site and degree of narrowing. The severe bronchospasm that develops in the bronchioles of the asthmatic during an acute exacerbation is high in pitch. Obstruction of the bronchi that develops with chronic bronchitis as copious amounts of tenacious sputum

narrow the airways may lead to a wheeze that is low in pitch.

During an asthma attack, wheezing is often heard upon auscultation. Wheezes are generated by the vibration of the wall of a narrowed or compressed airway as air passes through at high velocity. During an asthma attack, the diameter of the airway can be reduced due to mucosal edema, secretions, and bronchospasm. Wheezing is usually bilateral and diffuse and unilateral wheezing should always raise the suspicion of a mass or foreign body in the airway. When listening to breath sounds, note the pitch, intensity, and portion of the respiratory cycle occupied by the wheeze. For example, the patient may have a high-pitched wheeze throughout inspiration and expiration (the entire respiratory cycle). Following bronchodilator therapy, the wheezing may be heard only during the latter part of exhalation and may also decrease in pitch and intensity. Improvement in the patient's airway caliber can affect the pitch and intensity of the wheeze and the portion of the respiratory cycle occupied by the wheeze. High-pitched wheezes at end-expiration indicate less airflow obstruction than a lower-pitched wheeze throughout inspiration and expiration. However, wheezing can be an unreliable indicator of obstruction because cases of severe obstruction can result in "silent chest." Absent breath sounds in a patient with an acute episode of asthma is an ominous sign. It is also important to note that "all that wheezes is not asthma." Wheezing may also be caused by foreign body in one of the major bronchi, a bronchial tumor, or heart failure (e.g., cardiac asthma).

Crackles are discontinuous sounds associated with the sudden opening of small airways and alveoli during inspiration. Crackles may be described as fine or coarse. Coarse crackles may be due to mucus in the airways or opening of large or medium airways during inspiration. Fine, Velcro-like crackles are thought to be produced by the opening of collapsed alveoli. Fine crackles are more often heard at the lung bases and may be caused by pulmonary edema or interstitial lung disease.

Rhonchi are low-pitched gurgling sounds associated with secretions in a larger airway. Rhonchi may clear following an effective cough or suctioning.

A *pleural friction rub* is thought to be caused by the rubbing together of inflamed pleura as the lung expands and contracts during breathing.

Absent breath sounds indicate an absence of airflow that may occur with atelectasis, pneumothorax, or consolidation. *Diminished breath sounds* are often heard over a pleural effusion or with severe COPD.

Voice sounds are sometimes assessed during auscultation of the chest, and these may be helpful in clarifying a specific condition. E-A *egophony* refers to a technique in which the patient repeats the vowel "E" as the clinician moves the stethoscope from side to side across the chest. If the sound heard using the stethoscope changes from "E" to "A," this may be due to compression of the lung tissue below a pleural effusion or due to consolidation. *Whispered pectoriloquy* refers to a distinct increase in transmission of vocal sounds associated with early pneumonia, pulmonary infarction, or atelectasis. The following is a summary of the breath sounds heard with specific disorders:

- *Atelectasis*: Absent or diminished breath sounds. It should be noted that with *microatelectasis*, bronchial breath sounds with expiration equal or louder than inspiration are sometimes heard over the affected area (usually the lower lung zones). Microatelectasis is often seen in postop abdominal or thoracic surgery patients or others with an ineffective inspiration due to pain.
- *Bronchospasm*: Wheezing as seen in asthma. Wheezing may also be seen with tumor, heart disease, and foreign body inhalation.
- *Consolidation*: Bronchial breath sounds, crackles, E-A egophony, whispered pectoriloquy.
- *Interstitial fibrosis*: Bronchovesicular breath sounds, inspiratory crackles.
- *Pleural effusion*: Absent breath sounds over fluid; pleural rub may be heard above effusion; bronchial breath sounds may be heard over upper border of effusion.
- *COPD*: Often may exhibit diminished breath sounds.
- *Pneumothorax*: Absent or diminished breath sounds on affected side.

With respect to normal and abnormal breath sounds one should be cautious in the interpretation of findings. Often, there is little agreement between physicians as to the breath sounds being heard. In general, however, most would agree to the terms and possible implications described in **Table 5-15** when these sounds are present. **Figure 5-14** provides examples of normal (well) versus abnormal (ill) breath sounds heard during auscultation of the chest.

Cardiac Examination

The cardiac examination should be completed in a private and comfortable room, if possible. To complete a thorough examination, the patient's precordium should be exposed to allow visualization of the chest. Traditionally, the examiner is positioned on the patient's right side. Examination of a female may be a bit challenging due to breast tissue; if necessary, the examiner should move breast tissue to allow adequate exposure and stethoscope placement. As with all exams, the cardiac exam should be completed on bare skin and should never be completed over clothing or gowns.

Inspection and Palpation

To begin the cardiac exam, the clinician should observe and palpate the precordium.[33] The skin should be assessed for discoloration, scars, or lesions/rashes. Also, while inspecting the skin, the precordium should be inspected for pulsations on the chest wall. These impulses are generated from the pulsations of the heart itself and the great vessels. The examiner should be

BOX 5-15

Steps to Cardiac Auscultation

1. Begin with the aortic area, which is located along the right sternal border. Palpating for the right second intercostal space along the right sternal border will ensure the appropriate stethoscope location.
2. Next, move the stethoscope directly towards the patient's left sternal border at the left second intercostal space. This is clinically called the pulmonic area or left upper sternal border.
3. Moving down the left sternal border, next auscultate the tricuspid area. This area is located at the left lower sternal border at the left fourth intercostal space.
4. The final auscultatory site is the mitral area, which is located at the apex of the heart. The mitral area is anatomically located at the fifth intercostal space in the midclavicular line. Auscultating the mitral area can be accentuated by using the bell of the stethoscope and having the patient lie in the left lateral decubitus position.

accurately with the bell, as will be discussed below. The steps to the cardiac auscultation are outlined in **Box 5-15**.

Normal Cardiac Sounds

There are typically two "normal" heart sounds that are auscultated for during the cardiac examination, the S_1 and S_2.[33] The S_1 and S_2 represent the "lub" and "dub," respectively, that are heard by the clinician when listening to the heart. Both heart sounds represent portions of the normal cardiac cycle. Of note, while auscultating each of the anatomic locations discussed above, the clinician should note the quality of S_1 and S_2 in each location. Specifically, is S_1 loud or soft, or is there a split in S_1 or S_2?

Abnormal Heart Sounds

Aside from S_1 and S_2, extra heart sounds may be heard during cardiac auscultation that are typically indicative of a pathologic process.[33] Both extra heart sounds, termed S_3 and S_4, are associated with diastolic filling and blood striking the left ventricle. Both S_3 and S_4 are typically heard at the apex of the heart and can be appreciated best using the bell of the stethoscope

because they are typically low-pitched sounds. S_3 and S_4 may be caused by left ventricular dysfunction. S_3 is normal in young patients, but often implies ventricular stiffness in older patients. **Box 5-16** summarizes the primary (S_1 and S_2) and secondary (S_3 and S_4) heart sounds.

Heart murmurs are "whooshing" sounds caused by turbulent blood flow. Causes of heart murmurs include mitral valve regurgitation, aortic valve stenosis, and mitral valve stenosis. An abnormal opening between the left ventricle and the right heart or between the aorta or pulmonary arteries and a heart chamber may also cause a heart murmur. Box 5-15 describes the surface anatomy related to auscultation and palpation for heart sounds and thrills associated with valvular disease. Remember that a cardiac "thrill" is a vibration or a tremor felt upon palpation of the chest wall. **Box 5-17** provides a grading system for classifying heart murmurs from faint to loud.

Abdominal Examination

The abdominal exam is a multistep examination.[35] As with all physical examination procedures, the patient's comfort and modesty should be priorities. When beginning an abdominal exam, the patient should be placed comfortably in the supine position. If the patient is suffering from a cardiac or respiratory disorder that prevents the patient from lying in the supine position comfortably, the patient's head may be elevated to a comfortable level by either elevating the head of the exam table or utilizing pillows to prop the patient's head up to a comfortable level. Prior to laying the patient in the supine position, the examination table should be extended so the patient's legs will be parallel to ground. The patient should be draped to expose only the portions necessary for the exam. The patient should be supine and wearing a gown with the open portion to the back; the gown can be lifted to the level of the diaphragm to expose the abdominal region. Prior to exposing the abdominal region, the patient should be draped from pubic region and below. If the patient is wearing undergarments, the drape can be loosely tucked into the top of the undergarment to ensure modesty. The abdominal musculature may tense if the patient's head is not resting comfortably on the exam table. If the examiner notes abdominal tensing, the patient's legs may be bent to facilitate relaxation. Simply bending the leg at the knee and resting the patient's soles of the feet on the exam table should be sufficient to allow complete relaxation of the musculature. The clinician should discuss the exam techniques with the patient prior to doing the exam maneuvers.

Abdominal Anatomy

During all aspects of the abdominal exam, the examiner should be cognizant of the anatomic quadrants

BOX 5-16

Heart Sounds

The S_1 and S_2 "lub-dub" heart sounds are normal. The S_3 heart sound is usually abnormal, whereas the S_4 heart sound is always abnormal. Each sound is described below.

S_1, "Lub"

- S_1 marks the beginning of systole, or ventricular contraction.
- This is the sound that is created when the mitral and the tricuspid valves close.
- Best heard at the apex of the heart or along the left sternal border. It is normally a single sound.
- If the examiner is struggling to differentiate between S_1 and S_2, the carotid pulse can be located and palpated. S_1 just precedes the carotid upstroke, or the beginning of the carotid pulse.
- S_1 can be appreciated with either the bell or the diaphragm of the stethoscope, but because this is a higher-pitched heart sound, it can be more readily assessed with the diaphragm.
- S_1 should be assessed in all four auscultatory areas.

S_2, "Dub"

- S_2 marks the beginning of diastole or ventricular filling that directly follows ventricular ejection.
- S_2 is the heart sound created when the pressure between the atrium and ventricle changes to allow the aortic and pulmonic (semilunar) valves to close.
- S_2 is loudest and best heard at the base of the heart.
- As with S_1, S_2 correlates with the carotid pulse but directly follows the pulsation. S_2 should be assessed in all four auscultatory areas.

S_3

- S_3 is heard in early diastole, just following S_2 during the rapid ventricular filling phase.
- S_3 can be a normal finding in healthy athletic young people but is rarely normal after the age of 40.
- S_3 is most often a sign of a distended or floppy left ventricle and indicates some level of systolic dysfunction
- S_3 is commonly heard in patients with congestive heart failure.
- Timing of the S_3 follows directly after S_2 and before S_1.
- The S_3 is sometimes described as the "Kentucky gallop," where S_1 = Ken; S_2 = tuk; S_3 = y.
- "Lub-du-bub" is the typical sound heard with S_3.

S_4

- S_4 is heard in late diastole, just prior to S_1.
- S_4 is caused by atrial contraction or atrial kick.
- S_4 is also a low-pitched sound and is best heard best with the bell of the stethoscope at the apex of the heart.
- S_4 is never a normal finding and is caused by a still left ventricle.
- The mnemonic commonly utilized to describe an S_4 is "Ten-ne-see," where S_4 is the "Ten" syllable.
- "Dub-lub-dub" is the typical sound heard with S_4.

that are used for documentation as well as localization of findings. Typically the abdomen is separated into four quadrants: right and left upper quadrants and right and left lower quadrants, utilizing the umbilicus as the landmark for differentiation of left and right regions and upper and lower regions. The four-quadrant system is commonly utilized in clinical practice for documentation purposes.

Inspection

The first component of the abdominal exam is inspection.[35] The exam room should be well lit so that the clinician is able to observe small details that may otherwise be overlooked. First, the abdomen should be observed for general shape and contour. Skin color, distension, ascites, scars, pulsation, or ecchymoses (subcutaneous blood) should be noted. Jaundice may suggest liver disease due to increased bilirubin. Abdominal distension can be caused by obesity, excess abdominal gas, peritoneal fluid (ascites), enlarged liver (hepatomegaly), enlarged spleen, tumor, or obstruction.[35] **Ascites** can be caused by liver disease (e.g., portal hypertension), lymph obstruction, decreased plasma oncotic pressure, infection, or inflammation.[35] Visible abdominal peristalsis can sometimes be observed in patients with a thin abdominal wall.[35] Visible pulsation of the abdomen may be caused by the motion of the abdominal aorta.[35]

Auscultation

Auscultation of the abdomen should be performed prior to percussion or palpation.[35] The exam is completed using the diaphragm of the stethoscope. Typically, the examiner should listen for bowel sounds in all four anatomic locations. The clinician should place the prewarmed diaphragm of the stethoscope on the abdomen and listen for 15 or 20 seconds. Bowel sounds are created by intestinal motility and movement of digested food through the bowel. Bowel sounds should be evaluated for frequency and quality. Bowel sound descriptors include the following:

- *Hyperactive bowel sounds*: Loud, gurgling rushed sounds
- *Hypoactive bowel sounds*: Soft, low, widely separated sounds, such as one or two occurring in 2 minutes
- *Absent sounds*: Sounds are not heard for 3 to 5 minutes of auscultating in each quadrant

Decreased or absent bowel sounds may be caused by a decrease or absence of peristalsis. This may occur due to mechanical bowel obstruction (e.g., tumor, adhesions, hernia), inadequate blood supply (e.g., mesenteric artery obstruction), or paralytic ileus (e.g., blockage, hypokalemia, infection, trauma). Abnormal bowel sounds should be evaluated along with other symptoms such as nausea, vomiting, gas, and nature (or absence) of bowel movements.

Palpation

Palpation techniques are used to assess organ size and location of masses or abdominal pain.[35] Most commonly, the liver, spleen, and kidneys are assessed for enlargement, shape, and contour. When palpating the abdomen, it is important for the practitioner to remember the basics of adnominal anatomy in relation to the quadrant that is being assessed. If masses or tenderness are noted, the practitioner should be aware of the quadrant and begin thinking of possible causes. When palpating the abdomen, one should note the quality of the abdominal musculature. The average patient should have a soft, nonrigid abdomen. The term *guarding* is utilized to describe abdominal muscle spasm upon palpation, which is a sign of abdominal tenderness or inflammation. *Rigidity* describes a boardlike spasm that does not correlate to palpation. This is a more ominous sign, because it may indicate serious abdominal disorders, such as a perforated viscous, mesenteric infarction, or diffuse peritonitis. All four quadrants should be assessed utilizing light and deep palpation techniques. If the patient has known abdominal pain, that palpational area should be left until the very end of the assessment.

Percussion

Abdominal percussion is performed by using one hand as the base on the patient, typically the non-dominant hand, and the dominant hand as the "hammer." Commonly the dorsal aspect of the middle third phalanx is struck on the base with the dominant hand being the "hammer." When completing this technique, the base finger should be pressed firmly on the patient's bare skin while the dominant hand being the hammer delivers two blows to the base by bending at the wrist only. When using percussion techniques on the abdominal exam, all four quadrants should be percussed, noting the quality of the note elicited. Most areas of the abdomen will have a tympanic quality to them due to the gas located within the bowel. Important findings include excessive gas (e.g., tympanic percussion), pain, or pneumoperitoneum (air in the peritoneal space) caused by abdominal trauma or perforation.

Extremities

Assessing a patient's upper and lower extremities, including skin and nails, can give insight into the underlying disorder. When examining a patient's extremities, it is important to be aware of the patient's comfort. Drapes/sheets should be utilized to expose only the extremity being examined and to provide privacy when at all possible. Specifically for the extremities, the practitioner should compare findings bilaterally (i.e., side to side) and note if any abnormalities are unilateral or bilateral in nature.

The practitioner should inspect both upper and lower extremities, comparing both sides of the body and noting any sort of discoloration, such as redness, cyanosis, or skin changes or lesions.[26,27] **Table 5-17** provides a summary of skin changes seen with different disease states and conditions.

The next step in the examination of the extremities should be testing for temperature of the extremities. The temperature of the skin can be assessed by feeling the patient's skin on the lower and upper extremities with the back of the hand. It is important to compare both sides, specifically looking for temperature changes or differences.

Specific Exam Findings

When examining a patient's extremities care should be taken to assess capillary refill, color, temperature (warm vs. cool), skin condition (dry vs. moist), digital clubbing, and the presence of edema. Specific for a cardiopulmonary examination, inspection of the patient's fingers for the presence of nicotine stains should also be performed. Adequate capillary refill is an indication of adequate peripheral circulation and oxygenation. Peripheral cyanosis (as opposed to central cyanosis) may indicate poor peripheral circulation and oxygenation. Warm, moderately moist extremities generally indicate good peripheral perfusion and oxygenation. Cold, clammy extremities indicate poor perfusion and circulation.

Edema is swelling of the soft tissues due to excess fluid accumulation associated with cardiopulmonary disease, kidney failure, liver disease, or obstruction of venous or lymph drainage.[25,27] Edema may be generalized or present only in dependent portions of the body, such as the legs and ankles or back hip area of the patient confined in bed. Unilateral peripheral edema may be caused by venous flow obstruction as may occur with tight bandages or deep vein thrombosis.[25,35] Bilateral peripheral edema, particularly in the ankles, feet (pedal edema), and, in severe cases, arms and legs, is associated with CHF and fluid overload. Edema of the ankles and feet is often most prominent after the patient has been standing or sitting for a period of time and may be relieved following bed rest with elevation of the legs.[35] Edema of the lower legs, and particularly the ankles, is commonly seen in patients with right heart failure (cor pulmonale) due to chronic lung disease. With severe right side CHF, edema can lead to hepatomegaly (due to liver congestion) and ascites (collection of fluid in the abdomen).[35] The patient with left heart failure also often presents with pedal edema, and edema of the feet, legs, and arms is not uncommon in patients in multisystem organ failure. **Pitting edema** is present when the depression in the skin left by pressing on the edematous area does not refill immediately.[35] **Table 5-18** provides a scale for grading pitting edema.

Clubbing

Digital clubbing is associated with chronic pulmonary disease and, on occasion, lung cancer.[25,35] Clubbing is characterized by a bulbous swelling of the distal phalanges of the fingers and toes caused by proliferation of the connective tissue between the nail matrix and the distal phalanx. The exact etiology of this condition is unknown, but possible factors associated with the development of clubbing may include chronic infection, circulating vasodilators or unspecified toxins, and chronic hypoxemia.[25,35] Clubbing is sometimes

TABLE 5-17
Skin Appearance

Appearance	Suspected Disease State or Condition
Redness	Infection
Cyanosis	Hypoxia
Brown discoloration	Venous stasis
Pale	Arterial insufficiency
Mottled appearance	Underperfusion or arterial insufficiency
Petechia	Microvascular hemorrhage
Ulceration	Trauma, diabetes, vascular insufficiency
Black/eschar	Gangrene

TABLE 5-18
Grades of Pitting Edema

Grade	Description
Absent	Normal skin response following application and removal of pressure (e.g., indentation does not persist).
+	Mild pitting edema present in feet and ankles.
++	Moderate pitting edema present in feet, ankles, lower legs (also, maybe present in hands or lower arms).
+++	Severe generalized pitting edema including feet, ankles, legs, arms, and face.

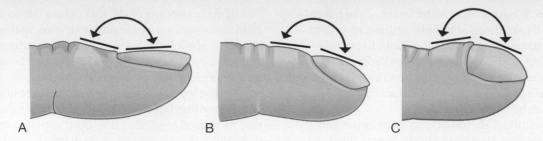

FIGURE 5-17 Digital clubbing.

seen with cystic fibrosis, bronchiectasis, interstitial lung disease, bronchogenic cancer, lung abscess, or chronic cardiovascular disease.[25,35] Digital clubbing may be associated with decreased oxygen delivery to the tissues; however, clubbing may or may not be associated with cyanosis, and COPD alone does not lead to clubbing.[25,35]

To assess for digital clubbing the clinician can look at various aspects of the digits, such as nail fold angles and the shape, depth, and width of the fingertips. A common technique utilized clinically is assessing for Schamroth's sign. To assess Schamroth's sign the clinician will ask the patient to place opposite forefinger (dorsal surface) nails together and will look between them. Normally, the clinician should observe a small diamond space between the nails called Schamroth's window. If this is observed, then the nails are not clubbed; if the window is not observed, then digital clubbing is present. Normal, mild, and severe digital clubbing are pictured in **Figure 5-17**.

Ancillary Equipment in Use

Always note the presence or absence of IVs, respirators, cardiac monitors, urinary catheters (Foley bags), oxygen or aerosol equipment, isolation equipment, incentive spirometry equipment, chest drainage systems, sputum cups, restraints, and so on. The presence or absence of *each* of these items tells you something about the patient's condition.

CLINICAL FOCUS 5-2

Patient Assessment

Maria Rodriguez, a 67-year-old female is admitted to the emergency department complaining of increasing shortness of breath over the last several days. Her dyspnea worsens at night or when lying down. She has not taken any medications to treat her illness, but has made an appointment for next week to see her primary care provider. The following information is collected by the respiratory care clinician as a part of a complete assessment:

Patient profile: The patient is married, and has two children and four grandchildren, all in good health. The patient does not smoke, though her husband smoked for 20 years and recently quit smoking. The patient worked for 40 years as an administrative secretary in the social security office downtown. Since retirement, she spends most of her time at home, caring for her family. She does not exercise on a regular basis and her diet is high in fat and carbohydrates. She sees her primary care provider on occasion, and she has had her flu and pneumococcal vaccines this past year. She states she has "high cholesterol" but is not taking medications at this time. She also says she has experienced some weight gain over the last week or so.

General appearance: The patient is sitting up in bed and is awake, alert and oriented to time and situation. She appears to be well nourished and her BMI is recorded as 30. She appears to be anxious and somewhat restless. The nurses have placed the patient on oxygen therapy by nasal cannula at 2 L/minute due to her dyspnea.

Vital signs:

Heart rate: 100 bpm; pulse slightly irregular
Respiratory rate: 22 breaths/min
BP: 150/100

(*continued*)

Temperature: 99° F

SpO$_2$: 90% on O$_2$ at 2 L/min

Pain: the patient states that "I do not have any chest pain, but I do feel short of breath right now" and "I don't have any pain in my abdomen, but it feels swollen".

HEENT: Jugular venous distention noted with patient seated at a 45-degree angle; no cyanosis of lips or gums; otherwise HEENT normal.

Chest: Chest resonant to percussion, no fremitus noted, no tracheal shift, equal bilateral chest expansion with increased respiratory rate and inspiratory accessory muscle contractions. Upon auscultation, vesicular breath sounds noted over most of the thorax with fine crackles (rales) at the bases and intermittent wheezing on expiration.

Cardiac: S$_1$ and S$_2$ noted with an S$_3$ gallop rhythm. The point of maximal impulse (apical impulse) is laterally displaced past the midclavicular line. No murmurs or thrills noted.

Abdomen: Liver and abdomen feel swollen

Extremities: Swelling noted in the ankles, legs and hands with ++ pitting edema; no peripheral cyanosis in nail beds.

What is the patient's chief complaint?

Answer: Increasing shortness of breath.

Describe the HPI.

Answer: The patient came to the emergency department because of increasing shortness of breath over the last several days. She has not taken any medications to treat her illness, but had made an appointment for next week to see her primary care provider. She breathes easier in the sitting position and becomes more short of breath when lying down (orthopnea). Symptoms worsen at night (paroxysmal nocturnal dyspnea). Recent weight gain noted.

Provide your assessment of the patient's vital signs.

Answer: Tachycardia, tachypnea, and hypertension are present. Temperature is within normal range and the patient is not in pain. SpO$_2$ suggests corrected hypoxemia on 2 L/min of O$_2$.

Provide your assessment of the patient's HEENT examination.

Answer: JVD is associated with fluid overload and CHF. The patient does not show central cyanosis while receiving O$_2$ therapy; however, she may become hypoxemic if switched to breathing room air.

Provide your assessment of the patient's chest examination.

Answer: Breath sounds suggest possible pulmonary edema (crackles) with wheezing, which could be due to airway narrowing or congestion. Chest assessment does NOT suggest a unilateral lung problem. Cardiac sounds suggest possible left ventricular enlargement.

Provide your assessment of the abdominal and extremities examinations.

Answer: Abdominal distention may be due to hepatomegaly and/or ascites, which may be associated with CHF and fluid retention. Peripheral edema suggests fluid overload.

What is your overall assessment of the patient's condition?

Patient history suggests factors that predispose to the development of CHF, including sedentary lifestyle, hyperlipidemia, and obesity (BMI = 31). Tachycardia, tachypnea, and hypertension suggest a cardiopulmonary problem. Physical examination suggests bilateral lung disease such as pulmonary edema based on chest expansion and breath sounds. Heart sounds are consistent with CHF. SpO$_2$ is 90% on O$_2$ therapy, suggesting hypoxemia on room air. CHF with cardiac pulmonary edema is a likely diagnosis. ECG, chest X-ray, echocardiogram, and laboratory studies (e.g., CBC, liver function test, BNP or NT-proBNP) should be considered to confirm or rule out this diagnosis. Fasting blood glucose should be obtained to screen for diabetes.

Treatment: Treatment of CHF with fluid overload includes administration of diuretics and sodium restriction. ACE inhibitors (or alternative medications) may be given to treat left ventricular dysfunction; β-blockers may be indicated in patients with markedly reduced left ventricular ejection fraction (LVEF ≤ 40). Smoking cessation, diet, exercise, and management of comorbid conditions (e.g., diabetes, obesity, hyperlipidemia) may be helpful in many patients.

BNP, brain natriuretic peptide, a hormone released from the heart (aka B-type natriuretic peptide)

TABLE 5-19
Physical Findings of Common Respiratory Diseases

Condition	Percussion Note Sounds	Fremitus	Breath Sounds	Adventitious Sounds
Normal	Resonant	Normal	Vesicular	None
Left heart failure	Resonant	Normal	Vesicular	Crackles or occasionally wheezes
Pleural effusion	Dull or flat	Absent or decreased	Decreased or absent	None or pleural rub
Consolidation	Dull	Increased	Bronchial	Crackles, rhonchi, or egophony
Bronchitis	Resonant	Normal or decreased	Prolonged exhalation	Wheezes, crackles, or rhonchi
Emphysema	Hyperresonant	Decreased	Decreased or absent	None
Pneumothorax	Hyperresonant	Decreased or absent	Decreased or absent	None
Atelectasis	Dull	Variable	Absent or diminished	None or crackles
Asthma	Resonant or hyperresonant	Normal or decreased	Vesicular	Wheezes
Pulmonary fibrosis	Resonant	Normal	Vesicular	Crackles

Putting It All Together

Being competent at physical examination is only one component of patient care. The respiratory care clinician must be able to correlate the patient's history, physical examination, and diagnostic test results to create a differential list and working diagnosis. This process begins as soon as the clinician determines the patient's chief complaint. For example, if a patient presents with a complaint of shortness of breath, the initial "idea" list (i.e., differential list) can be very broad, ranging from cardiac to pulmonary to neurologic disorders. As the clinician progresses with the history and physical exam, the differentials may narrow or broaden depending on what the patient says or findings on physical examination (Table 5-19).

For example, a patient with acute dyspnea may suffer from upper airway problems (e.g., aspiration, airway trauma, angioedema, or anaphylaxis); pulmonary problems (e.g., pulmonary embolism, pulmonary edema, infection, acute exacerbation of COPD, acute asthma, acute respiratory distress syndrome [ARDS]); neuromuscular disease (e.g., myasthenia gravis or Guillain-Barré syndrome); other ventilatory impairments (e.g., trauma or poisoning); or cardiac problems (e.g., arrhythmia, CHF, MI). Careful review of the findings on the physical examination may clarify the differential diagnosis and guide the selection of additional diagnostic studies. For example, the patient's general appearance may suggest acute distress but the vital signs may suggest hypoxia. The HEENT may identify swelling of the lips, tongue, or pharynx (angioedema) associated with allergy or anaphylaxis. Inspection of the thorax may reveal rib fractures, trauma, or surgical scars (e.g.,

postcardiac surgery). Chest examination (percussion, palpation, auscultation) may further suggest the presence of pulmonary edema, pleural effusion, consolidation, or bronchospasm. Cardiac arrhythmia may be suggested by an abnormal heart rhythm. Examination of the extremities may reveal peripheral edema related to heart failure.

In short, the physical examination provides vital clues as to the patient's diagnosis and guides further diagnostic studies. Last, the physical examination serves a vital role in the development and evaluation of the patient's respiratory care plan.

Key Points

▶ Physical assessment skills include inspection, palpation, percussion, and auscultation.
▶ A physical examination will include vital signs; skin; head, eyes, ears, nose, and throat (HEENT), thorax, abdomen, and extremities.
▶ Tachycardia (HR > 100 bpm) and bradycardia (HR < 60 bpm) can be caused by cardiopulmonary disease.
▶ Rapid shallow breathing is common with respiratory failure.
▶ Chronic hypertension is associated with the development of congestive heart failure, heart attack, stroke, and kidney disease.
▶ Risk factors for chronic hypertension include obesity, tobacco smoking, poor conditioning, and poor eating habits.
▶ Antihypertensive medications should be considered for patients with a persistent elevation in blood pressure.

▶ Hypotension may be caused by decreased cardiac output, peripheral vasodilation, or hypovolemia.

▶ Types of shock include cardiogenic, hypovolemic, and distributive shock.

▶ Most fevers are caused by infection, often viral in origin.

▶ Antipyretics include acetaminophen, aspirin, and NSAIDs (e.g., ibuprofen).

▶ Heat exhaustion may occur following exertion in a hot, humid environment.

▶ Signs of pain sometimes seen in the ICU patient include grimacing, writhing, tachycardia, hypertension, and diaphoresis.

▶ Body mass index (BMI) provides an indirect estimate of body fat.

▶ BMI > 25 indicates the patient is overweight; BMI ≥ 30 indicates obesity.

▶ Significant weight loss in a previously healthy person can signal serious health problems.

▶ Excessive sweating can be a sign of respiratory distress.

▶ Cyanosis is a variable finding with hypoxia.

▶ Assessment of mental status includes orientation to person, place, time, and situation.

▶ The following terms are used to describe levels of consciousness (LOC): awake and alert, sleepy, confused, lethargic, obtunded, stuporous, and comatose.

▶ The neurologic examination seeks to identify cognitive, sensory, motor, or coordination deficits.

▶ Normal pupils will contract when exposed to a bright light and dilate when the light is removed.

▶ Common general neurologic symptoms include headache, memory loss, spells, and insomnia.

▶ Cyanosis is often most apparent in the lips, gums, and oral mucosa.

▶ Jugular venous distension may suggest heart failure or fluid overload.

▶ An increased anteroposterior chest diameter suggests overinflation.

▶ Retractions may be caused by upper airway obstruction.

▶ Abdominal paradox is sometimes seen in patients in respiratory failure and may be associated with diaphragmatic fatigue.

▶ Tympany, or hyperresonance, is seen with pneumothorax.

▶ Dullness is seen with pleural effusion or consolidation.

▶ Abnormal breath sounds include wheezing, stridor, crackles, and rhonchi.

▶ S_1 and S_2 are normal heart sounds; S_3 and S_4 are abnormal heart sounds.

▶ Clubbing is associated with chronic respiratory disease and, on occasion, lung cancer.

▶ Abdominal disorders include distension, ascites, abnormal bowel sounds, and obstruction.

References

1. Price DH, Tracy CS, Upshur RE. Chaperone use during intimate examinations in primary care: postal survey of family physicians. *BMC Fam Pract*. 2005 Dec 21;6:52.

2. Gatty CM, Turner M, Buitendorp DJ, Batman H. The effectiveness of back pain and injury prevention programs in the workplace. *Work*. 2003;20(3):257–266.

3. Murphy TH, Labonte P, Klock M, Houser L. Falls prevention for elders in acute care: an evidence-based nursing practice initiative. *Crit Care Nurs Q*. 2008;31(1):33–39.

4. Lorenz K, Sherbourne CD, Shugarman LR, et al. How reliable is pain as the fifth vital sign? *J Am Board Fam Med*. 2009;22(3):291–298.

5. LeBlond RF, Brown DD, DeGowin RL. Vital signs, anthropometric data, and pain. In: LeBlond RF, Brown DD, DeGowin RL, eds. *DeGowin's Diagnostic Examination*, 9th ed. New York: McGraw-Hill; 2009: 88–114.

6. Wilkins RL, Heuer AJ. Vital signs. In: Wilkins RL, Dexter JR, Heuer AJ, eds. *Clinical Assessment in Respiratory Care*, 6th ed. St. Louis, MO: Elsevier-Mosby; 2010: 51–67.

7. Guyton AC, Hall JE. Cardiac arrhythmias and the electrocardiographic interpretation. In: Guyton AC, Hall JE, eds. *Textbook of Medical Physiology*. Philadelphia: Elsevier Saunders; 2006: 147–157.

8. Thompson BT, Hales CA. Diagnosis of acute pulmonary embolism. In: UpToDate. Basow DS (ed.), UpToDate, Waltham, MA, 2012.

9. Pickering TG, Hall JE, Appel LJ, et al. Recommendations for blood pressure monitoring in humans and experimental animals. Part 1: blood pressure measurement in humans: a statement for professionals from the Subcommittee of Professional and Public Education of the American Heart Association Council on High Blood Pressure Research. *Hypertension*. 2005;45(1):142–161.

10. Kaplan NM, Domino FJ. Overview of hypertension in adults. In: UpToDate, Basow DS (ed.), UpToDate, Waltham, MA, 2012.

11. Kaplan NM. Choice of therapy in essential hypertension: clinical trials. In: UpToDate, Basow DS (ed.), UpToDate, Waltham, MA, 2012.

12. Kaplan NM. Malignant hypertension and hypertensive encephalopathy in adults. In: UpToDate, Basow DS (ed.), UpToDate, Waltham, MA, 2012.

13. Gaieski D. Shock in adults: types, presentation, and diagnostic approach. In: UpToDate, Basow DS (ed.), UpToDate, Waltham, MA, 2012.

14. Rubia-Rubia J, Arias A, Sierra A, Aguirre-Jaime A. Measurement of body temperature in adult patients: comparative study of accuracy, reliability and validity of different devices. *Int J Nurs Stud*. 2011;48(7):872–880.

15. Ryan M, Levy MM. Clinical review: fever in intensive care unit patients. *Crit Care*. 2003;7(3):221–225.

16. Porat R, Dinarello CA. Pathophysiology and treatment of fever in adults. In: UpToDate, Basow DS, (ed.), UpToDate, Waltham, MA, 2012.

17. Longo DL, Fauci AS, Kasper DL, Hauser SL, Jameson JL, Loscalzo J. Abdominal pain. In: Longo DL, Fauci AS, Kasper DL, Hauser SL, Jameson JL, Loscalzo J, eds. *Harrison's Manual of Medicine*, 18th ed. New York: McGraw-Hill; 2013: 239–244.

18. Tietze KJ. Pain control in the critically ill adult patient. In: UpToDate, Basow DS (ed.), UpToDate, Waltham, MA, 2012.

19. Centers for Disease Control. About BMI for adults. Updated September 2011. http://www.cdc.gov/healthyweight/assessing/bmi/adult_bmi/index.html.

20. National Institutes of Health, National Heart Lung and Blood Institute. What are the health risks of overweight and obesity? July 13, 2012. http://www.nhlbi.nih.gov/health/health-topics/topics/obe/risks.html. Accessed February 1, 2013.

21. Byrd J. Scale consistency study: how accurate are in patient hospital scales? *Nursing*. 2011;41(11):21–24.

22. Longo DL, Fauci AS, Kasper DL, Hauser SL, Jameson JL, Loscalzo J. Weight loss. In: Longo DL, Fauci AS, Kasper DL, Hauser SL, Jameson JL, Loscalzo J, eds. *Harrison's Manual of Medicine*, 18th ed. New York: McGraw-Hill; 2013: 218–221.

23. Longo DL, Fauci AS, Kasper DL, Hauser SL, Jameson JL, Loscalzo J. Assessment of nutritional status. In: Longo DL, Fauci AS, Kasper DL, Hauser SL, Jameson JL, Loscalzo J, eds. *Harrison's Manual of Medicine*, 18th ed. New York: McGraw-Hill; 2013: 46–48.

24. Lainscak M, Filippatos GS, Gheorghiade M, Fonarow GC, Anker SD. Cachexia: common, deadly, with an urgent need for precise definition and new therapies. *Am J Cardiol.* 2008;101(11A):8E–10E.

25. Wilkins RL. Fundamentals of physical examination. In: Wilkins RL, Dexter JR, Heuer AJ, eds. *Clinical Assessment in Respiratory Care*, 6th ed. St. Louis, MO: Elsevier-Mosby; 2010: 68–94.

26. LeBlond RF, Brown DD, DeGowin RL. The screening physical examination. In: LeBlond RF, Brown DD, DeGowin RL, eds. *DeGowin's Diagnostic Examination*, 9th ed. New York: McGraw-Hill; 2009: 34–47.

27. LeBlond RF, Brown DD, DeGowin RL. The skin and nails. In: LeBlond RF, Brown DD, DeGowin RL, eds. *DeGowin's Diagnostic Examination*, 9th ed. New York: McGraw-Hill; 2009: 115–177.

28. Dugdale DC. Sweating. MedlinePlus Medical Encyclopedia. Updated May 29, 2011. http://www.nlm.nih.gov/medlineplus/ency/article/003218.htm. Accessed January 31, 2013.

29. Longo DL, Fauci AS, Kasper DL, Hauser SL, Jameson JL, Loscalzo J. Cyanosis. In: Longo DL, Fauci AS, Kasper DL, Hauser SL, Jameson JL, Loscalzo J, eds. *Harrison's Manual of Medicine*, 18th ed. New York: McGraw-Hill; 2013: 229–231.

30. DeGowin RL, Brown DD, LeBlond RF. The mental status, psychiatric, and social evaluations. In: DeGowin RL, Brown DD, LeBlond RF. *DeGowin's Diagnostic Examination*, 9th ed. New York: McGraw-Hill; 2009: 766–786.

31. DeGowin RL, Brown DD, LeBlond RF. The neurologic examination. In: DeGowin RL, Brown DD, LeBlond RF. *DeGowin's Diagnostic Examination*, 9th ed. New York: McGraw-Hill; 2009: 683–765.

32. DeGowin RL, Brown DD, LeBlond RF. The head and neck. In: DeGowin RL, Brown DD, LeBlond RF. *DeGowin's Diagnostic Examination*, 9th ed. New York: McGraw-Hill; 2009: 178–297.

33. DeGowin RL, Brown DD, LeBlond RF. The chest: chest wall, pulmonary, and cardiovascular systems; the breasts. In: DeGowin RL, Brown DD, LeBlond RF. *DeGowin's Diagnostic Examination*, 9th ed. New York: McGraw-Hill; 2009: 302–407.

34. Gardner DD, Wilkins RL. Cardiopulmonary symptoms. In: Wilkins RL, Dexter JR, Heuer AJ. *Clinical Assessment in Respiratory Care*, 6th ed. St. Louis, MO: Mosby-Elsevier; 2010: 28–50.

35. DeGowin RL, Brown DD, LeBlond RF. The abdomen, perineum, anus, and rectosigmoid. In: DeGowin RL, Brown DD, LeBlond RF. *DeGowin's Diagnostic Examination*, 9th ed. New York: McGraw-Hill; 2009: 445–527.

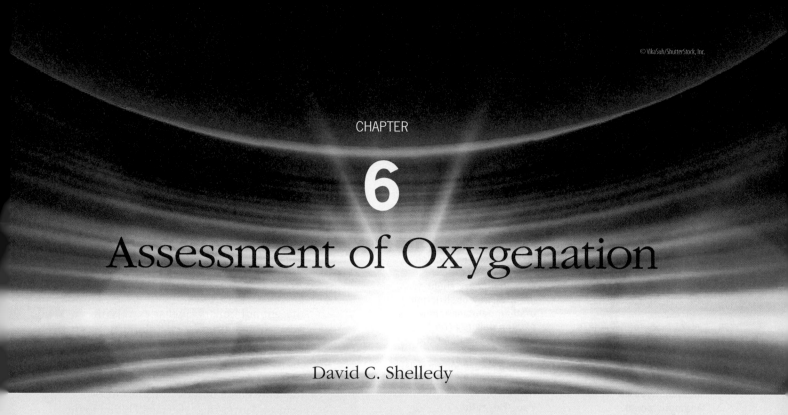

CHAPTER

6

Assessment of Oxygenation

David C. Shelledy

CHAPTER OUTLINE

CHAPTER OBJECTIVES

1. Describe the clinical manifestations (signs and symptoms) of hypoxia.
2. Contrast the findings associated with mild, moderate, and severe hypoxia.
3. Define *respiratory failure* and contrast lung failure and pump failure.
4. Given the needed information, calculate inspired and alveolar oxygen tension.
5. Define *altitude hypoxia* and explain when it might occur.
6. Describe the stages of altitude hypoxia.
7. Describe acute mountain sickness, including signs, symptoms, and treatment.
8. Explain why in-flight supplemental oxygen may be required by patients with lung disease.
9. Provide examples of other forms of ambient hypoxia.
10. List five causes of upper airway obstruction in adults.
11. Describe common causes of upper airway obstruction in children.
12. Contrast variable and fixed upper airway obstruction.
13. Describe the diagnosis and treatment of obstructive sleep apnea (OSA).
14. Describe causes of and common clinical findings associated with lower airway obstruction.
15. Explain the relationships among alveolar ventilation, CO_2 production, and arterial CO_2 tension.
16. Use the alveolar air equation to calculate alveolar oxygen tension (P_{AO_2}).
17. Describe the effects of hyperventilation and hypoventilation on P_{AO_2}.
18. Calculate the alveolar–arterial oxygen gradient [$P(A - a)_{O_2}$], the arterial–alveolar oxygen ratio (Pa_{O_2}/P_{AO_2}), and the arterial oxygen–oxygen concentration ratio (Pa_{O_2}/F_{IO_2}) and interpret the results.
19. Name disease states or conditions that may cause low $\dot{V}/\dot{Q}$, shunt, and dead space.
20. Contrast anatomic and intrapulmonary shunt and give examples of each.
21. Explain how low $\dot{V}/\dot{Q}$ affects oxygenation.
22. Calculate shunt fraction and explain how shunt affects oxygenation.
23. Contrast response to oxygen therapy in patients with low $\dot{V}/\dot{Q}$ versus shunt.
24. Describe the factors that affect diffusion across the lung.
25. Compare disease states or conditions that impair diffusion.
26. Calculate arterial blood oxygen content (Ca_{O_2}) and explain and interpret the results.
27. Explain the effect of hemoglobin (Hb) levels on Ca_{O_2} and describe the clinical consequences of anemia, polycythemia, and abnormal Hb on oxygenation.
28. Describe the oxyhemoglobin (HbO_2) dissociation curve and contrast the relationship between Pa_{O_2} and Sa_{O_2} on the flat and steep portions of the curve.
29. Describe the effects of the blood's chemical environment on the HbO_2 dissociation curve and explain why this is clinically important.
30. Explain the relationship between P_{50} and the affinity between Hb and O_2.
31. Describe carbon monoxide poisoning to include causes, diagnosis, and treatment.
32. List the causes of methemoglobinemia and describe its diagnosis and treatment.
33. Contrast adult hemoglobin (HbA) and fetal hemoglobin (HbF).
34. Calculate oxygen delivery ($\dot{D}_{O_2}$) and explain why it is important.
35. List causes and treatment of low cardiac output and shock.

36. Calculate the oxygen extraction ratio (O_2 ER) and interpret the results.
37. Describe cyanide poisoning to include causes, diagnosis, and treatment.
38. Identify the indications for oxygen therapy and recommend methods of administration.
39. Explain other techniques that may be used to improve oxygenation.
40. Perform a complete assessment of a patient's oxygenation and develop and implement an appropriate respiratory care plan.

KEY TERMS

2,3-diphosphoglycerate (2,3-DPG)
A-a gradient [$P(A - a)o_2$]
a-A oxygen ratio (Pao_2/PAo_2)
acute mountain sickness
altitude hypoxia
alveolar oxygen tension (PAo_2)
alveolar ventilation ($\dot{V}_A$)
ambient hypoxia
anatomic shunt
anemia
arterial oxygen content (Cao_2)
arterial oxygen saturation (Sao_2)
arterial oxygen tension (Pao_2)
Bohr effect
carboxyhemoglobin (COHb)
dead space
diffusion limited
HbO$_2$ dissociation curve
hypoxemia
hypoxia
hypoxic hypoxia

inspired oxygen tension (Pio_2)
intrapulmonary shunt
lower airway obstruction
methemoglobinemia
oxygen delivery ($\dot{D}o_2$)
oxygen extraction ratio (O_2 ER)
oxygen saturation by pulse oximetry (Spo_2)
P$_{50}$
Pao_2/Fio_2 ratio
perfusion without ventilation (shunt)
polycythemia
pulmonary capillary oxygen tension (P_co_2)
respiratory failure
sickle cell disease
stagnant or circulatory hypoxia
upper airway obstruction
venous admixture
ventilation–perfusion ratio $\dot{V}/\dot{Q}$
ventilation without perfusion

Overview

Ensuring adequate oxygenation is one of the most critical responsibilities of the respiratory care clinician. Assessment of the patient's oxygenation status requires a clear understanding of the causes of hypoxia, an in-depth knowledge of the associated clinical findings, and a strong grasp of the underlying pathophysiology of respiratory failure. After determining that a patient's oxygenation status is at risk, the respiratory care clinician must be able to design, implement, and evaluate an appropriate respiratory care plan to achieve and maintain adequate oxygenation.

Introduction

Adequate oxygenation is dependent on having sufficient inspired oxygen concentrations, clear and patent conducting airways, adequate alveolar ventilation, and good matching of gas and blood in the gas exchange units of the lung. There must then be adequate diffusion of oxygen across the alveolar–capillary (A–C) membrane in the lung and oxygen loading of the

BOX 6-1

Steps in the Oxygenation Process

Adequate tissue oxygenation requires the following:

1. Inspired oxygen tension (Pio_2) must be adequate.
2. The conducting airways must be clear and patent.
3. Adequate alveolar ventilation ($\dot{V}_A$) is required.
4. Matching of gas and blood in the alveoli and adjacent pulmonary capillaries must occur.
5. Oxygen must diffuse across the alveolar–capillary membrane into the blood.
6. The arterial blood oxygen content (Cao_2) must be adequate.
7. Adequate blood oxygen transport must occur to deliver the oxygenated blood to the tissues.
8. The systemic tissue beds must be adequately perfused, and oxygen must be unloaded from the blood and move to the tissues.
9. Tissue oxygen uptake and utilization must function properly.

hemoglobin resulting in adequate blood oxygen content. The oxygen-rich arterial blood must then be delivered to the tissues for utilization in aerobic metabolism. **Box 6-1** summarizes the steps in the oxygenation process. We will look at each step in the oxygenation process in order to understand the key elements that must be considered when assessing a patient's oxygenation status.

Initial Assessment of Oxygenation

Before describing the essential steps in the oxygenation process, we will review the initial assessment of a patient's oxygenation status and describe the clinical manifestations of hypoxia. **Hypoxia** is a term generally used to describe inadequate tissue oxygenation. **Hypoxemia** refers to low blood-oxygen levels. Other types of hypoxia include **ambient hypoxia**, alveolar hypoxia, **hypoxic hypoxia**, anemic hypoxia, circulatory hypoxia, and histotoxic hypoxia.[1] These and related terms are defined in **Box 6-2**.

Clinically, hypoxia is suspected when the clinical manifestations (signs and symptoms) of inadequate oxygen levels are present. In the presence of mild to moderate hypoxia, patients may experience excitement, overconfidence, restlessness, anxiety, nausea, headache,

BOX 6-2

Terms Used to Describe Types of Hypoxia

Altitude hypoxia: Form of ambient hypoxia due to reduced barometric pressure at high altitude.

Alveolar hypoxia: Decrease in alveolar oxygen levels (P_{AO_2}). Alveolar hypoxia may be caused by a decrease in P_{IO_2}, hypoventilation, airway obstruction, or atelectasis.

Ambient hypoxia: Hypoxia due to a reduction in inspired oxygen (decrease in P_{IO_2} or F_{IO_2}). Causes include breathing gas in a confined space without fresh gas replacement, resulting in consumption of the available oxygen, or decreased barometric pressure, as seen with high altitude.

Anemic hypoxia: Inadequate blood oxygen content due to decreased hemoglobin or alteration in the ability of the hemoglobin to carry oxygen (e.g., elevated carboxyhemoglobin or methemoglobinemia).

Anoxia: An older term used to indicate a complete absence of oxygen.

Cerebral hypoxia: Inadequate oxygen supply to the brain.

Circulatory hypoxia: Hypoxia due low cardiac output, low blood pressure, or inadequate circulation. The terms *stagnant hypoxia* and *circulatory hypoxia* are sometimes used interchangeably.

Histotoxic hypoxia: An inability of the tissues to utilize oxygen due to tissue poisoning (e.g., cyanide poisoning).

Hypoxemia: Low blood oxygen levels, usually assessed by measurement of P_{aO_2}, S_{aO_2}, and/or arterial blood oxygen content (C_{aO_2}).

Hypoxia: A general term meaning inadequate oxygen levels.

Hypoxic hypoxia: Hypoxia resulting from inadequate oxygenation of the blood by the lungs.

Ischemic hypoxia: Tissue hypoxia characterized by tissue oligemia (inadequate blood supply) caused by arteriolar obstruction or vasoconstriction.

Oxygen affinity hypoxia: Hypoxia due to reduced ability of hemoglobin to release oxygen.

Stagnant hypoxia: Inadequate tissue oxygenation due to inadequate local, regional, or systemic perfusion.

Tissue hypoxia: Inadequate tissue oxygenation.

Data from: Pierson DJ. Pathophysiology and clinical effects of chronic hypoxia. *Respir Care.* 2000;45(1):39–51.

---

and/or shortness of breath.[2] Upon physical examination, the respiratory care clinician will often see an increased heart and respiratory rate, increased blood pressure, and signs of respiratory distress.[2] The patient may be excited, exhibit impaired judgment, or be listless, disoriented, and confused. With severe hypoxia, tachycardia, hypertension, and tachypnea may progress to bradycardia; hypotension; slowed, irregular breathing; and loss of consciousness.[2] Cyanosis, although often associated with hypoxemia, is not a reliable indicator of the presence or severity of hypoxia for reasons that will be discussed below. Dyspnea is also a variable finding. Severe hypoxia may lead to respiratory arrest, cardiac arrest, and death. **Table 6-1** describes the clinical manifestations of hypoxia.

When the clinical manifestations of hypoxia are present, the respiratory care clinician should assess the patient's arterial blood oxygen levels.[3] The simplest and easiest test is measurement of **oxygen saturation by pulse oximetry (Sp$_{O_2}$)** of the hemoglobin. Sp$_{O_2}$ provides a noninvasive estimate of the **arterial oxygen saturation (Sa$_{O_2}$)** that is fast, safe, and convenient. Pulse oximetry, however, may not detect certain types of hypoxia (e.g., anemic hypoxia, circulatory hypoxia, ischemic hypoxia, or histotoxic hypoxia) and should not be relied upon in the presence of carbon monoxide poisoning or other abnormalities of the hemoglobin (e.g., methemoglobinemia).

Arterial blood gas studies allow for the direct measurement of a patient's **arterial oxygen tension (Pa$_{O_2}$)**, carbon dioxide tension (Pa$_{CO_2}$), and pH. When combined with co-oximetry (which also measures carboxyhemoglobin and methemoglobin), Sa$_{O_2}$ and hemoglobin (Hb) levels can be measured, which allows for the accurate calculation of the **arterial oxygen content (Ca$_{O_2}$)**. Arterial blood gas measurement requires an arterial blood sample and is more costly and time consuming than simple pulse oximetry. Assessment of arterial blood oxygenation is fairly straightforward, and normal values are listed in **Box 6-3**. Typically, classification of the degree of hypoxemia is based on Pa$_{O_2}$. A Pa$_{O_2}$ value of 80 to 100 mm Hg (when breathing room air) is considered normal; mild, moderate, and severe hypoxemia correspond to Pa$_{O_2}$ values of 60 to 79, 40 to 59, and < 40 mm Hg, respectively.[4,5] It should be noted that although many authors classify a Pa$_{O_2}$ in the range

TABLE 6-1
Signs and Symptoms of Hypoxia

Degree of Hypoxia	Respiratory	Cardiac/Cardiovascular	Cognitive/Neurologic
Mild hypoxia	Shortness of breath Increased respiratory rate Respiratory distress	Increased heart rate Mild hypertension Peripheral vasoconstriction	Overconfidence Restlessness Anxiety Excitement Euphoria Lightheadedness Nausea Dizziness Fatigue
Moderate hypoxia	Increased respiratory distress Tachypnea Increased minute volume/hyperventilation Accessory muscle use Intercostal retractions	Tachycardia Arrhythmias Hypertension	Agitation Impaired judgment Confusion Decreased night vision Disorientation Listlessness Headache Tingling Loss of coordination
Severe hypoxia	Severe dyspnea Slowed, irregular breathing Cyanosis Respiratory arrest	Hypertension followed by hypotension Tachycardia followed by bradycardia Cardiac arrest	Confusion Somnolence Severe headache Unconsciousness Vision disturbances (blurred vision, tunnel vision) Slowed reaction time Coma

of 40 to 59 mm Hg as moderate hypoxemia, we believe that a Pao_2 of 40 to 49 mm Hg represents a medical emergency that requires immediate attention. Consequently, we would suggest that a Pao_2 in the range of 40 to 49 mm Hg be considered moderately severe (rather than moderate) hypoxemia and that a $Pao_2 < 40$ mm Hg be considered very severe hypoxemia (see Box 6-3). It also should be noted that the expected Pao_2 declines

BOX 6-3

Assessment of Severity of Hypoxemia

Value	Normal[1] Range	Mild	Moderate	Moderate to Severe	Very Severe
Pao_2 (mm Hg)[2]	80–100	60–79	50–59	40–49	< 40
Sao_2 (%)[3]	96–98	91–95	85–90	75–84	< 75

[1]Expected Pao_2 declines with age. For subjects > 60 years, expected "normal" Pao_2 can be estimated as follows:
    Supine normal $Pao_2 = 109 - (0.43 \times age) \pm 8$ mm Hg
    Standing normal $Pao_2 = 104 - (0.27 \times age) \pm 12$ mm Hg
[2]Many authors list the range of Pao_2 for assessment of hypoxemia as follows:
    Mild: $Pao_2 = 60–79$ mm Hg
    Moderate: $Pao_2 = 40–59$ mm Hg
    Severe: $Pao_2 < 40$ mm Hg
We believe, however, that a $Pao_2 < 50$ mm Hg represents a medical emergency that should be treated as moderate to severe hypoxemia.
[3]Actual Sao_2 will vary with pH, Pao_2, and temperature.

with age. For example, a normal Pao_2 for an 80-year-old supine patient would be 75 mm Hg with a range of 67 to 83 mm Hg (see Box 6-3 for the formula).

The oxygen concentration (Fio_2, fraction of inspired O_2) provided should be taken into account when considering the severity of hypoxemia based on arterial blood oxygen levels. For example, a Pao_2 of 80 mm Hg while breathing room air ($Fio_2 = 0.21$) is considered within normal range, whereas a Pao_2 of 80 mm Hg while breathing 100% O_2 represents a severe oxygenation disturbance. In the past, the definition of acute lung injury (ALI) included a $Pao_2/Fio_2 \leq 300$ mm Hg but > 200 mm Hg, whereas the definition of acute respiratory distress syndrome (ARDS) required a $Pao_2/Fio_2 \leq 200$ mm Hg. More recently[6] it has been suggested that the **Pao_2/Fio_2 ratio** be used to classify the severity of ARDS when patients are receiving increased oxygen concentrations and positive end expiratory pressure (PEEP ≥ 5 cm H_2O):

- $Pao_2/Fio_2 > 300$ mm Hg but < 500 mm Hg: Normal
- $Pao_2/Fio_2 \leq 300$ mm Hg but > 200 mm Hg: Mild
- $Pao_2/Fio_2 \leq 200$ mm Hg but > 100 mm Hg: Moderate
- $Pao_2/Fio_2 \leq 100$ mm Hg: Severe

Thus, an ARDS patient with a Pao_2 of 80 mm Hg while breathing 100% O_2 with 5 cm H_2O PEEP would be classified as a *severe ARDS* ($Pao_2/Fio_2 = 80/1.0 = 80$). This patient would be severely hypoxemic if breathing room air. The Pao_2/Fio_2 ratio can also be used to predict the resultant Pao_2 with changes in Fio_2, as shown in **Clinical Focus 6-1**.

It should also be noted that although measurement of arterial blood oxygen levels (Pao_2 and Sao_2) are necessary to evaluate the presence and severity of hypoxemia, tissue hypoxia can be present due to many other reasons, including low cardiac output, anemia, other hemoglobin abnormalities, and poor tissue perfusion, which are discussed in the following sections of this chapter.

Respiratory Failure

As noted in Chapter 2, *respiration* refers simply to *gas exchange*. The two types of respiration of concern are external respiration and internal respiration:

- *External respiration* is the gas exchange (O_2 and CO_2) that occurs between the pulmonary capillaries and the alveoli.
- *Internal respiration* is the gas exchange (O_2 and CO_2) that takes place between the systemic tissue beds and the adjacent systemic capillaries.

Respiratory failure is a general term indicating the inability of the heart and lungs to deliver adequate levels of oxygen to the tissues and/or remove CO_2. Acute respiratory failure (ARF) may be defined as a sudden decrease in arterial blood oxygen levels (with or without elevated $Paco_2$). The term *hypoxemic respiratory failure* (i.e., lung failure) is sometimes used when the primary problem is inadequate oxygenation of the arterial blood as assessed by Pao_2, Spo_2, and/or Sao_2. Respiratory failure that includes hypoventilation (an elevated $Paco_2$) is sometimes described as *pump failure* (i.e., ventilatory failure; see Chapter 7).

It is important that assessment of a patient's oxygenation status involve much more than simply measuring arterial Pao_2, Spo_2, and/or Sao_2. In order to perform a complete assessment of oxygenation, the respiratory care clinician must understand and be able to assess each step the oxygenation process.

The Oxygenation Process

The oxygenation process begins with inspired oxygen tension and concentration and moves to the conducting airways, matching of gas and blood in the lung, diffusion of oxygen across the A–C membrane, and oxygen loading of the arterial hemoglobin. The oxygen-laden blood must then be delivered to tissues, and tissue uptake and utilization must be adequate. Tissue hypoxia may be caused by a number of conditions, and a complete patient assessment must include an assessment of inspired, alveolar, and arterial blood oxygen levels; cardiac output; peripheral perfusion; and tissue oxygen uptake and utilization. In this chapter, we will review the oxygenation process beginning with the inspired gas and ending with oxygen uptake and utilization by the tissues. We will also discuss problems that may occur at each step of the oxygenation process and outline the recognition and treatment of these problems.

Inspired Oxygen

Normal inspired gas at sea level has a fractional oxygen concentration (Fio_2) of 0.2095 (about 21% O_2) at a barometric pressure (P_B) of 760 mm Hg. The water vapor pressure (Ph_2o) in the inspired gas is about 47 mm Hg by the time the gas reaches the isothermic saturation boundary (ISB) in the airways below the carina, resulting in an **inspired oxygen tension (Pio_2)** of about 150 mm Hg:

$$Pio_2 = Fio_2 (P_B - Ph_2o)$$
$$= 0.21 (760 \text{ mm Hg} - 47 \text{ mm Hg}) = 150 \text{ mm Hg}^*$$

* Also often reported as torr, where 1 mm Hg = 1 torr.

The two major factors that determine Pio_2 are the inspired oxygen concentration (Fio_2) and the barometric pressure (P_B). Declines in Fio_2 or P_B will reduce Pio_2 and may cause hypoxia. An increase in Fio_2 (e.g., due to oxygen therapy) or P_B (e.g., due to underwater diving or hyperbaric therapy) will increase the Pio_2 and may

CLINICAL FOCUS 6-1

Severity of Oxygenation Problems: Hypoxemia

A patient with acute respiratory distress syndrome (ARDS) is receiving mechanical ventilatory support. The following data have been collected:

Ventilator mode: Assist/control
Respiratory rate: 12 breaths per minute
Tidal volume: 600 mL (8 mL/kg of ideal body weight)
FIO_2: 0.60 (60% O_2)
PEEP: 5 cm H_2O
Blood gases:
$P_B = 760$ mm Hg
FIO_2: = 0.60
pH = 7.42
$PaO_2 = 60$ mm Hg
$PaCO_2 = 38$ mm Hg
$HCO_3 = 22$ mEq/L
$SaO_2 = 90\%$

1. Based on the patient's PaO_2 and SaO_2, how would you classify the patient's level of hypoxemia?
   Hypoxemia is defined as low arterial blood oxygen levels, usually assessed by measurement of arterial oxygen tension (PaO_2), arterial oxygen saturation via pulse oximetry (SpO_2), or arterial blood oxygen saturation measurement (SaO_2). A PaO_2 of 60 mm Hg would be classified as *mild hypoxemia* using a conventional classification system while a $PaO_2 < 60$ mm Hg would be moderate hypoxemia (see Box 6-3).

2. Based on the patient's PaO_2/FIO_2 ratio, how severe is the patient's ARDS?
   The patient's PaO_2/FIO_2 ratio is 100 mm Hg ($PaO_2/FIO_2 = 60$ mm Hg/0.60 = 100 mm Hg). It has been suggested that the PaO_2/FIO_2 ratio be used to determine the *severity of ARDS* when patients are receiving increased oxygen concentrations and positive end expiratory pressure (PEEP ≥ 5 cm H_2O):
   Normal: $PaO_2/FIO_2 > 300$ mm Hg but < 500 mm Hg with PEEP
   Mild: $PaO_2/FIO_2 ≤ 300$ mm Hg but > 200 mm Hg
   Moderate: $PaO_2/FIO_2 ≤ 200$ mm Hg but > 100 mm Hg
   Severe: $PaO_2/FIO_2 ≤ 100$ mm Hg
   Using this classification, the patient has a *severe ARDS*.

3. What would happen to the patient's PaO_2 if he were allowed to breathe room air ($FIO_2 = 0.21$)?
   The PaO_2/FIO_2 ratio can be used as a rough estimate of the effect of changes in FIO_2 on PaO_2 where:
   Initial PaO_2/FIO_2 = Final PaO_2/FIO_2
   Entering the patient's initial and final data, we have: 60/0.60 = PaO_2/0.21
   Solving for the new or final PaO_2, we have: $PaO_2 = (60/0.60) × 0.21 = 21$ mm Hg
   If this patient was changed from an FIO_2 of 0.60 (60% O_2) to room air ($FIO_2 = 0.21$ or 21% O_2), it is likely that his PaO_2 would drop from 60 mm Hg to 21 mm Hg, which is *very severe hypoxemia*.

Data from: ARDS Definition Task Force, Ranieri VM, Rubenfeld GD, et al. Acute respiratory distress syndrome: the Berlin Definition. *JAMA*. 2012;307(23):2526–2533. doi: 10.1001/jama.2012.5669.

be used to treat hypoxia. Oxygen therapy may increase the FIO_2 up to 1.0 (100% O_2), depending on the delivery method used. At a normal barometric pressure of 760 mm Hg, breathing 100% O_2 will result in a PIO_2 of 713 mm Hg. **Box 6-4** illustrates the relationship between FIO_2 and PIO_2 known as the "Rule of Seven," which states that for each 0.01 (1%) change in oxygen concentration the PIO_2 will vary by about 7 mm Hg.

Problems with oxygenation due to an inadequate PIO_2 are known as *ambient hypoxia*. Normally, FIO_2 remains constant with changes in altitude up to an altitude of about 60 miles; however, P_B declines with increasing altitude, resulting in a decrease in PIO_2. The decrease in PIO_2 at high altitude may cause a form of ambient hypoxia known as **altitude hypoxia**, as well as generalized cardiovascular and neurologic problems.

BOX 6-4

Rule of Seven

The Rule of Seven states that for each 1% change in inspired oxygen percent (or change in F_{IO_2} of 0.01), the P_{IO_2} will change by 7 mm Hg.

Assuming a normal barometric pressure of 760 mm Hg:

$F_{IO_2} = 0.21 \rightarrow P_{IO_2} = F_{IO_2} (P_B - P_{H_2O}) = 0.21$
(760 mm Hg − 47 mm Hg) = 150 mm Hg
$F_{IO_2} = 0.50 \rightarrow P_{IO_2} = F_{IO_2} (P_B - P_{H_2O}) = 0.50$
(760 mm Hg − 47 mm Hg) = 357 mm Hg
$F_{IO_2} = 1.0 \rightarrow P_{IO_2} = F_{IO_2} (P_B - P_{H_2O}) = 1.0$ (760 mm Hg − 47 mm Hg) = 713 mm Hg

The Rule of Seven predicts that if you increase the F_{IO_2} from 0.50 to 0.60 (or 10%), the P_{IO_2} will increase approximately 70 mm Hg: 357 mm Hg + 70 mm Hg = 427 mm Hg.

Another form of ambient hypoxia may occur when inspired oxygen levels are reduced due to a decrease in F_{IO_2} at a normal P_B. This may occur due to consumption of the oxygen in the inspired air, such as occurs when people are trapped in a confined space with no fresh gas source or displacement of ambient oxygen by an asphyxiant gas. Generally, we will refer to oxygen problems due to a reduced P_{IO_2} as ambient hypoxia. Ambient hypoxia due to decreased P_B and decreased F_{IO_2}, as well as causes and related problems, are discussed below.

Altitude Hypoxia

Altitude hypoxia occurs when the barometric pressure (P_B) is reduced at high altitude, resulting in low inspired oxygen (P_{IO_2}) levels. Altitude hypoxia is a special case of ambient hypoxia due to a low P_B. It is interesting to note that the inspired oxygen concentration (F_{IO_2} or percentage) remains constant at about 0.21 (21%) until an altitude of 60 miles is reached. To put that in perspective, the elevation at the top of Mount Everest is 29,029 feet (about 5.5 miles), and a passenger airplane flying at 38,000 feet is at an altitude of about 7.2 miles. The F-22 Raptor Advanced Tactical Fighter aircraft can reach an altitude of over 50,000 feet, or about 11.36 miles. An altitude of 60 miles corresponds to about 316,800 feet above sea level. The orbital altitude of the International Space Station ranges from about 205 to 255 miles.

Although F_{IO_2} remains constant to a very high altitude, P_B and P_{IO_2} decline significantly at much lower altitudes (**Table 6-2**). For example, P_B and P_{IO_2} decline when one moves from Miami Beach, Florida (altitude = 0 feet; P_B = 760 mm Hg; P_{IO_2} = 150 mm Hg) to Denver (altitude = 5880 feet; P_B = 620 mm Hg; P_{IO_2} = 122 mm Hg) or Vail, Colorado (altitude = 8500 feet; P_B = 565 mm Hg; P_{IO_2} = 111 mm Hg). Acute altitude sickness is common in people who abruptly travel to above about 8200 feet.[7] Abrupt ascent to very high altitudes (> 11,400 feet) can be dangerous, and a gradual ascent to allow for acclimatization is recommended. Mountain climbers may suffer from altitude hypoxia and altitude sickness (mountain sickness), and those attempting to ascend very high mountains, such as Mount Everest, generally must use supplemental oxygen in order to survive the climb. Normal Pao_2 and Sao_2 at sea level are 80 to 100 mm Hg and 95% to 98%, respectively. Arterial hypoxemia is typically of concern when Pao_2 < 60 mm Hg (or Sao_2 < 90%), for reasons that will be discussed below. Arterial oxygen levels are somewhat diminished at altitudes of 5000 feet (resulting in a Pao_2 of 55 to 75 mm Hg), moderately diminished over 11,500 feet (resulting in a Pao_2 of 40 to 60 mm Hg), and greatly diminished at extreme altitudes of 18,000 to 29,000 feet (resulting in a Pao_2 of 28 to 40 mm Hg).[7]

Commercial aircraft often fly at altitudes of up to 40,000 feet (P_B = 140 mm Hg; P_{IO_2} − 4 mm Hg). In order to avoid profound hypoxia during flight, the Federal Aviation Administration (FAA) requires that airliner cabins be pressurized to simulate a cabin altitude of less than 8000 feet, and cabin pressures are typically maintained at the equivalent of an altitude of between 5000 to 8000 feet.[8] At these cabin pressures, P_{IO_2} will be about 108 to 122 mm Hg, which may result in hypoxemia in individuals with compromised lung function.[8] Because of this, patients with compromised cardiopulmonary function should be screened for the risk of developing in-flight hypoxemia. Patients with a resting Spo_2 < 92% on room air should be considered candidates for supplemental in-flight oxygen therapy.[8] Patients with a resting Spo_2 of 92% to 95% and certain risk factors, such as prior dyspnea, chest pain, hypercapnea, reduced pulmonary function (e.g., FEV_1 < 50% predicted or decreased diffusing capacity), obstructive or restrictive lung disease, cardiac disease, cerebrovascular disease, or pulmonary hypertension should receive further evaluation regarding the need for supplemental oxygen in-flight.[8] Generally, supplemental in-flight oxygen is recommended for patients whose in-flight Pao_2 is expected to be < 50 to 55 mm Hg.[8] A number of methods are available for predicting in-flight hypoxemia in patients, including regression equations, the hypoxia altitude simulation test (HAST), and use of a hypobaric chamber (though availability of hypobaric chambers is limited). In the event that hypoxia altitude testing is not available, an oxygen flow of 2 L/min has been recommended for most patients at risk for in-flight hypoxemia.[8] Patients receiving long-term oxygen therapy will generally need to have their

TABLE 6-2
Effect of Altitude on Barometric Pressure and Inspired Oxygen Levels

Location	Altitude (ft.)	F_{IO_2}	P_B (mm Hg)	Saturated P_{H_2O} (mm Hg)	P_{IO_2}[1] (mm Hg)	P_{aO_2}[2] (mm Hg)	S_{pO_2}[2] (% sat Hb)
Sea level	0	0.21	760	47	150	80–100	95–99
New Orleans, LA	4	0.21	759	47	150	80–100	95–99
Miami, FL	11	0.21	759	47	150	80–100	95–99
Chicago, IL	619	0.21	744	47	146	80–100	95–99
Atlanta, GA	1,026	0.21	733	47	144	80–100	95–99
Denver, CO	5,880	0.21	620	47	120	55–75	90–95
Mexico City, Mexico	7,350	0.21	590	47	114	55–75	90–95
Vail, CO	8,500	0.21	565	47	109	55–75	90–95
Mount Rainier	14,400	0.21	450	47	85	40–60	75–85
Mount Kilimanjaro	19,300	0.21	375	47	69	28–40	58–75
Mount McKinley	20,320	0.21	360	47	66	28–40	58–75
Mount Everest	29,029	0.21	250	47	43	28–40	58–75
Passenger airliner following cabin pressure loss	35,000	0.21	195	47	31	18–0	< 30

[1]$P_{IO_2} = F_{IO_2}(P_B - P_{H_2O})$; assumes P_{H_2O} of inspired gas at approximately 100% saturation; P_{H_2O} remains relatively constant with increasing altitude.
[2]Assumes normal lung function breathing room air to include compensatory hyperventilation with altitude and hypoxemia.

liter flow increased by 1 to 2 L/min during flight.[8] In addition, the reduced cabin pressures associated with aircraft ascent may cause expansion of trapped gases in the body. In the case of lung bullae (which are sometimes present in patients with emphysema), this expansion as the aircraft ascends to altitude has the potential to cause a pneumothorax.[8]

Stages of Altitude Hypoxia

Symptoms of altitude hypoxia include the general symptoms of hypoxia seen with other conditions (see Table 6-1), as well as specific findings seen with acute mountain sickness. The general findings of hypoxia may include dyspnea and changes in heart rate, respiratory rate and pattern, and blood pressure. Neurologic findings may include euphoria, behavioral changes, decreased ability to concentrate, poor judgment, confusion, or loss of consciousness. The effects of altitude hypoxia can be categorized into four stages corresponding to altitude:

- *Indifferent stage (5000 to 10,000 feet)*: Increased heart rate, respiratory rate, and tidal volume. Decreased night vision and impairment in

performing novel tasks (such as responding to an emergency) may occur.
- *Compensatory stage (10,000 to 15,000 feet)*: Marked increase in heart rate, respiratory rate, and tidal volume. Drowsiness, slowed mental processes, and increased reaction time may occur.
- *Disturbance stage (15,000 to 20,000 feet)*: Overt signs of hypoxia appear. Serious impairment in ability to perform tasks.
- *Critical stage (> 20,000 feet)*: Severe compromise of neurologic and cardiovascular function resulting in loss of consciousness and/or death.

Severe hypoxia at high altitude can cause life-threatening physiologic derangements as well as inappropriate or dangerous behavior. Severe hypoxia causes intellectual impairment, poor judgment, delayed reaction time, and inability to perform simple tasks, which may lead to life-threatening responses in an emergency situation. Inappropriate actions taken by aircraft pilots following loss of cockpit cabin pressure and poor or dangerous decisions made by mountain climbers ascending to very high altitude, such as Mount Everest, provide examples. In the event of aircraft cabin pressure loss at an altitude of 30,000 feet, an individual only has 1 to 2 minutes (or less) of "effective performance time" in which to take appropriate emergency actions, including putting on an emergency oxygen mask.[9] The oxygen levels needed to compensate for a reduced barometric pressure vary with altitude. For example, an F_{IO_2} of 0.45 (45% O_2) should be sufficient to correct hypoxemia at an altitude of 20,000 feet, whereas an F_{IO_2} of 1.0 (100% O_2) would be required to correct hypoxemia at an altitude of 34,000 feet.[9,10]

Acute Mountain Sickness (High-Altitude Illness)

Acute mountain sickness (often called *high-altitude illness*) is an illness that may affect hikers, skiers, mountain climbers, or travelers to high-altitude locations, generally over 6500 feet.[7] Symptoms of mild mountain sickness are similar to a hangover from excessive alcohol consumption. Symptoms may include headache, loss of appetite, nausea, vomiting, trouble sleeping, and feeling tired or out of sorts.[7] Symptoms may occur within the first day following ascent to high altitude and should subside in a day or two; further ascent to higher altitude should be avoided until symptoms recede.[7] Up to one-fourth of lowlanders who travel to altitude experience acute mountain sickness.[7] Most recover in a few days at altitude. Treatment of severe acute mountain sickness may include moving the patient to a lower altitude as soon as possible, oxygen therapy as needed, and medications for prevention or treatment of symptoms. The findings and treatment of acute mountain sickness are summarized in **Box 6-5**.

BOX 6-5

Symptoms of Altitude Sickness

Mountain Sickness

Occurs in about 25% of lowlanders who travel and stay at altitudes at or above about 6500 feet.
Hangover-like symptoms (e.g., headache, loss of appetite, nausea, vomiting, sleep disturbance, fatigue, exertional dyspnea).
May occur as early 1 to 2 hours on the first day at high altitude; typically occurs within the first 24 hours.
Generally subsides in a day or two.
Treatment:
- Rest.
- Limit physical activity.
- Avoid alcohol and respiratory depressants.
- Avoid further ascent until symptoms subside.
- Treat headache (aspirin, acetaminophen) and nausea (antiemetics such as ondansetron).
- Acetazolamide (Diamox) may be effective to treat or prevent mild acute mountain sickness.
- Dexamethasone (a corticosteroid) may be used to treat moderate to severe acute mountain sickness.
- Supply oxygen therapy, as needed.
- For severe acute mountain sickness, hyperbaric therapy using lightweight chambers or hyperbaric bags may be available as equipment on expeditions or in remote mountain clinics.

Prevention may include a gradual ascent over more than one day, avoidance of alcoholic beverages, avoidance of sedative and hypnotic drugs, and return to a lower altitude to sleep.

High-Altitude Cerebral Edema (HACE)

Symptoms may include anxiety, irritability, confusion, weakness, extreme tiredness, and drunken behavior.
May occur as early as the first day after ascent, but generally occurs sometime within the first 2 to 3 days.
Treatment:
- Transport to a lower altitude as soon as possible.
- Supply oxygen therapy, as needed.
- Provide hyperbaric therapy (see above).

High-Altitude Pulmonary Edema (HAPE)

Symptoms may include cough, shortness of breath, or frothy sputum.
Nifedipine (a calcium blocker used in the treatment of high blood pressure) may help prevent high-altitude pulmonary edema.

(continues)

Treatment:
- Administration of dexamethasone.
- Supply oxygen therapy, as needed.
- Provide hyperbaric therapy (above).
- Salmeterol/fluticasone (Advair) may have benefit in prevention of HAPE.

Data from: Gallagher, SA, Hackett, P. Acute mountain sickness and high altitude cerebral edema. In: UpToDate, Danzl DF (ed.). UpToDate, Waltham, MA, 2012.

In severe cases, acute mountain sickness may lead to high-altitude cerebral edema (HACE) and/or high altitude pulmonary edema (HAPE). HACE and HAPE represent medical emergencies, and treatment should include moving the patient to a lower altitude as soon as possible (see Box 6-5).[7]

Other Forms of Ambient Hypoxia

Ambient hypoxia may also be caused by decreased inspired oxygen concentrations (FIO_2) as may occur when a victim is enclosed in a confined space, such as a mine, submarine, or airtight enclosure without fresh gas replacement. This is a special threat to children, who are predisposed to using small, confined spaces, such as abandoned refrigerators or airtight storage chests, for play. Ambient hypoxia may also be a cause of death in mining accidents where individuals are trapped below the earth in confined spaces without adequate ventilation of fresh air. Victims of mining accidents may also be exposed to asphyxiant gases, such as methane, that may displace ambient oxygen and markedly decrease FIO_2. Other asphyxiant gases include nitrogen, helium, neon, argon, carbon dioxide, and propane. In high concentrations, these gases may displace oxygen and cause ambient hypoxia. Fatal industrial accidents, in which victims are exposed to high concentrations of asphyxiant gases, are not uncommon. There has also been at least one event in which a volcanic eruption resulted in the large-scale release of carbon dioxide, causing approximately 1800 deaths. This occurred in 1986, near Lake Nyos in Central Africa. Treatment of ambient hypoxia includes moving victims to a location with adequate ventilation and providing oxygen therapy, if indicated. In industrial settings, workers should use a self-contained breathing apparatus or airline respirator in areas where ambient oxygen concentrations may be deficient.[11]

Ventilation and the Conducting Airways

The next step in the oxygenation process is the delivery of oxygen-rich inspired gas to the alveoli for gas exchange. In order for this to occur properly, the conducting airways should be unobstructed and offer low resistance to gas flow. In addition, the ventilatory muscles and the neurologic drive to breathe must result in adequate alveolar ventilation. Last, the ventilated alveoli must have adequate pulmonary capillary perfusion for matching of gas and blood. We will discuss each of these essential steps in the oxygenation process below.

Conducting Airways

The conducting system of the respiratory tract extends from the external nares down to (and including) the terminal bronchioles. In order to achieve adequate oxygenation, these airways should be unobstructed and offer low resistance to gas flow. Problems with the oxygenation and ventilation can occur due to upper or lower airway obstruction, increased secretions, airway mucosal edema, and bronchospasm. **Box 6-6** summarizes problems related to the conducting airways that may interfere with the oxygenation process.

The upper airways are considered to be those that lie above the carina. Upper airway obstruction (UAO) may be caused by infection, trauma, edema, tumor, or aspiration of foreign bodies.[12] Trauma may result in airway swelling, as seen with inhalation of hot, noxious gases or flames. Laryngeal edema can be caused by infection, trauma, inhalation of noxious gases, and artificial airways (e.g., endotracheal tubes). Angioedema is swelling under the skin, mucosa, or submucosal tissue and may be caused by an allergic reaction. In severe cases, angioedema may result in laryngeal edema, which may compromise the patient's airway. Treatment of angioedema includes the administration of antihistamines, H_2 receptor blocking agents, corticosteroids, and epinephrine (in severe cases) and protection of the airway. Common causes of UAO in children include infection (e.g., epiglottitis, bacterial tracheitis, viral laryngotracheitis, retropharyngeal abscess), foreign body aspiration, trauma (e.g., neck trauma, burns), or anaphylaxis.[13]

UAO may be fixed or variable and intrathoracic or extrathoracic. Inspection of a flow-volume loop obtained during pulmonary function testing can help determine which type of UAO is present. *Fixed obstructions* may be intrathoracic or extrathoracic. An example

BOX 6-6

Problems Associated with the Conducting Airways

In order for oxygenation to be effective, the conducting airways should be unobstructed and offer low resistance to airflow. Common problems that may occur include:

- Airway obstruction
  - Infection (viral or bacterial)
  - Upper airway edema
  - Laryngeal abnormalities (croup, epiglottitis, postextubation laryngeal edema, vocal cord dysfunction, tumor)
  - Tracheal stenosis or tumor
  - Foreign body inhalation
  - Trauma (burns, inhalation of noxious gases)
  - Obstructive sleep apnea (OSA)
  - Lower airway inflammation and edema (asthma, infection, inhalation of irritants such as smoke)
  - Secretions
  - Bronchospasm
  - Loss of elastic tissue and loss of airway patency (emphysema)
- Increased airway resistance (R_{aw})
  - Bronchospasm
  - Mucosal edema
  - Increased secretions

BOX 6-7

Fixed Versus Variable Upper Airway Obstruction

Fixed Upper Airway Obstruction

Fixed upper airway obstruction (UAO) is characterized by decreased inspiratory and expiratory flow on the flow-volume loop. Fixed UAO may be extrathoracic or intrathoracic and includes:

- Postintubation or posttracheostomy tracheal stenosis (narrowing of the trachea due to scar tissue formation)
- Goiter (an enlarged thyroid gland) compressing the trachea
- Firm tracheal tumors or lesions

Variable Upper Airway Obstruction

Variable UAO may be extrathoracic or intrathoracic:

- Extrathoracic: Characterized by decreased inspiratory flow on the flow-volume loop.
  - Laryngeal abnormalities
    - Vocal cord paralysis
    - Paradoxical vocal cord motion
    - Glottic strictures
    - Subglottic stenosis (narrowing of the airway below the true vocal cords, but above the cricoid cartilage)
    - Laryngeal tumor
    - Laryngomalacia (supraglottic laryngeal cartilage collapses on inspiration)
  - Extrathoracic tracheomalacia (weakness or flaccidity of tracheal cartilage with partial tracheal collapse on inspiration)
- Intrathoracic: Characterized by decreased expiratory flow on the flow-volume loop.
  - Tracheomalacia of the intrathoracic airway (weakness or flaccidity of tracheal cartilage that leads to partial tracheal collapse on forced expiration)
  - Bronchogenic cysts
  - Tumor near the carina
  - Tracheal lesions (often malignant)

Data from: Braman SS, Gaissert HA. Upper airway obstruction. In: Fishman AP, Elias JA, Fishman JA, et al. (eds.). *Fishman's Pulmonary Diseases and Disorders*, 3rd ed. New York: McGraw-Hill; 1998: 783–801.

of a fixed UAO is tracheal stenosis (narrowing of the trachea), which may be caused by scar tissue formation following prolonged intubation. A firm tracheal tumor or goiter (an enlarged thyroid gland) compressing the trachea may also cause fixed UAO. *Variable extrathoracic obstruction* may be caused by vocal cord paralysis, vocal cord tumors, laryngomalacia, or tracheomalacia of the extrathoracic portion of the trachea. *Variable intrathoracic obstruction* may be caused by tracheal lesions of the intrathoracic portion of the trachea. This occurs because airways become larger during inspiration and smaller with expiration. A mass within the trachea moves closer to the opposite wall during expiration and thus the amount of obstruction increases.

Possible causes of variable intrathoracic UAO include tumor or bronchogenic cyst just above the carina and tracheomalacia (tracheal cartilage collapse) of the intrathoracic portion of the trachea. **Box 6-7** provides a summary of conditions associated with fixed and variable UAO.

Adults may also experience upper airway obstruction due to obstructive sleep apnea (OSA). OSA is caused by soft tissue obstruction during sleep and is characterized by repeated episodes of apnea or hypopnea and hypoxemia throughout the night. These recurring episodes of hypoxemia may cause cardiac arrhythmias, including bradycardia.[14] OSA victims often complain of daytime sleepiness and have an increased incidence of motor vehicle accidents, presumably due to somnolence while driving.[14] Generally, five or more episodes of apnea/hypopnea per hour in symptomatic patients (or $\geq$ 15 per hour without complaints) are diagnostic for sleep apnea in patients with sleep disturbances.

OSA affects up to 6% of middle-aged and older people and is associated with the development of systemic hypertension and increased incidence of stroke, diabetes, and coronary artery disease.[14] OSA is best evaluated in the sleep laboratory, whereas other forms of upper airway obstruction should be assessed in the pulmonary function laboratory via measurement of forced expiratory/inspiratory flow-volume loops. Treatment of OSA may include weight loss in the presence of obesity, avoidance of sedative drugs and alcohol, and use of continuous positive airway pressure (CPAP) via a well-fitted mask during sleep.[14] CPAP is effective for most patients; however, compliance is often an issue. In severe cases of OAS, tracheostomy may be considered.

In children, the most common cause of upper airway obstruction is croup (laryngotracheobronchitis).[13] Other common causes of upper airway obstruction in children include foreign body aspiration; decreased upper airway muscle tone, as seen with depressed levels of consciousness or neuromuscular disease; and upper airway infection (e.g., epiglottitis, bacterial tracheitis, or pharyngeal or peritonsillar abscess).[13]

Lower airway obstruction can be caused by respiratory tract infections resulting in inflammation, bronchospasm, and increased secretions. Other causes of lower airway obstruction include chronic obstructive pulmonary disease (COPD), chronic bronchitis, emphysema, asthma, cystic fibrosis, and bronchiectasis. Chronic progressive dyspnea, airway inflammation, and lung structural changes, often due to long-term inhalation of an irritant, such as cigarette smoke, are the hallmarks of COPD.[15] Obstruction in COPD may be irreversible or only partially reversible with administration of a bronchodilator. Asthma, in contrast, is an inflammatory lung disease characterized by intermittent cough, dyspnea, and bronchospasm due to bronchial smooth muscle hyperreactivity that is reversible following bronchodilator administration, although some cases of chronic asthma are only partially reversible.[15] Other obstructive lung diseases include immotile cilia syndrome and small airways disease (obstructive bronchiolitis). Recurrent infections due to hypogammaglobulinemia may lead to bronchiectasis.[15] Common clinical findings with obstructive lung disease include hypoxemia, an increased work of breathing, dyspnea, decreased expiratory flow rates on forced expiration, and increased lung volumes, which may be seen as a flattened diaphragm on imaging. **Table 6-3** lists the major features of the more common obstructive lung diseases.

Alveolar Ventilation

The next step in the oxygenation process is movement of the oxygen-rich inspired gas into the alveoli. This requires adequate **alveolar ventilation ($\dot{V}_A$)**. Clinically, a patient's level of ventilation is best assessed by measurement of the partial pressure of carbon dioxide in the arterial blood (Pa_{CO_2}; see also Chapter 7). Normally, alveolar CO_2 tension (PA_{CO_2}) is equal to arterial Pa_{CO_2},

TABLE 6-3
Characteristics of the Obstructive Lung Diseases

Disease	Clinical Manifestations	Pulmonary Function Test, Imaging, and Laboratory Findings
Asthma	Episodes of dyspnea, cough, wheezing	Airway hyperreactivity Response to bronchodilator
COPD	Progressive dyspnea	Decreased $FEV_{1.0}$ $FEV_{1.0}/FVC < 70\%$ postbronchdilator Decreased Pa_{O_2}, Sa_{O_2}, Sp_{O_2} Increased Pa_{CO_2} with end stage disease
Emphysema	Dyspnea, little sputum	Hyperinflation Decreased D_{LCO} α_1-antitrypsin deficiency with α_1 disease
Chronic bronchitis	Chronic cough, sputum production	May have normal D_{LCO} if emphysema is not present
Bronchiectasis	Large volume of sputum	Dilated, thick-walled bronchi on imaging Decreased $FEV_{1.0}$ Decreased $FEV_{1.0}/FVC$
Cystic fibrosis	Sinusitis, bronchiectasis, meconium ileus, malabsorption	Increased sweat chloride CFTR chloride channel mutation Elevated fecal fat

COPD, chronic obstructive pulmonary disease; $FEV_{1.0}$, forced expiratory volume in 1.0 second; $FEV_{1.0}/FVC$, ratio of the forced expiratory volume in 1.0 second to the forced vital capacity; Sa_{O_2}, arterial oxygen saturation; Sp_{O_2}, pulse oximetry oxygen saturation; Pa_{CO_2}, partial pressure of arterial carbon dioxide; D_{LCO}, diffusing capacity for carbon monoxide; CFTR, cystic fibrosis transmembrane conductance regulator.

This article was published in *Andreoli and Carpenter's Cecil Essentials of Medicine*, 8th ed. Andreoli TE, Benjamin IJ, Griggs RC, Wing EJ, eds., Obstructive lung disease by Jankowich MD. Pages 213–224, Copyright Saunders 2010.

and the relationship between alveolar ventilation and $PaCO_2$ is defined by the following equation:

$$\dot{V}_A = (0.863 \times \dot{V}CO_2) \div PaCO_2$$

where

> $\dot{V}A$ = Alveolar ventilation in L/min
> $\dot{V}CO_2$ = Carbon dioxide production in mL/min
> $PaCO_2$ = Partial pressure of arterial carbon dioxide in mm Hg
> 0.863 = Conversion factor

Thus, normal ventilation can be defined as a $PaCO_2$ of 35 to 45 mm Hg. *Hypoventilation* corresponds to a $PaCO_2 > 45$ mm Hg, whereas *hyperventilation* corresponds to a $PaCO_2 < 35$ mm Hg. For a complete discussion of assessment of ventilation, please refer to Chapter 7.

Alveolar oxygen levels are described by the *alveolar air equation*:

$$PAO_2 = PIO_2 - PACO_2 \left[FIO_2 + \frac{1 - FIO_2}{R} \right]$$

where

> PAO_2 = Calculated alveolar oxygen tension (mm Hg or torr)
> PIO_2 = Inspired oxygen tension;
> $PIO_2 = FIO_2 (P_B - PH_2O)$
> $PACO_2$ = Alveolar carbon dioxide tension (mm Hg or torr)
> FIO_2 = Fractional inspired oxygen
> R = Respiratory quotient where R is $\dot{V}CO_2/\dot{V}O_2$

Normal O_2 consumption ($\dot{V}O_2$) is about 250 mL/min, and normal CO_2 production ($\dot{V}CO_2$) is about 200 mL/min. This would result in a normal R value of about 0.80:

$$R = \dot{V}CO_2 / \dot{V}O_2 = 200/250 = 0.80$$

For clinical use, it is acceptable to use a simplified version of the alveolar air equation, which assumes that alveolar and arterial PCO_2 are equal (i.e., $PACO_2 = PaCO_2$), which is true under most conditions:

$$PAO_2 = PIO_2 - \frac{PaCO_2}{R}$$

Assuming a steady-state R value of 0.80, the simplified alveolar air equation becomes:

$$PAO_2 = PIO_2 - \frac{PaCO_2}{0.80} = PIO_2 - PaCO_2 \times 1.25$$

Note that R may vary with exercise, dietary changes, and increased metabolic rate, such as may occur with fever or sepsis. This should be taken into account when using the alveolar air equation. It should also be noted that the respiratory quotient (RQ) and the respiratory exchange ratio (RER) of CO_2 and O_2 across the lung are normally equal (i.e., R = RQ = RER); this may not be the case in non-steady-state situations, such as may occur during exercise. Finally, some authors have suggested that correction for R is not needed for the calculation of PAO_2 if the $FIO_2 \geq 0.60$:[16]

$$PAO_2 = PIO_2 - PaCO_2$$

Box 6-8 provides examples of the PAO_2 calculation while breathing different oxygen concentrations. A normal PAO_2 while breathing room air at sea level is approximately 104 mm Hg, with a range of 100 to 110 mm Hg; PAO_2 increases to approximately 663 mm Hg while breathing 100% oxygen at sea level.

Effect of Hyperventilation on Oxygenation

As can be seen by inspection of the alveolar air equation, an increase or decrease in $PaCO_2$ may have an important effect on PAO_2, and, in turn, arterial oxygen levels. For example, with hyperventilation and a

---

BOX 6-8

Alveolar Oxygen Tension (PAO_2) Calculation

Estimation of normal alveolar oxygen tension when breathing room air (with a normal $PaCO_2$) is as follows:

- Room air calculation of PAO_2:
  - Given a room air of $FIO_2 = 0.21$, $P_B = 760$, $PH_2O = 47$, and a normal $PaCO_2$ of 40 mm Hg or torr*, estimate PAO_2:
    $PAO_2 = PIO_2 - PaCO_2 \times 1.25$
      $= FIO_2 (P_B - PH_2O) - PaCO_2 \times 1.25$
    $PAO_2 = 0.21(760 - 47) - 40 \times 1.25$
    $PAO_2 = 149.73 - 50 = 99.73 = 100$ mm Hg
- Calculation of PAO_2 with increased FIO_2:
  - Given a normal subject breathing 50% oxygen, estimate PAO_2:
    $PAO_2 = PIO_2 - PaCO_2 \times 1.25$
      $= FIO_2(P_B - PH_2O) - PaCO_2 \times 1.25$
    $PAO_2 = 0.50(760 - 47) - 40 \times 1.25$
    $PAO_2 = 756.5 - 50 = 306.5$ mm Hg
  - Given a normal subject breathing 100% oxygen, estimate PAO_2:
    $PAO_2 = PIO_2 - PaCO_2 \times 1.25$
      $= FIO_2 (P_B - PH_2O) - PaCO_2 \times 1.25$
    $PAO_2 = 1.0 (760 - 47) - 40 \times 1.25$
    $PAO_2 = 713 - 50 = 663$ mm Hg

*Torr and mm Hg may be used interchangeably, where 1 torr = 1 mm Hg.

corresponding $PaCO_2$ of 18 mm Hg while breathing room air, the resultant PAO_2 would be:

$$PAO_2 = PIO_2 - \frac{PaCO_2}{0.80}$$

$$PAO_2 = FIO_2(P_B - PH_2O) - (PaCO_2 \times 1.25)$$

$$PAO_2 = 0.21(760 - 47) - (18 \times 1.25)$$

$$PAO_2 = 150 - 22.5 = 128 \text{ mm Hg}$$

Assuming a normal room air A-a gradient of 10 mm Hg (see below for discussion of the A-a gradient), then the resultant PaO_2 would be 118 mm Hg:

$$PAO_2 = 128 \text{ mm Hg}$$

$$PaO_2 = PAO_2 - \text{A-a gradient}$$

$$PaO_2 = 128 - 10 = 118 \text{ mm Hg}$$

Thus hyperventilation can have a small but sometimes significant benefit in terms of raising PAO_2 and, in turn, arterial oxygen levels. Two of the most common early responses to hypoxia are an increased heart rate (tachycardia) and increased respiratory rate (tachypnea). An increase in heart rate increases oxygen delivery to the tissues by increasing cardiac output. An increase in respiratory rate increases alveolar ventilation and reduces $PACO_2$ and $PaCO_2$, and thus increases PAO_2, as illustrated by the alveolar air equation. **Clinical Focus 6-2** provides an example of a commonly encountered clinical condition: hyperventilation secondary to hypoxemia. In short, hyperventilation is a normal physiologic response to hypoxia. **Clinical Focus 6-3** provides a second example of the effect of hyperventilation on PaO_2.

CLINICAL FOCUS 6-2

Hyperventilation Secondary to Hypoxemia

A 32-year-old male patient comes to the emergency department complaining of shortness of breath, cough, fever, and chills. The patient's vitals are as follows: temperature 38.9° C (102° F), respiratory rate 26 breaths/min, heart rate 112 beats/min, and blood pressure 126/86 mm Hg. A chest x-ray and arterial blood gases are ordered. Blood gases while breathing room air are as follows:

P_B = 760 mm Hg
FIO_2 = 0.21
pH = 7.50
PaO_2 = 55 mm Hg
$PaCO_2$ = 28 mm Hg
HCO_3 = 22 mEq/L
SaO_2 = 88%

1. What is your assessment of each of the patient's arterial blood gas values?

pH = 7.50	Overall alkalosis
PaO_2 = 55 mm Hg	Moderate hypoxemia
$PaCO_2$ = 28 mm Hg	Hyperventilation (respiratory alkalosis)
HCO_3 = 22 mEq/L	Within normal range of 22 to 28 mEq/L
SaO_2 = 88%	Hypoxemia

2. What is your overall assessment of the patient's arterial blood gases?

   This blood gas would be correctly interpreted as an uncompensated respiratory alkalosis with moderate hypoxemia. However, a more useful description of the patient's condition would be *acute alveolar hyperventilation secondary to hypoxemia.*

3. What would the patient's PaO_2 be if he was not hyperventilating?

   a. The patient's calculated PAO_2 while breathing room air while hyperventilating is:

   $$PAO_2 = PIO_2 - PaCO_2 \times 1.25 = 0.21(760 - 47) - 28 \times 1.25 = 115 \text{ mm Hg}$$

   b. The patient's calculated A-a gradient is:

   $$P(A - a)O_2 = PAO_2 - PaO_2 = 115 - 55 = 60 \text{ mm Hg}$$

   c. The patient's calculated PAO_2 while breathing room air with a normal $PaCO_2$ would be:

   $$PAO_2 = PIO_2 - PaCO_2 \times 1.25 = 0.21(760 - 47) - 40 \times 1.25 = 100 \text{ mm Hg}$$

d. Assuming a $P(A-a)O_2$ of 60 mm Hg (from b, above), the PaO_2 could be estimated as follows:

$PaO_2 = PAO_2 - P(A-a)O_2$
$PaO_2 = 100 - 60$ mm Hg
$PaO_2 = 40$ mm Hg

This calculation demonstrates the effect of hyperventilation in improving oxygenation. In the example, if the patient were breathing normally ($PaCO_2 = 40$ mm Hg), the resultant PaO_2 would be 40 mm Hg. If the patient were able to hyperventilate to reduce the $PaCO_2$ to 28 mm Hg, the PaO_2 would increase to 55 mm Hg. In other words, the patient is able to improve his PaO_2 from a low of about 40 mm Hg with normal ventilation ($PaCO_2 = 40$ mm Hg) to 55 mm Hg with hyperventilation ($PaCO_2 = 28$ mm Hg).

Effect of Hypoventilation on Oxygenation

Whereas hyperventilation can result in small increases in alveolar and arterial oxygen levels, hypoventilation can have a profound effect on oxygenation. For example, if a subject with otherwise normal lung function experienced an increase in $PaCO_2$ from 40 to 80 mm Hg while breathing room air, the PAO_2 would decline to about 50 mm Hg:

$$PAO_2 = PIO_2 - \frac{PaCO_2}{0.80}$$
$$PAO_2 = FIO_2(P_B - PH_2O) - (PaCO_2 \times 1.25)$$
$$PAO_2 = 0.21(760 - 47) - (80 \times 1.25)$$
$$PAO_2 = 150 - 100 = 50 \text{ mm Hg}$$

CLINICAL FOCUS 6-3

Effect of Hyperventilation on Oxygen Levels

The following data have been collected from the patient:
$P_B = 760$ mm Hg
$PaO_2 = 125$ mm Hg
$PaCO_2 = 12$ mm Hg

1. What would the patient's alveolar PAO_2 be if she were breathing room air ($FIO_2 = 0.21$) at a normal barometric pressure?
   Based on the following calculation, if the patient is breathing room air the PAO_2 is 135 mm Hg:

   $FIO_2 = 0.21$
   $P_B = 760$ mm Hg
   $PAO_2 = (P_B - PH_2O)FIO_2 - PaCO_2 \times 1.25$
   $PAO_2 = (760 - 47)0.21 - 12 \times 1.25$
   $PAO_2 = 150 - 15 = 135$ mm Hg

2. The patient's arterial PaO_2 is 125 mm Hg. Do you think the patient is receiving supplemental O_2?
   Although inexperienced clinicians often assume that a patient with a PaO_2 above the normal range of 80 to 100 mm Hg must be receiving oxygen therapy, this may not be the case in the presence of marked hyperventilation. This patient has a very low $PaCO_2$ due to significant hyperventilation ($PaCO_2 = 12$ mm Hg). This might occur for a number of reasons, including in response to a severe metabolic acidosis. In fact, the blood gas data provided are from a 17-year-old-patient with a severe diabetic ketoacidosis (pH = 7.18). The patient has normal lung function and is able to hyperventilate in order to partly compensate for the severe metabolic acidosis. As noted in the first calculation, if the patient were breathing room air, the calculated PAO_2 would be about 135 mm Hg. A PAO_2 of 135 mm Hg could result in a PaO_2 of 125 mm Hg (assuming a normal $P(A-a)O_2$ of 10 mm Hg and normal lung function). However, in this example, we cannot be sure whether the patient is breathing room air or not.

Assuming a normal room air A-a gradient of 10 mm Hg (see below for discussion of the A-a gradient), the patient's resultant PaO_2 would be only 40 mm Hg. Thus, hypoventilation alone may cause severe hypoxemia, even with otherwise normal lungs. The "Rule of 4 and 5" suggests that in patients breathing room air, with each increase in $PaCO_2$ of 4 mm Hg the PaO_2 will decrease by 5 mm Hg. Possible causes of acute, severe hypoventilation include trauma, sedative or narcotic drug overdose, central nervous system (CNS) or neuromuscular disease, and acute cardiopulmonary disease (see Chapter 7). Assuming normal lung function, if the patient just described had his or her ventilation restored to normal ($PaCO_2$ = 40 mm Hg), the patient's PAO_2 and PaO_2 should also return to normal. **Box 6-9** provides additional examples of the effects of ventilation on PAO_2 and PaO_2. **Clinical Focus 6-4** provides

---

RC Insights

Rule of 4 and 5

To estimate the effect of an increase in $PaCO_2$ on PaO_2 in a patient breathing room air, use the Rule of 4 and 5. According to the Rule of 4 and 5, for each increase in $PaCO_2$ of 4 mm Hg, the PaO_2 will decrease about 5 mm Hg (when breathing room air).

For example, in a patient breathing room air with a PaO_2 of 60 mm Hg, what would happen to the PaO_2 if the $PaCO_2$ increased to 48 mm Hg?

- If the arterial $PaCO_2$ increases from 40 to 48 mm Hg:
  - This is an increase of +8 mm Hg = 2 × 4 mm Hg
- Expect the PaO_2 to decrease to 2 × 5 mm Hg = 10 mm Hg:
  - PaO_2 = 60 − 10 = 50 mm Hg
  - The PaO_2 will decrease from 60 to 50 mm Hg.

BOX 6-9

Effects of Ventilation on Alveolar and Arterial Oxygen Levels

Hypoventilation Reduces Alveolar Oxygen Levels (as $PaCO_2$ rises, PAO_2 falls)

Example: Hypoventilation while breathing room air

FIO_2 = 0.21
$PaCO_2$ = 70 mm Hg
$PAO_2 = (P_B - PH_2O)FIO_2 - PaCO_2 \times 1.25$
$PAO_2 = [(713)0.21] - 70 \times 1.25 = 150 - 87.5$
PAO_2 = 62.5 mm Hg

If $P(A - a)O_2$ was 10 mm Hg (a normal value), then PaO_2 would be 52.5 mm Hg:

$PaO_2 = PAO_2$ − A-a gradient
$PaO_2 = PAO_2 - P(A - a)O_2$
PaO_2 = 87.5 − 10 = 52.5 mm Hg

This is the alveolar hypoxia (and arterial hypoxemia) caused by hypoventilation.

Hyperventilation Increases Alveolar Oxygen Levels (as $PaCO_2$ decreases, PAO_2 increases)

Example: Hyperventilation while breathing room air

FIO_2 = 0.21
$PaCO_2$ = 18 mm Hg
$PAO_2 = (P_B - PH_2O)FIO_2 - PaCO_2 \times 1.25$
$PAO_2 = [(713)0.21] - 18 \times 1.25$
PAO_2 = 150 − 22.5 = 127.5 mm Hg

If $P(A - a)O_2$ was 10 mm Hg, then PaO_2 would be 117.5 mm Hg:

$PaO_2 = PAO_2$ − A-a gradient
$PaO_2 = PAO_2 - P(A - a)O_2$
PaO_2 = 127.5 − 10 = 117.5 mm Hg

Thus, hyperventilation can cause a relatively small (but sometimes clinically important) increase in alveolar (and arterial) oxygenation.

CLINICAL FOCUS 6-4

Alveolar Oxygen Levels During Normal Ventilation

The following data have been collected from the patient:

P_B = 760 mm Hg
Pa_{O_2} = 130 mm Hg
Pa_{CO_2} = 40 mm Hg

This patient has a normal level of ventilation, as indicated by the Pa_{CO_2} of 40 mm Hg. However, the patient's arterial oxygen level is much higher than the normal clinical range of 80 to 100 mm Hg. The question may arise as to whether this patient is receiving oxygen therapy or if it is possible to have a Pa_{O_2} of 130 mm Hg while breathing room air (see Clinical Focus 6-2). The following steps can be used to determine if this patient is receiving supplemental oxygen.

1. Calculate what the patient's alveolar oxygen level (PA_{O_2}) would be if he were breathing room air (FI_{O_2} = 0.21)

   PA_{O_2} = 0.21(760 − 47) − 40 × 1.25
   PA_{O_2} = 150 − 50 = 100

2. Is this patient receiving supplemental O_2?
   This patient must be receiving supplemental oxygen. We know this because the arterial Pa_{O_2} cannot exceed the alveolar PA_{O_2}. *If* the patient were breathing room air (FI_{O_2} = 0.21), the calculated PA_{O_2} would be about 100 mm Hg (see step 1, above). Because the patient's Pa_{O_2} is 130 mm Hg, we know that the PA_{O_2} must be above 130 mm Hg—which would require supplemental oxygen administration. In fact, this patient is receiving 28% oxygen by air-entrainment mask:

   P_B = 760 mm Hg
   FI_{O_2} = 0.28
   Pa_{CO_2} = 40 mm Hg
   PA_{O_2} = 0.28(760 − 47) − 40 × 1.25
   PA_{O_2} = 200 − 50 = 150

   Oxygen therapy at 28% O_2 has resulted in a PA_{O_2} of 150 mm Hg. With normal ventilation (Pa_{CO_2} = 40 mm Hg), a Pa_{O_2} of 130 mm Hg is possible with an increased FI_{O_2}.

example of the relationship between FI_{O_2} and Pa_{O_2} with normal ventilation. As noted previously, the "Rule of 4 and 5" states that for each 4 mm Hg increase in Pa_{CO_2} the Pa_{O_2} will fall about 5 mm Hg; this provides a quick way to estimate the effect of increases in Pa_{CO_2} on Pa_{O_2} in patients breathing room air

Summary of Possible Problems with Alveolar Oxygenation

Problems that may reduce alveolar oxygen levels (and, in turn, Pa_{O_2}) include inadequate inspired oxygen tension, problems with the conducting airways, and reduced alveolar ventilation. An inadequate PI_{O_2} due to altitude or other forms of ambient hypoxia may result in a low **alveolar oxygen tension (PA_{O_2})**. Upper or lower airway obstruction or increased resistance to gas flow may affect the conducting airways and interfere with achieving an adequate PA_{O_2}. Hypoventilation and the resultant increase in arterial and alveolar carbon dioxide tensions may also result in decreased alveolar

oxygen tension. The term *alveolar hypoxia* refers to reduced PA_{O_2} and may be caused by decreased PI_{O_2}, obstruction of the airways, or alveolar collapse (atelectasis). Hypoxic hypoxia refers to inadequate oxygenation of the blood by the lungs.

Matching of Gas and Blood

So far, we have considered the oxygenation process down to the alveolar level. The next step is the matching of alveolar gas to pulmonary capillary blood flow and the diffusion of oxygen into the blood. The effectiveness of oxygen transfer across the lung is determined in large part by the relationship between alveolar ventilation and pulmonary capillary blood flow. The most common causes of reduced oxygen transfer are hypoventilation, ventilation–perfusion mismatch, right-to-left shunt, and diffusion limitations. Assessment of effective gas transfer across the lung includes measurement of arterial oxygen levels and calculation of several indices of oxygenation, which are described below.

Alveolar Versus Arterial Oxygen Levels

The effect of alveolar P_{AO_2} on arterial oxygen levels can be examined by several oxygenation indices. The first is the alveolar–arterial P_{O_2} difference [$\mathbf{P(A-a)O_2}$; aka the **A-a gradient**], which is calculated by subtracting the P_{aO_2} from the P_{AO_2}:

$$P(A-a)O_2 = \text{A-a gradient} = P_{AO_2} - P_{aO_2}$$

A normal A-a gradient for a healthy young adult breathing room air is 10 mm Hg with a range of 5 to 15 mm Hg. The A-a gradient increases with age, and a normal value for a healthy 60-year-old breathing room air is ≤ 25 mm Hg.[17] The A-a gradient also may increase with lung disease, and a change in the A-a gradient can be used to assess improvement or worsening in lung function (when F_{IO_2} is constant).

It is important to note that the A-a gradient varies with F_{IO_2} and increases to about 100 mm Hg when breathing 100% O_2 (range of about 80 to 120 mm Hg while breathing 100% O_2).[3] Because F_{IO_2} often varies due to treatment needs in acutely ill patients, two other measures of the effectiveness of oxygenation transfer across the lung are sometimes used: the P_{aO_2}/P_{AO_2} ratio and the P_{aO_2}/F_{IO_2} ratio. Both of these are relatively stable with changes in F_{IO_2}. A normal P_{aO_2}/P_{AO_2} ratio (aka **a/A oxygen ratio**) while breathing room air is about 0.80 (range: 0.77 to 0.82), whereas a normal P_{aO_2}/F_{IO_2} ratio is 380 to 500.[3]

A P_{aO_2}/F_{IO_2} ratio ≤ 300 has been used as one criterion in the definition of ALI (now called mild ARDS), whereas a P_{aO_2}/F_{IO_2} ratio ≤ 200 has been used as one criterion to identify ARDS.[18] More recently, the Berlin definition of ARDS has been proposed, in which the severity hypoxemia is based on the P_{aO_2}/F_{IO_2} ratio.[6]

In summary, the A-a gradient increases with increasing F_{IO_2}, whereas the P_{aO_2}/P_{AO_2} and P_{aO_2}/F_{IO_2} ratios remain fairly constant with changes in F_{IO_2}. Because of this, the P_{aO_2}/P_{AO_2} and P_{aO_2}/F_{IO_2} ratios are more useful clinical tools to assess lung function in acutely ill patients with varying oxygen therapy requirements. **Clinical Focus 6-5** provides an example of the calculation and use of the P_{aO_2}/P_{AO_2} and P_{aO_2}/F_{IO_2} ratios.

CLINICAL FOCUS 6-5

Calculation of the P_{aO_2}/P_{AO_2} and P_{aO_2}/F_{IO_2} Ratios

1. Given a patient with the following data, calculate the P_{aO_2}/P_{AO_2} and P_{aO_2}/F_{IO_2} ratios:

   P_{aO_2} = 80 mm Hg
   F_{IO_2} = 0.21
   P_{AO_2} = 100 mm Hg
   P_{aO_2}/P_{AO_2} = 80/100 = 0.80
   P_{aO_2}/F_{IO_2} = 80/0.21 = 381

   These values are at the low range of normal for a healthy adult.

2. Given a patient with the following normal values, calculate the P_{aO_2}/P_{AO_2} and P_{aO_2}/F_{IO_2} ratios.

   P_{aO_2} = 100 mm Hg
   F_{IO_2} = 0.21
   P_{AO_2} = 110 mm Hg
   P_{aO_2}/P_{AO_2} = 100/110 = 0.91
   P_{aO_2}/F_{IO_2} = 100/0.21 = 476

   These values are at the high range of normal for a healthy, young adult.

3. Given a patient with the following data, calculate the P_{aO_2}/P_{AO_2} and P_{aO_2}/F_{IO_2} ratios:

   P_{aO_2} = 80 mm Hg
   F_{IO_2} = 0.35
   P_{AO_2} = 200 mm Hg
   P_{aO_2}/P_{AO_2} = 80/200 = 0.40
   P_{aO_2}/F_{IO_2} = 80/0.35 = 229

   These values are consistent with oxygenation problems, as may be seen with acute lung injury (ALI; P_{aO_2}/F_{IO_2} ≤ 300 but > 200).[1]

4. Given a patient with the following data, calculate the Pao_2/Pao_2 and Pao_2/Fio_2 ratios:

Pao_2 = 60 mm Hg
Fio_2 = 0.50
Pao_2 = 307 mm Hg
Pao_2/Pao_2 = 60/307 = 0.20
Pao_2/Fio_2 = 60/0.50 = 120

These values are consistent with severe oxygenation problems, as may be seen with acute respiratory distress syndrome (ARDS; $Pao_2/Fio_2 \leq 200$).[2]

[1]The traditional definition of ALI includes $Pao_2/Fio_2 \leq 300$ but > 200.
[2]The proposed Berlin definition of ARDS includes severity based on the Pao_2/Fio_2 ratio as noted here: mild ARDS, $Pao_2/Fio_2 \leq 300$ but > 200; moderate ARDS, $Pao_2/Fio_2 \leq 200$ but > 100; and severe ARDS, $Pao_2/Fio_2 \leq 100$.
Data from: ARDS Definition Task Force, Ranieri VM, Rubenfeld GD, et al. Acute respiratory distress syndrome: the Berlin Definition. *JAMA.* 2012;307(23):2526–2533. doi: 10.1001/jama.2012.5669.

Ventilation–Perfusion Relationships

Figure 6-1 illustrates the six gas-to-blood matching arrangements possible in the lung: normal, underventilation to perfusion, pure shunt, overventilation to perfusion, alveolar dead space, and the silent unit.[19–21] For the "ideal" alveolar unit, ventilation matches perfusion and the **ventilation–perfusion ratio ($\dot{V}/\dot{Q}$)** is 1.0. Normal alveolar ventilation ($\dot{V}_A$) is about 4.2 L/min, whereas perfusion of the lung is equal to the cardiac output ($\dot{Q}_T$) at about 5 L/min. The resultant overall or average lung $\dot{V}_A/\dot{Q}_T$ is:

$$\dot{V}_A/\dot{Q}_T = 4.2/5.0 = 0.84$$

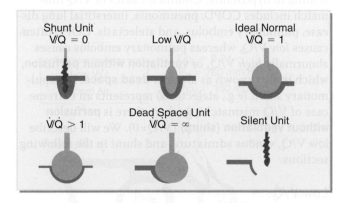

FIGURE 6-1 Ventilation perfusion relationships in health and disease. There are six possible relationships of ventilation and perfusion in the lung. Where ventilation matches perfusion, the $\dot{V}/\dot{Q}$ ratio is 1.0. Where ventilation exceeds perfusion, the $\dot{V}/\dot{Q}$ ratio is greater than 1.0. Ventilation without perfusion (aka alveolar dead space) represents an extreme case, where $\dot{V}/\dot{Q} = \dot{V}/0 = \infty$ (or undefined). With underventilation with respect to perfusion, $\dot{V}/\dot{Q}$ is less than 1.0 but greater than 0 (aka low $\dot{V}/\dot{Q}$). In cases of perfusion without ventilation (aka alveolar shunt) $\dot{V}/\dot{Q} = 0$.

Whereas the overall $\dot{V}_A/\dot{Q}_T$ in the normal lung is about 0.80, the actual $\dot{V}/\dot{Q}$ in each region of the lung varies due to regional differences in ventilation and the associated capillary blood flow. These regional differences are largely due to the effects of gravity and vary with position. **Figure 6-2** provides a description of the $\dot{V}/\dot{Q}$ values in different lung regions in an upright normal subject. Pulmonary capillary blood flow and ventilation are less in the apices of the lung than in the bases, and $\dot{V}/\dot{Q}$ tends to be greater at the apices of the lung and lower at the bases. For example, the $\dot{V}/\dot{Q}$ in the lung apices is about 3.3, whereas the $\dot{V}/\dot{Q}$ in the bases is about 0.63 (see Figure 6-2).[20,21] The $\dot{V}/\dot{Q}$ in the midportion of the lung may approach the ideal of 1.0, where there is a match between ventilation and perfusion.[20,21] In the normal lung, the inspired tidal volume tends to flow preferentially to dependent portions of the lung where there is the greatest perfusion. As illustrated in the Figure 6-2, as alveolar ventilation increases as we move from the apices to the bases in the upright lung; the differences in ventilation across the various lung regions are much less than the differences in perfusion.

Because regional differences in $\dot{V}/\dot{Q}$ are due to gravity, $\dot{V}/\dot{Q}$ will change with a patient's position. For example, a patient lying with his or her right side down will have greater perfusion of the dependent right lung. If a patient has unilateral pulmonary disease, the clinician may see oxygenation worsen when the affected side is placed down because of increased perfusion of the "bad" lung. **Figure 6-3** provides an illustration of the effects of position and exercise on the normal lung. At rest, the dependent part of the lung receives the most pulmonary capillary blood flow, as well as the larger part of the inspired tidal volume. The nondependent portions of the lung receive less pulmonary capillary blood flow, and although the nondependent

BOX 6-10

Methods of Administering Various Oxygen Concentrations

Low to Moderate Concentration of O_2 (22% to 40%)

Nasal cannula:

- 0.5 to 6 L/min will deliver approximately 22% to 40% O_2.
- Device of choice for most patients.
- Easy to use, well accepted by most patients.
- Does not interfere with eating, drinking fluids, or talking on the telephone.
- Humidification not needed at flows ≤ 4 L/min.
- FIO_2 will vary with ventilatory pattern.
- In the presence of an irregular ventilatory pattern or with rapid, shallow breathing, it will not deliver a stable FIO_2.

Air-entrainment mask:

- FIO_2 of 24%, 28%, 30%, 35%, and 40% available.
- High air flow with oxygen enrichment provides a relatively constant and stable FIO_2.
- May be the device of choice to deliver low to moderate concentrations of oxygen in the presence of a variable ventilatory pattern or rapid, shallow breathing.
- Patients may remove the mask to eat or to talk on the telephone or due to discomfort, resulting in a sudden and unwanted episode of hypoxemia.

Moderate to High Concentration of O_2 (40% to 100%)

Simple mask:

- 35% to 50% O_2 at 5 to 10 L/min.
- FIO_2 may vary with ventilatory pattern.
- Patients may remove the mask to eat or talk on the telephone or due to discomfort, resulting in a sudden and unwanted episode of hypoxemia.
- Good choice for short periods of time (e.g., emergency department) as assessment is made.

Partial rebreathing mask:

- 40% to 70% O_2 at 5 to 10 L/min.
- FIO_2 may vary with ventilatory pattern.
- Patients may remove the mask to eat or talk on the telephone or due to discomfort, resulting in a sudden and unwanted episode of hypoxemia.
- Good choice for short periods of time (e.g., emergency department) as assessment is made.

Nonrebreathing mask:

- 60% to 80% O_2 at 6 to 10 L/min.
- FIO_2 may vary with ventilatory pattern.
- Patients may remove the mask to eat or talk on the telephone or due to discomfort, resulting in a sudden and unwanted episode of hypoxemia.
- Good choice for short periods of time (e.g., emergency department) as assessment is made.

Air-entrainment nebulizers via aerosol mask, tracheostomy mask, or "T" piece:

- Provide stable oxygen concentration from 28% to 50%.
- Good choice to deliver a constant, stable FIO_2 with humidity and bland aerosol in the presence of artificial airways.
- May be heated to increase humidity output.
- Patients may remove the aerosol mask to eat or talk on the telephone or due to discomfort, resulting in a sudden and unwanted episode of hypoxemia. This is less of problem with an artificial airway (e.g., tracheostomy or endotracheal tube).

Misty-Ox High FIO_2–High Flow nebulizer:

- 60% to 96% oxygen with total gas flows of 42 to 80 L/min.
- High air flow with oxygen enrichment provides a relatively constant and stable FIO_2.

- May be effective at delivering moderate to high concentrations of oxygen in the presence of a variable ventilatory pattern or rapid, shallow breathing.
- Patients may remove the mask to eat or talk on the telephone or due to discomfort, resulting in a sudden and unwanted episode of hypoxemia.

Thera-Mist air-entrainment nebulizer:

- 36% to 96% O_2 at flows of 47 to 74 L/min.
- High air flow with oxygen enrichment provides a relatively constant and stable FIO_2
- May be effective at delivering moderate to high concentrations of oxygen in the presence of a variable ventilatory pattern or rapid, shallow breathing
- Patients may remove the mask to eat, talk on the telephone or due to discomfort, resulting in a sudden and unwanted episode of hypoxemia.

Anatomic Shunt and Venous Admixture

As noted earlier, normally there is complete equilibration of oxygen across the alveolar–capillary membrane and $PAO_2 = P_c'O_2$. If 100% of the cardiac output went to pulmonary capillaries that were normally ventilated, the resultant arterial oxygen tension would be the same as the pulmonary capillary oxygen tension. This does not occur, however, due to venous admixture.

A shunt is a circulatory path whereby oxygen-poor (venous) blood mixes with oxygenated blood, thus reducing arterial oxygen tension (PAO_2) and content (CaO_2). A right-to-left **anatomic shunt** occurs when the alveoli are bypassed as blood travels from the right side of the heart to the left side of the heart. Normally, a small amount of venous blood, the venous admixture, is carried from the bronchial veins, Thebesian veins (veins within the heart muscle), and pleural veins to the left side of the heart, where it mixes with the oxygenated blood from the pulmonary circulation (see **Box 6-11**). This normal anatomic shunt (the venous admixture) represents about 2% to 5% of the cardiac output.[20] Shunted venous blood has a low oxygen tension (normally $P\bar{v}O_2 = 40$ mm Hg), which explains why a normal arterial oxygen tension ($PaO_2 = 80$ to 100 mm Hg) is less than pulmonary capillary oxygen tension ($P_c'O_2 = 104$ mm Hg). Figure 6-4 illustrates a normal $\dot{V}/\dot{Q}$ with normal venous admixture and demonstrates why anatomic shunting causes $PaO_2 < P_c'O_2$.

BOX 6-11

Causes of Shunt

Anatomic Shunt

Normal anatomic shunt (2% to 5% of the cardiac output):

- *Bronchial veins*: The bronchial circulation nourishes the bronchial tree, and the pulmonary veins collect deoxygenated blood from the bronchi. Most of this venous blood (two-thirds to three-quarters) from the bronchial circulation empties into the pulmonary veins and is carried to the left atrium of the heart as venous admixture.
- *Thebesian veins*: Venous blood from the myocardium of the heart drains into the right atrium; however, a small amount of venous blood from the Thebesian veins drains into the left ventricle as venous admixture.
- *Pleural veins*: In addition to the oxygenated blood from the pulmonary capillaries, the pulmonary veins collect deoxygenated blood from the visceral pleura and carry it to the left atrium.

Abnormal anatomic shunt:

- Persistent fetal circulation
  - Patent ductus arterious (PDA)
  - Patent foramen ovale
- Congenital cardiac defects, such as tetralogy of Fallot and cardiac septal defects

(continues)

Capillary Shunt (intrapulmonary or physiologic shunt)

Atelectasis

Pulmonary edema (alveolar filling):

- Cardiogenic
- Noncardiogenic
  - Acute lung injury (ALI)
  - Acute respiratory distress syndrome (ARDS)
  - Neurogenic pulmonary edema
- Consolidation
  - Pneumonia
- Complete airway obstruction
- Pneumothorax

Certain pathologic conditions can cause an abnormal anatomic shunt, including persistent fetal circulation, sometimes seen in the neonate due to acute respiratory distress, and a hypoxic episode at birth, such as meconium aspiration. Certain congenital cardiovascular defects or anomalies may also cause anatomic shunting. These abnormal cardiovascular anatomic shunts can be right to left or left to right, depending on the nature of the defect; however, it is the right-to-left shunts that may cause severe hypoxemia.

Intrapulmonary Shunt

Intrapulmonary shunt (physiologic shunt or capillary shunt) occurs when venous blood is carried from the right side of the heart to the lungs (via the pulmonary arteries) to pulmonary capillaries adjacent to alveoli that are not ventilated. This oxygen-poor blood then returns, via the pulmonary veins, to the left side of the heart without participating in gas exchange. This represents an extreme case of $\dot{V}/\dot{Q}$ mismatch (perfusion without ventilation, $\dot{V}/\dot{Q} = 0.0$; see **Figure 6-6**).

Intrapulmonary shunting can cause severe hypoxemia (Figure 6-6A), and administration of high concentrations of O_2 may be ineffective in correcting this hypoxemia (Figure 6-6B). This phenomenon is known as *refractory hypoxemia*, which can be defined as a Pao_2 rise of < 5 mm Hg following an increase in $Fio_2 \geq$ 0.10. In contrast, hypoxemia in patients with low $\dot{V}/\dot{Q}$ (i.e., $\dot{V}/\dot{Q} < 1.0$ but > 0.0) is often very responsive to the administration of low to moderate concentrations of oxygen therapy. Thus, breathing 100% O_2 can be used to test for the presence of right-to-left shunt versus low $\dot{V}/\dot{Q}$ (see **Clinical Focus 6-6**). As a rough rule of thumb, with low $\dot{V}/\dot{Q}$ an increase in oxygen concentration of 1% will increase Pao_2 at least 5 mm Hg, whereas with shunt the Pao_2 will increase 1 mm Hg or less.

Causes of intrapulmonary shunting include atelectasis, consolidative pneumonia, ALI, ARDS, complete

RC Insights

Shunt Versus Low $\dot{V}/\dot{Q}$

With low $\dot{V}/\dot{Q}$, an increase in oxygen concentration of 1% will increase Pao_2 at least 5 mm Hg.

With shunt, an increase in oxygen concentration of 1% will increase Pao_2 1 mm Hg or less.

airway obstruction, and a large pneumothorax. As noted earlier, these clinical problems often do not respond well to low to moderate concentrations of oxygen administration and may require the use of CPAP or PEEP. Methods for delivering high oxygen concentrations in spontaneously breathing patients are described in Box 6-10. Box 6-11 describes the various causes of shunt.

Shunt Calculations

As illustrated in Clinical Focus 6-6, the percentage of intrapulmonary right-to-left shunt can be roughly estimated by calculating the alveolar to arterial oxygen difference [$P(A - a)o_2$] while breathing 100% oxygen:

$$\% \text{ shunt (estimated)} = \frac{P(A - a)O_2}{20}$$

However, placing a patient on 100% oxygen to estimate shunt fraction is not required when using the clinical shunt equation:

$$\dot{Q}_S / \dot{Q}_T = (C_c'O_2 - CaO_2) \div (C_c'O_2 - C\overline{v}O_2)$$

where

$\dot{Q}_S/\dot{Q}_T$ = Shunt fraction
$C_c'O_2$ = Pulmonary capillary O_2 content
CaO_2 = Arterial O_2 content
$C\overline{v}O_2$ = Mixed venous O_2 content

Alveolar Filling

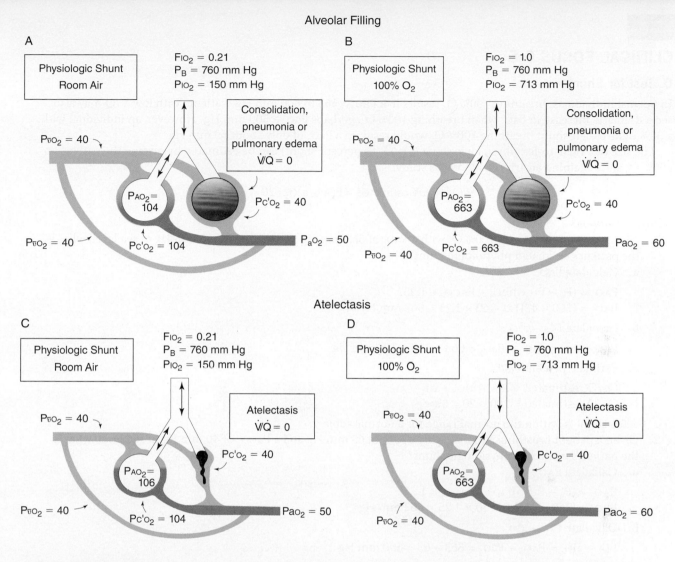

FIGURE 6-6 Matching of gas and blood with pulmonary capillary shunt ($\dot{V}/\dot{Q} = 0$). (A) The effects of alveolar filling and atelectasis on oxygenation while breathing room air ($F_{IO_2} = 0.21$). (B) With a large physiologic shunt, refractory hypoxemia is present and high concentrations of O_2 therapy may be relatively ineffective.

Clinical Focus 6-7 provides an example of the calculation of indices of oxygenation and shunt using the clinical shunt equation.

Diffusion of Oxygen

The next step in the oxygenation process is the diffusion of oxygen across the alveolar–capillary membrane and into the blood, where most of the oxygen is carried by the hemoglobin. **Box 6-12** lists the structures that oxygen must traverse as it diffuses from the alveoli into the pulmonary capillary blood and attaches to the red blood cell hemoglobin. As noted previously, under normal conditions P_{AO_2} completely equilibrates with the adjacent pulmonary capillary blood, and $P_{AO_2} = P_{c'O_2}$.

It is of interest to note that some gases are primarily perfusion limited, such as nitrous oxide, whereas others

are primarily **diffusion limited**, such as carbon monoxide.[21] Oxygen transfer is generally perfusion limited. This means that O_2 transfer across the alveolar–capillary membrane is normally only limited by the perfusion of the pulmonary capillaries. Diffusion limitation can occur during exercise, with alveolar hypoxia, or with thickening of the alveolar–capillary membrane.

With impaired diffusion, hypoxemia may occur, often only during exercise. Diffusion of oxygen from the alveoli into the adjacent pulmonary capillary can be impaired due to mismatch of ventilation and perfusion, a reduction in the available surface area for diffusion, or an increase in the diffusion distance, as may occur with thickening of the alveolar–capillary membrane or dilation of the capillary bed (e.g., hepatopulmonary syndrome). A common cause of a diffusion limitation is inflammation and fibrosis associated with interstitial

CLINICAL FOCUS 6-6

O_2 Test for Shunt

In normal individuals, breathing 100% O_2 results in a $Pao_2 > 563$ to 600 mm Hg. Patients with low $\dot{V}/\dot{Q}$ may also see a dramatic increase in Pao_2 when breathing 100% O_2, perhaps $Pao_2 \geq 500$ mm Hg. However, an individual with a 30% right-to-left shunt breathing 100% O_2 would result in a Pao_2 of only about 60 mm Hg.

The size of a right-to-left physiologic shunt ($\dot{Q}s/\dot{Q}_T$ as percent shunt) can be estimated by placing the patient on 100% O_2 and obtaining an arterial blood gas study:

$$\dot{Q}s / \dot{Q}_T \% \text{ estimated} = P(A - a)o_2 / 20$$

Sample Problems

1. Given a patient breathing 100% O_2 with a Pao_2 of 563 mm Hg and a $Paco_2$ of 40 mm Hg at sea level, what is the patient's estimated physiologic shunt?
    a. Calculate Pao_2:

    $Pao_2 = (P_B - Ph_2o)Fio_2 - Paco_2 \times 1.25$
    $Pao_2 = (760 - 47)1.0 - 40 \times 1.25 = 663$ mm Hg

    b. Calculate $P(A - a)o_2$:

    $P(A - a)o_2 = Pao_2 - Pao_2 = 663 - 563 = 100$ mm Hg

    c. Estimate percent $\dot{Q}s/\dot{Q}_T$:

    $\dot{Q}s/\dot{Q}_T$ estimated $= P(A - a)o_2 \div 20$
    $\dot{Q}s/\dot{Q}_T$ estimated $= 100 \div 20 = 5\%$

   A 5% shunt is within the normal range for a normal subject.

2. Given a patient breathing 100% O_2 with a Pao_2 of 63 mm Hg and a $Paco_2$ of 40 mm Hg at sea level, what is the patient's estimated physiologic shunt?
    a. Calculate Pao_2:

    $Pao_2 = (P_B - Ph_2o)Fio_2 - Paco_2 \times 1.25$
    $Pao_2 = (760 - 47)1.0 - 40 \times 1.25 = 663$ mm Hg

    b. Calculate $P(A - a)o_2$:

    $P(A - a)o_2 = Pao_2 - Pao_2 = 663 - 63 = 600$ mm Hg

    c. Estimate $\dot{Q}s/\dot{Q}_T$:

    $\dot{Q}s/\dot{Q}_T$ estimated $= P(A - a)o_2 \div 20$
    $\dot{Q}s/\dot{Q}_T$ estimated $= 600 \div 20 = 30\%$

   A 30% shunt is a very large shunt and represents refractory hypoxemia.

lung disease (ILD). Other causes of diffusion limitation include alveolar edema, interstitial edema, pulmonary vascular disease, and emphysema. Diffusion defects alone generally do not cause hypoxemia in most patients at rest (see discussion below). Problems that cause diffusion limitation, however, often alter lung compliance and $\dot{V}/\dot{Q}$, and it may be difficult to determine the precise cause of any resultant hypoxemia.

With ILDs, inflammation may cause the deposit of scar tissue in the interstitial space (interstitial fibrosis) between the alveolar epithelial basement membrane and the adjacent pulmonary capillary endothelium. ILDs include idiopathic pulmonary fibrosis, asbestosis, silicosis, coal workers' pneumoconiosis, and

sarcoidosis. ILDs cause restrictive lung disease, which is demonstrated by a reduction in lung volumes (total lung capacity and vital capacity).[22,23] With interstitial fibrosis, equilibration of alveolar and pulmonary capillary Po_2 may occur at rest; hypoxemia may become evident, however, during exercise.[22] During exercise with a diffusion limitation there may be inadequate time for equilibration of alveolar and capillary O_2 because of the increased rate of capillary blood flow. Hypoxemia that becomes evident (or worsens) with exercise is one finding associated with a diffusion limitation, such as may be seen with ILD.[3]

Other causes of an increased diffusion distance include fluid in the alveoli and/or interstitial space

CLINICAL FOCUS 6-7

Calculation of Indices of Oxygenation and Shunt

A 24-year-old man is in the intensive care unit following a traumatic motor vehicle accident. The following data have been collected on the patient:

P_B = 760 mm Hg

FIO_2 = 0.50

Hb = 10 grams

Pao_2 = 50 mm Hg

Sao_2 = 0.88

Cao_2 = 1.34 × Hb × SaO2 + 0.003 × Pao_2 = (1.34 × 10 × .88) + (0.003 × 50) = 11.94 vol%

$Paco_2$ = 40 mm Hg

$P\bar{v}o_2$ = 36 mm Hg

$S\bar{v}o_2$ = 0.66

$C\bar{v}o_2$ = 1.34 × Hb × $S\bar{v}o_2$ + 0.003 × $P\bar{v}o_2$ = (1.34 × 10 × 0.66) + (0.003 × 36) = 8.95 vol%

1. What is the patient's calculated $P(A − a)o_2$?

    a. Calculate PAo_2:

    $PAo_2 = (P_B − PH_2O)FIO_2 − Paco_2 × 1.25$
    $PAo_2 = (760 − 47)0.50 − 40 × 1.25 = 306.5$ mm Hg

    This is a normal PAo_2 in a patient breathing 50% O_2 at sea level.

    b. Calculate $P(A − a)o_2$:

    $P(A − a)o_2 = PAo_2 − Pao_2 = 306.5 − 50 = 256.5$ mm Hg

    A normal $P(A − a)o_2$ in a patient at sea level breathing 21% O_2 is about 10 mm Hg. It is about 100 mm Hg in a normal patient breathing 100% O_2. A normal $P(A − a)o_2$ when breathing 50% O_2 would be about 60 mm Hg; consequently, an actual $P(A − a)o_2$ of 256.5 mm Hg is much greater than would be expected and indicates abnormal gas exchange.

2. What is the patient's calculated Pao_2/PAo_2 ratio?

    $Pao_2/PAo_2 = 50/256.5 = 0.20$

    A normal Pao_2/PAo_2 ratio is about 0.80 (range of 0.77 to 0.82). A value of 0.20 is very low, probably due to a large intrapulmonary shunt.

3. What is the patient's calculated Pao_2/FIO_2 ratio?

    $Pao_2/FIO_2 = 50/0.50 = 100$

    A normal Pao_2/FIO_2 ratio is 300 to 500. A Pao_2/FIO_2 < 300 represents abnormal gas exchange, and a Pao_2/FIO_2 < 200 represents severe hypoxemia.

4. What is the patient's calculated shunt fraction $(\dot{Q}s/\dot{Q}_T)$?

    a. Estimate P_co_2 and S_co_2:

    • Assume $PAo_2 = P_co_2 = 306.5$ mm Hg
    • Estimate S_co_2 based on estimated P_co_2:
       ◦ P_co_2 of 306.5 mm Hg would achieve 100% saturation of the hemoglobin.
       ◦ $P_co_2 = 306.5 → S_co_2 = 1.0$

    b. Calculate C_co_2:

    $C_co_2 = 1.34 × Hb × S_co_2 + 0.003 × P_co_2$
    $C_co_2 = (1.34 × 10 × 1.0) + 0.003 × 306.5 = 14.32$ vol%

    c. Calculate shunt fraction:

5. $\dot{Q}s/\dot{Q}_T = (C_co_2 − Cao_2) ÷ (C_co_2 − C\bar{v}o_2)$
6. $\dot{Q}s/\dot{Q}_T = (14.32 − 11.94) ÷ (14.32 − 8.95)$
7. $\dot{Q}s/\dot{Q}_T = 0.44$, or 44%

P_B, barometric pressure; FIO_2, fractional concentration of oxygen; Hb, hemoglobin concentration (grams/100 mL blood); Pao_2, partial pressure of oxygen in the arterial blood (mm Hg); Sao_2, arterial oxygen saturation; Cao_2, arterial blood oxygen content (mL O_2 per 100 mL blood); $Paco_2$, partial pressure of carbon dioxide in the arterial blood; Pvo_2, partial pressure of oxygen in the mixed venous blood; Svo_2, mixed venous oxygen saturation; Cvo_2, mixed venous blood oxygen content (mL O_2 per 100 mL blood); $\dot{Q}s/\dot{Q}_T$, shunt fraction; C_co_2, pulmonary capillary O_2 content (mL O_2 per 100 mL blood); P_co_2, partial pressure of oxygen in the pulmonary capillary blood; $C\bar{v}o_2$, mixed venous O_2 content (volumes % or mL O_2 per 100 mL blood).

BOX 6-12

Diffusion of Oxygen from Alveoli to Pulmonary Capillary to the Hemoglobin

Normal diffusion for oxygen from the alveoli into the blood and attachment to hemoglobin (Hb) requires that the oxygen molecules cross the following structures:

1. Alveoli (requires adequate Pao_2)
2. Alveolar fluid, including surfactant (alveolar edema can impair diffusion)
3. Alveolar epithelium (thickening of the alveolar walls due to fibrosis can impair diffusion)
4. Basement membrane of alveolar epithelium
5. Interstitial space (interstitial fibrosis or interstitial edema can impair diffusion)
6. Basement membrane of capillary endothelium
7. Capillary endothelium
8. Capillary fluid
9. Red blood cell membrane
10. Red blood cell fluid
11. Hemoglobin

and pulmonary vascular disease. Interstitial and/or pulmonary edema may occur due to leaky capillaries or increased pulmonary vascular pressures. High pulmonary vascular pressures may be caused by congestive heart failure (CHF), increased pulmonary vascular resistance, or fluid overload. With damaged or leaky pulmonary capillaries, as occurs with ARDS, interstitial edema may be followed by alveolar filling (noncardiogenic pulmonary edema). Pulmonary vascular disease (e.g., pulmonary embolism) can reduce the available surface area for diffusion and result in hypoxemia, a common (but not universal) finding in patients with acute pulmonary embolus.

The presence and severity of a diffusion defect can be determined by measuring the patient's diffusion capacity for carbon monoxide (DLCO) in the pulmonary function laboratory (see Chapter 12). DLCO provides an overall measure of gas exchange and is affected by available surface area for gas diffusion, matching of ventilation and perfusion, thickness of the alveolar–capillary membrane, hemoglobin concentration, and the volume of red blood cells in the pulmonary capillaries.[23] DLCO is useful in the differential diagnosis of restrictive lung disease.[23] A reduced DLCO is often seen in patients with ILD, whereas patients with extrapulmonary causes of restriction (e.g., obesity, neuromuscular disease, or chest wall deformity) tend to have a normal DLCO.

Emphysema is an enlargement of the air spaces below the terminal bronchioles and represents a permanent anatomic change in the lung parenchyma.[15] With emphysema, there is destruction of the alveolar septal walls and obliteration of the adjacent pulmonary capillaries, which causes a reduction in the surface area available for diffusion. Emphysema also causes abnormal distribution of the inspired gases, which may result in hypoxemia due to low $\dot{V}/\dot{Q}$. A low DLCO in smokers who have reduced forced expiratory flow rates (e.g., due to obstruction) provides clear evidence of anatomic emphysema.[23] Measurement of DLCO can also be useful in COPD patients to determine if the patient has emphysema versus either asthma or "pure" chronic bronchitis (e.g., bronchitis associated with toxic gas inhalation). In patients with "pure" chronic bronchitis (no emphysema), the DLCO will be normal; however, emphysema will cause a reduction in DLCO. Most patients with COPD have a mixture of emphysema and chronic bronchitis, causing a reduction in their DLCO. Other causes of a low DLCO include anemia and decreased pulmonary blood volume, as may occur with pulmonary vascular disease (e.g., embolus, primary pulmonary hypertension, or pulmonary vascular involvement due to other conditions). A low DLCO also predicts hypoxemia and oxygen desaturation during exercise.[23] Smokers may exhibit a decreased DLCO due to an elevated carboxyhemoglobin (COHb) caused by the carbon monoxide found in cigarette smoke.[23]

Polycythemia, pulmonary hemorrhage, left-to-right intracardiac shunt, and increased pulmonary blood volume (as may occur with mild left-sided heart failure) may increase DLCO.[24] Asthma patients may have a normal or even elevated DLCO.

Hypoxemia and Diffusion Limitation

Patients with diffusion limitation often have other problems that contribute to the development of hypoxemia. During exercise, increased cardiac output and rapid pulmonary capillary blood flow may not allow adequate time for oxygenation to occur. Thus, hypoxemia that appears or worsens with exercise is a hallmark of diffusion limitation.[3] Hypoxemia due to a diffusion defect is typically reversible by the administration of low to moderate concentrations of oxygen. Treatment should include oxygen therapy to correct hypoxemia and therapy to correct the underlying cause of the diffusion limitation. Unfortunately, once interstitial fibrosis or emphysematous anatomic changes have occurred, they may not be reversible. In these cases, treatment should focus on avoidance of the causal agents and optimizing remaining lung function. Pulmonary rehabilitation may also be useful for advanced disease.[15,22] The specific management of ILD varies, depending on the cause.[22]

Blood Oxygen Content

The majority of oxygen is transported by the arterial blood from the lungs to the tissues in chemical combination with hemoglobin. The effectiveness of blood oxygen transport is dependent on the partial pressure of oxygen in the arterial blood (Pa_{O_2}), the hemoglobin level, and the percent saturation of the hemoglobin with oxygen.[25,26] Total arterial blood oxygen content (Ca_{O_2}) in mL/100 mL blood can be calculated as follows:

$$Ca_{O_2} = 1.34 \times Hb \times Sa_{O_2} + 0.003 \, Pa_{O_2}$$

where

  1.34 = The maximum amount of oxygen 1 gram of hemoglobin can carry in mL of O_2 (1.34 mL O_2 per gram of Hb)
  Hb = Hemoglobin level of the blood in grams per 100 mL of blood (reported as grams per deciliter [g/dL])
  Sa_{O_2} = Fractional percent saturation of hemoglobin
  0.003 = Bunson solubility coefficient for oxygen
  Pa_{O_2} = Arterial oxygen tension

Normal Ca_{O_2} is 19.8 mL O_2/100 mL of arterial blood, and often is reported as 19.8 volumes percent (vol%). Of this, 19.5 mL of O_2 is carried combined with the hemoglobin as oxyhemoglobin (HbO_2), and only 0.3 mL O_2 is dissolved in the plasma. **Box 6-13** provides an example of the calculation of Ca_{O_2}. The two main determinants of Ca_{O_2} are the hemoglobin and the Sa_{O_2}, which are described below.

Hemoglobin and Oxygen Content (Ca_{O_2})

The hemoglobin level in the blood can have a profound effect on total arterial blood oxygen carrying capacity and O_2 content (Ca_{O_2}). A reduced hemoglobin level will reduce Ca_{O_2}, whereas an elevated hemoglobin level will increase Ca_{O_2}. Two common conditions encountered clinically will serve to illustrate the importance of the hemoglobin level on Ca_{O_2}.

Anemia

Anemia is defined as a reduction in the number of circulating red blood cells (RBCs), the amount of hemoglobin, or the volume of packed red blood cells (i.e., hematocrit, HCT).[24] Causes of anemia include blood loss, excessive red blood cell destruction, and decreased red blood cell formation. Decreased Ca_{O_2} due to low hemoglobin or a hemoglobin dysfunction (such as seen in carbon monoxide poisoning) can cause anemic hypoxia.

Clinical Focus 6-8 illustrates the effect of low hemoglobin on Ca_{O_2}. It is important to note that anemic hypoxia can occur with a normal Pa_{O_2}, normal Sp_{O_2}, and normal Sa_{O_2}, even though the patient has other

---

BOX 6-13

Normal Arterial Oxygen Content (Ca_{O_2})

Given the following normal values, calculate the resultant Ca_{O_2}:
  Hb = 15 g/100 mL of blood (normal range is 12 to 16 g in females and 14 to 18 g in males)
  Pa_{O_2} = 100 mm Hg (normal clinical range is 80 to 100 mm Hg)
  Sa_{O_2} = 0.97 (normal range is 0.95 to 0.97)
  Normal arterial oxygen content in millimeters of oxygen per 100 milliliters of blood (aka volume %) would be:

Ca_{O_2} = 1.34 × Hb × Sa_{O_2} + 0.003 Pa_{O_2}
Ca_{O_2} = 1.34 × 15 × 0.97 + 0.003(100)
Ca_{O_2} = 19.5 mL O_2/100 mL blood + 0.3 mL O_2/100 plasma
Ca_{O_2} = 19.8 mL O_2/100 mL blood, or 19.8 vol%

CLINICAL FOCUS 6-8

Anemic Hypoxia

A male patient enters the emergency department following a gunshot wound with shortness of breath, headache, tachycardia, tachypnea, and fatigue. The patient is pale, but exhibits no cyanosis. The following data are collected:

Pao_2 = 100 mm Hg
Sao_2 = 0.97 or 97%
Hb = 5 g/100 mL (5 g/dL; about a one-third reduction from normal)

1. Calculate the patient's Cao_2:

   $Cao_2 = 1.34 \times Hb \times Sao_2 + 0.003 \times Pao_2$
   $Cao_2 = 1.34 \times 0.97 \times 5 + 0.3 = 6.5 + 0.3$
   $Cao_2 = 6.8$ mL O_2/100 mL blood, or 6.8 vol %

2. What is your interpretation of these results?

   A normal Cao_2 is 19.8 vol%; a normal Hb is about 15 g/dL. The normal Hb range is 13.5 to 16.5 g/dL in men and 12 to 15 g/dL in women. An Hb level of 5 g/dL is only about one-third of a normal Hb level of 15 g/dL and represents severe anemia. A Cao_2 of only 6.8 vol% represents severe anemic hypoxia.

3. Would review of the Pao_2 value obtained help identify the problem in this patient?

   The Pao_2 is 100 mm Hg, which is normal (clinical range is 80 to 100 mm Hg). Consequently, measurement of Pao_2 alone would not identify this patient's problem.

4. Would review of the Sao_2 indicate the presence of hypoxemia?

   The Sao_2 is 0.97, which is a normal value (normal range is about 0.95 to 0.97). Observation of Sao_2 or pulse oximetry (Spo_2) in this patient would not be helpful in identifying the cause of the hypoxia.

5. Would the patient's color indicate the presence of hypoxemia?

   Cyanosis is a distinctive blue tinge to the skin, gums, nail beds, or mucosa due to the presence of least 5 g/dL of desaturated Hb. This patient is pale, but shows no signs of cyanosis. It should be noted that the patient's Hb is only 5 g/dL. In order for cyanosis to be apparent, the patient would need a Sao_2 of zero; in other words, 5 g/dL of desaturated Hb, leaving no hemoglobin to carry oxygen. The patient would die long before he would turn blue.

6. How can the clinician identify anemic hypoxia in patients?

   This example illustrates the effect of low Hb on total blood oxygen content (Cao_2). Clinically, anemic hypoxia is detected by being alert to the clinical manifestations (signs and symptoms) of hypoxia and the laboratory measurement of red blood cell (RBC) count, Hb, and/or hematocrit. Direct measurement of Sao_2 and Hb can be achieved in the blood gas laboratory using a co-oximeter with the corresponding calculation of Cao_2.

This article was published in *Clinical Assessment in Respiratory Care*. 6th ed., Wilkins RL, Dexter JR, Heuer AJ, eds., Clinical laboratory studies, Pages 117–141, Copyright Mosby 2010.

signs and symptoms of hypoxemia. With anemia, oxygen delivery can sometimes be maintained by increased cardiac output or increased extraction of O_2 by the tissues. Clinical manifestations of anemic hypoxia include dyspnea, fatigue, increased heart rate, and increased respiratory rate.[26] Some patients may experience a full, bounding pulse, palpitations, angina, and a "roaring" in the ears due to increased cardiac output.[26] With severe anemic hypoxia, patients may become confused and lethargic, and cardiac arrhythmias and/or cardiac arrest may occur.[26] It should also be noted that cyanosis is not generally seen with anemic hypoxia. Cyanosis occurs when the concentration of deoxygenated hemoglobin in the arterial blood exceeds 5 g/dL.[27] With severe anemia, there may simply not be enough total hemoglobin present for this to occur.

Verification of anemic hypoxia requires the measurement of RBCs, hemoglobin, and/or hematocrit levels. These values are usually obtained as a part of the routine complete blood count (CBC). Although standard pulse oximeters do not measure hemoglobin, recently a new pulse oximeter has become available that measures Spo_2 and hemoglobin (Masima, Inc., Irvine, Calif.). A hemoglobin value of < 13.5 g/dL or a HCT < 41.0% in men or a hemoglobin value < 12 g/dL or a HCT < 36.0% in women is consistent with a diagnosis of anemia.[26] Generally, tissue O_2 delivery may become compromised when hemoglobin is < 8 or

TABLE 6-4
Normal Values for Red Blood Cell Count, Hemoglobin, and Hematocrit

Laboratory Test	Normal Range
RBC	
Men	$4.6–6.2 \times 10^6/mm^3$
Women	$4.2–5.4 \times 10^6/mm^3$
Hb	
Men	13.5–16.5 g/dL
Women	12.0–15.0 g/dL
HCT	
Men	40–54%
Women	38–47%

RBC, red blood cell; Hb, hemoglobin, HCT, hematocrit.
Values are affected by red blood cell mass and plasma volume. Subjects living at high altitude will have higher values. Hb values in African Americans are 0.5–1.0 g/dL lower.

9 g/dL.[26] The normal laboratory ranges for RBCs, hemoglobin, and hematocrit are listed in **Table 6-4**.

As noted above, causes of anemia include blood loss, decreased RBC production, and excessive RBC destruction. Blood loss may be due to trauma, surgery, or gastrointestinal (GI) tract bleeding. Bleeding secondary to inadequate blood clotting may be caused by drugs (e.g., aspirin or blood thinning agents, such as heparin or warfarin) or platelet disorders.[26] Decreased RBC production may be caused by a lack of nutrients (e.g., iron, B[12], or folate); iron deficiency is the most common cause of anemia. Other causes of decreased RBC production include bone marrow disorders (e.g., aplastic anemia), bone marrow suppression (as seen with chemotherapy or radiation), hormone deficiencies (such as thyroid hormone or androgens), and chronic disease with inflammation. Abnormal RBC destruction may be caused by genetic or acquired hemolytic anemias, such as sickle cell disease (which is genetic) or malaria (which is acquired).

Treatment of anemia depends on the cause. For example, oral iron supplements may be used to treat anemia due to an iron deficiency.[24] Traditionally, blood transfusion has been considered with a Hb < 10 g/dL or HCT < 30%, and transfusion probably should be given when Hb < 7 to 8 g/dL.[28] Unfortunately, transfused blood has a significantly reduced capacity to deliver oxygen to tissues. With anemia, oxygen therapy should be prescribed when symptoms of hypoxemia are present; however, O_2 administration will be of limited value until hemoglobin levels are restored.

Polycythemia

Polycythemia is defined as an abnormally high red blood cell count. Polycythemia is suspected if Hb > 16.5 g/dL or HCT > 48% in women and Hb > 18.5 g/dL or HCT > 52% in men.[29] Primary polycythemia, such as polycythemia vera, is caused by a gene mutation resulting in increased RBC production. Secondary polycythemia is often a response to chronic hypoxemia, which stimulates erythropoiesis and RBC production. The most common cause of secondary polycythemia is chronic pulmonary disease, such as COPD. Living for an extended period at high altitude or chronic exposure to carbon monoxide may also cause secondary polycythemia. Patients who smoke and those exposed to secondhand smoke may have an elevated hemoglobin and hematocrit bordering on polcythemia.[29,30]

Patients with chronic lung disease and secondary polycythemia are often able to maintain an adequate Cao_2 in the face of a low Pao_2 and low Sao_2. It is also interesting to note that patients with polycythemia tend to develop cyanosis easily, as blood viscosity increases and levels of desaturated hemoglobin rise. **Clinical Focus 6-9** provides an example of a COPD patient with polycythemia. In polycythemic patients, cyanosis can occur without profound tissue hypoxia. With severely anemic patients, however, profound hypoxia can exist without cyanosis.

Abnormal Hemoglobin

With an adequate hemoglobin level and Pao_2 and normal chemical environment, hemoglobin can carry sufficient O_2 (as HbO_2) in the arterial blood to maintain tissue oxygenation. However, several disease states or conditions can affect hemoglobin's oxygen-carrying capacity, three of which we will consider here.

Carboxyhemoglobin (HbCO) is formed by the combination of hemoglobin with carbon monoxide (CO), a colorless, odorless gas. Carbon monoxide is a natural byproduct of incomplete combustion, and exposure can occur due to use of internal combustion engines (e.g., motor vehicles or gas powered generators) in a poorly ventilated space, improperly functioning heating systems (e.g., kerosene space heaters or camping stoves), and inhalation of smoke, including tobacco smoke. Carbon monoxide has about 200 to 250 times the affinity for hemoglobin as O_2. Carbon monoxide binds very strongly to hemoglobin, reducing the HbO_2 carrying capacity. It also impairs unloading of hemoglobin at the peripheral tissues by causing a "left shift" in the HbO_2 dissociation curve (see below).

Carbon monoxide poisoning is one of the leading causes of poisoning deaths in the United States.[30] Smoke inhalation is the most common accidental cause, though cases of intentional carbon monoxide poisoning are not uncommon (e.g., suicide attempts).[31] The clinical effects of carbon monoxide poisoning

CLINICAL FOCUS 6-9

Secondary Polycythemia

A 68-year-old male with COPD presented to the clinic with chronic cough, sputum production, shortness of breath, dyspnea on exertion, and a history of cyanosis. The following data were collected:

Hb = 20 g
HCT = 60%
Pa_{O_2} = 50 mm Hg
Sa_{O_2} = 0.85
F_{IO_2} = 0.21

1. What is your interpretation of the clinical information provided?

    The patient has the clinical manifestations of COPD. A Pa_{O_2} of 50 mm Hg with an Sa_{O_2} of 0.85 while breathing room air indicates moderate hypoxemia. The Hb and HCT values are consistent with a diagnosis of polycythemia, probably secondary to chronic hypoxemia.

2. Calculate the patient's Ca_{O_2}:

    Ca_{O_2} = 1.34 × Hb × Sa_{O_2} + 0.003 × Pa_{O_2}
    Ca_{O_2} = 1.34 × 20 × 0.85 + 0.003 × 50
    Ca_{O_2} = 22.78 + 0.15 = 22.93 mL O_2/100 mL blood (often reported as vol%)

    The patient's Ca_{O_2} is 22.93 vol%, well above a normal Ca_{O_2} value of 19.8 vol%. Although the patient has a low Pa_{O_2} and Sa_{O_2}, the total oxygen content (Ca_{O_2}) is above normal due to the elevated Hb.

3. Would cyanosis develop in this patient?

    Based on the history and lab values, this patient has the potential to develop cyanosis easily. Cyanosis requires at least 5 g/dL of unsaturated Hb. Currently, the patient's Sa_{O_2} is 0.85 (or 85%), and the desaturated Hb is 0.15, or 15% (1.0 − 0.85 = 0.15). The desaturated Hb would be 3 g/dL (0.15 × 20 g/dL = 3 g/dL), which is not enough to cause cyanosis.

4. Would cyanosis develop if the patient's Pa_{O_2} and saturation (Sa_{O_2}) decline to 40 mm Hg and 0.75, respectively?

    A Sa_{O_2} of 0.75 would result in 5 g of unsaturated hemoglobin for this patient, as follows:

    Desaturated Hb = 0.25 (1.0 − 0.75 = 0.25)
    Desaturated Hb = 0.25 × 20 g/dL = 5 g/dL

    Consequently, if this patient's Sa_{O_2} drops to 0.75 (1.0 − 0.25 = 0.75), he would exhibit cyanosis, because the desaturated Hb would be 5 g/dL.

5. What would the patient's Ca_{O_2} be if the Pa_{O_2} and saturation (Sa_{O_2}) were 40 mm Hg and 0.75, respectively?

    Ca_{O_2} = 1.34 × Hb × Sa_{O_2} + 0.003 × Pa_{O_2}
    Ca_{O_2} = 1.34 × 20 × 0.75 + 0.003 × 40
    Ca_{O_2} = 20.1 + 0.12 = 20.22 vol%

    It is interesting to note that the patient would turn blue (cyanosis) even though the calculated Ca_{O_2} is above normal. Thus, patients with polycythemia may develop cyanosis, even though the Ca_{O_2} is adequate.

are dependent on how much HbCO is present and the resultant decrease in HbO_2. In nonsmokers, HbCO is generally less than 1% to 3%; however, HbCO may as high as 10% to 15% in tobacco smokers.[30] For reasons that are not clear, patients with severe COPD also may exhibit slightly elevated HbCO, even in the absence of exposure to tobacco smoke.[23,30]

Clinical manifestations of mild to moderate carbon monoxide poisoning include headache, nausea, dizziness, weakness, and discomfort.[30] An HbCO of 20% to 40% may cause moderate to severe hypoxemia with

the corresponding symptoms. HbCO of 50% may cause seizures and coma, and HbCO ≥ 60% may result in cardiopulmonary collapse and death. Suspected carbon monoxide poisoning should be confirmed by measurement of HbCO in the arterial blood using a co-oximeter. For example, if HbCO as measured by co-oximeter is 25%, the maximum possible HbO_2 would be 75% (i.e., Sa_{O_2} = 0.75; see also below).

It is important to note that measurement of oxygen saturation (Sp_{O_2}) using pulse oximetry in cases of elevated HbCO is useless and can in fact be very misleading. Conventional pulse oximeters do not detect HbCO and will give an incorrect and elevated value for SpO_2 in the presence of HbCO. It is of interest to note that a newer pulse oximeter is now available that uses eight wavelengths of light (Masima, Inc., Irvine, CA). This newer device can accurately measure HbO_2, HbCO, and methemoglobin (metHb), although false-positive and false-negative values have been reported, which suggests that confirmation by co-oximetry should be performed.[32] Also remember that PaO_2 only indicates the level of O_2 dissolved in the arterial blood, and PaO_2 may be normal or elevated with carbon monoxide poisoning (see **Clinical Focus 6-10**).

Treatment of carbon monoxide poisoning includes administration of high concentrations of oxygen and, in some cases, hyperbaric oxygen (HBO) administration. The half-life of HbCO while breathing room air is about 5 hours. This means that without treatment it will take about 5 hours for an HbCO of 20% to decline to 10%. The half-life of HbCO decreases to about 1 hour when breathing 100% O_2 and about 20 minutes at 100% O_2 at three atmospheres (ATA) of pressure administered using a hyperbaric chamber.

Patients with moderate to severe carbon monoxide poisoning should be assessed for the presence of myocardial ischemia by electrocardiogram (ECG) and

CLINICAL FOCUS 6-10

Carbon Monoxide Poisoning

A patient is admitted to the emergency department following smoke inhalation from a fire in her apartment. The patient is exhibiting signs and symptoms of moderate to severe hypoxia. She is receiving oxygen therapy via nonrebreathing mask at 10 L/min flow with a corresponding SpO_2 of 99% by pulse oximetry. The following arterial blood gas data are collected:

pH = 7.36
$PaCO_2$ = 28 mm Hg
PaO_2 = 300 mm Hg
SaO_2 = 0.68 as measured by co-oximeter
Hb = 15 g
CoHb = 0.30 as measured by co-oximeter

1. What are the clinical signs and symptoms of hypoxia?

   The clinical manifestations of moderate to severe hypoxia include tachypnea, tachycardia, hypertension, disorientation, and confusion. With severe hypoxia, tachycardia, hypertension and tachypnea may progress to bradycardia; hypotension; slowed, irregular breathing; and loss of consciousness.

2. What is your assessment of the patient's PaO_2, SaO_2, and SpO_2 values?

   The PaO_2 indicates hyperoxemia due to the administration of high concentrations of oxygen via nonrebreathing mask and indicates good oxygen transfer across the lung. The measured SaO_2 and SpO_2 are in conflict. Although the PaO_2 and SpO_2 indicate no problems with oxygenation, the clinical signs and symptoms of hypoxia are present and the SaO_2 is very low. Normally, a PaO_2 of > 200 mm Hg should result in 100% saturation of the Hb (i.e., SaO_2 = 1.0). Something must be interfering with hemoglobin function, because the SaO_2 is only 0.68 (68%) as measured by co-oximetry.

3. What is your assessment of the patient's oxygen content (CaO_2)?

   $CaO_2 = 1.34 \times Hb \times SaO_2 + 0.003 \times PaO_2$
   $CaO_2 = 1.34 \times 15 \times 0.68 + 0.003 \times 300$
   $CaO_2 = 13.7 + 0.9$
   $CaO_2 = 14.6$ mL O_2/100 mL blood, or 14.6 vol%

   The CaO_2 is very low, less than the normal value for venous blood due to the very low SaO_2. The Hb level is normal, but Hb function is impaired.

4. What is your assessment of the patient's oxygenation status?

   This patient has severe carbon monoxide poisoning as verified by measurement of carboxyhemoglobin via co-oximetry (HbCO = 0.30, or 30%). Note that the SpO_2 results are useless in assessing this patient's oxygenation status and that the PaO_2 values alone are misleading. Treatment should include high-concentration O_2 therapy, securing of the airway, and ventilatory support, if needed. Hyperbaric oxygen therapy should be considered, if available.

measurement of cardiac biomarkers if older than age 64 or in the presence of chest pain.[30] Patients with impaired mental status or coma should be intubated to secure the airway and mechanically ventilated, if needed. Patients with carbon monoxide poisoning due to smoke inhalation should also be evaluated for concurrent cyanide poisoning (see below). Generally, rapid initiation of HBO therapy should be considered when COHb > 25% to 40% and > 20% in pregnant women.[30] Loss of consciousness due to carbon monoxide poisoning in particular is associated with the development of cognitive deficits and other delayed neurologic problems seen after recovery that may persist for 12 months or longer.[30]

Methemoglobinenemia occurs when methemoglobin (metHb) is present. Methemoglobinemia can be congenital or acquired. Congenital methemoglobinemia is a relatively rare hereditary disease. Patients may be cyanotic, but are otherwise generally asymptomatic, and the disease is not life threatening. Acquired methemoglobinemia is most commonly caused by ingestion of certain drugs or chemicals. Acquired methemoglobinemia can be fatal.

Certain chemicals or oxidant drugs can cause hemoglobin to be oxidized from the ferrous (Fe^{2+}) to the ferric (Fe^{3+}) state. When this occurs, the resultant metHb cannot release its O_2 or combine with more O_2. Acquired methemoglobinemia can be caused by antibiotics such as dapsone and the sulfonamides (i.e., sulfa drugs), local anesthetics (e.g., benzocaine, lidocaine, prilocaine), and inhaled nitric oxide (NO).[33] Chemicals that may cause methemoglobinemia include nitrates, nitrobenzene, aniline and its derivatives (e.g., aniline dyes), and certain other chemical agents.[33] Symptoms of acquired methemoglobinemia include headache, fatigue, and dyspnea.[33] Respiratory depression, unconsciousness, shock, seizures, and death may occur with high levels of metHb.[33] Arterial Pao_2 may be normal with methemoglobinemia, and routine pulse oximetry for measurement of Spo_2 is inaccurate. For example, with significant methemoglobinemia, Spo_2 values plateau at about 85%. MetHb should be suspected when there is cyanosis in the presence of a normal Pao_2. The patient's blood may be brown, dark red, or blue in color.[33] Diagnosis is confirmed via co-oximetry followed by the Evelyn-Malloy method. It should be noted that co-oximetry cannot distinguish between metHb, sulfhemoglobin, and methylene blue, whereas the Evelyn-Malloy method is conclusive. MetHb levels > 20% typically cause clinical symptoms, and levels > 40% may be fatal.[32] Treatment of acquired methemoglobinenemia should include removal or discontinuation of the causal agent. Intravenous methylene blue should be administered in the presence of symptoms, although certain patients may worsen following administration of methylene blue. Ascorbic acid has also been suggested; however, it may not be effective. In cases of severe methemoglobinenemia, hyperbaric oxygen and/or exchange transfusion may be considered.[32]

Sickle cell disease is an inherited blood disorder caused by sickle cell hemoglobin (HbS). HbS is less soluble than normal adult hemoglobin (HbA) and tends to crystallize in the red blood cells, resulting in hypoxia, dehydration, or acidosis. With sickle cell disease, the RBCs become curved into a sickle or crescent shape (normal RBCs are biconcave), and an increase in deoxygenated hemoglobin tends to increase "sickling." With sickle cell disease, RBCs are fragile and may rupture, clump, and form clots.[31,34] Most of the complications of sickle cell disease are caused by microvascular occlusion by sickled RBCs or clot formation. Episodes of acute pain are the most common symptom and painful episodes are treated with analgesics, fluids, and O_2 therapy. Hydroxyurea has been shown to reduce the incidence of vaso-occlusive crises.[31,34] Infection is the most common cause of increased morbidity and mortality. Patients may have a reduced baseline Sao_2. Cardiac, hepatic, bone, cerebrovascular, and neurologic complications, including stroke, can occur.[31,34] Pulmonary complications include development of *acute chest syndrome*, which is characterized by chest pain, hypoxemia, and pulmonary infiltrates.[31,34] Clinically, acute chest syndrome is indistinguishable from bacterial pneumonia. As noted, sickling is exacerbated by hypoxemia. The development of pneumonia and pulmonary thrombosis and infarction in acute chest syndrome may lead to multiorgan failure and death.[31,34] Treatment of acute chest syndrome includes hospitalization, oxygen therapy, and antibiotics; emergent exchange transfusion should be considered.[31,34] Survival of patients with sickle cell disease has improved with proper immunizations, use of antibiotics, and comprehensive care.[31,34]

Fetal hemoglobin (HbF), similar to adult hemoglobin (HbA), contains a heme molecule and a globin molecule; however, the HbF globin molecule consists of two alpha and two gamma amino acid chains (versus two alpha and two beta chains in HbA). This results in an increased affinity for oxygen, allowing for greater oxygen saturation (Sao_2) at lower oxygen tensions (Pao_2). This is beneficial to the fetus, in that fetal Pao_2 levels are much lower than those seen in adults and children. HbF is replaced by HbA over the first year of life (see also Chapter 16).[35]

Oxygen Saturation

The hemoglobin molecule contains four heme groups, each consisting of four pyrrole rings with a ferrous iron ion (Fe^{2+}) in the center and globin, a protein.[35] Oxyhemoglobin (HbO_2) is hemoglobin combined with O_2, whereas deoxyhemoglobin (deoxyHb) does not contain O_2. Each hemoglobin molecule can combine with up to four O_2 molecules, and a single RBC contains about 280 million hemoglobin molecules. As O_2 is added to hemoglobin, the hemoglobin molecule changes shape, thus increasing its affinity for the next O_2 molecule (i.e., cooperative binding).[35] This change in shape affects the light absorption of hemoglobin and accounts for the color changes observed between HbO_2 (bright red) and deoxyHb (deep purple).[35] It also explains why spectrophotometry (e.g., oximetry) can be used to measure Sao_2 and Spo_2. Under normal circumstances, 1 gram of hemoglobin can bind with a maximum of 1.34 mL of O_2 when 100% saturated (Sao_2 = 1.0). However, this requires a Pao_2 of > 200 to 250 mm Hg, which cannot occur while breathing room air under normobaric conditions (i.e., normal barometric pressure). Normal Sao_2 is 0.975 (97.5%) at a Pao_2 of 100 mm Hg, and Sao_2 ranges from 0.95 (95%) to 0.98 (98%) when Pao_2 is in the clinical normal range of 80 to 100 mm Hg. Sao_2 is primarily determined by the Pao_2 and the chemical environment of the blood (i.e., temperature, $Paco_2$, 2,3-DPG, and pH). We will discuss each of these factors below.

Po_2 and So_2

The partial pressure of oxygen in the plasma (Po_2) is the primary determinant of the oxyhemoglobin saturation (So_2), and the effect of Po_2 on So_2 is described by the **HbO_2 dissociation curve** (see **Figure 6-7**). As illustrated by Figure 6-7, as Po_2 increases, so does So_2; however, the relationship is not linear. The sigmoid shape of the HbO_2 dissociation curve indicates that large changes in Po_2 result in small changes in So_2 when the Po_2 is > 60 mm Hg. This is known as the "flat" part of the curve and coincides with normal conditions in the lung where oxygen is "loaded" into the pulmonary capillary blood. A $Po_2 \geq 60$ mm Hg will result in an $So_2 \geq 0.90$ (90% saturation), and there is little gain in saturation with higher Po_2 values. This is physiologically beneficial in that adequate Sao_2 values are achieved within a large range of Pao_2 values. For example, people may travel and live at altitude where Pio_2 and Pao_2 are reduced and still maintain an adequate Sao_2. It also allows people to survive large decreases in Pao_2 due to cardiopulmonary disease. **Table 6-5** lists the corresponding Po_2 and So_2 values, assuming a normal HbO_2 dissociation curve.

On the "steep" part of the curve ($Po_2 < 60$ mm Hg), small changes in Po_2 result in large changes in So_2 and this facilitates unloading of the hemoglobin at the tissue level. Normal venous blood has a Pvo_2 of 40 mm Hg (range 34 to 45 mm Hg), which corresponds to an Svo_2 of 0.75 (75% saturation). Thus, the steep part of the HbO_2 dissociation curve is where "unloading" of oxygen at the peripheral tissue beds occurs, which is good for oxygen delivery to the tissues.

To summarize, on the flat part of curve ($Po_2 \geq 60$ mm Hg), large changes in Po_2 result in only small changes in So_2, and this promotes adequate loading of oxygen into the arterial blood within a wide range of

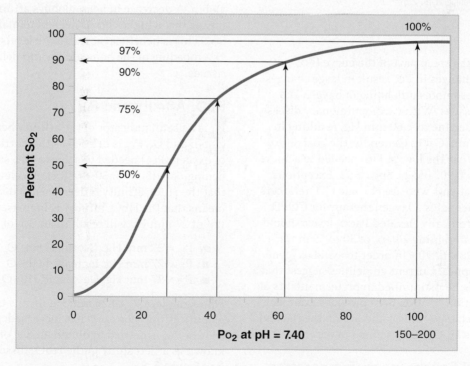

FIGURE 6-7 HbO_2 disassociation curve. Under normal conditions a Pao_2 > 60 mm Hg will result in Sao_2 > 90% and this is known as the "flat part" of the HbO_2 disassociation curve. On the flat part of the curve, large changes in Po_2 result in small changes in So_2. On the steep part of the curve (Po_2 < 60 mm Hg), small changes in Po_2 result in large changes in So_2. Key points on the curve include Pao_2 = 100 mm Hg, Sao_2 = 97% (ideal normal values); Pao_2 = 40 mm Hg, So_2 = 75% (normal values for venous blood); and Pao_2 = 27 mm Hg, So_2 = 50% (the normal value of P50). A Po_2 > 150–200 mm Hg is required to achieve So_2 = 100%. Hb, hemoglobin; So_2, oxygen saturation of the Hb; Po_2, oxygen partial pressure.

TABLE 6-5
Relationship Between Pa_{O_2} and Sa_{O_2}*

	Pa_{O_2} (mm Hg)	Sa_{O_2} (%)
Clinically acceptable values for most patients	100	98
	95	97
	90	96.9
	85	96.4
	80	95.7
	75	94.9
	70	93.8
	65	92.4
	60	90.6
Moderate hypoxemia	55	88.2
	50	85
Moderate to severe hypoxemia	45	80
	40	75

Pa_{O_2}, partial pressure of oxygen in the arterial blood; Sa_{O_2}, arterial hemoglobin saturation.
*Sa_{O_2} values are estimates and will vary depending on the blood's chemical environment (pH, Pco_2, temperature, 2,3-DPG).

Pa_{O_2} values. On the steep part of the curve ($Po_2 < 60$ mm Hg), small changes in Po_2 result in large changes in So_2, and this promotes unloading of oxygen and delivery to the tissues. With cardiopulmonary disease, Pa_{O_2} levels may decline to < 60 mm Hg, resulting in inadequate Sa_{O_2} and Ca_{O_2}. Generally, the goal of oxygen therapy is to use the lowest F_{IO_2} needed to achieve $Pa_{O_2} \geq 60$, $Sa_{O_2} \geq 0.90$, and/or $Sp_{O_2} \geq 92$. Exceptions include COPD patients who are chronic CO_2 retainers and premature neonates. Oxygen therapy for COPD patients with chronically elevated Pa_{CO_2} levels should be targeted at maintaining a Pa_{O_2} of 50 to 59 mm Hg with an Sa_{O_2} of 88% to 90% in order to avoid oxygen-induced hypercapnea. Current guidelines suggest that a $Pa_{O_2} \leq 80$ mm Hg be maintained in preterm infants of < 37 weeks gestation.[36,37] **Box 6-14** provides examples of the effects of changes in Po_2 and So_2 on the flat and steep parts of the HbO_2 dissociation curve.

The Chemical Environment: Temperature, pH, Pco_2, 2,3-DPG, and O_2 Saturation

Although Sa_{O_2} is primarily determined by the Pa_{O_2}, the chemical environment of the blood can have a marked effect on hemoglobin's affinity for oxygen,

the position of the HbO_2 dissociation curve, and the Sa_{O_2}. The major environmental factors affecting Hb–O_2 affinity and So_2 are temperature, pH, Pco_2 and **2,3-diphosphoglycerate (2,3-DPG)**. Temperature is determined by metabolic rate and may increase with activity or fever. CO_2 is a product of normal aerobic metabolism and production varies with metabolic rate. Pa_{CO_2} levels are primarily determined by the level of ventilation; hypoventilation increases Pa_{CO_2} and hyperventilation decreases it. The effect of Pco_2 on the HbO_2 dissociation curve is known as the **Bohr effect**, which states that the binding affinity of hemoglobin to O_2 is inversely related to blood acidity and CO_2 concentration. Acid-base balance and pH are determined by metabolic factors, as well as Pa_{CO_2}. Thus, acidosis (decreased pH) or alkalosis (increased pH) may be metabolic or respiratory in origin (see Chapter 8). The organic phosphate 2,3-DPG is manufactured by mature RBCs and decreases hemoglobin's affinity for oxygen. Increased 2,3-DPG may be beneficial for tissue O_2 uptake, and 2,3-DPG synthesis is increased in anemia, chronic hypoxemia, and in people living at high altitude.[35] Synthesis of 2,3-DPG also increases with vigorous exercise. Thus, temperature, pH, Pco_2, and 2,3-DPG all affect hemoglobin's affinity for oxygen.

As the affinity of hemoglobin for oxygen is increased, a lower Po_2 is needed to obtain a given O_2 saturation of the hemoglobin (So_2). This is beneficial in the lungs to facilitate oxygen loading of the hemoglobin. A decrease in hemoglobin's affinity for oxygen means that a higher Po_2 is needed to maintain a given So_2. This is beneficial at the tissue level to facilitate O_2 unloading of the hemoglobin and delivery to the tissues.

HbO_2 Affinity and P_{50}

P_{50} is a useful indicator of the affinity between hemoglobin and O_2. **P_{50}** is defined as the partial pressure of oxygen (Po_2) needed to achieve 50% saturation of hemoglobin ($So_2 = 0.50$, or 50%). An elevated P_{50} means that the HbO_2 affinity is decreased; a decreased P_{50} means that the HbO_2 affinity is increased. Normally, a Po_2 of 27 mm Hg will result in an So_2 of 0.50 (50%):

- $P_{50} = 27$ mm Hg: "Normal" Hb–O_2 affinity
- $P_{50} < 27$ mm Hg: Increased Hb–O_2 affinity
- $P_{50} > 27$ mm Hg: Decreased Hb–O_2 affinity

For example, a P_{50} of 25 mm Hg means that the hemoglobin's affinity for oxygen is increased; this means that a lower Po_2 is needed to obtain an So_2 of 50%. This is known as a "left shift" in the HbO_2 dissociation curve (see **Figure 6-8**):

- $P_{50} = 25$ mm Hg: Increased HbO_2 affinity leads to left shift
- Left shift ($P_{50} < 27$): Facilitates HbO_2 loading in the lung

BOX 6-14

Effects of Po$_2$ on So$_2$ and the HbO$_2$ Dissociation Curve

Flat Part of the Curve (Pao$_2$ > 60 mm Hg)

- Large changes in Po$_2$ result in only a small change in So$_2$.
- On the flat part of the curve, an increase in Pao$_2$ from 60 to 80 mm Hg results in an increase in Sao$_2$ from 0.90 to 0.95 (90% to 95%).
  - ↑ PaO$_2$ 20 mm Hg → ↑ SaO$_2$ 5%
- A Pao$_2$ drop from 100 to 80 mm Hg causes the Sao$_2$ to drop from 97.2% to 95.2%.
  - ↓ Pao$_2$ 20 mm Hg → ↓ Sao$_2$ 3%

The clinical goal for most patients in the hospital setting is a Pao$_2$ above 60 mm Hg, resulting in an Sao$_2$ of at least 0.90 (90%). There is a minimal gain in Sao$_2$ when increasing the Pao$_2$ significantly above 60 mm Hg; thus, most clinicians are satisfied as long as the Sao$_2$ is ≥ 0.90.

Steep Part of the Curve (Pao$_2$ < 60 mm Hg)

- Small changes in Po$_2$ result in large changes in So$_2$.
- On the steep part of the curve, a Pao$_2$ drop from 50 to 40 mm Hg results in an Sao$_2$ drop from 85% to 75%.
  - ↓ PaO$_2$ 10 mm Hg → ↓ SaO$_2$ 10%
- A Pao$_2$ increase from 50 to 60 mm Hg causes an Sao$_2$ increase from 85% to 90%.
  - ↑ Pao$_2$ 10 mm Hg → ↑ Sao$_2$ 5%

Clinically, a small drop in Pao$_2$ can cause a large drop in saturation when on the steep part of the curve, and this can result in a marked reduction in oxygen delivery. Thus, the clinical goal is generally to maintain Pao$_2$ ≥ 60 mm Hg to maintain adequate hemoglobin oxygen saturations. The exception is the COPD patient with carbon dioxide retention (high Paco$_2$). To avoid oxygen-induced hypercapnea in these patients, it is usually best to maintain the arterial Pao$_2$ values in the 50 to 60 mm Hg range.

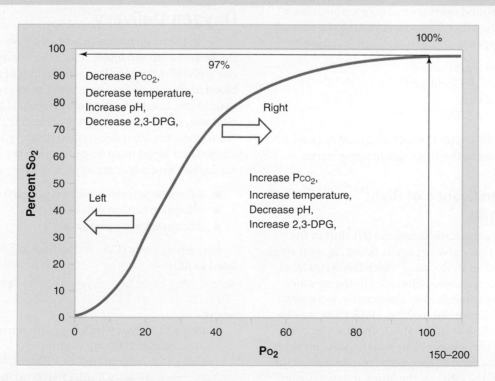

FIGURE 6-8 Right and left shifts in the HbO$_2$ disassociation curve. A decrease in Pco$_2$, decrease in temperature, increase in pH, or decrease in 2,3-DPG will shift the curve to the left. This occurs naturally as the blood enters the pulmonary capillaries and facilitates loading the hemoglobin with O$_2$ (↑HbO$_2$ affinity). An increase in Pco$_2$, increase in temperature, decrease in pH, or increase in 2,3-DPG will shift the curve to the right. This occurs naturally as the blood enters the peripheral tissue beds and facilitates unloading the hemoglobin (↓HbO$_2$ affinity) and O$_2$ delivery to the tissues. Hb, hemoglobin; So$_2$, oxygen saturation of the Hb; Po$_2$, oxygen partial pressure.

A left shift in the HbO_2 dissociation curve favors loading of oxygen into the blood in the lung. At the alveolar–capillary interface, there is a decreased metabolic rate (compared to the peripheral tissues), resulting in a lower temperature, while gas exchange lowers the carbon dioxide level. As blood travels from the right side of the heart into the pulmonary capillaries, it encounters a relatively lower temperature, decreased Pco_2, and increased pH. To summarize, a left shift in the HbO_2 dissociation curve at the lung is a normal physiologic response and is caused by:

- Decreased temperature
- Increased pH (alkalosis)
- Decreased Pco_2
- Decreased 2,3-DPG

A P_{50} of 30 mm Hg indicates that a higher than normal Po_2 is required to achieve a 50% So_2. This is known as a "right shift" in the HbO_2 dissociation curve (see Figure 6-6):

- P_{50} = 30 mm Hg: Decreased HbO_2 affinity, leading to right shift
- Right shift facilitates HbO_2 unloading of O_2 at the tissue level

A right shift in the HbO_2 dissociation curve favors unloading of oxygen from the blood at the tissue level. This corresponds with the conditions at the tissue level, where blood perfusing the tissues encounters an increased metabolic rate, relatively higher temperature, increased Pco_2, and decreased pH. To summarize, a right shift in the HbO_2 dissociation curve is a normal physiologic response at the tissues and is caused by:

- Increased temperature
- Decreased pH (acidosis)
- Increased Pco_2
- Increased 2,3-DPG

Figure 6-8 illustrates the factors that may cause a right or left shift in the HbO_2 dissociation curve.

Clinical Significance of Right and Left Shifts

A normal, physiologically beneficial left shift in the HbO_2 dissociation curve occurs as blood enters the pulmonary capillaries in the lung, which facilitates HbO_2 uptake and increases Sao_2. However, in the presence of alkalosis, hyperventilation, abnormally decreased body temperature, or reduced 2,3-DPG, there may be an abnormal left shift in the HbO_2 dissociation curve. Although this may appear to be beneficial in terms of the resultant increase in Sao_2 and CaO_2 because of the easy loading of the HbO_2 at the lungs, it may impair unloading of HbO_2 at the tissue level. Consequently, an abnormal left shift may actually be detrimental in terms of tissue oxygenation. Elevated carboxyhemoglobin or

methemoglobin can also cause a left shift in the HbO_2 dissociation curve (see discussion below).

A normal, physiologically beneficial right shift in the HbO_2 dissociation curve also occurs as oxygenated arterial blood enters the peripheral tissue capillary beds, which facilitates HbO_2 unloading and decreases So_2. An abnormal right shift, however, may make it difficult to achieve an adequate Sao_2 in the lung.

From a clinical standpoint, it is best to maintain a normal chemical environment in order maximize O_2 delivery and uptake by the tissues. Extreme right or left shifts in the HbO_2 dissociation curve are to be avoided, and the underlying causes of metabolic, acid-base, or ventilatory disorders that are causing an extreme right or left shift should be determined and treated, if appropriate. It is usually best to maintain temperature, pH, and $Paco_2$ at normal levels. Exceptions may include the use of hypothermia for certain types of complex surgery where the resultant decrease in tissue O_2 needs offset the reduction in O_2 release to the tissues due to the left shift in the HbO_2 dissociation curve. Some patients receiving mechanical ventilatory support are allowed to develop "permissive hypercapnea," resulting in a right shift in the HbO_2 dissociation curve. This may be necessary in order to avoid the lung damage that may occur because of otherwise high ventilation pressures required to maintain a normal $Paco_2$. In such cases, care is generally taken to ensure that the resultant pH does not fall below about 7.25.

Oxygen Delivery

So far in the oxygenation process we have considered the inspired oxygen levels (Pio_2), the conducting airways, alveolar oxygen (Pao_2), matching of gas and blood, diffusion of oxygen across the alveolar–capillary membrane, and O_2 loading of the arterial blood. The next step in the oxygenation process is O_2 transport to the tissues. For adequate oxygen delivery to occur, the oxygenated blood must be pumped to the systemic tissue beds. Thus, adequate oxygen delivery requires:

- Adequate arterial blood oxygen content (Cao_2)
- Adequate cardiac output ($\dot{Q}_T$)
- Adequate tissue perfusion

Oxygen delivery ($\dot{D}o_2$) to the tissues can be calculated as follows:

$$\dot{D}o_2 = Cao_2 \times \dot{Q}_T$$

where

$\dot{D}o_2$ = O_2 delivery (mL O_2/min); normal $\dot{D}o_2$ is about 1000 mL O_2/min.

Cao_2 = O_2 content (mL O_2/ 100 mL blood); normal Cao_2 is 19.8 mL O_2/100 mL blood.

$\dot{Q}_T$ = Cardiac output (mL/min); normal resting $\dot{Q}_T$ is about 5 L/min (5000 mL/min), with a range of 4 to 8 L/min.

The calculation of $\dot{D}o_2$ using normal values is shown in **Box 6-15**.

Cardiac Output

$\dot{D}o_2$ can be increased by an increase in Cao_2 or an increase in cardiac output ($\dot{Q}_T$). A decrease in Cao_2 can be overcome by an increase in $\dot{Q}_T$ in order to maintain tissue oxygen delivery. **Clinical Focus 6-11** provides an example of a patient with severe hypoxemia compensating for a low Cao_2 by increasing cardiac output. It is also important to note that even in cases where arterial oxygen levels are normal, a fall in $\dot{Q}_T$ can cause *circulatory hypoxia*. Cardiac output ($\dot{Q}_T$) is simply stroke volume (SV) multiplied by the heart rate (HR):

$$\dot{Q}_T = SV \times HR$$

Consequently, an increase in heart rate or stroke volume will increase cardiac output and vice versa. Heart rate is determined by physiologic needs, sympathetic nervous system activity, and electrical conductivity of the heart. With hypoxemia, the normal physiologic response is to increase heart rate in order to increase $\dot{Q}_T$, and tachycardia is one of the first responses to hypoxemia. Stroke volume is determined by ventricular preload, afterload, and contractility. Both stroke volume and heart rate are affected by a large number of different disease states and conditions, as well as many drugs and medications (see also Chapter 10). Common causes

of decreased cardiac output are listed in **Box 6-16**. **Clinical Focus 6-12** provides an example of how decreased cardiac output can reduce tissue oxygen delivery and cause circulatory hypoxia even though the patient's Pao_2, Sao_2, and Cao_2 are normal.

BOX 6-15

Calculation of Oxygen Delivery to the Tissues

Given the following normal values for O_2 content and cardiac output, calculate a normal O_2 delivery to the tissues.

$Cao_2 = 19.8$ mL O_2 / 100 mL blood

$\dot{Q}_T = 5$ L / min or 5000 mL / min

$\dot{D}o_2 = Cao_2 \times \dot{Q}_T$

$\dot{D}o_2 = \dfrac{O_2 \text{ content mL } O_2}{100 \text{ mL blood}} \times \dfrac{\text{Cardiac output (mL)}}{\text{min}}$

$\dot{D}o_2 = \dfrac{19.8 \text{ mL } O_2}{100 \text{ mL blood}} \times \dfrac{5000 \text{ mL}}{\text{min}}$

$Do_2 = 990$ mL O_2 / min

A normal O_2 delivery to the tissues is about 1000 mL per minute.

CLINICAL FOCUS 6-11

The Effect of Cardiac Output on Oxygen Delivery: Compensation for Hypoxemia

The following data were collected on a 38-year-old male patient with a diagnosis of acute respiratory distress:

$Fio_2 = 0.21$
$Pao_2 = 40$ mm Hg
$Sao_2 = 0.75$
$Hb = 15$ g/dL
$\dot{Q}_T = 5.0$ L/min = 5000 mL/min (normal range is 4 to 8 L/min)
$Cao_2 = 15$ mL O_2/100 mL of blood

1. Describe the patient's oxygenation status.

   The partial pressure of oxygen ($Pao_2 = 40$ mm Hg) and oxygen saturation ($Sao_2 = 0.75$) are very low, indicating severe hypoxemia. Cardiac output and hemoglobin are within normal range (though we would expect an increased heart rate and cardiac output due to the severe hypoxemia). The Cao_2 is 15 mL O_2 per 100 mL arterial blood, which is very low. To put this into perspective, a normal Cao_2 is about 20 mL O_2 per 100 mL of arterial blood, whereas normal *venous* blood oxygen content is 15 mL O_2 per 100 mL.

2. Calculate the patient's O_2 delivery ($\dot{D}o_2$).

   $\dot{D}o_2 = Cao_2 \times \dot{Q}_T$
   $\dot{D}o_2 = 15$ mL O_2/100 mL blood $\times$ 5000 mL/min
   $\dot{D}o_2 = 750$ mL O_2/min

   A normal $\dot{D}o_2$ is about 1000 mL O_2 per minute.

3. What would happen to the $\dot{D}o_2$ if the patient were able to increase his cardiac output ($\dot{Q}_T$) to 7 L/min (7000 mL/min) with no change in Cao_2?

$$\dot{D}o_2 = Cao_2 \times \dot{Q}_T$$

$$\dot{D}o_2 = 15 \text{ mL } O_2 / 100 \text{ mL blood} \times 7000 \text{ mL} / \text{min}$$

$$\dot{D}o_2 = 1050 \text{ mL } O_2 / \text{min}$$

If $\dot{Q}_T$ increases from 5 L/min to 7 L/min, O_2 delivery will increase from 750 mL/min to 1050 mL/min, which is a normal value.

This example demonstrates that it is possible to compensate for a large decrease in Cao_2 by increasing cardiac output to increase O_2 delivery.

BOX 6-16

Causes of Decreased Cardiac Output

Cardiac output ($\dot{Q}_T$) is simply stroke volume (SV) multiplied by heart rate (HR):

$$\dot{Q}_T = SV \times HR$$

- Normal $\dot{Q}_T$ is about 5 L/min (range is 4 to 8 L/min).
- Normal HR is 60 to 100 beats per minute (bpm).
- Normal SV is about 70 mL/stroke (range is 40 to 80 mL/stroke).
- Example where SV = 62.5 mL and HR = 80 bpm:

$$\dot{Q}_T = SV \times HR$$

$$\dot{Q}_T = 62.5 \text{ mL/stroke} \times 80 \text{ bpm}$$

$$\dot{Q}_T = 5000 \text{ mL/min, or } 5 \text{ L/min}$$

- HR is affected by physical activity, autonomic nervous system control, metabolic rate, temperature, drugs and medications, and disease.
  - *Bradycardia* (HR < 60 bpm) may occur due to ischemic heart disease, hypertension, myocardial infarction, inflammation, pericarditis, myocarditis, heart surgery or transplant, trauma, severe hypoxia, certain medications (e.g., antiarrhythmic drugs, cardiac glycosides, antihypertensive medications, others), excessive vagal stimulation, hypothyroidism, electrolyte imbalance, obstructive sleep apnea, hemochromatosis (iron overload), and other conditions.
  - *Sinus tachycardia* (HR > 100 bpm) may occur with exercise, fever, anxiety, pain, moderate hypoxemia, stimulant drugs (e.g., caffeine, alcohol, nicotine, epinephrine, sympathomimetics), and other sympathetic stimulation.
  - *Ventricular tachycardia* (VT) is due to extreme ventricular irritability; VT reduces stroke volume and cardiac output and should be considered life threatening.
- Stroke volume is determined by preload, afterload, and cardiac contractility.
  - *Preload* is the volume of blood in the ventricle at the end of diastole (e.g., left ventricular diastolic volume). It is primarily determined by venous return, total blood volume, intrathoracic pressures, and other factors.
  - *Afterload* is the force the ventricles must contract against. It is determined by arterial blood pressure, systemic vascular resistance (SVR), and other factors.
  - *Contractility* is the force of ventricular contraction. It is determined by sympathetic nerve activity, circulating catecholamines (e.g., epinephrine), inotropic drugs (e.g., digitalis, calcium), and other factors.

- Common causes of decreased cardiac output (decreased stroke volume and/or decreased heart rate) include:
  - Ischemic heart disease
  - Myocardial infarction
  - Cardiac arrhythmia (see Chapter 10)
  - Congestive heart failure (CHF; left ventricular failure)
  - Hypertension
  - Hypovolemia (blood or fluid loss)
  - Valvular disease
  - Cardiomyopathies
  - Late septic shock
  - Mechanical ventilatory support with PEEP

CLINICAL FOCUS 6-12

Circulatory Hypoxia

A 55-year-old female patient with a history of cardiac problems is exhibiting the clinical manifestations of hypoxia. The following data are collected:

$F_{IO_2} = 0.30$

$Pa_{O_2} = 100$ mm Hg

$Sa_{O_2} = 0.97$

$Hb = 15$

$Ca_{O_2} = 19.8$ mL O_2/100 mL of blood

BP = 60/40 mm Hg (normal range is 90 to 130/60 to 90 mm Hg)

$\dot{Q}_T = 2.5$ L/min (normal range is 4 to 8 L/min)

1. Describe the patient's oxygenation status.

   The partial pressure of oxygen ($Pa_{O_2} = 100$ mm Hg) and oxygen saturation ($Sa_{O_2} = 0.97$) are within normal range, though the patient is receiving supplemental oxygen ($F_{IO_2} = 0.30$). The Hb is also normal, and the resultant Ca_{O_2} is 19.8 mL O_2 per 100 mL arterial blood, which is also normal. Considering only the arterial blood oxygen levels, one might assume that this was corrected hypoxemia, and the patient is being adequately oxygenated. However, the patient is exhibiting the clinical manifestations of hypoxia, and her blood pressure and cardiac output are very low.

2. Calculate the patient's O_2 delivery ($\dot{D}_{O_2}$).

$$\dot{D}_{O_2} = Ca_{O_2} \times \dot{Q}_T$$

$$\dot{D}_{O_2} = 19.8 \text{ mL } O_2/100 \text{ mL blood} \times 2500 \text{ mL/min}$$

$$\dot{D}_{O_2} = 495 \text{ mL } O_2/\text{min}$$

   Normal $\dot{D}_{O_2}$ is about 1000 mL O_2 per minute; thus, this patient's $\dot{D}_{O_2}$ is only about 50% of a normal value. This patient is experiencing *circulatory hypoxia* (also known as stagnant hypoxia). Circulatory hypoxia can occur even in the presence of a normal arterial Pa_{O_2}, Sa_{O_2}, and Ca_{O_2}.

3. What would happen to the $\dot{D}_{O_2}$ if the patient were able to increase her cardiac output ($\dot{Q}_T$) to 5 L/min (5000 mL/min) with no change in Ca_{O_2}?

$$\dot{D}_{O_2} = Ca_{O_2} \times \dot{Q}_T$$

$$\dot{D}_{O_2} = 19.8 \text{ mL } O_2/100 \text{ mL blood} \times 5000 \text{ mL/min}$$

$$\dot{D}_{O_2} = 1050 \text{ mL } O_2/\text{min}$$

   If $\dot{Q}_T$ increases from 2.5 L/min to 5 L/min, O_2 delivery would increase from 495 mL/min to 990 mL/min, which is a normal value.

   This example demonstrates that $\dot{D}_{O_2}$ is dependent on an adequate cardiac output.

Blood Pressure

In addition to maintaining an adequate cardiac output, arterial blood pressure must be maintained in order to ensure tissue oxygen delivery. A normal arterial blood pressure (BP) is about 120/80 mm Hg (systolic over diastolic) with a range of 90 to 140/60 to 90 mm Hg. Pulse pressure is systolic pressure minus diastolic pressure, and mean arterial pressure (MAP) can be estimated where MAP = diastolic + 1/3 pulse pressure = 65–90 mm Hg. Blood pressure is determined primarily by stroke volume, heart rate, arterial compliance, and arterial resistance. The term **stagnant hypoxia (circulatory hypoxia)** is sometimes used to describe hypoxia due to low blood flow due to low cardiac output (pump failure) or low blood volume (hypovolemia). *Shock* can be defined as inadequate systemic tissue perfusion resulting in reduced O_2 delivery to the tissues, usually due to low blood pressure (BP < 90/60 mm Hg or a mean arterial pressure [MAP] < 65 to 70 mm Hg).[38,39] Shock causes cellular hypoxia, which may lead to cell and organ damage and death. Clinical findings in patients with shock include low blood pressure; oliguria (decreased urine output); cool, clammy skin; abnormal mental status; and metabolic acidosis.[38,39]

Types of shock include cardiogenic shock, hypovolemic shock, and distributive shock. *Cardiogenic shock* is caused by low cardiac output. *Hypovolemic shock* is caused by inadequate intravascular volume due to blood or fluid loss. *Distributive shock* (or redistributive shock) is caused by inappropriate peripheral vasodilatation resulting in decreased systemic vascular resistance (SVR) and low blood pressure. Types of distributive shock include septic shock, neurogenic shock, and anaphylactic shock. **Box 6-17** provides definitions and examples of each of these types of shock.

Treatment of shock includes aggressive fluid replacement and treatment of the underlying cause. In the case of cardiogenic shock, drugs to improve cardiac function may be administered. Mortality due to shock is high and varies with the type of shock and treatment. For example, 35% to 60% of patients with septic shock die, whereas 60% to 90% of patients with cardiogenic shock die.[39]

Uptake and Utilization of Oxygen in Tissues

The last step in the oxygenation process is the delivery of the oxygenated blood to the peripheral tissues and appropriate tissue uptake and utilization. This requires adequate perfusion of the tissues as well as adequate tissue uptake and utilization of oxygen.

BOX 6-17

Types of Shock

Anaphylactic shock: A form of distributive shock resulting in low blood pressure (< 90/60 mm Hg) due to an allergic reaction to a drug or other substance (e.g., insect stings, certain foods such as peanuts, shellfish, tree nuts, eggs, dairy products, or latex).

Cardiogenic shock: Low blood pressure (< 90/60 mm Hg) due to low cardiac output. Common causes include myocardial infarction, pericardial tamponade, cardiac arrhythmia (ventricular tachycardia, supraventricular tachycardia, ventricular fibrillation, bradycardia), and tear or rupture (myocardium, septum, valve tendons).

Hypovolemic shock: Low blood pressure (< 90/60 mm Hg) due to decreased intravascular volume. Common causes include blood loss due to trauma or internal bleeding or loss of fluids due to vomiting, diarrhea, burns, or excessive sweating.

Neurogenic shock: A form of distributive shock resulting in low blood pressure (< 90/60 mm Hg) and occasionally bradycardia. Causes include head trauma, brain injury, cervical or thoracic spinal cord injury resulting in a loss of sympathetic stimulation, vasodilation, and a decrease in peripheral vascular resistance.

Obstructive shock: A form of shock sometimes grouped with cardiogenic shock resulting in low blood pressure (< 90/60 mm Hg) due to obstruction of blood flow from the heart or major vessels. Causes include pulmonary embolus, cardiac tamponade, and narrowing of the aortic artery.

Septic shock: A form of distributive shock resulting in low blood pressure (< 90/60 mm Hg) due to decreased systemic vascular resistance as a result of an overwhelming infection. Common causes include gram-negative sepsis, although other bacteria or fungi may cause septic shock. The resulting hypotension is due to inappropriate peripheral vasodilation caused by toxins released by the offending microorganism. With early septic shock, cardiac output may be elevated; it may be depressed with late septic shock.

Peripheral Perfusion

Peripheral perfusion can be compromised by low cardiac output, low blood pressure, or blockage or disruption of blood flow to a particular tissue bed. Causes of low cardiac output and low blood pressure have been discussed briefly above and are further described in Chapters 10 and 14. Problems with perfusion of regional tissue beds can occur due to blockage (e.g., emboli, atherosclerosis), injury, infection, fibrosis, and other types of peripheral artery disease. For example, foot ulceration due to vascular disease is not uncommon in diabetics and, if untreated, may lead to amputation of the foot. Certain types of bacterial infections can cause abscess formation or soft tissue necrosis. For example, *Clostridial myonecrosis* (gas gangrene) is an anaerobic microorganism that can cause a life-threatening necrotizing muscle infection. Carotid artery stenosis (narrowing) or occlusion secondary to atherosclerosis and plaque buildup can occur and deprive the brain of blood flow and oxygen. Stroke can be classified as hemorrhagic or ischemic. Hemorrhagic stroke is characterized by bleeding in the brain.[40] Ischemic stroke may cause cerebral tissue hypoxia due to thrombosis, embolism, or systemic hypoperfusion.[40] In each of these cases where regional blood flow is disrupted, regional tissue oxygenation may be compromised.

Tissue Uptake and Utilization

The last step in the oxygenation process is tissue oxygen uptake and utilization. Adequate tissue oxygenation requires adequate O_2 delivery ($\dot{D}o_2$) and adequate regional tissue perfusion. Once the oxygenated blood is delivered to the peripheral tissues a number of things must happen. First, the hemoglobin must be unloaded. Then the O_2 must diffuse from within the RBC across the RBC membrane into the capillary plasma, across the capillary endothelium into the extracellular space, and then across the peripheral cell membrane into the intracellular space for utilization within the systemic tissue cells.

Several problems may occur in tissue uptake and utilization. First, the hemoglobin may fail to adequately release O_2. This can occur with extreme left shifts in the HbO_2 dissociation curve, such as may occur with severe alkalosis, severe hyperventilation, hypothermia, and carbon monoxide poisoning. Should an extreme left shift occur, steps should be taken to correct the cause of the abnormality. For example, in the case of extreme hyperventilation, the cause should be determined and corrected, if possible. In the case of metabolic alkalosis, any electrolyte abnormalities should be corrected (e.g., replace potassium and chloride, if needed) and any fluid volume lost due to vomiting, nasogastric suction, or diuretic therapy should be replaced.[41] For severe metabolic alkalosis, acetazolamide may be given and, in cases where acetazolamide is ineffective, an isotonic solution of hydrochloric acid (HCl) may be infused directly into a large vein (see Chapter 8).[41]

Once liberated from the hemoglobin, the O_2 must diffuse form the capillary to the peripheral tissue cells. Normally, the diffusion distance from the capillary to the tissue cells is small, and O_2 can diffuse in sufficient amounts to provide for aerobic metabolism. However, if cells are located far from the capillaries or capillary flow is reduced or absent, there may be problems in maintaining adequate diffusion of O_2 to the peripheral tissues.

Lastly, in order for oxygenation to be effective, the tissues must be able to adequately utilize the O_2 provided within the cell mitochondria as part of normal aerobic metabolism. Normally, tissue oxygen delivery ($\dot{D}o_2$) exceeds tissue oxygen requirements. Normal tissue oxygen delivery is about 1000 mL/min, whereas tissue oxygen consumption at rest is about 250 mL/min. This means that the O_2 tissue extraction rate is 25% (250 mL min/1000 mL min = 0.25 or 25%); that is, the tissues extract about 25% of the O_2 delivered to them by the arterial blood.[42] Another way to view O_2 tissue extraction is to compare arterial and mixed venous oxygen content to determine the **oxygen extraction ratio (O_2 ER):**

$$O_2\ ER = (CaO_2 - C\overline{v}o_2) \div CaO_2$$

Normal arterial oxygen content is about 20 mL O_2 per 100 mL of blood (20 vol% or 20 mL/dL); normal mixed venous O_2 content is about 15 mL of O_2 per 100 mL of blood (15 vol% or 15 mL/dL). This means that the tissues extract about 5 mL of O_2 from every 100 mL of blood delivered:

$$O_2\ ER = (CaO_2 - C\overline{v}o_2) \div CaO_2$$
$$O_2\ ER = (20\ mL/dL - 15\ mL/dL) \div 20\ mL/dL$$
$$O_2\ ER = 5\ mL/dL \div 20\ mL/dL = 0.25,\ or\ 25\%$$

The normal range for O_2 ER is 0.25 to 0.30 (25% to 30%).[42] In cases of low cardiac output or high tissue demand, the O_2 ER will increase. In extreme cases, $\dot{D}o_2$ may be inadequate to meet tissue O_2 requirements, and tissue hypoxia, anaerobic metabolism, and lactic acid production may ensue. Poor tissue perfusion is associated with an elevated arterial lactate concentration, an O_2 ER > 0.30, and a $\dot{D}o_2$ < 10 to 12 mL O_2/kg/min.[42]

Tissue Poisoning

Tissue poisoning may interfere with the ability of the cells to utilize oxygen, resulting in *histotoxic hypoxia*. One example of tissue poisoning that interferes with mitochondrial function and O_2 utilization is cyanide poisoning. Though relatively uncommon, cyanide poisoning is rapidly lethal and may cause death within minutes to hours of exposure.[43] It is a mitochondrial toxin produced in domestic fires, particularly where polyurethane (used in insulation, upholstery), other plastics, synthetic rubber, wool, or silk are burned.[43] Cyanide is used for executions in some U.S. states and has been used for intentional poisonings. Cyanide exposure can also occur due to certain industrial processes and medical treatments. Patients suffering from cyanide poisoning may experience headache, anxiety, confusion, vertigo, coma, and seizures.[43] Vomiting, abdominal pain, and renal failure may occur.[43] Some victims may describe a bitter, almond odor and complain of a metallic taste. Initial tachycardia and hypertension are followed by bradycardia and hypotension. A bright cherry-red color to the skin may be observed, and the patient's venous oxygen levels may be high because O_2 is not taken up by the tissues. Elevated plasma lactate concentration (≥ 8 to 10 mEq/L; normal range is 0.5 to 2 mEq/L) is correlated with cyanide poisoning in patients following smoke inhalation.[43]

Treatment of cyanide poisoning should include high-flow, high-concentration oxygen therapy. Intubation to secure the airway and resuscitation to maintain breathing and circulation may be required. Mouth-to-mouth resuscitation should *not* be performed in cases of suspected cyanide poisoning, and patients with skin exposure must be properly decontaminated.[43] Available antidotes are hydroxocobalamin (Cyanokit) and sodium thiosulfate and sodium nitrite (Nithiodote). Both are given intravenously. Hydroxocobalamin, routinely used in Europe, has been approved by the U.S. Food and Drug Administration (FDA) for treating known or suspected cyanide poisoning. If a diagnosis of cyanide toxicity is strongly suspected, administer hydroxocobalamin (Cyanokit) or the cyanide antidote kit without waiting for laboratory confirmation. Hydroxocobalamin combines with cyanide to form cyanocobalamin (vitamin B_{12}), which is renally cleared.

Mixed Venous Oxygen Levels and the Fick Equation

Measures of arterial blood oxygenation are summarized in **Box 6-18**. Mixed venous oxygen levels are sometimes measured in order to assess tissue oxygenation. To be of value, these measures must be obtained from a mixed venous blood sample from the pulmonary artery. This requires the placement of a pulmonary artery (Swan-Ganz) catheter. This is a relatively invasive procedure that is not without risk, but it allows for the continuous measurement of central venous pressures (CVP), pulmonary artery pressure (PAP), pulmonary capillary wedge pressure (PCWP) and provides a source for obtaining mixed venous blood for analysis. Values that may be measured using a mixed venous sample include mixed venous oxygen tension ($P\overline{v}o_2$), mixed venous saturation (Svo_2), and mixed venous oxygen content ($C\overline{v}o_2$). Normal values for mixed venous oxygen levels are listed in **Box 6-19**.

The relationships among tissue oxygen delivery, O_2 consumption, and arterial and venous oxygen content are described by the Fick equation:

$$\dot{Q}_T = \dot{V}o_2 \div (Cao_2 - C\overline{v}o_2)$$

BOX 6-18

Measures of Arterial Oxygenation

Arterial blood gas analysis and pulse oximetry are widely used to assess oxygenation. Normal values and clinically acceptable values are as follows:

Symbol	Description	Normal Value	Clinically Acceptable Values
Pao_2	Arterial O_2 tension	80–100 mm Hg	60–100 mm Hg
Sao_2	Arterial O_2 saturation	95–99%	$\geq 90\%$
Spo_2	O_2 saturation by pulse oximetry	95–99%	≥ 90–92%
Cao_2	Arterial O_2 content	20 vol%[1]	Men: ≥ 16.5 vol%[2] Women: ≥ 14.7 vol%

[1]Vol% = mL O_2/100 mL blood = mL O_2/dL
[2]Acceptable values are based on $Pao_2 \geq 60$ mm Hg, $Sao_2 \geq 0.90$, and a minimum normal Hb level (≥ 13.5 g/dL in men and ≥ 12 g/dL in women).

BOX 6-19

Mixed Venous Oxygen

A mixed venous blood sample is obtained from a pulmonary artery (Swan-Ganz) catheter. It contains venous blood that has been returned to the right side of the heart via the superior and inferior vena cava. A blood sample may be drawn from the distal port of the pulmonary artery catheter and analyzed to determine oxygen levels. Continuous measurement of mixed venous oxygen saturation is possible (e.g., fiber-optic Swan-Ganz catheter). Normal values, as well as clinically acceptable values, are as follows:

Symbol	Description	Normal Value	Clinically Acceptable Values
$P\bar{v}o_2$	Mixed venous O_2 partial pressure	40 mm Hg (range 35–40 mm Hg)	> 30 mm Hg
$S\bar{v}o_2$	Mixed venous Hb saturation	75% (range 70–75%)	> 65–70%
$C\bar{v}o_2$	Mixed venous O_2 content	15 mL/dL	> 10.0 mL/dL
$Cao_2 - C\bar{v}o_2$	Arterial–venous O_2 content difference	5 mL/dL (range 3.5–5.0)	< 7.0 mL/dL

Key Points

$P\bar{v}o_2$
- May decrease with:
  - Decreased cardiac output
  - Increased tissue O_2 consumption (increased activity)
- May increase with:
  - Increased cardiac output
  - Decreased tissue O_2 consumption (decreased activity)

  - Hyperthermia
  - Arterial hypoxemia

  - Skeletal muscle relaxation
  - Hypothermia
  - Cyanide poisoning

$S\bar{v}o_2$ and $C\bar{v}o_2$
- Changes generally follow changes in $P\bar{v}o_2$
- May decrease with:
  - Decreased cardiac output
  - Increased tissue O_2 consumption
- May increase with:
  - Increased cardiac output
  - Skeletal muscle relaxation

  - Hyperthermia
  - Arterial hypoxemia

  - Cyanide
  - Hypothermia

$Cao_2 - C\bar{v}o_2$
- May increase with:
  - Decrease in cardiac output
  - Increase in tissue O_2 consumption
  - Arterial hypoxemia
  - Exercise
- May decrease with:
  - Increase in cardiac output
  - Skeletal muscle relaxation (drugs)
  - Peripheral shunt

  - Seizures
  - Shivering in postop
  - Hyperthermia

  - Cyanide
  - Hypothermia

where
$\dot{Q}_T$ = Cardiac output in mL/min (normal is 5 L/min or 5000 mL/min)
$\dot{V}o_2$ = O_2 consumption in mL/min (normal is 250 mL/min)

Cao_2 = Arterial oxygen content in mL O_2/dL blood (normal is 20 mL O_2/dL and 1 dL = 100 mL)
$C\bar{v}o_2$ = Mixed venous oxygen content in mL O_2/dL blood (normal is 15 mL O_2/dL and 1 dL = 100 mL)

Placing normal values into the equation, we have:

$$\dot{Q}_T = \dot{V}O_2 \div (CaO_2 - C\overline{v}O_2)$$

$$\dot{Q}_T = 250 \text{ mL } O_2/\text{min} \div (20 \text{ mL}/\text{dL} - 15 \text{ mL}/\text{dL})$$

$$\dot{Q}_T = 250 \text{ mL } O_2/\text{min} \div (5 \text{ mL}/\text{dL})$$

$$\dot{Q}_T = 250 \text{ mL } O_2/\text{min} \div (5 \text{ mL}/100 \text{ mL})$$

$$= (250 \times 100) \div 5 = 5000 \text{ mL}/\text{min}$$

The Fick equation indicates that if cardiac output ($\dot{Q}_T$) and arterial oxygen content (CaO_2) are constant, then tissue utilization of O_2 is reflected by changes in mixed venous oxygen tension ($C\overline{v}O_2$). Specifically, an increase in $\dot{V}O_2$ will result in a decrease in $C\overline{v}O_2$ and a decrease in $\dot{V}O_2$ will result in an increase in an increase in $C\overline{v}O_2$ (assuming $\dot{Q}_T$ and CaO_2 are constant). Factors that increase $\dot{V}O_2$ include exercise, increased activity, increased temperature (e.g., fever or hyperthermia), stress, shivering, seizures, and hyperdynamic states (e.g., burns or trauma). Things that decrease $\dot{V}O_2$ include decreased levels of activity, skeletal muscle relaxation (e.g. sleep, sedation, and relaxation), hypothermia, increased peripheral shunt (e.g., sepsis, trauma) and certain poisons (e.g., cyanide)

If $\dot{V}O_2$ and CaO_2 are constant, $C\overline{v}O_2$ varies with changes in $\dot{Q}_T$. **Box 6-20** describes the relationships among $\dot{Q}_T$, $\dot{V}O_2$, CaO_2, and $C\overline{v}O_2$.

Overall Assessment of Oxygenation

Assessment of patients' oxygenation status should include obtaining a history and physical examination in order to identify the clinical manifestations (signs and symptoms) of hypoxia, review appropriate laboratory studies, and assess the possible causes of any oxygenation problems identified. Hypoxic patients may exhibit anxiety, excitement, restlessness, impaired judgment, and disorientation or confusion. Patients may complain of dizziness, headache, and/or blurred vision. Respiratory manifestations of hypoxia include dyspnea, tachypnea, hyperventilation, and use of accessory muscles. Cardiovascular manifestations of hypoxia include tachycardia, increased blood pressure, and cardiac dysrhythmias. Clinical manifestations of severe hypoxia may include slowed, irregular respirations; bradycardia; hypotension; loss of consciousness; somnolence; convulsions; and coma. Severe hypoxia can result in respiratory and/or cardiac arrest.

Laboratory studies should include routine use of pulse oximetry to measure SpO_2 and arterial blood analysis in cases where hypoxia may be moderate to severe or where there are questions about the patient's ventilatory or acid-base status. Hypoxemia may be classified based on measured PaO_2, SpO_2, and/or SaO_2 as mild, moderate, or severe, though classification systems vary. When reviewing oximetry or blood gas results, the clinician should always take into account the patient's inspired oxygen concentration (FIO_2); the PaO_2/FIO_2 ratio can be helpful in assessing the severity of hypoxemia present. Co-oximetry should be performed to assess for the presence of abnormal hemoglobin (e.g., HbCO or metHb), and many blood gas laboratories routinely perform co-oximetry as a part of routine arterial blood gas analysis. The most common cause of lactate acidosis in the acute care setting is tissue hypoxia, often due to tissue hypoperfusion. Normal

---

BOX 6-20

Flick Equation and O_2 Delivery and Utilization

The Fick equation describes the relationships among cardiac output ($\dot{Q}_T$), O_2 consumption ($\dot{V}O_2$), arterial oxygen content (CaO_2), and mixed venous oxygen content ($C\overline{v}O_2$):

$$\dot{Q}_T = \dot{V}O_2 \div (CaO_2 - C\overline{v}O_2)$$

The Fick equation establishes the following relationships:
- If $\dot{Q}_T$ is constant:
  - Then an increase in $\dot{V}O_2$ will cause an increase in $CaO_2 - C\overline{v}O_2$ and a decrease in $C\overline{v}O_2$ (assuming no change in CaO_2).
  - Then a decrease in $\dot{V}O_2$ will cause a decrease in $CaO_2 - C\overline{v}O_2$ and an increase in $C\overline{v}O_2$ (assuming no change in CaO_2).
- If $\dot{V}O_2$ is constant:
  - Then an increase in $\dot{Q}_T$ will cause a decrease in $CaO_2 - C\overline{v}O_2$ and an increase in $C\overline{v}O_2$.
  - Then a decrease in $\dot{Q}_T$ will cause an increase in $CaO_2 - C\overline{v}O_2$ and a decrease in $C\overline{v}O_2$.

Clinically, a decrease $C\overline{v}O_2$ or an increase in ($CaO_2 - C\overline{v}O_2$) with a constant $\dot{V}O_2$ is usually associated with a decrease in $\dot{Q}_T$.

plasma lactate concentration is 0.5 to 1.5 mEq/L; > 4 to 5 mEq/L is considered a lactic acidosis.

The primary causes of low arterial blood O_2 levels (hypoxemia) are hypoventilation, $\dot{V}/\dot{Q}$ mismatch, right-to-left shunt, diffusion limitations, and reduced inspired oxygen tension (decreased P_{IO_2}). Common causes of hypoventilation include CNS depression, obesity hypoventilation syndrome (OHS), impaired neuromuscular function, and chest wall abnormalities, such as flail chest or kyphoscoliosis.[3] Causes of $\dot{V}/\dot{Q}$ mismatch include underventilation with respect to perfusion caused by obstructive lung disease (e.g., asthma, emphysema, chronic bronchitis, COPD) and interstitial lung disease. Right-to-left shunt may be caused by atelectasis, pneumonia, pulmonary edema, ALI, and ARDS.[3] Anatomic right-to-left shunts may be caused by congenital cardiovascular anomalies and other abnormal arteriovenous abnormalities.[3] Pulmonary embolus (PE) may cause ventilation without perfusion (increased dead space) that often, but not always, results in hypoxemia. Pulmonary emboli may also induce bronchospasm and atelectasis. With PE, atelectasis is the most common chest x-ray finding, and platelets induce transient bronchospasm. Diffusion limitations may be caused by interstitial lung disease; however, oxygenation problems due to a diffusion limitation often only become apparent with exercise or at altitude. Reduced inspired oxygen tension can occur with altitude, aviation accidents (e.g., loss of cabin pressure), and confinement in enclosed spaces with inadequate ventilation and exposure to asphyxiant gases. Measures of adequate gas exchange in the lung include P_{aO_2}, Sp_{O_2}, Sa_{O_2}, A-a oxygen gradient, P_{aO_2}/F_{IO_2} ratio, and A-a ratio.

Oxygenation further requires adequate blood oxygen content (Ca_{O_2}), and this is dependent on P_{aO_2}, Sa_{O_2}, Hb level, and Hb function. There must be a sufficient P_{aO_2} to achieve an adequate Sa_{O_2}. Generally, a P_{aO_2} > 60 mm Hg results in a Sa_{O_2} > 0.90 (or 90%) and is on the "flat part" of the HbO_2 dissociation curve, where large changes in P_{aO_2} result in relatively small changes in Sa_{O_2}. A P_{aO_2} < 60 generally should be avoided as it results in an Sa_{O_2} < 0.90 (or 90%) and is on the "steep part" of the HbO_2 dissociation curve where small change in P_{aO_2} can result in large change in Sa_{O_2}. The chemical environment of the blood (temperature, Pa_{CO_2}, pH, 2,3-DPG) should be such that there are not wide shifts (left or right) in the HbO_2 dissociation curve. The hemoglobin level must be sufficient to carry an adequate amount of oxygen to the tissues, and abnormal or dysfunctional hemoglobin must be recognized (e.g., HbCO, metHb). Problems that may occur with Ca_{O_2} include low P_{aO_2}, low Sa_{O_2}, and low or dysfunctional hemoglobin.

Next, there must be adequate O_2 transport and delivery to the tissues, which requires adequate Ca_{O_2} and adequate cardiac output ($\dot{Q}_T$). Ca_{O_2} may be low due to any of the problems suggested above. Problems with cardiac output include CHF, ischemic heart disease, myocardial infarction, cardiac arrhythmia, cardiac valve disease, hypovolemia, shock, other cardiac myopathy, and ventilation with positive pressure and PEEP.

Lastly, there must be adequate peripheral tissue perfusion and oxygen uptake and utilization by the peripheral tissue cells. Problems that may occur include inadequate perfusion due to hypotension, peripheral vascular disease, blockage, increased diffusion distance, and tissue poisoning (e.g., cyanide). Additional measures that may be useful to assess tissue oxygen utilization include measurement of plasma lactate concentration, mixed venous oxygen content ($C\overline{v}_{O_2}$), calculation of the difference between Ca_{O_2} and $C\overline{v}_{O_2}$, and determination of the O_2 extraction ratio (O_2 ER). Poor tissue perfusion is associated with an elevated plasma lactate concentration (> 4 to 5 mEq/L), an O_2 ER > 0.30, and a $\dot{D}_{O_2}$ < 10 to 12 mL O_2/kg/min.[42] The most common cause of a lactic acidosis is tissue hypoxia.

In summary, the oxygenation process begins with inspired oxygen and moves to the conducting airways, matching of gas and blood in the lung, diffusion of oxygen across the alveolar–capillary membrane, and loading of the hemoglobin in the arterial blood. The oxygen-laden blood must then be delivered to tissues, and tissue uptake and utilization must be adequate. Problems with the oxygenation process that should be assessed include:

- Reduced P_{IO_2} due to altitude or other forms of ambient hypoxia
- Reduced P_{aO_2} due to problems with the conducting airways
- Hypoventilation resulting in decreased P_{aO_2}
- Problems with matching of gas and blood (low $\dot{V}/\dot{Q}$, shunt)
- Diffusion limitation
- Inadequate arterial blood oxygen content (Ca_{O_2})
  - Decreased P_{aO_2}
  - Decreased Sa_{O_2}
  - Decreased hemoglobin (anemia, blood loss)
  - Abnormal hemoglobin (COHb, metHb, other)
- Decreased O_2 transport
  - Decreased Ca_{O_2}
  - Decreased cardiac output
- Reduced peripheral perfusion
  - Decreased blood pressure
  - Decreased or blocked blood flow
- Impaired tissue uptake and utilization

Treatment

When hypoxemia and/or hypoxia are suspected or confirmed, oxygen therapy should be initiated. As noted above, common causes of hypoxemia are reduced inspired and alveolar O_2 tensions, hypoventilation, ventilation-perfusion mismatch, right-to-left shunt, and diffusion limitations. Common causes of reduced O_2 transport include decreased Sao_2, reduced or dysfunctional hemoglobin, and reduced cardiac output. Reduced blood flow to the tissues can be due to low blood pressure or poor perfusion. **Table 6-6** provides a summary of the assessment of oxygenation in patients.

Specific indications for O_2 therapy are documented or suspected hypoxemia, severe trauma, acute myocardial infarction (MI), and immediate postop recovery. O_2 therapy is also indicated to support the patient with chronic lung disease during exercise and to prevent or treat

right-side CHF (cor pulmonale) due to chronic pulmonary hypertension. A Pao_2 < 60 mm Hg and/or an Spo_2 < 90% to 92% are considered clear indications for oxygen therapy in most patients. Exceptions include patients with chronic CO_2 retention and the premature neonate.

With the exception of patients with chronic CO_2 retention and premature infants, O_2 therapy is generally titrated to achieve a Pao_2 of 60 to 100 mm Hg with an Spo_2 of 92% to 98% using the lowest concentration of oxygen possible.

TABLE 6-6
Assessment of Oxygenation

In order to perform a compete assessment of the patient's oxygenation status, the respiratory care clinician should review each for the following:

1. Are there clinical signs and symptoms of hypoxia/hypoxemia? (Check all that apply.)
   - ☐ Increased heart rate
   - ☐ Increased respiratory rate
   - ☐ Increased blood pressure
   - ☐ Shortness of breath
   - ☐ Excitement
   - ☐ Overconfidence
   - ☐ Restlessness
   - ☐ Anxiety
   - ☐ Nausea
   - ☐ Headache
   - ☐ Respiratory distress
   - ☐ Paleness
   - ☐ Cyanosis (variable finding)
   - ☐ Impaired judgment
   - ☐ Slowed reaction time
   - ☐ Confusion
   - ☐ Disorientation
   - ☐ Listless/lethargy
   - ☐ Somnolence
   - ☐ Blurred vision
   - ☐ Loss of coordination
   - ☐ Tunnel vision
   - ☐ Arrhythmias
   - ☐ Bradycardia
   - ☐ Hypotension
   - ☐ Slowed, irregular breathing
   - ☐ Loss of consciousness
   - ☐ Coma
   - ☐ Cardiac or respiratory arrest
   - Comments: _____

2. Are pulse oximetry values reduced (Spo_2 < 92)? Spo_2 = _____
   - ☐ Spo_2 < 92% may indicate hypoxemia[1]
   - ☐ Spo_2 < 90% is consistent with a Pao_2 < 60 mm Hg
   - ☐ Spo_2 < 85% is consistent with a Pao_2 < 50 mm Hg
   - ☐ Spo_2 < 80% is consistent with a Pao_2 < 45 mm Hg
   - ☐ Spo_2 < 75% is consistent with a Pao_2 < 40 mm Hg
   - Comments: _____

3. Is the patient receiving supplemental oxygen?   ☐ Yes   ☐ No
   - Device: _____   Liter flow or Fio_2: _____
   - For mechanical ventilatory support, list ventilator settings:
   - Mode: _____   Rate: _____   Tidal volume: _____ Fio_2: _____
   - Comments: _____

TABLE 6-6
Assessment of Oxygenation (*continued*)

4. Has an arterial blood gas been obtained?   ❑ Yes   ❑ No
   If yes, list results:
   F_{IO_2}: _____
   Pa_{O_2}: _____
   Sa_{O_2}: _____
   Hb (if known): _____
   Ca_{O_2}: _____
   CoHb (if measured): _____
   MetHb (if measured): _____
   pH: _____
   Pa_{CO_2}: _____
   HCO_3: _____
   Base excess (B.E.) _____
   or deficit (B.D.)
   Comments: _____

   Degree of hypoxemia is sometimes categorized based on Pa_{O_2}, where:
   ❑ $Pa_{O_2} > 100$ mm Hg: Hyperoxemia, generally due to supplemental O_2 administration (or, in some cases, hyperventilation).
   ❑ $Pa_{O_2} = 80$ to 100 mm Hg: Normal or corrected hypoxemia if the patient is receiving supplemental O_2.
   ❑ $Pa_{O_2} < 80$ mm Hg but ≥ 60 mm Hg: Mild hypoxemia (generally corresponds to an $Sa_{O_2} < 0.95$ but ≥ 0.90).
   ❑ $Pa_{O_2} < 60$ mm Hg but ≥ 50 mm Hg: Moderate hypoxemia (generally corresponds to an $Sa_{O_2} < 0.90$ but ≥ 0.85).
   ❑ $Pa_{O_2} < 50$ mm Hg but ≥ 40 mm Hg: Moderately severe hypoxemia (generally corresponds to an $Sa_{O_2} < 0.85$ but ≥ 0.75.
   ❑ $Pa_{O_2} < 40$ mm Hg: Very severe hypoxemia (generally corresponds to an $Sa_{O_2} < 0.75$).
   Comments: _____

5. Is Ca_{O_2} reduced? ❑ Yes   ❑ No Ca_{O_2}: _____
   $Ca_{O_2} = 1.34 \times Hb \times Sa_{O_2} + 0.003\ Pa_{O_2}$
   ❑ Normal Ca_{O_2} is approximately 20 mL O_2/dL of blood (20 vol%).
   ❑ $Ca_{O_2} < 18$ mL O_2/dL is equivalent to a $Pa_{O_2} < 60$ mm Hg and $Sa_{O_2} < 0.90$ with a Hb = 15 g/dL.
   ❑ $Ca_{O_2} < 15$ mL O_2/dL is equivalent to a $Pa_{O_2} < 40$ mm Hg and an $Sa_{O_2} < 0.75$ with Hb = 15 g/dL.
   Comments: _____

6. If hypoxemia (low arterial blood O_2 levels) or hypoxia (tissue hypoxia) are suspected or confirmed, determine the source of the oxygenation problem.
   a. Is inspired oxygen (P_{IO_2}) adequate? ❑ Yes   ❑ No
      Possible problems: Altitude, confined space, inhalation of asphyxiant gases.
      Comments: _____

   b. Are conducting airways functioning properly? ❑ Yes   ❑ No
      Possible problems: Upper airway obstruction, lower airway obstruction (inflammation, mucosal edema, bronchospasm, secretions).
      Comments: _____

   c. Is alveolar ventilation adequate? ❑ Yes   ❑ No
      Possible problems: Hypoventilation ($Pa_{CO_2} > 45$ mm Hg), hyperventilation ($Pa_{CO_2} < 35$ mm Hg).
      Comments: _____

   d. Is matching of gas and blood adequate? ❑ Yes   ❑ No
      Possible problems: Low $\dot{V}/\dot{Q}$ right-to-left shunt, increased dead space.
      Comments: _____

   e. Is O_2 diffusion adequate? ❑ Yes   ❑ No
      Possible problems: Increased diffusion distance (interstitial lung disease, fibrosis, alveolar or interstitial edema, pulmonary vascular disease), decreased surface area (e.g., emphysema). Diffusion problems generally do not cause hypoxemia in patients at rest. Diffusion problems may become apparent with exercise or at altitude.
      Comments: _____

   f. Are arterial blood oxygen content levels adequate? ❑ Yes   ❑ No
      Possible problems: Decreased Pa_{O_2}, Sa_{O_2}, Hb, or Ca_{O_2}; abnormal hemoglobin.
      Comments: _____

   g. Is oxygen delivery ($\dot{D}_{O_2}$) adequate?
      Possible problems: Decreased Ca_{O_2}, cardiac output, or blood pressure.
      Comments: _____

   h. Is tissue oxygen uptake and utilization adequate? ❑ Yes   ❑ No
      Possible problems: Strong HbO_2 attachment (left shift), poor or absent peripheral perfusion (blockage, vascular disease, low perfusion pressure, low blood pressure), or tissue poisoning (e.g., cyanide).
      Comments: _____

(continues)

TABLE 6-6
Assessment of Oxygenation (*continued*)

7. Are other indices of oxygenation reduced?   ❏ Yes   ❏ No
   a. $Pa_{O_2}/F_{I_{O_2}}$ ratio: _____
      For severity of ARDS (PEEP ≤ 5 cm H_2O; increased $F_{I_{O_2}}$):
      ❏ $Pa_{O_2}/F_{I_{O_2}}$ ≥ 300 mm Hg but < 500 mm Hg: Normal
      ❏ $Pa_{O_2}/F_{I_{O_2}}$ ≤ 300 mm Hg but > 200 mm Hg: Mild
      ❏ $Pa_{O_2}/F_{I_{O_2}}$ ≤ 200 mm Hg but > 100 mm Hg: Moderate
      ❏ $Pa_{O_2}/F_{I_{O_2}}$ ≤ 100 mm Hg: Severe
      Comments: _____

   b. $P(A - a)_{O_2}$ = _____
      ❏ $F_{I_{O_2}}$ = 0.21; $P(A - a)_{O_2}$ = 5 to 15 mm Hg: Normal
      ❏ $F_{I_{O_2}}$ = 1.0; $P(A - a)_{O_2}$ = 40 to 100 mm Hg: Normal
      $P(A - a)_{O_2}$ ÷ 20 when breathing 100% O_2 ($F_{I_{O_2}}$ = 1.0) provides a rough estimate of right to left shunt. For example, if $P(A - a)_{O_2}$ =
      100 mm Hg; and $F_{I_{O_2}}$ = 1.0, then the approximate shunt would be 5%: $P(A - a)_{O_2}$ ÷ 20 = 100 ÷ 20 = 5%
      Comments: _____

   c. $Pa_{O_2}/P_{A_{O_2}}$ ratio: _____
      Normal $Pa_{O_2}/P_{A_{O_2}}$ = 0.77 to 0.82 mm Hg
      Comments: _____

   d. Shunt fraction ($\dot{Q}s/\dot{Q}_T$) = _____

      $$\dot{Q}_S/\dot{Q}_T = (Cc'_{O_2} - Ca_{O_2}) \div (Cc'_{O_2} - C\bar{v}_{O_2})$$

      Normal $\dot{Q}_s/\dot{Q}_T$ is 0.02 to 0.05 (2% to 5%) (< 15% to 20% may be acceptable).
      Comments: _____

   e. O_2 delivery ($\dot{D}_{O_2}$) = _____ mL O_2/dL blood

      $$\dot{D}_{O_2} = Ca_{O_2} \times \dot{Q}_T$$

      Normal $\dot{D}_{O_2}$ = 1000 mL O_2/dL
      Comments: _____

   f. Mixed venous oxygen levels (if available):
      $P\bar{v}_{O_2}$ = _____
      $S\bar{v}_{O_2}$ = _____
      $C\bar{v}_{O_2}$ = _____
      Normal $P\bar{v}_{O_2}$ = 35 to 40 mm Hg (> 30 mm Hg may be acceptable).
      Normal $S\bar{v}_{O_2}$ = 0.75 (> 0.65 may be acceptable).
      Normal $C\bar{v}_{O_2}$ = 15 mL O_2/dL (> 10 mL/dL may be acceptable).
      Comments: _____

   g. Arterial-venous oxygen content difference ($Ca_{O_2} - C\bar{v}_{O_2}$): _____
      Normal $Ca_{O_2} - Cv_{O_2}$ = 5 mL O_2/dL (5 vol%)
      Comments: _____

   h. Oxygen extraction ratio (O_2 ER) = _____

      $$O_2 \, ER = (Ca_{O_2} - C\bar{v}_{O_2}) \div Ca_{O_2}$$

      Normal O_2 ER = 0.25, or 25%
      Comments: _____

8. Overall assessment of oxygenation:
   a. Clinical manifestations (signs and symptoms) of hypoxemia/hypoxia present?
      ❏ Yes   ❏ No
      If yes, indicate severity.
      ❏ Mild   ❏ Moderate   ❏ Severe
      Comments: _____

   b. Hypoxemia present?   ❏ Yes   ❏ No
      If yes, indicate severity.
      ❏ Mild   ❏ Moderate   ❏ Moderately severe   ❏ Very severe
      Comments: _____

   c. Cause of hypoxemia (check all that apply):
      ❏ Hypoventilation
      ❏ $\dot{V}/\dot{Q}$ mismatch
      ❏ Right-to-left shunt (↑ $\dot{Q}_S/\dot{Q}_T$)
      ❏ Diffusion limitation
      ❏ Reduced inspired oxygen tension ($P_{I_{O_2}}$)
      Comments: _____

TABLE 6-6
Assessment of Oxygenation (*continued*)

    d. Assess for blood oxygen transport (check if present):
- □ Anemia ($\downarrow$Hb)
- □ Polycythemia ($\uparrow$ Hb)
- □ Abnormal Hb ($\uparrow$ HbCO, $\uparrow$ metHb, other)
- □ Low oxygen saturation (Sao_2)
- □ HbO_2 disassociation curve shift (right or left)
- □ Inadequate cardiac output ($\dot{Q}_T$)
- □ Low blood pressure (BP < 90/60 mm Hg)
- Comments: _____

    e. Assess for adequate tissue O_2 uptake and utilization (check all that are present):
- □ Impaired peripheral perfusion
- □ Shifted HbO_2 dissociative curve (left shift)
- □ Impaired tissue utilization
- Comments: _____

9. Assessment for oxygen therapy (check all indications present):
- □ Documented hypoxemia (Spo_2 or arterial blood gases)
  - Adults and children: Pao_2 < 60 mm Hg and/or Spo_2 < 90%.
  - Neonates (< 28 days): Pao_2 < 50 mm Hg and/or SpO_2 < 88% or a capillary Po_2 < 40 mm Hg.
- □ Suspected hypoxemia based on patient condition and/or clinical manifestations of hypoxia (follow with Spo_2 or arterial blood gas measurement)
- □ Severe trauma
- □ Acute myocardial infarction
- □ Postoperative recovery
- □ Treat or prevent pulmonary hypertension secondary to chronic hypoxemia ($Pao_2 \leq$ 55 to 59 mm Hg and/or Spo_2 < 88% to 89%; see Chapter 2)
- Comments: _____

10. Select oxygen therapy device and liter flow and/or oxygen concentration.
- □ Low to moderate concentration of O_2 (22% to 40%)
  Hypoxemia due to low $\dot{V}/\dot{Q}$, hypoventilation, asthma, emphysema, chronic bronchitis, bronchiectasis, cystic fibrosis, congestive heart failure (CHF) without acute pulmonary edema and coronary artery disease (CAD) often responds well to low to moderate concentrations of oxygen.
- □ Nasal cannula at 0.5 to 6 L/min will deliver approximately 22% to 40% oxygen and is the device of choice for most patients.
- □ Air-entrainment mask if variable ventilatory pattern or rapid, shallow breathing to deliver a stable Fio_2 of 24%, 28%, 30%, 35%, and 40%.
- Comments: _____
- □ Moderate to high concentration of O_2 (40% to 100%)
  Hypoxemia due to pulmonary shunting (ARDS, severe pneumonia, alveolar filling), cardiogenic shock (severe acute MI), or trauma may require moderate to high concentrations of oxygen therapy.
  - □ Simple mask (35% to 50% O_2 at 5 to 10 L/min)
  - □ Partial rebreathing mask (40% to 70% at 5 to 10 L/min)
  - □ Nonrebreathing mask (60% to 80% at 6 to 10 L/min)
  - □ Air-entrainment nebulizers via aerosol mask, tracheostomy mask, or "T" piece to provide stable oxygen concentration of 28% to 50%.
  - □ Misty-Ox High Fio_2–High Flow nebulizer delivers 60% to 96% oxygen, with total gas flows of 42 to 80 L/min.
  - □ Thera-Mist air-entrainment nebulizer will provide 36% to 96% oxygen at flows of 47 to 74 L/min.
- Comments: _____

11. Consider other techniques to improve oxygenation.
- □ Respiratory care and/or ventilatory support
  - □ Bronchial hygiene
  - □ Humidity therapy
  - □ Suctioning and/or airway care for secretions
  - □ Bronchodilator therapy for bronchospasm
  - □ Cough and deep breathing instruction
  - □ Turning
  - □ PEEP/CPAP by mask for refractory/unresponsive hypoxemia
  - □ Mechanical ventilation for hypoventilation
  - □ Mechanical ventilation with PEEP/CPAP for refractory/unresponsive hypoxemia
  - □ Prone positioning (ARDS, mechanically ventilated patients)
- Comments: _____

(continues)

TABLE 6-6
Assessment of Oxygenation (*continued*)

12. Assess and revise care plan.
  □ Perform follow-up assessment and adjust therapy, as indicated.
    • Signs and symptoms of hypoxia: Assess for reversal or improvement.
    • Vital signs: Assess for improvement in pulse, respirations, and blood pressure.
    • Spo_2 measurement: Titrate therapy for improvement.
    • Arterial blood gases: Titrate therapy for improvement.
    • Improvement/reversal of cardiac arrhythmias.
  Comments: _____

[1]Spo_2 generally follows Sao_2. The relationship between Spo_2 and Pao_2 varies depending on the position of the HbO_2 disassociation curve.

RC Insights

Oxygen Therapy for COPD Patients
For most patients, the clinical goal of O_2 therapy should be to use the lowest possible Fio_2 to keep the Pao_2 above 60 mm Hg and the Sao_2 at least 0.90 (90%). The exception is the COPD patient with chronic CO_2 retention (chronic ventilatory failure). Excessive oxygen levels in patients who are chronic CO_2 retainers may lead to ventilatory depression and increased $\dot{V}/\dot{Q}$ mismatch when the Pao_2 exceeds 60 mm Hg. Oxygen therapy for the COPD patient with chronically elevated $Paco_2$ values should be targeted at maintaining a Pao_2 of 50 to 59 mm Hg with an Sao_2 of 0.88 to 0.90 (88% to 90%) in order to avoid further hypercapnea in these patients.

Hypoxemia due to low $\dot{V}/\dot{Q}$ or hypoventilation usually responds well to low to moderate concentrations of oxygen. Patients with right-to-left shunting may require moderate to high concentrations of oxygen and, in some cases, the use of mechanical ventilatory support with PEEP or CPAP. Other methods that may improve oxygenation include bronchial hygiene to mobilize secretions and bronchodilator therapy. Prone positioning and rotational therapy (turning the patient) may also be useful.

Attention to factors that affect Cao_2, $\dot{D}o_2$, and tissue uptake and utilization are essential. Body temperature, acid-base balance, and $Paco_2$ should be reviewed and abnormalities treated. Replacement of blood in patients with severe anemia should be considered. Attention to cardiac output and blood pressure is also required to ensure adequate oxygen delivery to the tissues. Chapter 2 provides a detailed description of the development of the respiratory care plan for patients requiring oxygen therapy.

Key Points

▶ Symptoms of hypoxia include excitement, overconfidence, restlessness, anxiety, nausea, headache, and shortness of breath.

▶ Signs of hypoxia include tachycardia, tachypnea, hypertension, impaired judgment, confusion, disorientation, and signs of respiratory distress.

▶ Severe hypoxia may cause bradycardia; hypotension; slowed, irregular breathing; and loss of consciousness.

▶ Cyanosis is not a reliable indicator for the presence or severity of hypoxia.

▶ Hypoxemic respiratory failure ("lung failure") is inadequate arterial oxygenation as assessed by Pao_2, Spo_2, and/or Sao_2.

▶ Factors that determine inspired oxygen tension are barometric pressure and oxygen concentration (Fio_2 or %O_2).

▶ Mountain sickness may affect hikers, skiers, mountain climbers, or travelers to high-altitude locations.

▶ Severe cases of mountain sickness may lead to high-altitude cerebral edema (HACE) and/or high-altitude pulmonary edema (HAPE).

▶ In-flight supplemental oxygen is recommended for patients who may otherwise develop a Pao_2 < 50 to 55 mm Hg.

▶ Ambient hypoxia may occur with industrial accidents and inhalation of asphyxiant gases.

▶ Causes of upper airway obstruction include secretions, edema, trauma, foreign bodies, and tumors.

▶ Bronchospasm, mucosal edema, and secretions in the lower airways may impair oxygenation.

▶ Upper airway obstruction may be classified as fixed or variable based on pulmonary function testing.

▶ Causes of airway obstruction in children include epiglottitis and croup.

▶ Obstructive lung diseases include asthma, COPD, emphysema, chronic bronchitis, bronchiectasis, and cystic fibrosis.

▶ $Paco_2$ is determined by alveolar ventilation and CO_2 production.

▶ Hypoventilation may cause hypoxemia, whereas hyperventilation may improve Pao_2.

▶ Causes of hypoxemia include reduced inspired oxygen tension, hypoventilation, low $\dot{V}/\dot{Q}$, shunt, and diffusion limitations.

▶ Other causes of hypoxia include inadequate arterial blood oxygen content, reduced cardiac output, inadequate tissue perfusion, and problems with tissue O_2 uptake and utilization.

▶ Pao_2/Fio_2 is a good index of effectiveness of oxygenation by the lung.

▶ Normal anatomic shunt or venous admixture accounts for about 2% to 5% of cardiac output.

▶ Causes of low $\dot{V}/\dot{Q}$ include asthma, COPD, emphysema, chronic bronchitis, bronchiectasis, and cystic fibrosis.

▶ Causes of intrapulmonary shunt include atelectasis, pulmonary edema, pneumonia, acute lung injury (ALI), and acute respiratory distress syndrome (ARDS).

▶ Hypoxemia due to low $\dot{V}/\dot{Q}$, hypoventilation, asthma, emphysema, chronic bronchitis, bronchiectasis, cystic fibrosis, congestive heart failure (CHF) without acute pulmonary edema, and coronary artery disease (CAD) often responds well to low to moderate concentrations of oxygen.

▶ Hypoxemia due to pulmonary shunting, cardiogenic shock, or trauma may require moderate to high concentrations of oxygen therapy.

▶ Interstitial lung disease (ILD) may cause hypoxemia by causing low $\dot{V}/\dot{Q}$ or by causing a diffusion limitation.

▶ Diffusion-limited diseases most commonly causes hypoxemia during exercise.

▶ Anemic hypoxia is associated with a low hemoglobin due to blood loss, excessive red blood cell destruction, or deceased red blood cell formation.

▶ Polycythemia sometimes develops as a compensatory response to chronic hypoxemia.

▶ A $Pao_2 \geq 60$ mm Hg generally results in an $Sao_2 \geq 90\%$—the flat part of the HbO_2 dissociation curve.

▶ On the steep part of the HbO_2 dissociation curve ($Pao_2 < 60$ mm Hg), small changes in Pao_2 result in large changes is Sao_2.

▶ Changes in temperature, pH, $Paco_2$ and 2,3-DPG can shift the HbO_2 dissociation curve to the right or left.

▶ A left shift favors O_2 loading and a right shift favors O_2 unloading.

▶ Cigarette smoke contains carbon monoxide.

▶ Carbon monoxide poisoning can occur due to exposure to internal combustion engine exhaust, fire, or smoke inhalation.

▶ Methemoglobinemia can be acquired through ingestion of certain drugs or chemicals.

▶ Sickle cell disease is a hereditary blood disease that may cause an acute chest syndrome.

▶ Low cardiac output may be due to decreased stroke volume or decreased heart rate.

▶ Peripheral perfusion may be compromised by low cardiac output, low blood pressure, or blockage or disruption of tissue blood flow.

▶ Increased plasma lactate levels and increased O_2 extraction ratio (O_2 ER) are associated with poor tissue perfusion and tissue hypoxia.

▶ Treatment of hypoxia includes O_2 therapy, techniques to improve lung function, and treatment of the underlying cause.

References

1. Pierson DJ. Pathophysiology and clinical effects of chronic hypoxia. *Respir Care.* 2000;45(1):39–51.
2. Adams AB. Monitoring and management of the patient in the intensive care unit. In: Wilkins RL, Stodler JK, Kacmarok RM (eds.). *Egan's Fundamentals of Respiratory Care*, 9th ed. St. Louis, MO: Mosby-Elsevier, 2009: 1115–1151.
3. Theodore AC. Oxygenation and mechanisms of hypoxemia. In: *UpToDate*, Basow DS (ed.). UpToDate, Waltham, MA, 2012.
4. Beachey W. Clinical assessment of acid-base and oxygenation status. In: Beachey W, (ed.). *Respiratory Care Anatomy and Physiology*, 2nd ed. St. Louis, MO: Elsevier-Mosby; 2007: 214–235.
5. Wettstein R, Wilkins RL. Interpretation of blood gases. In: Wilkins RL, Dexter JR, Heuer AJ (eds.). *Clinical Assessment in Respiratory Care*, 6th ed. St. Louis, MO: Elsevier-Mosby; 2010: 142–165.
6. ARDS Definition Task Force, Ranieri VM, Rubenfeld GD, et al. Acute respiratory distress syndrome: The Berlin Definition. *JAMA.* 2012;307(23):2526–2533. doi: 10.1001/jama.2012.5669.
7. Hackett PH, Roach, RC. High altitude categories and associated physiologic effects. In: *UpToDate*, Basow DS (ed.). UpToDate, Waltham, MA, 2012.
8. Stoller JK. Traveling with oxygen aboard commercial air carriers. In: *UpToDate*, Basow DS (ed.). UpToDate, Waltham, MA, 2012.
9. Federal Aviation Administration. Medical facts for pilots. Available at: http://www.faa.gov/air_traffic/publications/ATpubs/AIM/aim0801.html. Accessed January 16, 2013.
10. Federal Aviation Administration. Hypoxia. Available at: http://www.faa.gov/search/?omni=MainSearch&q=hypoxia&x=24&y=13. Accessed January 16, 2013.
11. U.S. Chemical Safety and Hazard Investigation Board. Safety bulletin: Hazards of nitrogen asphyxiation. No. 2003-10-B, June 2003. Available at: http://www.csb.gov/assets/document/SB-Nitrogen-6-11-03.pdf. Accessed January 16, 2013.
12. Braman SS, Gaissert HA. Upper airway obstruction. In: Fishman AP, Elias JA, Fishman JA, et al. (eds.). *Fishman's Pulmonary Diseases and Disorders*, 3rd ed. New York: McGraw-Hill; 1998: 783–801.
13. Loftis LL. Emergent evaluation of acute upper airway obstruction in children. In: *UpToDate*, Basow DS, (ed.). UpToDate, Waltham, MA, 2012.
14. Rounds S, Jankowich MD. Disorders of respiratory control. In: Andreoli TE, Benjamin IJ, Griggs RC, Wing EJ (eds.). *Andreoli and Carpenter's Cecil Essentials of Medicine*, 8th ed. Philadelphia: Elsevier Saunders; 2010: 245–247.
15. Jankowich MD. Obstructive lung disease. In: Andreoli TE, Benjamin IJ, Griggs RC, Wing EJ (eds.). *Andreoli and Carpenter's Cecil Essentials of Medicine*, 8th ed. Philadelphia: Elsevier Saunders; 2010: 213–224.
16. Beachey W. Gas diffusion. In: Beachey W (ed.). *Respiratory Care Anatomy and Physiology*, 2nd ed. St. Louis, MO: Elsevier-Mosby; 2007: 127–139.

17. Huang YCT, Lease E, Beachey WA. Gas exchange. In: Hess DR, MacIntyre NR, Mishoe SC, Galvin WF, Adams AB (eds.). *Respiratory Care: Principles and Practice*, 2nd ed. Sudbury, MA: Jones & Bartlett Learning; 2012: 21–40.

18. Bernard GR, Artigas A, Brigham KL, et al. The American–European Consensus Conference on ARDS. Definitions, mechanisms, relevant outcomes, and clinical trial coordination. *Am J Respir Crit Care Med*. 1994;149(3 Pt 1):818–824.

19. Beachey W. Ventilation–perfusion relationships and arterial blood gases. In: Beachey W (ed.). *Respiratory Care Anatomy and Physiology*, 2nd ed. St. Louis, MO: Elsevier-Mosby; 2007: 195–213.

20. West JB. Ventilation-perfusion relationships: how matching of gas and blood determines gas exchange. In: West JB (ed.). *Respiratory Physiology: The Essentials*, 8th ed. Philadelphia: Lippincott Williams & Wilkins; 2008: 55–74.

21. West JB. Diffusion: how gas gets across the blood-gas barrier. In: West JB (ed.). *Respiratory Physiology: The Essentials*, 8th ed. Philadelphia: Lippincott Williams & Wilkins; 2008: 25–34.

22. Aliotta JM, Jankowich MD. Interstitial lung diseases. In: Andreoli TE, Benjamin IJ, Griggs RC, Wing EJ (eds.). *Andreoli and Carpenter's Cecil Essentials of Medicine*, 8th ed. Philadelphia: Saunders Elsevier; 2010: 225–240.

23. Enright PL. Diffusing capacity for carbon monoxide. In: *UpToDate*, Basow DS, (ed.). UpToDate, Waltham, MA, 2012.

24. Schrier SL. Approach to the adult patient with anemia. In: *UpToDate*, Basow DS (ed.). UpToDate, Waltham, MA, 2012.

25. Guyton AC, Hall JE. Transport of oxygen and carbon dioxide in blood and tissue fluids. In: Guyton AC, Hall JE (eds.). *Textbook of Medical Physiology*, 11th ed. Philadelphia: Elsevier Saunders; 2006: 502–513.

26. West JB. Gas transport by the blood: how gases are moved to the peripheral tissues. In: West JB (ed.). *Respiratory Physiology: The Essentials*, 8th ed. Philadelphia: Lippincott Williams & Wilkins; 2008: 75–93.

27. Stack AM. Etiology and evaluation of cyanosis in children. In: *UpToDate*, Basow DS (ed.). UpToDate, Waltham, MA, 2012.

28. Kleinman S, Carson JL. Indications for red cell transfusion in the adult. In: *UpToDate*, Basow DS (ed.). UpToDate, Waltham, MA, 2012.

29. Tefferi A. Diagnostic approach to the patient with polycythemia. In: *UpToDate*, Basow DS (ed.). UpToDate, Waltham, MA, 2012.

30. Clardy PF, Manaker S, Perry H. Carbon monoxide poisoning. In: *UpToDate*, Basow DS (ed.). UpToDate, Waltham, MA, 2012.

31. Rose MG, Berliner N. Disorders of red blood cells. In: Andreoli TE, Benjamin IJ, Griggs RC, Wing EJ (eds.). *Andreoli and Carpenter's Cecil Essentials of Medicine*, 8th ed. Philadelphia: Elsevier Saunders; 2010: 520–532.

32. Weaver KL, Churchill SK, Deru K, Cooney D. False positive rate of carbon monoxide saturation by pulse oximetry of emergency department patients. *Respir Care*. 2013;58(2):232–240.

33. Prchal JT. Clinical features, diagnosis, and treatment of methemoglobinemia. In: UpToDate, Schrier SL, Mahoney DH, (eds.). UpToDate, Waltham, MA, 2012.

34. Vichinsky EP. Overview of the clinical manifestations of sickle cell disease. In: *UpToDate*, Basow DS (ed.). UpToDate, Waltham, MA, 2012.

35. Beachey W. Oxygen equilibrium and transport. In: Beachey W (ed.). *Respiratory Care Anatomy and Physiology*, 2nd ed. St. Louis, MO: Elsevier-Mosby; 2007: 140–156.

36. Myers TR, American Association for Respiratory Care (AARC). AARC Clinical Practice Guideline: selection of an oxygen delivery device for neonatal and pediatric patients—2002 revision & update. *Respir Care*. 2002;47(6):707–716.

37. Kallstrom TJ, American Association for Respiratory Care (AARC). AARC Clinical Practice Guideline: oxygen therapy in the acute care hospital—2002 revision & update. *Respir Care*. 2002;47(6):717–720.

38. Casserly B, Rounds S. Essentials in critical care medicine. In: Andreoli TE, Benjamin IJ, Griggs RC, Wing EJ (eds.). *Andreoli and Carpenter's Cecil Essentials of Medicine*, 8th ed. Philadelphia: Elsevier Saunders; 2010: 259–265.

39. Gaieski D. Shock in adults: types, presentation, and diagnostic approach. In: *UpToDate*, Basow DS (ed.). UpToDate, Waltham, MA, 2012.

40. Caplan LR. Etiology and classification of stroke. In: *UpToDate*, Basow DS (ed.). UpToDate, Waltham, MA, 2012.

41. Rose BD. Treatment of metabolic alkalosis. In: *UpToDate*, Basow DS (ed.). UpToDate, Waltham, MA, 2012.

42. Rosen IM, Manaker S. Oxygen delivery and consumption. In: *UpToDate*, Parsons PE (ed.). UpToDate, Waltham, MA, 2012.

43. Desai S, Su M. Cyanide poisoning. In: *UpToDate*, Basow DS (ed.). UpToDate, Waltham, MA, 2012.

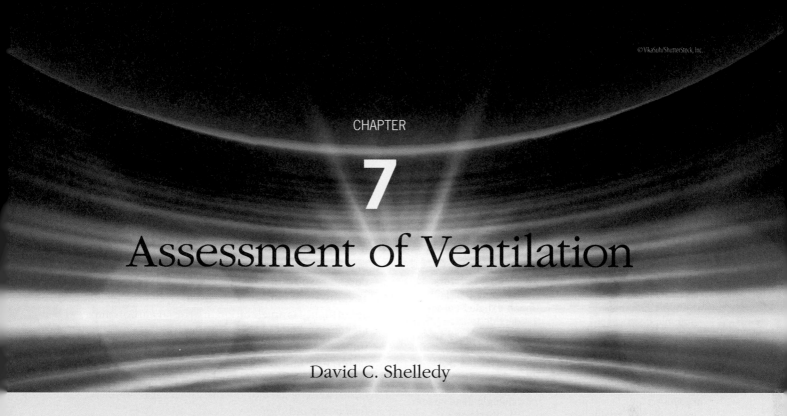

CHAPTER

7

Assessment of Ventilation

David C. Shelledy

CHAPTER OUTLINE

Introduction to Assessment of Ventilation
Factors Associated with Normal Ventilation
Ventilatory Failure
Indications for Mechanical Ventilatory Support
Ventilator Discontinuance

CHAPTER OBJECTIVES

1. Define *respiratory failure* and contrast hypoxemic and hypercapnic respiratory failure.
2. Define *ventilatory failure* and contrast acute and chronic ventilatory failure.
3. Explain the relationships among tidal volume (V_T), respiratory rate (f), minute volume ($\dot{V}_E$), dead space (V_D), and alveolar ventilation ($\dot{V}_A$).
4. Explain how anatomic, physiologic, alveolar, and mechanical dead space differ.
5. Use the Bohr equation to calculate V_D/V_T and physiologic dead space.
6. Define each of the following conditions based on Pa_{CO_2} and pH: normal ventilation, acute ventilatory failure, chronic ventilatory failure, acute alveolar hyperventilation, and chronic alveolar hyperventilation.
7. Describe the normal pattern of ventilation and possible consequences of shallow breathing without sigh.
8. Define each of the following lung volumes and capacities: tidal volume (V_T), inspiratory capacity (IC), vital capacity (VC), functional residual capacity (FRC), and total lung capacity (TLC).
9. Describe the normal sequence of events and pressure changes that occur during spontaneous breathing.
10. Evaluate bedside measures of ventilatory muscle strength including maximal inspiratory pressure (MIP), maximal expiratory pressure (MEP), and vital capacity (VC).
11. Explain the relationships among total compliance, lung compliance, and thoracic (chest wall) compliance.
12. Evaluate possible causes of changes in total compliance, lung compliance, thoracic compliance, and airway resistance.
13. Explain the relationships among lung recoil, thoracic recoil, and FRC.
14. Describe the evaluation of a patient with pneumothorax.
15. Calculate static and dynamic compliance and evaluate the results.
16. Explain the use of pressure–volume curves in the intensive care unit.
17. Explain the relationship between surface tension and elastic recoil of the lungs.
18. Explain the role of surfactant and identify factors that may disrupt surfactant function.
19. Describe elastic and nonelastic resistance in the lungs and explain factors that may alter each.
20. Calculate airway resistance and contrast airflow and resistance in the upper and lower airways.
21. Discuss the effects of each of the following on airway resistance: bronchospasm, mucosal edema, secretions, and endotracheal tubes.
22. Explain the relationship between the nature of the gas flow (e.g., laminar or turbulent) and breath sounds.
23. Describe the effects of specific disease states on work of breathing and the relationship between work of breathing and ventilatory pattern.
24. Recognize the causes and clinical signs of diaphragmatic fatigue.
25. Contrast factors that determine ventilatory capacity, ventilatory demand and respiratory drive.
26. Describe the risk factors for and clinical manifestations of ventilatory failure.
27. Explain each of the indications for mechanical ventilation and bedside measures that may be predictive of the need for mechanical ventilatory support.
28. Contrast acute ventilatory failure and impending ventilatory failure to include clinical recognition of each.
29. Describe the assessment and treatment of severe oxygenation problems (e.g., refractory hypoxemia).
30. Explain the assessment of patients for ventilator discontinuance and list criteria (e.g., indices) that may be helpful in evaluating patients for ventilator discontinuance.
31. Explain factors that may contribute to ventilator dependence.

32. Describe assessment of the patient's airway for extubation to include the cuff-leak test.
33. Explain how to perform readiness testing in patients being considered for ventilator discontinuance and preferred values for specific weaning indices.
34. Explain how to perform a spontaneous breathing trial (SBT).
35. Explain how to monitor and assess a patient during ventilator weaning and possible causes of weaning failure.

KEY TERMS

acute alveolar hyperventilation
acute ventilatory failure
airway resistance (R_{aw})
alveolar dead space (V_D alveolar)
alveolar ventilation
anatomic dead space (V_D anatomic)
apnea
apneustic breathing
aspiration
Biot's breathing
bradypnea
carbon dioxide production ($\dot{V}CO_2$)
Cheyne-Stokes breathing
chronic alveolar hyperventilation
chronic ventilatory failure
cuff-leak test
dead space to tidal volume ratio (V_D/V_T)
dynamic compliance ($C_{dynamic}$)
dyspnea
eupnea
functional residual capacity (FRC)
hypercapnic respiratory failure
hyperventilation
hypopnea
hypoventilation
hypoxemic respiratory failure
hysteresis
inspiratory capacity (IC)
Kussmaul breathing

laminar flow
lung compliance (C_L)
maximal expiratory pressure (MEP)
maximal inspiratory pressure (MIP)
mean exhaled carbon dioxide tension ($P\bar{E}CO_2$)
mechanical dead space
metabolic rate
minute volume ($\dot{V}_E$)
orthopnea
oxygen consumption ($\dot{V}O_2$)
physiologic dead space (V_D physiologic)
ponopnea
refractory hypoxemia
residual volume (RV)
respiratory drive
respiratory failure
respiratory rate (f)
static total compliance (C_{ST})
surface tension
surfactant
tachypnea
thoracic compliance (chest wall compliance, C_c)
tidal volume (V_T)
total compliance (C_T)
total lung capacity (TLC)
transitional flow
trepopnea
turbulent flow
upper airway obstruction
ventilator discontinuation
ventilator weaning
ventilatory failure
vital capacity (VC)
work of breathing (WOB)

Overview

Two of the most important activities the respiratory care clinician can perform are assessment of oxygenation and assessment of ventilation. Chapter 6 described assessment of oxygenation. This chapter will describe the assessment of ventilation. The chapter begins with review of the basic concepts related to ventilation and then moves on to describe the disorders of ventilation to include acute and chronic ventilatory failure. Physical findings associated with ventilatory disorders will be discussed, and measures of pulmonary function, arterial blood gases, capnography, and other methods to assess the patient's ventilatory status will

be reviewed. The chapter closes with a discussion of the treatment of disorders of ventilation and indications for mechanical ventilatory support.

Before beginning this chapter, a review of commonly used nomenclature used to describe aspects of respiratory failure and ventilatory failure is needed. **Respiratory failure** can be broadly defined as an inability of the heart and lungs to provide adequate tissue oxygenation and carbon dioxide removal (see Chapter 6).[1–3] Respiratory failure is sometimes divided into two categories: hypoxemic respiratory failure and hypercapnic respiratory failure.[2,4] **Hypoxemic respiratory failure** refers to inadequate oxygenation of the arterial blood. **Hypercapnic respiratory failure**, which is often referred to as **ventilatory failure**, is failure in which the primary abnormality is an elevation in arterial carbon dioxide tension ($PaCO_2$).[4] Hypoxemic respiratory failure is sometimes referred to as *lung failure*, and hypercapnic respiratory failure is sometimes known as *pump failure*. For the remainder of this chapter, the term *ventilatory failure* will be used to refer to an elevation in $PaCO_2$ (i.e., pump failure).

Introduction to Assessment of Ventilation

Ventilation can be defined as the process that exchanges gases between the external environment and the alveoli:

> *Ventilation is the bulk movement of gas into and out of the lungs.*

When referring to ventilatory volumes, the symbol V is often used for volume, whereas $\dot{V}$ ("V dot") refers to volume per unit of time (usually per minute). Ventilation has several components, and these include tidal volume, respiratory rate, and minute volume.

Tidal volume (V_T) can be defined as the volume of gas exhaled passively following a normal inspiration.[5,6] Normal adult tidal volume is about 500 mL, or approximately 7 mL per kilogram of ideal body weight (IBW).* The normal range for adult tidal volume is about 400 to 700 mL. Occasionally, inspiratory tidal volume (V_I) is measured and compared to expiratory tidal volume (V_E). Normally, these two values are almost identical, though there is often a very small difference between V_I and V_E due to differences in **oxygen consumption ($\dot{V}O_2$)** and **carbon dioxide production ($\dot{V}CO_2$)**. Normal $\dot{V}O_2$ is about 250 mL per minute, whereas normal $\dot{V}CO_2$ is

---

*Formulas for estimating IBW vary (e.g., Broca formula, Devine formula, Hamwi formula). The ARDS Network uses the term *predicted body weight* (PBW) where:

- Males: PBW (kg) = 50 + 2.3(height in inches – 60)
- Females: PBW (kg) = 45.5 + 2.3(height in inches – 60)

The ARDS Network recommendation is based on the Devine formula for IBW calculation (i.e., PBW = IBW; see http://www.ardsnet.org).

about 200 mL per minute. Consequently, normal V_I is slightly greater than V_E. This will, of course, vary as O_2 consumption and CO_2 production varies. For example, if $\dot{V}O_2$ is 250 mL/min and $\dot{V}CO_2$ is 200 mL/min, then the difference between inhaled and exhaled volumes would be 50 mL/min (250 − 200 = 50), or less than 5 mL per breath (assuming a normal respiratory rate). However, if $\dot{V}O_2$ and $\dot{V}CO_2$ are equal, then there should be no difference in inspired and expired tidal volumes. To summarize:

- Average V_T is 500 mL (approximately 7 mL/kg IBW, or about 3 to 4 mL/lb of IBW). Actual V_T will vary depending on the patient's size, sex, and overall condition.
- V_T ranges from 400 to 700 mL.
- V_I and V_E should be approximately equal, except for the small differences in O_2 consumption versus CO_2 production.

Mechanically ventilated patients may occasionally show a clinically measurable difference between inspired and expired tidal volume. For example, an intubated adult patient receiving mechanical ventilation may have inspired tidal volume of 600 mL and an expired tidal volume of only 400 mL due to a large air leak. Causes of air leaks sometimes seen in the intensive care unit (ICU) on ventilated patients include problems with the endotracheal tube cuff and pneumothorax with air leakage through the chest tubes. If an endotracheal tube cuff does not seal the airway (i.e., cuff leak), gas delivered to the endotracheal tube will exit the patient's mouth and will not be measured by the ventilator's volume-sensing system. Patients receiving mechanical ventilation who experience a pneumothorax will often have chest tubes inserted into the pleural space to remove fluid and gas. If there is a tear in the lung tissue, gas delivered by the ventilator during inspiration may exit via the tear into the pleural space and then out the chest tube. In both cases, measured V_I will be greater than V_E.

Children have smaller tidal volumes than adults, and infants have much smaller tidal volumes. Tidal volumes in children increase as they grow. For example, tidal volume for a normal full-term newborn is about 15 to 20 mL, whereas a 5-year-old child may have a tidal volume of 100 mL, depending in his or her size. By age 12 to 16 years, tidal volumes begin to approach adult values.

Respiratory rate (f) is the next component of ventilation. Respiratory rate is simply the number of breaths taken by the patient per minute. A normal respiratory rate for an adult is approximately 12 breaths per minute, with a range of about 12 to 18 or 20 breaths per minute. **Tachypnea** refers to an elevated respiratory rate, whereas **bradypnea** refers to an abnormally slow respiratory rate. Normal respiratory rates in infants and children are higher. For example, the normal newborn's respiratory rate is between 30 and 60 breaths per minute.

Minute volume ($\dot{V}_E$) is simply the tidal volume (V_T) multiplied by the respiratory rate, or frequency (f):

$$\dot{V}_E = V_T \times f$$

A normal adult minute volume is approximately 6 L/min with a range of about 5 to 10 L/min.

Alveolar Ventilation and Dead Space

Alveolar ventilation refers to the volume of gas reaching alveoli that are ventilated *and* perfused. Dead space refers to that portion of ventilation that does not participate in gas exchange (i.e., ventilation *without* perfusion). Generally, there are three types of dead space: anatomic, physiologic, and alveolar.

Anatomic dead space (V_D anatomic) refers to the volume of gas in the conducting airways.[7] Anatomic dead space is made up of the airways from the external nares (nostrils) down to and including the terminal bronchioles. Normal anatomic dead space is approximately 1 mL per pound of IBW. This is about 150 mL in a normal adult; however, anatomic dead space will vary based on the patient's size.

Alveolar dead space (V_D alveolar) refers to the volume of ventilation received by alveoli that are ventilated but not perfused.[5,7] An important cause of an increase in alveolar dead space is emphysema (where the capillaries are destroyed by the toxic effects of cigarette smoking). Pulmonary embolus (PE) is sometimes cited as a good example of dead space–causing disease. With PE, severe $\dot{V}/\dot{Q}$ problems may occur with partial occlusion of a pulmonary vessel; when there is complete occlusion of the vessel, alveolar dead space will increase.

Physiologic dead space (V_D physiologic) refers to the total functional dead space and consists of the alveolar dead space plus the anatomic dead space:[5,7]

$$V_D \text{ physiologic} = V_D \text{ anatomic} + V_D \text{ alveolar}$$

In normal subjects, V_D physiologic is approximately the same as V_D anatomic. With dead space–causing diseases (e.g., emphysema, PE), V_D physiologic > V_D anatomic.

Physiologic dead space can be measured fairly easily at the bedside using the Bohr equation,* which requires arterial blood gas analysis for measurement of Pa_{CO_2} and collection of expired gas from which **mean exhaled carbon dioxide tension ($P\bar{E}_{CO_2}$)** is measured.[5,7,8] This allows for calculation of the **dead space to tidal volume ratio (V_D/V_T)** and, in turn, the calculation of physiologic dead space:

$$V_D/V_T = \frac{Pa_{CO_2} - P\bar{E}_{CO_2}}{Pa_{CO_2}}$$

Physiologic dead space $= V_D / V_T \times V_T$

---

* Note that the original Bohr equation used alveolar CO_2 tension (i.e., PA_{CO_2}) in place of Pa_{CO_2}. Estimating PA_{CO_2} requires an end-tidal gas sample; in normal subjects $PA_{CO_2} = Pa_{CO_2}$.

Using normal values for $Paco_2$ (40 mm Hg), $P\overline{E}co_2$ (28 mm Hg), and V_T (500 mL), we can calculate the normal V_D/V_T and dead space volume:

$$V_D/V_T = \frac{Paco_2 - P\overline{E}co_2}{Paco_2}$$

$$V_D/V_T = \frac{40 \text{ mm Hg} - 28 \text{ mm Hg}}{40 \text{ mm Hg}}$$

$$= 0.30 \text{ (i.e., 30\% dead space ventilation)}$$

$$\text{Dead space volume} = V_D/V_T \times V_T = 0.30 \times 500 \text{ mL} = 150 \text{ mL}$$

A normal V_D/V_T ranges from about 0.20 to 0.40 (20% to 40% dead space ventilation), though it is not unusual to have a V_D/V_T of up to 0.50 (50% dead space ventilation) in mechanically ventilated patients with normal lungs.

A fourth type of dead space, **mechanical dead space**, refers to the volume of rebreathed gas due to a mechanical device. Examples of mechanical dead space include the volume of rebreathed gas associated with an oxygen face mask. Tubing is sometimes placed between the patient "Y" (or "wye") and the endotracheal or tracheostomy tube in intubated patients. This added volume of rebreathed gas is another form of mechanical dead space. The addition of mechanical dead space may cause an increase in $Paco_2$ if there is no change in the patient's tidal volume or respiratory rate.

Alveolar Ventilation

Alveolar ventilation refers to the actual volume of ventilation received by the alveoli per breath (V_A) and per minute ($\dot{V}_A$).[5,7] Alveolar ventilation is sometimes referred to as *effective ventilation* and normally is about 4.2 L per minute in a typical adult. Assuming a normal adult anatomic dead space of about 150 mL, alveolar ventilation would be:

- V_A per breath: $V_A = V_T - V_D = 500 - 150 = 350$ mL
- $\dot{V}_A$ per minute: $\dot{V}_A = (V_T - V_D)f = (500 - 150)12 = 4200$ mL = 4.2 L/min

Clinically, alveolar ventilation can be calculated per minute based on measured tidal volume, respiratory rate, and V_D/V_T, as follows:

$$\dot{V}_A = (V_T - V_D) \times f$$

$$\dot{V}_A = [V_T - (V_T \times V_D/V_T)] \times f$$

$$\dot{V}_A = \left[V_T - \left(V_T \times \frac{(Paco_2 - P\overline{E}co_2)}{Paco_2} \right) \right] \times f$$

Inserting normal values we have:

$$\dot{V}_A = \left[V_T - \left(V_T \times \left(\frac{Paco_2 - P\overline{E}co_2}{Paco_2} \right) \right) \right] \times f$$

$$\dot{V}_A = \left[500 - \left(500 \times \left(\frac{40 - 28}{40} \right) \right) \right] \times 12$$

$$\dot{V}_A = [500 - (500 \times 0.30)] \times 12$$

$$= [500 - 150] \times 12$$

$$= 350 \times 12$$

$$\dot{V}_A = 4200 \text{ mL/min, or } 4.2 \text{ L/min}$$

Alveolar Ventilation and $Paco_2$

$Paco_2$ and alveolar ventilation are closely related:

$$\dot{V}_A = \frac{0.863 \times \dot{V}co_2}{Paco_2}$$

where the $\dot{V}co_2$ is the CO_2 production per minute, $Paco_2$ is the arterial CO_2 tension, and 0.863 is a factor to convert the results of the calculation into liters per minute.[5,7] Normal CO_2 production will vary with the level of activity and the metabolic rate. For example, exercise or fever will increase $\dot{V}co_2$, whereas sedation or sleep may reduce $\dot{V}co_2$. Normal $\dot{V}co_2$ in the adult is approximately 200 mL/min, normal $Paco_2$ is 40 mm Hg, and 0.863 is a constant.* Inserting these values into the equation we can determine the normal alveolar ventilation:

$$\dot{V}_A = \frac{0.863 \times \dot{V}co_2}{Paco_2}$$

$$\dot{V}_A = \frac{0.863 \times 200}{40} = 4.3 \text{ L/min}$$

Best Index of Ventilation

Alveolar ventilation and $Paco_2$ are inversely proportional; that is, as alveolar ventilation decreases, $Paco_2$ increases, and vice versa. Thus, clinically $Paco_2$ *is the single best index of alveolar ventilation.*[5,7,8] This allows us to define the level of ventilation based on $Paco_2$:

- $Paco_2$ of 35 to 45 mm Hg: Normal ventilation
- $Paco_2$ > 45 to 50 mm Hg: **Hypoventilation** (ventilatory failure)
- $Paco_2$ < 35 mm Hg: Alveolar **hyperventilation**

Further, this allows us to define acute and chronic ventilatory failure based on the $Paco_2$ and pH. Because CO_2 is a volatile acid, a sudden increase in $Paco_2$ will result in a corresponding decrease in pH. Also, a chronic elevation on $Paco_2$ will allow time for the kidneys to attempt to normalize the pH by excreting HCO_3^-. There is generally a partial renal response to an elevated $Paco_2$ in 12 to 24 hours; maximal renal response occurs in 48 to 72 hours (see also Chapter 8). Definitions of acute and chronic ventilatory failure can be based on the degree of renal compensation and resultant pH:

- **Acute ventilatory failure:** An acute (sudden) increase in $Paco_2$ with a corresponding decrease in pH.
- **Chronic ventilatory failure:** A chronically elevated $Paco_2$ with a normal or near-normal pH (due to renal compensation).

---

* 0.863 (sometimes written as k) is a conversion factor to convert mm Hg and mL/min to L/min.

In a similar fashion, we can define acute and chronic alveolar hyperventilation:

- **Acute alveolar hyperventilation:** An acute (sudden) decrease in $Paco_2$ with a corresponding increase in pH.
- **Chronic alveolar hyperventilation:** A chronic decrease in $Paco_2$ with a normal or near-normal pH (due to renal compensation).

To reiterate, the single best index of alveolar ventilation is $Paco_2$, and the level of ventilation can be quantified based on $Paco_2$ values.

Factors Associated with Normal Ventilation

Most people tend to think that normal breathing is quiet, regular, and fairly static and consistent from breath to breath. In fact, normal breathing is quite dynamic and varies as subjects sit, stand, eat, drink, talk, and move about. In addition, normal subjects take a deep breath or sigh approximately every 6 minutes (or 9 to 10 sighs per hour), and the sigh volume is generally two to three times the tidal volume. It has been shown that constant, shallow tidal breathing (< 7 mL/kg of IBW) without an intermittent deep breath will cause progressive atelectasis and that intermittent sigh breaths reverse this trend.[5,7,9]

In addition to taking intermittent deep breaths to keep the lungs open, coughing helps clear air passageways and maintain pulmonary function. An adequate cough requires the ability to take a deep breath and adequate expiratory (abdominal) muscle strength. **Inspiratory capacity (IC)** is the maximum volume of air a person can inhale following a passive exhalation and is about 50 mL/kg IBW (or about 3600 mL) in a normal adult.[6] **Vital capacity (VC)** is the maximum volume of gas a person can exhale following a maximal inspiration and is normally about 60 to 70 mL/kg IBW (or about 4800 mL) in a normal adult.[6] In the pulmonary laboratory, predicted values for lung volumes and capacities are based on the patient's sex, age, and height (see Chapter 12). Patients who are unable to take a deep breath on their own (e.g., < one-third predicted IC) are at risk for developing atelectasis, pneumonia, and respiratory failure.[5,7,9]

It should also be noted that a normal tidal volume (i.e., 500 mL) represents only a relatively small portion of the **total lung capacity (TLC)**, which is about 6000 mL in a typical adult.[6] Further, it is not possible to exhale all of the gas in the lung. Following a forced maximal exhalation, about 1200 mL remains in the normal adult lung, and this is the **residual volume (RV)**.[6] The volume of gas in the lungs following a passive exhalation is about 2400 mL, and this is the **functional residual capacity (FRC)**. Chapter 12 describes the various lung volumes and capacities in more detail. **Figure 7-1** compares tidal volume, respiratory rate, minute volume, dead space, and alveolar ventilation.[8]

As noted in Chapter 6, there are regional differences in ventilation in the normal lung largely due to the effects of gravity. In the normal upright lung (i.e., subject in the sitting or standing position), ventilation and perfusion are greater in the bases than the apices. Ventilation and perfusion gradually decrease from the bases (greatest ventilation) toward the apices (least ventilation) in the upright lung. In the supine and prone positions, the differences between apical and basal ventilation and perfusion are not present. When patients are placed in the supine position, there is preferential

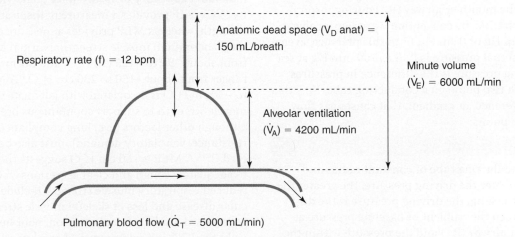

Respiratory rate (f) = 12 bpm

Anatomic dead space (V_D anat) = 150 mL/breath

Minute volume ($\dot{V}_E$) = 6000 mL/min

Alveolar ventilation ($\dot{V}_A$) = 4200 mL/min

Pulmonary blood flow ($\dot{Q}_T$ = 5000 mL/min)

A normal adult tidal volume (V_T) is about 500 mL with a respiratory rate (f) of about 12 bpm resulting in a minute volume ($\dot{V}_E$) of 6000 mL/min ($\dot{V}_E = V_T \times f$). Normally, anatomic and physiologic dead space are equal at about 150 mL resulting in an alveolar ventilation ($\dot{V}_A$) of 4200 mL/min ($\dot{V}_A = (V_T - V_D) \times f$).

bpm = breaths per minute

FIGURE 7-1 **Tidal volume, minute volume, and dead space.**

ventilation and blood flow to the dependent (posterior) portions of the lung, whereas in the prone position there is more blood flow and ventilation directed to the anterior portions of the lung. In the prone or supine positions, apical and basal ventilation and blood flow are similar.

The major muscle of ventilation is the diaphragm. The normal sequence of events that occurs during spontaneous ventilation is as follows:

1. The diaphragm contracts.
2. The intrathoracic space enlarges.
3. The intrathoracic pressure decreases due to Boyle's law (i.e., an increase in volume leads to a decrease in pressure).
4. The alveolar pressure decreases, creating a pressure gradient between the mouth and the alveoli.
5. Gas flows into the lung (i.e., inspiration)
6. During exhalation, the diaphragm relaxes and the elastic recoil of the lung causes the alveolar pressure to rise above the mouth pressure and gas flows out (i.e., expiration).

Factors that determine the adequacy of ventilation include the magnitude of the pressure gradient (ΔP) between the mouth and the alveoli, lung compliance, and airway resistance. In addition, surface tension plays an important role in ventilation. We will discuss each of these factors briefly, as they relate to assessment of ventilation.

Pressure Gradients in the Lung

Normal barometric pressure (P_B) at sea level is 760 mm Hg or 1 atmosphere of pressure, though this value varies with the weather and with altitude (see also Chapter 6). During normal breathing, P_B is the baseline pressure at the mouth or airway (P_{aw}) during inspiration and expiration; by convention we assign a value of zero (0 mm Hg or 0 cm H_2O)* to this pressure, even though the actual pressure is P_B (i.e., 760 mm Hg at sea level). Driving pressure is the difference in pressures (ΔP) between two points in a conducting tube.[7] It is this pressure difference, or gradient, that causes gas flow between two points:

$$\Delta P = P_1 - P_2$$

Given a conducting tube of constant radius and length, the greater the driving pressure, the greater the gas flow. In the lung, the driving pressure is the difference between the ambient or baseline pressure at the mouth or airway (P_{aw}) and the pressure within the alveoli (P_A). The pressure gradients in the lung vary between inspiration and expiration, which causes gas flow in and out. As noted, the diaphragm is the most important muscle of ventilation. During inspiration,

the diaphragm contracts and intrathoracic pressure decreases, resulting in an alveolar pressure of about −5 cm H_2O below mouth or ambient pressure (P_{aw}). During expiration, the diaphragm relaxes and the natural elastic recoil of the lungs causes the alveolar pressure to rise to about +5 cm H_2O above P_{aw} and gas flows out of the lung. To summarize:

- Inspiration
  - $P_{aw} = P_1 = 0$ cm H_2O
  - $P_A = P_2 = -5$ cm H_2O
  - $\Delta P = P_1 - P_2 = 0 - (-5) = +5$ cm H_2O (gas flows into the lung)
- Expiration
  - $P_{aw} = P_1 = 0$ cm H_2O
  - $P_A = P_2 = +5$ cm H_2O
  - $\Delta P = P_1 - P_2 = 0 - 5 = -5$ cm H_2O (gas flows out of the lung)

When the pressure gradient (ΔP) is zero, gas flow ceases.[7] This occurs at end inspiration and end expiration. By considering the effects of disease states or conditions on pressure gradients in the lung, we can predict their effects on ventilation. For example, an increase in diaphragmatic force of contraction may generate a larger pressure gradient and increase gas flow during inspiration. A weak or damaged diaphragm may result in a lower pressure gradient and less gas flow during inspiration. We can see that by raising the mouth or airway pressure above ambient values, inspiration may be supported, as occurs during positive-pressure ventilation. We can also see that the elastic recoil of the lung will affect the pressures in the alveoli when the diaphragm relaxes during expiration.

Bedside measures of ventilatory muscle strength include the **maximal inspiratory pressure (MIP)**,* **maximal expiratory pressure (MEP)**, and vital capacity (VC). MIP provides a measure of inspiratory muscle strength, whereas MEP provides a measure of expiratory (abdominal) muscle strength. Normal MIP ranges from about −90 to −125 cm H_2O, and normal MEP ranges from about +150 to 230 cm H_2O.[7] A MIP < −20 to −30 cm H_2O is associated with adequate ventilatory muscle strength to support spontaneous breathing, although other factors (e.g., lung compliance, airway resistance, ventilatory demand) must also be considered.[7,10,11] A MEP ≥ +60 cm H_2O suggests the ability to adequately cough and clear secretions.[7,10] Causes of reduced respiratory muscle strength include neuromuscular disease and loss of skeletal muscle strength (e.g., generalized weakness, malnutrition, poor health).

In the ICU, it is common to observe pressure–time curves taken at the airway displayed on ventilator monitors in patients receiving invasive mechanical ventilation.[7,12,13] These curves provide a dynamic display of

---

*P_B is often reported in mm Hg whereas airway pressures are often reported in cm H_2O where cm H_2O = mm Hg × 1.36.

*Other terms sometimes used (in place of MIP) include negative inspiratory force (NIF) and P_{Imax}.

airway pressure (P_{aw}) throughout the ventilatory cycle and can be used to compare various modes of ventilation (e.g., continuous positive airway pressure [CPAP], volume control, pressure support, pressure control, positive end-expiratory pressure [PEEP]). Observation of these curves can also identify the degree with which the patient's breathing efforts are in synchrony with breaths provided by the ventilator. The use of ventilator graphics for monitoring ventilation is described in Chapter 14.

Compliance and Elastance

Compliance can be defined as the "stretchability" of the lungs and thorax.[7,8] Compliance is the inverse of elastance. As the lungs and thorax become more compliant (i.e., elastance decreases), they become easier to inflate. As the lungs and thorax become less compliant (i.e., elastance increases), they become more difficult to inflate. *Elastic recoil* of the lungs refers to their tendency to deflate following inflation, whereas *elastance* represents the elastic resistance of the lungs and thorax to inflation. The elastic recoil of the lungs is due to the collagen fibers of the lung parenchyma and the surface tension generated by the fluid lining of the alveoli.[7]

Compliance (C) can be defined as the volume change divided by the pressure change:

$$C = \frac{\Delta V}{\Delta P} = \frac{mL}{cm\ H_2O} \quad or \quad \frac{L}{cm\ H_2O}$$

where ΔV is the inspired volume and ΔP is the pressure change required to achieve that volume.

To illustrate the effect of compliance on ventilation, let's look at two different patients. The first patient (A) has a normal inspiratory pressure gradient (ΔP of 5 cm H_2O) resulting in an inspired tidal volume (V_T) of 500 mL. The second patient (B) makes a similar inspiratory effort and also generates an inspiratory pressure gradient of 5 cm H_2O; however, the resultant tidal volume is only 250 mL. We can calculate the total compliance (C_T) of the lungs and thorax together for each patient:

Patient A

$$\Delta V = 500\ mL$$

$$\Delta P = 5\ cm\ H_2O$$

$$C_T A = \frac{500\ mL}{5\ cm\ H_2O} = 100\ mL/cm\ H_2O,\ or\ 0.1\ L/cm\ H_2O$$

Patient B

$$\Delta V = 250\ mL$$

$$\Delta P = 5\ cm\ H_2O$$

$$C_T A = \frac{250\ mL}{5\ cm\ H_2O} = 50\ mL/cm\ H_2O,\ or\ 0.05\ L/cm\ H_2O$$

In this example, Patient A has a normal total compliance (100 mL/cm H_2O), normal ΔP (5 cm H_2O), and normal tidal volume (500 mL). Both patients have a normal inspiratory effort as demonstrated by the inspiratory pressure gradient (ΔP = 5 cm H_2O). Patient B, however, has a total compliance of only 50 mL/cm H_2O. This patient's lungs and thorax together are less "stretchable," and a normal ΔP (5 cm H_2O) results in a reduced tidal volume (250 mL). In other words, at the same level of effort (ΔP = 5 cm H_2O) Patient B has a much smaller tidal volume due to a reduction in compliance. In order for Patient B to achieve a normal tidal volume (i.e., 500 mL), the patient would have to double the inspiratory pressure gradient (i.e., ΔP = 10 cm H_2O), and this would require an increase in the work of breathing (WOB). This example illustrates the effect of reductions in compliance on tidal volume when the same level of inspiratory effort is present. To summarize:

1. *decreased* C → *decreased* volume at the same ΔP → lungs and/or thorax are "stiff" or less stretchable → *increased* ΔP (increased inspiratory effort) and *increased* WOB required to maintain the same volume.
2. *increased* C → *increased* volume at the same ΔP → lungs and/or thorax are more "stretchable" or more compliant → *decreased* ΔP (decreased inspiratory effort) and *decreased* WOB required to maintain the same volume.
3. $C_A > C_B$ → C_A is more compliant and less elastic → C_B is less compliant and more elastic.
4. $C_A < C_B$ → C_A is less compliant and more elastic → C_B is more compliant and less elastic.

As noted, total compliance represents the ability of the lungs to stretch within the thorax as a system. Total compliance can be further divided into lung compliance and thorax compliance. **Lung compliance (C_L)** represents the stretchability of the lung tissue. **Thoracic compliance** (also called **chest wall compliance**, or C_c) represents the stretchability of the thorax. **Total compliance (C_T)**, also called *total thoracic compliance*, represents the compliance of the lungs within the thoracic cage. Normal lung compliance is about 200 mL/cm H_2O:

$$C_L = \frac{\Delta V}{\Delta P} = \frac{500\ mL}{2.5\ cm\ H_2O} = \frac{200\ mL}{cm\ H_2O} = or \frac{0.2\ L}{cm\ H_2O}$$

Normal thoracic or chest wall compliance is also about 200 mL/cm H_2O:

$$C_c = \frac{\Delta V}{\Delta P} = \frac{500\ mL}{2.5\ cm\ H_2O} = \frac{200\ mL}{cm\ H_2O} = or \frac{0.2\ L}{cm\ H_2O}$$

Normal (static) total compliance, however, is only 100 mL/cm H_2O. This makes sense when one considers that the lungs by themselves are more stretchable than

CLINICAL FOCUS 7-1

Calculation of Dynamic and Static Compliance

It is relatively easy to calculate static (C_{ST}) and dynamic ($C_{dynamic}$) compliance on patients receiving mechanical ventilation in the volume-control mode:

$$C_{ST} = \frac{V_T}{P_{plateau} - P_{baseline}}$$

$$C_{dynamic} = \frac{V_T}{PIP - P_{baseline}}$$

where

V_T = Delivered tidal volume
$P_{plateau}$ = Plateau pressure measured after a 1-second inspiratory hold
PIP = Peak inspiratory pressure
$P_{baseline}$ = Baseline pressure (e.g., PEEP or CPAP)

Given a patient receiving mechanical ventilatory support in the volume-control mode with the following data collected, calculate static and dynamic compliance:

V_T: 600 mL
PIP: 35 cm H_2O
$P_{plateau}$: 28 cm H_2O
PEEP ($P_{baseline}$): 5 cm H_2O

Static compliance:

$$C_{ST} = \frac{V_T}{P_{plateau} - P_{baseline}}$$

$$C_{ST} = \frac{600}{(28 - 5)} = 26 \text{ mL/cm } H_2O$$

Dynamic compliance:

$$C_{dynamic} = \frac{V_T}{PIP - P_{baseline}}$$

$$C_{dynamic} = \frac{600}{(35 - 5)} = 20 \text{ mL/cm } H_2O$$

As would be expected, the patient's static compliance (26 mL/cm H_2O) is greater than the dynamic compliance (20 mL/cm H_2O). Dynamic compliance is measured while air is flowing and represents lung and chest wall compliance and airway resistance. In contrast, static compliance is measured under conditions of no flow. The difference between the measured static and dynamic compliance is due to airway resistance. Airway pressures during inspiration (i.e., PIP) are a reflection of the elastic (compliance) and nonelastic (resistance) forces opposing lung inflation. Specifically, the difference between PIP and $P_{plateau}$ for this patient is 7 cm H_2O (35 − 28 = 7). The difference is due to the resistance to gas flow (i.e., airway resistance). Airway resistance increases (and dynamic compliance decreases) with bronchospasm, mucosal edema, secretions, and artificial airways (e.g., endotracheal tubes).

law states that the tension developed when an elastic structure is stretched is proportional to the degree of deformation produced.[5,7,8] In other words, an elastic structure changes dimension in direct proportion to the amount of force applied. For a spring, one unit of force results in one unit of stretch within the spring's functional range. When applied to the lung, Hooke's law

suggests that each unit of pressure (i.e., force) applied to the lung causes a unit of volume to be added. Further, as lung volume increases, recoil forces also increase in a linear fashion, up to the elastic limit of the lung. If the elastic limit is exceeded, the lung is in danger of rupture or tear. This linear relationship between pressure and volume in the lung is generally true within the

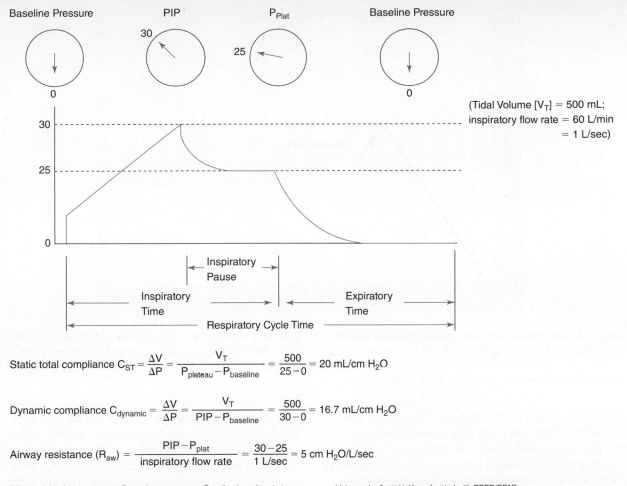

$$\text{Static total compliance } C_{ST} = \frac{\Delta V}{\Delta P} = \frac{V_T}{P_{plateau} - P_{baseline}} = \frac{500}{25 - 0} = 20 \text{ mL/cm } H_2O$$

$$\text{Dynamic compliance } C_{dynamic} = \frac{\Delta V}{\Delta P} = \frac{V_T}{PIP - P_{baseline}} = \frac{500}{30 - 0} = 16.7 \text{ mL/cm } H_2O$$

$$\text{Airway resistance } (R_{aw}) = \frac{PIP - P_{plat}}{\text{inspiratory flow rate}} = \frac{30 - 25}{1 \text{ L/sec}} = 5 \text{ cm } H_2O/L/sec$$

PIP - peak inspiratory pressure; P_{plat} - plateau pressure. Baseline is end expiratory pressure, which may be 0 cm H_2O or elevated with PEEP/CPAP

FIGURE 7-2 Pressure-time curves during volume-control mechanical ventilation with an inspiratory pause.

normal range of tidal breathing. At larger or smaller volumes the curve tends to be more sigmoid in shape. **Figure 7-3** illustrates an ideal pressure–volume curve following Hooke's law. **Figure 7-4** illustrates the actual relationship between pressure and volume in the lung when measured during expiration in a normal subject. **Figure 7-5** compares the effects of reduced compliance (e.g., fibrosis) and increased compliance (e.g., emphysema) on the pressure–volume curve.

In the laboratory, a pressure–volume curve can be generated for an excised cat lung to compare the differences between inspiration and expiration and to compare differences between an air-filled and fluid-filled lung (see **Figure 7-6**). Note in the figure that the inspiratory pressure–volume curve and expiratory pressure–volume curve are not the same in the air-filled lung. This is due to **hysteresis**, which refers to a physical manifestation that lags behind the application of force.[7,8] Hysteresis in the air-filled lung is caused by nonuniform opening of collapsed alveoli during early inflation, changes in surface tension as lung volume

changes, and the fact that it takes more pressure to open alveoli than to keep them open.[5,7,8] **Figure 7-6** also demonstrates the effects of filling the lung with liquid (e.g., saline). The liquid-filled lung is much more compliant, and hysteresis is minimal.[5,7,8] The differences between the air-filled and liquid-filled lung will be discussed below.

Surface Tension and the Lung

In normal subjects, surface tension is a major contributor to the lung's elastic recoil (i.e., lung elasticity).[7,8] **Surface tension** refers to the force of attraction between molecules of a fluid at the surface of an air–liquid interface. Surface tension causes water droplets to bead when placed on a waxed metal surface, such as a car. Surface tension can be directly experienced by jumping into a swimming pool in an awkward fashion resulting in a "belly flop." More specifically, surface tension can be thought of as the force required in overcoming intermolecular forces that attract like molecules of a fluid (e.g., water) to one another.

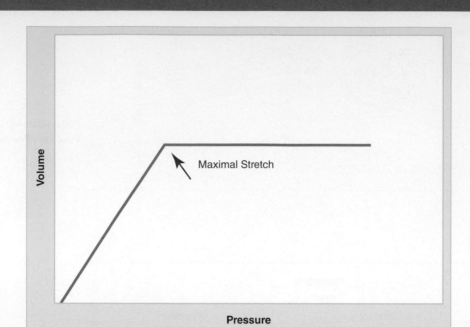

FIGURE 7-3 Ideal pressure—volume relationship in the lung. Ideally, the lung would behave much like a spring that obeys Hooke's law. As force increases (e.g., pressure), distance increases (e.g., volume) until the elastic limit (e.g., maximal stretch) is reached. In the normal lung, volume increases in a somewhat linear fashion as pressure increases in the normal tidal volume range. When the elastic limit is reached, additional pressure will result in no increase in volume.

Moisture (largely water) lines the 300 million alveoli. Because the alveoli are filled with air and lined with fluid, the surface water molecules attract each other, crowd together, and exert a force to contract the alveolar surface. If the alveoli were lined with pure water, they would collapse due to the high surface tension exerted.

Specifically, the law of Laplace tells us that if surface tension is constant, small spheres (e.g., alveoli) will require higher distending pressures to remain inflated than large ones.[7] In other words, if surface tension is the same for two different size alveoli, the pressure in the small alveolus will be greater than the pressure in the larger alveolus. If the two alveoli are connected, gas will flow from the smaller alveolus into the larger one.

To summarize, assuming surface tension to be constant, small alveoli will empty into larger ones because of the pressure differences. Fortunately, in normal subjects this does not occur due to the presence of a special

FIGURE 7-4 Normal compliance curve. An esophageal balloon is inserted to measure esophageal pressure, which provides and estimate of pleural pressure (P_{pl}). The subject inhales a full breath and then exhales slowly. At specific points during exhalation, the subject holds his or her breath with the glottis open. Lung volume and the corresponding esophageal pressure (as a surrogate for P_{pl}) are measured at each point during exhalation and an expiratory compliance curve is plotted.

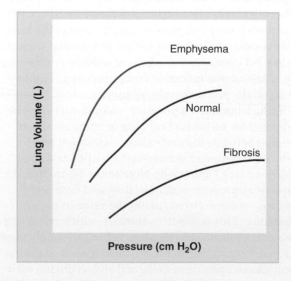

FIGURE 7-5 Compliance curves with disease.

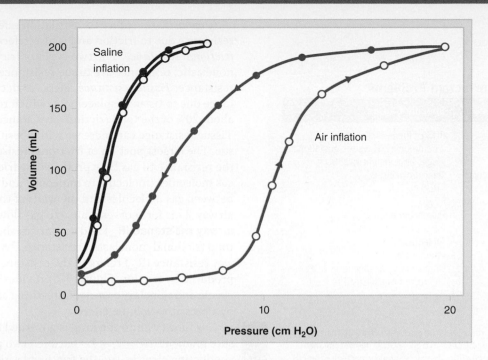

FIGURE 7-6 Inspiratory and expiratory pressure volume curves and hysteresis. Comparison of pressure–volume curves of air-filled and saline-filled lungs. Open circles, inflation; closed circles, deflation. Note that the saline-filled lung has a higher compliance and much less hysteresis than the air-filled lung.

Reproduced from: West JB. Mechanics of Breathing. In West JB: *Respiratory Physiology: The Essentials.* 9th ed. Philadelphia, PA: Wolters Kluwer Health/Lippincott Williams & Wilkins; 2008:101. http://www.lww.com/Product/9781609136406

surface active agent called **surfactant**. This substance was first postulated by the Swiss physiologist Dr. Kurt von Neergaard in 1929 when he compared pressure–volume curves of air-filled versus saline-filled cat lungs (see **Figure 7-6**).[7,8] The air-filled lung was more difficult to inflate, suggesting that there was something about the air–liquid interface in the alveoli that opposed lung inflation. It became clear that while only elastic forces opposed inflation of the saline-filled lung, the forces opposing inflation of the air-filled lung included both elastic forces and forces generated by the surface tension of the liquid film lining the lung. It has been subsequently shown that surface tension accounts for over half of the lung's elastic recoil.

Surfactant is secreted by Type II alveolar cells. Surfactant is made up of 90% polar phospholipids and 10% protein.[7] Dipalmitoyl phosphatidlycholine (DPPC; more commonly known as lecithin) is the phospholipid in surfactant primarily responsible for its surface tension–lowering properties.[7] Other phospholipids present in surfactant include sphingomyelin and phosphatidylglycerol. Surfactant acts by floating to the surface of the air–liquid interface in the alveoli, thus shielding the liquid below from contact with air and reducing surface tension. The effect of surfactant is variable, depending on alveolar size; there is greater surface-tension reduction for smaller alveoli. DPPC is normally present in the fetal lung at week 24 of gestation; DPPC levels continue to increase as the fetus progresses to term.

Infants born prematurely may have inadequate surfactant production and be at risk for the development of respiratory distress syndrome (RDS) of the neonate (surfactant deficiency disorder [SDD]; see also Chapter 16).* The lecithin-to-sphingomyelin ratio (L/S ratio) and phosphatidylglycerol concentrations in amniotic fluid are sometimes measured as predictors of fetal lung maturation.[7] Surfactant replacement therapy may be administered to preterm infants born with immature lungs. RDS of the neonate is more common in babies born at a gestational age < 30 weeks and low birth weight (< 1500 grams); risk of RDS declines with increasing gestational age. Genetic defects affecting surfactant metabolism have been identified that may account for about 10% of interstitial lung disease seen in children. For example, congenital pulmonary alveolar proteinosis is a genetic surfactant dysfunction disorder that causes diffuse lung disease.

A number of disease states and conditions can disrupt surfactant in adults. Disease states in which surfactant may be inactivated include pneumonia, pulmonary edema, ARDS, lung transplantation, and leakage of plasma proteins into the lung. Severe starvation may affect surfactant production, and surfactant dysfunction may occur with chronic lung disease (e.g.,

*Older terms used to describe RDS of the neonate include hyaline membrane disease (HMD) and infant respiratory distress syndrome (IRDS).

BOX 7-3

Causes of Surfactant Problems

General Causes	Specific Causes
Acidosis	RDS of the neonate: more
Hypoxia	common < 30 weeks gestational
Hyperoxia	age, birth weight < 1500 g
Pulmonary vascular	Near drowning
congestion	ARDS
	ECMO
	Pulmonary edema
	Pulmonary embolus
	Atelectasis
	Pneumonia
	Chronic lung disease (e.g. COPD,
	chronic bronchitis, CF)
	Asthma

RDS, respiratory distress syndrome; ARDS, acute respiratory distress syndrome; ECMO, extracorporeal membrane oxygenation; COPD, chronic obstructive pulmonary disease; CF, cystic fibrosis.

chronic bronchitis, chronic obstructive pulmonary disease [COPD], cystic fibrosis, asthma). Surfactant replacement therapy has been tried in the treatment of adult ARDS, but has not been shown to be effective.

To summarize, surfactant is synthesized in the lung from fatty acids and secreted by Type II alveolar cells, which are formed late in fetal life. Type II cells appear at about 22 to 26 weeks of gestation, but are not prominent until approximately week 34 (39 to 40 weeks of gestation is considered full term). Surfactant reduces surface tension in alveoli of all sizes, enabling small alveoli to remain inflated at low volumes. Surfactant stabilizes alveoli, improves compliance, and reduces the work of breathing. Surfactant also helps prevent pulmonary edema. Surfactant replacement therapy is used to treat neonatal RDS; it reduces the severity of disease by increasing lung compliance, reducing work of breathing, and decreasing the requirement for mechanical ventilatory support and oxygen therapy. **Box 7-3** lists causes of surfactant problems in infants and adults.

Resistance to Ventilation

Resistance to ventilation can be classified as elastic or nonelastic.[5,7] *Elastic resistance* and compliance are inversely related. As discussed previously, as compliance decreases, elastance (i.e., elastic resistance) increases. Normally, elastic resistance is much greater than nonelastic resistance. Causes of increased elastic resistance include decreased lung compliance and decreased thoracic compliance.

Nonelastic resistance to ventilation refers to the resistance due to friction and is also referred to as *frictional resistance*. The two types of frictional, or nonelastic, resistance are tissue resistance and airway resistance. *Tissue resistance* refers to frictional resistance due to tissue displacement, which represents about 20% of the total frictional resistance present.[5,7] Tissue resistance can increase with obesity and scar tissue. The largest portion of frictional resistance is due to the resistance to gas flow produced by friction between gas molecules (molecule to molecule) and the friction between gas molecules and the walls of the conducting airway. This form of resistance to gas flow is known as **airway resistance (R_{aw})** and comprises about 80% of the total frictional (nonelastic) resistance.[5,7] Simply put, airway resistance (R_{aw}) refers to the resistance to gas flow produced by friction. **Figure 7-7** provides an example of elastic and nonelastic work of breathing as illustrated by a pressure–volume curve.

Gas flow ($\dot{V}$) into the lung is governed by the pressure gradient ($\Delta P = P_1 - P_2$) between two points in the conducting airways and the frictional resistance to gas flow, which is mostly due to airway resistance (R_{aw}). Simply put, gas flow ($\dot{V}$) is equal to pressure (ΔP) over resistance (R_{aw}):

$$\dot{V} = \frac{\Delta P}{R_{aw}}$$

Rearranging this equation for airway resistance we have:

$$R_{aw} = \frac{\Delta P}{\dot{V}}$$

Airway Resistance

Airway resistance is typically reported in cm H_2O (pressure or ΔP) per liter per second (gas flow, or $\dot{V}$). Normal airway resistance in adults is about 1 to 2 cm H_2O/L/sec, though R_{aw} varies with lung volume and airway radius. For example, as lung volume increases, the radius of conducting airways increases and airway resistance decreases. It is also of interest to note that about 80% of total R_{aw} occurs in the upper and large airways, whereas less than 20% of R_{aw} is due to the small airways (diameter < 2 mm).[5,8] Gas flow in the small airways is normally smooth (i.e., laminar) and slow. This is because the very large number of small airways results in a very large total cross-sectional surface area that more than offsets the small radius of each airway. In contrast, airflow in the upper airways, trachea, and primary bronchi tends to be very turbulent. This is because the gas velocity is high and the total cross-sectional surface area for gas flow is small. It is also interesting to note that the upper airways (i.e., nose, pharynx, and larynx) contribute 25% to 40% of total airway resistance.[5,8] Consequently, endotracheal intubation adds resistance due to the relatively smaller

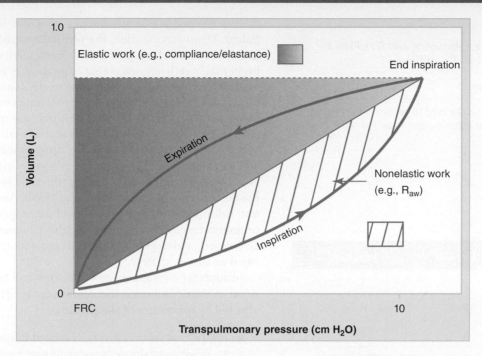

FIGURE 7-7 Pressure–volume curve and WOB. The area under the pressure–volume curve can be calculated to determine WOB. The shaded area represents the work to overcome elastic resistance to ventilation (e.g., compliance/elastance). The striped area represents the work to overcome the nonelastic resistance to ventilation (e.g., R_{aw}). WOB, work of breathing; R_{aw}, airway resistance.

diameter of the endotracheal tube while eliminating some resistance by bypassing the upper airway.

Laminar and Turbulent Flow

Airway resistance is affected by the nature of the gas flow in the lung. **Laminar flow** is smooth flow with little turbulence or eddy formation. Laminar flow is largely present in the distal small airways (i.e., bronchioles). Laminar flow is governed by Poiseuille's law, which describes the relationship among gas flow, pressure gradient, airway radius, gas viscosity, and length of the conducting tube:[5,7]

$$\dot{V} = \frac{\Delta P \pi r^4}{8nl}$$

where r = radius; l = length, n = gas viscosity, and $\dot{V}$ = flow.

Holding the length of the conducting tube and gas viscosity constant, Poiseuille's law can be simplified:

$$\dot{V} \approx \Delta P r^4$$

and

$$\Delta P \approx \frac{\dot{V}}{r^4}$$

Gas flow varies with r^4 of the airway. Thus, in the presence of laminar flow, a small change in airway radius (r) results in a large change in flow at the same driving pressure. If the radius of the conducting tube is decreased by half, the resistance to flow will increase

16-fold. By the same token, small changes in airway radius will require very large changes in the pressure gradient to maintain the same gas flow.

Poiseuille's law also illustrates the importance of gas viscosity when flow is laminar.[5,7] Helium–oxygen mixtures have a higher viscosity than air or oxygen, but lower density. Flow-volume loops generated following inhalation of a helium–oxygen gas mixture compared to those generated following inhalation of air demonstrate an increase in expiratory peak flow rates (i.e., upper airways) but no improvement in terminal gas flow (i.e., small airways) with helium mixtures. In the past, *helium isoflow studies* were used to try and differentiate between central and peripheral airway obstruction; however, these have not been shown to provide additional information beyond conventional flow-volume loops. Poiseuille's law illustrates that, at least theoretically, breathing helium–oxygen mixtures should have minimal benefits in terms of improving gas flow when flow is laminar, but may be beneficial when gas flow is turbulent.

Turbulent flow refers to gas flow that is rough and chaotic with a great deal of eddy formation. Turbulent gas flow occurs in the upper airways, larynx, trachea, and major bronchi.[5,7] Turbulence tends to increase as gas flow rate increases and decreases as gas flow rate decreases. Thus, high inspiratory gas flows tend to be more turbulent. With laminar flow, the pressure gradient and gas flow are directly proportional. Under conditions of laminar flow, an increase in pressure by a factor of two will approximately double gas flow.

TABLE 7-1
Relationship Between Pressure and Gas Flow for Laminar and Turbulent Conditions

Required Driving Pressure

The following equations can be used to determine the required driving pressure (ΔP) to achieve a given gas flow under laminar and turbulent conditions:

Laminar:

$$\Delta P = K\dot{V}$$

Turbulent:

$$\Delta P = K\dot{V}^2$$

Flow ($\dot{V}$)	Laminar	Turbulent
1	1	1
2	2	4
4	4	16
8	8	64
16	16	256

- To double gas flow under laminar conditions, increase pressure × 2.
- To double gas flow under turbulent conditions, increase pressure × 4.
- To increase gas flow 4-fold under turbulent conditions, increase pressure × 16.
- To increase gas flow 16-fold under turbulent conditions, increase pressure × 256.

In order to double gas flow under turbulent conditions, pressure may need to be increased fourfold. As noted, gas viscosity is relatively unimportant in the presence of turbulent flow. However, gas density becomes very important. In the presence of turbulent flow, breathing a helium–oxygen mixture may significantly increase flow. **Table 7-1** compares driving pressures and gas flow with laminar and turbulent flow.

Transitional flow refers to gas flow that combines aspects of laminar and turbulent flow.[5,7] Transitional flow occurs where airways branch, such as the bifurcation of the trachea and larger bronchi. Another name for transitional flow is *tracheobronchial flow*. The *Reynolds number* is a calculation that incorporates airway radius, velocity, gas density, gas viscosity, and gas velocity. The Reynolds number is designed to discriminate between laminar and turbulent flow. Reynolds number is greatest at the mouth, trachea, and primary bronchi and smallest in the terminal bronchioles. If Reynolds number exceeds 2000, turbulent gas flow is present.

Breath Sounds and Gas Flow

Breath sounds are affected by the nature of gas flow. Tracheal or bronchial breath sounds are heard over the trachea and primary bronchi where flow is turbulent. Upon auscultation, the resultant sounds are loud, coarse, and high pitched. A characteristic of bronchial breath sounds is that expiration is equal or louder than inspiration. Vesicular breath sounds are heard over peripheral areas of normal lungs where flow is laminar. Vesicular breath sounds are quiet, soft, and low-pitched. A characteristic of vesicular breath sounds is that expiration is diminished and less audible. With lung consolidation or pleural effusion, bronchial breath sounds may sometimes be heard over the periphery, and this is one of the physical examination findings associated with consolidative pneumonia or nonobstructive atelectasis (see also Chapter 5). Decreased or absent breath sounds indicate diminished or absent airflow.

In summary, resistance to ventilation can be classified as elastic or nonelastic. Nonelastic resistance is affected by the nature of the gas flow:[5,7,8]

- Elastic resistance is inversely related to compliance.
  - Elastic resistance is normally much greater than nonelastic resistance.
  - Elastic resistance increases with decreases in compliance.
- Nonelastic resistance is the frictional resistance.
  - Tissue resistance is due to friction between moving tissues in the thorax, which represents a small part of the total nonelastic resistance.
    - Normally, tissue resistance is about 20% of total frictional (nonelastic) resistance.
    - Obesity and fibrosis may increase tissue resistance.
  - Airway resistance (R_{aw}) makes up about 80% of total frictional (nonelastic) resistance.
    - 80% of R_{aw} is in the upper airways and large lower airways.
      - 25% to 40% of R_{aw} occurs in the nose, pharynx, and larynx.
      - R_{aw} of the upper airways can be up to up to one-half of the total during mouth breathing and up to two-thirds of the total during nasal breathing.
      - Endotracheal tubes (ET) bypass the upper airways, but introduce some additional resistance to gas flow due to the ET tube.
    - < 20% of R_{aw} is due to the small airways (< 2 mm).
  - Turbulent gas flow occurs mostly in the upper airways.
    - An increase in turbulence increases R_{aw}.
    - A decrease in turbulence decreases R_{aw}.
  - Laminar gas flow occurs in the small airways.
  - Transitional (tracheobronchial) flow occurs as large airways branch.

Box 7-4 provides examples of common causes of increased airway resistance. Of these, perhaps the

BOX 7-4

Causes of Increased Airway Resistance (R_{aw})

Upper airway obstruction
- Edema
  - Epiglottitis
  - Croup
  - Angioedema
- Upper airway tumor
- Foreign bodies

Lower airway disease
- Bronchospasm
- Mucosal edema
- Secretions

Asthma (may have a two- to three-fold increase in R_{aw} without symptoms)

Emphysema

Decreased lung volume

Artificial airways
- Endotracheal tubes
  - Decrease in tube diameter, increase in R_{aw}.
  - Increase in tube diameter, decrease in R_{aw}.
  - An endotracheal tube with a 9 mm internal diameter at 60 L/min inspiratory flow has a resistance of approximately 6 cmH_2O/L/sec.
- Tracheostomy tubes
  - Decrease in tube diameter, increase in R_{aw}.
  - Increase in tube diameter, decrease in R_{aw}.

Ventilator demand flow systems (e.g., demand valves)

Ventilator circuits

Increased inspiratory flow rates

---

most common are bronchospasm, mucosal edema, and increased secretions. Airway resistance may improve following treatment of bronchospasm and mucosal edema (e.g., bronchodilators and anti-inflammatory agents) and removal of airway secretions (e.g., cough, suctioning, bronchial hygiene, therapeutic bronchoscopy). Insertion of artificial airways (e.g., endotracheal or tracheostomy tubes) adds some additional airway resistance. For example, an endotracheal tube with a 9-mm internal diameter (ID) at a normal inspiratory flow rate of 60 L/min will impose approximately 6 cm H_2O/L/sec of additional airway resistance while at the same time eliminating a small amount of airway resistance by bypassing the upper airway. The net change, however, is an increase in R_{aw} for most patients following intubation.

Clinical Focus 7-2 provides an example of the calculation of airway resistance in patients receiving invasive mechanical ventilation and contrasts the effects of endotracheal tube size.

Work of Breathing

Work of breathing (WOB) refers to the work done by the ventilatory muscles to overcome elastic and nonelastic (i.e., resistive) forces opposing ventilation. Work is the product of force times distance. The units of work are kilogram × meter (kg × m) or joules (1 joule = 0.1 kg × m).[5,8] Pressure is the force per unit surface area (force/surface area), whereas volume is distance cubed (m^3 or cm^3). Thus, work of breathing can be calculated as the pressure change multiplied by the volume change ($\Delta P \times \Delta V$):

- Work = force × distance
- Work of breathing = $\Delta P \times \Delta V$
  - P is pressure (force per unit surface area).
  - Surface area is distance squared (often reported as cm^2).
  - V is volume (often recorded in cm^3, "ccs," or mL).
- Work of breathing = $\Delta P \times \Delta V$ = (Force/cm^2) × (cm^3) = Force × cm = Force × Distance

CLINICAL FOCUS 7-2

Calculation of Airway Resistance

In patients who have an artificial airway in place such as an endotracheal tube, the smaller the tube diameter, the greater the airway resistance (R_{aw}). Airway resistance can easily be calculated for patients receiving conventional volume-control mechanical ventilation via an endotracheal or tracheostomy tube:

$$R_{aw} = \frac{PIP - P_{plateau}}{\dot{V}}$$

where

R_{aw} = Airway resistance
PIP = Peak inspiratory pressure
$P_{plateau}$ = Plateau pressure obtained after a 1-second inspiratory pause or hold
$\dot{V}$ = Inspiratory flow rate in L/sec using a constant inspiratory flow pattern (e.g., square wave)

Given a patient with a 9.0-mm endotracheal tube in place and the following data, calculate airway resistance:

PIP: 36 cm H_2O
$P_{plateau}$: 30 cm H_2O
$\dot{V}$: 60 L/min = 1 L/sec

$$R_{aw} = \frac{PIP - P_{plateau}}{\dot{V}}$$

$$R_{aw} = \frac{36 - 30}{1} = 6 \text{ cm } H_2O/L/\text{ sec}$$

This example illustrates why it is always best to place an endotracheal tube with the largest diameter that can be inserted without difficulty or trauma. In the example, the patient has a fairly large endotracheal tube in place (9.0 mm), and the airway resistance is 6 cm H_2O/L/sec. Recall that normal airway resistance is approximately 1 to 2 cm H_2O/L/sec. Thus, even a relatively large endotracheal tube diameter may increase airway resistance up to six-fold.

Thus, when you factor in the units of measurement, $\Delta P \times \Delta V$ is equivalent to force × distance or work. WOB can be measured as pressure units (cm H_2O) × volume units (L) and then converted to kg × m or joules or normalized to volume (i.e., joules/L) where:

One joule = 0.1 kg × m
One joule per liter = joule/L = 0.1 kg × m/L

Normal WOB normalized to volume is approximately 0.05 kg × m/L, or about 0.5 joules per liter.

WOB is performed during inspiration; at rest expiration is normally passive and requires no work. About 65% of WOB is elastic work, and about 35% is frictional work (i.e., nonelastic work).[5,8] Of the frictional work performed, about 80% is to overcome airway resistance and about 20% is to overcome frictional tissue resistance.[5,8] To summarize:

- WOB is composed of work to overcome elastic and nonelastic (resistive) forces during breathing. Normally:
  - 65% of WOB is elastic work.
  - 35% of WOB is nonelastic (frictional) work.

- 80% of nonelastic (frictional) work is to overcome R_{aw}.
- 20% of nonelastic (frictional) work is to overcome tissue resistance.
- Normally, WOB occurs during inspiration and is the work performed by the diaphragm and accessory muscles of inspiration. Expiration is usually passive, requiring only the elastic recoil of the lung tissue (i.e., no work required). With severe obstructive lung disease, the accessory muscles of expiration may be engaged, increasing WOB during exhalation.

Measurement of Work of Breathing

Currently, it is not possible to directly measure total work of breathing of the thorax and lungs in spontaneously breathing patients. This is because the respiratory muscles lie within the thorax, and pleural or esophageal pressure measurements do not reflect the force required to distend the chest wall. With the help of an esophageal balloon, it is relatively easy to measure the WOB required to inflate the lungs alone (i.e., lung work).

TABLE 7-2
Normal Values for Work of Breathing (Lung Work)*

	Volume		Power	
	kg × m/L	joules/L	kg × m/min	joules/min
W_{total}	0.07–0.10	0.7–1.0	0.42–0.60	4.2–6.0
W_L	0.035–0.05	0.35–0.5	0.21–0.30	2.1–3.0
W_C	0.035–0.05	0.35–0.5	0.21–0.30	2.1–3.0

Work (W) = Force (F) × Distance (D) = kg × m or joules; 1 joule = 0.1 kg × m/L
Typically, work of breathing is reported as joules/L (normalized to volume) or joules/min (i.e., power). Power is work per unit time (e.g., joules/min).
*Total work of breathing (W_T) is lung work (W_L) plus thoracic or chest wall work (W_C):

$$W_T = W_L + W_C$$

Only W_L is measured clinically in spontaneously breathing patients. Total work can be estimated in relaxed or anesthetized subjects receiving mechanical ventilatory support.

Values for WOB are typically normalized to volume or time (i.e., joules/L or joules/min). Generally, spontaneous WOB should be in the range of 0.5 to 1.0 joules/L; prolonged values $\geq$ 1.5 joules/L may be excessive.[5,8,11,12] It also must be noted that WOB may not reflect patient effort, because a very large effort (ΔP) resulting in little or no volume change (ΔV) would be calculated as little or no work performed. Normal values for WOB are listed in **Table 7-2**.

Total Work of Breathing

It is relatively easy to measure total WOB provided during mechanical ventilation with positive pressure when the patient is making no effort to breathe (i.e., apnea). During mechanical ventilation, pressure–volume curves can be generated to compare total work and elastic and nonelastic work.[6,13] **Figure 7-7** illustrates a pressure–volume curve obtained during a positive pressure breath provided by a mechanical ventilator. Recall that WOB is simply $\Delta P \times \Delta V$. Thus, the area under the pressure–volume curve represents WOB. In the figure, the work performed to overcome elastic and nonelastic resistance to ventilation is identified.

Oxygen Cost of Breathing

Oxygen cost of breathing provides another method for assessing WOB.[5,8] To calculate oxygen cost of breathing, total oxygen consumption with full ventilatory support ($\dot{V}_{O_2}$ during apnea) is subtracted from total oxygen consumption during spontaneous breathing ($\dot{V}_{O_2}$ spontaneous). The difference represents the $\dot{V}_{O_2}$ of the ventilatory muscles:

$$O_2 \text{ cost of breathing} = \dot{V}_{O_2} \text{ spontaneous} - \dot{V}_{O_2} \text{ apnea}$$

Normal oxygen consumption of the ventilatory muscles in subjects at rest is about 12 mL/min or about 5% of total $\dot{V}_{O_2}$.[5,8] With hyperventilation, the oxygen cost of breathing can increase to 30%.[5,8] The oxygen cost of breathing increases with obstructive lung disease (e.g., COPD), restrictive disease (e.g., ARDS, pneumonia, pulmonary fibrosis), and obesity. For example, with severe COPD the oxygen cost of breathing may limit exercise and interfere with activities of daily living.

Ventilatory Pattern and Work of Breathing

Normally the body chooses a breathing pattern that minimizes WOB. Increased respiratory rate results in increased inspiratory gas flows and increased airway resistance (i.e., increased frictional or nonelastic resistance). Increased tidal volumes increase elastic work. Patients with increased airway resistance (e.g., obstructive lung disease) may breathe slowly to reduce work expended to overcome airway resistance. Patients with decreased lung compliance (e.g., pulmonary fibrosis) may reduce their tidal volume to reduce WOB. Patients with acute restrictive lung disease (e.g., ARDS or severe pneumonia) may exhibit rapid, shallow breathing, which is a common finding in these patients. COPD patients tend to breathe slowly to minimize frictional work and deeply because they have increased lung compliance and lower elastic recoil forces to overcome. With severe obstruction, COPD patients may expend energy to exhale by contracting their accessory muscles of expiration. Patients with severe pulmonary fibrosis, on the other hand, tend to employ a rapid, shallow breathing pattern due to the increase in elastic recoil (i.e., decreased compliance), which makes smaller tidal volumes less costly in terms of energy expenditure.

Muscular Weakness and Fatigue

Ventilatory muscle strength can be adversely affected by such things as electrolyte imbalance, malnutrition, starvation, or overall poor health.[9,10] A high ventilatory workload can fatigue the respiratory muscles. Fatigue occurs when the force-generating capacity of the diaphragm decreases. Fatigue may be reversible by allowing for muscle rest. Causes of an increased workload include an increased level of ventilation, reduced pulmonary or thoracic compliance, or increased airway resistance. Ventilatory muscle endurance requires adequate nutrient supply to the ventilatory muscles.

Diaphragmatic fatigue predisposes patients to acute ventilatory failure. For example, patients with severe COPD have a chronically elevated work of breathing, which may be just below the threshold that causes diaphragmatic fatigue. An acute exacerbation (e.g., infection) can push these patients into a fatigued state, resulting in acute hypercapnea, acidosis, and hypoxemia.[4,14]

Transdiaphragmatic Pressure

Measurement of transdiaphragmatic pressure (P_{di}) provides a method for evaluating the force-generating capacity of the diaphragm.[5,8] To measure the transdiaphragmatic pressure, a balloon catheter is placed in the esophagus and in the stomach to allow for measurement of esophageal (P_{es}) and gastric (P_g) pressures:

$$P_{di} = P_g - P_{es}$$

Although P_{di} provides a useful measure of the strength of the diaphragm, its use is primarily confined to experimental settings.

Clinical Signs of Impending Diaphragmatic Fatigue

Clinical findings associated with diaphragmatic fatigue include rapid, shallow breathing, inspiratory accessory muscle use (e.g., scalenes, sternomastoids, and pectoralis major muscle), intercostal retractions, and other signs of respiratory distress.[3,4,14–16] Specifically, an increased respiratory rate, respiratory alternations, and abdominal paradox are associated with diaphragmatic fatigue leading to acute ventilatory failure.[16] *Respiratory alternation* refers to the alternation between abdominal and rib cage breathing. *Abdominal paradox* refers to paradoxical inward abdominal motion during inspiration. Normally, as the chest rises the diaphragm descends and the chest and abdomen move synchronously. With abdominal paradox, the abdomen moves inward during inspiration (i.e., asynchronously). With ventilatory muscle fatigue, volumes will decline, the patient will begin to hypoventilate, and ventilatory failure will ensue. Clinical manifestations of ventilatory failure are described in more detail in the following section.

Ventilatory Failure

As previously noted, *acute ventilatory failure* can be defined as a sudden increase in $Paco_2$ with a corresponding decrease in pH, whereas *chronic ventilatory failure* refers to a chronically elevated $Paco_2$.[1,2] Because it can be life threatening, the respiratory care clinician must be able to promptly recognize acute ventilatory failure and take appropriate action, which may include mechanical ventilatory support. Factors associated with the development of ventilatory failure, including clinical manifestations, will be discussed next.

Ventilatory Capacity Versus Ventilatory Demand

Adequate ventilation requires that *ventilatory capacity* exceed *ventilatory demand* or *workload*. Adequate ventilatory capacity requires intact and functional respiratory control centers (i.e., brainstem, peripheral chemoreceptors, and central nervous system [CNS] drive) and sufficient ventilatory muscle strength and endurance.[1,3,17] Simply put, ventilatory capacity refers to the patient's ability to breathe, which includes maintaining an adequate spontaneous tidal volume and respiratory rate. Ventilatory demand or workload is determined by the level of ventilation required to remove CO_2, compliance and resistance of the respiratory system, and respiratory drive. When ventilatory demand exceeds ventilatory capacity, ventilatory failure ensues.

Ventilatory Demand or Workload

Ventilatory workload is the work the respiratory muscles must perform to provide adequate ventilation. Workload is determined by the level of ventilation required, compliance (lungs and thorax), and resistance to gas flow and any imposed work of breathing due to mechanical factors (e.g., endotracheal tubes).

Level of Ventilation Required

The level of ventilation required is determined by the **metabolic rate**, **respiratory drive**, and ventilatory dead space.[14,17] For example, fever, shivering, agitation, trauma, sepsis, and hypermetabolic states will increase CO_2 production (i.e., increase metabolic rate) and increase the level of ventilation required to remove CO_2. Metabolic acidosis, severe hypoxemia, pain, and anxiety will all increase respiratory drive and increase the level of ventilation. Pulmonary emboli and COPD may increase physiologic dead space and increase the level of ventilation required to remove CO_2. **Clinical Focus 7-3** provides an example of the effect of increased dead space on level of ventilation required to maintain a normal $Paco_2$.

Respiratory drive (also referred to as the *ventilatory drive*) refers to the stimulus to breathe provided by stimulation of the respiratory centers in the pons and medulla of the brainstem. Factors that increase respiratory drive include stimulation of the central chemoreceptors (e.g., decrease in cerebrospinal fluid [CSF] pH due to increase in Pco_2), peripheral chemoreceptors (e.g., $Pao_2 < 50$ mm Hg, decrease in pH, increase in $Paco_2$) or lung receptors (e.g., stimulation of J receptors, bronchial C receptors). Exercise, pain, anxiety, and low blood pressure can also stimulate ventilation.

CLINICAL FOCUS 7-3

The Effect of Increased Dead Space

A patient with normal physiologic dead space (V_D physiologic = 150 mL) develops an acute pulmonary embolus (PE) resulting in a sudden increase in physiologic dead space (V_D physiologic = 300 mL). Ventilatory values for this patient are listed below:

	Initial Values	Values Immediately Following PE	Values Following a Compensatory Increase in $\dot{V}_E$
V_T (mL)	500	500	600
f (breaths/min)	12	12	16
$\dot{V}_E$ (L/min)	6	6	9.6
$\dot{V}_A$ (L/min)	4.2	2.4	4.8
$Paco_2$ (mm Hg)	40	70	35

1. *Initially, what is the effect of a pulmonary embolus on $\dot{V}_A$ and $Paco_2$ if there is no increase in minute volume?*

Alveolar ventilation can be calculated as follows:

$$\dot{V}_A = (V_T - V_D) \times f$$

Initially, the patient's $\dot{V}_A$ is 4.2 L/min:

$$\dot{V}_A = (500 - 150) \times 12 = 4200 \text{ L/min, or } 4.2 \text{ L/min}$$

A PE will increase physiologic dead space. In this example, immediately following a PE physiologic dead space increases to 300 mL. If the tidal volume and respiratory rate remain constant, $\dot{V}_A$ will fall to 2.4 L/min:

$$\dot{V}_A = (V_T - V_D) \times f$$
$$\dot{V}_A = (500 - 300) \times 12 = 2400 \text{ L/min, or } 2.4 \text{ L/min}$$

This reduction in $\dot{V}_A$ would result in an immediate increase in $Paco_2$, which in this example rises to 70 mm Hg.

2. *What would be the expected compensatory response to a sudden increase in $Paco_2$ due to PE?*

The patient will attempt to increase minute volume to return $Paco_2$ to normal values. In this example, the patient increases his tidal volume, respiratory rate, and minute volume in order to lower $Paco_2$ to a normal value. This requires an increase in minute ventilation and an increase in WOB.

Most patients seen by the respiratory care clinician have a normal or increased ventilatory drive. Metabolic alkalosis, sleep deprivation, hypothyroidism, and CNS disorders can reduce ventilatory drive.[17] Respiratory drive can also be reduced or abolished by the administration of sedatives, narcotics, or neuromuscular blocking agents. Neuromuscular blocking agents can cause apnea and may also cause residual and prolonged ventilatory muscle weakness. Other factors that may reduce respiratory drive include decreased metabolic rate and very high carbon dioxide levels. The airway pressure a patient is able to generate during inspiration against a momentarily closed airway is sometimes used as a measure of ventilatory drive (i.e., pulmonary occlusion pressure, or PO.1). **Box 7-5** lists factors that may affect respiratory drive.

Compliance and Resistance

Decreases in compliance or increases in airway resistance will increase ventilatory workload. Lung compliance may be reduced because of atelectasis, pneumonia, pulmonary edema, or ARDS. Thoracic compliance may be reduced due to obesity, ascites, or abdominal

BOX 7-5

Respiratory Drive

Causes of Increased Respiratory Drive

- Hypoxemia
- Metabolic acidosis
- Increased CO_2 production (e.g., exercise, fever, agitation, seizures, shivering)
- Lung receptor stimulation (e.g., J receptors, bronchial C receptors)
- Pain
- Anxiety
- Decreased blood pressure

Causes of Decreased Respiratory Drive

- Alkalosis (e.g., respiratory alkalosis, metabolic alkalosis)
- CNS depressants (e.g., sedatives, tranquilizers, narcotics)
- Chronic elevation in $Paco_2$ (e.g., COPD patients with chronic CO_2 retention)
- Neurologic disease (brain injury)
- Neuromuscular disease
- Decreased metabolic rate
- Muscle fatigue
- Electrolyte disorders
- Pain

distension. Airway resistance (R_{aw}) is determined by the nature of the conducting airways. Causes of increased R_{aw} include bronchospasm, excessive secretions, and mucosal edema. R_{aw} may also increase due to insertion of artificial airways (e.g., endotracheal and tracheotomy tubes), ventilator circuits, mechanical demand flow systems, inappropriate ventilator flow and sensitivity settings, and auto-PEEP. Factors that may increase ventilatory workload are summarized in **Box 7-6**.

Ventilatory Capacity

Having an adequate ventilatory capacity requires functional conducting airways and gas exchange units, an intact and effective respiratory control system (i.e., CNS drive), and adequate ventilatory muscle strength and endurance.[17] Factors affecting ventilatory muscle strength or endurance include overall health, sex, muscle bulk, nutritional status, electrolytes (e.g., potassium, magnesium, phosphate, calcium), and neuromuscular transmission.[17] Increased ventilatory workloads (e.g., decreased compliance or increased airway resistance) can adversely affect ventilatory muscle strength and endurance.

Ventilatory Muscle Weakness

Ventilatory muscle strength is a function of energy supply versus energy demand.[17] Energy supply is determined by nutritional status, perfusion of the muscle tissue, and cell use, whereas energy demand is determined by the amount of work the respiratory muscles must perform.[17] Poor health, malnutrition, starvation, advanced age, and electrolyte disturbances can cause ventilatory muscle weakness.[2,17] High levels of ventilatory work over prolonged periods of time due to increased minute ventilation, decreased compliance, or increased airway resistance may also result in ventilatory muscle fatigue.[17] Once fatigue occurs, the respiratory muscles must be rested in order to recover, and this may require mechanical ventilatory support.[17] Major causes of ventilatory muscle weakness in the ICU include critical illness polyneuropathy, critical illness myopathy, and prolonged use of neuromuscular blocking agents.[17] Ventilatory muscle discoordination and atrophy can occur in patients receiving controlled mechanical ventilation for prolonged periods of time.[17]

Neuromuscular Disease

Neuromuscular disease can impair neuromuscular transmission to the ventilatory muscles. Ventilatory muscle weakness due to neuromuscular disease can be acute, chronic, intermittent, or progressive.[9] For example, Guillain-Barré syndrome typically (but not always) manifests as an acute, ascending muscle weakness that may rise to level of the diaphragm or above.[18] Myasthenia gravis and multiple sclerosis (MS) may cause relapsing, chronic respiratory muscle weakness, whereas muscle weakness due to amyotrophic lateral sclerosis (ALS) is chronic and relentlessly progressive.[9,18] Weakness of the diaphragm and accessory muscles of inspiration can result in reduced tidal volume accompanied by increased respiratory rate (i.e., rapid shallow breathing).[9] The resultant alveolar hypoventilation may require mechanical ventilatory support. It should be noted that significant respiratory muscle weakness may occur even when there is little or no peripheral muscle weakness; tests of respiratory muscle strength should be employed in the evaluation of neuromuscular disease patients.[9]

Risk Factors for Development of Ventilatory Failure

Many disease states or conditions predispose patients to the development of ventilatory failure. These include conditions that affect:[1-4]

- The conducting airways (e.g., upper airway obstruction, laryngeal edema [croup], epiglottitis, upper airway trauma [inhaled smoke, flames, or noxious gases])

BOX 7-6

Increased Ventilatory Workload

Factors that may increase ventilatory workload include:

- Increased Level of Ventilation
  - Hypoxia
    - Decreased F_{IO_2}
    - Low $\dot{V}/\dot{Q}$
    - Increased shunt
    - Diffusion defect
    - Decreased Pa_{O_2} and/or Sa_{O_2}
    - Decreased Ca_{O_2} ($\downarrow Pa_{O_2}$, $\downarrow Sa_{O_2}$, $\downarrow$ Hb, impaired Hb, anemia)
    - Decreased D_{O_2} ($\downarrow Ca_{O_2}$ $\downarrow$ cardiac output)
  - Metabolic acidosis
    - Diabetic ketoacidosis
    - Renal failure
    - Lactic acidosis (e.g., severe hypoxia, $\downarrow \dot{Q}_T$)
    - Other causes
  - Fear and anxiety
  - Pain
  - Pulmonary disease (e.g., lung receptor stimulation, hypoxemia)
  - Increased CO_2 production (e.g., fever, shivering, trauma, infection, sepsis)
  - Increased ventilatory dead space (e.g., COPD, pulmonary embolus)
  - Increased level of activity (e.g., agitation, fighting the ventilator, struggling against restraints)
- Decreased Respiratory System Conductance
  - Decreased system compliance
    - Decreased lung compliance (e.g., atelectasis, pneumonia, pulmonary edema, ARDS, pulmonary fibrosis)
    - Decreased thoracic (chest wall) compliance (e.g., thoracic deformity, obesity, ascites, pregnancy)
  - Increased resistance
    - Increased airway resistance (e.g., secretions, bronchospasm, mucosal edema)
    - Mechanical factors
      - Artificial airways (e.g., endotracheal tubes, tracheostomy tubes)
      - Ventilation equipment (e.g., ventilator circuits, demand flow systems, inappropriate ventilator flow or sensitivity settings)

$\dot{V}/\dot{Q}$ – ventilation perfusion ratio
Pa_{O_2} – arterial O_2 tension
Sa_{O_2} – arterial O_2 saturation
Ca_{O_2} – arterial O_2 content
Hb – hemoglobin
D_{O_2} – O_2 delivery
$\dot{Q}_T$ – Cardiac output

Data from: Shelledy DC. Discontinuing ventilatory support. In: Wilkins RL, Stoller JK, Kacmarek RM (eds.). *Egan's Fundamentals of Respiratory Care*, 9th ed. St. Louis, MO: Elsevier-Mosby; 2009: 1153–1184.

- Alveolar gas exchange (e.g., ARDS, pneumonia, pulmonary edema, aspiration, near drowning, pulmonary embolus)
- Respiratory drive (e.g., excessive sedation, anesthesia, narcotic or sedative drug overdose, head trauma, stroke)
- Neuromuscular function (e.g., Guillain-Barré, ALS, myasthenia gravis, multiple sclerosis, polio, spinal cord injury, botulism, tetanus)
- Mechanics of breathing (e.g., increased workload)
  - Decreased lung compliance (e.g., atelectasis, pneumonia, pulmonary edema, ARDS)

- Decreased thoracic compliance (e.g., obesity, ascites, thoracic deformity)
- Airway resistance (e.g., acute asthma exacerbation, COPD, airway inflammation, mucosal edema, bronchospasm)
- Thoracic or abdominal surgery (e.g., cardiac surgery)

■ Ventilatory demand or workload (e.g., increased respiratory drive due to hypoxia or acidosis, increased ventilatory requirements for CO_2 removal)

■ Ventilatory capacity (e.g., diaphragmatic fatigue, increased work of breathing)

In addition, patients with congestive heart failure (CHF), myocardial infarction (MI), shock, sepsis, severe burns, and trauma are at increased risk for development of acute ventilatory failure. Increased WOB resulting in respiratory muscle fatigue is associated with acute exacerbation of COPD, acute asthma exacerbation, and other acute pulmonary disease superimposed on chronic cardiopulmonary conditions.

Treatment of acute ventilatory failure may include initiation of mechanical ventilatory support. **Table 7-3** describes the most common diagnoses requiring mechanical ventilatory support. The most common diagnosis is acute respiratory failure, often due to postoperative complications, sepsis, pneumonia, heart failure, trauma, ARDS, or **aspiration**.[1,4] Other common diagnoses requiring mechanical ventilatory support include coma, acute exacerbation of COPD, and neuromuscular disease.[1,4]

Clinical Manifestations of Ventilatory Failure

The respiratory care clinician should be on the alert for the possibility of ventilatory failure in any patient with a diagnosis associated with increased risk. Often patients in acute ventilatory failure or those with impending ventilatory failure will display certain signs and symptoms. Clinical signs of ventilatory failure include increased heart rate, increased respiratory rate, accessory muscle use, intercostal retractions, nasal flaring (especially in infants and children), diaphoresis, and oxygen desaturation (i.e., decreased SpO_2).[1-3] Rapid shallow breathing is a common finding, often accompanied by anxiety and **dyspnea**.[1-3] Slowed or irregular respirations, reduced chest expansion, and hypotension are late findings associated with severe ventilatory failure.[1-3] Cyanosis is a variable finding that is dependent, in part, on the patient's hemoglobin level. For example, patients with anemia may be severely hypoxemic without showing cyanosis. CNS findings associated with ventilatory failure include restlessness, anxiety, headache, and altered mental status, followed by confusion, somnolence, and coma.

The term **eupnea** is used to describe normal spontaneous breathing, while a number of different terms are sometimes used to describe breathing disorders. **Hyperpnea** refers specifically to deep or rapid breathing, while **hypopnea** refers to shallow breathing, a reduced respiratory rate, or a transient decrease in airflow for more than 10 seconds (see Chapter 15). **Apnea** refers to the complete cessation of breathing (i.e., no spontaneous ventilation), while the term **dyspnea** is used to describe a patient's sensation of difficult breathing. Other terms sometimes employed to describe a patient's breathing include **orthopnea** (breathing is easier when upright), **trepopnea** (breathing is easier in a specific position), and **ponopnea** (painful breathing). Deep, gasping breathing with an inspiratory pause is referred to as **apneustic breathing**, while **Cheyne-Stokes breathing** and **Biot's breathing** refer to breathing patterns interrupted by periods of apnea. **Box 7-7** provides definitions of terms used to describe disorders of ventilation.

RC Insights

A respiratory rate > 30 breaths per minute with a tidal volume < 300 mL is associated with the need for mechanical ventilatory support.

Specific signs of increased work of breathing and possible ventilatory muscle fatigue include accessory muscle use, intercostal retractions, and asynchronous chest wall to diaphragm movement (i.e., abdominal paradox, the inward movement of the abdomen on inspiration). Often, hypoxemia develops first, accompanied by **hyperventilation** and respiratory alkalosis. As the severity of illness worsens, ventilatory muscle fatigue may set in and the patient may begin to hypoventilate. **Figure 7-8** illustrates this common progression, which if not interrupted may result in severe hypercapnea and respiratory acidosis.

RC Insights

Elevated respiratory rates (e.g., > 35 breaths per minute), severe distress with air hunger, diaphoresis, and accessory muscles use may signal impending respiratory arrest.

TABLE 7-3
Common Causes of Acute Respiratory Failure Requiring Mechanical Ventilation

Acute respiratory distress syndrome (ARDS)
Aspiration
Heart failure
Pneumonia
Postoperative respiratory failure
Sepsis
Trauma

BOX 7-7

Disorders of Ventilation

Eupnea: Normal, spontaneous breathing.

Apnea: Cessation of breathing.

Tachypnea: Increased respiratory frequency. Note that tachypnea is not synonymous with hyperventilation. In fact, many patients with tachypnea will exhibit rapid shallow breathing and elevation in $Paco_2$ (i.e., hypoventilation).

Bradypnea: Decreased respiratory frequency. This is fairly uncommon; sometimes seen with head injury, hypothermia, or drug overdose.

Hyperventilation: $Paco_2 < 35$ mm Hg; occurs with increased $\dot{V}_A$.

Hypoventilation: $Paco_2 > 45$ to 50 mm Hg; occurs with decreased $\dot{V}_A$.

Dyspnea: Conscious sensation of difficulty in breathing.

Orthopnea: Breathing is most comfortable in upright position.

Trepopnea: Breathing is more comfortable in a particular position.

Ponopnea: Painful breathing.

Biot's breathing: Tidal breathing interrupted by regular or irregular periods of apnea. Sometimes seen in meningitis or injuries to the pons.

Cheyne-Stokes breathing: Tidal breathing increases to a crescendo, then decreases, followed by a period of apnea. Fairly common; occurs with cerebral disorders.

Kussmaul breathing: Increased tidal volumes with increased frequency; occurs with diabetic ketoacidosis.

Apneustic breathing: Breathing that is stuck in inspiration; caused by surgical removal of the pons.

Hyperpnea: Increased depth of breathing or increased respiratory rate.

Hypopnea: abnormally shallow breathing, decreased rate or a transient decrease in airflow for more than 10 seconds which may be occur while the patient is asleep.

Oligopnea: Infrequent respirations (f = 6 to 10). Respirations may be shallow or abnormally deep. Occurs with increased intracranial pressure, head trauma, or cerebral hemorrhage.

Polypnea: Rapid breathing.

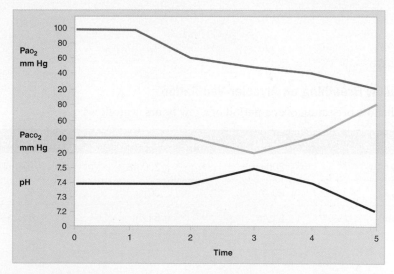

FIGURE 7-8 Progression of ventilatory failure. Ventilatory failure often progresses over time in a typical fashion, often in a few hours to days. Time 0 provides an example of a patient with normal Pao_2, $Paco_2$ and pH. Beginning at time 1, the patient's Pao_2 begins to decline due to lung disease. When the patient's Pao_2 decreases to about 60 mm Hg (Time 2), the patient begins to hyperventilate due to hypoxemia (i.e., the peripheral chemoreceptors are stimulated). As the patient's Pao_2 continues to decline (Times 2 to 3), the patient continues to hyperventilate and pH rises (i.e., acute respiratory alkalosis). By Time 3, the patient begins to tire and $Paco_2$ rises with a corresponding decrease in pH (Times 3 to 4). As the patient's condition worsens, Pao_2 continues to fall, $Paco_2$ continues to rise and an acute respiratory acidosis ensues (Times 4 to 5). At this time, the patient has developed acute ventilatory failure (Time 5).

Data from: Shelledy DC. Initiating and Adjusting Ventilatory Support. In: Wilkins RL, Stoller JK, Kacmarek RM. *Egan's Fundamentals of Respiratory Care.* 9th ed. St. Louis, MO: Elsevier-Mosby; 2009:1045-1090.

Certain physiologic variables can be measured at the bedside that may be predictive of the need for mechanical ventilatory support. These include spontaneous respiratory rate and tidal volume, rapid, shallow breathing index (RSBI), maximal inspiratory pressure (MIP), and vital capacity (VC). Generally speaking, a respiratory rate > 30 breaths per minute with a tidal volume < 300 mL is associated with the need for support. A calculated RSBI > 105 (f/V_T > 105) is also associated with the need for ventilatory support. MIP provides a measure of diaphragmatic strength, whereas VC measurement provides a measure of the patient's ability to cough and deep breathe. MIP > –20 to –30 cm H_2O and/or VC < 15 to 20 mL/kg IBW (or VC < 1.0 L) are associated with impeding or actual ventilatory failure. Arterial blood gases consistent with the need for mechanical ventilatory support include elevated $Paco_2$ with a corresponding respiratory acidosis (e.g., $Paco_2$ > 45 mm Hg and pH ≤ 7.25) and severe hypoxemia while receiving supplemental oxygen therapy (e.g., Pao_2 < 60 mm Hg and/or Sao_2 < 90% with Fio_2 > 0.40). **Clinical Focus 7-4** provides an example of the effect of rapid, shallow breathing on $Paco_2$.

> ### RC Insights
>
> MIP > –20 to –30 cm H_2O and/or VC < 15 to 20 mL/kg IBW (or VC < 1.0 L) are associated with impeding or actual ventilatory failure.

Respiratory muscle strength should be assessed in patients with neuromuscular disease.[9,10] Patients with respiratory muscle weakness will often show a restrictive pattern on pulmonary function testing (e.g., decreased VC, FVC, and TLC and normal FEV_1/FVC).[9] Vital capacity (VC and FVC) may decline by > 10% (compared to upright values) when the patient is placed in the supine position. Other measures of pulmonary function will also be reduced (e.g., decreased MVV, MIP, and MEP), though diffusion capacity (D_{LCO}) is often normal.[9] The ability to cough and deep breathe should also be assessed in these patients.[9]

> ### RC Insights
>
> Arterial blood gases consistent with the need for mechanical ventilatory support include elevated $Paco_2$ with a corresponding respiratory acidosis (e.g., $Paco_2$ > 45 mm Hg and pH ≤ 7.25).

Indications for Mechanical Ventilatory Support

The purpose of mechanical ventilatory support is to maintain tissue oxygenation and provide for removal of carbon dioxide. Mechanical ventilation supports or replaces the normal ventilatory pump; the goal is to ventilate, and the primary indication is inadequate or absent spontaneous breathing. The decision to initiate mechanical ventilation must considered carefully,

CLINICAL FOCUS 7-4

The Effect of Rapid, Shallow Breathing on Alveolar Ventilation

A patient develops rapid, shallow breathing over a period of a few hours, as follows:

	9 am	10 am	11 am	12 noon
V_T	500 mL	300 mL	200 mL	150 mL
f	12	20	30	40
$\dot{V}_E$	6 L/m	6 L/m	6 L/m	6 L/m
$\dot{V}_A$	4.2 L	3.0 L	1.5 L	0
$Paco_2$	40	58	115	—

What are the effects of these changes on $\dot{V}_E$, $\dot{V}_A$, and $Paco_2$?
This patient has experienced a decrease in V_T with a compensatory increase in respiratory rate. Although $\dot{V}_E$ is maintained, $\dot{V}_A$ is markedly decreased due to the increasing proportion of ventilation taken up by dead space ventilation. Thus, rapid shallow breathing represents tachypnea with hypoventilation.

because the potential complications and hazards can be life threatening.[1,14] Hazards include barotrauma, airway injury, infection, ventilator-associated pneumonia, pulmonary embolus, gastrointestinal bleeding, and increased morbidity and mortality.[11,17] In addition, catastrophic failures related to the ventilator or artificial airway can occur. Indications for mechanical ventilation can be summarized as follows:[1–3,14–19]

- Apnea
- Acute ventilatory failure
- Impending ventilatory failure
- Severe oxygenation problems (e.g., refractory hypoxemia)

Each of these indications will be discussed in the following sections.

Apnea

Failure to provide mechanical ventilatory support in the face of the complete cessation of breathing (i.e., apnea) will rapidly lead to death of the patient. **Apnea** may be caused by cardiac arrest, respiratory failure (e.g., severe hypoxemia), trauma (e.g., head injury, chest trauma, near drowning, electrical shock), drug overdose (e.g., sedatives, tranquilizers, narcotics), cervical spine injury (e.g., C2, C3, or C4 spinal cord damage), or neuromuscular disease. Administration of anesthesia or paralytic drugs may also cause apnea. In the absence of ventilatory support, apnea will be followed by cardiac arrest and brain death in minutes.

Acute Ventilatory Failure

As noted, acute ventilatory failure refers to a sudden increase in $Paco_2$ with a corresponding decrease in pH (i.e., acute respiratory acidosis). Though specific cut points should not be imposed, mechanical ventilation should be considered in patients with an acute increase in $Paco_2$ > 45 mm Hg resulting in a pH ≤ 7.25.

Impending Ventilatory Failure

Impending ventilatory failure refers to situations where ventilation may be adequate for the moment, but elevations in $Paco_2$ and a corresponding decline in pH are imminent.[1,2] Under these conditions, the decision to intubate and begin mechanical ventilation is sometimes made prior to the appearance of a significant respiratory acidosis. This decision is based on the clinical judgment that the patient will progress to acute ventilatory failure at some point in the near future. Mechanical ventilation is initiated prior to the appearance of significant hypercapnia.

One example where mechanical ventilation may be initiated prior to acute failure is impending respiratory arrest. Elevated respiratory rates (e.g., > 35 breaths per minute), severe distress with air hunger, diaphoresis, and accessory muscles use may signal impending respiratory arrest. Intubation and mechanical ventilation may be started in such patients prior to assessment by blood gases.

Another example in which the decision to intubate and begin mechanical ventilation prior the development of acute respiratory acidosis (i.e., acute ventilatory failure) is Guillain-Barré syndrome.[1,9] Development of Guillain-Barré may occur following a flulike illness in otherwise healthy adults. Guillain-Barré typically, though not always, causes ascending neuromuscular paralysis. A rapid decline in VC and MIP may occur as muscle weakness ascends from the legs towards the thorax. In about 20% to 30% of cases, this will result in respiratory muscle weakness requiring mechanical ventilatory support.[9] Patients are admitted to the hospital and monitored carefully for declines in VC and inspiratory muscle strength (e.g., MIP). When measures of pulmonary function decline to critical values, endotracheal intubation may be performed and mechanical ventilatory support begun. Critical values for institution of mechanical ventilation in patients with neuromuscular disease (especially acute illness) have been suggested:[9]

- VC declines to < 1 L (or < 15 to 20 mL/kg IBW or < 60% predicted).
  - Mechanical ventilation may also be indicated if there is a significant decrease in VC (e.g., > 30% to 50%) between the two most recent measures.
- MIP ≥ –30 cm H_2O (i.e., "less negative" than –30 cm H_2O).
- MEP < 40 cm H_2O.

Others have recommended that these measures be considered in combination. The so called "20-30-40 rule" suggests institution of mechanical ventilation when VC is < 20 mL/kg, MIP is > –30 cm H_2O, and MEP is < 40 cm H_2O.[9]

Thus, with impending ventilatory failure intubation may be performed and mechanical ventilation initiated prior to the onset of acute respiratory acidosis. Because the patient is not yet in acute distress, the process of establishing an artificial airway and beginning ventilatory support can proceed in an orderly and controlled fashion. The decision to proceed is based on the judgment of the clinician that ventilatory failure is impending and delay would place the patient at increased risk.

Severe Oxygenation Problems

Inadequate arterial oxygen levels (e.g., $Pao_2 < 60$ mm Hg, $Sao_2 < 90\%$) while breathing increased oxygen concentrations (e.g., $Fio_2 > 0.40$) signal severe oxygenation problems. Hypoxemia that fails to improve following conventional oxygen therapy is a severe oxygenation problem referred to as **refractory hypoxemia**. Specifically, an improvement in Pao_2 of < 5 mm Hg following an increase in Fio_2 of 0.10 (or more) indicates refractory hypoxemia. The Pao_2/Fio_2 ratio (P/F ratio) is sometimes used to assess the severity of hypoxemia. A P/F ratio ≤ 300 mm Hg is associated with oxygenation problems, whereas P/F ratios ≤ 200 mm Hg and ≤ 100 mm Hg are associated with moderate and severe oxygenation problems, respectively. Severe oxygenation problems are often seen in patients with ARDS or when other causes of significant intrapulmonary shunting are present (e.g., consolidative pneumonia, significant atelectasis, pulmonary edema; see also Chapter 6).

> ### RC Insights
>
> The "20-30-40 rule" suggests institution of mechanical ventilation when VC < 20 mL/kg, MIP > -30 cm H_2O, and MEP < 40 cm H_2O.

PEEP and CPAP

Severe oxygenation problems may require the use of positive end-expiratory pressure (PEEP), continuous positive airway pressure (CPAP), or the use of other techniques best applied using invasive mechanical ventilation. Modern mechanical ventilators allow for the application of PEEP, CPAP, prolonged inspiratory times, and elevated mean airway pressures, all of which may improve oxygenation in patients with severe oxygenation problems. PEEP is generally indicated when $PaO_2 < 60$ mm Hg on an $Fio_2 > 0.40$.[1,19] PEEP is applied during expiration following pressure or volume-controlled inspiration provided by a mechanical ventilator. CPAP is defined as spontaneous breathing with an elevated baseline pressure. Both PEEP and CPAP are thought to improve oxygenation by increasing FRC, "holding small airways open" and preventing end-expiratory alveolar collapse.[19]

> ### RC Insights
>
> An improvement in Pao_2 of < 5 mm Hg following an increase in Fio_2 of 0.10 (or more) indicates refractory hypoxemia.

Increased WOB is common in patients with severe oxygenation problems, often due to decreased lung compliance (e.g., severe pneumonia, ARDS). Although some patients with refractory hypoxemia are able to adequately breathe on their own for a while, they often tire and hypoventilation ensues. Because of this eventuality, some clinicians may choose to begin mechanical ventilatory support early. Early initiation of mechanical ventilation allows for the use of PEEP or CPAP, pressure support, pressure control, or other techniques and introduces the sophisticated alarm and monitoring systems incorporated in modern critical care ventilators.

The indications for CPAP include refractory hypoxemia in the presence of adequate spontaneous ventilation. CPAP improves oxygenation and may reduce WOB. Although CPAP assumes that spontaneous breathing is present, it is most commonly applied using a conventional mechanical ventilator in the "spontaneous" mode. CPAP may also be applied using a spontaneous-breathing apparatus and face mask. It should be noted that CPAP by face mask may not be effective in avoiding intubation or improving outcomes in patients with acute lung injury and hypoxemia, even if CO_2 levels are not elevated.[1]

To summarize, the four primary indications for initiation of mechanical ventilatory support are apnea, acute ventilatory failure, impending ventilatory failure, and severe oxygenation problems. The most common diagnosis requiring mechanical ventilatory support is acute respiratory failure. Other common diagnoses include acute exacerbation of COPD, coma, and neuromuscular disease. Clinical manifestations of respiratory failure include respiratory distress, dyspnea, accessory muscle use, retractions, and increased respiratory rate (often with rapid, shallow breathing). Early cardiac signs of distress include tachycardia and other arrhythmias; bradycardia is an ominous finding. Initially, patients may be restless and anxious, followed by confusion, somnolence, and coma. Physiologic measures associated with ventilatory failure and the need for mechanical ventilatory support include elevated respiratory rate (f > 30 breaths/min); spontaneous $V_T < 300$ mL; RSBI (V_T/f) > 105; VC < 15 to 20 mL/kg or 1.0 L; and MIP > -30 mm Hg. Arterial blood gas analysis will allow for identification of severe oxygenation problems (e.g., $Pao_2 < 60$ mm Hg [$Sao_2 < 90\%$] and $Fio_2 > 0.40$) and the development of acute respiratory acidosis (e.g., $Paco_2 > 45$ and pH ≤ 7.25).

> ### RC Insights
>
> A P/F ratio ≤ 300 mm Hg is associated with oxygenation problems. P/F ratios ≤ 200 mm Hg and ≤ 100 mm Hg are associated with moderate and severe oxygenation problems, respectively.

Ventilator Discontinuance

The process of removing mechanical ventilatory support is termed **ventilator discontinuation**. Patients receiving mechanical ventilatory support should have that support removed as quickly and safely as possible in order to reduce the risks and complications associated with mechanical ventilation. The primary criterion for discontinuing ventilatory support is the *improvement or reversal of the disease state or condition that required the need for mechanical ventilation.*[17,20] Once the problem requiring support is resolved, most patients can be quickly removed from the ventilator. Some patients, however, may require a structured discontinuation process referred to as **ventilator weaning**. Weaning is the process of gradually reducing mechanical ventilatory support and allowing the patient to assume a greater proportion of the required ventilation in an incremental fashion.[17,20] The need for a gradual reduction in the level of ventilatory support provided is limited to a small number of patients.

RC Insights

Patients who have only been receiving mechanical ventilation for brief periods of time (i.e., < 72 hours) can often be quickly removed from the ventilator when their primary problem has resolved.

Success with ventilator discontinuation is dependent on the patient's oxygenation status, cardiovascular function, and the relationship between ventilatory workload and ventilatory capacity.[17,20] Some patients may be ventilator dependent, or "unweanable." Ventilator dependence most commonly occurs when ventilatory demand or workload continues to exceed ventilatory capacity. Other factors that may contribute to ventilator dependence include oxygenation problems (e.g., hypoxemia, poor tissue oxygen delivery), cardiac problems (e.g., myocardial ischemia, arrhythmias, low cardiac output, cardiovascular instability), neurologic problems (e.g., decreased CNS drive to breathe, impaired nerve transmission), or psychological issues (e.g., anxiety, stress, depression, sleep deprivation).[17,20] **Box 7-8** summarizes factors contributing to ventilator dependence.

Patient Assessment

A careful patient assessment is required in order to determine when patients can be safely removed from mechanical ventilation and to determine the methods that will be used for ventilator discontinuance. As noted, mechanical ventilation is hazardous, and unnecessary delays in ventilator discontinuance may increase the frequency of complications.[17] However, premature termination of mechanical ventilatory support may result in acute hypoventilation, compromise of the patient's cardiovascular status, and difficulty reestablishing the artificial airway.[17]

Patients who have only been receiving mechanical ventilation for brief periods of time (i.e., < 72 hours) can often be quickly removed from the ventilator when their primary problem has resolved. Others may require a more structured weaning process. In order to assess a patient's readiness for ventilator discontinuance, the respiratory care clinician should:[17,20]

1. Determine if the disease state or condition requiring mechanical ventilatory support has been resolved or is significantly improved.
2. Ensure that the patient's oxygenation and acid-base status are adequate.
   a. $Pao_2/Fio_2 \geq 150$ mm Hg or
   b. $Pao_2 \geq 60$ mm Hg and/or $Sao_2 \geq 90\%$ and $Fio_2 \leq 0.40$ and PEEP ≤ 5 cm H_2O
   c. pH > 7.25
3. Ensure that the patient is medically and hemodynamically stable.
   a. Adequate blood pressure (systolic BP > 90 but < 180 mm Hg)
   b. Low dose or no vasopressors needed to maintain BP
   c. Absence of myocardial ischemia
   d. Adequate hemoglobin levels (≥ 7 g/dL)
   e. Absence of fever
4. Ensure that the patient can breathe spontaneously and has adequate CNS drive to breathe. Ideally, the patient will be awake and alert or easily arouseable.

Physical Assessment

Physical assessment techniques can be very helpful in prediction of weaning success. For example, the presence of tachypnea ($f \geq 30$ breaths/min) is a sensitive marker of respiratory distress.[17] Irregular or asynchronous breathing, periods of apnea, or rapid, shallow breathing suggest that difficulty with weaning may be encountered.[17] Palpable scalene muscle use during inspiration suggests an increased inspiratory WOB, whereas palpable abdominal muscle tensing during expiration suggests increased expiratory work associated with obstruction.[17] Ventilator to patient breathing dyssynchrony as assessed by review of ventilator graphics is also associated with poor weaning outcomes (see Chapter 14).

RC Insights

Tachypnea ($f \geq 30$ breaths/min) is a sensitive marker of respiratory distress.

BOX 7-8

Ventilator Dependence

The following factors contribute to ventilator dependence:

- Ventilatory Factors
  - Workload exceeds capacity
  - Decreased system compliance (e.g., decreased lung compliance or decreased thoracic [chest wall] compliance) increases workload
  - Increased airway resistance (e.g., bronchospasm, mucosal edema, secretions, artificial airways) increases workload
  - Increased pulmonary dead space (e.g., pulmonary embolus, COPD) requires increased ventilation and increased workload
  - Ventilatory muscle weakness or fatigue decreases ventilatory capacity
- Oxygenation Problems
  - Decreased $\dot{V}/\dot{Q}$
  - Increased shunt
  - Diffusion problems
  - Hypoventilation
  - Decreased O_2 delivery ($\downarrow$Hb, $\downarrow$Cao_2, $\downarrow \dot{Q}_T$)
- Cardiovascular Problems
  - Myocardial ischemia
  - Myocardial infarction
  - Arrhythmias
  - Coronary artery disease (CAD)
  - Congestive heart failure (CHF)
  - Hypotension
  - Hemodynamic instability
- Neurologic Problems
  - Abnormal central respiratory drive (e.g., increased drive to breathe, decreased drive to breathe)
  - Decreased nerve transmission (e.g., tetanus, botulism, neuromuscular blocking agents)
- Psychological Factors
  - Fear and anxiety
  - Confusion
  - Altered mental status
  - Psychological depression
  - CNS depression (e.g., sedatives, narcotics, brain injury)
- Nutritional Status
- Comorbidities
- Mechanical Factors
  - Inappropriate ventilator settings
  - Ventilator circuits
  - Demand flow systems
  - Inadequate ventilator inspiratory flow rate
  - Inappropriate ventilator trigger sensitivity

Data from: Shelledy DC. Discontinuing ventilatory support. In: Wilkins RL, Stoller JK, Kacmarek RM (eds.). *Egan's Fundamentals of Respiratory Care*, 9th ed. St. Louis, MO: Elsevier-Mosby; 2009: 1153–1184.

Assessment of Medical Condition

Assessment of oxygenation, acid-base balance, metabolic factors, renal function, electrolytes, cardiovascular function, and CNS function should be completed prior to attempting ventilator discontinuance. Poor oxygenation is associated with weaning failure, and arterial blood gas analysis, pulse oximetry, and calculation of the Pao_2/Fio_2 ratio should be completed and reviewed. Blood gases may identify acid-base abnormalities such as metabolic acidosis that will increase ventilatory drive and may make weaning more difficult. Patients with metabolic alkalosis, in contrast, may have a reduced drive to breathe. This may occur in patients who have been mechanically hyperventilated for several days. The patient's overall medical condition, oxygenation, ventilation, and cardiovascular status should be optimized prior to ventilator discontinuance.[17]

Respiratory Muscle Strength

Respiratory muscle strength is dependent, in part, on adequate nutrition. Malnutrition is a complication of critical illness, and hypermetabolic states may occur. Nutritional issues should be reviewed, such as nutritional support provided (e.g., parenteral or enteral), formula composition (e.g., carbohydrates, amino acids, fat, vitamins, and minerals), liver function, and blood glucose levels. For example, excessive carbohydrate feeding can increase CO_2 production. Fever, sepsis, shivering, seizures, or agitation can all increase metabolic rate, CO_2 production, and oxygen demand. Renal function should be assessed, and urine output should be appropriate (≥ 0.5 mL/kg/hr). There should be no inappropriate weight gain or peripheral edema associated with fluid retention. Fluid overload can lead to congestive heart failure, pulmonary edema, and oxygenation problems. Electrolytes should be reviewed, because electrolyte disorders may impair ventilatory muscle function.[17]

Cardiovascular Function

Cardiovascular function should be adequate to maintain tissue oxygen delivery. Heart rate and blood pressure should be in the normal range, and tachycardia, bradycardia, hypotension, or severe hypertension should be evaluated carefully. The electrocardiogram (ECG) should be reviewed for the presence of arrhythmia. If available, cardiac output and cardiac index values should be reviewed, as well as pulmonary artery pressures. Myocardial ischemia, cardiovascular instability, and left ventricular dysfunction are all associated with poor weaning outcomes.[17,20]

Central Nervous System

CNS function should be assessed to ensure a stable and adequate ventilatory drive, protection of the airway (e.g., gag and swallow reflex), and secretion clearance.[17] The patient should be alert, responsive, and able to follow instructions. Patients with reduced levels of consciousness are at increased risk for **upper airway obstruction**, aspiration, and secretion retention following extubation. Sedation, narcotic drugs, neuromuscular blocking agents, brainstem strokes, and electrolyte disturbances may impair neurologic control of ventilation.[17] If possible, CNS depressants should be discontinued prior to weaning and extubation. Daily cessation of sedative medications may improve weaning success.

Psychological Factors

Anxiety, depression, and motivation can affect weaning success. Patients who receive mechanical ventilation for extended periods of time may be extremely anxious regarding the prospect of having the ventilator removed. Frequent and supportive communication to the patient and patient's family can be helpful in reducing fear, anxiety, and stress.[21]

Factors that should be optimized prior to ventilator discontinuance are summarized in **Box 7-9**.

Airway Assessment

Although not the same, the decision to discontinue mechanical ventilation and the decision to extubate are closely linked. The ability of the patient to maintain an adequate natural airway following extubation must be assessed, because inability to protect the natural airway is a contraindication to extubation.[17] Measures of weaning readiness are not predictive of airway patency nor the need for airway protection.[17]

Artificial airways may increase airway resistance and imposed work of breathing, especially at high spontaneous minute volumes and when using small internal diameter (ID) endotracheal tubes (i.e., ID < 7 mm in adults).[17] Airway resistance can also increase dramatically if the endotracheal tube becomes partially occluded by dried secretions; adequate humidification should be provided. The presence of an endotracheal tube may cause reflex bronchoconstriction, and bronchodilator therapy may be justified in intubated patients.[17] Any imposed work of breathing (WOB_I) due to the endotracheal tube will be eliminated following extubation. Pressure support ventilation (PSV) or automatic tube compensation (ATC) provided during weaning may help alleviate WOB_I, and the use of low-level PSV (e.g., PSV of 5 to 8 cm H_2O) or ATC during weaning trials has become standard practice at many institutions.

BOX 7-9

Factors to Optimize Prior to Ventilator Discontinuance

1. Ensure adequate oxygenation (i.e., Pao_2, Spo_2, Sao_2, Cao_2, Do_2).
   a. Treat acute pulmonary disease (e.g., infection, pneumonia, atelectasis).
   b. Hemoglobin (treat anemia if present).
2. Ensure adequate ventilation.
   a. Provide adequate humidification.
   b. Ensure secretion clearance by providing bronchial hygiene (e.g., suctioning, turning, chest physiotherapy).
   c. Provide bronchodilator therapy to treat or prevent present bronchospasm.
   d. Avoid artificially hyperventilating the patient and creating a respiratory alkalosis.
   e. Reduce imposed work of breathing (provide adequate ventilator inspiratory flow rate and trigger sensitivity).
   f. Rest ventilatory muscles to avoid respiratory muscle fatigue or atrophy.
3. Assess acid-base balance and electrolytes.
   a. Treat metabolic acidosis (e.g., kidney failure, lactic acidosis, ketoacidosis).
   b. Treat metabolic alkalosis (e.g., treat low potassium, low chloride, nasogastric tube HCI loss, vomiting).
   c. Treat low phosphate or magnesium and any other electrolyte disorders.
4. Assess cardiovascular status.
   a. Maintain blood pressure and cardiac output.
   b. Assess for myocardial ischemia.
   c. Treat arrhythmias, if present.
   d. Optimize left ventricular function.
5. Assess renal function.
   a. Assess kidney function and fluid balance.
6. Treat fever, infection, or sepsis.
7. Minimize pain without oversedation.
8. Avoid sleep deprivation.
9. Increase exercise tolerance (up in chair, if possible).
10. Review medications that may affect ventilation.
    a. Narcotics, sedatives, tranquilizers, hypnotics.
    b. Aminoglycosides.
    c. Neuromuscular blocking agents.
11. Assess psychological status.
    a. Level of consciousness (delirium, coma).
    b. Agitation, anxiety.
    c. Motivation.
12. Assess for possible hypothyroidism.
13. Consider nutritional factors.
    a. Avoid overfeeding (increases CO_2 production).
    b. Adjust for malnutrition, protein loss.
    c. Consider high-fat, low-carbohydrate diet to minimize CO_2 production.
14. Assess gastrointestinal or abdominal factors.
    a. Bleeding or obstruction.
    b. Abdominal distension, ascites.
15. Optimize procedural factors.
    a. Time of day (avoid evenings, nights, shift change).
    b. Ensure adequate staffing.
    c. Avoid interruptions and disruptions.

16. Review technical factors.
   a. Compensate for endotracheal tube resistance (e.g., pressure support [PSV] or automatic tube compensation [ATC]).
   b. Assess intrinsic PEEP and use of PEEP/CPAP to "balance" intrinsic PEEP.

Data from: Shelledy DC. Discontinuing ventilatory support. In: Wilkins RL, Stoller JK, Kacmarek RM (eds.). *Egan's Fundamentals of Respiratory Care*, 9th ed. St. Louis, MO: Elsevier-Mosby; 2009: 1153–1184.

Some evidence suggests that tracheostomy tubes may reduce the work of breathing as compared to endotracheal tubes.[17] Tracheostomy tube placement may also reduce anatomic dead space, which, in theory, may be beneficial in borderline patients.[17]

The decision to extubate should be based on an objective review of specific criteria. These include adequate oxygenation and ventilation during spontaneous breathing, no anticipated need for continued mechanical ventilation, absence of upper airway obstruction, minimal risk of aspiration, and adequate pulmonary secretion clearance. Compression of the tissue of the larynx by the endotracheal tube may cause laryngeal edema, which can result in partial or complete airway obstruction following extubation. The potential for airway obstruction following extubation may be assessed by performance of a **cuff-leak test**, though the predictive value of this test has not been well established. Hoarseness and sore throat are common complaints following extubation, and patients should be advised that these symptoms may occur.[17] Patients may also experience mild to severe stridor, which may be managed by use of a cool aerosol with supplemental oxygen by mask, nebulized racemic epinephrine (0.5 mL of 2.25% racemic epinephrine in 3 mL of normal saline),

or nebulized dexamethasone (1 mg in 4 mL normal saline). If stridor is present, the patient should be carefully monitored and steps in preparation for possible reintubation should be taken. It should also be noted that glottic sensation and function may be impaired in patients who have been intubated for more than 6 days, and these patients may be at risk of aspiration.[17] **Box 7-10** describes the cuff-leak test for laryngeal edema. **Box 7-11** reviews the criteria to consider prior to extubation.

Most patients will be extubated shortly following ventilator discontinuance. Some patients, however, require continued intubation to protect the airway following successful discontinuance of ventilatory support. Tracheotomy should be considered in patients requiring an artificial airway for prolonged periods of time. Tracheostomies are generally well tolerated, improve patient comfort, improve access to secretions (e.g., suctioning), decrease airway resistance, enhance mobility, and may allow the patient to eat and speak.[17]

Occasionally, mechanical ventilation is discontinued and the patient's ventilatory status deteriorates. In such cases, if the patient is able to maintain a patent natural airway, a trial of noninvasive positive pressure ventilation (NPPV) may be considered.

BOX 7-10

Cuff-Leak Test

Prior to extubation, a cuff-leak test may be performed in an attempt to ensure that laryngeal edema is not present. To perform a cuff-leak test, the respiratory care clinician should:

1. Assess the patient to ensure that he or she can adequately breathe without mechanical ventilatory support.
2. Suction the patient's mouth and airway.
3. Deflate the endotracheal tube cuff.
4. Briefly occlude the endotracheal tube and assess ventilation.
5. Suspect laryngeal edema if the patient is unable to breathe around the occluded endotracheal tube with the cuff deflated.

Data from: Shelledy DC. Discontinuing ventilatory support. In: Wilkins RL, Stoller JK, Kacmarek RM (eds.). *Egan's Fundamentals of Respiratory Care*. 9th ed. St. Louis, MO: Elsevier-Mosby; 2009: 1153–1184; Sharar SS. Weaning and extubation are not the same. *Respir Care.* 1995;40:239.

BOX 7-11

Extubation Criteria*

1. Ensure that the patient does not require continued mechanical ventilatory support.
   a. Indications for mechanical ventilation have resolved (or improved significantly).
   b. Procedures requiring intubation (e.g., general surgery) are *not* planned.
2. Ensure that adequate oxygenation can be achieved using conventional oxygen therapy (e.g., face mask, air-entrainment device, or nasal cannula).
3. Ensure that adequate spontaneous ventilation is present.
   a. Spontaneous V_T, f, and $\dot{V}_E$ are adequate.
   b. Ventilatory pattern is stable.
   c. Rapid, shallow breathing is *not* present.
   d. Minute volume is *not* abnormally elevated.
   e. Respiratory distress is *not* present (e.g., dyspnea, tachypnea, fatigue, diaphoresis, accessory muscle use, intercostal retractions, abdominal paradox).
4. Ventilator weaning indices are positive.
   a. Reversal or improvement of the problem requiring ventilatory support.
   b. Adequate oxygenation is present.
   c. Hemodynamic stability.
   d. No evidence of myocardial ischemia.
   e. pH > 7.25.
   f. $f/V_T \leq 105$.
   g. MIP < −20 to −30 cm H_2O.
5. Upper airway obstruction or airway compromise is unlikely.
   a. Adequate level of consciousness.
      - Patient is awake and alert.
      - Patient is *not* unconscious or obtunded.
      - Neuromuscular function is good.
   b. Cuff-leak test passed.
   c. Oral and upper airway anatomy is normal.
   d. Gag reflex is present.
   e. Minimal risk of aspiration.
   f. Cough adequate to clear secretions.
   g. Gastric contents are minimized by discontinuation of tube feedings for at least 4 hours before extubation.

*Many patients who do not meet specific criteria may be successfully extubated.

Data from: Shelledy DC. Discontinuing ventilatory support. In: Wilkins RL, Stoller JK, Kacmarek RM (eds.). *Egan's Fundamentals of Respiratory Care.* 9th ed. St. Louis, MO: Elsevier-Mosby; 2009: 1153–1184; Sharar SS. Weaning and extubation are not the same. *Respir Care.* 1995;40:239.

Readiness Testing

Techniques for predicting when patients are ready for ventilator discontinuation are referred to as *readiness testing.*[11] Clinical judgment alone has been shown to be a poor predictor of success, and a number of more specific indicators have been suggested.[11,17] Patients receiving mechanical ventilation should have their readiness for ventilator discontinuance assessed daily.

Weaning Indices

A number of weaning indices have been suggested. Unfortunately, the predictive power of any single index is minimal. That said, the respiratory care clinician should be aware of each indicator and values that have been recommended in order to predict weaning success:

- *Measures of oxygenation*: Specific measures of oxygenation when used alone tend to be poor predictors of weaning success. However, clinicians must assess adequacy of oxygenation, and values that are reassuring include $PaO_2/FiO_2 \geq 150$ mm Hg; $PaO_2 \geq 60$ mm Hg; $SaO_2 \geq 90\%$; $FiO_2 \leq 0.40$; and PEEP ≤ 5 to 8 cm H_2O. A $PaO_2/FiO_2 \geq 120$ mm Hg and PaO_2 of 50 to 60 mm Hg may be acceptable in patients with chronic hypoxemia.[11]

- *Measures of acid-base balance*: Arterial pH should be > 7.25. Gastric mucosal acidosis (e.g., gastric mucosal ischemia) has been associated with weaning failure, but requires a special nasogastric tube for measurement.[11,17]

- *Measures of ventilation*: Specific measures of ventilation include spontaneous respiratory rate (f), tidal volume (V_T), RSBI (f/V_T), minute volume ($\dot{V}_E$), $PaCO_2$, maximum voluntary ventilation (MVV), and vital capacity (VC). Values that suggest successful weaning include:[17]
  - $f < 30$ and > 6 breaths/min
  - $V_T > 5$ mL/kg
  - $f/V_T < 105$
  - $\dot{V}_E < 10$ L/min
  - MVV $\geq 2 \times \dot{V}_E$ (as a measure of ventilatory reserve)
  - VC > 10 to 15 mL/kg (to ensure the ability to cough and deep breathing)

- *Measures of ventilatory muscle strength*: Adequate inspiratory muscle strength is required to maintain adequate ventilation, and adequate expiratory muscle strength is needed to have an effective cough. MIP and MEP assess inspiratory and expiratory muscle strength, respectively. Preferred values are:
  - MIP < -20 to -30 cm H_2O.
  - MEP $\geq +60$ cm H_2O suggests the ability to adequately cough and clear secretions.

- *Measures of ventilatory workload*: Static total compliance and airway resistance measured while on the ventilator provide an estimate of ventilatory workload. These measures, however, have not been shown to be predictive of weaning success when used in isolation. WOB can be estimated based on tidal volume and esophageal pressure measurement, though acceptable values for weaning have not been delineated. Oxygen cost of breathing provides another surrogate measure for WOB.[11]
  - Total static compliance approaching normal range ($C_{ST} = 60$ to 100 cm H_2O)
  - Airway resistance (R_{aw}) approaching normal (e.g., R_{aw} 1 to 2 cm H_2O/L/sec + endotracheal tube resistance)
  - WOB and oxygen cost of breathing (OCB) approaching normal values (e.g., spontaneous WOB = 0.5 to 1.0 joules/L; values ≥ 1.5 joules/L may be excessive). Normal OCB is $< 5\%$ of $\dot{V}O_2$; OCB $\leq 15\%$ may be acceptable as a goal for weaning.

- *Measures of respiratory drive*: Respiratory drive can be assessed by measurement of the pulmonary occlusion pressure (PO.1), which is the pressure generated upon inspiration in the first 10th of a second (0.10 second) following complete airway occlusion.[11]
  - PO.1 < 4 to 6 cm H_2O (normal PO.1 < 2 cm H_2O).
  - PO.1/MIP has greater predictive power than PO.1 alone.

Integrated Indices

Combined or integrated indices have been developed in an attempt to improve prediction of weaning success.[11,17] These include the CROP index, which combines measures of compliance, respiratory rate, oxygenation, and pressure (MIP).[11,17] Other combined indices include the inspiratory effort quotient (IEQ), the CORE index, the weaning index (WI), and the integrative weaning index (IWI).[11] These integrative indices use various combinations of measures that may include compliance, MIP, tidal volume, PaO_2/FiO_2, f/V_T, and/or pressure–time index, with varying degrees of predictive success.[11,22]

The most popular and well-studied measure is the RSBI (f/V_T).[22] Although RSBI may be a predictor of weaning success in patients requiring mechanical ventilatory support, there is little evidence that its use improves clinical outcomes.[17,22] We believe that use of specific weaning indices, as part of a comprehensive patient evaluation, can be helpful in guiding clinical decisions. *It must be stressed that many patients are successfully weaned from mechanical ventilation in spite of suboptimal results on specific weaning readiness tests.* Reliance on "getting the right numbers" may inappropriately delay ventilator discontinuance.

Weaning Methods

A number of techniques are available to facilitate ventilator weaning. These include spontaneous breathing trials (SBTs), pressure support ventilation (PSV), and intermittent mandatory ventilation (IMV and synchronized IMV [SIMV]).[20] Newer techniques include adaptive support ventilation (ASV), proportional assist ventilation (PAV), and proportional pressure support (PPS). Although all of these methods have been used to successfully discontinue mechanical ventilation, once daily SBTs are the technique most commonly used.

Spontaneous Breathing Trials

An SBT may be performed using a T-piece or by having the patient breathe in the "spontaneous" mode while attached to the mechanical ventilator. Automatic tube compensation (ATC) or low levels of PSV may be applied to help overcome the resistance imposed by the endotracheal tube. As an alternative, low levels of

CPAP may be applied. Generally, the SBT continues for 30 minutes, during which time the patient is carefully monitored for dyspnea, anxiety, agitation, diaphoresis, change in mental status, or distress. Heart rate, respiratory rate, SpO_2, and blood pressure are monitored.[17,20] The SBT is terminated if there are specific signs of distress (e.g., f > 30 to 35 breaths/min; SpO_2 < 90%; HR > 120 to 140 bpm; HR increases > 20%; BP systolic < 90 or > 180 mm Hg).[17,20]

An SBT of 30 minutes is usually sufficient to determine if mechanical ventilation can be discontinued, though the SBT may be continued for up to 120 minutes.[17,20] Patients who "pass" the SBT are removed from the ventilator and extubation is considered. Patients who "fail" continue to receive mechanical ventilatory support for 24 hours, and the SBT is then repeated. Daily SBTs are appropriate for most patients who are candidates for weaning. It should be noted that SBTs are better predictors of weaning success in patients who have been intubated < 1 week and in younger patients (age < 65 years).

Weaning Trial Monitoring

Regardless of the technique chosen for weaning from mechanical ventilation, the patient's oxygenation, ventilatory, and cardiovascular status should be monitored carefully. Respiratory rate and pattern are reliable indicators of patient progress. Increased respiratory rate, respiratory distress, fatigue, dyspnea, diaphoresis, accessory muscle use, intercostal retractions, or abdominal paradox suggest intolerance of a weaning trial.[17] Vital signs should be monitored to include heart rate, blood pressure, and SpO_2. For example, a 20% or greater increase in heart rate or a significant tachycardia (HR >120 bpm) may signal the need to terminate the weaning trial. Similarly, a significant fall in systolic blood pressure (i.e., BP < 90 mm Hg) may suggest that the trial be terminated. ECG monitoring should be in place, as the development of arrhythmias may also suggest weaning intolerance. SpO_2 monitoring provides a sensitive indicator of oxygenation status. Arterial blood gases may be obtained to access $PaCO_2$ and pH if the patient does not appear to be doing well. Capnography probably has no role in monitoring a weaning trial. Mental status should be monitored; anxiety, agitation, and discomfort are associated with difficulty in weaning. Somnolence, lethargy, or loss of consciousness may signal serious hypoxia or hypercapnea. Patients should not be overtired or pushed beyond their physiologic limits because this may result in diaphragmatic fatigue, which will further delay the weaning process.[17]

Weaning Failure

Possible causes of weaning failure should be investigated and problems identified corrected, if possible.[11,17,20] The most common reason for weaning failure is an imbalance between ventilatory load (e.g., WOB) and ventilatory capacity (e.g., respiratory muscle strength).[11,17,20] Other common reasons for weaning failure include volume overload, cardiac dysfunction, metabolic disturbances, neuromuscular problems, anxiety, delirium, and/or adrenal insufficiency.[11,17,20]

Key Points

▶ Respiratory failure can be broadly defined as the inability of the heart and lungs to provide adequate tissue oxygenation and carbon dioxide removal.

▶ Hypoxemic respiratory failure refers to inadequate oxygenation of the arterial blood while hypercapnic respiratory failure refers to an elevation in $PaCO_2$.

▶ Minute volume ($\dot{V}_E$) is tidal volume times rate ($\dot{V}_E = V_T \times f$).

▶ Dead space is the portion of ventilation that does not participate in gas exchange (i.e., ventilation without perfusion); types of dead space include anatomic (V_D anatomic), alveolar (V_D alveolar), physiologic (V_D physiologic) and mechanical.

▶ Alveolar ventilation is the volume of ventilation received by the alveoli per breath (V_A) and per minute ($\dot{V}_A$); $PaCO_2$ is the single best index of alveolar ventilation.

▶ $PaCO_2$ > 45 mm Hg is hypoventilation, or ventilatory failure, while $PaCO_2$ < 35 mm Hg is alveolar hyperventilation.

▶ Acute ventilatory failure is a sudden rise in $PaCO_2$ with a corresponding decrease in pH, while chronic ventilatory failure is a chronically elevated $PaCO_2$ with a normal or near-normal pH (due to renal compensation).

▶ Acute alveolar hyperventilation is an acute decrease in $PaCO_2$ with a corresponding increase in pH, while chronic alveolar hyperventilation is a chronic decrease in $PaCO_2$ with a normal or near-normal pH (due to renal compensation).

▶ Shallow, constant tidal breathing (< 7 mL/kg of IBW) without an intermittent deep breath will cause progressive atelectasis; intermittent sigh breaths reverse this trend.

▶ An adequate cough requires the ability to take a deep breath and adequate expiratory (abdominal) muscle strength.

▶ Inspiratory capacity (IC) is the maximum volume of air a person can inhale following a passive exhalation and is about 50 mL/kg IBW.

▶ Vital capacity (VC) is the maximum volume of gas a person can exhale following a maximal inspiration and is normally about 60 to 70 mL/kg IBW.

▶ Bedside measures of ventilatory muscle strength include maximum inspiratory pressure (MIP), maximum expiratory pressure (MEP), and ventilatory capacity (VC).

- Compliance can be defined as the "stretchability" of the lungs and thorax; compliance is the inverse of elastance.
- Lung compliance (C_L) represents the stretchability of the lung tissue while thoracic compliance (chest wall compliance, or C_C) represents the stretchability of the thorax and normal (static) total compliance is 60 to 100 mL/cm H_2O; a reduction in C_T can be caused by a reduction in C_L, a reduction in C_C, or both.
- Causes of reduced C_L include atelectasis, pneumonia, pulmonary fibrosis, and pulmonary edema (including ARDS); lung compliance increases with aging and emphysema.
- Causes of reduced thoracic compliance include obesity, ascites, chest wall deformity, and abdominal distension.
- The relationship between lung recoil (lung elastance) and thoracic recoil determines the functional residual capacity (FRC).
- Causes of pneumothorax include a spontaneous tear in the lung tissue or traumatic stab or puncture wound; tension pneumothorax may occur in patients receiving mechanical ventilatory support with positive pressure.
- Dynamic compliance is calculated by dividing the delivered tidal volume by the peak inspiratory airway pressure (PIP) adjusted for the baseline pressure.
- Barotrauma (a form of ventilator-induced lung injury) describes injury due to the application of excessive pressures.
- Surfactant reduces surface tension in alveoli of all sizes, enabling small alveoli to remain inflated at low volumes.
- The lecithin-to-sphingomyelin ratio (L/S ratio) and phosphatidylglycerol concentrations in amniotic fluid are predictors of fetal lung maturation.
- Respiratory distress syndrome (RDS) of the neonate is more common in babies born at a gestational age < 30 weeks and low birth weight (< 1500 grams).
- Diseases states in which surfactant may be inactivated include pneumonia, pulmonary edema, acute respiratory distress syndrome (ARDS), lung transplantation, and leakage of plasma proteins into the lung.
- Resistance to ventilation can be classified as elastic or nonelastic; elastic resistance and compliance are inversely related; two types of nonelastic, or frictional, resistance are tissue resistance and airway resistance.
- Causes of increased airway resistance include bronchospasm, mucosal edema, secretions, and small-diameter endotracheal tubes.
- Laminar flow is smooth with little turbulence or eddy formation; R_{aw} is reduced with laminar flow.
- Turbulent flow refers to gas flow that is rough and chaotic with a great deal of eddy formation; R_{aw} is increased with turbulent flow.
- Airflow in the upper airways, trachea, and primary bronchi tends to be very turbulent.
- Tracheal or bronchial breath sounds are heard over the trachea and primary bronchi where flow is turbulent; sounds are loud, coarse, and high-pitched.
- Vesicular breath sounds are heard over periphery of normal lungs where flow is laminar; sounds are quiet, soft, and low-pitched.
- With consolidation or pleural effusion, bronchial breath sounds may be heard over the periphery.
- Decreased or absent breath sounds indicate diminished or absent airflow.
- WOB is performed during inspiration; expiration is normally passive and requires no work.
- WOB and oxygen cost of breathing increase with obstructive disease, (e.g., COPD), restrictive disease (e.g., ARDS, pneumonia, pulmonary fibrosis), and obesity.
- Patients with restrictive lung disease may exhibit rapid, shallow breathing.
- COPD patients tend to breathe slowly to minimize frictional work; COPD patients may expend energy to exhale by contracting their accessory muscles of expiration.
- A high ventilatory workload can fatigue the respiratory muscles; diaphragmatic fatigue predisposes patients to acute ventilatory failure.
- The level of ventilation required is determined by the metabolic rate, respiratory drive, and ventilatory dead space.
- Metabolic alkalosis, sleep deprivation, hypothyroidism, CNS disorders, and administration of sedatives, narcotics, or neuromuscular blocking agents can reduce or abolish respiratory drive.
- The airway pressure a patient generates during the first part of inspiration against a closed airway provides a measure of ventilatory drive (i.e., pulmonary occlusion pressure, or PO.1).
- R_{aw} may increase due to insertion of artificial airways, ventilator circuits, mechanical demand flow systems, inappropriate ventilator flow and sensitivity settings, and auto-PEEP.
- Causes of ventilatory muscle weakness in the intensive care unit include critical illness polyneuropathy, critical illness myopathy, and prolonged use of neuromuscular blocking agents.
- The most common diagnosis requiring mechanical ventilatory support is acute respiratory failure, often due to postoperative complications, sepsis, pneumonia, heart failure, trauma, ARDS, or aspiration.
- Clinical signs of ventilatory failure include increased heart rate, increased respiratory rate, accessory muscle use, intercostal retractions, nasal flaring (especially in infants and children),

diaphoresis, and oxygen desaturation (i.e., decrease in Sp_{O_2}). Rapid shallow breathing is a common finding with acute ventilatory failure.

▶ Physiologic variables measured at the bedside that may be predictive of the need for mechanical ventilatory support include spontaneous f and V_T, RSBI, MIP, and VC.

▶ Indications for mechanical ventilation are apnea, acute ventilatory failure, impending ventilatory failure, and severe oxygenation problems.

▶ With impending ventilatory failure, intubation may be performed and mechanical ventilation initiated prior to the onset of acute respiratory acidosis.

▶ Severe oxygenation problems may require the use of PEEP, CPAP or techniques best applied using invasive mechanical ventilation.

▶ The primary criterion for discontinuing ventilatory support is the improvement or reversal of the disease state or condition that required the need for mechanical ventilation.

▶ Weaning is the process of gradually reducing mechanical ventilatory support; the need for gradual weaning is limited to a small number of patients.

▶ Ventilator dependence most commonly occurs when ventilatory demand or workload continues to exceed ventilatory capacity.

▶ Factors that may contribute to ventilator dependence include oxygenation problems, cardiac problems, neurologic problems, or psychological issues.

▶ Inability to protect the natural airway is a contraindication to extubation.

▶ Airway resistance can increase dramatically if the endotracheal tube becomes partially occluded by dried secretions; adequate humidification should be provided.

▶ The presence of an endotracheal tube may cause reflex bronchoconstriction, and bronchodilator therapy may be justified in intubated patients.

▶ Pressure support ventilation (PSV) or automatic to compensation (ATC) provided during weaning may help alleviate imposed work of breathing (WOB_I).

▶ Tracheostomy tubes may reduce the work of breathing as compared to endotracheal tubes; tracheostomy tube placement may reduce anatomic dead space.

▶ If stridor is present following extubation, the patient should be carefully monitored.

▶ Trachostomy should be considered in patients requiring an artificial airway for prolonged periods of time.

▶ Tracheostomies are generally well tolerated, improve patient comfort, improve access to secretions, decrease airway resistance, enhance mobility, and may allow the patient to eat and speak.

▶ Generally, an SBT of 30 minutes is sufficient to determine if mechanical ventilation can be discontinued.

▶ Increased respiratory rate, respiratory distress, fatigue, dyspnea, diaphoresis, accessory muscle use, intercostal retractions, or abdominal paradox suggest intolerance of a weaning trial.

References

1. Shelledy DC, Peters JP. Initiating and adjusting ventilatory support. In: Wilkins RL, Stoller JK, Kacmarek RM (eds.). *Egan's Fundamentals of Respiratory Care*, 9th ed. St. Louis, MO: Elsevier-Mosby; 2009: 1045–1090.

2. Aboussouan LS. Respiratory failure and the need for ventilatory support. In: Wilkins RL, Stoller JK, Kacmarek RM (eds.). *Egan's Fundamentals of Respiratory Care*, 9th ed. St. Louis, MO: Elsevier-Mosby; 2009: 949–964.

3. Longo DL, Fauci AS, Kasper DL, Hauser SL, Jameson JL, Loscalzo J. Respiratory failure. In: Longo DL, Fauci AS, Kasper DL, Hauser SL, Jameson JL, Loscalzo J (eds.). *Harrison's Manual of Medicine*, 18th ed. New York: McGraw-Hill; 2013: 83.

4. Matthay MA, Atabai K. Acute hypercapnic respiratory failure: Neuromuscular and obstructive diseases. In: George RB, Light RW, Matthay MA, Matthay RA (eds.). *Chest Medicine Essentials of Pulmonary and Critical Care Medicine*, 4th ed. Philadelphia: Lippincott Williams & Wilkins; 2000: 561–575.

5. Ruppel GL. Ventilation. In: Wilkins RL, Stoller JK, Kacmarek RM (eds.). *Egan's Fundamentals of Respiratory Care*, 9th ed. St. Louis, MO: Elsevier-Mosby; 2009: 215–236.

6. Beachey W. Pulmonary function measurements. In: Beachey W (ed.). *Respiratory Care Anatomy and Physiology*, 3rd ed. St. Louis, MO: Elsevier-Mosby; 2013: 95–109.

7. Beachey W. Mechanics of ventilation. In: Beachey W (ed.). *Respiratory Care Anatomy and Physiology*, 3rd ed. St. Louis, MO: Elsevier-Mosby; 2013: 44–82.

8. West JB. Mechanics of breathing. In: West JB (ed.). *Respiratory Physiology: The Essentials*, 8th ed. Philadelphia: Lippincott Williams & Wilkins; 2008: 95–122.

9. Epstein SK. Respiratory Muscle weakness due to neuromuscular disease: Clinical manifestations and evaluation. In: *UpToDate*, Shefner JM, Parsons PE, Morrison RS, Finlay G. (eds.), UpToDate, Waltham, MA, 2014.

10. Moxham J. Tests of respiratory muscle strength. In: *UpToDate*, Stoller JK, Finlay G. (eds.), UpToDate, Waltham, MA, 2013.

11. Epstein SK. Weaning from mechanical ventilation: Readiness testing. In: *UpToDate*, Parsons PE, Finlay G (eds.), UpToDate, Waltham, MA, 2013.

12. Adams AB. Monitoring and management of the patient in the intensive care unit. In: Wilkins RL, Stoller JK, Kacmarek RM (eds.). *Egan's Fundamentals of Respiratory Care*, 9th ed. St. Louis, MO: Elsevier-Mosby; 2009: 1115–1152.

13. Op T, Holt TB. Physiology of ventilatory support. In: Wilkins RL, Stoller JK, Kacmarek RM (eds.). *Egan's Fundamentals of Respiratory Care*, 9th ed. St. Louis, MO: Elsevier-Mosby; 2009: 1001–1043.

14. Brown III CA. The decision to intubate. In: *UpToDate*, Walls RM, Grayzel J. (eds.), UpToDate, Waltham, MA, 2014.

15. Casserly B, Rounds S. Essentials in critical care medicine. In: Andreoli TE, Benjamin IJ, Griggs RC, Wing EJ (eds.). *Andreoli and Carpenter's Cecil Essentials of Medicine*, 8th ed. Philadelphia: Saunders Elsevier; 2010: 259–265.

16. Cohen CA, Zagelbaum G, Gross D, Roussos C, Macklem PT. Clinical manifestations of inspiratory muscle fatigue. *Am J Med.* 1982;73(3):308–316.

17. Shelledy DC. Discontinuing ventilatory support. In: Wilkins RL, Stoller JK, Kacmarek RM (eds.). *Egan's Fundamentals of Respiratory Care*, 9th ed. St. Louis, MO: Elsevier-Mosby; 2009: 1153–1184.

18. Schilz R. Neuromuscular and other diseases of the chest wall. In: Wilkins RL, Stoller JK, Kacmarek RM (eds.). *Egan's Fundamentals of Respiratory Care*, 9th ed. St. Louis, MO: Elsevier-Mosby; 2009: 609–623.

19. Courey AJ, Hyzy RC. Overview of mechanical ventilation. In: *UpToDate*, Parsons PE, Finlay G (eds.), UpToDate, Waltham, MA, 2014.

20. Epstein SK, Walkey A. Methods of weaning from mechanical ventilation. In: *UpToDate*, Parsons PE, Finlay G (eds.), UpToDate, Waltham, MA, 2014.

21. Wilkins RL. Patient safety, communication, and recordkeeping. In: Wilkins RL, Stoller JK, Kacmarek RM (eds.). *Egan's Fundamentals of Respiratory Care*, 9th ed. St. Louis, MO: Elsevier-Mosby; 2009: 35–52.

22. Epstein SK. Weaning from mechanical ventilation: The rapid shallow breathing index. In: *UpToDate*, Parsons PE (ed.), UpToDate, Waltham, MA, 2014.

CHAPTER

8

Blood Gas Analysis, Hemoximetry, and Acid-Base Balance

J. Brady Scott, Brian K. Walsh, and David C. Shelledy

CHAPTER OUTLINE

Introduction to Blood Gases and Acid-Base Balance
Blood Gas Analysis
Arterial Line Insertion and Sampling
Venous Blood Gas Sampling
Sample Analysis
Acid-Base Chemistry
Arterial Blood Gas Interpretation
Expected Respiratory and Renal Compensation
Clinical Interpretation of Arterial Blood Gases
Noninvasive Oximetry

CHAPTER OBJECTIVES

1. List the indications for arterial blood gas analysis.
2. Describe the advantages and disadvantages of radial, brachial, and femoral sampling.
3. Describe the equipment, procedure, and complications associated with radial, brachial, and femoral artery punctures.
4. Explain the technique and purpose for the modified Allen test.
5. Describe the equipment, procedure, complications, and monitoring associated with radial artery cannulation.
6. Describe the equipment, procedure, and complications associated with arterialized capillary sampling.
7. Describe the technique for mixed venous blood gas sampling and interpret the results.
8. Explain blood gas analysis in terms of preanalytic errors, analytic errors, postanalytic errors, quality assurance, and quality control.
9. Explain methods to quantify hydrogen ion concentration and pH.
10. Use the Henderson equation to derive the Henderson-Hasselbalch equation.
11. Demonstrate methods to calculate bicarbonate ion concentration.
12. Describe the regulation of blood acid and blood base.

13. Define terms associated with arterial blood gas interpretation.
14. Perform arterial blood gas interpretation using traditional nomenclature.
15. Describe patients' oxygenation and ventilatory status based on arterial blood gas results.
16. Estimate maximal compensation and classify blood gas results as maximally or submaximally compensated.
17. Describe the causes and treatment of metabolic acidosis and alkalosis.
18. Describe the indications for and limitations of pulse oximetry.
19. Explain how pulse oximetry obtains its values.

KEY TERMS

acid-base status
acidemia
acidosis
acute alveolar
  hyperventilation
acute alveolar
  hyperventilation
  superimposed on chronic
  ventilatory failure
acute ventilatory failure
acute ventilatory failure
  superimposed on chronic
  ventilatory failure
alkalemia
alkalosis
anion gap
arterial blood gas study
arterialized capillary
  sampling
base excess/deficit (BE/
  BD)
chronic alveolar
  hyperventilation

chronic ventilatory failure
electrolytes
fully compensated
hemoximetry
Henderson-Hasselbalch
  equation
maximal compensation
metabolic acidosis
metabolic alkalosis
mixed venous blood gas
  study
modified Allen test
oxygenation status
partially compensated
plasma bicarbonate (HCO_3^-)
pulse oximetry
respiratory acidosis
respiratory alkalosis
submaximal and maximal
  compensation
uncompensated

Overview

This chapter describes blood gas analysis and interpretation, hemoximetry, and acid-base balance. The respiratory care clinician must have solid knowledge of the technical aspects of blood gas sampling and analysis to accurately assess blood gas values. Interpretation of blood gas study results requires a thorough knowledge of the principles of oxygenation, ventilation, and acid-base balance. This chapter presents information on the indications, sampling techniques, quality assurance, and possible errors in blood gas reporting. Oxygenation, ventilation, and acid-base chemistry are then reviewed and clinical nomenclatures that are commonly used in the interpretation of blood gases are explained. Causes and treatment of acid-base disturbances are discussed, with an emphasis on the clinical application of blood gas study results. Finally, noninvasive pulse oximetry techniques to monitor blood oxygen levels are described.

Introduction to Blood Gases and Acid-Base Balance

The **arterial blood gas study** is a tremendously useful laboratory test for the assessment of acid-base balance, **oxygenation status**, and ventilatory status. Accurate analysis of blood gas values can aid the clinician in identifying physiologic disturbances and clinical conditions. The data gathered from analysis provide valuable information to quantitate the response to therapeutic interventions and provide diagnostic evaluation in both the acute and chronic care setting.[1] The process of obtaining samples requires technical skill and knowledge of anatomy and physiology. Although simple in terms of acquisition, the complexity of the blood gas test lies within the indications, complications, hazards, interpretation, and clinical decision making.[2]

The typical arterial blood gas study includes measures of oxygenation, ventilation, and acid-base balance. The modern blood gas analyzer directly measures oxygen tension (Po_2), carbon dioxide tension (Pco_2), and pH. With the addition of **hemoximetry**, oxygen saturation (Sao_2), hemoglobin (Hb), methemoglobin (metHb), and carboxyhemoglobin (COHb) can be measured. Calculated values for **plasma bicarbonate (HCO_3^-)** and **base excess/deficit (BE/BD)** are also routinely reported. Oxygen content (Cao_2) may also be calculated and reported, as well as of other measures related to acid-base balance (e.g., standard bicarbonate and T_{40} bicarbonate). Normal arterial blood gas values are listed in **Table 8-1**.

Blood Gas Analysis

Prior to obtaining an arterial blood sample, the respiratory care clinician should review the indications,

TABLE 8-1
Normal Arterial Blood Gas Values

Analyte (units)	Description	Normal (range)
pH	$-\log$ [H⁺]	7.40 (7.35–7.45)
$Paco_2$ (mm Hg)	Arterial carbon dioxide tension	40 (35–45)
Pao_2 (mm Hg)	Arterial oxygen tension	95 (80–100)
Sao_2 (%)[1]	Arterial oxygen saturation	97.5 (95–98)
COHb (%)[1]	Carboxyhemoglobin	0.5–1.5
metHb (%)[1]	Methemoglobin	0.0–1.5
Hb (g/dL)[1]	Hemoglobin	15 (men: 13.5–16.5; women: 12–15)
Cao_2 (mL/dL or vol%)[1]	Arterial oxygen content	19.8 (17–21)
Plasma HCO_3^- (mEq/L)[2]	Plasma bicarbonate	24 (22–28)[3]
BE/BD (mEq/L)[2]	Base excess or deficit	0 (±2)
TCO_2 (mmol/L or mEq/L)[2,4]	Total CO_2	25 (22–30)

[1]Requires hemoximetry for measurement (e.g., co-oximetry).
[2]Calculated values, usually based on algorithms incorporated into the blood gas analyzer.
[3]Clinical range for plasma bicarbonate varies by reference source; HCO_3^- range of 21 to 27 mEq/L has been suggested [Emmett M. Simple and mixed acid-base disorders. UpToDate, 2013]. Others have suggested a normal HCO_3^- range of 22 to 26 and 22 to 28 mEq/L [Post TW, Burton RD. Approach to the patient with metabolic acidosis. UpToDate, 2013].
[4]Total CO_2 range based on the Siggaard-Andersen nomogram would be 23 to 27 mmol/L (arterial blood) and 24 to 29 mmol/L (venous blood).

contraindications, and hazards of the procedure. The clinician must also be well versed in sampling techniques and errors that can occur during sample collection, analysis, and reporting.

Indications for Blood Gas Analysis

Indications for arterial blood gas and pH analysis and hemoximetry include the need to:[3]

- Evaluate the adequacy of a patient's ventilatory, acid-base, and/or oxygenation status.[4–6]
- Evaluate oxygen-carrying capacity and intrapulmonary shunt.[4–6]
- Quantify the response to therapeutic intervention and/or diagnostic evaluation (e.g., exercise desaturation).[2,5–7]

- Assess goal-directed therapy in patients with cardiopulmonary disease.[8]
- Monitor severity and progression of documented disease processes.[2]

Arterial Percutaneous Sampling

When obtaining an arterial blood gas sample, it is important for the clinician to use a puncture site that is safe and accessible.[4] Many variables associated with the arterial puncture can make a given site difficult to use. The lack of palpable pulses, wound or intravenous catheter dressings, absence of collateral circulation (e.g., radial artery puncture), and overlying skin infection are reasons clinicians may choose alternate anatomic locations. Recently, bedside sonography devices have been introduced that may aid in visualizing the artery prior to performing arterial puncture. Arterial blood gas samples may be obtained from the radial, brachial, femoral, dorsalis pedis, or axillary artery, with the radial arterial puncture being most common. **Box 8-1** summarizes the procedure for radial, brachial, and femoral arterial percutaneous sampling.

BOX 8-1

Procedure for Radial, Brachial, and Femoral Sampling

All three sampling procedures have elements in common. Common procedural elements prior to obtaining the sample include:
- Review the medical record:
  - Order
  - Respiratory care (O_2 therapy, mechanical ventilatory support)
  - Recent hemoglobin (Hb)
  - Patient temperature
  - Blood pressure (if > 200 mm Hg systolic, reconsider procedure)
  - Patient allergy to iodine or Betadine, if used (most sites use chlorhexidine instead)
  - Patient receiving anticoagulants (e.g., heparin, warfarin, other)
  - Patient receiving dialysis
- Gather the equipment needed:
  - Syringe
    - Prepackaged blood gas kit with vented, preheparinzed syringe is commonly used.
    - Low-diffusion plastic or glass syringe may be prepared using liquid sodium heparin (1000 unit/mL or 10 mg/mL).
  - Needles (21-to 25-gauge × 1-inch, short bevel, transparent plastic hub)
    - Femoral artery punctures may require a longer needle (e.g., 1.5 inch).
  - Gauze pads (2 × 2 or 4 × 4)
  - Antiseptic wipe (chlorhexidine [preferred] or iodine)
  - Alcohol pads
  - Ice and sample bag
  - Bandage and/or surgical tape (3/4 inch)
  - Local anesthetic (optional): 0.5% to 1% lidocaine, 25-gauge needle, and 1-mL syringe
- Enter room, identify self, and explain the procedure.
- Complete proper hand hygiene and put on gloves.
- Properly identify the patient.
- Note if the patient is breathing room air or O_2 therapy (device, liter flow, and/or FIO_2) and record information.
- Note and record ventilator settings (e.g., mode, rate, tidal volume, FIO_2).
- Inspect site for suitability (e.g., rash, tissue damage, burns, infection, presence of surgical arteriovenous anastomosis, dialysis fistulas).
- Choose appropriate-sized needle, depending on site.
- Assemble the equipment (i.e., syringe, needle, disinfectant, gauze pads, tape, bandage).
- Clean and disinfect the site.
- Follow universal precautions (gloves, mask, and safety glasses/goggles).

(continues)

Site-Specific Elements: Radial Artery Puncture

- Assess for collateral circulation (see modified Allen test).
- Position the patient so he or she is comfortable and site is accessible; position should allow the wrist to be slightly hyperextended.
  - Use a rolled towel or arm board to assist in keeping the wrist extended, if needed.
  - Hyperextension of the wrist lifts the artery superficially, or more towards the skin.
- Clean and prep the site according to institutional standards (e.g., clean site with chlorhexidine or alcohol wipe followed by prep using an iodine wipe). Iodine should be allowed to dry on the skin for at least 15 seconds in order to be most effective.
- Consider local anesthesia. This may improve patient compliance and be helpful for difficult or repeated punctures.
- Carefully palpate the artery 1 to 2 cm from the wrist to determine the exact location.
- Anesthetize the site, if desired, by raising a small skin weal using 0.5% to 1% lidocaine, a 25-gauge needle and 1-mL syringe.
- Continue palpating the artery and prepare to perform arterial puncture.
  - Be sure you have a good feel for the location of the artery prior to inserting the needle.
- Hold the syringe in a comfortable and stable manner. Clinicians often hold the syringe like a pencil using their dominant hand.
- Puncture the skin at a 45-degree angle with the needle bevel up, facing the flow of blood.
- Advance the needle and syringe slowly, until a flash of blood enters the syringe. Then hold the syringe stable until it fills with blood.
  - Avoid jabbing or probing for the artery.
  - Allow the syringe to self-fill.
  - Avoid aspirating the sample, as this may introduce bubbles or venous blood.
- When the syringe contains an adequate sample (e.g., 2 to 3 mL of blood), withdraw the needle and apply firm pressure over the now exposed puncture site with a sterile dressing.
- Seal the syringe and place in sample bag with ice.
  - Promptly expel any air bubbles if present.
  - Dispose of needle in proper container.
- Hold pressure to the site manually for at least 3 to 5 minutes to ensure bleeding has ceased.
  - Large hematomas may develop if this step is not following carefully.
  - Patients with clotting problems or receiving anticoagulants may require additional time.
  - Inspect the site to ensure bleeding has stopped.
- Place adhesive bandage strip over the site.
- Transport the sample to the blood gas laboratory for analysis.

Site-Specific Elements: Brachial Artery Puncture

- Position the patient so he or she is comfortable and the site is accessible; position should allow the arm to lay flat with antecubital fosse exposed and accessible.
  - Position the arm in a hyperextended fashion with the palm up.
  - Use towel under the arm at the elbow to aid in keeping the area extended.
- Palpate the brachial artery medial to the bicep tendon in the antecubital fossa.
- Clean and prep the site according to institutional standards (e.g., clean site with alcohol wipe followed by prep using an iodine wipe). Iodine should be allowed to dry on the skin for at least 15 seconds in order to be most effective.
- Consider local anesthesia. This may improve patient compliance and be helpful for difficult or repeated punctures.
- Carefully palpate the artery to determine the exact location.
- Continue palpating the artery and prepare to perform arterial puncture.
  - Be sure you have a good feel for the location of the artery prior to inserting the needle.
- Hold the syringe in a comfortable and stable manner. Clinicians often hold the syringe like a pencil using their dominant hand.
- Insert the needle just above the antecubital crease at about a 60-degree angle with the bevel facing the flow of blood.

- Advance the needle and syringe slowly, until a flash of blood enters the syringe. Then hold the syringe stable until it fills with blood.
  - The needle is advanced slowing, maintaining an angle close to 60 degrees.
  - Avoid jabbing or probing for the artery.
- Allow the syringe to self-fill.
  - Avoid aspirating the sample, as this may introduce bubbles or venous blood.
- When the syringe contains an adequate sample (e.g., 2 to 3 mL of blood), withdraw the needle and apply firm pressure over the now exposed puncture site with a sterile dressing.
- Seal the syringe and place in sample bag with ice.
  - Promptly expel any air bubbles if present.
  - Dispose of needle in proper container.
- Hold pressure to the site manually for at least 3 to 5 minutes to ensure bleeding has ceased.
  - Large hematomas may develop if this step is not following carefully.
  - Patients with clotting problems or receiving anticoagulants may require additional time.
  - Inspect the site to ensure bleeding has stopped.
- Place adhesive bandage strip over the site.
- Transport the sample to the blood gas laboratory for analysis.

Site-Specific Elements: Femoral Artery Puncture

- Position the patient in the supine position with the leg externally rotated.
- Locate the femoral artery by palpating approximately 1 inch below the midpoint of the inguinal ligament.
- Clean the site according to institutional standards.
- Insert the needle at a 90-degree angle to the femoral artery.
- Advance the needle slowly until blood begins to fill the syringe, then hold syringe stable and allow blood to fill syringe.
- Once the desired volume (usually 2 to 3 mL) is obtained withdraw the needle and immediately apply pressure with a gauze pad to the puncture site.
- Ensure that the sample is free of air bubbles, as this may cause erroneous sample values.
- Seal the cap immediately and dispose of needle in proper container.
- Hold pressure for a minimum of 5 minutes until bleeding has completely stopped.
  - Patients in a hypocoagulable state may require additional time to stop bleeding completely.
- Inspect the site to ensure that there is no continued bleeding.
- Place the sample in ice or ice slush per institutional policy.
- Transport sample to blood gas laboratory.

Radial Arterial Puncture

The radial artery is usually the puncture site of choice for obtaining an arterial blood sample. The "thumb side" forearm location is usually easily accessible, easy to palpate, and easy to stabilize.[6] This location is the also commonly used to palpate a patient's pulse during assessment of vital signs. Collateral circulation to the hand provided by the ulnar artery makes this site relatively safe.

The equipment and supplies used to perform a radial arterial puncture may vary between institutions. Some facilities purchase preassembled kits that contain all of the necessary supplies, whereas other facilities may have clinicians assemble the needed supplies. In either case, the equipment needed to successfully collect an arterial blood gas sample includes:

- Preheparinized, low-diffusibility plastic blood gas syringe (dry lyophilized heparin or lithium heparin is generally used)
  - A sterile glass syringe (2 to 5 mL) and < 1 mL of liquid sodium heparin (1000 units/mL) may be used, as an alternative. Excess heparin must be expelled prior to use.
- Short-bevel 21- to 23-gauge × 1-inch needle with a transparent, clear plastic hub
  - A 23-gauge × 1-inch needle should suffice for most adult radial punctures.
  - A 21- or 22-gauge × 1-inch needle may be used for brachial or femoral punctures (femoral punctures may require a 1.5-inch needle).
  - A smaller needle is required for children and infants (23-to 25-gauge).

- Topical antiseptic wipes (e.g., chlorhexadine or providone iodine [Betadine]) and isopropyl alcohol [70%]). CDC guidelines currently recommend the use of a 2% chlorhexidine solution, which is available in single-use, latex-free, hands-off applicators. The solution can be removed with a ChloraPrep clear applicator, alcohol, or soap and water.
  - Check the medical record and ask the patient about sensitivity or allergy prior to application.
- Equipment to provide optional local analgesia (e.g., 0.25 to 1.0 mL of 0.5% to 2% lidocaine, syringe, 25-gauge × 5/8-inch needle) (optional)
- Sterile gauze squares (2 × 2 or 4 × 4), tape, bandages
- Patient sample label
- Gloves and face shield or safety goggles
- Needle-capping device
- Biohazard plastic bag for sample
- Ice (optional)

For the arterial puncture, the clinician should use the smallest needle that is practical. Typically, a 23-gauge, 1-inch needle is selected, though a smaller needle may sometimes be used (e.g., 25 gauge × 1 inch). The needle radius must be large enough for blood flow to fill the syringe without having to aspirate the sample, yet small enough to reduce the likelihood of vessel damage. The syringe is first heparinized to prevent blood clotting. The amount and type of heparin used in prepackaged, preheparinized plastic blood gas syringes varies by manufacturer.[9] If the clinician is using an empty glass syringe, about 1 mL of liquid sodium heparin (1000 units/mL) is drawn up and used to lubricate the syringe; the excess heparin is then expelled. The blood sample volume obtained for analysis should be large enough to meet the needs of the blood gas analyzer and to allow for retesting if needed, generally about 2 to 3 mL. **Figure 8-1** illustrates the location of the radial artery and the technique for radial arterial sampling.

Brachial Artery

The brachial artery provides a secondary site for arterial puncture. When performed properly by an experienced clinician, brachial artery punctures are safe, reliable, and relatively painless.[10] The brachial artery does not have collateral circulation and is a higher risk sampling site if the artery is damaged. The clinician performing the procedure should be mindful of the close proximity of the brachial artery and median

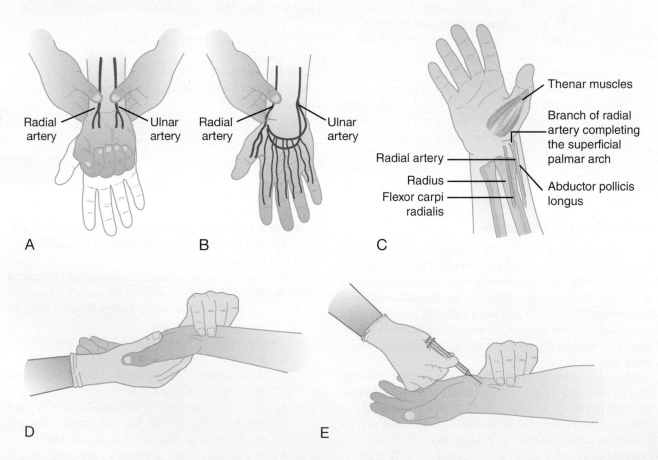

FIGURE 8-1 Allen test (A and B) and radial artery sampling (C–D).

Courtesy of Hess DR, MacIntyre NR, Mishoe SC, Galvin WF and Adams AB.

nerve. In the event that the needle touches the nerve or the underlying bone, the patient may experience a sudden, sharp, neuropathic pain. This sudden feeling of pain, not unlike an electric shock, may cause the patient to move or jerk his or her arm suddenly. Should this occur, the needle should be immediately withdrawn and an alternative site for arterial puncture considered. **Figure 8-2** illustrates the location of the brachial artery.

Femoral Artery

The femoral artery can also be used to obtain an arterial blood sample, particularly when the patient is very hypotensive and the radial and brachial pulses are not easily palpable (e.g., severe sepsis or cardiac resuscitation). This site is used less frequently, and many clinicians have limited experience in femoral artery punctures. The procedure should be performed by those personnel most familiar with the technique and only when necessary. Technically, the procedure can be challenging because the patient is required to be in a supine position and the artery may be difficult to locate. It is also difficult because of the close proximity of the femoral artery, vein, and nerve (see **Figure 8-3**).

Because the femoral artery is located in close proximity to the femoral vein, it is possible to inadvertently obtain a venous sample. Special care should be taken to ensure that arterial blood has been obtained, because medical decision making may be misinformed if the results of analysis of a venous or mixed venous/arterial sample are believed to be arterial.

Complications Associated with Arterial Punctures

Although most arterial punctures can be performed safely, the procedure is not without risks. These include significant complications such as vessel laceration, vessel spasm, excessive bleeding, infection, and vessel obstruction. Vessel laceration may occur due to needle manipulation and can be avoided with proper technique. Spasm of the vessel can occur, which may result in transient decline of blood flow to the distal tissues. In the case of the radial artery, this decline in blood flow may be offset by collateral circulation. The risk of excessive bleeding can be mitigated by identifying patients at risk prior to the procedure. Patients receiving anticoagulant medications (e.g., heparin, warfarin

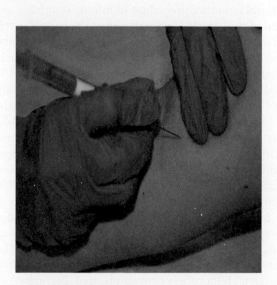

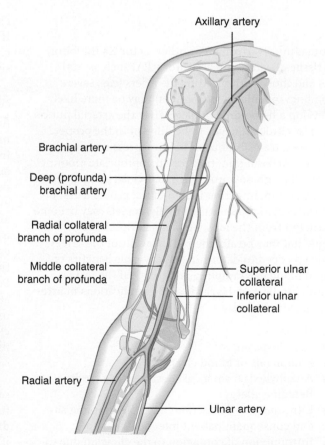

Axillary artery

Brachial artery

Deep (profunda) brachial artery

Radial collateral branch of profunda

Middle collateral branch of profunda

Superior ulnar collateral

Inferior ulnar collateral

Radial artery

Ulnar artery

FIGURE 8-2 Brachial artery puncture. Position the arm in an extended fashion with the palm up and assess for potential contraindications not discovered in the medical record. Palpate the brachial artery medial to the bicep tendon in the antecubital fossa. Clean the site and palpating finger(s) according to institutional standards. Insert the needle just above the antecubital crease and congruent with the humerus bone at a 45°–60° angle.

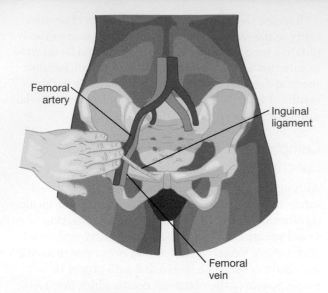

FIGURE 8-3 Femoral artery puncture. Locate the femoral artery by palpating approximately 1 inch below the midpoint of the inguinal ligament. Clean the site and palpating finger(s) according to institutional standards. Insert the needle at a 90° angle with the femoral artery.

[Coumadin], rivaroxaban or other factor Xa inhibitor, or a tissue plasminogin activator [tPA] such as Activase) and those with bleeding disorders (e.g., severe thrombocytopenia or hemophilia) may be more likely to develop a hematoma or bleed after the arterial puncture. The clinician needs to be diligent in the proper postprocedure technique of holding pressure over the site of the arterial puncture for an appropriate amount of time. As with any procedure that violates the integrity of the skin, infection is a potential problem associated with arterial puncture. Finally, vessels may become obstructed from the loosening of arteriosclerotic plaque that may be attached to the walls of the artery. Clinicians need to determine risks versus benefits of arterial blood gas sampling and decide if the test is clinically indicated. Hazards and complications of arterial puncture include:[3]

- Hematoma
- Arteriospasm
- Emboli (air or blood clot)
- Anaphylaxis from local anesthetic (e.g., iodine/ Betadine allergy)
- Introduction of infectious agent at sampling site and consequent patient infection
- Introduction of contagion to the clinician due to inadvertent "needlestick"
- Bleeding/hemorrhage
- Trauma to the vessel
- Arterial occlusion

- Vasovagal response (e.g., fainting)
- Pain

Assessing Collateral Circulation

In the past, the Allen test was used to assess for collateral circulation by occluding the radial artery for 3 minutes and then comparing the hand color to the opposite hand; if no change in color was noted, it was assumed that the ulnar artery was providing sufficient collateral circulation. Today, the **modified Allen test** is commonly performed just prior to the radial artery puncture procedure. The technique for the modified Allen test is illustrated in **Figure 8-4**.

Despite the widespread use of the modified Allen test, there is little data to suggest that it is a reliable method to properly identify potential complications associated with cessation of radial arterial blood flow. The modified Allen test is also used to evaluate patency of the ulnar artery before radial artery cannulation. The diagnostic accuracy of the test is reported to be greatest at a cutoff time of 5 to 6 seconds.

Evaluating hand perfusion by assessing blanching and flushing is highly subjective. Critically ill patients may not be able to participate because of sedation, confusion, or other clinical reasons. It is up the individual clinician to assess the results of the modified Allen test. If there is a question about the presence of collateral circulation to the hand, it is appropriate to seek another site for arterial puncture.[11,12]

Arterialized Capillary Sampling

Arterialized capillary sampling provides an alternative method of obtaining blood gas values without performing an arterial puncture on neonates and infants. An arterial puncture procedure in infants requires a great deal of skill due to the small size of the vessels. Arterialized capillary samples are technically easier to obtain, and the procedure is indicated when blood gas analysis is needed but access to an arterial site is limited.[13] The capillary blood gas offers valuable clinical information that generally reflects arterial P_{CO_2} and pH, though P_{O_2} values obtained via capillary samples are problematic. In infants, abnormal monitor readings (e.g., pulse oximetry, transcutaneous carbon dioxide), a change in clinical status, or the need to assess the progression of illness may suggest the need for arterialized capillary sampling.

In neonates and small infants, a capillary blood sample is typically obtained from the heel of the foot (i.e., a "heel stick"), though capillary samples may be drawn from fingers or toes in older infants and children if arterial puncture is contraindicated. Perfusion of the sample site can be improved by "arterializing" the site prior to sampling. Arterializing the capillary sample site is performed by warming the location with a warm towel or commercially available chemical heating pad;

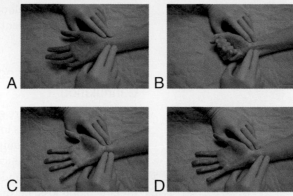

The steps of the modified Allen test
1. Locate the radial and ulnar arteries. (A)
2. Clench the fist.(B)
3. Apply pressure to both the radial and ulnar artery. (B)
4. Relax the hand. Do not allow the patient to fully extend the hand. (C)
5. The hand should appear blanched (indicating a lack of adequate perfusion).
6. The pressure on the ulnar artery is released, which should result in the flushing (or return of color) to the hand. (D)
7. The hand should appear normal in color within 10 seconds. This is a *positive modified Allen test*.
8. If 10 or more seconds elapse before color returns, the test is considered abnormal or a *negative modified Allen test*.

FIGURE 8-4 The steps of the modified Allen test.

this, in turn, increases capillary blood flow by dilating blood vessels. The P_{CO_2} and pH values obtained via an arterialized capillary sample are similar to arterial samples; however, it must be emphasized that the capillary P_{O_2} does not accurately reflect the actual arterial P_{O_2}. Clinicians making decisions based on arterialized capillary samples must understand the limitations of this technique. **Figure 8-5** illustrates the "heel stick." Typical arterialized capillary blood gas values in the neonate are reported in **Box 8-2**.

A number of hazards and complications are associated with obtaining an arterialized capillary sample. These include pain, bleeding, nerve damage, infection, scarring, and burns to the skin as a result of inappropriate skin warming. The risk of possible complications may be warranted if the test results are expected to have significant clinical implications.

Arterial Line Insertion and Sampling

Indwelling arterial catheters provide valuable information for the medical team by supporting continuous monitoring of arterial blood pressure and providing a route for repeated blood gas sampling. The need for

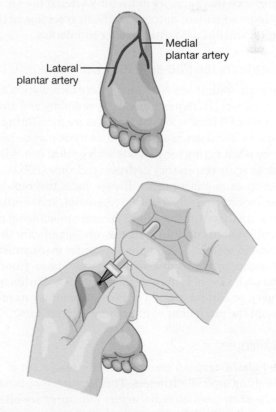

FIGURE 8-5 Arterialized capillary sampling. When performing an arterialized capillary sampling procedure, a highly vascular area of the heel such as the lateral or medial plantar surface is used.

continuous monitoring of blood pressure is a major indication for artery cannulation. In addition to blood gas samples, blood specimens for other laboratory studies can be drawn from an indwelling arterial catheter. The use of indwelling arterial catheters is relatively common in today's intensive care unit (ICU) environment, with 6 to 8 million used in the United States annually.[14,15] Although arterial lines are used frequently in the ICU, there is considerable debate regarding the necessity, cost, potential for complications, and the lack of evidence that suggests indwelling arterial lines actually improve patient outcomes. The next section of this chapter will discuss radial artery cannulation.

Indications for Radial Artery Cannulation

The main indications for radial artery cannulation are the need for: (1) frequent blood gas sampling and analysis and/or (2) continuous blood pressure monitoring. Frequent blood gas sampling and analysis may be necessary when caring for patients with critical conditions such as acute respiratory distress syndrome (ARDS), severe pneumonia, or other disease states that require close monitoring of patients' oxygenation and ventilation status. Continuous blood pressure monitoring may be indicated in conditions that involve significant fluctuation in systemic blood pressure or for management of patients with unstable hemodynamic status. Conditions such as shock, hypertensive crisis, cardiothoracic surgery, or administration of vasoactive infusions often prompt the placement of indwelling arterial lines.

Techniques

The radial artery is a common site for placement of indwelling arterial catheters. This location is optimal for the same reasons radial artery punctures are often utilized. The radial artery is easily accessed, palpated, and stabilized. The ulnar artery typically provides adequate collateral circulation to the palmer arch, thus

providing sufficient blood flow to the hand. **Figure 8-6** illustrates the placement of an indwelling arterial catheter.[14-16]

Complications Associated with Arterial Cannulation

Radial arterial lines are generally preferred because the rate of complication is low and the location is easily accessed. Although complication rates are low, radial arterial lines can produce considerable morbidity. Serious complications of radial arterial line placement include blood loss, permanent ischemic damage, pseudoaneurysm formation, and infection.[16] For this reason, arterial lines should be placed in the nondominant hand whenever possible. It is essential that the medical team continuously monitor the hand and fingers to ensure adequate perfusion. If infection is suspected, it may be necessary to remove the arterial catheter.

Blood Pressure Monitoring

For continuous blood pressure monitoring, radial artery catheters are attached to a pressure transducer and monitoring system. The catheter is attached to the transducer by noncompliant tubing. This tubing must be rigid enough to prevent inaccurate readings on the monitor. The length of the tubing should be kept as short as possible. The transducer responds to changes in pulsatile blood pressure within the artery and translates these to an electrical signal. The transducer must to be positioned at the level of the heart (i.e., the midaxillary line at the fourth intercostal space at the level of the right atrium [the phlebostatic axis]). If the transducer is positioned below the heart, the blood pressure will be artificially high. If the transducer is positioned above the heart, the blood pressure will be artificially low.

The transducer is connected to the patient monitoring system by a cable. This cable relays the electrical signal to the monitor, where it is converted into numeric values and waveform displays. Blood pressure is displayed digitally on the monitor as numeric values for systolic and diastolic pressure (mm Hg) and a graphic waveform display of pressure versus time (see **Figure 8-7**). Mean arterial blood pressure may be displayed and is the most accurate because arterial lines may overestimate the systolic and underestimate the diastolic blood pressure. It is important for the clinician to understand the components of the arterial pressure monitoring system in case troubleshooting is required. Hemodynamic monitoring is discussed in Chapter 14.

Arterial Line Sampling

The three-way stopcock closest to the cannulation site is used to draw arterial blood samples. This source of blood gas samples is advantageous for both the clinician and patient as multiple arterial sticks are avoided.

SEPARATE-GUIDEWIRE TECHNIQUE

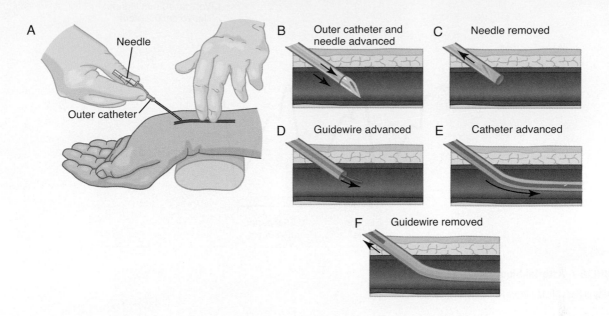

A Needle

Outer catheter

B Outer catheter and needle advanced

C Needle removed

D Guidewire advanced

E Catheter advanced

F Guidewire removed

INTEGRAL-GUIDEWIRE TECHNIQUE

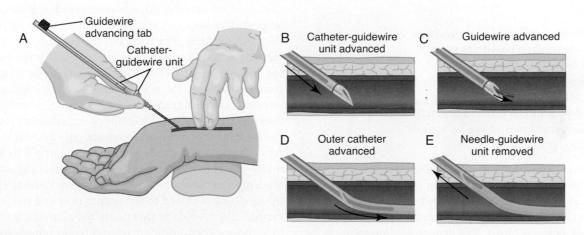

A Guidewire advancing tab

Catheter-guidewire unit

B Catheter-guidewire unit advanced

C Guidewire advanced

D Outer catheter advanced

E Needle-guidewire unit removed

FIGURE 8-6 Two methods for the insertion of the arterial line catheter placement. *Separate-guidewire approach**: The nondominant hand palpates the artery while the dominant hand manipulates the catheter, which is inserted and advanced slowly until pulsatile blood return is observed. The catheter is advanced slightly, ensuring the outer catheter has also entered the lumen. Care must be taken to avoid puncturing the posterior wall of the vessel when advancing the catheter. The nondominant hand then stabilizes the catheter while the dominant hand removes the needle from the intravascular catheter. If pulsatile blood return is observed after the needle is removed, the guidewire is advanced until its tip is beyond the distal end of the catheter. Finally, the catheter is advanced into the artery over the guidewire and the guidewire is removed. *Integral-guidewire approach**: The guidewire of this specialized device is integrated with the needle and catheter. The nondominant hand palpates the artery, while the dominant hand manipulates the needle-guidewire-catheter unit, which is inserted and advanced slowly until pulsatile blood return is observed. The nondominant hand then stabilizes the needle-guidewire-catheter unit, while the dominant hand advances the guidewire tab to push the wire into and through the needle and catheter. The outer catheter is advanced over the needle and wire into the artery. Finally, the needle-guidewire unit is removed. *For illustration purposes, full barrier precautions are not pictured.

Data from Clermont G, Theodore AC. Arterial cathererization techniques for invasive monitoring. *UpToDate* 2012; http://www.uptodate.com/contents/arterial-catheterization-techniques-for-invasive-monitoring/contributors. Accessed February 16, 2013.

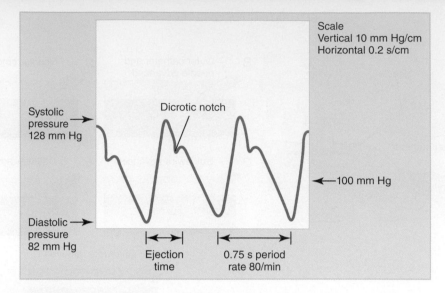

FIGURE 8-7 Arterial blood pressure waveform.

Courtesy of Hess DR, MacIntyre NR, Mishoe SC, Galvin WF, Adams AB.

The equipment needed for the arterial line sampling includes:

- Alcohol pads and chlorhexidine swab
- Heparinized blood gas syringe
- 5 to 10 mL "waste" syringe
- Sterile gauze squares (2 × 2 or 4 × 4)
- Patient sample label
- Gloves and face shield or safety goggles
- Biohazard plastic bag for sample
- Ice (optional)

Arterial line sampling is technically simple, but may be complicated by the operation of the three-way stopcock and flush system (see **Figure 8-8**). With the stopcock in the proper position for pressure monitoring, it provides a channel for a slow drip of a saline solution from a pressurized reservoir bag to enter the catheter to prevent clot formation. In the past, the saline flush solution was routinely heparinized; however, the addition of heparin to the saline flush solution is no longer considered necessary. The reservoir bag is typically pressurized to 300 mm Hg, resulting in a solution flow of about 3 mL/hour. A flush valve is incorporated into the system to allow the flush solution to rapidly flow through the tubing when the valve is activated to clear blood from the arterial catheter. The stopcock generally has three positions:

- Upright or 12 o'clock for pressure monitoring (sampling port "off")
- Pointing away from the arterial catheter for blood sampling (flush solution and transducer port "off")
- Pointing towards the catheter to allow flush solution to purge the stopcock sampling port (tubing to arterial catheter "off")

To obtain an arterial sample, a waste syringe is first inserted into the three-way stopcock sample outlet port. The stopcock is then *closed* or turned *off* to the flush solution. The clinician then withdraws the mixture of saline and diluted blood that fills the tubing and arterial catheter, otherwise known as "waste," from the tubing. The intent of this step is to eliminate any flush solution from the line between the cannulation site and the stopcock output port, ensuring that the sample for analysis will contain only arterial blood. After the waste is withdrawn (approximately 3 to 5 mL or until blood enters the syringe, depending on the length of tubing between the stopcock and site), the stopcock is closed to the output port and the waste syringe is removed. At this point, the clinician is ready to withdraw the undiluted arterial blood sample from the system. Next, the blood gas syringe is attached to the output port and the stopcock is closed to the flush solution. The desired amount of arterial blood (generally 2 to 3 mL) is then drawn into the syringe. The stopcock to the output port is then closed and the syringe is removed. The clinician should ensure that no bubbles are in the sample, and then immediately cap the syringe. Finally, the tubing and stopcock output port will need to be flushed to prevent blood clotting and bacterial colonization. Closed systems are also now available that allow the "waste" to be drawn into sterile tubing and flushed back to the patient after the blood gas sample is taken.

Maintenance, Troubleshooting, and Removal of Radial Arterial Catheters

Clinicians should be diligent in the assessment and care of radial arterial catheters. This will ensure patient

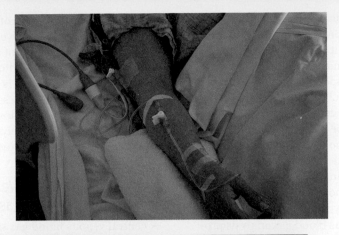

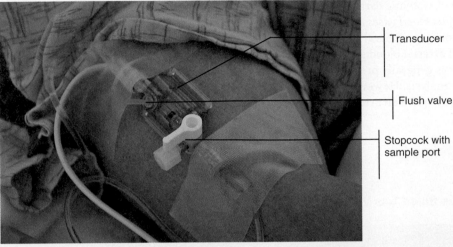

Transducer

Flush valve

Stopcock with
sample port

FIGURE 8-8 **(A) Radial artery monitoring system for a patient in the intensive care unit. (B) Close-up of transducer, flush valve, and stopcock with sample port.**

comfort and safety and the accuracy of the blood pressure readings. The distal extremity (hand in the case of radial arterial lines) should be routinely assessed for signs of adequate perfusion such as appropriate skin temperature, color, and capillary refill. The insertion site itself should be observed for redness or drainage, which may indicate infection. If the arterial line dressing needs to be changed, it should be performed using sterile technique.

If the radial arterial catheter system blood pressure readings fail to correlate with the patient's condition, it may be necessary to troubleshoot the system. Inaccurate readings are due to either human or monitoring system error. Inspect the insertion site to ensure that the catheter is still inserted properly and the connection to the pressure tubing is intact. Check all connections, stopcocks, flush solution pressure bag (300 mm Hg), transducer level, and pressure line. If all efforts to troubleshoot the system fail, it may be necessary to remove the arterial catheter and replace it using an alternative site.

Radial artery catheters should be removed when no longer clinically needed. Removal may also be required

because of infection, lack of perfusion of the distal extremity, or because of failure, as previously mentioned. In some institutions, policy may dictate that indwelling lines be replaced after a certain amount of time has elapsed. When arterial catheters are removed, the clinician should be aware that bleeding may occur. Clean gloves and sterile gauze should be used to hold firm pressure on the site for a minimum of 5 minutes (or longer in some patients). Always monitor the site after catheter removal to ensure that bleeding has ceased.

Venous Blood Gas Sampling

Three types of venous blood gas analysis are possible, depending on the source of the venous blood: mixed venous, central venous, and peripheral venous blood gas analysis.[17–22] Of these, the central venous study and the **mixed venous blood gas study** may provide information useful in evaluation of oxygen delivery to the tissues, as well as assessment of acid-base balance and systemic carbon dioxide.[22] Chapter 6 describes the use of mixed venous blood gas analysis for measurement of mixed venous oxygen tension, saturation, and content and calculation of oxygen consumption, oxygen extraction ratio, and cardiac output using Fick's equation. Use of mixed venous oximetry may also reduce morbidity and mortality in patients undergoing major surgery or in patients with septic shock.[18-20]

Mixed venous sampling requires a pulmonary artery catheter, which should *not* be placed for the sole purpose of obtaining mixed venous blood samples (see below).[22] As an alternative, *central venous blood gases* are measured in the ICU using a sample from a central venous catheter. Central venous oxygen saturation reflects peripheral tissue oxygen extraction and O_2 consumption, and central venous blood gas analysis provides an estimate of systemic carbon dioxide and pH.

Peripheral venous blood gases are measured using a blood sample from a peripheral vein. Given the general availability of arterial blood gas analysis, arterial blood gas analysis is generally preferred over peripheral venous blood gas analysis. However, peripheral venous blood gases do not require an arterial puncture and

can be measured as a part of routine laboratory venous blood analysis. Peripheral venous blood gases can be helpful in the assessment of acid-base balance (e.g., pH) and systemic carbon dioxided. Central venous and peripheral venous pH is highly correlated (usually +/− 0.03), even with severe sepsis or septic shock. If the peripheral venous P_{CO_2} is low (e.g., P_{CO_2} < 45 to 50 mm Hg), hypercapnea is unlikely. Normal peripheral venous blood gas values are reported in **Box 8-3**.

Indications for Mixed Venous or Central Venous Blood Gas Measurement

A central venous blood gas sample is drawn from a central venous catheter, whereas a mixed venous blood sample is obtained from the distal port of a pulmonary artery catheter. The central venous pH and P_{CO_2} are similar to mixed venous values. Properly drawn mixed venous blood samples should reflect the oxygen tension, saturation, and oxygen content of the blood returning from all areas of the body, and this

BOX 8-3

Normal Venous Blood Gas Values

	Analyte (unit)	Description	Blood Gas Values (range)
Peripheral venous blood gases[1]	**pH**	−log [H⁺]	**7.37 (7.31–7.43)**
	P_{VCO_2} (mm Hg)	Venous carbon dioxide tension	46 (38–53)
	P_{VO_2} (mm Hg)	Venous oxygen tension	40 (35–50)
	S_{VO_2} (%)	Venous oxygen saturation	75 (60–80)
	C_{VO_2} (mL/dln vol²)	Venous oxygen content	15 (10–16)
	HCO_3^- (mEq/L)	Venous plasma bicarbonate	24 (19–25)
	TCO_2 (mml/L)	Venous total carbon dioxide	25 (22–26)
Mixed venous blood gas values[2]	**pH**	−log [H⁺]	**7.36 (7.30–7.42)**
	$P\bar{v}_{CO_2}$	Mixed venous CO_2 tension	46 (39–50)
	$P\bar{v}_{O_2}$	Mixed venous O_2 tension	40 (35–40)
	$S\bar{v}_{O_2}$	Mixed venous O_2 saturation	75 (70–75)
	$C\bar{v}_{O_2}$	Mixed venous O_2 content	15 (10–16)

[1]Peripheral venous pH is 0.02 to 0.04 lower than arterial pH; HCO_3^- is 1 to 2 mEq/L higher and P_{CO_2} is 3 to 8 mm Hg higher.
[2]Mixed venous blood pH is usually 0.03 to 0.05 units lower than arterial; P_{CO_2} is 4 to 5 mm Hg higher; HCO_3^- is approximately the same as arterial. Mixed venous and central venous pH and P_{CO_2} are very similar. Central venous oxygen saturation can be 16% higher than mixed venous saturation, and thus central venous O_2 may overestimate mixed venous O_2.
Data from: Theodore, AC. Venous blood gases and other alternatives to arterial blood gases. *Up to Date*, 2013.

may be useful in calculation of indices of oxygenation. Blood within the pulmonary artery is fully mixed and includes blood from the superior vena cava (normally 70% saturated with oxygen), inferior vena cava (normal 80% saturated with oxygen), and coronary sinus (normal 56% saturated with oxygen). If a blood sample is drawn from the right atrium only (e.g., central venous sampling), it may mostly reflect the saturation of oxygen from the superior vena cava. Central venous oxygen saturation can be 16% higher than mixed venous saturation, and thus central venous O_2 may overestimate mixed venous O_2.[20,21] Current guidelines for management of septic shock suggest a target central venous oxygen saturation ≥ 70% or a mixed venous saturation ≥ 65%.

In addition to providing a source for mixed venous blood samples, the pulmonary artery catheter allows for direct measurement of central venous pressure, pulmonary arterial pressure, and pulmonary capillary wedge pressure (which can be used to estimate left ventricular end-diastolic pressure; i.e., preload).[22] A pulmonary artery catheter also can allow for measurement of cardiac output using the thermal dilution technique and calculation of pulmonary vascular resistance. Possible indications for pulmonary artery catheterization include use in determining causes of shock (e.g., cardiogenic, hypovolemic, septic/distributive, or obstructive shock), determining causes of pulmonary edema (e.g., cardiogenic vs. noncardiogenic), and diagnosis of cardiac disease (e.g., pericardial tamponade, left-to-right cardiac shunt).[21,22] Pulmonary artery catheterization may also be of value in fluid management (e.g., blood loss, hypovolemia) and in the management of ICU patients with burns, sepsis, heart failure, or complicated myocardial infarction (MI).[22] In spite of this impressive list of indications, pulmonary artery catheters are used much less often today than was the case in the past. Complications, more difficult site access, lack of evidence that information gathered from the pulmonary artery catheter improves outcomes, and the development of less invasive technology have contributed to the decline in use of the pulmonary artery catheter.[22] Newer technologies using noninvasive systems that calculate cardiac output, stroke volume, and systemic vascular resistance from arterial waveforms have also contributed to the decline in the use of pulmonary artery catheters. Central venous blood gases obtained from a central venous line have also proven to be useful alternatives for the management of conditions such as septic shock. Normal values for venous blood gases are listed in Box 8-3.

Technique for Mixed Venous Blood Gas Sampling

After following proper hand hygiene and identifying the patient according to institutional policy, the clinician should assemble the following equipment:

- Heparinized blood gas syringe
- 3- to 5-mL syringe for discharge sample (waste)
- Chlorhexidine 2% and 70% alcohol swab
- Gloves and face shield or goggles
- A functional pulmonary artery line (Swan-Ganz catheter)

Mixed venous blood is drawn from the pulmonary artery port of the catheter. The stopcock connector should be cleaned with chlorhexidine and alcohol per institutional policy and procedure. The clinician will next connect the waste syringe on the appropriate lumen and turn the stopcock off to the fluid line and on to the patient. Depending on the length or size of the pulmonary artery catheter, 3 to 5 mL of blood should be drawn to clear all fluid from within the catheter. The stopcock should next be closed to the patient, but not open to the fluids, and the waste syringe removed. Prior to drawing the mixed venous sample, the clinician should ensure that the pulmonary artery catheter is not wedged. The blood gas sample syringe should be connected to the stopcock sample port and the stopcock opened to the patient once again so that 2 to 3 mL of mixed venous blood can be gently aspirated for the blood gas sample.

Complications

Complications of central venous lines include bleeding, infection, pneumothorax, collapse of the vessel, interruption of infusions that may maintain blood pressure, and forgetting to restart a medication after obtaining a blood sample. If infection is suspected, it may be necessary to remove the catheter. Possible serious complications of pulmonary artery catheters include bleeding, arrhythmia, air embolism, pneumothorax, hemothorax, infection, tricuspid valve and pulmonary valve complications, myocardial or pulmonary artery perforation, nerve injury, and clot formation.[22] Knotting of the catheter can occur during insertion, and catheter migration can lead to pulmonary infarction.[22] The decision to insert a pulmonary artery catheter should be made based on the potential benefits versus the risks and associated cost.[22]

Sample Analysis

The modern blood gas analyzer directly measures oxygen tension (Po_2 via the Clark electrode), carbon dioxide tension (Pco_2 via the Severinghaus electrode), and pH (via the Sanz electrode).[6,23] With the addition of a multiwavelength blood oximeter (i.e., co-oximeter), oxygen saturation (Sao_2), hemoglobin (Hb), methemoglobin (metHb), and carboxyhemoglobin (COHb) can also be measured.[6,23] Oxygen content (Cao_2) may also be reported based on Hb and measured or calculated Sao_2. Calculated values for plasma bicarbonate (HCO_3^-) and base deficit (BE) or excess (BE) are also routinely reported. Additional measures related to acid-base balance may also be calculated and reported (e.g., standard bicarbonate and T_{40} bicarbonate).[6,23]

In order for the respiratory care clinician to make good clinical decisions based on the results of blood gas analysis, the clinician should be aware of specific problems that can cause the information provided to be inaccurate or misleading. For example, the conditions under which the sample was collected may not be properly recorded or the sample may not represent arterial blood due to the collection technique. Error can also occur during the analysis stage and reporting error can also occur. Last, the respiratory care clinician must be able to interpret the results of an arterial or mixed venous blood gas study with a high degree of confidence in order to ensure that appropriate clinical decisions are made.

Errors in Blood Gas Analysis

Errors in blood gas analysis are sometime classified as preanalytic, analytic, or postanalytic. Preanalytic errors refer to those arising before the blood sample is analyzed. Preanalytic errors are usually related to the methods used in obtaining the sample or handling the sample prior to analysis. Analytic errors are those errors that occur during sample analysis. Postanalytic errors are typically errors in documentation, errors in reporting, or inappropriate action (or inaction) taken by the clinician with respect to the results of the blood gas analysis.

Sample Collection

Preanalytic errors in sample collection include unintentionally collecting a sample that contains venous blood, bubbles in the sample, or excess liquid heparin in the sample. Mislabeling the sample, failure to record the corresponding oxygen concentration or correct mechanical ventilatory support parameters (if applicable), or entering incorrect or inaccurate data into the patient medical record may also be sources of preanalytic error.

Before any blood gas sample is analyzed, it should be properly labeled with the patient's name, location, date/time, and the identity of the person who collected the sample. It must be noted whether the patient is breathing room air or supplemental oxygen. If the patient is receiving oxygen therapy, the oxygen concentration or liter flow being delivered to the patient must be recorded to include oxygen therapy delivery device settings (e.g., liter flow or FIO_2). If the patient is receiving mechanical ventilatory support, the ventilator settings should also be recorded (e.g., mode, respiratory rate, tidal volume, FIO_2). Any needed paperwork should be completed prior to the sampling procedure in order to reduce the time to analysis after the sample is collected. Recording this information prior to obtaining the sample also helps to reduce the opportunity for sample mix-up and incorrect reporting of results. Information

regarding the exact tests to be performed should accompany the sample to the laboratory.

Generally, the respiratory care clinician should determine that there have been no changes in delivered FIO_2 (or ventilator settings for those receiving ventilatory support) for 20 to 30 minutes prior to drawing a blood gas sample in order to ensure that the results reflect the patient's condition. If there have been very recent changes in oxygen administration or level of ventilatory support, the blood gas results may not accurately reflect the patient's response to those changes. In some cases, it may not be possible to wait for 20 to 30 minutes; the clinician needs to be aware of the situation in which the sample was drawn and interpret the results accordingly. It is also important to remember that an arterial blood gas study only represents a snapshot in time. A patient's condition can change rapidly, and it may be necessary to redraw a sample if the clinical situation has changed.

Use of Heparin

Blood gas samples should be obtained using a heparinzed glass or plastic syringe. Plastic syringes may allow gas to diffuse across the wall of the syringe, altering the results of the analysis. This potential source of error can be avoided by prompt sample analysis (within 15 minutes) or use of a glass or plastic syringe designed for blood gas sampling.[23] Heparin is used to prevent coagulation; however, if acidic heparin is used (e.g., liquid sodium heparin), excessive heparin may decrease the sample's measured pH. When used for blood gas sampling, liquid sodium heparin is generally drawn into the sample syringe in sufficient quantity to lubricate the syringe (e.g., 1 to 2 mL of a 1000 unit per mL solution) and then completely ejected so that there is less than 0.5 mL remaining in the needle and needle hub. The use of prepackaged blood gas syringes that include lyophilized (freeze-dried) heparin or lithium heparin will avoid this potential source of error; however, dry heparin may fail to dissolve quickly or sufficiently to prevent clot formation. Most prepackaged arterial sampling syringes today contain lithium heparin. Lithium heparin syringes are preferred over sodium heparin when electrolytes are measured; however, they should not be used when lithium levels are being measured. It is important to know the type of heparin being used and the minimum volume of blood needed per sample (generally 2 to 3 mL).

Bubbles in the Sample

Arterial blood gas samples should be free of air bubbles and any bubbles in the sample should be expelled immediately. At sea level, the partial pressure of oxygen (PO_2) in room air is approximately 150 mm Hg, and the partial pressure of carbon dioxide (PCO_2) is very close to zero. If an arterial blood gas sample contains air bubbles, the blood sample PO_2 and PCO_2 will attempt to equilibrate with the gas tensions of the bubble. This problem will be exacerbated with larger bubbles, a longer time of exposure of the blood to the air in the bubble, or agitation of the sample. Air bubbles may cause the analyzed blood to indicate a falsely decreased P_{CO_2} because CO_2 in the blood sample will diffuse out of the blood and into the bubble. An air bubble's effect on analyzed P_{O_2} will vary depending on whether the actual blood P_{O_2} is higher or lower than the P_{O_2} of the air bubble. At sea level (bubble $P_{O_2} \approx 150$ mm Hg), if the patient's actual P_{O_2} is < 150 mm Hg, the analysis may indicate a falsely elevated P_{O_2}, whereas if the patient's actual P_{O_2} is > 150 mm Hg, the results of the analysis may indicate a falsely low P_{O_2}. To summarize, an air bubble in the sample will cause the analyzed P_{CO_2} to be lower than actual and usually cause the analyzed P_{O_2} to be greater than actual, because the actual patient P_{O_2} is usually less than the P_{O_2} of the bubble, which contains room air. In cases where the patient's Pa_{O_2} is greater than the air bubble P_{O_2}, blood gas analysis may indicate a falsely lower Pa_{O_2} than normal.

Cooling the Sample

Cooling samples with ice or ice slush is performed to slow oxygen consumption by blood cells, which may occur over time if the sample is not analyzed promptly. There is some debate and practice variability regarding the use of ice prior to sample analysis. Although it is probably not necessary to cool samples if analysis is performed immediately, we suggest that all samples be placed on ice prior to transport to the lab in case there is a delay. In particular, very high leukocyte count (leukocytosis [elevated white blood cell count]) or high platelet count may result in a reduction in Pa_{O_2} due to O_2 consumption by these cells.[3,23] A prolonged time to analysis (> 30 minutes) may also adversely affect the analysis if samples are not cooled.

Temperature Correction

Blood gases are measured at 37° C, and temperature correction of the blood gas values is performed to adjust the results based on the patient's actual body temperature. In cases where the patient's body temperature is > 37° C, the analyzed values for P_{O_2} and P_{CO_2} will be lower than the patient's actual values and the pH will be higher. If the patient's actual body temperature is < 37° C, the analyzed values for P_{O_2} and P_{CO_2} will be higher than the patient's actual values and the pH will be lower. The following example indicates how the actual patient values will vary from the analyzed values when the patient's body temperature is low (35° C), normal (37° C), or elevated (38° C):

Patient temperature	35° C	37° C	38° C
Analyzed P_{O_2} (mm Hg)	80	80	80
Actual P_{O_2} (mm Hg)	70	80	85
Analyzed P_{CO_2} (mm Hg)	40	40	40
Actual P_{CO_2} (mm Hg)	37	40	42
Analyzed pH	7.4	7.4	7.4
Actual pH	7.43	7.4	7.39

The practice of temperature correction is somewhat complex and controversial. In general, temperature correction provides information that may not be particularly clinically important when the patient's temperature is in the range of 35° C to 39° C.[6,23,24] In cases of severe hypothermia or hyperthermia (< 35° C or > 39° C), the blood gas results may be inaccurate enough to warrant temperature correction, as shown in these two examples of hypothermia and elevated temperature:

- Patient temperature: 30° C (86° F)

	Values analyzed at 37° C	Values corrected to 30° C
P_{O_2}	100 mm Hg	88 mm Hg
P_{CO_2}	40 mm Hg	27.7 mm Hg
pH	7.40	7.499

In the case of hypothermia, the actual P_{O_2} and P_{CO_2} are lower than the analyzed values and the pH is higher. In this first example, the differences may be clinically important.

- Patient temperature: 41° C (105.8° F)

	Values analyzed at 37° C	Values corrected to 41° C
P_{O_2}	100 mm Hg	106 mm Hg
P_{CO_2}	40 mm Hg	47 mm Hg
pH	7.40	7.343

In this case of elevated temperature, the actual P_{O_2} and P_{CO_2} are higher than the analyzed values and the pH is lower; these differences may be clinically important.

To make the most informed clinical judgment, both the temperature-adjusted values and nonadjusted values should be reported. Though different temperature-correction formulas will generate slightly different results, as a rough guide, the P_{O_2} will vary directly with temperature about 5% to 7% for each 1° C, P_{CO_2} will vary directly about 5% for each 1° C, and pH will vary inversely by about 0.015 for each 1° C. Temperature-adjusted values must be clearly labeled as such on any laboratory report.

Quality Assurance and Control

A careful quality assurance (QA) and quality control (QC) program for arterial blood gas analysis includes the routine analysis of known control values and monitoring of the results. The accuracy and reliability of arterial blood gas results is absolutely essential because important, often critical, decisions are made based on these results.

The basics of a successful QA/QC program include:

- Assurance of proper sampling technique and handling
- Analyzer function and accuracy determinations
- Result reporting procedures

Many different arterial blood gas analyzers are available on the commercial market. Each manufacturer may have a different calibration procedure for their analyzer. Operators of the equipment must follow the specific calibration procedure, use specified material, and follow the frequency for quality control procedures detailed by the manufacturer. Documenting when the procedures have been completed is also important.

Acid-Base Chemistry

A normal acid-base balance is needed for most body functions to proceed properly. In order to properly interpret the results of blood gas analysis, the clinician must have a firm grounding in acid-base chemistry, particularly as it affects the body and homeostasis.

Solutions and Ions

The following definitions are helpful when discussing solutions and ions:

- *Solvent*: The major component of a solution. In biology, it is water (H_2O).
- *Solute*: The minor component of a solution. It is usually a chemical substance, drug or medication, weak acid, weak base, or salt.
- *Un-ionized*: A molecular substance that has not dissociated into its ionized components. Table salt is un-ionized sodium chloride (NaCl); that is, sodium bound to chloride to form the salt molecule (NaCl).
- *Ionized*: Dissociated. When placed in solution, salt dissociates into sodium ions and chloride ions:

$$NaCl \rightarrow Na^+ \; Cl^-$$

Brønsted-Lowry Definitions

In order to understand acid-base chemistry, the respiratory care clinician must understand a few additional definitions:

- *Acid*: A substance (molecule or ion) that tends to donate protons (hydrogen ions, or H^+) in solution (i.e., a proton donor). This is the Brønsted-Lowry definition of an acid.
- *Base*: A substance that tends to accept protons (remove H^+) from solution (i.e., a proton acceptor). This is the Brønsted-Lowry definition of a base.
- *Buffer*: A weak acid or base that accepts or donates hydrogen ions in response to the availability of free hydrogen ions in solution. Buffers in solutions help avoid extremes in hydrogen ion concentration ([H^+], note that the brackets indicate hydrogen ion concentration).

BOX 8-4

Strong and Weak Acids and Bases

Substance	In Solution
Strong acid: Hydrochloric acid (HCl)	$HCl \rightarrow H^+ + Cl^-$
Strong base: Sodium hydroxide (NaOH)	$NaOH \rightarrow N^+ + OH^-$
Salt: Sodium chloride (NaCl)	$NaCl \rightarrow Na^+ + Cl^-$
Weak acid: Carbonic acid (H_2CO_3)	$H_2CO_3 \rightarrow H^+ + HCO_3^-$
Weak base: Sodium bicarbonate ($NaHCO_3$)	$NaHCO_3 \rightarrow Na^+ + HCO_3^-$

Examples of strong and weak acids and bases are found in **Box 8-4**.

Quantifying Hydrogen Ion Concentration

In order to understand acid-base chemistry, the clinician must know how quantities of acids and bases are reported. Quantities of a chemical substance in solution are typically expressed in moles/L or millimoles/L, where 1 mole is 6.023×10^{23} molecules of the substance (6.023×10^{23} is Avogadro's number). One mole of a substance has a mass of 1 gram molecular weight (gmw), which is the sum of the atomic weights of the elements that make up the substance. For instance, oxygen (O) has an atomic weight of 16 grams (g). For molecular oxygen (O_2), the gram molecular weight would be 32 g (2×16). Thus, 32 g of oxygen at standard temperature and pressure dry (STPD) would constitute 1 gram molecular weight, contain 6.023×10^{23} oxygen molecules (1 mole), and have a volume of 22.4 L. Carbon dioxide (CO_2) has a gram molecular weight of 44, or 44 grams per mole.

Because hydrogen ions are charged particles, hydrogen ion concentration ([$H+$]) is often reported using *equivalent weights*. The gram equivalent weight of a substance is the gram mass that contains, replaces, or reacts (directly or indirectly) with 1 mole of hydrogen ions. For our purposes, 1 mole of H^+ = 1 Equivalent (Eq). A common unit of measure for ions found in the body is mEq/L, where:

$$1 \text{ mEq/L} = 0.001 \text{ Eq/L}$$

Water dissociates slightly into hydrogen ions and hydroxyl ions:

$$H_2O \rightarrow H^+ + OH^-$$

The hydrogen ion concentration [H$^+$] for water is very small:

$$[H^+] = \frac{1 \times 10^{-7} \text{ moles}}{\text{Liter}} = \frac{1 \times 10^{-7} \text{ Eq}}{L} = \frac{0.0000001 \text{ mole of } H^+}{L}$$

Because such small quantities of H$^+$ are often dealt with in solutions, the Scandinavian scientist S. P. L. Sorensen referred to hydrogen ion concentrations for values such as 1×10^{-7} as 7 puissance hydrogen. Karl Hasselbalch liked this system and formalized it into what has become known as *Sorenson's expression*:

$$pH = -\log [H^+]$$

The pH scale ranges from a low of 1.0 (extremely acid) to a high of 14.0 (extremely alkaline or basic). Water has a pH of 7.0, which is considered to be neutral. Normal arterial blood pH is 7.40 with a range of 7.35 to 7.45. **Box 8-5** provides examples of hydrogen ion concentration reported as pH and in Eq/L for various acids and bases.

An alternate method sometimes used to report [H$^+$] is nanoequivalents per liter (nEq) or nanomoles per liter (nM/L). One nanomole of H$^+$ is equal to one nanoequivalent; *nano* refers to a billionth. A normal arterial pH of 7.4 represents a hydrogen ion concentration ([H+]) of 40 nEq/L. For each 0.1 change in pH, [H+] varies indirectly by approximately 10 nEq/L. Thus, a pH of 7.3 is equivalent to a hydrogen ion concentration of about 50 nEq/L, and a pH of 7.5 is a hydrogen ion concentration of about 30 nEq/L. **Box 8-6** compares pH and [H+] concentration in nEq/L in the range sometimes seen clinically.

BOX 8-6

Hydrogen Ion Concentration in the Physiologic Range (pH Units and Nanoequivalents per Liter [nEq/L])

For each 0.1 decrease in pH, [H$^+$] increases approximately 10 nEq/L. Using this rule, hydrogen ion concentration can be estimated from pH as follows:

pH	Hydrogen Ion Concentration (nEq/L)	
	Estimated	Actual
7.60	20	25
7.55	25	28
7.50	30	32
7.45	35	35
7.40	40	40
7.35	45	45
7.30	50	50
7.25	55	56
7.20	60	63
7.15	65	71
7.10	70	79

Using this rule, the estimated [H$^+$] is fairly close to actual [H$^+$] for the pH range of 7.20 to 7.55. The rule tends to fail at extreme values of pH (pH < 7.2 or > 7.55).

BOX 8-5

Hydrogen Ion Concentration in Eq/L and pH Units

[H$^+$] Eq/L	pH	Acidity/Alkalinity
1×10^{-1}	1.0	Extreme acid
1×10^{-6}	6.0	Acidic
1×10^{-7}	7.0	Neutral (water)
1×10^{-8}	8.0	Alkaline (basic)
1×10^{-14}	14.0	Extreme base

Henderson Equation for Carbonic Acid

The Henderson equation is used to describe the disassociation of any weak acid or base in solution. For carbon dioxide in water, the reaction is:

$$CO_2 + H_2O \leftrightarrow H_2CO_3 \leftrightarrow [H^+] + [HCO_3^-]$$

where H_2CO_3 is carbonic acid and HCO_3^- is the bicarbonate ion.

Now for the system $H_2CO_3 \leftrightarrow [H+] + [HCO_3^-]$ in solution, the following two reactions are ongoing:

$$R_1 \quad H_2CO_3 \rightarrow [H^+] + [HCO_3^-]$$

and

$$R_1 \quad [H^+] + [HCO_3^-] \rightarrow [H_2CO_3]$$

where R_1 is the disassociation of carbonic acid into hydrogen ions and bicarbonate ions and R_2 is the reformation of carbonic acid from hydrogen ions and bicarbonate ions. In solution, both R_1 and R_2 are occurring simultaneously. When the reactions are equal ($R_1 = R_2$), the system is said to be at equilibrium. At equilibrium, the ratio of the product of the hydrogen ion concentration and the bicarbonate ion concentration to the carbonic acid concentration will be a constant:

$$K_a = \frac{[H^+]\,[HCO_3^-]}{[H_2CO_3]}$$

This is known as the *Henderson equation*, where K_a is the dissociation constant, $[H^+]$ is the hydrogen ion concentration, $[HCO_3^-]$ is the bicarbonate ion concentration, and $[H_2CO_3]$ is the carbonic acid concentration. Under normal conditions in the body, $K_a = 1 \times 10^{-6.1}$ and normal arterial $[H^+]$ is 40 mEq/L. Carbonic acid concentration ($[H_2CO_3]$) can be calculated based on $Paco_2$ levels, as follows:

$$[H_2CO_3] = Paco_2 \times 0.03$$

Given a normal $Paco_2$ of 40 mm Hg, normal $[H_2CO_3]$ would be calculated as follows:

$$[H_2CO_3] = Paco_2 \times 0.03 = 40 \times 0.03 = 1.2\ \text{mEq/L}$$

The Henderson equation can be rearranged to calculate $[HCO_3^-]$:

$$K_a = \frac{[H^+]\,[HCO_3^-]}{[H_2CO_3]}$$

$$[HCO_3^-] = \frac{[H_2CO_3]}{[H^+]} \times K_a$$

Substituting normal values for arterial blood this becomes:

$$[HCO_3^-] = \frac{[H_2CO_3]}{[H^+]} \times K_a = \frac{(Paco_2 \times 0.03)}{[H^+]} \times 10^{-6.1}$$

$$= \frac{Paco_2}{40} \times 24^* = 24\ \text{mEq/L}$$

* Includes factor to convert from nEq/L to mEq/L.

Henderson-Hasselbalch Equation

Clinically, hydrogen ion concentration is commonly reported in pH units. The **Henderson-Hasselbalch equation** explains the relationship among pH, $[HCO_3^-]$, $[H_2CO_3]$, and $Paco_2$:

$$pH = pK_a + \log\frac{[HCO_3^-]}{[H_2CO_3]}$$

and

$$pH = pK_a + \log\frac{[HCO_3^-]}{Pco_2 \times 0.03}$$

where pK_a is the $-\log(K_a) = 6.1$; $[HCO_3^-]$ is the bicarbonate ion concentration (mEq/L); $[H_2CO_3]$ is the carbonic acid concentration; Pco_2 is the partial pressure of carbon dioxide in mm Hg; and 0.03 is the solubility constant for CO_2 in plasma ($H_2CO_3 = Pco_2 \times 0.03$).

Box 8-7 provides the derivation of the Henderson-Hasselbalch equation. **Figure 8-9** illustrates the "acid-base balance" and demonstrates how the ratio of $[HCO_3^-]$ to $Paco_2$ (as $[H_2CO_3]$) determines the pH. As long as the ratio is 20:1, the pH will be normal (pH = 7.40). Figure 8-9 also illustrates that an increase in volatile acid (e.g., increase in $Paco_2$) can be balanced by a corresponding increase in base (e.g., increase in HCO_3^-). In a similar fashion, a decrease in volatile acid (e.g., decrease in $Paco_2$) can be balanced by a corresponding decrease in base (e.g., decrease in HCO_3^-).

Calculation of Bicarbonate

Bicarbonate concentration $[HCO_3^-]$ and base excess/deficit (BE/BD) are not directly measured; these values must be calculated. Total CO_2 (TCO_2) may be measured in the clinical laboratory or calculated (see below). An older method of deriving the plasma bicarbonate and related values is the Siggaard-Andersen alignment nomogram (**Figure 8-10**) that allows for determination of plasma HCO_3^-, TCO_2, and BE/BD. based on the patient's measured pH, $Paco_2$, and hemoglobin (Hb). The bicarbonate level may also be calculated using a variation of the Henderson-Hasselbalch equation:

$$[HCO_3^-] = \text{antilog}\,(pH - 6.1) \times 0.003\ Paco_2$$

Box 8-8 provides examples of plasma bicarbonate (HCO_3^-) calculation using Henderson-Hasselbalch; **Box 8-9** provides examples of plasma HCO_3^- calculation using a modification of the Henderson equation. In clinical practice, plasma bicarbonate and related values are typically calculated using algorithms built into the blood gas analyzer.

Regulation of Blood Acids

The major volatile acid in the body is carbonic acid, which is formed from carbon dioxide and water. Carbon dioxide ($Paco_2$) is transported in the blood and regulated by the level of ventilation, as discussed in Chapter 7. Increased levels of carbon dioxide may result in a **respiratory acidosis** (hypoventilation or ventilatory failure), whereas decreased levels of carbon dioxide may result in a **respiratory alkalosis** (alveolar hyperventilation).

Nonvolatile acids in the body include dietary acids, lactic acids, and ketoacids. Dietary acids are the result of the metabolism, which generates organic and inorganic acids. The kidneys must excrete 50 to 100 mEq of these organic and inorganic acids per day. A normal diet in the presence of inadequate kidney function will result in a renal acidosis.

BOX 8-7

Derivation of the Henderson-Hasselbalch Equation

The Hasselbalch derivation of the Henderson equation is as follows:

1. $K_a = \dfrac{[H^+]\,[HCO_3^-]}{[H_2CO_3]}$

2. $[H^+] = (K_a)\dfrac{[H_2CO_3]}{[HCO_3^-]}$

3. $\log[H^+] = \log\left[K_a\dfrac{[H_2CO_3]}{[HCO_3^-]}\right]$

4. The $\log(ab) = \log a + \log b \rightarrow \log[H^+] = \log\left[K_a\dfrac{H_2CO_3}{HCO_3^-}\right] = \log K_a + \log\dfrac{[H_2CO_3]}{HCO_3^-}$

5. $(-1)\log[H^+] = (-1)\log(K) + (-1)\log\dfrac{[H_2CO_3]}{[HCO_3^-]}$

6. $-\log[H^+] = -\log K + -\log\dfrac{[H_2CO_3]}{[HCO_3^-]}$

7. $-\log(a/b) = +\log(b/a) \rightarrow -\log[H^+] = -\log K + \log\dfrac{[HCO_3^-]}{[H_2CO_3]}$

8. $-\log[H^+] = pH$ *AND* $-\log K = pK \rightarrow pH = pK + \log\dfrac{[HCO_3^-]}{[H_2CO_3]}$

9. Finally, $K = 10^{-6.1} \rightarrow pK = 6.1$
   AND
   $[H_2CO_3] = P_{CO_2} \times 0.03$ (solubility coefficient for CO_2)

10. $pH = 6.1 + \log\dfrac{[HCO_3^-]}{P_{CO_2} \times 0.03}$

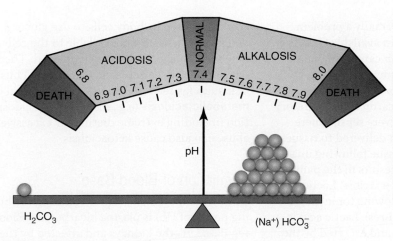

pH	Ratio
7.8	50:1
7.6	30:1
7.4	20:1
7.3	15:1
7.2	13:1
7.1	10:1

FIGURE 8-9 Acid–base balance.

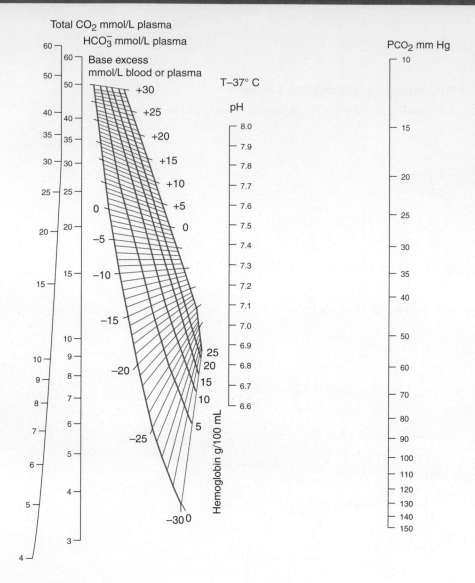

FIGURE 8-10 **Siggaard-Andersen alignment nomogram.**

Modified with permission from Mahoney JJ, Hodgkin J, Van Kessel A. Arterial blood gas analysis. In: Burton G, Hodgkin J, Ward J, eds. *Respiratory Care: A Guide to Clinical Practice.* Lippincott Williams & Wilkins; 1997, p. 263 (Figure 9.6).

Lactic acid production is not normally a problem. However, with a marked decrease in available O_2 at the cellular level, anaerobic metabolism can occur. The major waste product of anaerobic metabolism is lactic acid. A lactic acidosis often accompanies severe hypoxemia, such as is found following a cardiac or respiratory arrest. Lactic acid also occurs in severe sepsis where tissues are unable to utilize oxygen delivered to tissues. Lactic acid also forms in muscle tissue following unaccustomed strenuous exercise and results in the pain felt the next day by many weekend warriors. Lactic acid may also form in muscle tissue following tonic-clonic seizures (epileptic generalized seizures). Lactic acid is metabolized primarily by the liver and excreted by the kidneys.

Normal aerobic metabolism uses glucose to produce energy. Insulin is a hormone secreted by the pancreas

that is required by body cells to use glucose. If insulin is deficient, glucose is not available to the cells, and alternate metabolic pathways are employed. These alternate pathways produce keto acids (ketones). Thus, a lack of insulin (as seen in diabetes) is a potential cause of a **metabolic acidosis** (e.g., diabetic ketoacidosis). Starvation (including extreme dieting) or excessive alcohol abuse can also cause ketoacidosis.

Regulation of Blood Base

The primary blood base (not counting the buffering power of Hb) is plasma bicarbonate. Blood base is regulated via the kidneys and affected by the body's electrolytes. The kidneys have the ability to increase or decrease the bicarbonate ion concentration in body fluids. This is done through a complex series of reactions

BOX 8-8

Calculation of Bicarbonate Using the Henderson-Hasselbalch Equation

The modern blood gas analyzer directly measures:

- Po_2 via the Clark electrode
- Pco_2 via the Severinghaus electrode
- pH via the Sanz electrode

With the addition of a blood oximeter (e.g., co-oximeter), oxygen saturation (Sao_2), hemoglobin (Hb), methemoglobin (metHb), and carboxyhemoglobin (COHb) can be measured using multiple wavelength spectrophotometry and O_2 content (Cao_2) calculated.

Bicarbonate, base excess, and total CO_2, however, must be calculated. Examples of calculation of bicarbonate concentration using the Henderson-Hasselbalch equation follow.

Example 1: Given pH = 7.4 and Pco_2 = 40 mm Hg, calculate HCO_3^-.

1. $pH = pK + \log \dfrac{[HCO_3^-]}{[H_2CO_3]}$

2. $7.4 = 6.1 + \log \dfrac{[HCO_3^-]}{(Paco_2 \times 0.03)}$

3. $7.4 = 6.1 + \log \dfrac{[HCO_3^-]}{(40 \times 0.03)}$

4. $7.4 = 6.1 + \log \dfrac{[HCO_3^-]}{1.2}$

5. $7.4 - 6.1 = \log \dfrac{[HCO_3^-]}{1.2}$

6. $1.3 = \log \dfrac{[HCO_3^-]}{1.2}$

7. The antilog of $1.3 = 20$ or $\log(20) = 1.3$

$1.3 = \log \dfrac{[HCO_3^-]}{1.2} \; AND \; 1.3 = \log(20)$

8. By substitution: $\log(20) = \log \dfrac{[HCO_3^-]}{1.2}$

9. If the $\log(a) = \log(b)$, then $a = b$

$20 = \dfrac{[HCO_3^-]}{1.2}$

10. $[HCO_3^-] = 20 \times 1.2 = 24$ mEq/L

Example 2: Given pH = 7.28 and $Paco_2$ = 40, calculate HCO_3^-.

1. $pH = pK + \log \dfrac{[HCO_3^-]}{[H_2CO_3]}$

2. $7.28 = 6.1 + \log \dfrac{[HCO_3^-]}{(40 \times 0.03)}$

3. $7.28 - 6.1 = \log \dfrac{[HCO_3^-]}{(1.2)}$

4. $1.18 = \log \dfrac{[HCO_3^-]}{(1.2)}$

5. A log table or scientific calculator must be used to find the antilog of 1.18:

Antilog of $1.18 = 15$

OR

$\log(15) = 1.18$

6. $\log \dfrac{[HCO_3^-]}{[1.2]} = 1.18$

AND

$\log(15) = 1.18$

7. $\log(15) = \log \dfrac{[HCO_3^-]}{[1.2]}$

8. $15 = \dfrac{[HCO_3^-]}{1.2}$

9. $[HCO_3^-] = 15 \times 1.2 = 18$ mEq/L

BOX 8-9

Bicarbonate Calculation Based on the Modified Henderson Equation

Because the Henderson-Hasselbalch equation requires the use of logarithms, some clinicians prefer to use a variation on the original Henderson equation to calculate bicarbonate:

1. $K_a = \dfrac{[H^+][HCO_3^-]}{[H_2CO_3]}$

3. $[HCO_3^-] = \dfrac{10^{-6.1}(P_{CO_2} \times 0.03)}{[H^+]}$

2. $[HCO_3^-] = \dfrac{K_a[H_2CO_3]}{[H^+]}$

4. $[HCO_3^-] = \dfrac{24 \times P_{CO_2}^*}{[H+]}$

Example 1: Given pH = 7.5 and Pa_{CO_2} = 30, what is the approximate $[HCO_3^-]$?

1. First we must estimate the hydrogen ion concentration. Using the rule of thumb discussed in **Box 8-7**, we have:

pH	[H+] Approximate (nEq/L)
7.2	60
7.3	50
7.4	40
7.5	30

Consequently, a pH of 7.5 is equivalent to a $[H^+]$ of approximately 30 nEq/L.

2. The data are entered into our formula:

$$[HCO_3^-] = \frac{24 \times P_{CO_2}}{[H^+]}$$

$$[HCO_3^-] = \frac{24 \times 30}{30} = 24 \text{ mEq/L}$$

Example 2: Given pH = 7.2 and P_{CO_2} = 80, estimate HCO_3^-.
A pH of 7.2 represents a $[H^+]$ of approximately 60 nEq/L.

$$[HCO_3^-] = \frac{24 \times P_{CO_2}}{[H^+]}$$

$$[HCO_3^-] = \frac{24 \times 80}{60} = 32 \text{ mEq/L}$$

*The factor (24) includes the conversion from nEq to mEq.

in the renal tubules, including reactions for hydrogen ion secretion, sodium ion reabsorption, bicarbonate absorption into the urine, and ammonia secretion into the renal tubules. Simply put, the kidneys can excrete HCO_3^- in order to lower plasma HCO_3^- and pH and retain HCO_3^- to increase plasma HCO_3^- and pH. Older texts suggest it takes 24 to 48 hours for this renal mechanism to adjust for a pH disorder in the blood; however, full renal compensation may take 3 to 5 days to complete.[23,25] In addition to plasma and erythrocyte bicarbonate, nonbicarbonate buffers are present in the

blood. These include hemoglobin, organic phosphates, inorganic phosphates, and plasma proteins.[25]

Electrolytes

Electrolytes are free ions (i.e., charged particles of acids, bases, or salts) found in body fluids. These electrolytes can have a profound effect on acid-base balance. The major electrolytes in the plasma are potassium (K^+), sodium (Na^+), chloride (Cl^-), and bicarbonate (HCO_3^-). Other important electrolytes include calcium (Ca^{2+}), magnesium (Mg^{2+}), and phosphorus (HPO_4^{-2}, PO_4^{-3}). Normal values for serum electrolytes are described in Chapter 9. A brief discussion of the effects of electrolyte disturbances on acid-base balance follows.

Potassium (K^+) is a major intracellular cation (positive charge). Normal values for K^+ in the plasma are 3.5 to 5.0 mEq/L. A loss of extracellular potassium will cause K^+ to be pulled from within the cells in exchange for hydrogen ions, lowering the plasma hydrogen ion concentration and raising the pH. *Hypokalemia* refers to a reduction in serum potassium that may be caused by K^+ loss in the urine or body fluids, decreased K^+ intake, or a shift from extracellular to intracellular K^+. A decrease in serum K^+ will cause the kidneys to conserve K^+ in exchange for H^+ excretion. The result is a *hypokalemic alkalosis*. Specific causes of hypokalemia include inadequate K^+ intake in the diet, administration of loop or thiazide diuretics (e.g., furosemide [Lasix] or hydrochlorothiazide [Aquazide H, HydroDIURIL]), loss through the gastrointestinal (GI) tract (e.g., diarrhea, vomiting), excessive sweating, and K^+ loss during dialysis or plasmapheresis. Certain potassium-sparing diuretics (e.g., aldosterone inhibitors) may cause an abnormal increase in K^+ (hyperkalemia).

Chloride (Cl^-) is a major extracellular anion (negative charge). Normal values for Cl^- in the plasma are 98 to 105 mEq/L. A decrease in plasma Cl^- (hyporchloremia) will cause an increase in plasma HCO_3^- to maintain electrical balance and a corresponding increase in pH (alkalosis). A decrease in Cl^- in the renal tubules will also cause additional K^+ loss, further contributing to an alkalosis. The net result is a **metabolic alkalosis** (*hypochloremic alkalosis*). Ammonium chloride is sometimes used in the treatment of patients with a metabolic alkalosis. Although low Cl^- may cause metabolic alkalosis, elevated Cl^- may cause a metabolic acidosis (*hyperchloremic acidosis*). Possible causes of a metabolic acidosis include loss of gastrointestinal HCO_3^-, renal tubular failure to reabsorb HCO_3^-, ingestion or administration of ammonium chloride, and intravenous nutrition (e.g., hyperalimentation).

Plasma bicarbonate (HCO_3^-) is the major body anion responsible for maintaining acid-base balance; the ratio of HCO_3^- to carbonic acid (H_2CO_3) determines pH. A metabolic acidosis may be defined as decreased plasma HCO_3^-. Causes of HCO_3^- loss include diarrhea, loss via pancreatic fistula, and renal tubular loss. Other causes of low plasma HCO_3^- include lactic acid accumulation (e.g., lactic acidosis), ketoacidosis (e.g., diabetes, starvation), renal failure (e.g., failure to excrete dietary acids), and ingestion of acids (e.g., salicylate [aspirin] overdose, ingestion of methanol or ethylene glycol). Causes of elevated plasma HCO_3^- include loss of acid (H^+) through vomiting or nasogastric (NG) drainage (e.g., NG suction) or the urine (e.g., diuretics). Other causes of increased HCO_3^- include hypochloremia

(decrease in Cl^-), hypokalemia (decrease in K^+), hypovolemia (low blood volume), and ingestion or administration of $NaHCO_3$. To summarize, accurate assessment of an acid-base disorder should include measurement of serum electrolytes.[25] Alterations in K^+, Cl^-, or HCO_3^- may all contribute to acid-base disturbances.

Anion Gap

The routine measurement of serum electrolytes includes the measurement of sodium (Na^+), potassium (K^+), chloride (Cl^-), and bicarbonate (HCO_3^-). Electrolytes that may not be routinely measured and reported include calcium (Ca^{2+}), magnesium (Mg^{2+l}), and phosphorus (PO_4). Normally, the values for plasma anions (negative charge) and cations (positive charge) must balance in order to maintain electrical neutrality (electroneutrality):

Cations	Value	Anions	Value
Na+	140 mEq/L	Cl-	105 mEq/L
K+	4 mEq/L	HCO3-	24 mEq/L
Unmeasured cations	10 mEq/L	Unmeasured anions	25 mEq/L
Total cations	154 mEq/L	Total anions	154 mEq/L

Even though the sum of charges for body anions and cations is zero, for clinical assessment of acid-base balance the **anion gap** is often calculated:

$$\text{Anion gap (mEq/L)} = [Na^+] - ([Cl^-] + [HCO_3^-])$$

For the purposes of the calculation, the potassium and unmeasured anions and cations are ignored. Using normal values for sodium, chloride, and bicarbonate, a calculated anion gap would be:

$$\text{Anion gap (mEq/L)} = [Na^+] - ([Cl^-] + [HCO_3^-])$$
$$\text{Anion gap (mEq/L)} = 140 - (105 + 24) = 11 \text{ mEq/L}$$

In fact, the "normal" anion gap is dependent on the methods used for electrolyte measurement. Historically, the normal range for the anion gap has been reported at 8 to 16 mEq/L; newer technology in use in today's clinical laboratories suggests that a normal anion gap is < 11 mEq/L.

Certain types of acidosis will cause an increase in the calculated anion gap (> 11 mEq/L), whereas other types of acidosis will occur with a normal anion gap. This fact can be used to help identify the cause of a metabolic acidosis. Causes of high anion gap acidosis include lactic acidosis (e.g., severe tissue hypoxia), ketoacidosis (e.g., diabetic crisis), or ingestion of acids (e.g., methanol, ethylene glycol, and salicylate [aspirin] overdose, which in adults causes a lactic acidosis). Causes of a normal anion gap acidosis include diarrhea, pancreatic fistula, and ingestion of certain substances (e.g., ammonium chloride or hyperalimentation). Kidney disease can cause an increased anion gap acidosis (e.g., renal failure with failure to excrete acid) or a normal anion gap acidosis (e.g., renal tubular acidosis with failure to reabsorb HCO_3^-).

Arterial Blood Gas Interpretation

Interpretation of the results of arterial blood gas analysis requires a solid understanding of respiratory physiology and the ability to clinically apply the information. The respiratory care clinician must understand oxygenation, ventilation, and acid-base chemistry and be able to interpret blood gas results in light of the patient's condition. Appropriate interpretation of arterial blood gas study results can give provide insight to the underlying clinical condition and may positively impact clinical decision making; inaccurate or incorrect interpretation of results can lead to harmful, even catastrophic, patient outcomes.[25-27]

Interpretation of arterial blood gases is best done systematically. Before any blood gas can be clinically interpreted, the clinician must have adequate information regarding the patient's condition and have conducted a clinical assessment. The value of the arterial blood gas study relies on the clinician's ability to interpret the results appropriate to the situation and apply clinical interventions accordingly. A typical arterial blood gas report contains the following measured values:

- Arterial pH
- Pa_{O_2} (arterial oxygen tension in mm Hg)
- Pa_{CO_2} (arterial carbon dioxide tension in mm Hg)

If the blood gas laboratory employs co-oximetry as a part of routine blood gas analysis, the following additional measured values may be reported:

- Sa_{O_2} (arterial oxygen saturation)
- Hb (hemoglobin in g/dL)
- COHb (% carboxyhemoglobin)
- metHb (% methemoglobin)

The blood gas report also typically includes a number of calculated values:

- Plasma bicarbonate (HCO_3^-)
- Base excess or deficit (BE or BD)
- Sa_{O_2} (if calculated)
- Ca_{O_2} (if calculated; calculation of Ca_{O_2} may be based on measured or calculated Sa_{O_2})

When interpreting the results of an arterial blood gas study, the clinician will typically review the patient's oxygenation, ventilation, and acid-base balance using a standardized approach.

Assessment of Oxygenation

Chapter 6 provides a detailed description of the assessment of a patient's oxygenation. This should include physical assessment to identify clinical manifestations (signs and symptoms) of hypoxia and review of the factors that affect the oxygenation process. The effectiveness of oxygenation begins with an adequate inspired oxygen tension ($P_{I_{O_2}}$). The conducting airways must be free of obstruction and offer low resistance to gas flow. Alveolar ventilation must be sufficient, and there must be adequate matching of gas and blood in the lung. Effective diffusion of oxygen across the alveolar–capillary membrane must occur, resulting in adequate arterial blood oxygen tension (Pa_{O_2}), saturation of the hemoglobin (Sa_{O_2}), and blood oxygen content (Ca_{O_2}). The oxygen-laden blood must then be delivered to tissues; this requires adequate cardiac output and blood pressure and good tissue perfusion. Finally, tissue uptake and utilization of oxygen must occur.

For basic blood gas interpretation, Pa_{O_2} and Sa_{O_2} are typically reviewed and classification of severity of hypoxemia is based on the Pa_{O_2} value. For classifying severity of hypoxemia, we suggest the following guidelines for patients breathing room air ($F_{I_{O_2}} = 0.21$):

- Pa_{O_2} 80 to 100 mm Hg: Normal
- Pa_{O_2} < 80 but ≥ 60 mm Hg: Mild hypoxemia
- Pa_{O_2} < 60 mm Hg but ≥ 50 mm Hg: Moderate hypoxemia
- Pa_{O_2} < 50 but ≥ 40 mm Hg: Moderate to severe hypoxemia
- Pa_{O_2} < 40 mm Hg: Severe hypoxemia

These values must be interpreted based on the patient's age, condition, and care received. For example, whereas a Pa_{O_2} of ≥ 80 mm Hg (Sa_{O_2} ≥ 0.95 or 95%) is considered normal for individuals breathing room air, these values would be very low for patients breathing 100% oxygen ($F_{I_{O_2}} = 1.0$). Expected normal values for Pa_{O_2} also decline with age. For example, for an 80-year-old patient in the supine position, the expected "normal" Pa_{O_2} would be approximately 75 mm Hg with a range of 76 to 83 mm Hg (see **Clinical Focus 8-1**).

Clinically, a Pa_{O_2} ≥ 60 mm Hg usually results in oxygen saturation (Sa_{O_2}) ≥ 90%, and this is generally considered to be an acceptable clinical goal for most patients. It also must be noted that assessment of a patient's oxygenation status should always include assessment of oxygen saturation (Sa_{O_2}), oxygen content (Ca_{O_2}), oxygen delivery ($\dot{D}_{O_2}$), and tissue oxygen uptake and utilization. It must also be noted that the alveolar air equation describes the relationship between ventilation and oxygenation. As ventilation decreases (Pa_{CO_2} increases), alveolar and arterial oxygen decrease ($P_{A_{O_2}}$ and Pa_{O_2} decrease) This relationship can be simplified for patients breathing room air: if P_{CO_2} increases by 4 mm Hg, then Pa_{O_2} decreases by about 5 mm Hg. These and other aspects of assessment of oxygenation are discussed in Chapter 6.

Assessment of Ventilation

Chapter 7 provides a detailed description of the assessment of a patient's ventilation. For purposes of blood gas interpretation, suffice it to note that for clinical

CLINICAL FOCUS 8-1

Expected Changes in Pa_{O_2} with Age

Arterial oxygen tension (Pa_{O_2}) varies with age and can be estimated as follows when the patient is breathing room air:

$$Pa_{O_2} = 104 - (0.27 \times age)$$

Using this formula to calculate expected normal values:

- Pa_{O_2} for a 70-year-old would be 85 mm Hg
- Pa_{O_2} for an 80-year-old would be 82 mm Hg
- Pa_{O_2} for a 90-year-old would be 80 mm Hg

As an alternative, the following method has been suggested to estimate expected values for patients older than 60 years:

- For each year above 60 years of age, subtract 1 mm Hg from the low normal Pa_{O_2} of 80 mm Hg. This is sometimes known as the 70-70 rule, because it predicts a Pa_{O_2} of 70 for a patient age 70 years.*
  - The expected minimum Pa_{O_2} for an 80-year-old patient is:
    - $80 - 60 = 20$ mm Hg
    - Normal Pa_{O_2}: 80 to 100 mm Hg
    - Adjust Pa_{O_2} for age 80 years: $80 - 20 = 60$ mm Hg; $100 - 20 = 80$ mm Hg
    - Expected minimum Pa_{O_2} for an 80-year-old patient would be 60 to 80 mm Hg
- Example:
  - Age < 60 years: Pa_{O_2} < 80 mm Hg = hypoxemia
  - Age 70: Pa_{O_2} < 70 mm Hg = hypoxemia
  - Age 80: Pa_{O_2} < 60 mm Hg = hypoxemia

* It should be noted that this rule is somewhat controversial, and there is evidence that the rule is unreliable for older patients in the age range of 80–90 years.

Generally, for patients of any age Pa_{O_2} < 60 mm Hg should be considered hypoxemia.*

Alternative calculations have been suggested for age based on the patient's position:

- Supine: Normal $Pa_{O_2} = 109 - (0.43 \times Age) \pm 8$ mm Hg
- Prone: Normal $Pa_{O_2} = 104 - (0.27 \times Age) \pm 12$ mm Hg

*Beachy W. Clinical assessment of acid-base and oxygenation status. In: Beachy W (ed.). *Respiratory Care Anatomy and Physiology*, 2nd ed. St. Louis, MO: Mosby-Elsevier; 2007: 214–235.

purposes, the single best index of ventilation is the arterial carbon dioxide tension (Pa_{CO_2}). Consequently, we can assess a patient's ventilatory status based on blood gas analysis of Pa_{CO_2} using the following definitions:

- Pa_{CO_2} of 35 to 45 mm Hg: Normal ventilation
- Pa_{CO_2} > 45 mm Hg: Hypoventilation (ventilatory failure)
- Pa_{CO_2} < 35 mm Hg: Hyperventilation (alveolar hyperventilation)

Hypoventilation (ventilatory failure) and hyperventilation can be characterized as acute, subacute, or chronic, depending on how long the condition has been present. Typically, acute conditions are of very recent occurrence, whereas chronic conditions have been present for a number of days, weeks, months, or even years. A respiratory acidosis (or acidemia) is caused by

an abnormal elevation in Pa_{CO_2}, whereas a respiratory alkalosis (or alkalemia) is caused by an abnormally low Pa_{CO_2}. *Acidosis* and *alkalosis* are generalized terms, whereas *acidemia* and *alkalemia* refer to conditions in the blood.

Assessment of Acid-Base Balance

The respiratory care clinician should first assess the patient's overall **acid-base status** by reviewing the arterial blood pH. We will define normal (or fully compensated) arterial pH as 7.40 with a range of 7.35 to 7.45. A pH < 7.35 may be defined as an **acidosis** (or **acidemia**). A pH > 7.45 may be defined as an **alkalosis** (or **alkalemia**). As noted earlier, the terms acidemia and alkalemia are used to indicate that these values are measured in the blood, whereas the terms acidosis and alkalosis are used to describe the overall condition. For the purposes of our discussion, we will use these terms interchangeably. To summarize:

- pH of 7.35 to 7.45: Normal (fully compensated)
- pH < 7.35: Acidosis (acidemia)
- pH > 7.45: Alkalosis (alkalemia)

Causes of Observed pH

The pH of the arterial blood is determined in large part by the relationship between the plasma HCO_3^- (the major blood base) and the $Paco_2$ (the volatile blood acid):

$$pH \approx \frac{HCO_3^-}{Paco_2}$$

Plasma bicarbonate is primarily regulated by the kidneys and represents the *metabolic component* of acid-base balance. An abnormal pH caused by a change in HCO_3^- is defined a metabolic disorder (e.g., *metabolic acidosis* or *metabolic alkalosis*). Derived measures that reflect changes in HCO_3^- include base excess (BE) and base deficit (BD), which are described below. Carbon dioxide (as represented by $Paco_2$) is primarily regulated by the lungs and is considered the *respiratory component* of acid-base balance. An abnormal pH caused by a change in $Paco_2$ is defined a respiratory disorder (e.g., respiratory acidosis or respiratory alkalosis).

Because pH is determined by the ratio of HCO_3^- to Pco_2, an abnormal HCO_3^- can be compensated for by a change in Pco_2 and vice versa. For example, if HCO_3^- increases with no change in $Paco_2$, this will result in an *uncompensated metabolic alkalosis*. If HCO_3^- increases with a corresponding (compensatory) increase in $Paco_2$, this will result in a *partially compensated metabolic alkalosis* if the pH is not normalized and a *fully compensated metabolic alkalosis* if the pH is normalized. If HCO_3^- decreases with no change in $Paco_2$, this will result in an *uncompensated metabolic acidosis*. If HCO_3^- decreases with a corresponding (compensatory) decrease in $Paco_2$, this will result in a *partially compensated metabolic acidosis* if the pH is not normalized and a *fully compensated metabolic acidosis* if the pH is normalized.

If $Paco_2$ increases with no change in HCO_3^- this will result in an *uncompensated respiratory acidosis.* If $Paco_2$ increases with a corresponding (compensatory) increase HCO_3^-, this will result in a *partially compensated respiratory acidosis* if the pH is not normalized and a *fully compensated respiratory acidosis* if the pH is normalized. If $Paco_2$ decreases with no change in HCO_3^-, this will result in an *uncompensated respiratory alkalosis.* If $Paco_2$ decreases with a corresponding (compensatory) decrease HCO_3^-, this will result in a *partially compensated respiratory alkalosis* if the pH is not normalized and a *fully compensated respiratory*

alkalosis if the pH is normalized. Figure 8-9 illustrates the fact the pH is determined by the ratio of HCO_3^- to CO_2 (as H_2CO_3).

To summarize, plasma HCO_3^- and BE/BD are used to quantify the metabolic component of acid-base balance. Carbon dioxide (as represented by $Paco_2$) is used to quantify the respiratory component of acid-base balance. The following conditions can be defined using conventional nomenclature:

- $Paco_2$ of 35 to 45 mm Hg: Normal
- $Paco_2$ > 45 mm Hg: Respiratory acidosis (hypoventilation or ventilatory failure)
- $Paco_2$ < 35 mm Hg: Respiratory alkalosis (alveolar hyperventilation)
- HCO_3^- of 22 to 28 mEq/L: Normal
- HCO_3^- < 22 mEq/L: Metabolic acidosis
- HCO_3^- >28 mEq/L: Metabolic alkalosis
- BE/BD ± 2 mEq/L: Normal
- BD < −2.0: Metabolic acidosis
- BE > +2.0: Metabolic alkalosis

Conventional Nomenclature for Blood Gas Interpretation

Using conventional nomenclature, any blood gas result can quickly be classified using the following steps:

1. Classify the overall acid-base status based on pH:
   - Normal or fully compensated (pH = 7.35 to 7.45)
   - Acidosis (pH < 7.35)
   - Alkalosis (pH > 7.45)
2. Classify the respiratory condition based on $Paco_2$:
   - Normal ($Paco_2$ = 35 to 45 mm Hg)
   - Respiratory acidosis ($Paco_2$ > 45 mm Hg)
   - Respiratory alkalosis ($Paco_2$ < 35 mm Hg)
3. Classify the metabolic condition based on plasma (HCO_3^-) and BE/BD:
   - Normal (HCO_3^- = 22 to 28 mEq/L; BE/BD ±2 mEq/L)
   - Metabolic acidosis (HCO_3^- < 22 mEq/L; BD < −2.0)
   - Metabolic alkalosis (HCO_3^- > 28 mEq/L; BE > +2.0 mEq/L)
4. Describe the cause of the pH abnormality based on steps 2 and 3:
   - pH abnormalities caused by an increase or decrease in $Paco_2$ are classified as respiratory acidosis or respiratory alkalosis.
   - pH abnormalities caused by an increase or decrease in HCO_3^- (and increase or decrease in BE/BD) are classified as metabolic alkalosis or metabolic acidosis.
   - pH abnormalities in which you have both a metabolic and respiratory acidosis *or* a metabolic and respiratory alkalosis are classified as combined conditions.

5. Determine the degree of compensation (if any). An increase in respiratory acid (increase in $Paco_2$) can be compensated by an increase in metabolic base (increase in HCO_3^-, increase in BE). Conversely, a decrease in respiratory acid (decrease in $Paco_2$) can be compensated by a decrease in metabolic base (decrease in HCO_3^-, decrease in BD). By the same token, an increase in metabolic base may be compensated by an increase in $Paco_2$ and a decrease in metabolic base may be compensated by a decrease in $Paco_2$. Compensation for respiratory and metabolic disorders is summarized below:

Primary Problem	Compensation
↑ HCO_3^- (metabolic alkalosis)	↑ $Paco_2$ (respiratory acidosis)
↓ HCO_3^- (metabolic acidosis)	↓ $Paco_2$ (respiratory alkalosis)
↑ $Paco_2$ (respiratory acidosis)	↑ HCO_3^- (metabolic alkalosis)
↓ $Paco_2$ (respiratory alkalosis)	↓ HCO_3^- (metabolic acidosis)

To determine whether compensation is occurring, examine the $Paco_2$ and bicarbonate levels for trending in the appropriate direction to return the pH towards normal. For example, if the arterial pH is acidic due to an elevated $Paco_2$, the body will attempt to correct the problem by elevating the bicarbonate level. The degree of compensation (full or partial) is determined by the pH value. If the pH value is < 7.35 but trending towards normal, it would be partially compensated. If the pH value is normal, it may be classified as fully compensated. Full compensation may occur with mild to moderate respiratory alkalosis and with mild to moderate respiratory acidosis.[23,25] With these exceptions, compensatory responses tend not to return the arterial pH to normal, and what may appear to be full compensation may instead represent a mixed acid-base disturbance (see below).[25]

The body also does not overcompensate for an acid-base distrubance.[23,25-27] This means that for an acidosis with complete compensation, the pH would tend to remain on the acidotic side of 7.40. With complete compensation, an alkalosis would tend to remain on the alkalotic side of 7.40. This fact can be helpful when trying to determine the cause of a fully compensated condition. If the pH is in the range of 7.35 to 7.40, the condition may be classified as a fully compensated acidosis; if the pH is in the range of 7.40 to 7.45, the condition may be classified as a fully compensated alkalosis. This guideline should *not* be applied indiscriminately, because it may lead to errors. The patient history and prior blood gas studies (if available) should always be reviewed when classifying an acid-base disturbance, as well as the likely compensatory response.

To review, using conventional nomenclature an acid-base disorder can be classified as uncompensated, partially compensated, or fully compensated:

- **Uncompensated:** There is an abnormality in HCO_3^- but no corresponding (compensatory) change in $Paco_2$ *or* there abnormality in $Paco_2$ but no corresponding (compensatory) change in HCO_3^-.
- **Partially compensated:** There is an increase $Paco_2$ and HCO_3^- *or* there is a decrease in $Paco_2$ and HCO_3^- and pH is abnormal.
- **Fully compensated:** There is an increase in $Paco_2$ and HCO_3^- *or* there is a decrease in $Paco_2$ and HCO_3^- and pH is normal.

Table 8-2 provides examples of changes in pH, HCO_3^-, BE/BD and the corresponding blood gas classification using conventional nomenclature. **Box 8-10** provides examples of basic blood gas interpretation using conventional nomenclature. **Clinical Focus 8-2** provides examples of partially and fully compensated blood gases for metabolic acid-base disturbances. Compensation for respiratory acid-base disturbances is discussed below.

Other Measures of the Metabolic Component of Acid-Base Balance

Whereas plasma HCO_3^- is thought to primarily represent the metabolic component of acid-base balance, acute changes in $Paco_2$ directly affect HCO_3^- levels:

$$CO_2 + H_2O \rightleftarrows H_2CO_3 \rightleftarrows H^+ + HCO_3^-$$

An acute increase in $Paco_2$ of 10 mm Hg will increase plasma HCO_3^- by about 1 mEq/L.[25] Conversely, an acute reduction in $Paco_2$ of 10 mm Hg ($Paco_2$ < 35 mm Hg) will reduce HCO_3^- about 2 mEq/L.[25] This relationship between HCO_3^- and CO_2 does *not* represent renal compensation.

A chronically elevated $Paco_2$ will result in an increased HCO_3^- of about 5 mEq/L per 10 mm Hg elevation in $Paco_2$.[25] A chronic reduction in $Paco_2$ will result in a decrease in HCO_3^- of about 4 to 5 mEq/L for every 10 mm Hg decrease in $Paco_2$.[25] This change in HCO_3^- is caused by renal compensation, and generally takes 3 to 5 days to complete.

Although the direct effects of acute changes in $Paco_2$ on HCO_3^- are small, other measures that better reflect the metabolic component of acid base disorders have been sought. These include standard bicarbonate, base excess/deficit (BE/BD), and T_{40} bicarbonate.

Standard Bicarbonate

One attempt to better quantify the metabolic component of an acid-base disturbance is the calculation of *standard bicarbonate*. Standard bicarbonate is defined as the plasma bicarbonate concentration when the blood has been equilibrated to achieve a $Paco_2$ of 40 mm Hg, a temperature of 37° C, and an Sao_2 of 100%.[6,25-28] Normal values for standard bicarbonate are 24 mEq/L with a range of 22 to 26 mEq/L. Because

TABLE 8-2
Traditional Conventional Nomenclature for Blood Gas Interpretation

Respiratory Acidosis	pH	Paco$_2$	HCO$_3^-$	BE
Uncompensated	↓	↑	N	N
Partially compensated	↓	↑	↑	↑
Fully compensated*	N	↑	↑	↑
Respiratory Alkalosis	**pH**	**Paco$_2$**	**HCO$_3^-$**	**BD**
Uncompensated	↑	↓	N	N
Partially compensated	↑	↓	↓	↓
Fully compensated*	N	↓	↓	↓
Metabolic Acidosis	**pH**	**Paco$_2$**	**HCO$_3^-$**	**BD**
Uncompensated	↓	N	↓	↓
Partially compensated	↓	↓	↓	↓
Fully compensated*	N	↓	↓	↓
Metabolic Alkalosis	**pH**	**Paco$_2$**	**HCO$_3^-$**	**BE**
Uncompensated	↑	N	↑	↑
Partially compensated	↑	↑	↑	↑
Fully compensated*	N	↑	↑	↑

N, normal (pH: 7.35 to 7.45; Paco$_2$: 35 to 45 mm Hg; BE/BD ± 2 mEq/L); BE, base excess (abnormal > + 2.0); BD, base deficit (abnormal < −2.0).
*Normally, the body does not fully compensate for an acid-base disturbance. Full compensation may occur with mild to moderate respiratory alkalosis and with mild to moderate respiratory acidosis. With these exceptions, compensatory responses tend not to return the arterial pH completely back to normal and what may appear to be full compensation may instead represent a mixed acid-base disturbance. That said, conventional nomenclature as taught in many settings retains the term *fully compensated* to describe a normal pH with increased Paco$_2$ and HCO$_3^-$ or a normal pH with decreased Paco$_2$ and HCO$_3^-$, as illustrated in this table.

BOX 8-10

Examples of Blood Gas Interpretation Using Traditional Conventional Nomenclature

	pH	Paco$_2$	HCO$_3^-$	BE/BD
Respiratory acidosis				
Uncompensated	7.20	70	26	−1.0
Partially compensated	7.30	65	31	+4.6
Fully compensated	7.36	55	30	+4.7
Respiratory alkalosis				
Uncompensated	7.55	26	22	−0.2
Partially compensated	7.50	25	19	−4
Fully compensated	7.44	25	16.4	−6.9

	pH	Paco$_2$	HCO$_3^-$	BE/BD
Metabolic acidosis				
Uncompensated	7.20	40	15	−11
Partially compensated	7.30	28	13	−12
Fully compensated	7.36	26	14	−10
Metabolic alkalosis				
Uncompensated	7.55	40	34	+11
Partially compensated	7.50	50	38	+14
Fully compensated	7.45	55	37	+12
Combined states				
Metabolic and respiratory alkalosis	7.58	32	29	+7
Metabolic and respiratory acidosis	7.15	50	17	−11

Paco$_2$, arterial partial pressure of carbon dioxide; HCO$_3^-$, plasma bicarbonate; BE/BD, base excess/base deficit.

CLINICAL FOCUS 8-2

Conventional Nomenclature: Partially and Fully Compensated Metabolic Acidosis and Alkalosis[1]

Example 1

A hospitalized patient suffered a cardiac arrest and was successfully resuscitated. Postresuscitation arterial blood gases were drawn and analyzed with the following results:

pH: 7.28
Paco$_2$: 32 mm Hg
HCO$_3^-$: 14.5 mEq/L
BD: −10.8

Using conventional nomenclature, what is your interpretation of this patient's acid-base status?

Step 1: Classify the pH. The blood pH indicates an *overall acidosis.*

Step 2: Classify the respiratory condition based on the Paco$_2$. The Paco$_2$ of 32 mm Hg indicates a *respiratory alkalosis* (hyperventilation).

Step 3: Classify the metabolic condition based on the HCO$_3^-$ and BE/BD. The HCO$_3^-$ (14.5 mEq/L) and BD (−10.8) indicate a *metabolic acidosis.*

Step 4: Describe the cause of the pH abnormality based on steps 2 and 3. The overall condition (step 1) is acidosis and the source is metabolic (step 3). Thus, the patient has a *metabolic acidosis* caused by the low HCO$_3^-$.

Step 5: Determine the degree of compensation (if any). Compensation for a metabolic acidosis is a respiratory alkalosis, which has occurred; however, the pH has *not* normalized. Using traditional nomenclature, this blood gas result would be described as *partially compensated metabolic acidosis.*

The patient suffered a cardiac arrest that caused severe tissue hypoxia resulting in a lactic acidosis. Following successful resuscitation, the patient was able to hyperventilate in order to partially compensate for the metabolic acidosis.

Several hours later, blood gases are repeated on this patient with the following results:

pH: 7.35
Paco$_2$: 30 mm Hg

(continues)

HCO_3^-: 16 mEq/L
BD: −8.5

Using traditional conventional nomenclature, how should the patient's acid-base status now be described?

Step 1: Classify the pH. The pH is now *normal* or *fully compensated*.

Step 2: Classify the respiratory condition based on the $Paco_2$. The $Paco_2$ of 30 mm Hg indicates a *respiratory alkalosis* (hyperventilation).

Step 3: Classify the metabolic condition based on the HCO_3^- and BE/BD. The HCO_3^- (16 mEq/L) and BD (−8.5) indicate a *metabolic acidosis*.

Step 4: Describe the cause of the pH abnormality based on steps 2 and 3. This patient has a normal pH and a metabolic acidosis combined with a respiratory alkalosis. The primary abnormality can often be determined according to which condition occurred first. Because the metabolic (lactic) acidosis occurred first, this blood gas would be classified as a *metabolic acidosis*.

Step 5: Determine the degree of compensation (if any). The postresuscitation blood gases indicated a partially compensated metabolic acidosis. Several hours later, the pH has returned to normal (full compensation). Using traditional conventional nomenclature, this blood gas result would now be described as a *fully compensated metabolic acidosis*.[2]

Normally, respiratory compensation for a metabolic acid-base disturbance occurs very quickly. The response generally begins within 30 minutes and is complete within 12 to 24 hours.

Example 2

A hospitalized postoperative abdominal surgery patient is in the intensive care unit (ICU). Blood chemistry testing indicates a hypokalemia (low K^+), probably secondary to intravenous fluid (IV) administration without potassium replacement. Arterial blood gases were drawn and analyzed with the following results:

pH: 7.50
$Paco_2$: 48 mm Hg
HCO_3^-: 36 mEq/L
BD: +12

Using conventional nomenclature, what is your interpretation of this patient's acid-base status?

Step 1: Classify the pH. The blood pH indicates an *overall alkalosis*.

Step 2: Classify the respiratory condition based on the $Paco_2$. The $Paco_2$ of 48 mm Hg indicates a *respiratory acidosis* (hypoventilation).

Step 3: Classify the metabolic condition based on the HCO_3^- and BE/BD. The HCO_3^- (36 mEq/L) and BD (+12) indicate a *metabolic alkalosis*.

Step 4: Describe the cause of the pH abnormality based on steps 2 and 3. The patient has a *metabolic alkalosis* caused by the increased HCO_3^-.

Step 5: Determine the degree of compensation (if any). Compensation for a metabolic alkalosis is a respiratory acidosis, which has occurred; however, the pH has not normalized. Using traditional conventional nomenclature, this blood gas result would be described as a *partially compensated metabolic alkalosis*.

The patient had major surgery and is in the ICU with intravenous IV fluid administration resulting in a reduced potassium level. The reduced potassium level has caused a *hypokalemic alkalosis*.

Several hours later, blood gases are repeated on this patient with the following results:

pH: 7.45
$Paco_2$: 50 mm Hg
HCO_3^-: 34 mEq/L
BD: +9.2

Using traditional conventional nomenclature, how should the patient's acid-base status now be described?

Step 1: Classify the pH. The blood gas results now indicates a *normal (or fully compensated) pH*.

Step 2: Classify the respiratory condition based on the $Paco_2$. The $Paco_2$ of 50 mm Hg indicates a *respiratory acidosis* (hypoventilation).

Step 3: Classify the metabolic condition based on the HCO_3^- and BE/BD. The HCO_3^- (34 mEq/L) and BD (+9.2) indicate a *metabolic alkalosis*.

Step 4: Describe the cause of the pH abnormality based on steps 2 and 3. The patient has a metabolic alkalosis and a respiratory acidosis resulting in a normalized pH. The primary abnormality can often be determined according to which condition occurred first in time. Because the metabolic alkalosis occurred first, this blood gas would be classified as a *metabolic alkalosis*.

Step 5: Determine the degree of compensation (if any). The initial blood gas study indicated a partially compensated metabolic alkalosis. Several hours later, the pH has returned to normal (full compensation). Using traditional conventional nomenclature, this blood gas result would now be described as a *fully compensated metabolic alkalosis.*[2]

As noted above, respiratory compensation for a metabolic acid-base disturbance usually occurs very quickly. The response generally begins within 30 minutes and is complete within 12 to 24 hours.

[1]The terms *acidosis* and *alkalosis* refer to overall, or extracellular, fluid pH, whereas the terms *acidemia* and *alkalemia* refer to arterial blood pH, $Paco_2$, and HCO_3^-. For the purposes of this exercise, we will use the terms loosely.

[2]In cases of a fully compensated alkalosis or acidosis, another indicator of the possible cause is based on which side of 7.40 the pH value falls. For example, if pH is < 7.40 but > 7.35, the condition may represent a *fully compensated acidosis*; if the pH is > 7.40 but < 7.45, the condition may represent a *fully compensated alkalosis*. The source of the acidosis or alkalosis is then used to describe the primary condition (e.g., *respiratory* or *metabolic*). This guideline is based on the fact that the body tends not to overcompensate for an acidosis or alkalosis. The guideline should be used with caution, and the clinician should review the patient's history and previous blood gases (if available) before drawing a conclusion as to the primary cause of a fully compensated acid-base disturbance.

standard bicarbonate is calculated as if the $Paco_2$ were normal, it is thought to better represent the metabolic component of an acid-base disorder than plasma bicarbonate. It may work well in adjusting for the effect of $Paco_2$ on HCO_3^- when $Paco_2$ is low, but may be unreliable in cases of elevated $Paco_2$ because it does not account for the differences in actual body response (in vivo) versus what occurs in the laboratory (in vitro).[28] In the body, HCO_3^- can diffuse out of the blood into the extracellular fluid, whereas other blood buffers (e.g., blood proteins, including hemoglobin) cannot.

Base Excess or Deficit

Base excess (BE) or deficit (BD) is defined as the amount of acid or base needed to return the pH to normal with a normal $Paco_2$ (e.g., $Paco_2$ = 40 mm Hg). Base excess of blood is an in vitro measure done in the laboratory, which probably does not reflect changes in the body (in vivo) in the presence of hypercapnea (increased $Paco_2$).[6,25–28] BE/BD of extracellular fluid is easy to calculate and is probably a better measure of metabolic status than plasma HCO_3^-. BE/BD of extracellular fluid takes into account the buffering effect of the red blood cell and is thought to better reflect the entire extracellular fluid, not just the blood.[25-28] In cases where the HCO_3^- value is normal but the BE/BD value is not (or vice versa), we recommend that for the purposes of classification the BE/BD be used. **Box 8-11** illustrates a method for calculation of BE/BD.

T$_{40}$ Bicarbonate

T_{40} bicarbonate is an additional calculation that may be performed to quantify the metabolic component of an acid-base disorder in the event of an acute increase in $Paco_2$. T_{40} bicarbonate is simply the observed plasma bicarbonate minus the bicarbonate expected to occur due to acute changes in $Paco_2$. Normal T_{40} bicarbonate

is 24 mEq/L with a range of 22 to 26 mEq/L. T_{40} bicarbonate is thought to be a good measure of the metabolic component of an acid-base disorder in the presence of hypercapnea (increased $Paco_2$).[28] **Box 8-12** illustrates calculation of T_{40} bicarbonate.

Total CO$_2$

Total CO_2 (TCO_2) is often directly measured in the clinical laboratory and reported as a part of routine blood chemistry testing. TCO_2 may also be calculated:

$$TCO_2 = HCO_3^- + Paco_2 \times 0.03$$

Given a normal $Paco_2$ of 40 mm Hg with a normal HCO_3^- of 24 mEq/L:

$$TCO_2 = 24 \text{ mEq/L} + 40 \times 0.03$$

$$TCO_2 = 24 \text{ mEq/L} + 1.2 \text{ mEq/L} = 25.2 \text{ mEq/L}$$

Problems with Conventional Nomenclature

Classifying an arterial blood gas result using conventional nomenclature has several shortcomings. Assuming for a moment that full compensation is possible, it may be difficult to distinguish between a fully compensated metabolic alkalosis and a fully compensated respiratory acidosis. It also may not be easy to distinguish between a fully compensated metabolic acidosis and a fully compensated respiratory alkalosis. Although prior blood gases and a review of the patient's history and other assessment findings may help, a single blood gas result may not discriminate between these conditions. It also must be remembered (with the exception of mild to moderate respiratory acidosis and alkalosis) that compensatory mechanisms generally tend *not* to return the arterial pH to normal; what appears to be full compensation may in fact be a mixed disorder (see below).[25]

BOX 8-11

Estimation of Base Excess or Base Deficit (BE/BD)

Base excess or deficit can be estimated using the following formula:[1,2]

$$BE/BD \cong (0.90 \times HCO_3^-) + (14 \times pH) - 125$$

Example 1: Given a patient with pH = 7.04, $Paco_2$ = 76, and HCO_3^- = 19.9, estimate BE/BD.

$$BE/BD = (0.90 \times HCO_3^-) + (14 \times pH) - 125$$
$$= (0.90 \times 19.9) + (14 \times 7.04) - 125$$
$$= -8.5 \ (actual \ BD^1 = -9.2)$$

Example 2: Given a patient with pH = 7.21, $Paco_2$ = 90, and HCO_3^- = 34.8, estimate BE/BD.

$$BE/BD = (0.90 \times HCO_3^-) + (14 \times pH) - 125$$
$$= (0.90 \times 34.8) + (14 \times 7.21) - 125$$
$$= +7.3 \ (actual \ BE^1 = +7.0)$$

Example 3: Given a patient with pH = 7.47, $Paco_2$ = 18, and HCO_3^- = 12.7, estimate BE/BD

$$BE/BD = (0.90 \times HCO_3^-) + (14 \times pH) - 125$$
$$= (0.90 \times 12.7) + (14 \times 7.47) - 125$$
$$= -9.0 (actual \ BE = -10.0)$$

Example 4: Given a patient with pH = 7.54, $Paco_2$ = 29, and HCO_3^- = 24, estimate BE/BD.

$$BE/BD = (0.90 \times HCO_3^-) + (14 \times pH) - 125$$
$$= (0.90 \times 24) + (14 \times 7.54) - 125$$
$$= +2.2 \ (actual \ BE = +1.5)$$

[1]Actual formula is: BE/BD = (0.9287 × HCO_3^-) + (13.77 × pH) − 124.50
[2]BE/BD will vary with hemoglobin levels. Estimate is approximately ±1 units.

BOX 8-12

Calculation of T_{40} Bicarbonate

1. ***To estimate T_{40} bicarbonate for an acute increase in $Paco_2$:***

$$T_{40} \ bicarbonate = Observed \ HCO_3^- - \left(\frac{Paco_2 - 40}{15} \right)$$

Example 1: Given a patient with pH = 7.14, $Paco_2$ = 85, HCO_3^- = 28 mEq/L, and BE/BD = 0, estimate T_{40} bicarbonate.

$$T_{40} \ bicarbonate = Observed \ HCO_3^- - \left(\frac{Paco_2 - 40}{15} \right)$$
$$= 28 - \left(\frac{85 - 40}{15} \right)$$
$$= 28 - 3 = 25 \ mEq/L$$

The patient has an uncompensated respiratory acidosis (i.e., acute ventilatory failure).

2. ***To estimate T_{40} bicarbonate for an acute decrease in $Paco_2$:***

$$T_{40} \ bicarbonate = Observed \ HCO_3^- - \left(\frac{40 - Paco_2}{5} \right)$$

Example 2: Given a patient with pH = 7.58, $Paco_2$ = 22, HCO_3^- = 20 mEq/L, and BE/BD = −7, estimate T_{40} bicarbonate.

$$T_{40} \ bicarbonate = Observed \ HCO_3^- - \left(\frac{40 - Paco_2}{5} \right)$$
$$= 20 + 3.6 = 23.6 \ mEq/L$$

The patient has an uncompensated respiratory alkalosis (acute alveolar hyperventilation).

The second problem with conventional nomenclature is that it does not do a good job of describing certain disorders often seen in patients with pulmonary disease. For example, a patient with chronic obstructive pulmonary disease (COPD) with a history of chronic CO_2 retention (chronic ventilatory failure) may present to the emergency department with an acute exacerbation. Blood gases may then be drawn and analyzed:

Oxygen: Nasal cannula at 2 L/min
Pao_2: 48 mm Hg

pH: 7.28
$Paco_2$: 72 mm Hg
HCO_3^-: 38 mEq/L
BE: +10 mEq/L

Using conventional nomenclature, the clinician may classify this blood gas result as partially compensated respiratory acidosis with moderate to severe hypoxemia. However, if this blood gas represents an acute change superimposed on a chronic condition, the clinical picture could be described differently. A better assessment based on the patient's history would be *acute ventilatory failure superimposed on chronic ventilatory failure.*[6] This approach to clinical interpretation will be discussed further below.

A third problem with conventional nomenclature is that it assumes that full compensation is possible. In fact, respiratory compensation for a metabolic condition is limited. Metabolic acidosis may be compensated (in part) by hyperventilation (respiratory alkalosis). Respiratory compensation for a severe metabolic acidosis, however, will not achieve a $Paco_2$ of less than 8 to 12 mm Hg in patients with good lung function.[25] Patients with lung disease will have a more limited response. Respiratory compensation for a metabolic alkalosis is hypoventilation (respiratory acidosis). This respiratory response is limited to a maximum $Paco_2$ of about 55 mm Hg in most patients.[25] Though limited, respiratory compensation usually occurs rapidly. Respiratory compensation begins within 30 minutes and is complete within 12 to 24 hours.[25]

Metabolic compensation for a respiratory condition is slower and may also be limited. The initial response to a respiratory disturbance involves buffering by the blood, extracellular fluid, and cells.[25] This response, though modest, occurs within a few minutes.[25] The kidneys provide the majority of metabolic compensation for a respiratory disorder. In the case of a respiratory acidosis, the kidneys increase acid excretion and HCO_3^- reabsorption.[25] For a respiratory alkalosis, the kidneys decrease acid excretion and HCO_3^- reabsorption.[25] Renal compensation for a respiratory disorder begins quickly but takes 3 to 5 days to be complete.[25] Compensation for a mild to moderate chronic respiratory alkalosis or acidosis may return the pH to normal (e.g., fully compensated respiratory alkalosis or full compensated respiratory acidosis).[25]

Expected Respiratory and Renal Compensation

As previously described, the body attempts to regulate pH through compensation. Bicarbonate (HCO_3^-) is normally maintained by the kidneys at a level of 22 to 26 mEq/L (though we will consider the normal range 22–28 mEq/L). $Paco_2$ levels are normally maintained between 35 and 45 mm Hg by the lungs. The relationship between the HCO_3^- and $Paco_2$ determines the pH. Metabolic disorders that cause increases or decreases in HCO_3^- are typically accompanied by an appropriate response from the respiratory system (e.g., increase or decrease in $Paco_2$). Respiratory disorders that cause increases or decreases in $Paco_2$ are typically accompanied by an appropriate renal response (e.g., increase or decrease in HCO_3^-). The expected respiratory response to a metabolic disorder causes the $Paco_2$ to change in the same direction as the HCO_3^-. For respiratory disorders, renal compensation occurs and causes the HCO_3^- to change in the same direction as the $Paco_2$. Using conventional nomenclature for an

acid-base disturbance, when pH is returned to a normal it is referred to as being *fully compensated*. When pH is trending towards normal but is not within normal limits, it is termed *partially compensated*. When no changes have occurred, this is termed *uncompensated*.

Conventional nomenclature assumes that acid-base disturbances may be fully compensated, when in fact this may not occur. Respiratory and metabolic compensation may be limited, and pH may not be completely restored to normal by these mechanisms. Because of this problem, some clinicians prefer to calculate expected compensation for metabolic and respiratory disorders and to classify the response as *maximal* or *submaximal*. General rules can be applied when considering expected or **maximal compensation**.

Expected Maximal Compensation for Respiratory Disorders

Calculation of expected or maximal metabolic compensation for a respiratory acid-base disorder can be very helpful in distinguishing between acute and chronic conditions and clarifying the degree of compensation.

Respiratory Acidosis

For an *acute respiratory acidosis*, a 10 mm Hg increase in $Paco_2$ will increase the HCO_3^- about 1 mEq/L. This small increase in HCO_3^- is due to increased CO_2 and does *not* represent renal compensation:

$$CO_2 + H_2O \rightarrow H_2CO_3 \rightarrow H^+ + HCO_3^-$$

As an example, a patient with an acute respiratory acidosis may have the following blood gas results:

pH: 7.20
$Paco_2$: 70 mm Hg
HCO_3^-: 27 mEq/L
BE/BD: 0 mEq/L

Based on the slightly elevated HCO_3^- (27 mEq/L), the clinician might be tempted to suggest that renal compensation has begun. However, an increase in $Paco_2$ from 40 to 70 mm Hg (+30 mm Hg) acutely, will result in an increase in HCO_3^- of about 3 mEq/L:

- Increase of 1 mEq/L HCO_3^- per 10 mm Hg acute increase in $Paco_2$
- Normal $HCO_3^- = 24$ mEq/L
- Expected HCO_3^- due to an acute increase in $Paco_2$ of 30 mm Hg = 24 + 3 = 27 mEq/L

The patient's actual HCO_3^- is 27 mEq/L, which would be expected with an acute increase in $Paco_2$ of 30 mm Hg. The blood gas results, as described, represent an acute increase in $Paco_2$ without renal compensation. The blood gas interpretation would be *uncompensated respiratory acidosis* (acute ventilatory failure).

In conditions where CO_2 is chronically elevated (i.e. *chronic respiratory acidosis*), renal compensation should occur and may return the pH to normal or near normal values.[25] In these cases, expected renal compensation for a 10 mm Hg increase in $Paco_2$ should result in an increase of 4 to 5 mEq/L in HCO_3^-. Renal compensation takes 3 to 5 days to complete. As an example, a patient with a chronic respiratory acidosis (chronic ventilatory failure) may have the following blood gas results:

> pH: 7.40
> $Paco_2$: 50 mm Hg
> HCO_3^-: 29 mEq/L
> BD: +4 mEq/L

Using conventional nomenclature, this blood gas result could be interpreted as *fully compensated respiratory acidosis* (chronic ventilatory failure). A chronic increase in $Paco_2$ from 40 to 50 mm Hg (+10 mm Hg) will result in a compensatory renal mediated increase in HCO_3^- of 4 to 5 mEq/L:

- Increase of 4 to 5 mEq/L HCO_3^- per 10 mm Hg increase in $Paco_2$

- Normal HCO_3^- = 24 mEq/L
- Expected HCO_3^- due to an chronic 10 mm Hg increase in $Paco_2$= 24 + (4 to 5) = 28 to 29 mEq/L

The patient's actual HCO_3^- is 29 mEq/L, which we would expect for maximal renal compensation. Based on this assessment, we might describe the blood gas results as *chronic respiratory acidosis (chronic ventilatory failure) with maximal compensation.*

To summarize, in patients with an acute increase in $Paco_2$ (acute ventilatory failure) we will see a small increase in HCO_3^-, and this does not represent metabolic (i.e., renal) compensation. These patients typically have an elevated $Paco_2$, decreased pH, and slightly increased HCO_3^- (about 1 mEq/L increase per 10 mm Hg acute increase in $Paco_2$). Patients with a chronic elevation in $Paco_2$ should demonstrate renal compensation, and the expected increase in HCO_3^- can be estimated at about 4 to 5 mEq/L per 10 mm Hg chronic increase in $Paco_2$ Clinical Focus 8-3 provides examples of acute and chronic changes in HCO_3^- (e.g., metabolic compensation) due to a respiratory acidosis.

CLINICAL FOCUS 8-3

Expected Metabolic Compensation for a Respiratory Acidosis

The expected metabolic compensation for a respiratory acidosis is an increase in plasma bicarbonate (HCO_3^-). It is important, however, to separate the effects of an acute respiratory acidosis (acute ventilatory failure) from those that occur with a chronic respiratory acidosis (chronic ventilatory failure).

Acute Respiratory Acidosis (Acute Ventilatory Failure)

With an acute increase in $Paco_2$ there is a small increase in plasma HCO_3^-:

$$CO_2 + H_2O \rightarrow H_2CO_3 \rightarrow H^+ + HCO_3^-$$

This increase is rapid and is *not* due to renal compensation. The expected increase in HCO_3^- due to an acute increase in CO_2 can be quantified as follows:

- For acute increases in $Paco_2$, an increase in $Paco_2$ of 10 mm Hg leads to an increase in HCO_3^- of 1 mEq/L. Thus, an acute increase in $Paco_2$ from 40 to 50 mm Hg (10 mm Hg increase in $Paco_2$) will result in an increase in HCO_3^- from 24 mEq/L (normal) to 25 mEq/L (1 mEq/L increase in HCO_3^-). As noted, this occurs rapidly and does not represent renal compensation.

Example: A patient is admitted to the emergency department due to a narcotic drug overdose. Arterial blood gases are obtained with the following results:

> pH: 7.21
> $Paco_2$: 70 mm Hg
> HCO_3^-: 27 mEq/L
> BD: −0.2

Using conventional nomenclature, classify this blood gas result.

Step 1: Classify the pH. The pH indicates an *overall acidosis*.

Step 2: Classify the respiratory condition based on the $Paco_2$. The $Paco_2$ indicates a *respiratory acidosis* (hypoventilation or ventilatory failure).

Step 3: Classify the metabolic condition based on the HCO_3^- and BE/BD. At 27 mEq/L, the HCO_3^- is normal, but slightly elevated if we assume a normal range of 22 to 26 mEq/L; however, the base deficit is clearly normal. Using the BD value (−0.2), the metabolic component would be classified as *normal* (see also below); many laboratories suggest a normal plasma HCO_3^- range of 22 to 28 mEq/L.

Step 4: Describe the cause of the pH abnormality based on steps 2 and 3. The overall condition in acidosis and the source of the acidosis is respiratory (step 2). Consequently, the cause of the pH abnormality is a *respiratory acidosis* ($Paco_2$ = 70 mm Hg).

Step 5: Determine the degree of compensation (if any). A respiratory acidosis is compensated for by a metabolic alkalosis. The inexperienced clinician may be tempted to classify this blood gas result as a partially compensated respiratory acidosis, due to the slight increase in plasma bicarbonate (HCO_3^- = 27 mEq/L). As we have seen, however, a sudden (acute) increase in $Paco_2$ will result in an immediate, but small, increase in HCO_3^- and this is *not* due to renal compensation. Renal compensation is a relatively slow process that takes 3 to 5 days to complete.

In this case, the $Paco_2$ is 30 mm Hg higher than normal (70 − 40 = 30 mm Hg). A 30 mm Hg increase in $Paco_2$ will result in an immediate increase in HCO_3^- of approximately 3 mEq/L:

- Normal HCO_3^- = 24 mEq/L (range 22 to 28 mEq/L)
- With an acute increase in $Paco_2$, an increase in $Paco_2$ of 10 mm Hg leads to an increase in HCO_3^- of 1 mEq/L.
- An increase in $Paco_2$ of 30 mm Hg (70 − 40 = 30 mm Hg) would lead to an increase in HCO_3^- of 3 mEq/L.
- The adjusted HCO_3^- value based on the increased $Paco_2$ would be 27 mEq/L (24 +3 = 27 mEq/L) with a range of 25 to 31 mEq/L.

For this patient, we would expect the HCO_3^- to be about 27 mm Hg (i.e., 24 + 3 = 27 mEq/L) due to the acute increase in $Paco_2$. It also should be noted that the BE/BD is normal. Consequently, the correct interpretation of this blood gas would be an *uncompensated respiratory acidosis* (acute ventilatory failure).

Chronic Respiratory Acidosis (Chronic Ventilatory Failure or Chronic Hypercapnea)

Renal compensation (increase in HCO_3^-) in response to a respiratory acidosis may begin in 24 to 48 hours but takes 3 to 5 days to complete. The expected increase in HCO_3^- due to a chronic increase in CO_2 can be quantified as follows:

- A chronic increase in $Paco_2$ of 10 mm Hg leads to an increase in HCO_3^- of 4 to 5 mEq/L.

Thus, a chronically elevated $Paco_2$ of 50 mm Hg (increase in $Paco_2$ of 10 mm Hg) will result in an increase in HCO_3^- from 24 mEq/L (normal) to 28 to 29 mEq/L (increase in HCO_3^- of 4 to 5 mEq/L). This occurs slowly and will take 3 to 5 days to be complete.

Example: A patient is hospitalized due to an acute exacerbation of COPD. After 2 days of treatment, the patient is evaluated for discharge. Arterial blood gases are obtained with the following results:

pH: 7.36
$Paco_2$: 55 mm Hg
HCO_3^-: 30 mEq/L
BD: +4.7

Using conventional nomenclature, classify this blood gas result.

Step 1: Classify the pH. The pH is *normal* or *fully compensated*.

Step 2: Classify the respiratory condition based on the $Paco_2$. The $Paco_2$ indicates a *respiratory acidosis* (ventilatory failure).

Step 3: Classify the metabolic condition based on the HCO_3^- and BE/BD. The HCO_3^- of 30 mEq/L indicates a metabolic alkalosis, which is confirmed by the base excess of +4.7.

Step 4: Describe the cause of the pH abnormality based on steps 2 and 3. The patient has a metabolic alkalosis and respiratory acidosis resulting in a normalized pH. The primary abnormality can often be determined according to which condition occurred first. Based on the patient's history of COPD, this is probably a *respiratory acidosis*. The pH is < 7.40 but > 7.35, which also suggests the primary problem is an acidosis. Previous blood gases would be very helpful in classifying the current blood gas results.

Step 5: Determine the degree of compensation (if any). The expected renal compensation for a chronically elevated $Paco_2$ would be an increase in HCO_3^- of 4 to 5 mEq/L for each 10 mm Hg increase in $Paco_2$. This patient's $Paco_2$ is 10 mm Hg above normal (i.e., 50 − 40 = 10 mm Hg). Consequently, if the condition is chronic, we would expect renal compensation to increase the patient's HCO_3^- about 4 to 5 mEq/L:

- Normal HCO_3^-: 24 mEq/L (normal range: 22 to 28 mEq/L)
- With complete renal compensation, expected HCO_3^- values increase 4 to 5 mEq/L for each 10 mm Hg increase in $Paco_2$ in chronic respiratory acidosis. For a 10 mm Hg increase in $Paco_2$, we would have:
  - Expected HCO_3^- − Normal value + 4 to 5 mEq = 24 + 4 = 28 mEq/L; 24 + 5 = 29 mEq/L
  - Expected range for HCO_3^- = Normal range + 4 to 5 mEq/L = 26 to 33 mEq/L

(continues)

The patient's actual HCO_3^- of 30 mEq/L is within the expected range for metabolic (i.e., renal) compensation for a chronic respiratory acidosis as calculated above (i.e., 26 to 33 mEq/L). Based on the patient's history and the expected compensation as described, the most likely explanation of these results would be a *fully compensated respiratory acidosis* (chronic ventilatory failure).

Respiratory Alkalosis

For an acute respiratory alkalosis, for every 10 mm Hg decrease in $Paco_2$, the HCO_3^- will decrease by about 2 mEq/L.[25] This is because a decrease in $Paco_2$ causes a small decrease in HCO_3^-; this decrease does *not* represent renal compensation. For a chronic respiratory alkalosis, expected compensation is such that a decrease of 10 mm Hg in $Paco_2$ will decrease the HCO_3^- by about 4 to 5 mEqL.[25] Renal compensation for mild to moderate respiratory alkalosis may return the arterial pH to normal (fully compensated).[25] Renal compensation takes 3 to 5 days to be complete.

To summarize, in patients with an acute decrease in $Paco_2$ (acute alveolar hyperventilation), a small decrease in HCO_3^- will occur, and this does not represent metabolic (i.e., renal) compensation. These patients typically have a decreased $Paco_2$, increased pH, and slightly decreased HCO_3^- (about 2 mEq/L decrease per 10 mm Hg acute decrease in $Paco_2$). Patients with a chronically decreased $Paco_2$ (chronic alveolar hyperventilation) should demonstrate renal compensation, and the expected decrease in HCO_3^- can be estimated at about 4-5 mEq/L per 10 mm Hg chronic decrease in $Paco_2$. **Clinical Focus 8-4** provides examples of expected metabolic compensation for respiratory alkalosis.

Expected Maximal Compensation for Metabolic Disorders

Respiratory compensation for a *metabolic acidosis* consists of hyperventilation, generally limited to a minimum $Paco_2$ of 8 to 12 mm Hg in individuals with good lung function (e.g., healthy lungs); respiratory compensation is less effective in patients with ventilatory impairment.[25] Respiratory compensation for a *metabolic alkalosis* consists of hypoventilation, generally limited to a maximum $Paco_2$ of about 55 mm Hg.[25] It also must be noted that respiratory compensation for a metabolic acid-base disorder is most effective for acute changes. The respiratory response is fast, but may not be as effective with chronic conditions. Expected

CLINICAL FOCUS 8-4

Expected Metabolic Compensation for a Respiratory Alkalosis

The expected metabolic compensation for a respiratory alkalosis is a decrease in plasma bicarbonate (HCO_3^-). It is important, however, to separate the effects of an acute respiratory alkalosis (acute alveolar hyperventilation) from those that occur with a chronic respiratory alkalosis (chronic alveolar hyperventilation).

Acute Respiratory Alkalosis (Acute Alveolar Hyperventilation)

With an acute decrease in $Paco_2$ there is a small decrease in plasma HCO_3^-:

$$\downarrow CO_2 \rightarrow \downarrow H_2CO_3 \rightarrow \downarrow H^+ + \downarrow HCO_3^-$$

This decrease is rapid and is *not* due to renal compensation. The expected decrease in HCO_3^- due to an acute decrease in CO_2 can be quantified as follows:

- For acute decreases in $Paco_2$, a decrease in $Paco_2$ of 10 mm Hg leads to a decrease in HCO_3^- of 2 mEq/L. Thus, an acute decrease in $Paco_2$ from 40 to 30 mm Hg (a 10 mm Hg decrease in $Paco_2$) will result in a decrease in HCO_3^- from 24 mEq/L (normal) to 22 mEq/L (a decrease in HCO_3^- of 2 mEq/L). As noted, this occurs rapidly and does not represent renal compensation.

   Example: A patient is admitted to the emergency department with pneumonia and a corresponding hypoxemia based on pulse oximetry results. Arterial blood gases are obtained with the following results:

   pH: 7.52

$Paco_2$: 28 mm Hg
Pao_2: 48 mm Hg
Sao_2: 83%
HCO_3^-: 22 mEq/L
BD: −0.5

Using conventional nomenclature, classify this blood gas result.

Step 1: Classify the pH. The pH indicates an *alkalosis*.

Step 2: Classify the respiratory condition based on the $Paco_2$. The $Paco_2$ indicates a *respiratory alkalosis* (alveolar hyperventilation).

Step 3: Classify the metabolic condition based on the HCO_3^- and BE/BD. The HCO_3^- and BE/BD are within normal range.

Step 4: Describe the cause of the pH abnormality based on steps 2 and 3. The patient has a *respiratory alkalosis.*

Step 5: Determine the degree of compensation (if any). The expected compensation for a chronically decreased $Paco_2$ would be a decrease in HCO_3^- of 4 to 5 mEq/L for each 10 mm Hg decrease in $Paco_2$. Consequently, if the condition is chronic, we would expect renal compensation to decrease the patient's HCO_3^- about 4 to 5 mEq/L. On the other hand, an acute decrease in $Paco_2$ will result in a small decrease in HCO_3^-:

- Normal HCO_3^-: 24 mEq/L (normal range: 22 to 28 mEq/L)
- With an acute decrease in $Paco_2$, HCO_3^- values decrease about 2 mEq/L for each 10 mm Hg decrease in $Paco_2$. For a 10 mm Hg decrease in $Paco_2$, we would have:
  - Expected HCO_3^- = Normal value − 2 mEq/L = 24 − 2 = 22 mEq/L
  - Expected range for HCO_3^- = Normal range − 2 mEq/L = 20 to 26 mEq/L

The patient's actual HCO_3^- of 22 mEq/L is within the expected range for an acute decrease in $Paco_2$ and does *not* represent renal compensation. Based on the patient's history and the blood gas results, this represents an *uncompensated respiratory alkalosis* (acute alveolar hyperventilation) probably secondary to acute hypoxemia (Pao_2 = 48 mm Hg).

Chronic Respiratory Alkalosis (Chronic Alveolar Hyperventilation)

The expected renal compensation for a chronic respiratory alkalosis is to decrease HCO_3^-. This response may begin in 24 to 48 hours but take 3 to 5 days to complete. The expected decrease in HCO_3^- due to a chronic decrease in $Paco_2$ can be quantified as follows:

- With a chronic decrease in $Paco_2$, a decrease in $Paco_2$ of 10 mm Hg leads to a decrease in HCO_3^- of 4 to 5 mEq/L.

Thus with renal compensation, a chronic decrease in $Paco_2$ to 30 mm Hg (decrease in $Paco_2$ of 10 mm Hg) will result in a decrease in HCO_3^- from 24 mEq/L (normal) to 19 to 20 mEq/L (a 4 to 5 mEq/L decrease in HCO_3^-: 24 − 4 = 20; 24 − 5 = 19). As noted previously, this occurs slowly and will take 3 to 5 days to be complete.[27]

Example: A patient is admitted to the hospital with chronic alveolar hyperventilation secondary to an ongoing, chronic hypoxemia. Arterial blood gases are obtained with the following results:

pH: 7.44
$Paco_2$: 30 mm Hg
Pao_2: 55 mm Hg
Sao_2: 88 mm Hg
HCO_3^-: 20 mEq/L
BD: −3.8

Using conventional nomenclature, classify this blood gas result.

Step 1: Classify the pH. The pH is *normal* or *fully compensated*.

Step 2: Classify the respiratory condition based on the $Paco_2$. The $Paco_2$ indicates a *respiratory alkalosis* (hyperventilation).

Step 3: Classify the metabolic condition based on the HCO_3^- and BE/BD. The HCO_3^- is slightly below the normal range of 22 to 28 mEq/L and the base deficit is reduced. The metabolic component would be classified as a *metabolic acidosis*.

Step 4: Describe the cause of the pH abnormality based on steps 2 and 3. We have both a metabolic acidosis and a respiratory alkalosis resulting in a normal (fully compensated) pH. The primary abnormality can often be determined according to which condition occurred first in time. Hypoxemia often causes hyperventilation

(continues)

due to stimulation of the peripheral chemoreceptors. Based on the patient's history of chronic hypoxemia, this is probably a *respiratory alkalosis.* The pH is > 7.40 but < 7.45, which also suggests that the primary problem is an alkalosis. Previous blood gases would be very helpful in classifying the current blood gas results. However, based on the available information, the likely cause of the abnormalities seen suggest a *respiratory alkalosis* ($Paco_2$ = 30 mm Hg).

Step 5: Determine the degree of compensation (if any). A respiratory alkalosis is compensated for by a metabolic acidosis, which has occurred resulting in a normalized pH. Consequently, the most likely classification of this blood gas result is *fully compensated respiratory alkalosis* secondary to chronic hypoxemia.

In this case, the $Paco_2$ is 10 mm Hg lower than normal (40 – 30 = 10 mm Hg). With renal compensation, a 10 mm Hg decrease in $Paco_2$ will result in a decrease in HCO_3^- of approximately 4 to 5 mEq/L:

- Normal HCO_3^- = 24 mEq/L (range 22 to 28 mEq/L)
- With a chronic decrease in $Paco_2$, a decrease in $Paco_2$ of 10 mm Hg results in a decrease in HCO_3^- of 4 to 5 mEq/L.
- If $Paco_2$ decreased 10 mm Hg (40 – 30 = 10 mm Hg), then the HCO_3^- would decrease by 4 to 5 mEq/L.
- With renal compensation, the expected HCO_3^- value based on the decreased $Paco_2$ would be 19 to 20 mEq/L (24 – 4 to 5 = 19 – 20 mEq/L) with a range of 17 to 24 mEq/L.

With renal compensation in this patient, we would expect the HCO_3^- to decrease to somewhere in the range of 17 to 24 mEq/L. The patient's actual HCO_3^- is 20 mEq/L, which is in the expected range for complete renal compensation for a chronic respiratory alkalosis. Renal compensation is a relatively slow process that takes 3 to 5 days to complete.

respiratory compensation, however, can be estimated in order to better determine the nature and extent of a metabolic acid-base disorder.

Respiratory Compensation for a Metabolic Acidosis

Respiratory compensation for a metabolic acidosis results in a decrease in $Paco_2$ of about 1.2 mm Hg for each 1 mEq/L decrease in HCO_3^-.[25] This decline in $Paco_2$ usually begins within 30 minutes and is complete within 12 to 24 hours.[25] As noted, the lowest possible $Paco_2$ for patients is 8 to 12 mm Hg. This assumes excellent lung function, and most patients with cardiopulmonary disease will be unable to hyperventilate to this extreme. It should also be noted that an uncompensated respiratory acidosis is rare. In cases where there is no respiratory compensation for a metabolic acidosis, there is probably a ventilatory defect present (e.g., respiratory center depression, mechanical inability to hyperventilate, or other pulmonary or neuromuscular problem). Winter's formula may also be used to calculate expected respiratory compensation for a metabolic acidosis:

$$\text{Expected } Paco_2 = (1.5 \times HCO_3^-) + 8 \pm 2$$

For example, a patient with a metabolic acidosis may have the following blood gas values:

pH: 7.27
$Paco_2$: 23 mm Hg
HCO_3^-: 10 mEq/L
BD: –15 mEq/L

Using conventional nomenclature, we might classify this blood gas as a *partially compensated metabolic acidosis.* However, if we calculated the maximum expected respiratory compensation, we may come to a different conclusion:

$$\text{Expected } Paco_2 = (1.5 \times HCO_3^-) + 8 \pm 2$$

$$\text{Expected } Paco_2 = (1.5 \times 10) + 8 \pm 2 = 23 \text{ mm Hg } (\pm 2)$$

Thus, with an HCO_3^- of 10 mEq/L, the expected (maximal) respiratory compensation would result in a $Paco_2$ of about 23 mm Hg (± 2). A better assessment of the patient's blood gases would be *metabolic acidosis with maximal respiratory compensation.* We should not expect further improvements in the pH due to additional respiratory compensation for the observed metabolic acidosis.

As a fast estimate, the expected respiratory compensation for a metabolic acidosis is roughly equal to the last two digits of the pH. For example, if a metabolic acidosis results in a pH of 7.20, one might expect a compensatory hyperventilation resulting in a $Paco_2$ of 20 mm Hg. **Clinical Focus 8-5** provides additional examples of expected respiratory compensation for a metabolic acidosis.

Respiratory Compensation for Metabolic Alkalosis

Respiratory compensation for a metabolic alkalosis results in an increase in $Paco_2$ of about 0.7 mm Hg for each 1 mEq/L increase in HCO_3^-.[25] This response is rapid, but $Paco_2$ generally does not exceed 55 mm Hg in

CLINICAL FOCUS 8-5

Expected Respiratory Compensation for a Metabolic Acidosis

Respiratory compensation for a metabolic acidosis is hyperventilation (decrease in $Paco_2$). In patients with good lung function, this is generally limited to a $Paco_2$ of not less than 8 to 12 mm Hg. Maximal respiratory compensation can be estimated as follows:

$$\text{Expected } Paco_2 = 1.5 \times [HCO_3^-] + 8 \pm 2 \text{ mm Hg (Winter's equation)}$$

Alternative methods to estimate maximal respiratory compensation include:

Method 1. For each decrease in HCO_3^- of 1 mEq, $Paco_2$ decreases by 1.2 mm Hg.

Method 2. Expected $Paco_2 \cong [HCO_3^-] + 15$.

Method 3. Expected $Paco_2 \cong$ last two digits of the pH.

Example: A patient presents to the emergency department with an acute, diabetic ketoacidosis. An arterial blood gas is drawn and analyzed.

pH: 7.18
$Paco_2$: 18 mm Hg
Pao_2 : 105 mm Hg (breathing room air)
HCO_3^-: 6.5 mEq/L
BE/BD: −19.7 mEq/L

1. Classify this patient's arterial blood gas results using conventional nomenclature.
   Overall condition: Acidosis (pH = 7.18)
   Respiratory condition: Respiratory alkalosis ($Paco_2$ = 18 mm Hg; hyperventilation)
   Metabolic condition: Metabolic acidosis (HCO_3^- = 6.5 mEq/L; BD = −19.7 mEq/L)
   Conventional classification: *Partly compensated metabolic acidosis*

2. Estimate maximal (expected) respiratory compensation for this patient's metabolic acidosis using Winter's equation:

$$\text{Expected } Paco_2 = 1.5 \times [HCO_3^-] + 8 \pm 2$$

$$= 17.8 \text{ mm Hg} \pm 2 \text{ (i.e., 15.8 to 19.8 mm Hg)}$$

Based on Winter's equation, maximal respiratory compensation would be in the range of $Paco_2 \cong 16$ to 20 mm Hg. The patient's $Paco_2$ is 18 mm Hg, which probably represents a *metabolic acidosis with maximal respiratory compensation.*

3. Estimate maximal (expected) respiratory compensation for this patient's metabolic acidosis using the other techniques suggested above.
   Method 1: For each decrease in HCO_3^- of 1 mEq, $Paco_2$ decreases by 1.2 mm Hg. The patient's HCO_3^- is 6.5 mEq/L. This represents a decrease from normal (HCO_3^- = 24 mEq/L) of 17.5 mEq/L (i.e., 24 mEq/L − 6.5 mEq/L = 17.5 mEq/L).

$$\text{Expected decrease in } Paco_2 \cong \frac{1.2 \text{ mm Hg}}{1 \text{ mEq/L } HCO_3^-} \times 17.5 \text{ mEq/L} = 21 \text{ torr}$$

If the patient's initial $Paco_2$ were normal (e.g., $Paco_2$ = 40); maximal compensation would cause the $Paco_2$ to decrease 21 torr to 19 mm Hg (i.e., 40 − 21 = 19 mm Hg). The patient's actual $Paco_2$ is 18 mm Hg, again maximal expected respiratory compensation.

Method 2: Expected $Paco_2 = [HCO_3^-] + 15$. In this case:

$$\text{Expected } Paco_2 = 6.5 + 15 = 21.5 \text{ mm Hg}$$

The estimate suggests maximal respiratory compensation for the patient would be a $Paco_2 \cong 22$ mm Hg.

Method 3: Expected $Paco_2$ is the last two digits of the pH. A pH of 7.18 suggests the maximal respiratory compensation would be a $Paco_2$ = 18 mm Hg. The patient's actual $Paco_2$ is 18 mm Hg, again suggesting maximal respiratory compensation.

compensation for a metabolic alkalosis.[25] The expected maximal respiratory compensation for a metabolic alkalosis can also be estimated:

$$\text{Expected } Pa_{CO_2} = 0.7\,(HCO_3^-) + 20\,(\pm 2)$$

For example, a patient with a metabolic alkalosis may have the following blood gas values:

pH: 7.55
Pa_{CO_2}: 52 mm Hg
HCO_3^-: 44 mEq/L
BD: +20 mEq/L

Using conventional nomenclature, we might classify this blood gas as a *partially compensated metabolic alkalosis*. However, if we calculated the maximum expected respiratory compensation we may come to a different assessment:

$$\text{Expected } Pa_{CO_2} = 0.7\,(HCO_3^-) + 20$$

$$\text{Expected } Pa_{CO_2} = 0.7\,(44) + 20 = 50.8 \text{ mm Hg}$$

Thus, with an HCO_3^- of 44 mEq/L, the expected (maximal) respiratory compensation would result in a Pa_{CO_2} of about 51 mm Hg (± 2). A better assessment of this patient's blood gases would be *metabolic alkalosis with maximal respiratory compensation*. We should not expect further improvements in the pH due to further respiratory compensation. **Clinical Focus 8-6** provides additional examples of expected respiratory compensation for a metabolic alkalosis.

Clinical Interpretation of Arterial Blood Gases

Traditional conventional blood gas classification nomenclature is widely used and understood by many clinicians. As noted earlier, this approach has a number of drawbacks. One drawback is the classification of respiratory abnormalities. In order to better describe respiratory disorders, an alternative approach to the clinical interpretation of arterial blood gas results

CLINICAL FOCUS 8-6

Expected Respiratory Compensation for a Metabolic Alkalosis

Respiratory compensation for a metabolic alkalosis is hypoventilation. This response is generally limited to a maximum Pa_{CO_2} of about 55 mm Hg. Maximum respiratory compensation for a metabolic alkalosis can be estimated as follows:

- For each increase in HCO_3^- of 1 mEq/L, expect Pa_{CO_2} to increase 0.7 torr.

Example: A patient with a metabolic alkalosis has the following arterial blood gas results:
pH: 7.50
Pa_{CO_2}: 50
HCO_3^-: 38
BE: 13.7 mEq/L

1. Classify the patient's arterial blood: gas results using conventional nomenclature.
   Overall condition: Alkalosis (pH = 7.50)
   Respiratory condition: Respiratory acidosis (Pa_{CO_2} = 50 mm Hg; hypoventilation)
   Metabolic condition: Metabolic alkalosis (HCO_3^- = 38 mEq/L; BE = +13.7)
   Conventional classification: *Partly compensated metabolic alkalosis*

2. Estimate maximum (expected) respiratory compensation for the patient's metabolic alkalosis.
   Expected Pa_{CO_2} = Increase of 0.7 mm Hg for each 1 mEq/L increase in HCO_3^-.
   The HCO_3^- increase above normal (i.e., 24 mEq/L) is 14 mEq/L:
   - Actual HCO_3^- = 38 mEq/L
   - Normal HCO_3^- = 24 mEq/L
   - Increase in HCO_3^- = 38 − 24 = 14 mEq/L
   The expected increase in Pa_{CO_2} would be:

   $$\frac{\uparrow 0.7 \text{ mm Hg } Pa_{CO_2}}{\uparrow HCO_3 - mEq/L} \times 14 \text{ mEq/L} = 9.8 \text{ mm Hg}$$

3. Based on the expected maximum respiratory compensation, how would you describe this blood gas result?
   The expected respiratory compensation for this metabolic alkalosis would be an increase in Pa_{CO_2} about 10 mm Hg to a value of approximately 50 mm Hg. The blood gas (pH = 7.50, Pa_{CO_2} = 50, HCO_3^- = 38, BE = +13.7) suggests a *metabolic alkalosis with maximum respiratory compensation*.

has been suggested[6] that incorporates the following terminology:

- **Acute ventilatory failure**: A sudden rise in $Paco_2$ with a corresponding decrease in pH.
- **Chronic ventilatory failure**: A chronically elevated $Paco_2$ with a normal (compensated) or near normal pH.
- **Acute ventilatory failure superimposed on chronic ventilatory failure**: A sudden rise in $Paco_2$ in a patient with chronic ventilatory failure.
- **Acute alveolar hyperventilation**: A sudden fall in $Paco_2$ with a corresponding increase in pH.
- **Chronic alveolar hyperventilation**: A chronically decreased $Paco_2$ with a normal (compensated) or near normal pH.
- **Acute alveolar hyperventilation superimposed on chronic ventilatory failure**: A sudden decrease in $Paco_2$ in a patient with chronic ventilatory failure.

RC Insights

The Effect of Acute Changes in $Paco_2$ on pH[1]
- For every 10 mm Hg increase in $Paco_2$ (acutely), the pH decreases approximately 0.08 units.
  - A sudden rise in $Paco_2$ from 40 to 60 mm Hg would lower the pH from 7.40 to 7.24.
- For every 10 mm Hg decrease in $Paco_2$ (acutely), the pH increases approximately 0.08 units.
  - A sudden decrease in $Paco_2$ from 40 to 30 mm Hg will raise the pH from 7.40 to 7.48.

*For acute changes in $Paco_2$, an increase in $Paco_2$ of 1 mm Hg decreases pH by 0.008; a decrease in $Paco_2$ of 1 mm Hg increases pH by 0.008.

It is thought that the above terminology describes respiratory conditions more effectively.[6] We believe it is important for the bedside clinician to understand both traditional conventional nomenclature and the above clinical terminology when describing a respiratory disorder. **Table 8-3** provides the definitions and criteria for classification of blood gas values for acute and chronic ventilatory failure, alveolar hyperventilation (acute and chronic), and related disturbances. We will now review the clinical interpretation of arterial blood gases.

Ventilatory Failure (Respiratory Acidosis)

Ventilatory failure can be defined as an abnormally elevated $Paco_2$ (respiratory acidosis or hypercapnea). Ventilatory failure is caused by a reduction in alveolar ventilation (hypoventilation). Acute ventilatory failure is a sudden rise in $Paco_2$ with a corresponding decrease in pH (uncompensated respiratory acidosis). Common causes of acute ventilatory failure include reduced lung compliance (e.g., atelectasis, pneumonia, ARDS, pulmonary edema), increased airway resistance (e.g., asthma, airway obstruction), reduced drive to breathe (e.g., sedative or narcotic drugs, head trauma), or a reduced ability to breathe due to neuromuscular disease (e.g., Guillain-Barré, myasthenia gravis).

Chronic ventilatory failure is a chronic elevation in $Paco_2$ (chronic hypercapnea) with a normal or near normal pH (partially or fully compensated respiratory acidosis). Generally, with chronic hypercapnea the kidneys will not return the pH to much beyond 7.32 to 7.35. Common causes of chronic ventilatory failure are COPD and other forms of chronic lung disease. Patients

---

TABLE 8-3
Clinical Interpretation of Ventilatory Disorders

Disorder	$Paco_2$	pH	Base Excess/Deficit
Acute ventilatory failure	↑	↓	N BD/BE and HCO_3^-
Chronic ventilatory failure	↑	Normal or near normal	↑BE and ↑HCO_3^-
Acute ventilatory failure superimposed on chronic ventilatory failure[1]	↑↑	↓	↑BE and ↑HCO_3^-
Acute alveolar hyperventilation	↓	↑	N BD/BE and HCO_3^-
Chronic alveolar hyperventilation	↓	Normal or near normal	↓BE and ↓HCO_3^-
Acute alveolar hyperventilation superimposed on chronic ventilatory failure[2]	N or ↑	N or ↑	↑BE and ↑HCO_3^-

N, normal.

[1]The blood gas results seen in acute ventilatory superimposed on chronic ventilatory failure are similar to those seen with a partially compensated respiratory acidosis. The best way to identify this disorder is to review the patient's history and previous blood gas studies. If the patient has a history of chronic lung disease (e.g., COPD) with documented chronic CO_2 retention (e.g., chronic ventilatory failure) and now presents with an acute exacerbation of chronic lung disease, the most like cause of the blood gas abnormality is acute ventilatory failure superimposed on chronic ventilatory failure.

[2]The blood gas results seen with acute alveolar hyperventilation superimposed on chronic ventilatory failure are similar to those seen with a metabolic alkalosis. To identify this disorder, a patient history is needed documenting a baseline state of chronic ventilatory failure. In such patients, an episode of acute distress may result in a relative decrease in $Paco_2$ and corresponding increase in pH.

with COPD sometimes suffer an acute exacerbation of their chronic lung disease. In these cases, the respiratory clinician must be on the alert for the development of *acute ventilatory failure superimposed on chronic ventilatory failure*. Causes and treatment of ventilatory failure are discussed in Chapter 7. A summary of causes of ventilatory failure are listed in **Box 8-13**. **Clinical Focus 8-7** and **Clinical Focus 8-8** provide examples of acute and chronic ventilatory failure. **Clinical Focus 8-9** provides an example of acute ventilatory failure superimposed on chronic ventilatory failure.

Treatment of ventilatory failure must address the underlying cause of alveolar hypoventilation. For example, work of breathing may be increased due to a reduction in pulmonary or thoracic compliance or an increase in airway resistance. Examples of disease states or conditions that may increase the work of breathing and reduce alveolar ventilation include pneumonia, ARDS, cardiogenic pulmonary edema, and COPD or asthma exacerbation. The drive to breathe may be affected by drugs or medications or neurologic disease (e.g., head trauma). Neuromuscular disease may affect a patient's ability to maintain adequate spontaneous ventilation (e.g., Guillain-Barré syndrome, myasthenia gravis).

Treatment is also dictated by whether the condition is acute or chronic. Acute ventilatory failure may represent a medical emergency requiring noninvasive or invasive mechanical ventilatory support. The severity of acute ventilatory failure is assessed, in part, by the severity of the resultant decline in pH. For example, an acute rise in $Paco_2$ that results in a decrease in arterial pH to < 7.25 is generally considered the point at which mechanical ventilation should be considered. Chronic ventilatory failure, as seen in COPD, may suggest oxygen therapy, administration of bronchodilators, and pulmonary rehabilitation. Chapter 7 describes the recognition and treatment of ventilatory failure.

Alveolar Hyperventilation (Respiratory Alkalosis)

Acute alveolar hyperventilation is defined as a sudden decrease in $Paco_2$ with a corresponding increase in pH. Clinically, alveolar hyperventilation can be caused by hypoxemia, pain, anxiety, respiratory distress (e.g., alveolar congestion or filling), or neurologic disorders; in the ICU, it is often a sign of early sepsis where bacterial toxins lead to hyperventilation. Hyperventilation may also be in response to an acute metabolic acidosis as a compensatory response. Acute hyperventilation syndrome is sometimes associated with anxiety and panic attacks. Patients receiving mechanical ventilatory support may be overventilated unintentionally (iatrogenic hyperventilation) due to inappropriate ventilator settings. Patients with cerebral edema in the ICU who are receiving invasive mechanical ventilation may also be intentionally overventilated in order to reduce $Paco_2$, cause cerebral vasoconstriction, and reduce cerebral edema, though this strategy has limited usefulness.

BOX 8-13

Causes of Respiratory Acidosis (Hypoventilation)

Respiratory acidosis is also known as *hypercapnea*, *hypoventilation*, and *ventilatory failure*. Common causes of respiratory acidosis include:

- Increased work of breathing
  - Decreased lung compliance (e.g., atelectasis, postop respiratory failure, pneumonia, cardiogenic pulmonary edema, ARDS, chest trauma, pneumothorax, fibrotic lung disease).
  - Increased airway resistance (e.g., asthma, COPD exacerbation, upper airway obstruction, secretions, mucosal edema).
  - Decreased chest wall compliance (e.g., obesity, kyphoscoliosis, chest wall deformity).
- Decreased ventilatory drive
  - Sedative or narcotic drugs
  - Brainstem lesions
  - Morbid obesity
- Neurologic disease
  - Spinal cord injury
  - Amyotrophic lateral sclerosis
  - Poliomyelitis
  - Guillain-Barr syndrome

- Head trauma
- Sleep apnea
- Metabolic alkalosis

- Myasthenia gravis
- Botulism
- Muscular dystrophy
- Critical care myopathy

CLINICAL FOCUS 8-7

Acute Ventilatory Failure

A 37-year-old male arrived in the emergency department unresponsive. He was suspected of taking an overdose of an unknown substance. An arterial blood gas sample taken on room air reveals:

pH: 7.15
$Paco_2$: 80 mm Hg
HCO_3^-: 28 mEq/L
BE: 0
Pao_2: 42 mm Hg
Sao_2: 80%

1. Using conventional nomenclature, classify this blood gas result.
   This blood gas study represents an *uncompensated respiratory acidosis with moderate to severe hypoxemia*.
2. Using clinical nomenclature, describe this patient's ventilatory status.
   This patient is in acute ventilatory failure with moderate to severe hypoxemia.
3. Describe the metabolic response to the respiratory acidosis.
   With an acute increase in $Paco_2$, there will be a small increase in HCO_3^- (about 1 mEq/L for each 10 mm Hg increase in $Paco_2$). The 40 mm Hg increase in $Paco_2$ (80 – 40 = 40 mm Hg) above normal would cause a 4 mEq/L decrease in HCO_3^- acutely, which is what has occurred (i.e., HCO_3^- = 24 + 4 = 28 mEq/L). This does *not* represent renal compensation, which occurs more slowly Based on the pH and BE = 0, this acidosis is uncompensated.
4. Describe the relationship between pH and $Paco_2$.
   With acute increases in $Paco_2$ of 20 mm Hg, the pH will fall approximately 0.10 points. If the $Paco_2$ suddenly increases from 40 to 80 mm Hg (a 40 mm Hg increase), the pH will fall approximately 0.20. That means that the expected decrease in pH for this patient would be 7.40 – 0.20 = 7.20, which is what has occurred and is consistent with an acute rise in $Paco_2$ (acute ventilatory failure). The effect of acute changes in $Paco_2$ on pH has been suggested as:
   - Increase in $Paco_2$ of 20 mm Hg decreases pH by 0.10.
   - Decrease in $Paco_2$ of 10 mm Hg increases pH by 0.10.
   It should be noted that other sources suggest a simplified rule:
   - For each 1 mm Hg change in $Paco_2$ (acutely), pH will vary 0.008 units in the opposite direction.
5. Describe the relationship between the increased $Paco_2$ and the decreased Pao_2 in this patient.
   The alveolar air equation describes the relationship between ventilation and oxygenation:

$$P_Ao_2 \approx Pio_2 - (Paco_2 \div 0.8)$$

where P_Ao_2 is the alveolar oxygen tension, Pio_2 is the inspired oxygen tension, and $Paco_2$ is the arterial carbon dioxide tension. Thus, as $Paco_2$ increases, alveolar and arterial oxygen tensions decrease (i.e., decrease in P_Ao_2 and Pao_2). For patients breathing room air, this relationship can be simplified as follows:
   - Increase in Pco_2 of 4 mm Hg leads to a decrease in Pao_2 of 5 mm Hg.
   In our example, the patient has an acute increase in $Paco_2$ to 80 mm Hg (an increase of 40 mm Hg above normal) while breathing room air. The expected effect on Pao_2 would be:
   - Increase in $Paco_2$ of 4 mm Hg leads to a decrease in Pao_2 of 5 mm Hg.
   - Decrease in $Paco_2$ of 40 mm Hg leads to a decrease in Pao_2 of 50 mm Hg.
   If the patient's Pao_2 was 90 mm Hg prior to the acute episode of ventilatory failure, the expected decrease in Pao_2 due to the increase in $Paco_2$ would be:

$$Pao_2 = 90 - 50 = 40 \text{ mm Hg}$$

The patient's actual Pao_2 is 42 mm Hg which is what would be expected due to the severe hypoventilation present ($Paco_2$ = 80 mm Hg).

CLINICAL FOCUS 8-8

Chronic Ventilatory Failure

A stable, 62-year-old male with COPD is to be enrolled in a pulmonary rehabilitation program. A baseline arterial blood gas sample is obtained on room air:

pH: 7.38
$Paco_2$: 52 mm Hg
HCO_3^-: 30 mEq/L
BE: + 5.0
Pao_2: 55 mm Hg
Sao_2: 88%

1. Using conventional nomenclature, classify this blood gas result.
   This blood gas study represents a *fully compensated respiratory acidosis with moderate hypoxemia*.
2. Using clinical nomenclature, describe this patient's ventilatory status.
   This patient has chronic ventilatory failure with moderate hypoxemia.
3. Describe the metabolic response to the respiratory acidosis.
   With a chronically elevated $Paco_2$, there will be a compensatory increase in HCO_3^- (4 to 5 mEq/L for each 10 mm Hg increase in $Paco_2$). The patient's $Paco_2$ is 12 mm Hg above an ideal normal of 40 mm Hg (i.e., 52 – 40 = 12 mm Hg). Renal compensation for this elevated $Paco_2$ would cause HCO_3^- to increase 4.8 to 6 mEq/L:

$$\frac{Paco_2 - 40}{10} \times 4 \text{ mEq / L} = 4.8 \text{ mEq / L}$$

$$\frac{Paco_2 - 40}{10} \times 5 \text{ mEq / L} = 6.0 \text{ mEq / L}$$

   The patient's actual HCO_3^- is 30 mEq/L, which is a 6 mEq/L increase above an ideal normal of 24 mEq/L. Thus the patient's HCO_3^- level is consistent with full renal compensation for a respiratory acidosis.
4. Describe the relationship between pH and $Paco_2$.
   For acute increases in $Paco_2$, for each 20 mm Hg increase in $Paco_2$, the pH will fall approximately 0.10 points. However, this patient has a 12 mm Hg increase in $Paco_2$ above an ideal normal of 40 mm Hg with no corresponding decline in pH. This is because renal compensation has occurred, increasing the HCO_3^- to 30 mEq/L. The effect of acute changes in $Paco_2$ on pH has been suggested as:
   ○ Increase in $Paco_2$ of 20 mm Hg results in a 0.10 decrease in pH.
   ○ Decrease in $Paco_2$ of 10 mm Hg results in a 0.10 increase in pH.
   It should be noted that other sources suggest a simplified rule:
   ○ For each 1 mm Hg change in $Paco_2$ (acutely), pH will vary 0.008 units in the opposite direction.

CLINICAL FOCUS 8-9

Acute Ventilatory Failure Superimposed on Chronic Ventilatory Failure

A 72-year-old female patient with a long history of COPD with documented chronic CO_2 retention is admitted to the emergency department with a diagnosis of acute exacerbation of her chronic lung disease. Arterial blood gases are drawn while the patient is receiving oxygen therapy via nasal cannula at 2 L/min:

pH: 7.28   BE: +6.0
$Paco_2$: 72 mm Hg Pao_2: 50 mm Hg
HCO_3^-: 33 mEq/L Sao_2: 86%

1. Using conventional nomenclature, classify this blood gas result.
   This blood gas study appears to be a *partly compensated respiratory acidosis with moderate hypoxemia*.
2. Using clinical nomenclature, describe this patient's ventilatory status.

The key to understanding this patient's current blood gas results is based on her prior history and past blood gas results. The patient has a documented and long-standing history of COPD with chronic CO_2 retention. The respiratory care clinician may inquire about previous blood gases for this patient and find that she had been admitted to the hospital about a year ago. At that time, her stable discharge blood gases while breathing room air were:

pH: 7.37   BE: +6.5

$Paco_2$: 57 mm Hg Pao_2: 58 mm Hg

HCO_3^-: 32 mEq/L Sao_2: 90%

The stable, baseline blood gases from the patient's last admission (above) indicate *chronic ventilatory failure with moderate hypoxemia.*

The patient currently is suffering an acute exacerbation of her COPD. Her $Paco_2$ has increased from the previous baseline value of about 57 to 72 mm Hg, and this has caused a corresponding decrease in her pH. The patient now has *acute ventilatory failure superimposed on chronic ventilatory failure with moderate hypoxemia.*

3. Describe the metabolic response to the respiratory acidosis.

   This patient's current HCO_3^- is elevated (HCO_3^- = 33 mEq/L); however, this is due to her long-standing chronically elevated $Paco_2$ (i.e., chronic ventilatory failure). Given time, additional metabolic compensation may occur, but this has not yet happened.

4. Describe the relationship between pH and $Paco_2$.

   In patients with a baseline normal $Paco_2$ of 40 mm Hg, an acute increase in $Paco_2$ to over 70 mm Hg would result in a significant fall in pH, probably to near 7.2. This patient's pH has not fallen as much as expected, indicating an underlying condition (metabolic alkalosis in compensation for the chronic respiratory acidosis).

Chronic alveolar hyperventilation is defined as a chronic decrease in $Paco_2$ with a normal or near normal pH. Chronic hypoxemia is a potential cause of chronic alveolar hyperventilation. A patient may also be stimulated to chronically hyperventilate due to a persistent metabolic acidosis.

Treatment should address the underlying cause of alveolar hyperventilation. For example, if the patient is experiencing acute hyperventilation syndrome, mild anxiolytic therapy and reassurance may be warranted. Patients with acute hyperventilation syndrome associated with severe anxiety may also find some benefit to rebreathing exhaled gas using a paper bag. Hyperventilation secondary to hypoxemia must address the cause of the patient's hypoxemia. Common causes of respiratory alkalosis are listed in **Box 8-14**. **Clinical Focus 8-10** provides an example of acute alveolar hyperventilation. **Clinical Focus 8-11** provides an example of chronic alveolar hyperventilation. **Clinical Focus 8-12** provides an example of acute alveolar hyperventilation superimposed on chronic ventilatory failure.

Metabolic Acidosis

Normal metabolism produces 50 to 100 mEq of nonvolatile acids daily, most of which is sulfuric acid

---

BOX 8-14

Common Causes of Respiratory Alkalosis (Hyperventilation)

Hypoxia/hypoxemia (e.g., hyperventilation secondary to hypoxemia)

Anxiety/pain

Early sepsis

Hepatic encephalopathy

Other neurologic disorders

- Trauma
- Infection
- Stroke

Pulmonary emboli

Metabolic acidosis (e.g., salicylate toxicity [aspirin overdose], ketoacidosis, lactic acidosis, kidney failure, other)

Hyperventilation due to excessive mechanical ventilatory support (e.g., iatrogenic hyperventilation)

*Hyperventilation is a normal response to hypoxemia. The peripheral chemoreceptors are stimulated when $P_{A}O_2$ < 60 mm Hg, resulting in an increase in ventilation.

CLINICAL FOCUS 8-10

Acute Alveolar Hyperventilation

A 62-year-old female patient with a history of congestive heart failure presents to the clinic with a "chest cold," cough, and shortness of breath. Her heart rate is 110 beats per minute, and her respiratory rate is 28 breaths per minute. An arterial blood gas sample taken on room air reveals:

pH: 7.54
$Paco_2$: 25 mm Hg
HCO_3^-: 22 mEq/L
BE: +2.0
Pao_2: 48 mm Hg
Sao_2: 85%

1. Using conventional nomenclature, classify this blood gas result.
   This blood gas study would be classified as an *uncompensated respiratory alkalosis with moderate to severe hypoxemia.*

2. Using clinical nomenclature, describe this patient's ventilatory status.
   The patient has a history of congestive heart failure. She has come to the clinic with a "chest cold," cough, and shortness of breath, which may indicate a respiratory tract infection. Her Pao_2 and Sao_2 while breathing room air show moderate to severe hypoxemia. The normal physiologic response to hypoxemia (Pao_2 < 60 mm Hg) is increased heart rate, increased respiratory rate, and hyperventilation. The patient's blood gas values would be best described as *acute alveolar hyperventilation secondary to moderate to severe hypoxemia.*

3. Describe the metabolic response to the respiratory acidosis.
   This patient's current HCO_3^- is 22 mEq/L with a BE of +2. These values are within the normal range and suggest that renal compensation has not yet occurred.

4. Describe the relationship between pH and $Paco_2$.
   With acute decrease in $Paco_2$, we would expect an increase in pH of about 0.10 units for each 10 mm Hg decrease in $Paco_2$. Assuming a baseline $Paco_2$ of 40 mm Hg, an acute decrease in $Paco_2$ to 25 mm Hg would result in an increase in pH of about 0.15 to about 7.55:

$$\text{Expected pH (acute hyperventilation)} = 7.40 + \left(\frac{(40 - Paco_2 \ \text{actual})}{10} \times 0.10 \right)$$

$$\text{Expected pH (acute hyperventilation)} = 7.40 + \left(\frac{(40 - 25)}{10} \times 0.10 \right) = 7.55$$

The patient's actual pH is 7.54, which is consistent with an acute decrease in $Paco_2$, or *acute alveolar hyperventilation.*

CLINICAL FOCUS 8-11

Chronic Alveolar Hyperventilation

A 24-year-old man with severe chest wall deformity (pectus excavatum) is admitted to the hospital with pneumonia. His current arterial blood gas values while receiving oxygen therapy are:

Fio_2: 40%
pH: 7.44
$Paco_2$: 25 mm Hg
HCO_3^-: 16 mEq/L
BE: −7.0

Pao_2: 72 mm Hg

Sao_2: 93%

1. Using conventional nomenclature, classify this blood gas result.

    This blood gas study would be classified as a *fully compensated respiratory alkalosis with mild hypoxemia.* Based on a Pao_2 value of only 70 mm Hg while breathing 40% O_2, the patient would be severely hypoxemic if he were breathing room air. The Pao_2 and Sao_2 values, however, have been corrected to clinically acceptable levels (i.e., $Pao_2 \geq 60$ mm Hg; $Sao_2 \geq 90\%$).

2. Using clinical nomenclature, describe this patient's ventilatory status.

    This patient has a chest wall deformity, which causes a restrictive ventilatory defect and may impact his ventilatory and oxygenation status on a chronic basis. He now suffers from pneumonia, which further impacts his oxygenation status. Although it would be very helpful to have previous (baseline) blood gas results, the patient's current blood gas values would probably be best described as *chronic alveolar hyperventilation,* which may be due to a chronic hypoxemia associated with his chronic restrictive ventilatory disorder.

3. Describe the metabolic response to the respiratory acidosis.

    This patient's current HCO_3^- is 16 mEq/L with a BE of −7.0. These values suggest that full compensation has occurred in response to the chronic respiratory alkalosis. Renal compensation generally takes several days to complete and results in a 4 to 5 mEq/L decrease in HCO_3^- for every 10 mm Hg decrease in $Paco_2$. This patient's current $Paco_2$ is 25 mm Hg. Assuming this represents a 15 mm Hg decrease (40 − 25 = 15 mm Hg), with complete metabolic compensation we would expect the HCO_3^- to decrease by about 6 to 7.5 mEq/L (i.e., HCO_3^- expected range = 14.5 to 22 mEq/L). The patient's actual HCO_3^- is 16 mEq/L, which is well within the expected range for complete renal compensation (fully compensated respiratory alkalosis).

4. Describe the relationship between pH and $Paco_2$.

    With acute decrease in $Paco_2$, we would expect an increase in pH of about 0.10 units for each 10 mm Hg decrease in $Paco_2$. With a chronic decrease in $Paco_2$, we would expect renal compensation to lower the HCO_3^-, returning the pH towards a normal value, which has occurred in this case.

CLINICAL FOCUS 8-12

Acute Alveolar Hyperventilation Superimposed on Chronic Ventilatory Failure

A 68-year-old male patient is admitted to the hospital with an acute exacerbation of his long standing COPD. The patient has documented chronic hypercapnea (chronic ventilatory failure) based on prior blood gas reports. An arterial blood gas study is drawn and analyzed for this patient while breathing oxygen via nasal cannula at 2 L/min:

pH: 7.54

$Paco_2$: 44 mm Hg

HCO_3^-: 37 mEq/L

BE: +14

Pao_2: 48 mm Hg

Sao_2: 83%

1. Using conventional nomenclature, classify this blood gas result.

    This blood gas study appears to represent an uncompensated metabolic alkalosis. However, this interpretation would be incorrect based on the patient's history and previous blood gases.

2. Using clinical nomenclature, describe the patient's ventilatory status.

    The key to understanding the current blood gas results is based on the patient's history and prior blood gases. Stable baseline blood gases for this patient are obtained from a previous admission while breathing room air:

    pH: 7.38

    $Paco_2$: 55 mm Hg

    HCO_3^-: 31 mEq/L

    BE: +6

(*continues*)

Pao_2: 55 mm Hg

Sao_2: 88%

These prior blood gases reflect chronic ventilatory failure with moderate hypoxemia. Thus, the current $Paco_2$ of 44 mm Hg represents a *relative hyperventilation* when compared to the patient's previous stable baseline $Paco_2$ of 55 mm Hg. The best description of the patient's current blood gases could be *acute alveolar hyperventilation superimposed on chronic ventilatory failure*. Although a $Paco_2$ of 44 mm Hg would not represent hyperventilation in a normal patient, in this case it may, relative to the patient's baseline chronic ventilatory failure.

resulting from the breakdown of amino acids.[29] Normally, renal excretion of these fixed acids maintains body homeostasis and pH. Metabolic acidosis may be is defined as a decrease in the concentration of bicarbonate (HCO_3^-) in the plasma to < 22 mEq/L. This can be caused by increased fixed acid production, ingestion of acids, decreased renal excretion of acids, or loss of bicarbonate.[29]

Examples of *increased fixed acid production* include lactic acidosis and ketoacidosis. Anaerobic metabolism due to insufficient cellular oxygen levels produces lactic acid. Lactic acidosis is caused by tissue hypoxia, usually associated with circulatory collapse or shock (see Chapter 6). Ketoacidosis may be caused by uncontrolled diabetes mellitus (diabetic ketoacidosis), excessive alcohol consumption (alcoholic ketoacidosis), or fasting (starvation). With ketoacidosis, alteration in normal metabolic pathways result in the production of ketones formed from the breakdown of fatty acids and the deamination of amino acids. Increased fixed acid production typically causes an *increased anion gap acidosis* (see below).

Ingestion of acids such as methanol, ethylene glycol, aspirin (acetylsalicylic acid), or toluene may also cause metabolic acidosis. Methanol and ethylene glycol are found in automotive antifreeze and de-icing solutions, windshield wiper fluid, and certain other chemical solvents, cleaners, and industrial products.[29] Aspirin overdose (i.e., salicylate poisoning) is occasionally seen in children who ingest excessive aspirin in an unsupervised environment. Accidental or intentional inhalation of products containing toluene (e.g., glue sniffing) may also cause metabolic acidosis.[30] Toluene is found in various glues, adhesives, acrylic paints, paint thinners, and other products.[30] Ingestion of acids typically causes an *increased anion gap acidosis* (see below).

Decreased renal excretion of acid occurs with renal failure. With kidney disease, a reduction in kidney function leads to hydrogen ion retention, decreased plasma HCO_3^-, and acidosis. When the kidneys fail to excrete fixed organic and inorganic acids (e.g., retained sulfate, urate, phosphate, hippurate), there is usually an increase in the anion gap value (> 16 mEq/L; see below).[29,31]

Renal tubular acidosis (RTA) may involve impaired distal tubular H^+ secretion (Type 1 RTA), a reduction in proximal tubular reabsorption of HCO_3^- (Type 2 RTA), or decreased aldosterone secretion (hypoaldosteronism; Type 4 RTA).[32,33] RTA is associated with a wide variety of disorders, most of which are rare. Examples include certain autoimmune diseases (e.g., Sjgren syndrome, lupus, and rheumatoid arthritis), RTA caused by certain drugs and chemicals (e.g., amphotericin B; ifosfamide, a cancer drug), excessive urinary calcium excretion (e.g., hypercalciuria sometimes seen in sarcoidosis, hyperparathyroidism, and vitamin D intoxication), genetic disease, heavy metal exposure (e.g., lead, mercury), and renal transplant rejection.[32,33] Fanconi syndrome is seen most frequently in children and includes Type 2 RTA, vitamin D deficiency, and abnormal excretion of glucose.[32,33]

RTA Types 1, 2, and 4 typically cause a *normal anion gap acidosis* (see below). Hypokalemia (decreased K^+) is common with both Type 1 and Type 2 RTA.[32] Aldosterone is a steroid hormone secreted by the adrenal gland. Causes of low aldosterone (hypoaldosteronism, Type 4 RTA) include adrenal insufficiency, congenital disease (e.g., adrenal hyperplasia), and certain medications (e.g., nonsteroidal anti-inflammatory drugs [NSAIDs], ACE inhibitors).

Metabolic acidosis due to loss of HCO_3^- can occur due to loss via GI tract fluids (e.g., diarrhea), pancreatic fistula, ureteral diversion, or failure to reabsorb HCO_3^- in the proximal tubules of the kidney (e.g., Type 2 renal tubular acidosis). Lower GI tract sections are alkaline, and loss due to diarrhea or removal of GI fluids (e.g., tube drainage or fistula) can cause acidosis (often with hypokalemia). A pancreatic fistula is an abnormal opening that may allow alkaline pancreatic fluid to be lost through the GI tract. A ureteral diversion (e.g., ileal loop) is created as part of a surgical procedure to remove the bladder and divert urine flow. A "dilution acidosis" may also occur when an expansion of extracellular fluid volume (e.g., I.V. fluid administration) results in a relative decrease in plasma HCO_3^-. Loss of HCO_3^- typically causes a *normal anion gap acidosis* (e.g., *hyperchloremic acidosis*, see below).

Evaluation of patients with a metabolic acidosis should include measurement of serum electrolytes to determine if there is an increased or normal anion gap present. Certain types of metabolic acidosis are associated with an increased anion gap, whereas other types of metabolic acidosis are associated with a normal anion gap. Calculation of the anion gap can sometimes help identify the cause of a metabolic acidosis

Anion Gap Evaluation

Assessment of the anion gap can be helpful in determining if an acidosis is caused by a gain in fixed acids or a loss of HCO_3^-. Measurement of serum electrolytes allows for calculation of the anion gap. Plasma has no net electrical charge; however, all plasma ions are not included in the calculation of the anion gap:

$$\text{Anion gap (mEq/L)} = [Na^+] - ([Cl^-] + [HCO_3^-])$$

Historically, the normal range for the anion gap was considered to be 8 to 16 mEq/L. The normal range may vary by clinical laboratory, depending on type of analyzers used; some sources suggest a normal range of 7 to 13 mEq/L or as low as 3 to 11 mEq/L.[29] We suggest that an anion gap > 11 mEq/L be considered elevated. Common causes of normal or elevated anion gap acidosis are listed in **Box 8-15**.

Increased Anion Gap Acidosis

An increased anion gap acidosis indicates an elevation of fixed acids in the body, either from overproduction of acids, ingestion of acids, or inadequate removal of acids. As noted previously, causes of high anion gap acidosis include lactic acidosis (e.g., severe tissue hypoxia), ketoacidosis (e.g., diabetic crisis), or ingestion of acids (e.g., salicylate [aspirin] overdose or methanol or ethylene glycol ingestion). Most, but not all, patients with renal failure develop an increased anion gap acidosis due to a failure to excrete acid. A rare cause of increased anion gap acidosis in adults is due to accumulation of 5-oxoproline (pyroglutamic acid) associated with genetic or acquired problems with glutathion metabolism or depletion.[29]

RC Insights

Increased Anion Gap Acidosis
An elevated anion gap (>11 mEq/L) acidosis means that the fixed acid concentration in the body has increased.

Normal Anion Gap Acidosis

Metabolic acidosis with a *normal anion gap* is associated with HCO_3^- loss, failure to reabsorb HCO_3^-, or ingestion of certain substances. HCO_3^- loss does not elevate the anion gap because it is typically associated

with chloride (Cl⁻) gain, sometimes referred to as *hyperchloremic acidosis*. Causes of a normal anion gap acidosis include diarrhea, pancreatic fistula, ureteral diversion, and ingestion of certain substances (e.g., ammonium chloride or hyperalimentation). Ammonium chloride is sometimes administered to treat hypochloremic states (low Cl⁻) and metabolic alkalosis. A normal anion gap is also seen with renal tubular acidosis (Type 1 RTA and Type 2 RTA) and hypoaldosteronism (Type 4 RTA).[29]

RC Insights

Normal Anion Gap Metabolic Acidosis
A normal anion gap acidosis is associated with loss of HCO_3^-, failure to reabsorb HCO_3^-, or ingestion of base.

Overlap Acidosis (Normal or Increased Anion Gap)

Some types of metabolic acidosis can present with a normal or increased anion gap. As noted, most patients with renal failure and metabolic acidosis have an increased anion gap, though some do not. Most patients with diarrhea and metabolic acidosis have a normal anion gap, but patients with severe diarrhea may have an increased anion gap. With diabetic ketoacidosis, the anion gap is usually increased, but will return to normal during insulin therapy, if volume status and kidney function are good. Similarly, lactic acidosis and toluene-induced metabolic acidosis typically present with an increased anion gap, though with good kidney function the anion gap may be normal.

Total Parenteral Nutrition and Acid-Base Balance

Malnutrition is a complication of critical illness, and nutritional support should be provided. Critical illness often results in increased caloric needs, catabolic states (e.g., trauma, burns, sepsis), and skeletal muscle loss. During recovery from critical illness, anabolic states (e.g., tissue repair) may also require nutritional support.[34] Nutritional support may be provided enterally (by mouth or feeding tube) or parenterally (by intravenous [IV] administration). The term *total parenteral nutrition* (TPN) refers to IV hyperalimentation. Although enteral nutrition is generally preferred, parenteral nutrition should be considered in patients who are malnourished and who have contraindications to enteral nutrition (e.g., hemodynamic instability, bowel obstruction [ileus], upper GI tract bleeding, fistulas, or severe vomiting or diarrhea). Clinical practice guidelines suggest that parenteral nutrition be started in patients unable to tolerate enteral nutrition within 5 to 7 days.[35]

BOX 8-15

Causes of Metabolic Acidosis

Increased Anion Gap Acidosis[1]

Lactic acidosis (e.g., acute, severe hypoxia; shock; tissue hypoperfusion)

Ketoacidosis[2] (e.g., diabetes mellitus [diabetic ketoacidosis], fasting, starvation, alcoholic ketoacidosis)

Most patients with renal failure[3] (e.g., retention of hydrogen ions, sulfate ions, phosphate, and urate ions)

Salicylate (aspirin) overdose

Ingestion of methanol (e.g., methyl alcohol [wood alcohol], antifreeze, solvents)

Ingestion of ethylene glycol (e.g., automotive radiator antifreeze, brake fluid)

Ingestion of large quantities of propylene glycol (e.g., newer automotive antifreeze, airport de-icers, cosmetic products)

Ingestion of toluene, a solvent used in paint thinners and for other industrial uses (metabolic acidosis is an early finding or seen with impaired kidney function)

Accumulation of pyroglutamic acid (5-oxoproline) associated with genetic glutathione synthetase deficiency or acquired glutathione depletion

Normal Anion Gap Acidosis

Diarrhea (loss of HCO_3^-)

Pancreatic fistula (loss of HCO_3^-)

Distal (Type 1) renal tubular acidosis[3]

Proximal (Type 2) renal tubular acidosis (failure to reabsorb HCO_3^-)

Hypoaldosteronism (Type 4 renal tubular acidosis)[3]

Post treatment ketoacidosis[2]

Ureteral diversion (e.g., ileal loop) performed as part of surgery to remove the bladder

Ingestion or administration of ammonium chloride (sometimes used to treat severe metabolic alkalosis)

Administration of carbonic anhydrase inhibitors (e.g., acetazolamide [Diamox], a diuretic sometimes used to treat metabolic alkalosis)

Intravenous hyperalimentation

Ingestion of toluene (late finding or with good kidney function)

[1]Low albumin may cause a decrease in anion gap (AG). To adjust for this, some suggest calculation of "corrected anion gap" = AG + 2.5 × (4 − Measured albumin). If the corrected AG > 16, then increased anion gap acidosis is present; if corrected AG < 16, then normal anion gap acidosis is present.

[2]During the treatment phase of diabetic ketoacidosis the anion gap may return to normal.

[3]With renal failure, some patients may have a normal anion gap, though most do not.

[4]Type 1 renal tubular acidosis (RTA) or hypoaldosteronism (Type 4 RTA) generally present with a normal anion gap.

Data from: Beachy W. Clinical assessment of acid-base and oxygenation status. In: Beachy W (ed.). *Respiratory Care Anatomy and Physiology*, 2nd ed. St. Louis, MO: Mosby-Elsevier; 2007: 214–235; and Post TW, Rose BD. Approach to the adult with metabolic acidosis. In: *UpToDate*, Basow DS (ed.), UpToDate, Waltham, MA, 2013.

Parenteral nutrition provides carbohydrate (dextrose), fat (lipids), protein (amino acids), electrolytes (Na^+, Cl^-, K^+, Ca^{2+}, Mg^{2+l}, PO_4, acetate), vitamins, minerals, trace elements, and fluids. TPN solutions are acidic (in order to ensure stability) and contain both preformed acids and nutrients that are metabolized to acids.[34-36] For example, certain amino acids produce sulfuric acid when metabolized, and phosphorus-containing compounds generate phosphoric acid.[36] In patients with normal respiratory and renal function, these acids are excreted and acid-base balance is maintained.[36] Certain conditions, however, may lead to incomplete glycolysis (sugar metabolism), which may produce pyruvic and lactic acids. Lipolysis (fat metabolism) produces ketones, which in large quantities can produce acidosis (e.g., ketoacidosis).

Metabolic acidosis is a potential complication in patients receiving TPN, especially in patients with hypoxia, poor tissue perfusion, and hypermetabolism.[36] The majority of TPN amino acids are acidic. TPN associated acidosis may be due to an increase in chloride (i.e., hyperchloremia) following infusion, increased renal or GI tract loss of HCO_3^-, decreased renal excretion of H^+, or increased production of acids.[36] Depending on the cause, TPN-induced acidosis may be associated with a normal or increased anion gap.[36]

In ventilator-dependent patients, it is generally recommended that calories provided be 40% to 50% carbohydrate, 30% to 40% fat, and 20% to 25% protein.[35] In addition to metabolic acidosis, complications of TPN include electrolyte abnormalities, hyperglycemia, infection, and problems with venous access.[34] Overfeeding can cause hypercapnea, resulting in acidosis due to elevated CO_2. Refeeding syndrome may occur with TPN in which patients develop fluid and electrolyte disturbances and other cardiopulmonary, neuromuscular, and neurologic complications.[34] Low serum phosphorus (PO_4; hypophosphatemia) can lead to respiratory muscle weakness, further exacerbating respiratory failure.[35] Pneumothorax is a potential complication of parenteral nutrition associated with gaining and maintaining central venous access, which is needed when administering higher dextrose concentrations (e.g., > 10%).[35]

In stable patients, acid-base balance during parenteral nutrition can usually maintained by ensuring that equal amounts of chloride and acetate are provided.[35] Acetate is metabolized as bicarbonate, and in patients with metabolic acidosis chloride should be minimized and acetate maximized. Critically ill patients receiving TPN should probably have blood gases (pH, $Paco_2$, and HCO_3^-), electrolytes (calcium, magnesium, and phosphate), and glucose levels monitored daily until stable.[34]

In summary, metabolic acidosis associated with TPN may be associated with an increased or normal anion gap. Increased anion gap acidosis can occur with parenteral nutrition using alternative carbohydrates (such as fructose or sorbitol) or alternative lipids.[36] Infusion with amino acids without carbohydrates (e.g., protein-sparing therapy) can result in a ketoacidosis with increased anion gap.[36] A normal anion gap acidosis is associated with loss of HCO_3^- (e.g., diarrhea, fistula drainage, and proximal [Type 2] renal tubular acidosis).[36]

Clinical Manifestations

Clinical manifestations of metabolic acidosis will vary with the underlying cause. Hyperventilation is the normal compensatory response, and patients may exhibit tachypnea, increased minute volume, and increased tidal volume (hyperpnea). Respiratory distress, dyspnea, and accessory muscle use may be present. For example, Kussmaul breathing refers to hyperventilation with deep, labored breathing sometimes seen in diabetic ketoacidosis. With extreme acidosis, patients may become lethargic, stuporous, or comatose. Severe acidosis may cause hemodynamic instability, and ventricular arrhythmias may develop when pH falls to less than about 7.10 in subjects with normal cardiac function; patients with cardiovascular instability may

develop arrhythmias at a higher pH (e.g., pH ≤ 7.20). Acidosis also may cause arterial vasodilation, venous vasoconstriction, and blunt the body's response to catecholamines (e.g., epinephrine, other catecholamine vasopressors).[25]

Treatment

Treatment should focus on the underlying cause of the metabolic acidosis. For example, lactic acidosis due to poor tissue perfusion secondary to shock may be treated by providing oxygen therapy and restoring circulation, blood pressure, and cardiac output (see Chapter 6). A patient with a diabetic ketoacidosis may be given insulin to correct hyperglycemia and fluid and potassium replacement, if indicated. Treatment of metabolic acidosis should aim to restore extracellular pH to a normal value. Generally, once the underlying cause has been resolved, the acidosis will improve rapidly.

Hyperventilation can be effective in improving arterial pH. In spontaneously breathing patients with good lung function, hyperventilation may achieve a $Paco_2$ as low as 8 to 12 mm Hg.[25,36] If a patient's ventilatory response is less than expected, it may be due to a ventilatory disorder (e.g., lung disease, muscle weakness, or impaired ventilatory drive).

RC Insights

Metabolic Acidosis and Expected $Paco_2$

For metabolic acidosis, the expected $Paco_2$ (maximal compensation) will usually be the last two digits of the pH. For example, if the pH is 7.30, then the $Paco_2$ is 30 mm Hg; if the pH is 7.20, then the $Paco_2$ is 20 mm Hg; if the pH is 7.15, then the $Paco_2$ is 15 mm Hg (patients usually cannot sustain a $Paco_2$ below 15 mm Hg for prolonged periods).

Bicarbonate Administration

Sodium bicarbonate ($NaHCO_3$) may be administered to correct a metabolic acidosis under certain circumstances. Bicarbonate administration in the treatment of *acute metabolic acidosis* is generally not considered unless the acidemia is severe (e.g., pH < 7.20; HCO_3^- < 10 mEq/L).[37] With severe metabolic acidosis, the intravenous HCO_3^- dosage (given as $NaHCO_3$) can be estimated as follows:[37]

$$HCO_3^- \text{ (mEq/L)} = 0.5 \times \text{Weight (kg)} \\ \times \text{Desired increase in plasma } HCO_3^-$$

For most patients, the goal is to return the pH to about 7.20 with HCO_3^- of 10 to 12 mEq/L.[29] For example, a patient weighing 70 kg may have the following blood gas values:

pH: 7.10
$Paco_2$: 20 mm Hg

of gastric secretions in patients with low or absent gastric secretion of HCl (achlorhydria).[39]

Treatment of Metabolic Alkalosis

Treatment of metabolic alkalosis should be aimed at the underlying cause. For example, GI tract loss of H^+ due to vomiting or NG tube suction should be appropriately addressed. Antiemetic medications may be helpful in controlling nausea and vomiting, and stopping NG suction (if present) should be considered. The acid content of gastric secretions can also be reduced by administration of H_2 blockers (e.g., cimetidine [Tagamet], ranitidine [Zantac]) or proton pump inhibitors (e.g., omeprazole, [Prilosec], esomeprazole [Nexium]).[40]

Treatment of renal loss of H^+ should be targeted, depending on the cause. For example, loop or thiazide diuretics may be stopped and K^+ replaced. Administration of base (e.g., $NaHCO_3$, calcium carbonate) or substances that are metabolized to bicarbonate (e.g., citrate, lactate) should be discontinued. Hypercalcemia may be treated by removing sources of excess calcium.

Renal excretion of excess HCO_3^- can be improved by attention to factors that impair renal function. Hypochloremia and hypokalemia may be corrected by administration of solutions containing sodium chloride (NaCl) and potassium chloride (KCl); potassium may be given orally in patients able to take oral medications.[40] Hypovolemia should be treated to restore blood volume and renal perfusion. True volume depletion can be caused by bleeding, GI tract loss of fluids, and diuretics. With true volume depletion, fluid administration may restore circulating blood volume. These patients also typically have low Cl^-, and the resulting hypochloremic alkalosis is often responsive to chloride-containing solutions (e.g., normal saline [0.9% NaCl]). Fluid repletion with normal saline with a target volume of about 100 mL/hour > urine output has been suggested.[40] Alkalosis that is responsive to this therapy is often associated with conditions such as severe vomiting or gastric suctioning. These patients are often volume depleted and have low potassium levels. An increase in HCO_3^- excretion can be detected by measuring urine pH (e.g., pH > 7.0).[40] Metabolic alkaloses that are unresponsive to chloride (saline) administration are characterized by normal or elevated extracellular fluid level and increased chloride level in the urine.

Fluids should be given cautiously, if at all, in patients with heart failure, cor pulmonale, cirrhosis, or nephrotic syndrome, because fluids may worsen these patients' condition.[40] Treatment with saline solutions is contraindicated in patients with generalized edema, because it will not correct the alkalosis and it may exacerbate edema, ascites, or effusions.[40] In these patients, K^+ depletion (if present) should be corrected by administration of KCL. If diuresis is required, a potassium-sparing diuretic (e.g., amiloride) may be used.[40] Heart failure and systemic vasodilatation (as may occur with cirrhosis) should be treated to improve or maintain adequate renal perfusion, blood pressure, and cardiac output.[40] Potassium-sparing diuretic aldosterone agonists (e.g., spironolactone, eplerenone) are sometimes used in patients with edematous states (e.g., heart failure, cirrhosis); however; use caution to avoid increased K^+ (hyperkalemia) in these patients.[40]

Posthypercapnic alkalosis in patients receiving mechanical ventilation should be prevented by selecting appropriate ventilator settings to avoid a relative hyperventilation (e.g., lower respiratory rates in an SIMV mode). Posthypercapnic alkalosis may also respond to administration of IV normal saline solution, and patients requiring diuresis can be treated with acetazolamine (see below).[40]

Acetazolamide (Diamox) is a carbonic anhydrase inhibitor and diuretic that increases $Paco_2$ and renal HCO_3^- excretion.[40] This therapy is only effective in patients with normal potassium levels because hypokalemia results in potassium-H+ exchange in the distal tubule in hypokalemic patients. Dosage for treatment of metabolic alkalosis is 250 to 500 mg 1 to 2 times per day.[40] Although acetazolamide increases HCO_3^- excretion, it may also cause an increase in K^+ excretion, and potassium replacement therapy may be needed. In general, it is not used until hypokalemia and volume depletion are corrected. Renal dialysis for patients with acute or chronic kidney disease using a low bicarbonate bath concentration can rapidly improve an alkalosis is these patients.[40]

In cases of severe metabolic alkalosis (e.g., HCO_3^- > 50 mEq/L; pH > 7.55) where kidney function is compromised and dialysis is not an option, administration of ammonium chloride NH_4Cl or a dilute solution of hydrochloric acid (HCl) may be considered.[40] Formulas are available for calculation of total excess plasma HCO_3^- concentrations based on the generalization that total body water is 50% to 60% of ideal body weight (IBW), depending on gender:[40]

- Rough estimate of total body water (men) = 0.6 × IBW
- Rough estimate of total body water (women) = 0.5 × IBW

The total body base deficit or excess can then be estimated using the BE/BD value obtained from an arterial blood gas report:

$$\text{Total BE/BD} = \text{BE/BD} \times \text{Total body water}$$

Clinical Focus 8-13 provides an example of the estimate of total body base deficit.

As noted, in rare cases of acute severe metabolic alkalosis, the direct administration of acid may be considered. For HCl administration, a 0.1 to 0.15 normal solution is infused via a central venous catheter over a period of 8

CLINICAL FOCUS 8-13

Calculation of Total Base Excess or Deficit

A rough estimate of total excess or deficit of plasma HCO_3^- can be based on the generalization that total body water is 50% to 60% of ideal body weight (IBW), depending on gender:[1]

- Rough estimate of total body water (men) = 0.6 × IBW
- Rough estimate of total body water (women) = 0.5 × IBW

The total body base deficit or excess can then be estimated:

$$\text{Total base excess/deficit} = \text{Base excess/deficit in mEq/L} \times \text{Total body water}$$

Example: A male patient with an IBW of 70 kg has the following arterial gas results:

pH: 7.60
$Paco_2$: 55 mm Hg
Plasma HCO_3^-: 52 mEq/L
BE: +28.5 mEq/L

This represents a severe metabolic alkalosis with a compensatory (expected) respiratory acidosis. The total body HCO_3^- deficit can be roughly estimated as follows:

$$\text{Total base excess/deficit} = \text{BE/BD} \times \text{Total body water} = 28.5 \times (0.6 \times \text{IBW})$$

$$\text{Total base deficit} = 28.5 \times (0.6 \times \text{IBW})$$

$$\text{Total base deficit} = 28.5 \times (0.6 \times 70) = 1197 \text{ mEq}$$

Thus, to return the pH to normal with a $Paco_2$ of 40 would require the administration of about 1200 mEq of acid or the excretion of about 1200 mEq of base. In the rare cases where acid would be administered for a severe metabolic alkalosis (e.g., NH_4Cl or HCl), the dose would be about 100 mEq at a time, followed by measurement of blood gases, pH, and HCO_3^- in 30 to 60 minutes. The dose could then be repeated, if the therapeutic goal was not achieved.

An alternative calculation has been suggested for estimating total HCO_3^- excess with metabolic alkalosis:[*]

- Men: Total excess plasma HCO_3^- (mEq) = 0.6 × IBW × (plasma HCO_3^- – 24)
- Women: Total excess plasma HCO_3^- (mEq) = 0.5 × IBW × (plasma HCO_3^- – 24)

Using our same patient and this alternative calculation, the total HCO_3^- excess would be:

$$\text{Excess plasma } HCO_3^- = 0.6 \times \text{IBW} \times (\text{plasma } HCO_3^- - 24)$$

$$\text{Excess plasma } HCO_3^- = 0.6 \times 70 \text{ kg} \times (52 - 24) = 1176 \text{ mEq}$$

Regardless of formula used, these calculations provide only a rough estimate of the total body base excess or deficit.

Data from: Mehta A, Emmett M. Treatment of metabolic alkalosis. In: *UpToDate*, Basow, DS (ed.), UpToDate, Waltham, MA, 2013.

---

to 24 hours.[40] HCl can cause tissue necrosis and it reacts with plastic, making its use problematic.[40] IV administration of ammonium chloride (NH_4Cl) is a good alterative, using 100 to 200 mEq NH_4Cl in 1000 mL of 0.9% NaCl.[40] Generally, not more than 100 mEq of NH_4Cl would be infused followed by measurement of arterial blood gases, pH, and plasma HCO_3^-.[40] The dose would be then repeated, if the therapeutic goal is not achieved.

In summary, metabolic alkalosis is most commonly caused by excess H^+ loss from the GI tract or in the urine. Other causes include administration of base, H^+ movement into cells, and volume contraction. Treatment of metabolic alkalosis should be aimed at the underlying cause. Renal excretion of HCO_3^- should be supported by maintaining renal perfusion and blood volume and correcting hypochloremia and hypokalemia. Except in certain cases, fluid repletion with normal saline may be beneficial. Treatment of vomiting and stopping interventions that may cause or worsen alkalosis (e.g., diuretics, NG suction, alkali therapy) should occur. Common causes of metabolic alkalosis are listed in **Box 8-16**.

BOX 8-16

Causes of Metabolic Alkalosis

GI tract loss of hydrogen ions
- Vomiting (loss of HCl, stomach acid)
- Nasogastric (NG) tube suction (loss of HCl via NG tube)
- Unusual cases of diarrhea with potassium loss[1]

Renal loss of hydrogen ions
- Loop or thiazide diuretics (loss of Cl^-, K^+, fluid volume)
- Genetic renal tubular disorder (e.g., Bartter and Gitelman syndromes)
- Posthypercapnic increase in HCO_3^- (e.g., chronic ventilatory failure) followed by mechanical ventilation and a relative hyperventilation
- Excess mineralocorticoid (e.g., primary aldosteronism)
- Hypochloremia (increased Cl^-, H^+ secretion, and HCO_3^- reabsorption)
- Hypokalemia (decreased K^+ and increased H^+ secretion and HCO_3^- reabsorption)
- Hypercalcemia due to ingestion of calcium containing substances (milk-alkali syndrome)

Intracellular shift of hydrogen ions
- Hypokalemia (decreased plasma K^+ pulls potassium from cells in exchange for H^+)

Contraction of blood volume
- Hypovolemia (resulting in a relative increase in HCO_3^-)
  - Fluid loss (bleeding, excessive sweating)
  - Loop or thiazide diuretics[2]

Administration of base
- Sodium bicarbonate ($NaHCO_3$) administration for severe metabolic acidosis
- Ingestion of base ($NaHCO_3$, citrate salts) in the presence of inadequate renal function
- Crack cocaine or freebase cocaine (contains $NaHCO_3$)

GI, gastrointestinal; HCl, hydrochloric acid; Cl^-, chloride ions; K^+, potassium ions; H^+, hydrogen ions; HCO_3^-, bicarbonate ions; $NaHCO_3$, sodium bicarbonate

[1]Lower GI tract secretions are alkaline, and diarrhea more commonly causes a metabolic acidosis. Unusual cases of diarrhea (e.g., laxative abuse) with potassium loss may cause a metabolic alkalosis.

[2]Loop or thiazide diuretics may cause hypokalemia. Potassium diuretics (e.g., amiloride, spironolactone, eplerenone) may conserve K^+.

Mixed and Combined Disorders

In many critically ill patients, respiratory and metabolic disturbances coexist. For example, a patient may have a combined respiratory and metabolic acidosis due to concurrent hypoventilation and lactic acidosis. With combined respiratory and metabolic conditions in the same direction (i.e., acidosis or alkalosis), the pH may reach extreme values. It is also possible to have concurrent metabolic problems that push the pH in opposite directions. For example, it is possible to have a loss of gastric acid (metabolic alkalosis) in combination with a lactic acidosis due severe hypoxia. Identification of mixed blood gas disorders begins with determining the major disorder and subsequent evaluation of expected compensation. If compensation is submaximal on the one hand, or more than expected on the other hand, a coexisting disorder may be present.[25] The patient history and prior blood gas studies (if available) should always be reviewed when assessing an acid-base disturbance. It also is important to note that compensatory responses often do not return the arterial pH to normal.[25,27] What may appear to be full compensation may instead be a mixed acid-base disturbance. **Clinical Focus 8-14**, **Clinical Focus 8-15**, and **Clinical Focus 8-16** provide examples of combined respiratory and metabolic acid-base disturbances.

In summary, arterial blood gas interpretation requires a thorough understanding of factors that affect oxygenation, ventilation, and acid-base balance. The respiratory care clinician must then apply this knowledge in light of a specific patient's history, prior blood gas studies (if available), and clinical condition. Conventional classification of acid-base status describes blood gas results as uncompensated, partly compensated, or fully compensated metabolic or respiratory alkalosis or acidosis. Although conventional blood gas nomenclature is often used to classify blood gas study results, it has limitations that must be acknowledged. There are limits to both respiratory and metabolic compensation, and these can be estimated using simple

CLINICAL FOCUS 8-14

Combined Metabolic and Respiratory Acidosis

A patient in the emergency department with thoracic trauma following a motor vehicle accident has the following blood gas values while receiving O_2 therapy via simple mask at 8 L/min.

pH: 7.12
$Paco_2$: 60 mm Hg
Pao_2: 40 mm Hg
Sao_2: 75%
HCO_3^-: 19 mEq/L
BE/BD: −9

Interpret this patient's arterial blood gas results.

1. pH: Overall acidosis.
2. $Paco_2$: Ventilatory failure (respiratory acidosis).
3. HCO_3^- and BE/BD: Metabolic acidosis.
4. Cause of pH abnormality: This is a combined respiratory and metabolic acidosis.
5. Compensation: None.

This patient has a combined respiratory and metabolic acidosis. The respiratory acidosis (hypoventilation/ventilatory failure) is probably due to a problem related to lung function secondary to thoracic trauma (e.g., flail chest, lung contusions, possible aspiration). The metabolic acidosis could be caused by a number of concurrent conditions, such as lactic acidosis (due to severe hypoxemia).

CLINICAL FOCUS 8-15

Combined Metabolic and Respiratory Alkalosis

A patient in the intensive care unit has the following arterial blood gas values while receiving oxygen therapy via nasal cannula at 6 L/min:

pH: 7.58
$Paco_2$: 32 mm Hg
Pao_2: 48 mm Hg
Sao_2: 75%
HCO_3^-: 30 mEq/L
BE/BD: +7

Interpret this patient's arterial blood gas results.

1. pH: Overall severe alkalosis.
2. $Paco_2$: Alveolar hyperventilation (respiratory alkalosis), possibly secondary to hypoxemia.
3. HCO_3^- and BE: Metabolic alkalosis.
4. Cause of pH abnormality: This is a combined metabolic and respiratory alkalosis.
5. Compensation: None.

The patient has a combined metabolic and respiratory alkalosis. The respiratory alkalosis (alveolar hyperventilation) is probably caused by hypoxemia. The patient's Pao_2 and Sao_2 are very low, especially in a patient receiving O_2 therapy at 6 L/min (approximately 40% O_2). The cause of the respiratory alkalosis should be identified and the hypoxemia should be corrected, if possible.

The metabolic alkalosis could be caused by a number of conditions, including GI tract loss of hydrogen ions (e.g., nasogastric tube suction, vomiting), renal loss of hydrogen ions (e.g., decrease in Cl^- or K^+) or administration of base (e.g., $NaHCO_3$). In cases of severe metabolic alkalosis (e.g., $HCO_3^- > 50$ mEq/L; pH > 7.55) where kidney function is compromised and dialysis is not an option, administration of ammonium chloride (NH_4Cl) or a dilute solution of hydrochloric acid (HCl) may be considered.

CLINICAL FOCUS 8-16

Blood Gas Interpretation Exercises*

Interpret each of the following blood gas reports using conventional nomenclature for metabolic disorders and clinical nomenclature for ventilatory disorders.*

	1	2	3	4	5	6	7
pH	7.26	7.52	7.60	7.44	7.38	7.20	7.56
Pa_{CO_2}	56	28	55	24	76	25	44
HCO_3^-	24	22	52	16	43	9	38
BE/BD	−2	−1	+29	−8	+17	−17	+14

	8	9	10	11	12	13	14
pH	7.36	7.60	7.35	7.56	7.55	7.20	7.46
Pa_{CO_2}	25	25	90	40	58	78	26
HCO_3^-	15	24	49	34	49	30	18
BE/BD	−10	−2	+15	+11	+20	0	−4

	15	16	17	18	19	20	21
pH	7.35	7.58	7.14	7.18	7.52	7.19	7.45
Pa_{CO_2}	55	26	90	35	55	80	27
HCO_3^-	30	23	30	13	43	30	19
BE/BD	+4	+2	+1	−14	+19	−1	−4

	22	23	24	25	26	27	28
pH	7.39	7.45	7.40	7.24	7.54	7.55	7.24
Pa_{CO_2}	25	28	56	44	25	52	36
HCO_3^-	15	20	34	18	21	44	14
BE/BD	−7	−4	+7	−7	0	+17	−13

	29	30	31	32	33	34	35
pH	7.35	7.52	7.45	7.16	7.28	7.44	7.55
Pa_{CO_2}	25	44	20	83	20	58	28
HCO_3^-	14	39	16	29	9	40	18
BE/BD	−11	+14	−7	−2	−17	+11	−2

Answers:

1. Acute ventilatory failure (uncompensated respiratory acidosis)
2. Acute alveolar hyperventilation (uncompensated respiratory alkalosis)
3. Partly compensated metabolic alkalosis
4. Chronic alveolar hyperventilation (fully compensated respiratory alkalosis)
5. Chronic ventilatory failure (fully compensated respiratory acidosis)
6. Partly compensated metabolic acidosis

7. Uncompensated metabolic alkalosis
8. Fully compensated metabolic acidosis
9. Acute alveolar hyperventilation (uncompensated respiratory alkalosis)
10. Chronic ventilatory failure (fully compensated respiratory acidosis)
11. Uncompensated metabolic alkalosis
12. Partly compensated metabolic alkalosis
13. Acute ventilatory failure. (uncompensated respiratory acidosis)
14. Chronic alveolar hyperventilation (fully compensated respiratory alkalosis)
15. Chronic ventilatory failure (fully compensated respiratory acidosis)
16. Acute alveolar hyperventilation (uncompensated respiratory alkalosis)
17. Acute ventilatory failure (uncompensated respiratory acidosis)
18. Uncompensated metabolic acidosis
19. Partly compensated metabolic alkalosis
20. Acute ventilatory failure (uncompensated respiratory acidosis)
21. Chronic alveolar hyperventilation (fully compensated respiratory alkalosis)
22. Fully compensated metabolic acidosis
23. Chronic alveolar hyperventilation (fully compensated respiratory alkalosis)
24. Chronic ventilatory failure (fully compensated respiratory acidosis)
25. Uncompensated metabolic acidosis
26. Acute alveolar hyperventilation
27. Partly compensated metabolic alkalosis
28. Uncompensated metabolic acidosis
29. Fully compensated metabolic acidosis
30. Uncompensated metabolic alkalosis
31. Chronic alveolar hyperventilation (fully compensated respiratory acidosis)
32. Acute ventilatory failure (uncompensated respiratory acidosis)
33. Partly compensated metabolic acidosis
34. Fully compensated metabolic alkalosis
35. Acute alveolar hyperventilation (uncompensated respiratory alkalosis)

This system was published in Clinical application of blood gases. Vol 5th ed., Shapiro BA PW, Kozelowski-Templin R., Copyright Mosby 1994.
*Classification of blood gas results based on a single blood gas analysis may lead to errors. Patient history, clinical course, and previous blood gases (if available) will often be helpful when interpreting blood gas results. Note that fully compensated metabolic acidosis and fully compensated respiratory alkalosis (hyperventilation) cannot clearly be distinguished on the basis of a single blood gas result alone. Fully compensated respiratory acidosis (chronic ventilatory failure) and fully compensated metabolic alkalosis also cannot be distinguished on the basis of a single blood gas result alone. In order to distinguish between causes of fully compensated acid-base disorders, previous blood gases (if available) and a review of the patient's history and clinical course are generally required. Reviews of formulas or other guidelines for maximal compensation may also be helpful.

rules to determine if maximal or **submaximal compensation** has occurred. Ventilatory disorders can often be better described using terms such as acute ventilatory failure, chronic ventilatory failure, and alveolar hyperventilation (acute and chronic). Finally, understanding the assessment and treatment of metabolic acidosis and alkalosis is essential, because these disorders are frequently encountered in the acute care setting.

Noninvasive Oximetry

Oxygen binds to hemoglobin in red blood cells when moving through the pulmonary vascular bed. It is transported from the lungs to the rest of the body by the arterial blood vessel system. Multiwavelength blood oximeters use spectrophotometric absorption of a blood specimen to determine the percentage of hemoglobin saturated with oxygen and the percentage of dyshemoglobins.[42] The varieties of hemoglobins that can be detected by the multiwavelength laboratory blood oximeters may vary by model, but generally include oxyhemoglobin, deoxyhemoglobin, carboxyhemoglobin, and methemoglobin. The blood oximeters use a minimum of seven light-emitting diodes (LEDs) to accomplish this.

Multiwavelength laboratory oximeters calculate fractional oxygen saturation among other parameters (e.g., Hb):

Fractional oxygen saturation

$$= \frac{Oxyhemoglobin}{(Oxyhemoglobin + Deoxyhemoglobin + COHb + metHb + SulfHb)} \times 100$$

Pulse oximetry is a noninvasive method of estimating the arterial oxygen saturation and pulse rate from pulsatile absorption signals derived from a sensor placed on the skin. The principle is based on the fact that oxy- and deoxyhemoglobin have different absorption spectra.

The sensor consists of light sources at the red and infrared wavelengths and a photodetector. When light from the sensor passes into the tissue, a portion is absorbed and the photodetector measures the residual. A fixed amount of light (DC) is absorbed by tissue, including nonpulsatile blood, and a modulating amount (AC) is absorbed by the pulsating arterial inflow. The percentage of absorption is called blood oxygen saturation, or SpO_2. A pulse oximeter also measures and displays the pulse rate at the same time it measures the SpO_2 and is a standard of care in most healthcare facilities. Most pulse oximeters use only two LEDs and are able to distinguish between oxyhemoglobin and deoxyhemoglobin, but not other forms of hemoglobin. **Figure 8-11** provides an illustration of oximetry for the measurement of oxyhemoglobin and deoxyhemoglobin.

Regardless of their ability to distinguish abnormal hemoglobin species, all pulse oximeters only estimate functional oxygen saturation:

Fractional oxygen saturation

$$= \frac{\text{Oxyhemoglobin}}{(\text{Oxyhemoglobin} + \text{Deoxyhemoglobin})} \times 100$$

Thus, it is apparent that pulse oximeter estimates of SpO_2 will not be accurate in the presence of dyshemoglobins. For example, in cases of carbon monoxide poisoning (elevated carboxyhemoglobin), conventional pulse oximeters will provide dangerously misleading results, because they cannot distinguish between oxyhemoglobin and carboxyhemoglobin.

Some newer pulse oximeters have recently become available that do measure oxyhemoglobin, deoxyhemoglobin, carboxyhemoglobin, methemoglobin, and hemoglobin. These newer devices have been used in emergency departments to detect cases of carbon monoxide poisoning.[43] It is important to note that one such device (Masimo, Irvine, Calif.) has an accuracy of ± 3%. This means that a measure carboxyhemoglobin of 10% could actually be as low as 7% and as high as 13%.[43,44] The respiratory care clinician should also be aware of the potential for false-positive and false-negative results and consequently should not rule out carbon monoxide poisoning without confirmation by blood co-oximetry. **Figure 8-12** illustrates oximetry for the measurement of oxyhemoglobin, deoxyhemoglobin, carboxyhemoglobin, and methemoglobin.

Indications

The purpose of pulse oximetry is to noninvasively assess blood oxygenation in order to aid in the prevention of hypoxemia or hyperoxemia. Pulse oximetry is used across the spectrum of patient ages. The areas of known utility of pulse oximetry within a hospital or patient care facility include, but are not limited to:

- Emergency department
- Intensive care
- Acute care
- Long-term care
- Clinics
- Home care
- Emergency medical services
- Patient transport
- Wherever an anesthetic is in use
- Diagnostic laboratories

Pulse oximetry does not provide assessment of ventilation (e.g., $PaCO_2$) or acid-base balance and should not be substituted for arterial blood gas analysis in patients where these may be compromised.

Technique

The amount of oxygen dissolved in the blood is proportional to the partial pressure of oxygen. The amount of oxygen bound to hemoglobin will increase as the partial pressure of oxygen increases. In contrast, the amount of oxygen bound to hemoglobin does not increase in proportion to the partial pressure of oxygen. The increase may be indicated by the S-shaped oxygen dissociation curve (see **Figure 8-13**). The oxygen dissociation curve is standardized to a body temperature of 37° C and a pH of 7.4; however, this curve may shift to the right or the left depending on the patient's

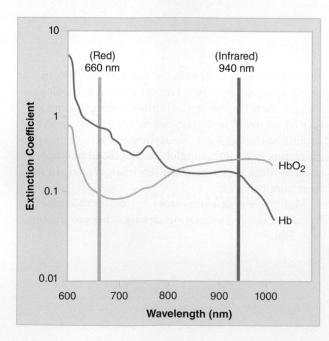

FIGURE 8-11 Oximetry for measurement of oxyhemoglobin and deoxyhemoglobin.

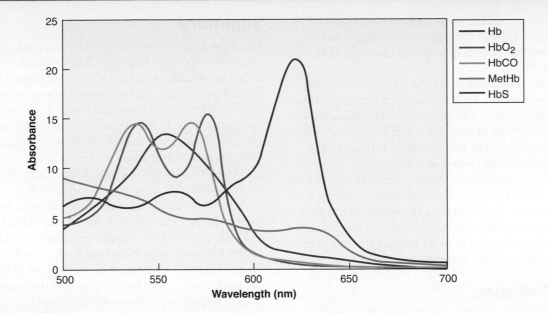

FIGURE 8-12 Oximetry for measurement of oxyhemoglobin, deoxyhemoglobin, carboxyhemoglobin, sickle-cell hemoglobin, and methemoglobin.

Modified from Radiometer Medical ApS. *Blood Gas, Oximetry, and Electrolyte Systems Reference Manual.* Radiometer Medical;1996.

condition. For example a patient who has a normal pH and body temperature with a SpO_2 of 90% will have estimated PaO_2 of 60 mm Hg. However, a patient with a respiratory alkalosis and SpO_2 of 90 may have a much lower PaO_2, depending on the severity of the alkalosis.

The performance of a pulse oximeter can be adversely affected by the patient/sensor interface. It is essential to select a sensor that is appropriate for the chosen monitoring site and that the sensor is correctly aligned and securely fitted to the site. The site should also be well perfused and free of known artifact sources (e.g., deep skin pigmentation, nail polish, tattoos, extraneous light, intravascular dyes, venous congestion, motion). Because the devices utilize different

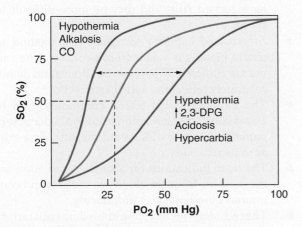

FIGURE 8-13 Oxyhemoglobin dissociation curve.

Modified from Baum GL, et al. *Textbook of Pulmonary Diseases.* 6th ed. Lippincott Williams & Wilkins; 1998.

algorithms and sensor placements, it is vitally important that the manufacturer's recommendations for setup and monitoring be followed.

Monitoring

The basic relationship between optical signals and the displayed value of SpO_2 and pulse rate is determined by the manufacturer for a given combination of pulse oximeter and sensor, which is stored permanently in the device. To prevent damage, soaking or immersing the pulse oximeter sensor in any liquid should be avoided unless specifically recommended by the sensor manufacturer. If a sensor is damaged in any way, it should be replaced.

Transmittance-type sensors have the advantage of ease of user placement and use of sites that are generally well perfused. However, they can be a source of patient entanglement and are prone to motion artifact. When placed in a central body position, the reflectance-type sensors are typically more responsive, less prone to motion, and well tolerated by the patient, but are faced with inherently weaker signals from which to detect patient values. Ideally, the extremity should be free of a blood pressure cuff and intravenous or intra-arterial catheters. This will minimize the problems related to weak arterial pulse signals and venous congestion at the sensor site.

Safety

Pulse oximetry has been a relatively safe device since clinical use.[42] However, off-label use and inappropriate clinical application can increase the hazards. Known safety concerns include pressure ischemia, burns,[42,44–47] burns associated with photodynamic therapy, and burns associated with inappropriate use in an MRI scanner.[44–48]

Pulse oximeter sensors may be a source of contamination.[49] Sensors are available in sterile packaging from some manufacturers. The adhesives and materials used in the construction of disposable and reusable sensors are generally latex-free, but should be verified by the user in conditions of known sensitivity.

As with any patient-monitoring device that uses wire leads, there can be a risk of entanglement. There is a need for ongoing assessment of the sensor site, type of sensor used, methods used to capture and display the values, and device used in order to limit the complications and optimize the performance of pulse oximetry.

Signal Averaging

Signal averaging is the process of averaging instantaneous values over a given interval, usually in seconds. The technique of signal averaging can reduce artifactual fluctuations in Spo_2, but an unintended effect is that the display of real changes in Spo_2 is blunted.[48] Particularly in apnea of prematurity, but also in adult sleep apnea, episodes of hyperventilation often follow each apnea, leading to acute resaturation/desaturation epochs. The result is that long signal averaging times during assessment of desaturation events can lead to underestimating the number of events by up to 60% when compared to a control.[48] The signal-averaging interval should be adjusted by the user to minimize nuisance alarms while maintaining the desired sensitivity to changes in Spo_2.

Signal Quality

Assessment of the quality of the signal is paramount to interpretation of the data. Poor signal quality occurs when the arterial pulsations are small compared to the background of physiologic components and nonphysiologic noise. These may be the result of vasoconstriction, venous congestion, low blood pressure, and/or high noise levels, which would include motion, ambient light, electrical interference, or other factors.[48–53]

The pulse oximeter estimates how much of the hemoglobin in arterial blood is saturated with oxygen, but it does not directly indicate how much oxygen is contained in the arterial blood. Because almost all the oxygen carried in the blood is bound to hemoglobin, a reduction in the concentration of hemoglobin in the blood (anemia) will reduce the oxygen content just as decreased saturation does. It must be emphasized that knowing the Spo_2 does not provide information about oxygen delivery to tissue, which is the product of arterial oxygen content (Cao_2) and cardiac output; that is, the pulse oximeter does not indicate whether an adequate amount of oxygen is reaching the vital organs or other tissues.

Summary

Blood gas analysis and interpretation is a complex and clinically important endeavor. The respiratory care clinician must understand the various methods to obtain a blood gas sample and be aware of potential complications of arterial punctures and errors associated with sample analysis. Proper labeling, steady-state assurance, air bubble–free samples, sample cooling, coagulation prevention, and attention to quality assurance and quality control procedures will help ensure that the results of analysis are accurate and reliable.

Arterial blood gas interpretation requires assessment of factors that affect oxygenation, ventilation, and acid-base balance. Assessment must consider the patient's history, prior blood gas studies, and clinical condition. Conventional classifications of blood gas study results have limitations, and there are limits to both respiratory and metabolic compensation for acid-base disorders. Ventilatory disorders may be best described using terms such as ventilatory failure and alveolar hyperventilation. Understanding the assessment and treatment of metabolic acid-base disorders is essential, because these disorders are frequently encountered in the acute care setting.

Finally, noninvasive technology can enable clinicians to collect objective data on patients with the minimum risk. Risks include misinterpretation of the values and misunderstanding the limitations of the technology.

Key Points

▶ Indications for blood gas and pH analysis include, but are not limited to, the need for further evaluation of a patient's ventilatory, acid-base, and/or oxygenation status.

▶ The radial artery is often the site of choice for arterial blood gas punctures.

▶ Brachial and femoral arteries may be utilized for obtaining blood gas samples; however, these sites have certain risks and may be more difficult to access.

▶ Arterialized capillary sampling is a method to obtain blood gas values from neonates. The values are clinically important, but Po_2 values do not accurately reflect the actual arterial Po_2.

▶ The modified Allen test is commonly used to assess collateral circulation prior to a radial artery puncture. Despite widespread use, little data exist as to its reliability.

▶ The main indications for arterial cannulation are the need for frequent blood gas samples and continuous blood pressure monitoring.

▶ The technique for inserting indwelling radial artery catheter often includes the use of a guide wire.

▶ Arterial cannulation may be helpful but is not without risks. It is important to understand that ischemic damage, pseudoaneurysm, and infection

- are very serious risks associated with arterial line placement.

▶ Central venous and mixed venous blood gases may offer valuable information regarding oxygen extraction and consumption.

▶ Preanalytic issues must be considered during blood gas analysis. Labeling, steady state, and uncontaminated samples are key to ensuring proper values that will be interpreted.

▶ Clinical interpretation of blood gases is best done systematically and requires knowledge of respiratory physiology and clinical application.

▶ The normal values for blood gases are:
  - pH: 7.35 to 7.45
  - Pa_{CO_2}: 35 to 45 mm Hg
  - HCO_3^-: 22 to 28 mEq/L
  - Pa_{O_2}: 80 to 100 mm Hg (adults < 60 years)
  - Base excess (BE): −2 to +2

▶ The body attempts to regulate pH through compensation. The kidneys normally regulate HCO_3^-, and the lungs normally maintain Pa_{CO_2}.

▶ The Henderson-Hasselbalch equation describes the relationship among pH, Pa_{CO_2}, and HCO_3^- and can be used to calculate bicarbonate if two of the values are known.

▶ Respiratory acidosis is a condition that describes an increase in Pa_{CO_2}.

▶ Respiratory alkalosis is a condition that describes a decrease in Pa_{CO_2}.

▶ Estimating the expected maximal renal compensation for a respiratory acid-base disorder can be helpful in assessing the patient's response.

▶ Metabolic acidosis is a condition that describes a decrease in HCO_3^- concentration in the plasma.

▶ A metabolic acidosis can be caused by severe tissue hypoxia (lactic acidosis), accumulation of ketones (ketoacidosis), renal failure, ingestion of acids, and GI tract loss of base.

▶ The cause of a metabolic acidosis sometimes can be identified by calculation of the anion gap.

▶ Metabolic alkalosis is a condition that describes an increase in HCO_3^- concentration in the plasma.

▶ A metabolic alkalosis can be caused by loss of stomach acid (vomiting or NG tube suction), loss of bicarbonate in the urine (diuretics), hypochloremia (decrease in Cl^-), hypokalemia (decrease in K^+), and ingestion or administration of base ($NaHCO_3$, other).

▶ Estimating the expected maximal respiratory compensation for a metabolic acid-base disorder can be helpful in assessing the patient's response.

▶ The terms acute ventilatory failure, chronic ventilatory failure, and acute ventilatory failure superimposed on chronic ventilatory failure are useful clinical terms to describe various states of hypercapnea (i.e., elevated Pa_{CO_2}).

▶ The terms acute alveolar hyperventilation and chronic alveolar hyperventilation are very useful clinical terms to describe various state of hypocapnea (i.e., decreased Pa_{CO_2}).

▶ The treatment of these acid-base imbalances typically involves correction of the underlying condition.

▶ Pulse oximetry is a noninvasive method of estimating arterial oxygen saturation.

▶ Although pulse oximetry aids in determining hemoglobin saturation, it does not provide information regarding oxygen delivery to the tissues.

References

1. Clinical Laboratory Standards Institute (CLSI). *Blood Gas and pH Analysis and Related Measurements; Approved Guideline*, 2nd ed. Vol. C46-A2. Wayne, PA: CLSI; 2009.

2. Criner GJ, Barnette, RE, D'Alonzo GE (Eds.). *Critical Care Study Guide: Text and Review*, 2nd ed. New York: Springer; 2010.

3. AARC clinical practice guideline. In-vitro pH and blood gas analysis and hemoximetry. American Association for Respiratory Care. *Respir Care*. 1993;38(5):505–510.

4. Clinical Laboratory Standards Institute (CLSI). *Procedures for the Collection of Arterial Blood Specimens; Approved Standard*, 4th ed. Vol. H11-A4. Wayne, PA: CLSI; 2004.

5. Breen PH. Arterial blood gas and pH analysis. Clinical approach and interpretation. *Anesthesiol Clin North America*. 2001;19(4):885–906.

6. Shapiro BA, Peruzzi WT, Kozelowski-Templin R. *Clinical Application of Blood Gases*, 5th ed. St. Louis, MO: Mosby; 1994.

7. Chuang ML, Lin IF, Vintch JR, Ho BS, Chao SW, Ker JJ. Significant exercise-induced hypoxaemia with equivocal desaturation in patients with chronic obstructive pulmonary disease. *Intern Med J*. 2006;36(5):294–301.

8. Lynch F. Arterial blood gas analysis: Implications for nursing. *Paediatr Nurs*. 2009;21(1):41–44.

9. Dev SP, Hillmer MD, Ferri M. Videos in clinical medicine. Arterial puncture for blood gas analysis. *N Eng J Med*. 2011;364(5):e7.

10. Okeson GC, Wulbrecht PH. The safety of brachial artery puncture for arterial blood sampling. *Chest*. 1998;114(3):748–751.

11. Brzezinski M, Luisetti T, London MJ. Radial artery cannulation: A comprehensive review of recent anatomic and physiologic investigations. *Anesth Analg*. 2009;109(6):1763–1781.

12. Barone JE, Madlinger RV. Should an Allen test be performed before radial artery cannulation? *J Trauma*. 2006;61(2):468–470.

13. AARC clinical practice guideline. Capillary blood gas sampling for neonatal and pediatric patients. American Association for Respiratory Care. *Respir Care*. 1994;39(12):1180–1183.

14. Scheer B, Perel A, Pfeiffer UJ. Clinical review: Complications and risk factors of peripheral arterial catheters used for haemodynamic monitoring in anaesthesia and intensive care medicine. *Crit Care*. 2002;6(3):199–204.

15. Maki DG, Kluger DM, Crnich CJ. The risk of bloodstream infection in adults with different intravascular devices: a systematic review of 200 published prospective studies. *Mayo Clin Proc*. 2006;81(9):1159–1171.

16. Clermont G, Theodore AC. Arterial cathererization techniques for invasive monitoring. In: UpToDate, JF Edit, JL Mills (eds.). UpToDate, Waltham, MA. (Accessed February 16, 2013).

17. Blasco V, Leone M, Textoris J, Visintini P, Albanese J, Martin C. [Venous oximetry: physiology and therapeutic implications]. *Ann Fr Anesth Reanim*. 2008;27(1):74–82.

18. Walkey AJ, Farber HW, O'Donnell C, Cabral H, Eagan JS, Philippides GJ. The accuracy of the central venous blood gas for acid-base monitoring. *J Intensive Care Med*. 2010;25(2):104–110.

19. Christensen M. Mixed venous oxygen saturation monitoring revisited: Thoughts for critical care nursing practice. *Aust Crit Care*. 2012;25(2):78–90.

20. van Beest PA, van Ingen J, Boerma EC, et al. No agreement of mixed venous and central venous saturation in sepsis, independent of sepsis origin. *Crit Care.* 2010;14(6):R219.

21. Jalonen J. Invasive haemodynamic monitoring: Concepts and practical approaches. *Ann Med.* 1997;29(4):313–318.

22. Weinhouse GL. Pulmonary artery catherization. In: UpToDate, Parsons PE (ed.), UpToDate, Waltham, MA, 2013.

23. Theodore AC. Arterial blood gases. In: UpToDate, Basow DS (ed.), UpToDate, Waltham, MA, 2013.

24. Hansen JE, Sue DY. Should blood gas measurement be corrected for the patient's temperature? *N Eng J Med.* 1980;303(6):341.

25. Emmett M. Simple and mixed acid-base disorders. In: UpToDate, Basow DS, (ed.), UpToDate, Waltham, MA, 2013.

26. Berend K, Engels R. Analysis of acid-base disorders in patients with chronic respiratory failure. *Respir Care.* 2011;56(3):367–368; author reply 368.

27. Haber RJ. A practical approach to acid-base disorders. *West J Med.* 1991;155(2):146–151.

28. Peters JA, Hodgkin JE, Collier CR. Blood gas analysis and acid-base physiology. In: Burton GG, Hodgkin JE, Ward JJ, (eds.). *Respiratory Care: A Guide to Clinical Practice.* 3rd ed. Philadelphia: J. B. Lippincott Company; 1991: 181–209.

29. Post TW, Rose BD. Approach to the adult with metabolic acidosis. In: UpToDate, Basow DS, (ed.), UpToDate, Waltham, MA, 2013.

30. Endom EE, Perry H. Inhalant abuse in children and adolescents. In: UpToDate, Basow DS (ed.), UpToDate, Waltham, MA, 2013.

31. Rose BD. Pathogenesis and treatment of metabolic acidosis in chronic kidney disease. In: UpToDate, Basow DS (ed.), UpToDate, Waltham, MA, 2013.

32. Emmett M. Etiology and diagnosis of distal (type 1) and proximal (type 2) renal tubular acidosis. In: UpToDate, Basow DS (ed.), UpToDate, Waltham, MA, 2013.

33. Emmett M. Pathophysiology of renal tubular acidosis and the effect on potassium balance. In: UpToDate, Basow DS (ed.), UpToDate, Waltham, MA, 2013.

34. Seres D. Nutrition support in critically ill patients: An overview. In: UpToDate, Basow DS (ed.), UpToDate, Waltham, MA, 2013.

35. Stralovich-Romani A, Mahutte CK, Matthay MA, Luce JM. Administrative, nutritional, and ethical principles for the management of critically ill patients. In: George RB, Light RW, Matthay MA, Matthay RA (eds.). *Chest Medicine: Essentials of Pulmonary and Critical Care Medicine*, 4th ed. Philadelphia: Lippincott Williams & Wilkins; 2000: 517–538.

36. Kushner RF. Total parenteral nutrition-associated metabolic acidosis. *JPEN J Parenter Enteral Nutr.* 1986:10(3):306–310.

37. Wiederkehr M, Emmett M. Bicarbonate therapy in lactic acidosis. In: UpToDate, Basow DS (ed.), UpToDate, Waltham, MA, 2013.

38. Lexi-Comp, Inc. Sodium bicarbonate: Drug information. In: UpToDate, Basow DS (ed.), UpToDate, Waltham, MA, 2013.

39. Emmet M. Causes of metabolic alkalosis. In: UpToDate, Basow DS (ed.), UpToDate, Waltham, MA, 2013.

40. Mehta A, Emmett M. Treatment of metabolic alkalosis. In: UpToDate, Basow DS (ed.), UpToDate, Waltham, MA, 2013.

41. Agus ASA. The milk-alkali syndrome. In: UpToDate, Goldfarb S, Forman JP (eds.), UpToDate, Waltham, MA, 2013.

42. AARC (American Association for Respiratory Care) clinical practice guideline. Pulse oximetry. *Respir Care.* 1991;36(12):1406–1409.

43. Weaver LK, Churchill SK, Deru K, Cooney D. False positve rate of carbon monoxide saturation by pulse oximetry of emergency department patients. *Respir Care.* 2013;58(2):232–240.

44. Thilo EH, Andersen D, Wasserstein ML, Schmidt J, Luckey D. Saturation by pulse oximetry: Comparison of the results obtained by instruments of different brands. *J Pediatr.* 1993;122(4):620–626.

45. Monitoring your adult patient with bedside pulse oximetry. *Nursing.* 2008;38(9):42–44.

46. Farber NE, McNeely J, Rosner D. Skin burn associated with pulse oximetry during perioperative photodynamic therapy. *Anesthesiology.* 1996;84(4):983–985.

47. Barker SJ, Tremper KK. Pulse oximetry: Applications and limitations. *Int Anesthesiol Clin.* 1987;25(3):155–175.

48. Severinghaus JW, Kelleher JF. Recent developments in pulse oximetry. *Anesthesiology.* 1992;76(6):1018–1038.

49. Wilkins MC. Residual bacterial contamination on reusable pulse oximetry sensors. *Respir Care.* 1993;38(11):1155–1160.

50. Brouillette RT, Lavergne J, Leimanis A, Nixon GM, Ladan S, McGregor CD. Differences in pulse oximetry technology can affect detection of sleep-disorderd breathing in children. *Anesthes Analg.* 2002;94(1 Suppl):S47–S53.

51. Webb RK, Ralston AC, Runciman WB. Potential errors in pulse oximetry. II. Effects of changes in saturation and signal quality. *Anaesthesia.* 1991;46(3):207–212.

52. Shamir M, Eidelman LA, Floman Y, Kaplan L, Pizov R. Pulse oximetry plethysmographic waveform during changes in blood volume. *Br J Anaesth.* 1999;82(2):178–181.

53. Urschitz MS, Von EV, Seyfang A, Poets CF. Use of pulse oximetry in automated oxygen delivery to ventilated infants. *Anesth Analg.* 2002;94(1 Suppl):S37–S40.

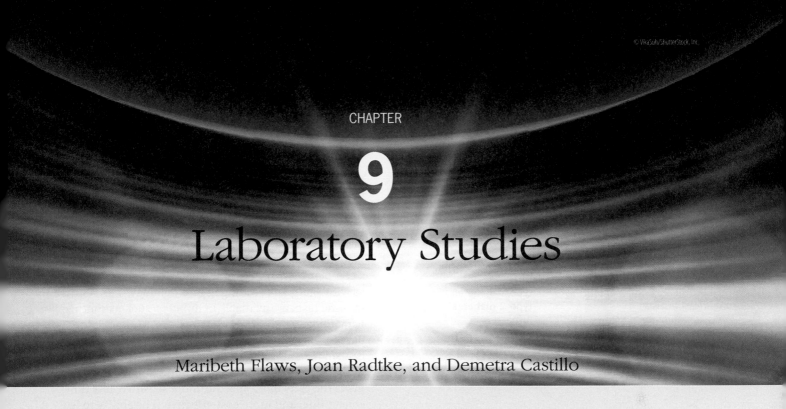

CHAPTER

9

Laboratory Studies

Maribeth Flaws, Joan Radtke, and Demetra Castillo

CHAPTER OUTLINE

Introduction to the Diagnostic Laboratory
Hematology
Clinical Chemistry
Microbiology
Skin Testing
Histology and Cytology
Molecular Diagnostics
Summary

CHAPTER OBJECTIVES

1. List the components of the blood that are measured in a complete blood count (CBC) and explain the function of each.
2. Discuss the relationship of red blood cell (RBC) count, hemoglobin, and hematocrit to each other and to the analysis of RBCs.
3. List the causes of anemia.
4. Classify anemias given the MCV, MCHC, and RDW.
5. List and describe the function of the five types of leukocytes.
6. Describe the tests that are used to assess platelets and coagulation function.
7. List the major analytes measured in a clinical chemistry laboratory.
8. Discuss the laboratory tests that are used in the diagnosis and monitoring of patients with diabetes mellitus to include fasting glucose and hemoglobin A_{1C}.
9. Describe the laboratory tests that are used to assess renal function.
10. Describe the tests that are used to assess risk of cardiovascular disease.
11. Explain the utility of troponin in assessing patients with suspected myocardial infarction.
12. Name the electrolytes that are measured in a routine metabolic panel and list normal values and causes of abnormal values.
13. Describe the most common microorganisms that cause pneumonia and other lower respiratory tract infections.

14. Describe the proper collection of an expectorated sputum sample and determine whether the specimen is representative of the lower respiratory tract.
15. State the type of sputum smear that would be used for a particular group of microorganisms.
16. List the types of analyses that are performed in a urinalysis and interpret the results.
17. Name the respiratory tract pathogens that can be identified by laboratory tests performed on urine.
18. Describe the two types of immune responses that are measured in skin testing and identify the target of each response.
19. Interpret purified protein derivative results on a patient along with patient history to determine if a patient has been exposed to *Mycobacterium tuberculosis*.
20. State the type of disease that is diagnosed and characterized as the major application of histology and cytology.
21. Describe the purpose of and steps involved in the polymerase chain reaction (PCR).
22. Define *viral load* and describe how it is determined in the laboratory.
23. Name the viruses that can cause respiratory tract infections.
24. Discuss the laboratory detection of respiratory viruses in terms of the appropriate specimen to collect and most common methodology.

KEY TERMS

activated partial
  thromboplastin time
  (aPTT)
albumin
basophils
bilirubin
blood urea nitrogen (BUN)
complete blood count (CBC)
coagulation
creatinine
creatinine clearance (CrCl)

diabetes mellitus
delayed-type
  hypersensitivity (DTH)
eosinophils
erythrocytes
false-negative
false-positive
gestational diabetes
  mellitus (GDM)
glomerular filtration rate
  (eGFR)

© VikaSuh/ShutterStock, Inc.

hematocrit (HCT)
hemoglobin (Hb)
hemoglobin A$_{1c}$
hemolysis
hemostasis
immediate hypersensitivity
interferon-gamma-release
 assays (IGRA)
leukemia
leukocytes
lymphocytes
macrocytic
mean cell (or corpuscular)
 volume (MCV)
mean cell (or corpuscular)
 hemoglobin (MCH)
mean cell (or corpuscular)
 hemoglobin content
 (MCHC)
mean platelet volume (MPV)
microalbumin
microcytic
monocytes
normochromic

normocytic
oral glucose tolerance test
 (OGTT)
platelets
polymerase chain reaction
 (PCR)
polymorphonuclear
 neutrophil (PMN,
 segmented neutrophil,
 Seg)
prothrombin time (PT)
RBC count
red blood cell distribution
 width (RDW)
thrombocytes
thrombocytopenia
thrombocytosis
type 1 diabetes
type 2 diabetes
urinalysis
viral load
white blood cells (WBCs)
WBC count
WBC differential

Overview

This chapter describes tests that are performed in a diagnostic laboratory and are used to diagnose, monitor, and make treatment decisions on patients. Although laboratory testing is more diverse than what is described in this chapter, the laboratory tests that are described herein were chosen based on their relevance to the practicing respiratory care clinician. The discussion will focus on tests performed in hematology, clinical chemistry, and microbiology laboratories. A brief description of each test and its utility will be provided, together with some causes and effects of abnormal results. Although reference ranges are given for some analytes, it is important to note that reference ranges vary greatly from laboratory to laboratory based on patient populations and the methodology used to measure the analyte. Thus, reference ranges are only given as a general guide, not as absolutes. All healthcare professionals are encouraged to consult the scientists in the diagnostic laboratory when there are questions about acceptable specimen types for tests, the methodology of a test, as well as the interpretation of laboratory test results.

Introduction to the Diagnostic Laboratory

The diagnostic laboratory plays an essential role in the assessment of the cardiopulmonary patient. Often seen as the unsung heroes, scientists in the laboratory are responsible for performing complex tests, interpreting results, reporting those results in a timely manner, and ensuring quality throughout the process in order for healthcare providers to make sound judgments regarding the diagnosis, treatment, and monitoring of

their patients. Medical laboratory scientists are highly qualified individuals who maintain national certification and hold advanced degrees in medical laboratory science. The respiratory care clinician should consider these laboratory personnel a part of the interprofessional patient care team.

The diagnostic laboratory conducts many different tests in a variety of disciplines. Hematology, chemistry, and microbiology will be discussed in this chapter, but tests in immunohematology, also known as blood banking, and immunology also are performed in the diagnostic laboratory. Laboratory tests may be automated, with many different tests being performed on a complex instrument, or they may be manual, such as with agar plate reading in microbiology. The results of some tests are available in minutes, such as routine hematology or chemistry tests, whereas others take days to weeks, such as when the growth of a microorganism is required in order to identify it. Technology in the diagnostic laboratory is continually changing to make the tests more specific, more sensitive, less time consuming, and more cost-effective. The ability to isolate, amplify, and characterize nucleic acids has driven much of the change in the diagnostic laboratory over the last 10 years, improving the diagnosis of viral infections, characterization of tumor cells, and identification of inherited diseases. This chapter will discuss some of the tests that are performed in the diagnostic laboratory, with an emphasis on those that are most relevant to the cardiopulmonary patient.

Hematology

Blood is involved in the transport of many vital components that are essential for life. The blood has two main compartments: the cellular portion and the liquid portion. The cellular portion of the blood consists of cells that are responsible for transporting oxygen to the tissues (**erythrocytes**), cells that fight infection (**leukocytes**), and cells involved in tissue repair (**thrombocytes**). The liquid portion of the blood is responsible for transporting proteins that are essential in maintaining cells and organs and tissue repair. The main screening test used to assess the cellular constituents of the blood is the complete blood count (CBC). Hematologic tests that focus on assessing the functionality of proteins responsible for tissue repair (coagulation) include the **prothrombin time (PT)** and **activated partial thromboplastin time (aPTT)**. A PT test may also be called an INR test. INR (international normalized ratio) stands for a way of standardizing the results of prothrombin time tests, no matter the testing method.

In order to ensure quality results, specimen collection must occur with minimum damage to the cellular constituents of the blood. Red blood cell destruction (**hemolysis**) due to improper specimen collection can compromise specimen integrity and lead to inaccurate test results, which can impact the care and treatment of the patient.

Complete Blood Count

The **complete blood count (CBC)** is the major screening test used to evaluate the quantity and quality of the cellular constituents of the blood: that is, erythrocytes (**red blood cells [RBCs]**), leukocytes (**white blood cells [WBCs]**), and thrombocytes (**platelets**). Information is obtained about the appearance and distribution of the red blood cells in relation to other plasma components and other blood cells. CBCs are performed on complex instruments that rely on multiple methodologies and calculations to produce clinically relevant information. Tests used to assess erythrocyte distribution and functionality are: **red blood cell (RBC) count, hemoglobin (Hb), hematocrit (HCT), mean cell volume (MCV), mean cell hemoglobin (MCH), mean cell hemoglobin content (MCHC)**, and **red blood cell distribution width (RDW)**. Each test assesses a different component of the red blood cell. Although each single test (e.g., RBC count) carries significant information, the entire panel can provide a more complete diagnostic picture. For leukocytes, the CBC is a report of the absolute and relative numbers of total WBCs, as well as the numbers of each type of WBC. Thrombocytes or platelets are enumerated in the CBC and assessed for their size and morphology.[1]

Red Blood Cell Parameters

The RBC count enumerates the amount of RBCs in a blood specimen (in million cells per microliter ($\times 10^6/\mu L$). RBCs are described in terms of their size, shape, and hemoglobin content. Normal RBCs are non-nucleated biconcave discs that stain pink with Romanowsky-type stains. They range from 6 to 8 microns in diameter and show a faint central pallor (see **Figure 9-1**). Normal RBCs can be classified as **normocytic, normochromic**,

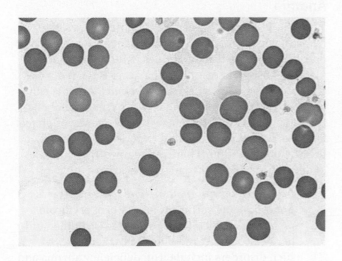

FIGURE 9-1 Normal red blood cells.

but it is important to mention that a classification of normocytic normochromic can also be applied to anemias, as discussed below. Classifying the relative color and size of an erythrocyte is designated through the different classification systems, as follows:

- Normocytic, normochromic
- Microcytic, hypochromic
- Macrocytic (usually normochromic)

To classify a RBC as *normocytic, normochromic*, the RBC will be about the same size as the nucleus of a lymphocyte and the central pallor will be less than half the diameter of the red blood cell. A **microcytic** *hypochromic* RBC will be smaller than the nucleus of a lymphocyte with a central pallor that is more than half the diameter of the red blood cell. Finally, a **macrocytic** RBC will be larger than the nucleus of a lymphocyte and typically normochromic.[2]

Hemoglobin and Hematocrit

Hemoglobin is the protein found inside red blood cells that is responsible for oxygen transport to the tissues. The hemoglobin (Hb) test measures the quantity (in grams per deciliter [g/dL]) of hemoglobin inside the red blood cells. The hematocrit (HCT) is the percentage of the blood that is composed of red blood cells. This is different from the RBC count in that it is a reflection of the total blood volume rather than the actual quantity of cells in a blood sample. These three parameters (RBC, Hb, and HCT) are directly measured by the analyzer, and the results of the rest of the tests are derived from these parameters. Consequently, the RBC, Hb, and HCT are most sensitive to quantitative changes in red blood cells, such as acute blood loss or polycythemia (see **Table 9-1**).[3]

Hemoglobin Measurement

The quantity of Hb is measured by most analyzers through spectrophotometry. Because Hb is found inside RBCs, the first step in its measurement requires lysing the RBCs to release the Hb into solution. Whole blood is mixed with a lysing reagent, and the turbidity of the lysate is measured in a spectrophotometer at 540 nm. The amount of turbidity in the sample is directly related to the concentration of Hb. Because whole blood is used, highly colored plasma can interfere and cause falsely elevated Hb results. The three main causes of highly colored plasma are icteria (brown-green color), due to excessive bilirubin in the sample; lipemia (milky-white color), due to excessive chylomicrons in the sample; and hemolysis (red-pink color), due to excessive RBC destruction in the sample. Inaccuracies in Hb measurement cause inaccuracies in the derived indices as well (e.g., elevated MCH and MCHC). Corrective measures are performed by the laboratory professional to correct

TABLE 9-1
Clinical Relevance of RBC Count, Hemoglobin, and Hematocrit

Test	Definition	Units	Clinical Significance	Reference Range	Correlated to
RBC count	Number of red blood cells in a sample	millions/μL ($\times 10^6$/μL)	Low numbers: anemic patients; blood loss High numbers: polycythemic patients	Males: 4.8–6.2×10^6/μL Females: 4.4–6.2×10^6/μL	Hb and HCT (Rule of 3) MCV and MCH (derived from RBC count)
Hemoglobin (Hb)	Amount of oxygen-carrying protein in the blood	g/dL	Low numbers: anemic patients; blood loss High numbers: polycythemic patients or infants	Males: 14–16 g/dL Females: 13–15 g/dL	RBC count and HCT (Rule of 3) MCH and MCHC (derived from Hb)
Hematocrit (HCT)	Percentage of blood that is composed of red blood cells	%	Low numbers: anemic patients; blood loss High numbers: polycythemic patients or infants	Males: 40–50% Females: 37–47%	RBC count and Hb (Rule of 3) MCV and MCHC (derived from HCT)

RBC, red blood cell; MCV, mean corpuscular volume; MCH, mean corpuscular hemoglobin; MCHC, mean corpuscular hemoglobin concentration.

for falsely elevated Hb results and thereby provide reliable results to the healthcare provider.

Hematocrit and Other Indices

The HCT is the percentage of the total blood volume that is composed of RBCs. This provides valuable information to the healthcare provider about the overall composition of the blood. As a general rule of thumb, the HCT is roughly three times the Hb measurement. For example: a HCT of 45% will correspond to Hb of approximately 15 g/dL ($15 \times 3 = 45\%$).

The rest of the parameters are collectively termed "indices" because they are a reflection of the relationship between the RBC count, Hb, and HCT. Examples include mean corpuscular volume (MCV), mean corpuscular hemoglobin (MCH), mean corpuscular hemoglobin content (MCHC), and red blood cell distribution width (RDW). Because of the relationship between RBC, Hb, HCT, and these indices, results should not deviate greatly from day to day. CBCs are a routine component of a patient workup and are heavily employed as a means of monitoring treatment effectiveness, so it is common to see daily CBCs on many different types of patients. If there is a deviation in these indices of ± 3 units, it may indicate an error in patient identification. Each parameter provides information about the size of the RBC (MCV), the weight of Hb inside the RBC (MCH), and the percentage of Hb in the RBC (MCHC). The calculations for these indices are provided in Table 9-2. These provide better correlation to clinical conditions than measuring the RBC count, Hb, and HCT alone. Another

index that can provide valuable information about the amount of variation in the RBC population is the red blood cell distribution width (RDW). There is approximately less than 12% variation in RBCs in healthy individuals. The RDW is most sensitive to recent transfusion or maintenance of blood volume through supportive therapies such as erythropoietin (EPO). Transfusion can cause deviations in the indices, but it will also cause significant changes in the RDW value as well. Employing the RDW along with the indices can help provide a differential to erroneous deviation as a result of therapeutic interventions.[4]

Anemia

The CBC is a robust screening tool used to evaluate hematologic disorders. These disorders can range from one cell line to all three cell lines (RBC, WBC, and platelet). Disorders resulting in a decrease in red blood cells or hemoglobin are termed *anemias*. Anemia can reduce oxygen delivery and adversely affect metabolic function. As a result, patients who are anemic often feel fatigued, have skin pallor, and experience shortness of breath upon exertion. There are many different causes of anemia, but the four main causes are:

- *Insufficient erythropoiesis:* The bone marrow is not producing sufficient numbers of erythroid precursors, which leads to a decrease in the number of circulating red blood cells. Examples of such disorders include iron deficiency anemia and bone marrow failure.

TABLE 9-2
Clinical Relevance of Indices

Test	Definition	Units	Reference Range	Clinical Significance	Derived from
Mean cell volume (MCV)	Numerical value describing RBC size	Femtoliters (fL)	80–100 fL	Low numbers: IDA or thalassemia High numbers: megaloblastic or pernicious anemia	RBC count Hematocrit Calculation: (HCT/RBC) × 10
Mean cell hemoglobin (MCH)	Numerical value describing weight of hemoglobin in RBC count	Picograms (pg)	27–31 pg	Low numbers: IDA or thalassemia High numbers: megaloblastic or pernicious anemia	RBC count Hemoglobin Calculation: (Hb/RBC) × 10
Mean cell hemoglobin content (MCHC)	Percentage of RBC count that is hemoglobin	% or g/dL	32–36%	Low numbers: IDA or thalassemia	Hemoglobin Hematocrit Calculation: (Hb/HCT) × 100
Red blood cell distribution width (RDW)	Amount of variation in the red blood cell population	%	< 12%	High numbers: Mostly indicative of recent transfusion or supportive therapy for severe anemia	Coefficient of variation of red blood cells

RBC, red blood cell; IDA, iron deficiency anemia.

- *Ineffective erythropoiesis:* The bone marrow has the capability to produce sufficient numbers of circulating red blood cells, but the resulting cells are defective. Examples of such disorders include hemoglobinopathies, thalassemias, and megaloblastic anemia.
- *Increased destruction of RBCs:* The bone marrow produces sufficient numbers of circulating red blood cells, but the cells are destroyed by intrinsic or extrinsic defect mechanisms. Examples of such disorders include hemolytic anemia, *Plasmodium* infection (e.g., malaria) and autoimmune destruction.
- *Chronic blood loss:* The body loses blood chronically and the bone marrow cannot compensate effectively for the loss. Examples of such disorders include trauma, surgery, menorrhagia, and chronic gastrointestinal bleeding.

Anemia can be classified morphologically by using the MCV and the MCHC, with the RDW providing a differential diagnosis between anemias that are classified similarly. When the MCV and the MCHC are within their respective reference ranges, the classification of anemia is termed normocytic, normochromic. When the MCV and MCHC values are below the reference interval, the classification is termed microcytic, hypochromic. Lastly, when the MCV is above the reference interval, the classification is termed macrocytic.

Macrocytic anemias are typically normochromic. Higher-than-normal MCHCs are not associated with anemias, and instead often indicate the presence of spherocytes in a patient sample or a problem with specimen integrity (see **Table 9-3**).

TABLE 9-3
Morphologic Classification System of Anemias

Classification System	Parameter Results	Clinical Correlation
Normocytic, normochromic	MCV: 80–100 fL MCHC: 32–36%	Normal Hemolytic anemia Aplastic anemia Hemoglobinopathies Renal disease Infectious RBC conditions
Microcytic, hypochromic	MCV < 80 fL MCHC < 32%	Iron deficiency anemia Thalassemia
Macrocytic (normochromic)	MCV > 100 fL	Megaloblastic anemia Pernicious anemia Liver disease Alcoholism

MCV, mean corpuscular volume; MCHC, mean corpuscular hemoglobin concentration; RBC, red blood cell.

TABLE 9-4
Morphologic Description of Circulating Leukocytes

Cell Type	Nuclear shape	Chromatin	Cytoplasm	Cellular Texture
Neutrophil	Lobed (3–5 lobes)	Condensed; pronounced heterochromatin	Granular with light dusting of pink	Grainy cytoplasm; smooth nucleus
Lymphocyte	Round; takes up most of the cytoplasm	Condensed; pronounced heterochromatin	Scanty; agranular and basophilic	Smooth, glossy appearance
Monocyte	Free-form	Open chromatin pattern; may have nucleoli	Grainy with pink granules; amoeboid cytoplasm	Has a rough appearance like a sponge or crushed glass
Eosinophil	Lobed (2–3 lobes)	Condensed; pronounced heterochromatin	Large, refractile prominent pink-orange granules	Granular cytoplasm; smooth nucleus
Basophil	Lobed (speculated)	Cannot be described	Large purple-black granules	Abundant granules that obscure nucleus

Morphology is another key assessment tool in identifying anemic conditions. To provide a more thorough understanding of the pathology of anemic conditions, the ultrastructure of the cells is closely examined for changes in appearance. These changes are much more prominent in RBCs than in other cells. Assessment of morphology is performed through peripheral blood smear evaluation. A drop of blood is placed on a slide, spread with another slide, stained typically with a Wright-Giemsa stain, and reviewed. Table 9-3 illustrates the broadness of the classification of anemias, but it is a starting point, because peripheral blood review can provide a differential for these conditions. For example, a hemolytic anemia, whether it has an immune or nonimmune cause, will display schistocytes (RBC fragments) on the peripheral blood smear. In some instances, the peripheral blood smear is considered diagnostic. For example, sickle cell disease, a type of hemoglobinopathy, is the only condition in which sickle-shaped cells (called drepanocytes) are observed on the peripheral blood smear. The presence of drepanocytes is thus pathognomonic for sickle cell disease.[3]

White Blood Cell Parameters

The assessment of white blood cells (WBCs) involves enumerating their amount in the blood (**WBC count**) and determining their identity (e.g., lymphocytes versus monocytes) by conducting a peripheral blood examination (known as a **WBC differential**). WBCs, or leukocytes, are the cells that are responsible for maintaining immunity against infectious agents, such as bacteria, viruses, fungi, and parasites. A patient's immune system is a highly organized system where each cell carries out a specific function through a specific mechanism, so identifying the cell type is an indirect indicator of the type of infection that may be present. This can be important in early detection of infection and can

suggest appropriate therapy, because it takes several days to identify the causative agent of infection but only minutes to identify the defending cell. There are five types of leukocytes that normally circulate in peripheral blood. They are the **polymorphonuclear neutrophil (PMN), segmented neutrophil (Seg)**, lymphocyte (lymph), monocyte (mono), eosinophil (eos), and basophil (baso). Morphologic descriptions of these leukocytes are provided in **Table 9-4** and pictured in **Figures 9-2** through **9-6**.[5]

WBC percentages are expressed as relative percentages (e.g., lymph %) or absolute counts (e.g., lymph #). When a qualified medical laboratory scientist performs a differential, he or she counts 100 white blood cells and identifies them. The number obtained will be the relative percentage. This can identify singular increases in a particular cell line, but because they are relative to the other cells, it will falsely decrease the other cell lines. The absolute count takes the WBC count into consideration.

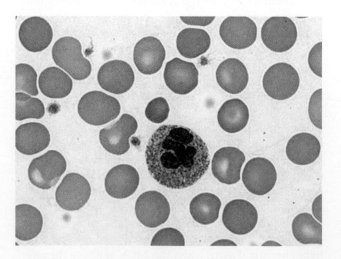

FIGURE 9-2 Segmented neutrophil.

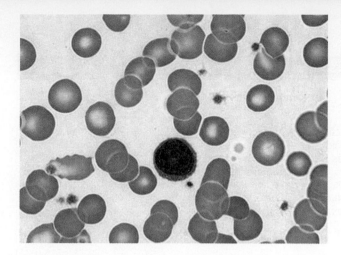

FIGURE 9-3 **Lymphocyte.**

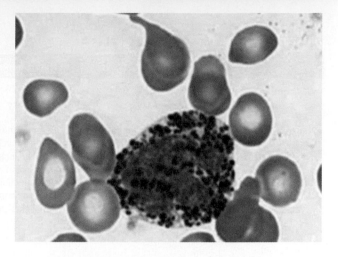

FIGURE 9-6 **Basophil.**

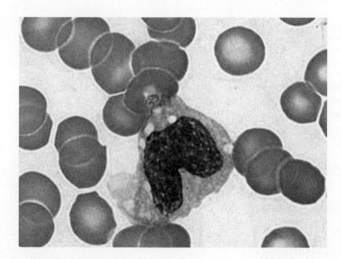

FIGURE 9-4 **Monocyte.**

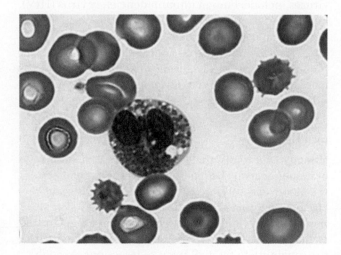

FIGURE 9-5 **Eosinophil.**

It is calculated by taking the percentage of the cell line and multiplying it by the WBC count. For example:

65% PMNs with a WBC count of $8.5 \times 10^3/\mu L$
$= 0.65 \times 8500 = 5525$ PMNs/μL

A normal WBC count is 4,500 to 10,000 WBCs per microliter of blood (abbreviated as μL or mcL). A low WBC count is *leukopenia,* whereas an elevated WBC count is *leukocytosis.* The absolute count is a much more reliable indicator of disease and is often utilized in treatment regimens to determine dosages of chemotherapeutic agents for the treatment of malignancies.

Leukemia

The WBC count and differential can also provide clinically relevant information in the workup of malignancies of the blood (see **Table 9-5**). Malignancies of the blood and bone marrow are termed *leukemias.* Malignancies can be classified as acute or chronic and further subclassified based on the cell type affected—myeloid or lymphoid. Malignancies of the blood are derived from changes in the bone marrow that spill over into the blood. The general pathology of **leukemia** involves excessive proliferation of precursors in the bone marrow that cause a "crowding out" effect on the normal constituents of the blood. Leukemic patients often present with signs of anemia (i.e., fatigue, skin pallor, or shortness of breath) due to lack of RBC production, susceptibility to infections due to the crowding out of normal blood leukocytes and increase in nonfunctional leukocytes, and sporadic bleeding and bruising due to lack of platelets. Morphology and identification of lineage-specific cells is key to identifying these disorders and to determining whether they are acute or chronic. In general, acute malignancies present with primarily immature cells and very few mature cells, whereas chronic malignancies have all stages of lineage-specific maturation present.[6]

TABLE 9-5
Clinical Relevance of White Blood Cells

Test	Used for	High Counts Seen in:	Low Counts Seen in:	Reference range
WBC count	Infections Malignancy	Infections Malignancy	Infections Malignancy	4–10 × 10³/µL
Neutrophil Terminology: neutrophilia (increase), neutropenia (decrease)	Bacterial infections	Bacterial infections Chronic myeloid malignancies	Bacterial infections Acute malignancies Lymphoid malignancies	50–70% of the total blood differential Abs #: 2000–7000/µL
Lymphocyte Terminology: lymphocytosis (increase), lymphocytopenia (decrease)	Viral infections	Viral infections Chronic lymphoid malignancies	Viral infections Acute malignancies Bacterial infections	20%–40% of the total blood differential Abs #: 800–4000/µL
Monocyte Terminology: monocytosis (increase), monocytopenia (decrease)	Tubercular infections Fungal infections	Tubercular or fungal infections Selected chronic myeloid premalignancies	Viral infections Bacterial infections Acute malignancies	2–10% of the total blood differential Abs #: 80–1000/µL
Eosinophil Terminology: eosinophilia (increase)	Allergic reactions Parasitic infections	Allergic reactions Parasitic infections Chronic eosinophilic malignancies	Bacterial infections Viral infections Tubercular infections Fungal infections	2–4% of the total blood differential Abs #: 80–400/µL
Basophil Terminology: basophilia (increase)	Allergic reactions	Allergic reactions Chronic myeloid malignancies	All infections Most malignancies	0–1% of the total blood differential Abs #: 0–10/µL

WBC, white blood cell; Abs #, absolute number.

Segmented Neutrophil

The segmented neutrophil (PMN; see Figure 9-2) accounts for roughly 50% to 70% of total blood differential and is responsible for fighting bacterial infections. Examples of bacteria include: *Staphylococcus aureus*, *Streptococcus pyogenes*, *Escherichia coli*, *Listeria monocytogenes*, and *Pseudomonas aeruginosa*. These organisms cause many different types of infections, ranging from skin and wound infections to intestinal, respiratory, blood, and urine infections. Neutrophils may exhibit quantitative and morphologic changes in the presence of bacteria. These changes include toxic granulation, in which the neutrophil contains primary basophilic granules in their cytoplasm; vacuolization, which may contain bacteria; and Dohle bodies, which are pockets of ribosomal RNA that appear faint blue in the cytoplasm. Quantitative changes include neutrophilia and a "left shift." Left shift is a term used to describe the presence of younger neutrophilic precursors in the blood. Neutrophilic precursors include band neutrophils, metamyelocytes, and myelocytes. Under normal circumstances, you may see up to 5% bands in circulation, but in the presence of bacteria that number will typically increase, and younger metamyelocytes and myelocytes may also be present. The term *neutrophilia* refers to an increased neutrophil count, whereas *neutropenia* refers to a decreased neutrophil count (see Table 9-5).

Lymphocytes

Approximately 20% to 40% of the differential is composed of **lymphocytes** (see Figure 9-3). These are the cells responsible for providing immunity against viral agents, as well as other microorganisms. Examples of viruses include: human immunodeficiency virus (HIV), hepatitis A virus, Epstein-Barr virus, cytomegalovirus, and coronavirus. Lymphocytes transform their appearance from a common to an activated morphology in the presence of viruses. The term *lymphocytosis* refers to an increased lymphocyte count; *lymphocytopenia* refers to a decreased lymphocyte count (Table 9-5).

Monocytes

Monocytes (monos) (see Figure 9-4) are derivations of mononuclear cells/macrophages that circulate in the blood. Macrophages are nonspecific cells that can circulate but that are also fixed in organs, body cavities, and body fluids. Monocytes account for 2% to 10% of the peripheral blood differential. Monocytes have the capability to fight all types of infections through phagocytosis and intracellular superoxide killing mechanisms, but elevations are predominantly seen in tuberculosis and fungal infections. The term *monocytosis* refers to an increased monocyte count; the term *monocytopenia* refers to a decreased monocyte count (see Table 9-5).

Eosinophils

Eosinophils (see Figure 9-5) are named as such because of their high affinity for the eosin component of the stain. This is reflective in the appearance of bright orange-pink refractile granules in their cytoplasm. Eosinophils account for 2% to 4% of the total blood differential and are responsible for eliciting responses against allergens and parasitic infections. The term *eosinophilia* refers to an increased eosinophil count (see Table 9-5).

Basophils

Basophils (see Figure 9-6) are the least prevalent of all the cell types, only accounting for up to 1% of the total blood differential. This is mainly because basophils undergo subsequent maturation into mast cells and are localized in the mucosal membranes and epithelial layers of the skin. Like eosinophils, basophils play a role in both parasitic infections and allergies. Basophils are highly granular, and often the granules obscure the nucleus, making it difficult to ascertain nuclear structure information. The granules contain histamine and heparin and are responsible for hypersensitivity reactions associated with contact with allergens. The term *basophilia* refers to an increased basophil count (see Table 9-5).

Platelet Parameters

Platelets, or thrombocytes, are small, anucleated, granular cells (see **Figure 9-7**) that are responsible for repairing tissue after injury. For the purposes of arresting bleeding after injury (**hemostasis**), platelets are involved in clot formation (coagulation). Coagulation is done through a series of biochemical interactions between platelets and clotting proteins. It is vital that these interactions only occur when there is a physiologic need. Deficiencies in platelets and/or clotting proteins can cause bleeding episodes; conversely, increases in platelet quantity or functionality or increased activation of clotting proteins can cause exacerbated thrombosis, or clot formation.[7] Inappropriate clot formation has been implicated in conditions such as myocardial infarction, transient ischemic attacks, pulmonary embolus, and deep vein thrombosis. Assessment of thrombocytes mainly involves determining the number of platelets in a sample and comparing it to a reference interval. Results below the reference interval are termed **thrombocytopenia** and above are termed **thrombocytosis**. Additional tools on the CBC that evaluate the appearance of the platelets are the **mean platelet volume (MPV)**, which measures the average size of the platelet and platelet morphology on the peripheral blood smear. Younger platelets usually appear a little larger than mature platelets.

It is important to note that although the CBC is primarily a screening test, it provides valuable information to the healthcare provider about the overall health of the patient and may lead to the need for follow-up tests based on the results of the CBC. Although the CBC focuses on the cellular constituents of the blood, changes in organ systems can affect these numbers, so it has become a widespread screening for the overall health of a patient. These cellular constituents are all produced in the bone marrow, so if abnormalities are detected in the CBC they could be an indirect indicator of bone marrow dysfunction. It is important that analysis of these results include direct comparison to bone marrow or other organ systems.

Coagulation Studies

Coagulation is the process by which the body elicits repair after trauma. It is a complex biochemical process involving platelets and activatable clotting proteins that culminate in the formation of a thrombus (clot).[8] The process is tightly regulated because improper activation or neutralization of these constituents can cause bleeding or clotting episodes, either of which can be life threatening. Bleeding episodes can be caused by low platelet counts (*thrombocytopenia*) or deficiencies in clotting proteins. Clotting episodes can be caused by elevated platelet counts (*thrombocytosis*) or improper platelet or clotting protein activation. Testing for these impairments involves both the quantity and functionality of the platelets and clotting proteins.

Testing for the functionality of the platelets involves exposing the patient's platelets to agonists, or substances that induce platelet activation. The majority of agonists mimic constituents that activate platelets in vivo. These include thrombin, adenosine diphosphate

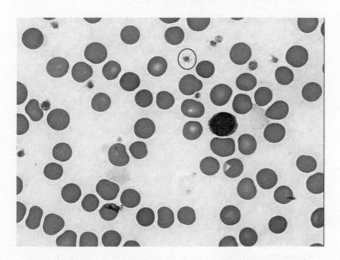

FIGURE 9-7 **Platelet (circled cell at top of picture).**

(ADP), arachidonic acid, epinephrine, collagen, and ristocetin. Testing for the clotting proteins involves maintaining a blood-to-anticoagulant ratio that is stable to ensure that coagulation will occur in vitro. Several methodologies are employed to test the functionality of clotting proteins, but all are considered to be clot-based assays, meaning that the endpoint detection is the formation of a clot. Stimulants biochemically similar to agonists are added to patient's plasma, and clot formation is observed usually in terms of the time it takes the blood to clot. Prolongation of clotting times is an indirect measure of clotting protein dysfunctionality. The biochemical activation of clotting proteins involves a "waterfall" or "cascade" approach, where an activated factor becomes the substrate (or cofactor) for the subsequent factor. On a larger scale, there are two pathways that eventually merge to form a common pathway, and selected factors are activated in each pathway. The two pathways are called intrinsic and extrinsic. The intrinsic pathway involves activation of the following factors (in sequential order): Factor XII, XI, IX, and VIII. The extrinsic pathway is responsible for activation of Factor VII. The common pathway involves activation of the following factors (also in sequential order): Factor X, V, II, and I. Screening tests involve assessment of one or more of these pathways. The two main screening tests are the prothrombin time (PT) and the activated partial thromboplastin time (aPTT). The PT monitors factor activity in the extrinsic and common pathway, whereas the aPTT monitors factor activity in the intrinsic and common pathway. If prolongation is seen in one or more of these test results, selected factor assays can be performed to confirm the deficiency. Factor deficiencies are highly correlated to several hemorrhagic clotting disorders. Clinical relevance can be found in **Table 9-6**.[8]

In closing, the CBC is an excellent screening test for identifying many different hematologic disturbances as well as to evaluate blood homeostasis. When used appropriately, it can provide the respiratory care clinician with the tools needed to identify blood cell abnormalities and monitor the stability of the patient. It is important to work together with the laboratory professionals to ensure quality results and minimize errors in testing that can affect overall patient care.

Clinical Chemistry

In clinical hematology, the blood is analyzed in terms of the number of cells of each type that are present. Clinical chemistry, in contrast, analyzes the noncellular components, reporting the concentration of atoms and molecules present in the plasma.

Approximately 70% to 80% of the data used to diagnose and treat patients comes from the medical laboratory, and the highly automated section, clinical chemistry, is the largest contributor. Scientists in the chemistry section perform hundreds of different types of tests to detect the rise and fall of atoms and molecules in serum and body fluids. Significant ones include carbohydrates (e.g., glucose), cardiac makers (e.g., troponin), proteins, lipids (e.g., cholesterol, HDL), therapeutic drugs and drugs of abuse, tumor markers, electrolytes, hormones, and toxins (e.g., lead, carbon monoxide). Frequently ordered chemistry tests and those of interest to patients with respiratory disorders will be emphasized in this section. **Table 9-7** lists the analytes that are described in this chapter, their relative reference ranges, as well as major causes of elevated and decreased results.[9]

A comprehensive chemistry panel containing tests that give the healthcare provider a quick assessment of a patient's overall health status is frequently ordered. Performed on serum, the comprehensive panel may include glucose, calcium, total protein, albumin, electrolytes (Na^+, K^+, Cl^-, HCO_3^-), blood urea nitrogen (BUN), creatinine, bilirubin, and enzymes. Together, these tests are an effective and cost-efficient way to detect and monitor common disorders such as diabetes, heart disease, cancers, acid-base problems, liver and kidney disease, and even some endocrine disorders.[10]

Carbohydrates: Diabetes Tests

Along with fats and proteins, carbohydrates are a source of energy. A major breakdown product of carbohydrate metabolism is glucose, which is absorbed in the gastrointestinal (GI) tract and then circulates to cells for metabolism. **Insulin** is released in response to elevation in plasma glucose and functions to allow glucose to enter cells where glycolysis, glycogenesis, and gluconeogenesis can then occur. Glucose has a number of different metabolic pathways. The pathway chosen will depend on the energy needs of the body at a particular time. When the body requires energy, glycolysis will occur. When the energy needs of the body are met, glucose will be converted to glycogen. When the glycogen stores are filled, excess glucose will be stored in the form of fat.

Diabetes mellitus is a common and serious group of disorders that involves insulin and the inability to

TABLE 9-6
Clotting Deficiencies

Deficient Factor	Condition
Factor VIII	Hemophilia A (classic hemophilia)
Factor IX	Hemophilia B
Factor XI	Hemophilia C
Factor X	Stuart-Prower deficiency
Von Willebrand factor	Von Willebrand disease
Factor II	Prothrombin deficiency

TABLE 9-7

References Ranges and Major Causes of Elevated and Decreased Results for Some Serum Analytes

Serum Analyte	Adult Reference Interval*	Elevated Results	Decreased Results
Bilirubin			
Total	0–2.0 mg/dL	Liver disease Hemolytic disorder Biliary obstruction	—
Direct	0–0.2 mg/dL	Biliary obstruction	—
Calcium, total	8.6–10.2 mg/dL	Hyperparathyroidism Malignancies	Tetany Renal failure
Creatinine	Male: 0.62–1.10 mg/dL Female: 0.45–0.75 mg/dL	Kidney disease Muscle breakdown	
Electrolytes			
Sodium (Na+)	136–145 mEq/L	Cushing syndrome Diabetes insipidus Dehydration	Addison disease SIADH
Potassium (K+)	3.5–5.1 mEq/L	Addison disease Alkalosis Renal failure	Cushing syndrome Acidosis
Chloride (Cl−)	98–107 mEq/L	Metabolic acidosis	Respiratory acidosis Metabolic alkalosis Vomiting
Bicarbonate (HCO$_3^-$) Total CO$_2$ (tCO$_2$)	22–32 mEq/L	Alkalosis	Acidosis
Glucose, fasting	74–100 mg/dL	Diabetes mellitus Cushing syndrome Hyperthyroid	Excessive insulin Addison disease Hypothyroid
Proteins			
Total	6.4–8.3 mg/dL, ambulatory	Multiple myeloma Dehydration	Renal failure Liver failure
Albumin	3.5–5.2 mg/dL	Dehydration	Renal failure Liver failure
Urea nitrogen (BUN)	6–20 mg/dL	Kidney disease Dehydration High-protein diet	Pregnancy Overhydration Liver failure
Uric acid	Males: 3.5–7.2 mg/dL Females: 2.6–6.0 mg/dL	Gout Renal disease	—

SIADH, syndrome of inappropriate antidiuretic hormone secretion; BUN, blood urea nitrogen.

*The reference intervals presented in the table are for **general information purposes** only. Individual laboratories link test results to their own reference intervals, which should be used to interpret a particular test result.

Data from: Burtis CA, Ashwood ER, Bruns DE (eds.). *Tietz Fundamentals of Clinical Chemistry*, 6th ed. St. Louis, MO: Saunders; 2008.

maintain normal levels of circulating glucose. There are three commons types of diabetes mellitus. **Type 1 diabetes** is characterized by low or absent insulin levels resulting from autoimmune destruction of the pancreas. Due to insufficient insulin, type 1 diabetics cannot utilize dietary carbohydrates. Glucose in the circulation remains elevated and alternative processes—gluconeogenesis and lipolysis—take over.

Treatment of diabetes mellitus is directed at maintaining a circulating glucose level that approaches that found in the nondiabetic population (i.e., 74 to 100 mg/dL). A serious consequence of insulin deficiency is metabolic acidosis. Because glucose is not entering the cells, alternate metabolic processes take over. Lipids and proteins are broken down to supply the energy needs of the body. Ketoacids (ketone bodies) are breakdown

a sequence of biochemical processes that lead to the release of aldosterone. Aldosterone functions to elevate Na^+ in the plasma. An elevated Na^+ attracts water, which, in turn, elevates the plasma blood volume. Blood volume is also adjusted by the body's thirst mechanism and release of ADH. Osmoreceptors in the hypothalamus sense changes in osmolality (Na^+ concentration). An elevation in plasma osmolality triggers the thirst mechanism, which signals the body to drink more water. An elevated plasma osmolality (elevated Na^+) also stimulates release of ADH from the pituitary, which signals the kidneys to retain water.

Dehydration is the most common cause of an elevated Na^+ level. Loss of water may result from vomiting and/or diarrhea, excess sweating, or burns or when a patient with uncontrolled diabetes mellitus undergoes osmotic diuresis due to an extremely high glucose level in the urine. An elevated sodium level is also a finding in diabetes insipidus. In this condition, water loss is due to decreased levels of ADH or the failure of the kidneys to respond to ADH. Because aldosterone functions to retain sodium, a patient diagnosed with primary hyperaldosteronism (Conn syndrome) will have an elevation in serum sodium. Elevated sodium is also a finding in another type of adrenal hyperfunction, Cushing syndrome. Sodium will also elevate when there is excess ingestion or infusion of sodium.

Sodium levels in plasma will decrease due to processes that deplete or dilute it. Some diuretics remove water by eliminating sodium into the urine, and, because Na^+ attracts water, urine volume will increase. Decreased secretion of aldosterone, as seen in adrenal hypofunction (Addison disease), will also decrease serum sodium levels. Syndrome of inappropriate antidiuretic hormone (SIADH) includes conditions that produce excess ADH or ADH-like molecules (e.g., malignancies, pulmonary and central nervous system [CNS] disorders, drugs, or pituitary gland hyperfunction). Because ADH works to retain water, serum sodium is diluted when the hormone elevates. Edema, which is seen in chronic renal failure, is another condition associated with water retention and decreased sodium levels.[18]

Potassium

Potassium (K^+) plays a role in transmission of nerve impulses that affect muscle contraction and is also an activator of cellular enzymes. Because it serves as the main intracellular cation, K^+ concentration in extracellular fluids, such as plasma, is relatively low (3.5 to 5.0 mEq/L). Nevertheless, K^+ plays a significant role in acid-base balance and has a dramatic effect on muscle contraction, including heart and lung muscles. Indeed, when a serum K^+ result on a patient is critically low or high, the healthcare provider is contacted immediately by the analyst so that the life-threatening imbalance can be corrected. It is also important to note that

falsely elevated potassium levels are a frequent problem. Hemolyzed specimens are always rejected because the sample is diluted with intracellular fluid, which is high in K^+. Over time, potassium will leak out of the cells, so serum must be separated from cellular components. *Hyperkalemia* is defined as having a serum K^+ level greater than 5.0 mEq/L. Symptoms of hyperkalemia include muscle weakness and paralysis. Levels greater than 6 mEq/L are associated with cardiac arrhythmias, and levels over 10 mEq/L lead to ventricular fibrillation. Hyperkalemia is seen in acute and chronic renal failure, hypoaldosteronism, and with excessive use of diuretics that retain potassium. Serum potassium elevates in acidosis to compensate for the elevated H^+ in this acid-base disturbance. K^+ moves out of the cell in exchange for H^+ moving into the cell, thus lowering the number of H^+. A normal serum K^+ level in a patient in acidosis would indicate the presence of potassium depletion, and a low serum K^+, as seen in acidosis, would indicate a very severe one. Patients recovering from respiratory acidosis should have their potassium stores replenished in order to avoid the effect of low potassium levels on lung muscle contraction. Potassium is also elevated in crush injuries due to the excessive amount of cell lysis.

Symptoms of *hypokalemia* ($K^+ < 3.5$ mEq/L) include muscle aches and weakness and irregular heartbeat, which can lead to dangerous disturbances in heart rhythm. Along with other muscles of the body, the diaphragm and lung muscles will be affected by low potassium levels. Hypokalemia can be due to renal mechanisms that lower potassium by excretion into the urine, as seen when aldosterone and cortisol (Cushing syndrome) become elevated, or with the use of some diuretics. Excessive loss of potassium-containing body fluids from vomiting and diarrhea will also lead to hypokalemia. Decreased potassium is found in alkalosis.[18]

Serum Chloride and Sweat Chloride

Chloride (Cl^-) is the major extracellular anion. It is important for the maintenance of electrolyte balance, hydration, and osmotic pressure. Conditions that cause retention or loss of chloride are generally the same as those that cause retention or loss of sodium. *Hyperchloremia* can be caused by excess loss of bicarbonate from the gastrointestinal tract or when there is a decrease in bicarbonate in acid-base imbalances, such as with metabolic acidosis. *Hypochloremia* may be due to prolonged vomiting or the presence of a kidney disease. Chloride will also decrease when serum bicarbonate increases to compensate for acid-base disturbances, such as respiratory acidosis or metabolic alkalosis.

Cystic fibrosis is a genetic disorder affecting the exocrine glands. A diagnostic finding is an elevated chloride level in sweat (i.e., elevated sweat chloride test), which can be incorporated into a diagnostic algorithm that includes family history and disease symptoms.

Blood immunoreactive trypsin, with positive results followed by direct gene analysis, is used to screen newborns for cystic fibrosis.[19,20]

Bicarbonate

Bicarbonate (HCO_3^-) is the second most predominant anion in the plasma and is a major component of the bicarbonate/carbonic acid buffer system that functions to maintain plasma pH. The anion is measured to evaluate a patient's acid-base status. A number of methods are used to determine HCO_3^- concentration. A blood gas analyzer calculates the HCO_3^- concentration most accurately. The instrument directly measures pH and P_{CO_2} and calculates the bicarbonate concentration using the Henderson-Hasselbalch equation (see Chapter 8). The carbonic acid concentration can be calculated from the P_{CO_2} and is used to further diagnose and classify an acid-base problem. Blood gas analysis is expensive and involves skillful anaerobic collection and stat processing. To roughly evaluate a patient's acid-base status, the medical laboratory offers a bicarbonate test, which is usually measured as total CO_2 content (TCO_2). The TCO_2 is roughly equivalent to the sum of the bicarbonate plus the carbonic acid (H_2CO_3). Serum that has not been handled anaerobically is used so that carbonic acid in the form of CO_2 is drawn out of the specimen, making the TCO_2 content less accurate than the TCO_2 calculated from blood gas electrode analysis. However, because the bicarbonate concentration is normally 20 times that of carbonic acid, the TCO_2 content performed on serum reflects the bicarbonate concentration.[21]

The Anion Gap

The anion gap is a calculated value and equals the routinely measured anions minus the cations. The most common formula is $(Na^+ + K^+) - (Cl^- + HCO_3^-)$. Anion gap is a misnomer, because there is not an actual physiological gap between anions and cations. The gap is actually an analytical one, because not all of the anions and cations are routinely measured. Abnormal anion gaps provide nonspecific information. The calculation is most useful for detection of acidosis due to an accumulation of organic acids, such as ketone bodies, lactic acid, and phosphate/sulfate and certain drugs and toxic alcohol metabolites. The anion gap increases when these anions accumulate.[21] For additional discussion of the anion gap, see Chapter 8.

Calcium

Calcium exists in three forms in the plasma, and measurement of all forms is reported as total calcium. Serum total calcium is frequently ordered, and the test is included on a comprehensive chemistry test panel. Some blood gas analyzers have an additional calcium electrode that measures the ionized fraction of the plasma calcium (Ca^{++}). The ionized form of calcium is regulated primarily by the parathyroid gland and activated vitamin D. The parathyroid gland secretes parathyroid hormone (PTH) when there is a drop in ionized calcium and signals the bone and kidney to increase the calcium level. Vitamin D also functions to maintain an increased ionized calcium. In the plasma, calcium controls neuromuscular activity. Tetany (i.e., muscle constriction) results when ionized calcium drops, whereas muscle weakness is a symptom of elevated calcium. Calcium is also a cofactor for plasma enzyme reactions such as those involved in coagulation. Disorders associated with *hypercalcemia* include primary hyperparathyroidism and some types of cancer. *Hypocalcemia* will occur in conditions associated with a low PTH level, such as post removal or damage to the parathyroid gland or in renal failure when the kidneys no longer respond to PTH control. A deficiency of vitamin D will also result in low serum calcium levels.[22]

Hormones and Therapeutic Drug Monitoring

The chemistry section of the laboratory also offers tests that measure the concentration of various hormones in order to evaluate endocrine problems. Thyroid hormones (TSH, thyroxine) and hormones synthesized by the adrenal gland (cortisol, aldosterone) are frequently ordered, as are tests to evaluate the fertility status of a couple (progesterone, estrogen, LH, FSH). Drug testing is also performed in the chemistry laboratory. Some prescribed drugs have a very narrow therapeutic range, so it is important to determine serum levels in order to avoid toxicity. The antiasthmatic drug theophylline is one of these.

In summary, clinical chemistry encompasses a diverse array of analyses that are performed on serum and help the respiratory care clinician determine if the patient has an abnormality in almost any body system. The tests are all performed on complex analyzers that offer the sensitivity, specificity, and timeliness required to make an accurate diagnosis in a fast-paced healthcare environment.

Microbiology

In the clinical microbiology laboratory, microorganisms that infect patients are isolated, identified, and, if necessary, tested for their susceptibility to antimicrobial agents that are used to eliminate the causative organism. Bacteria (aerobic and anaerobic), mycobacteria, yeast, molds, parasites, and viruses can all infect humans and cause disease. Many of these same organisms can be found in certain places on the body as normal flora, which may complicate the interpretation of culture results. Thus, it is important to know which sites harbor normal flora and what organisms are typically found as normal flora as opposed to those that are considered pathogens when isolated. It is the isolation, identification, and treatment of the pathogenic organisms that should be targeted with appropriate laboratory tests.[23] Even though there are millions of different microorganisms in the environment, only relatively few organisms are isolated from humans at great frequency. Further, particular organisms are only found in certain environments, whereas others only infect patients with underlying disease. Thus, by knowing some information about the history of the patient along with the most likely causative agents, predicting the organism infecting a particular site, especially the lower respiratory tract, can be fairly straightforward.[24] **Table 9-12** lists the most common causative agents of pneumonia isolated from patients of different ages and underlying disease.

Laboratory tests that are used to detect microorganisms range from traditional culture-based methods in which an organism is placed in an artificial medium and allowed to grow and then identified by interpreting its reaction in biochemical tests to molecular methods in which only the nucleic acid of the microorganism is isolated and then analyzed to determine which organism is present.

Specimens of the Lower Respiratory Tract

Specimens that are representative of the lower respiratory tract include sputum, aspirates of the trachea and bronchi, pleural fluid, and biopsies or aspirates of the lung. These specimens are collected in order to determine the causative agent of bronchitis or pneumonia. In order to get clinically relevant results from laboratory tests, obtaining the highest quality specimen is critical. In general, high-quality specimens are representative of the site of infection and are collected so as to minimize contamination with surrounding sites. Aspirates, pleural fluid, and biopsies are collected by healthcare professionals following specified protocols to maximize integrity of the specimen and minimize discomfort to the patient. Sputum is a specimen that is collected by the patient, who must receive good instructions so as to deliver a high-quality specimen that is not contaminated with oropharyngeal secretions. The best specimen to submit to the clinical microbiology laboratory is one that is collected early in the morning, a "first morning" specimen that is collected soon after the patient gets up. This specimen is the most concentrated in terms of the number of organisms present because secretions have accumulated and much of the excess fluid was reabsorbed overnight.

Sputum Collection

In order to collect a sputum specimen that has minimal contamination with oropharyngeal flora, the patient should be instructed to brush his or her teeth and/or rinse his or her mouth with water to wash away as much bacteria as possible out of the mouth. The patient should then be instructed that saliva is not the specimen to collect. The patient should be told to breathe deeply

TABLE 9-12

Most Common Organisms Causing Pneumonia in Different Types of Patients

Patient Characteristics	Most Common Causes of Pneumonia
Neonates and Infants (up to 5 months of age)	Respiratory syncytial virus, parainfluenza viruses, adenovirus, *Chlamydia trachomatis*
Children (5 to 18 months)	*Streptococcus pneumoniae*, *Haemophilus influenzae*
Children (2 years to teens)	*Mycoplasma pneumoniae*, *Staphylococcus aureus*, parainfluenza viruses, adenovirus
Young adults	*Chlamydia pneumoniae*, *Mycoplasma pneumoniae*
Older adults	*Streptococcus pneumoniae*, *Legionella pneumophila*, influenza virus, respiratory syncytial virus
Older adults in long-term care institutions	*Streptococcus pneumoniae*, *Staphylococcus aureus*, gram-negative bacilli
Cystic fibrosis patients	*Pseudomonas aeruginosa*, *Burkholderia cepacia*, *Staphylococcus aureus*, *Haemophilus influenzae*
Hospitalized patients	*Pseudomonas aeruginosa*, *Klebsiella pneumoniae*, other gram-negative bacilli, *Staphylococcus aureus*
Community acquired	*Streptococcus pneumoniae*, *Haemophilus influenzae*, *Klebsiella pneumoniae*, *Legionella pneumophila*, *Chlamydophila* (*Chlamydia*) *pneumoniae*, *Mycoplasma pneumoniae*, *Moraxella catarrhalis*, *Bordetella pertussis*, *Mycobacterium tuberculosis*
Immunocompromised	*Candida* spp. *Cryptococcus* spp., *Pneumocystis jiroveci*, *Mycobacterium avium*, Cytomegalovirus
Occupational or geographic-associated organisms	Ohio and Mississippi River Valleys: *Histoplasma capsulatum* Southwest U.S. (California and Arizona): *Coccidioides immitis* Exposure to pigeons, parakeets, bats: *Chlamydia psittaci* and *Cryptococcus neoformans* Exposure to cattle, pigs, sheep, horses: *Coxiella burnetii* Exposure to rodents and rodent body fluids: Hantavirus Exposure to birds and pigs: Influenza virus

Data from: Carroll KC. 2002. Laboratory diagnosis of lower respiratory tract infections: controversy and conundrums. *J Clin Microbiol.* 40(9):3115–3120.

and cough from down deep in the lungs. If the patient cannot cough deeply enough, coughing can be induced by inhaling an aerosolized solution of saline. The material that is produced after coughing should be put directly into a sterile container and sent to the clinical microbiology laboratory as soon as possible.[25]

Direct Examination

When sputum or other specimen of the lower respiratory tract is received in the microbiology laboratory, direct examination of the specimen can be performed, which will give information about the possible cause of the pneumonia before the culture results will be available. Direct examination will also give information about the suitability of the specimen for culture as well as indicate the presence of host cells in the specimen.

Because sputum can easily be contaminated with saliva, and because saliva is not a specimen representative of the lower respiratory tract, when sputum is received in the clinical microbiology laboratory it will be screened for its suitability for culture. Typically, a portion of the sputum will be put onto a microscope slide and then a Gram stain will be performed. The Gram stain is a differential stain in which crystal violet (primary stain), iodine (mordant), acetone-alcohol (decolorizer), and safranin (counter stain) are used sequentially to stain host cells and bacteria present in the specimen. After Gram staining the slide, only the gram-positive bacteria will have retained the primary crystal violet and appear purple. The gram-negative bacteria, as well as all host cells, will lose the primary stain and will be stained pink due to the safranin.

To screen sputum for suitability, the slide is placed onto a microscope and the smear is examined on low power (10×) for the presence of epithelial cells and white blood cells. The cells are counted per low power field and reported. If the specimen is representative of the lower respiratory tract, very few epithelial cells will be present, and the specimen will be tested further according to what tests have been ordered. If the specimen is saliva, there will be numerous epithelial cells, and the specimen is not suitable for culture or further testing. Because aspirates, pleural fluid, and lung biopsies are collected by healthcare professionals directly from the site, these specimens should not be contaminated by oropharyngeal flora; thus, these types of lower respiratory tract specimens will not be screened for suitability.

The most common direct smear performed in clinical microbiology is a Gram stain. When a Gram stain is reported on a specimen, the report will include whether host cells are present in the specimen (e.g., RBCs, WBCs and epithelial cells) and whether bacteria are seen. Typically these components will be reported along with the quantity seen. "Rare," "few," "moderate," or "many" are terms used to quantitate the number of cells or organisms seen, depending on how many cells or organisms are seen per oil immersion field.

TABLE 9-13

Gram-Stain Reactions of Selected Organisms That May be Isolated from Lower Respiratory Tract Specimens

Gram Reaction and Morphology	Examples of Organisms (genus only)
Gram-positive cocci	*Staphylococcus, Streptococcus*
Gram-positive bacilli	*Corynebacterium*
Gram-negative cocci	*Neisseria, Moraxella*
Gram-negative bacilli	*Escherichia, Pseudomonas, Klebsiella*

If a specimen is representative of the site of infection and the patient has an infection, then it is expected that WBCs will be present. Thus the lack of WBCs in a specimen suggests that either the specimen is not representative of the site of infection or that the patient may not have an infection. The bacteria are reported as the Gram-stain reaction (positive or negative), along with the morphology of the organism (i.e., cocci [round] or bacilli [rod-shaped]). Some examples of bacteria that may be seen in lower respiratory tract specimens according to their Gram stain are listed in **Table 9-13**.

Other types of direct smears that can be performed on lower respiratory tract specimens include a fluorochrome stain, Ziehl-Neelsen or Kinyoun, Calcofluor white, and direct fluorescence antibody stains. The organisms detected in these smears are listed in **Table 9-14**.

Information obtained from the direct smear can be used to determine if the patient has an infection and what the cause may be. Empirical antimicrobial therapy can be prescribed as appropriate. The results of direct smears have to be evaluated carefully, however, keeping in mind the following important factors:

1. The sensitivity of direct smears is dependent on the quality of the specimen as well as the number of organisms per milliliter of specimen and averages at about 70%.[26] Thus the patient could have pneumonia, but organisms will not be seen in the direct smear if there are not enough of them in the specimen.

2. Sputum contains normal flora, so the presence of bacteria is expected unless the patient is already on antimicrobial agents and the flora has been eradicated. Many different organisms have the same Gram stain appearance, and it is impossible to tell between a potential pathogen, such as *Streptococcus pneumoniae*, and viridans *Streptococcus*, which is normal flora, just by the Gram stain results. Only the testing of organisms growing in culture can determine what they are, and thus sometimes decisions on therapy have to wait until the results of the cultures are reported.

TABLE 9-14
Direct Smears That Can Be Performed on Lower Respiratory Tract Specimens and the Organisms That Are Detected

Stain Type	Organisms Detected	Appearance of Organisms in Stain
Fluorochrome	*Mycobacterium* (mycobacteria or acid-fast bacilli)	Yellow-orange fluorescing rods
Ziehl-Neelsen or Kinyoun	*Mycobacterium* spp. (mycobacteria or acid-fast bacilli)	Red rods
Calcofluor white	Yeasts (e.g., *Candida* or *Cryptococcus*) or molds (e.g., *Aspergillus* or *Rhizopus*)	Whitish-bluish fluorescing yeast cells or fungal elements
Direct fluorescence antibody (targeted organism must be specified by the physician)	Examples of organisms that can be detected: *Legionella*, *Pneumocystis*	Fluorescing organisms

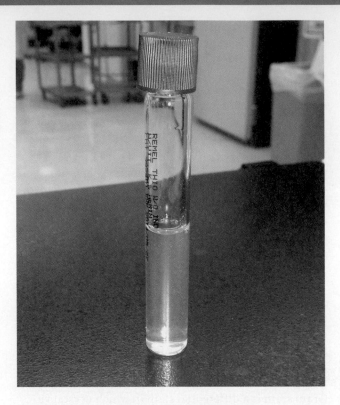

FIGURE 9-8 **Thioglycollate broth in a tube.**

3. The direct smears for mycobacteria cannot differentiate between the pathogen *Mycobacterium tuberculosis* and other nonpathogenic species of *Mycobacterium*. If the clinical suspicion that the patient has tuberculosis is high and the direct smear for mycobacteria is positive, it may be appropriate to consider that the patient has tuberculosis until the culture results suggest otherwise.

4. Bronchial aspirates, pleural fluid, and lung aspirates or biopsies are more likely to be sterile specimens than sputum, thus the presence of any organisms suggests infection.

Isolation and Identification of Microorganisms

Direct smears can give a certain amount of information about whether the patient has an infection, but the definitive method for determining whether a patient has an infection is to isolate and identify a pathogenic organism in culture. Although direct smears can typically be performed and reported within hours of the specimen being collected, cultures for microorganisms will not yield results for at least 24 hours and can take from days to weeks, depending on the organism.

Isolation of bacteria and fungi is accomplished by inoculating the specimen onto a solid agar medium, usually in the form of a plate. Alternatively, a liquid medium can be used (see **Figure 9-8**) or solid agar in a

tube can be inoculated. Numerous types of media are commercially available to support the growth of microorganisms in vitro. Selection of media depends on the specimen source submitted for culture and what type of organisms the physician wants to rule out (e.g., aerobic bacteria versus mycobacteria). Media are classified into three different groups:

■ *Enrichment media* that will support the growth of most microorganisms and includes trypticase soy agar with 5% sheep red blood cells (blood agar) (**Figure 9-9**) and chocolate agar (**Figure 9-10**).

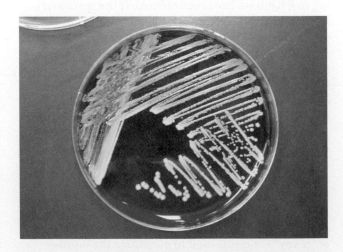

FIGURE 9-9 *Staphylococcus aureus* **colonies on Trypticase soy agar with 5% sheep RBCs (blood agar plate).**

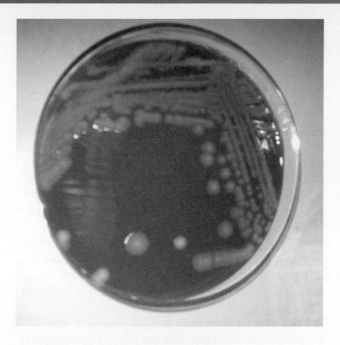

FIGURE 9-10 *Haemophilus* colonies on chocolate agar.

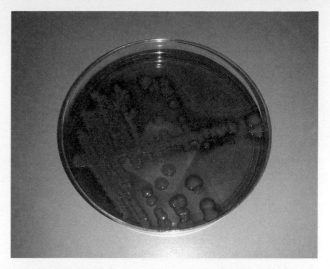

FIGURE 9-11 Lactose-fermenting gram-negative bacilli on MacConkey agar.

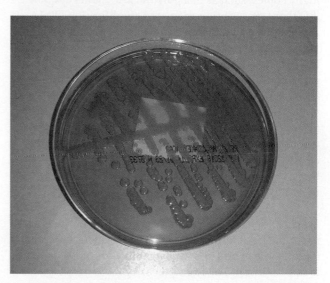

FIGURE 9-12 Lactose nonfermenting gram-negative bacilli on MacConkey agar.

- *Selective media* that will inhibit the growth of some organisms (the normal flora) and allow for the growth of other organisms (the pathogens). Modified Thayer Martin is a selective medium for *Neisseria gonorrhoeae*, and Middlebrook 7H10 is a selective medium for *Mycobacterium* spp.
- *Selective-differential media* that will inhibit the growth of some organisms and allow for the growth of other organisms similar to selective media, but, in addition, has additional ingredients that will differentiate between the organisms that do grow. For example, MacConkey agar is selective for gram-negative bacilli and differentiates between the gram-negative bacilli based on the presence or absence of lactose fermentation. Lactose-fermenting gram-negative bacilli will appear as dark pink-purple colonies on MacConkey (**Figure 9-11**), whereas lactose nonfermenting gram-negative bacilli will appear as "colorless" colonies, although they may take on the color of the medium, which is a light pink-purple color (**Figure 9-12**).

Once an organism is isolated (i.e., grows on media in vitro), the organism is identified by performing a Gram stain and biochemical tests. Biochemical tests measure whether the organism produces certain enzymes (e.g., catalase, coagulase, and urease); how it breaks down a certain substrate (e.g., the production of indole from tryptophane); or if it can use a particular substrate (e.g., citrate). Performance of most biochemical tests requires actively metabolizing cells and is measured after an 18- to 24-hour period of incubation. The results from multiple biochemical tests are compiled and compared

to known results in order to identify the organism, which is then reported as genus and species for most organisms. For example, a gram-positive coccus that is catalase-positive and coagulase-positive is identified as *Staphylococcus aureus*, and a gram-negative bacillus that is oxidase-negative, indole-positive, citrate-negative, Voges-Proskauer-negative, and ferments lactose is identified as *Escherichia coli*. A new method for identifying microorganisms called Matrix-Assisted Laser Desorption/Ionization Time of Flight Mass Spectrometry (MALDI-TOF MS) is being used in some clinical microbiology laboratories.[27] In MALDI-TOF MS, sample material is ionized and accelerated by a laser and the time of flight is measured. The spectra of ribosomal proteins are measured. Particular molecules and organisms have particular spectra, and so the spectrum of an unknown is compared to a known that has been saved in a database. Some of the advantages of this procedure are that organisms can be identified in a matter of minutes and many different organisms can be identified, such as fastidious bacteria (e.g., *Neisseria* and *Mycobacterium)*, anaerobes (e.g., *Clostridium*), nonfastidious bacteria (e.g., *Staphylococcus*), and even yeast (e.g., *Candida*). The potential also exists to identify organisms directly from a body fluid, negating the need to isolate the organism, thereby saving at least 24 hours of time to report the cause of an infection.[27] The disadvantages of MALDI-TOF MS at this time include a limited database thus far, the lack of ability to determine susceptibility of the organism to antimicrobial agents, and a high initial investment in instrumentation.

A third method by which microorganisms may be identified in the clinical microbiology laboratory is to isolate and analyze the nucleic acid (DNA or RNA) in the organism. Isolated nucleic acid can be amplified to make many copies, such as in a **polymerase chain reaction (PCR)** or transcription-mediated amplification (TMA). Alternatively, the nucleic acid can be hybridized to a probe to be detected or a portion of the nucleic acid can be sequenced and compared to sequence data of known genes contained in a database.[28] Targets for molecular-based analyses are still limited, and the assays remain very expensive, which limits their availability and utility for routine use. However, organisms can be identified in a few hours and often directly from a clinical specimen. Many of the originally very time-consuming steps are being automated, which will lead to the increased implementation of these procedures over time.

After a microorganism has been identified, for most organisms the antimicrobial susceptibility of the organism must be determined. The antimicrobial susceptibility for some organisms can be predicted, and thus testing is not required. For example, *Streptococcus pyogenes* (also known as Group A *Streptococcus*) is predictably susceptible to penicillin, which is commonly used to treat infections caused by *S. pyogenes*. Many organisms, however, vary in their susceptibility to antimicrobial agents, and thus must be tested. In order to determine if an organism is susceptible or resistant to a particular antimicrobial agent, the organism is grown in the presence of a certain concentration of agent, and its ability to grow is measured 18 to 24 hours later. Susceptibility results are usually reported as the minimum inhibitory concentration (MIC) of the agent along with an interpretation of whether the organism is susceptible or resistant to that agent. The MIC is the least amount of agent that will inhibit the growth of the organism. If the organism is resistant to an agent, in general, that agent is not given to the patient. To choose between agents to which the organism is susceptible, in general, the agent with the lowest MIC is chosen for treating the patient, provided other considerations are met, such as whether that agent can travel to the site of infection or whether the patient can tolerate any possible side effects of the agent. Consultation with a pharmacist and/or infectious disease specialist may be needed in complex situations.[29]

Urine

Urine is analyzed in the laboratory to determine if the renal system is functioning appropriately and to ensure that the patient does not have a urinary tract infection or renal system malignancy. Analysis of urine can also reveal if a patient has diabetes or is dehydrated or has a poor diet. Urine is collected into a clean cup as a midstream clean catch sample preferably. If a culture of the urine is to be performed, then the container used to collect the urine has to be sterile. Urine has to be examined within 2 hours of passage or it should be refrigerated or put into a boric acid preservative if a culture is going to be performed and there is a delay in processing.

Urinalysis involves macroscopic, chemical, and microscopic examinations of the urine. Macroscopic or visual analysis of the urine involves assessing the color, smell, and clarity of the urine. In the chemical analysis, the following properties are measured: specific gravity, pH, protein, ketones, glucose, nitrites, leukocyte esterase, blood, urobilinogen, and bilirubin. The presence of RBCs, WBCs, bacteria, and other cellular components, such as casts and crystals, are determined in the microscopic analysis of the urine.[30]

Macroscopic Analysis of Urine

The first part of the urinalysis is to assess the color, clarity, and odor of the urine. The urine in the container should be viewed under a good light against a white background. Normal urine is a pale yellow color, like the color of straw or amber. Urochrome (yellow), uroerythrin (red), and urobilin (orange-red) are pigments that combine in urine to produce its color. Lighter yellow-colored urine or colorless urine indicates a dilute specimen and is seen in patients who drink more fluids. Darker urine colors of dark yellow, orange, or brown indicate more concentrated urine or the presence of bilirubin. Blood, hemoglobin, or myoglobin in the urine will cause the urine to turn a reddish color. Patients on certain medications or who have eaten certain foods may have urine that appears bright orange, green, or even blue.[31]

With regards to clarity, normal urine is clear. If the urine appears hazy, cloudy, or turbid, the patient has substances in the urine, such as WBCs, RBCs, bacteria, phosphates, casts, or crystals. Amorphous crystals tend to form as the urine sits at room temperature, making clear urine at collection appear cloudy as it sits. Thus it is critical to perform this analysis as soon as possible after collection. Some substances that cause the urine to appear hazy or cloudy can be normal, such as amorphous phosphates in alkaline urine, whereas others indicate pathology, such as WBCs. In order to determine the cause of a cloudy urine specimen and thereby whether the abnormal clarity is clinically significant, microscopic examination would need to be performed.

As for the odor, urine has a distinctive odor due to the presence of volatile acids. Urine can begin to smell more ammoniacal as it sits at room temperature and bacteria break down the urea to ammonia. Diabetic patients who have increased ketones will have urine that smells "fruity." A pungent or putrid odor may be associated with the presence of bacteria. Ingestion of certain foods, especially asparagus, can change the smell of urine. As with abnormal clarity, abnormal odors require the performance of chemical and microscopic analyses to determine the cause and clinical significance.

Chemical Analysis of Urine

The chemical analysis of urine is typically performed by a dipstick method in which a small stick containing pads with reagents used to detect the various analytes is dipped into fresh, well-mixed, uncentrifuged urine. This is a common point-of-care test and relatively easy to perform, but it must be performed correctly in order to obtain accurate results. **Table 9-15** lists the urine analytes measured by a dipstick along with their reference (normal) values and some conditions that will cause abnormal values.[31]

TABLE 9-15
Analytes Measured in the Chemical Analysis of Urine

Analyte	Overview	Reference Values	Conditions Resulting in Lower Levels	Conditions Resulting in Higher Levels
Specific gravity	Measurement of dissolved substances in urine Relates to the function of the kidney with regards to its ability to concentrate urine and to hydration status	1.003–1.030	Use of diuretics Diabetes insipidus Lack of adrenal hormone Decreased renal function	Glycosuria Dehydration
pH	Knowing the urine pH assists with identification of crystals in the urine sediment and resolving discrepancies between chemical and microscopic analyses Limited relationship to systemic acid-base status	4.5–8 (usually 5–6)	Starvation Diabetes mellitus Respiratory tract disease	Severe vomiting Respiratory hyperventilation Urinary tract infection
Glucose	Detected in urine when the blood glucose level is > 180–200 mg/dL and excess glucose cannot be reabsorbed into the blood Measurement of metabolic function	Negative (≤ 130 mg/dL)	N/A	Diabetes mellitus Cushing syndrome
Ketones	Measurement of metabolic function Found in urine when excess fat is broken down for energy	Negative	N/A	Diabetes mellitus Starvation Pregnancy Low-carbohydrate diet
Nitrite	Found when bacteria break down nitrate to nitrite in the urinary tract	Negative	N/A	Bacteriuria (especially gram-negative bacteria)
Leukocyte esterase	An enzyme found in granulocytes that is used as an indirect measurement of the amount of WBCs in urine	Negative	N/A	Urinary tract infection Glomerulonephritis Bladder tumors

(continues)

TABLE 9-15
Analytes Measured in the Chemical Analysis of Urine (*continued*)

Analyte	Overview	Reference Values	Conditions Resulting in Lower Levels	Conditions Resulting in Higher Levels
Bilirubin (conjugated)	Product of RBC breakdown when the heme portion of hemoglobin is converted to bilirubin and conjugated to glucuronic acid in the liver Measurement of metabolic (liver) function	Negative	N/A	Hepatitis Biliary obstruction
Urobilinogen	Produced by bacteria acting on bilirubin in the intestine Measurement of metabolic (liver) function	≤ 1 mg/dL	Bile duct obstruction Antibiotic use decreasing intestinal bacteria	Liver disease Excessive hemolysis Congestive heart failure
Protein	Found in urine when the glomerulus has increased permeability and the renal tubules have decreased resorption Measure of renal function	Negative, Trace	N/A	Pyelonephritis Polycystic kidney disease Wilson disease Fanconi syndrome
Blood (RBCs)	Detects RBCs, hemoglobin, or myoglobin in urine by measuring peroxidase activity of heme	Negative, Trace	N/A	Hematuria: Urinary tract bleeding Renal tumor Glomerulonephritis Hemoglobinuria: Intravascular or intrarenal hemolysis Myoglobinuria: Strenuous exercise or trauma to muscles

WBC, white blood cell; RBC, red blood cell.
Data from: Simmerville JA, Maxted WC, Pahira JJ. Urinalysis: a comprehensive review. *Am Fam Physician.* 2005;71(6):1153–1162.

Microscopic Analysis of Urine

The microscopic analysis of the urine is the final step in a urinalysis. The sediment or solid material present in the urine is examined under the microscope to determine its identity. Microscopic analysis does not need to be performed on every urine specimen that is submitted to the laboratory, but rather is an important adjunct to determine the cause and clinical significance of abnormal macroscopic and/or chemical analyses. Whereas a chemical analysis of urine is a "waived" test and can be performed by minimally trained personnel, the microscopic analysis is a moderately complex procedure that must be performed by well-educated and skilled laboratory professionals.[31]

To perform the microscopic analysis, a consistent volume of fresh, well-mixed urine must be centrifuged to concentrate the sediment, which is then resuspended in a consistent volume of urine remaining in the centrifuge tube. Typically 12 mL (ranging from 10 to 15 mL) of urine is concentrated to 1 mL. Next the sediment is examined under low (10×) and high (40×) power as an unstained wet mount in a brightfield

(typical) microscope. Phase contrast microscopy may be used to help identify translucent materials such as hyaline casts and other cells. Under low power, casts, crystals, squamous epithelial cells, and mucus are observed and counted. The amounts of the structures seen are reported in relative amounts as few, moderate, or many per low-power field. RBCs, WBCs, crystals, epithelial cells, bacteria, yeast, *Trichomonas*, and sperm are visualized under high power and reported in relative amounts per high-power field with similar designations as above for structures seen at low power.

Normally, none to very few RBCs, WBCs, hyaline casts, epithelial cells, and crystals are present in urine. RBCs and WBCs look the same in urine as they do in blood, but their presence in numbers greater than few are abnormal in urine. The presence of RBCs indicates glomerulonephritis or bleeding, and the presence of WBCs indicates infection or inflammation in the urinary tract. If the RBCs are not shaped normally, it could indicate glomerular disease where the RBCs are being distorted by moving through a glomerulus that has changed in some way.

Squamous epithelial cells in urine typically indicate that the specimen was contaminated by contact with the lower urethral tract or vaginal tract. However, the presence of renal tubule cells in urine indicates serious renal disease, and thus is clinically significant. Casts are made up of protein and contents of a tubule that complex together and are passed into the urine. The type of cast is determined by the type of cell found in the cast (e.g., hyaline, RBC, WBC, waxy, or fatty). The cast will have an elongated morphology, like a sausage, due to the structure of the tubule in which it was formed. The presence of casts suggests pyelonephritis, advanced renal disease, or nephritic syndrome.

A variety of crystals may be seen in urine, but most of the time their presence is not associated with pathology. Normal crystals can be formed by calcium oxalate, uric acid, and triple phosphate. Cystinuria is diagnosed by the presence of cystine crystals in acidic urine. With urinary tract infections, especially when *Proteus* is the causative organism, triple-phosphate crystals in the alkaline urine may be seen.

The presence of bacteria, yeast, and *Trichomonas* can be detected in the microscopic analysis of urine and will indicate that the patient has an infection with that kind of organism. Although it might be possible to determine if the bacteria have a coccal or bacillary morphology, no other information about the identity of the organism can be determined from the wet mount. Urine culture will have to be performed to isolate and identify the bacterial pathogen. Yeast are not a common cause of urinary tract infection, and if the patient is a woman it may indicate that she has a vaginal yeast infection rather than a urinary tract infection. *Trichomonas* is a sexually transmitted protozoan that causes genitourinary infections. In a wet mount of urine such as is performed for microscopic analysis, *Trichomonas* appears as a round, motile structure about the size of a WBC, but with flagella that propel the organism around the slide.

Although discussion of urinalysis may seem less important to the respiratory care clinician, analysis of the urine not only reveals problems with the urinary tract system, but also metabolic problems that may impact the cardiopulmonary system (e.g., ketoacidosis in patients with uncontrolled diabetes mellitus). In addition, urine can be used as a diagnostic specimen to identify respiratory tract infections caused by *Legionella pneumophila* and *Streptococcus pneumoniae*.[32,33] In these assays, antibodies are used to bind to *L. pneumophila* serogroup 1 antigens or *S. pneumoniae* capsular antigens present in urine. Although a respiratory specimen is the specimen of choice for the diagnosis of *L. pneumophila*, patients often will not be able to produce a sputum specimen, and more invasive methods will be required to collect respiratory tract secretions. Urine is an easy, noninvasive specimen to collect.

Studies performed shortly after the first identified outbreak of *L. pneumophila* in Philadelphia in 1979 demonstrated that *L. pneumophila* antigens are excreted in urine shortly after symptoms appear and persist after treatment.[34] The sensitivity of these tests is about 85%; their specificity is about 99%. The main advantage of the urine antigen tests compared to culture is that they can be performed in minutes, compared to days for culture results, and they give reliable presumptive evidence that a patient has *L. pneumophila* if the test is positive.[35] One study performed on the urine antigen detection tests for *S. pneumoniae* showed similar sensitivities (around 80%) and specificities (97%) as studies found for *L. pneumophila* urine antigen tests with a similar advantage (i.e., being able to detect the cause of pneumonia in a shorter time frame than culture).[32] These applications demonstrate that urine analysis can reveal valuable information regarding respiratory function and/or infection.

Skin Testing

Skin testing is performed to measure the host immune response against an organism or allergen as a sign of either past exposure to the organism, current infection with that organism, or allergic response to a noninfectious allergen.

A skin test that measures either past exposure to or current infection with an organism detects the presence of a **delayed-type hypersensitivity (DTH)** reaction to that organism. A DTH reaction is measured when a suspension of antigen from an organism is injected intradermally into a patient. If the patient has been infected with that organism either in the past or currently, T cells, in particular, T_H1 cells, will recognize the injected antigen, become activated, and secrete cytokines, primarily interferon-gamma, which will, in turn, activate macrophages. Macrophages respond by migrating to the site of the antigen and releasing additional cytokines that will promote inflammation such that fluids and cells accumulate at the site of injection, resulting in an induration that is measured in millimeters. The reaction is measured 48 to 72 hours after inoculation. A positive reaction indicates that the patient was either infected with that organism in the past or that the patient is currently infected. A negative reaction occurs in patients who were never infected with the organism, who were very recently infected and have not had time to mount a detectable immune reaction, or who are immunosuppressed and cannot mount an immune response.

Skin Testing for Tuberculosis or Fungi

In the past, skin testing was performed for some fungi, such as *Histoplasma* and *Coccidioides*, but this form of testing is not performed for these organisms any longer.

DTH testing is primarily performed when a patient is suspected to have tuberculosis (TB) as well as to screen people for exposure to *Mycobacterium tuberculosis* (MTB). Another name used for this test is the Mantoux tuberculin skin test (TST). It is the gold standard for identifying if someone has latent tuberculosis in particular. It was first developed by Koch in 1890, refined by Mantoux in 1912, and further developed into what is used today by Seibert in 1934.[36] For this purpose, purified protein derivative (PPD) (more specifically called PPD-S for standard), which is a suspension of primarily protein extracted from cultures of MTB, is injected intradermally into the forearm. The patient returns to a healthcare practitioner for the reaction to be read 48 to 72 hours after injection. Redness at the site of inoculation by itself is common but not a positive reaction. A positive reaction is indicated by the presence of induration (swelling) at the site of inoculation. The diameter of induration is measured in millimeters and interpreted in conjunction with patient history as positive or negative.[37]

TST reactions that are 15 mm or greater are interpreted as positive in people who have no known risk factors for MTB. A TST that is 10 mm or greater is interpreted as positive in people who have come from a country with a high prevalence of MTB, intravenous drug users, personnel who work in mycobacteriology laboratories, children exposed to adults in high-risk groups for MTB, as well as people who live and work in group settings (e.g., healthcare workers) such as prisons, nursing homes, and homeless shelters. Patients who are HIV positive, have had known contact with someone with active TB, or who are immunosuppressed and who have a TST induration of only 5 mm or greater are interpreted as being TST positive.[37]

It must be realized with interpreting TST results that there are many causes of both **false-positives** and **false-negatives**. If the TST is not administered properly or interpreted properly, the result can be falsely positive or negative. People who are infected with other species of *Mycobacterium* and those who have received the Bacillus Calmette-Guerin (BCG) vaccine may have false-positive TST results. The most common causes of false-negative reactions are anergy (the inability to mount an immune response) and very recent or very old infections. To reduce the number of false-negative results due to these reasons, a two-step TST has been implemented in which a second TST is performed shortly (optimal is 1 to 5 weeks) after the first TST. It is thought that the first placement of the antigen suspension will boost the immune response such that there is a detectable response when the second TST is placed.

Because the TST is a fairly invasive test that requires trained personnel to administer and interpret it and patients have to return to the healthcare provider's office for interpretation of the test, in vitro methods for assessing the immune response against MTB have been developed, commonly called **interferon-gamma-release assays (IGRA)**.[38] WBCs isolated from whole blood drawn from the patient are cultured in vitro in the presence of MTB-specific antigens and the amount of interferon-gamma released from stimulated T lymphocytes is measured. Currently, results from the IGRAs are accepted in lieu of TST in many situations, offering a more patient-friendly, reliable, and more standardized test for assessing infection with MTB, although it is still not without challenges in interpretation.[39]

Allergy Testing

Allergies are caused by an exaggerated immune response against a benign antigen found in the environment. Identifying the cause of a patient's allergy is important so the patient can avoid exposure to the cause if at all possible. One way to determine the cause of the allergy is to inject the allergen into the skin and look for a reaction. Skin testing for allergies is performed typically in an allergist's office because the reactions are measured within minutes and there is a risk of anaphylactic shock while undergoing skin testing for allergens. Reactions against almost any allergen, ranging from food items (e.g., nuts, dairy, and shellfish) to environmental agents (e.g., molds and pollens), drugs (e.g., penicillin), and insect venom (e.g., bees and wasps), can be determined by skin testing.[40]

Controlled suspensions of allergens are injected either percutaneously in a prick or scratch test or injected intradermally, similar to the skin test for MTB. Unlike the immune reaction against MTB, however, allergens illicit an **immediate hypersensitivity** response in which IgE bound to mast cells and basophils subsequently binds to an allergen, causing the mast cells and basophils to release their intracellular contents, which include vasoactive agents such as histamine, leukotrienes, and prostaglandins. There is an almost immediate accumulation of fluid at the site of the allergen as the blood vessels at the local site increase their permeability. Redness and swelling (wheal and flare) within 15 minutes is measured and compared to a negative control response. A positive reaction is noted when the reaction to a particular allergen is ≥ 3 mm the reaction to the negative control. Skin testing for food allergens lacks specificity because of some cross-reactions; a better laboratory test to confirm food allergens in particular and also some airborne pathogens is a test in which allergen-specific IgE is measured. Measurement of allergen-specific IgE requires collection of blood and is performed whenever skin tests cannot be performed or when skin test results need confirmation.

Histology and Cytology

Histology narrowly refers to the examination and characterization of tissues from biopsies, whereas *cytology* involves the examination of cells derived from secretions or aspirates. Often the difference between the two fields is blurred and/or combined in the same laboratory. Histology involves examination of tissue by preparing very thin sections of the tissue and staining it with various stains depending on the type of analysis that has been requested. Histological and cytological procedures primarily aim to determine if abnormal host cells (i.e., cells that have changed into tumor cells) are present and then characterize any abnormal cells that are found to refine the diagnosis. For example, the most common type of lung cancer is non-small cell lung cancer, which must be differentiated from small cell lung cancer because of differing treatment regimens. Sometimes, tumor cells that have originated in another tissue may metastasize to the lungs, and determining the origin of those cells will be important for diagnosis and treatment. Another distinction that needs to be made with regard to abnormal cells is whether they are malignant or benign. Malignant cells need to be eliminated, whereas benign abnormal cells may not warrant any treatment.

Histology and cytology are very specialized fields that involve personnel who have undergone extensive training in preparing tissues or cells for staining, performing staining procedures, and examining the stained tissues to find and identify abnormal cells. A technician or technologist will prepare the tissue sections for staining, stain the section, and then perhaps complete an initial review of the slide. An anatomic pathologist, a physician who has specialized in the examination of tissues and cells in order to diagnose disease, reviews all slides and determines whether the tissue is normal or contains abnormal cells.

Techniques used in histology and cytology laboratories include electron microscopy, stains to differentiate between different types of cells, and analysis of DNA or RNA from isolated cells. Electron microscopy and examination of stained tissue determines whether cells are normal or abnormal based on their morphology. Common stains used in histology laboratories include:

- *Hematoxylin and eosin (H&E):* Stains cytoplasm and connective tissue pink and nuclei blue.
- *Periodic acid Schiff (PAS):* stains polysaccharides and is used to stain the glomeruli in a kidney section and glycogen in a liver section.
- *Silver stains:* Stain fungi, spirochetes, basement membranes, and melanin.

Immunohistochemical stains often are used in histology laboratories to assist with the identification of cells based on the expression of different surface markers or antigens on the cells. In an immunohistochemical stain, antibodies with known specificity (called *primary antibodies*) are selected based on the analysis requested and type of tissue submitted and used to identify cells in a tissue section. Chosen antibodies are allowed to bind to corresponding antigens in a tissue section, and unbound antibodies are washed off the tissue. Bound antibody is detected using a labeled secondary antibody that will bind to the primary antibody bound to the tissue. The substrate for the label (typically an enzyme, such as horseradish peroxidase) on the secondary antibody will be added, and the label will convert the substrate to a colored product wherever the antibody was bound. Examination of the tissue under the microscope will reveal the distribution of the antigen and the identity of the cells.

Molecular Diagnostics

Molecular diagnostics refers to the analysis of nucleic acids—DNA and RNA—in order to determine the cause of disease or to refine the diagnosis of disease. A variety of diseases are now targeted by nucleic acid analysis, from inherited diseases, such as Huntington disease and fragile X syndrome, to cancer and infectious diseases, especially viral diseases. Molecular diagnostics encompasses isolation, amplification, and/or sequencing of nucleic acids. Clinical applications of nucleic acid analysis exploded after Kary Mullis envisioned the enzymatic amplification of DNA, which became known as the polymerase chain reaction (PCR), in 1983 and published the first description and application in 1985,[41] followed by a publication describing the method in detail.[42] From that innocuous beginning to 30 years later, there are hundreds of nucleic acid—based tests that have been approved for clinical use by the Food and Drug Administration (FDA)[43] and many more that have been developed and are employed in individual laboratories as "home-brew" assays.

In the early days of molecular-based tests, procedures were manual, time consuming, and cost prohibitive for almost everyone. Now, these tests are highly automated and performed with results obtained more likely in minutes than days, although they are still among the most expensive tests performed in the clinical laboratory. The high specificity and sensitivity of molecular-based tests, together with the ability to obtain rapid results that can be used to quickly make decisions about patient care, however, have driven the incorporation of these methodologies into almost all medium- and large-sized laboratories, if not small-sized laboratories. Cost savings are realized when overall treatment and hospitalization costs are decreased due to faster realization of actual causes of disease with concomitant implementation of appropriate treatment.

PCR involves copying DNA using DNA polymerase similarly to how a cell replicates DNA in vivo. The process starts by denaturing double-stranded DNA to single-stranded DNA. Next, primers (short pieces of DNA) that have been designed to bind specifically to a sequence of nucleotides either in or around a sequence of interest bind to the target sequence if present in the sample. After the primers bind to the target sequence, DNA polymerase adds nucleotides to the primers that are complementary to bases in the target (template) DNA, thereby making a single-stranded piece of DNA double stranded. When the newly synthesized double-stranded DNA is denatured, the primers bind (anneal) to the target sequence and DNA polymerase adds nucleotides, making another copy of double-stranded DNA. Each of the three steps, denaturation, annealing, and extension, comprise one cycle and are driven by changing temperature in the reaction vial in an instrument called a thermal cycler. After each cycle, the amount of DNA doubles, with millions of copies of target DNA being made after the 25 to 35 cycles that are performed in a typical PCR reaction.

Since Mullis first described PCR, other scientists have developed methods to amplify DNA, for example, transcription-mediated amplification (TMA), nucleic acid sequence–based amplification (NASBA), and branched DNA signal amplification. Modifications to the original PCR procedure have also been created to expand the functionality of the assay. For example, in reverse transcriptase PCR (RT-PCR), reverse transcriptase is used to make a DNA copy of an RNA template and then the complementary DNA is put through PCR; in multiplex PCR, multiple sets of primers are added to DNA or RNA isolated from the sample so as to amplify multiple target genes; and, in real-time or quantitative PCR (qPCR), the amplification of nucleic acid is measured at the same time new copies of nucleic acid are produced, decreasing the time and eliminating extra procedural steps needed to detect product nucleic acid.[44,45] Also, with qPCR the amount of target nucleic acid originally in the specimen is calculated based on the rate of amplicon production. For patients with HIV, cytomegalovirus, hepatitis B virus, and hepatitis C virus, in particular, the **viral load**—the quantity of nucleic acid in a sample—is used for prognosis as well as monitoring the effectiveness of antiviral treatment and has significantly changed patient care for these infections.[46–49]

Although the sensitivity and specificity of PCR and other nucleic acid amplification procedures approach 100%, it is important to know that false-positive and false-negative results can occur in molecular-based tests just as they do in other laboratory methods. False-positive results occur when samples become contaminated with previously produced PCR products (amplicons), and so methods have been developed to minimize contamination by separating the activities involved in setting up PCR reactions and assaying for the production of amplicons. Another common cause of false-positive PCR results is the presence of nucleic acid from dead or dying microorganisms. A patient who is undergoing treatment for infection will remain positive by molecular-based tests longer than by culture-based tests because the nucleic acid from the dying microorganism can still be amplified and give a positive result. False-negative results occur when there is less than the detectable limit of nucleic acid present in the sample or the nucleic acid gets degraded by poor specimen collection, storage, or processing conditions. Although molecular-based assays have high sensitivity and theoretically only one copy of target DNA or RNA is needed to start the amplification process, in reality there still needs to be hundreds of copies of nucleic acid in the sample for amplification to occur.

For the respiratory care clinician, the most relevant molecular-based tests are those that are used to diagnose infectious disease of the respiratory tract. Interestingly, this is an area of laboratory testing that has seen the most improvement in terms of detection of microorganisms, especially viruses, and the speed at which they are detected. Multiplex nucleic acid amplification assays have been developed and successfully implemented in the clinical laboratory to detect multiple respiratory pathogens, either bacterial or viral or both, from a single nasal aspirate, nasopharyngeal swab, or bronchoalveolar lavage sample.[50,51]

Nineteen different viruses are known to cause acute respiratory disease. Some are well-known pathogens: influenza A and B viruses, adenovirus, parainfluenza virus (PIV) types 1 through 4, rhinovirus, coronavirus, and respiratory syncytial virus (RSV). Others are newly recognized or emerging viruses: human metapneumovirus (hMPV), bocavirus, parvovirus types 4 and 5, and mimivirus. Whereas some viruses are more associated with causing serious respiratory tract disease (e.g., influenza A virus), and others are generally ignored because disease is typically not significant (e.g., rhinovirus), all of the respiratory viruses can cause significant respiratory tract disease in the right host, requiring hospitalization and respiratory support. Occasionally these viruses may cause death. In addition, newly described antigenic variants of some of the respiratory viruses emerge regularly, challenging the laboratory community to keep up with changing viruses. For example, recently described variants of influenza A virus (e.g., novel H1N1[52], H5N1[53], and H7N9[54]), as well as new variants of coronavirus, (e.g., severe acute respiratory syndrome [SARS])[55] and MERS-CoV[56]), have required adjustments in laboratory methods to detect these new variants.

Nineteen or more different virus types or subtypes may cause respiratory tract disease, but in reality only a fraction of those are isolated with any frequency; laboratory tests do not need to routinely detect 19 viruses, although those tests are available.[57] Commonly used assays in the clinical laboratory simultaneously detect either 12 viruses (xTAG™ Respiratory Viral Panel, Luminex Molecular Diagnostics, Toronto, Canada); 17 viruses along with 3 bacteria (FilmArray Respiratory Panel, Idaho Technology, Inc., Salt Lake City, UT); or 18 viruses (ResPlex II plus panel PRE version 2.0, Qiagen, Hilden, Germany).[58] Multiplex molecular-based assays for the detection of bacterial respiratory pathogens detect, at a minimum, *Chlamydophila pneumoniae*, *Mycoplasma pneumoniae*, and *Legionella pneumophila*, the most common bacterial pathogens in the respiratory tract (Chlamylege, bioMerieux Argene, Verniolle, France)[59] and may also include *Bordetella pertussis* and *L. micdadei* (Pneumoplex, Prodesse, Waukesha, WI).[50] Implementation of molecular-based assays in general has significantly decreased the turnaround time as well as increased the detection and identification of respiratory pathogens, making a significant impact on patient care.[51]

Finally, diagnosis and management of MTB has also been significantly improved with the implementation of molecular-based tests in the clinical laboratory.[60] Before molecular-based tests were available for the direct detection of MTB in clinical specimens, laboratory tests for the detection of MTB relied on the isolation of the organism in culture, which took weeks, followed by identification using biochemical tests, which also took about a week, and then a few weeks to determine the antimicrobial susceptibility of the isolate, for a total of at least 3 to 4 weeks. In the early 1990s, DNA-based probes (AccuProbe, GenProbe, San Diego, CA) became available to identify colonies of MTB, eliminating the biochemical testing of colonies suspected of being MTB and saving a week of time, because the DNA-based probes only take a few hours to perform once colony growth is noted. In the mid to late 1990s, nucleic acid amplification assays were approved by the FDA to detect MTB directly in smear-positive respiratory specimens initially and are currently approved for all specimen types. The direct detection of MTB in clinical specimens saves weeks of time that had been needed for the organism to grow to detectable levels. Now, in just a few hours, the nucleic acid of the organism can be amplified and detected. In addition, genes associated with resistance to antitubercular drugs, (e.g. Rifampin and isoniazid) can be detected in a few hours using nucleic amplification procedures and provide information to the clinician about the appropriate treatment modality for the patient.[61]

In conclusion, scientists in the clinical microbiology laboratory perform procedures designed to detect and identify microorganisms, bacteria, mycobacteria, viruses, fungi, and parasites present in clinical specimens. The procedures used include stains, cultures, and nucleic acid amplification and analysis. As with all types of laboratory tests, the analysis of results provided by the clinical microbiologist need to be interpreted along with information derived from the patient history, symptoms, physical exam, and other diagnostic tests in order to determine the clinical relevance of a result. Remember that many microorganisms can be found as normal flora or contaminants of body fluids and secretions and these organisms should not be the focus of antimicrobial therapy. Determination of whether an infectious process is present, the cause, and the appropriate antimicrobial therapy is complex and requires cooperation between many different healthcare professionals.

Summary

To summarize, tests performed in the diagnostic clinical laboratory are used to diagnose, monitor, and make treatment decisions on patients requiring respiratory care. Laboratory studies related to hematology, clinical chemistry, microbiology, assessment of sputum, urinalysis, skin testing, histology and cytology, and molecular diagnostics provide invaluable information to the respiratory care clinician. Laboratory testing can identify a large number of disease states and conditions that affect the cardiopulmonary system ranging from blood disorders, fluid and electrolyte problems, impaired kidney or liver function, cardiac disorders, cancer, allergy, and infection. The respiratory care clinician should be able to identify needed laboratory studies and interpret the associated results in order to provide the best and most appropriate care to patients.

Key Points

▶ Scientists in the diagnostic laboratory perform and interpret complex tests that are used in the diagnosis, treatment, and monitoring of disease.

▶ Hematology involves the analysis of the cellular components of blood.

▶ Erythrocytes, leukocytes, and thrombocytes are cells found in blood.

▶ The complete blood count (CBC) is a screening test used to assess quantity and quality of cells in the blood.

▶ Prothrombin time (PT; INR) and activated partial thromboplastin time (aPTT) are tests used to assess coagulation function.

▶ Hemoglobin is a protein found in red blood cells (RBCs) that transports oxygen.

▶ Hematocrit is a laboratory determination of the percentage of the blood volume that is red blood cells and is different from the RBC count.

▶ The mean corpuscular volume (MCV) is a measurement of the size of the red blood cells.

▶ The weight of hemoglobin in a RBC count is measured as the mean corpuscular hemoglobin (MCH).

▶ The MCH content is a measurement of the percentage of hemoglobin in the RBC.

▶ The inability to transport oxygen because of reduced or defective red blood cells results in anemia.

▶ Leukocytes are either neutrophils, lymphocytes, monocytes, eosinophils, or basophils.

▶ Segmented neutrophils (PMN/Seg) are the most numerous and are primarily responsible for getting rid of bacteria.

▶ Lymphocytes are primarily involved in antiviral immune responses.

▶ Monocytes are the major cell type that engages in phagocytosis to eliminate pathogens and abnormal cells.

▶ Eosinophils are primarily responsible for immediate hypersensitivity reactions (allergies) and antiparasitic immune responses.

▶ Basophils are a minor cell type involved in allergies and antiparasitic immune responses.

▶ Thrombocytes (platelets) function in coagulation.

▶ Defects in coagulation can either cause the abnormal production of thrombi or lack of clotting, leading to bleeding.

▶ The three forms of diabetes mellitus—type 1, type 2, and gestational—are diagnosed by measuring serum glucose and finding elevated levels.

▶ Hemoglobin A_{1C} (A1C) is measured to indicate the overall blood glucose level over a 2- to 3-month period.

▶ Kidney disease is indicated by elevations in blood urea nitrogen (BUN) and creatinine.

▶ The presence of albumin in urine (microalbuminuria) is a more sensitive indicator of kidney disease.

▶ Cardiac troponin is measured at least twice (spaced several hours apart) in the diagnosis of myocardial infarction.

▶ Respiratory tract infections can be caused by bacteria, viruses, fungi, or parasites.

▶ *Pseudomonas aeruginosa* and *Klebsiella pneumoniae* are the most common causes of pneumonia in hospitalized patients.

▶ *Legionella pneumophila*, *Chlamydophila pneumoniae*, *Mycoplasma pneumoniae*, and *Bordetella pertussis* are the most common causes of community-acquired pneumonia.

▶ The Gram stain is the most common stain used for the direct detection of bacteria in a clinical specimen.

▶ The Fluorochrome, Ziehl-Neelsen, and Kinyoun stains are used for the direct detection of mycobacteria.

▶ Expectorated sputum that is representative of the lower respiratory tract will have very few epithelial cells.

▶ Direct smears will only give a certain amount of information about the cause of an infection, and definitive culture or molecular-based assays will be required to identify an organism.

▶ Sputum contains oropharyngeal flora and thus is not a sterile specimen.

▶ Various types of media—enriched, selective, and selective-differential—are used to isolate bacteria from clinical specimens.

▶ Bacteria that are isolated from specimens are identified as well as tested for susceptibility to antimicrobial agents to assist with treatment decisions.

▶ Urinalysis includes macroscopic, microscopic, and chemical analyses.

▶ Normal urine is the color of straw or amber and is clear, not cloudy.

▶ Chemical analysis of urine involves the measurement of the specific gravity, pH, protein, ketones, glucose, nitrites, leukocyte esterase, blood, urobilinogen and bilirubin.

▶ The identification of cells, crystals, and casts is made in the microscopic analysis of urine.

▶ Urine can be used as the specimen of choice for the diagnosis of pneumonia caused by *Streptococcus pneumoniae* and *Legionella pneumophila* using antigen detection tests.

▶ Delayed-type hypersensitivity (DTH) is measured when assessing exposure to *Mycobacterium tuberculosis*.

▶ Gamma-interferon release assays are an alternative to DTH tests for MTB.

▶ Immediate hypersensitivities (allergies) can be identified by skin tests in which the immune response to individual allergens is measured.

▶ Tumors are detected and described in histology and cytology laboratories.

▶ Molecular-based tests involve the isolation, amplification, detection, and/or characterization of DNA and RNA.

▶ The first nucleic acid amplification assay to be developed was the polymerase chain reaction (PCR) in which DNA is denatured and bound by primers. Nucleotides are then added by DNA polymerase, making a new piece of double-stranded DNA.

▶ Multiplex nucleic acid amplification assays are used to identify the presence of viruses and/or bacteria in specimens.

CLINICAL FOCUS 9-1

Acute Respiratory Tract Infection

A previously healthy 55-year-old woman presents to her primary care physician in February complaining of cough, shortness of breath, malaise, and headaches over the past 3 days. She has been running a fever over that time that has been between 100° and 102° F. She has tried ibuprofen and cold medicine with limited relief. The woman works as a home health nurse and enjoys relaxing in the evenings in her hot tub. A few of her patients have had respiratory tract infections without specific cause, which is not unusual given the time of year. The patient lives with her husband, who has been healthy.

What could be causing this woman's symptoms?

Answer: Because it is February, respiratory viruses, especially influenza virus, should be considered. Given that she was previously healthy, causes of community-acquired pneumonia should also be considered. Typical causes of community-acquired pneumonia include *Streptococcus pneumoniae, Haemophilus influenzae, Legionella pneumophila, Staphylococcus aureus,* Group A streptococci, *Moxacella catarrhalis*, certain anaerobes, and gram-negative bacteria. Atypical causes of community-acquired pneumonia include *Mycoplasma pneumoniae, Chlamydophila pneumonia,* and *Coxiella burnetii.* Hypersensitivity pneumonitis can result from environmental exposures (e.g., pet birds or hot tubs).

What laboratory tests would you order to identify the causative agent?

Answer: To detect respiratory viruses, a nasopharyngeal swab or aspirate should be collected and sent for a respiratory virus panel test involving amplification of viral nucleic acid. For suspected community acquired pneumonia, a complete blood count (CBC) and chest x-ray should be obtained. Most patients with community-acquired pneumonia are treated without laboratory isolation of the offending organism. Sputum cultures, blood cultures, and urinary antigen testing may be of value, depending on the patient's presentation. For example, patients admitted to the intensive care unit (ICU) and those with pleural effusion may have blood and sputum cultures performed, as well as urinary antigen testing for *Legionella* and pneumococcal antigens. For *Legionella*, a sputum or bronchoalveolar lavage (BAL) specimen should be sent for culture. It should be noted that BAL dilutes the number of organisms and suctioned sputum may have higher yield. *Mycoplasma* and *Chlamydophila* (chlamydia) may be diagnosed by collecting blood and requesting that antibodies to these organisms (IgM and IgG) be measured; however, PCR of upper airway specimens is now becoming available. New viral PCR swabs now include mycoplasma, chlamydia, and pertussis.

What information given in the history suggests where she may have acquired this organism?

Answer: She could have acquired an infection from her patients given that some of them were also sick with lower respiratory tract disease. Hot tubs can be a source of *Legionella* or a cause of hypersensitivity pneumonitis (allergic response to *Mycobacterium avium* complex [MAC]).

CLINICAL FOCUS 9-2

Persistent Cough

The patient is a 44-year-old African American male who is incarcerated in an Illinois state prison for murder. He has already served 10 years of his life sentence. He acquired HIV and hepatitis C virus from his fellow inmates shortly after he arrived at the prison. He has been a smoker for 30 years and trades sex for smokes and other favors from inmates and guards.

He presents to the prison infirmary complaining of a persistent and productive cough over the last month. It is January, and although all the inmates got the "flu" vaccine in November, he still thinks that he has the "flu." He also complains of fever and waking up in the morning with his sheets all wet because he has been sweating profusely all night. He has lost 15 pounds in the last month and had to get new clothes because his other clothes were too big.

What could be causing this inmate's symptoms?

Answer: Given the time of year, a respiratory virus is possible although the patient states that he has had the symptoms for a month, which would likely rule out a respiratory virus given that those infections are generally more self-limiting. He could have a bacterial pneumonia caused by *Streptococcus pneumoniae, Haemophilus influenzae, Legionella pneumophila, Staphylococcus aureus,* or gram-negative bacteria; however, these also cause symptoms for days to a week prior to presentation. Atypical causes of pneumonia include *Mycoplasma pneumonia, Chlamydophila psittaci,* and *Coxiella burnetii. Mycobacterium tuberculosis* should also be considered given the duration of symptoms and presence of a productive cough, night sweats, and weight loss. In HIV-positive patients, opportunistic infections such as *Pneumocystis* pneumonia, atypical mycobacteria, cytomegalovirus (CMV), and fungi must be included in the differential.

What laboratory tests would you order to identify the causative agent?

Answer: To detect respiratory viruses, a nasopharyngeal swab or aspirate should be collected and sent for a respiratory virus panel test involving amplification of viral nucleic acid. For suspected community-acquired pneumonia, a chest radiograph and complete blood count (CBC) should be obtained. Sputum and blood cultures for evaluation of community-acquired pneumonia remain controversial. A positive tuberculin test (PPD) will indicate exposure to tuberculosis (TB), but not necessarily active disease. HIV patients with a positive tuberculin test, however, are much more likely to have active disease. Note that many labs now run interferon-gamma release assays in lieu of PPD.

For *Legionella,* a sputum or bronchoalveolar lavage (preferred) specimen may be sent for culture for *Legionella. Mycoplasma* and *Chlamydophila* are best diagnosed by collecting blood and requesting that antibodies to these organisms (IgM and IgG) be measured or by PCR of airway secretions.

Sputum or bronchoalveolar lavage may also be cultured for unusual causes of pneumonia (e.g., aerobic culture, fungi, CMV, *Pneumocystis* pneumonia, or atypical mycobacteria) as well as for *Mycobacterium tuberculosis.*

What information given in the history suggests where he may have acquired this organism?

Answer: Living in a prison puts inmates at risk for acquiring any of the organisms considered here, but compared to people living in other group situations inmates are particular at risk for acquiring *Mycobacterium tuberculosis.* Inmates and prison employees should be screened at least annually for TB, and infected personnel should be treated appropriately and put on respiratory precautions until they are determined to be no longer infectious.

CLINICAL FOCUS 9-3

Fungal Lung Disease

The patient is a 65-year-old retired man living in Phoenix, Arizona, who presents to his primary care physician in October complaining of cough, fever, chest pain, headache, muscle aches, and fatigue over the last month. The man has type 2 diabetes and hypertension, both of which are being controlled by medication and diet. The man and his wife retired to Phoenix 2 years ago from Minnesota and are enjoying the hot, dry weather so much that they are rarely inside. The man enjoys golfing, gardening, and swimming. Only the dust storms could convince him to go inside, and that was only after he couldn't take the dust in his eyes any longer.

What could be causing this man's symptoms?

Answer: Respiratory viruses are not likely in this case given the time of year and the duration of symptoms. He could have a community-acquired bacterial pneumonia. In addition, given that he lives in Arizona and is outside during dust storms, *Coccidioides immitis* should also be considered.

What laboratory tests would you order to identify the causative agent?

Answer: Sputum or bronchoalveolar lavage should be examined for usual bacterial causes of pneumonia as well as for fungi to rule out *Coccidioides* or *Histoplasma.* Fungi will grow in specialized laboratory media. Gram stains of respiratory tract secretions will not identify coccidioides sphericals, although a silver stain (GMS) or calcofluor stain may allow for visualization of fungi.

What information given in the history suggests where he may have acquired this organism?

Answer: The fact that he lives in Phoenix, Arizona, is mostly healthy, and spends a great deal of time outdoors strongly suggests that he could have Valley Fever caused by *Coccidioides immitis* (e.g., coccidiomycosis). The organism is acquired by inhaling spores from the soil that are aerosolized during dust storms.

CLINICAL FOCUS 9-4

Aspiration

The patient is a 45-year-old man who has been intubated for 7 days in cardiac intensive care following a presumed heart attack due to significant cardiovascular disease. Although the patient aspirated during intubation, chest x-rays were negative 2 days later. Seven days after intubation, the patient's temperature increased to 100° F. A complete blood count (CBC) and differential showed an overall increase in white blood cells, with an increased percentage of neutrophils in particular. Other indices measured in the CBC were normal. Chest x-ray at this time showed presence of a pulmonary infiltrate. Tracheobronchial secretions were noted to be purulent. Ventilator settings required adjustment due to increased respiratory rate, decreased tidal volume, and decreased oxygenation.

What could be causing this man's symptoms?

Answer: This man has a ventilator-associated pneumonia (VAP). This is a nosocomial infection due to the presence of the mechanical ventilator. The most common organisms causing VAP are the gram-negative bacilli, including *Pseudomonas aeruginosa*, *Acinetobacter* spp., *Stenotrophomonas maltophilia*, and *Klebsiella pneumoniae*.

What laboratory tests would you order to identify the causative agent?

Answer: Tracheobronchial secretions should be sent to the clinical microbiology laboratory for aerobic culture. Blood cultures could also be collected and sent to microbiology. The organism causing a respiratory tract infection will not only be isolated in respiratory tract secretions but also in a blood culture (10% to 15%) and the finding of the same organism in both specimens helps confirm that the organism is the causative agent.

What information given in the history suggests where he may have acquired this organism?

Answer: The man has been intubated and spikes a fever after 7 days on the ventilator. Given that there was no suggestion of respiratory tract disease when he was admitted and ventilated, the source of the infection is due to the prolonged ventilation, a fairly common event.

CLINICAL FOCUS 9-5

Cystic Fibrosis

The patient is a 10-year-old girl who was diagnosed with cystic fibrosis (CF) when she was 1 month old. She lives in Houston, Texas, with her parents and older brother, who does not have CF. Her father is a quarterback for the Houston Texans NFL team. Her mother is a socialite/homemaker.

The girl has received the best care from the best CF specialists in the country. She has been reasonably healthy her whole life and has enjoyed a relatively normal life. She takes her medications religiously, and her mother gives her the "chest/back thumping" therapy every night to reduce the congestion that is always present.

The patient was getting prepared to go to Girl Scout camp with her troop when she woke up one morning with increased congestion in her lungs and a temperature of 38° C. She started coughing and having trouble breathing. She was sick for about 2 days, missing her camping trip, and then her mom brought her to the physician.

What could be causing this girl's symptoms?

Answer: Infections in patients with CF are typically caused by *Pseudomonas aeruginosa* or *Burkholderia cepacia*, although they may also have *Staphylococcus aureus* or *Haemophilus influenzae*. *Pseudomonas* infection usually occurs after CF patients are treated with multiple courses of antibiotics.

What laboratory tests would you order to identify the causative agent?

Answer: Sputum should be submitted for aerobic culture with specification that the patient has CF, because many laboratories have a specific protocol for processing CF sputa due to their typically thick mucus, which requires special processing such that bacteria present are liberated in order to be able to grow on artificial media. In addition, CF sputa protocols will include the utilization of additional culture media directed at isolating *Burkholderia cepacia* and *Haemophilus influenzae* in particular.

What information given in the history suggests where she may have acquired this organism?

Answer: The only relevant information seems to be the fact that she has CF, which makes her more susceptible to respiratory tract infections with difficult-to-treat organisms (e.g., *Pseudomonas aeruginosa*, *Burkholderia cepacia*, and methicillin-resistant *Staphylococcus* [MRSA]).

CLINICAL FOCUS 9-6

Viral Infection

The patient is a 32-year-old woman who presented to the Urgent Care Center in suburban Chicago in December complaining of fever, malaise, fatigue, sore throat, headache, fever, nausea, and aches. The woman is a trader on the Chicago Option Exchange and has been working extra hours because it seems as if everyone else has been out sick. She has no underlying disease and has been healthy prior to this presentation. She is single and works out at a gym near her house, although she has had having difficulty even getting out of bed the last few days.

What could be causing this woman's symptoms?

Answer: Since it was December, respiratory viruses, especially influenza virus, should be considered. Since she was previously healthy, causes of community-acquired pneumonia should also be considered.

What laboratory tests would you order to identify the causative agent?

Answer: To detect respiratory viruses, a nasopharyngeal swab or aspirate should be collected and sent for a respiratory virus panel test involving amplification of viral nucleic acid. Sputum cultures for bacterial pneumonia remain controversial. For suspected *Legionella*, a sputum or bronchoalveolar lavage specimen may be sent for culture for *Legionella*. *Mycoplasma* and *Chlamydophila* are diagnosed by collecting blood and requesting that antibodies to these organisms (IgM and IgG) be measured or by PCR of upper airway secretions.

What information given in the history suggests where she may have acquired this organism?

Answer: Given the time of year and the fact that many of her coworkers were out sick, it is likely that she has influenza virus or other respiratory virus. Traders who engage in open exchange pits where saliva is being aerosolized from constant yelling are at risk of acquiring respiratory tract infections. Treatment with antiviral therapy within 48 hours of symptoms reduces the duration of influenza.

CLINICAL FOCUS 9-7

Dyspnea, Cough, and Sputum Production

The patient is a 70-year-old male who presents to his primary care physician for his annual physical. The man has a history of type 2 diabetes, hypertension, and chronic cough with production of sputum. The man had smoked cigarettes for 40 years of his life, but for the last 20 years had not smoked at all. He is a social alcohol drinker. The man has lived a fairly sedentary life since retiring from teaching. He has lived in Chicago, Illinois, his entire whole life and has only traveled either within the United States, mostly to places within short driving distances in the last 20 years, or on cruises to Panama and Europe more recently.

   The man is sedentary because of extreme knee pain and because even slight exertion leaves him breathless and makes his chest hurt. Breathlessness, productive cough, and chest pain seem to be increasing over the last 3 months.

What could be causing this man's symptoms?

Answer: Given that his history suggests more of a chronic disease than an acute one, most infectious organisms would be ruled out. There is nothing in his history to suggest fungal or mycobacterial causes of infection. His symptoms are more consistent with chronic obstructive pulmonary disease (COPD) that seems to be progressing.

What laboratory tests would you order to identify the cause?

Answer: Although not a clinical laboratory test, spirometry should be performed to assess lung function. Chest x-ray can provide some information about progression of the disease. Arterial blood gases can provide information about how severe his disease is and can be compared to previous results to determine if the disease is progressing. Alpha-1 antitrypsin (AAT) levels can be measured because a deficiency in AAT is associated with an increased development of COPD as well as emphysema. Chest x-ray and spirometry would also help assess interstitial lung disease secondary to collagen vascular disorders (e.g., rheumatoid arthritis).

CLINICAL FOCUS 9-8

Chest Discomfort

A 58-year-old woman went to the local emergency department (ED) because of shortness of breath even when she was sitting and feeling more tired than usual over the last few days, along with some back pain. The woman was a professor of biology at the University of Minnesota. She was morbidly obese and known to have type 2 diabetes.

   The woman reported that she felt like an elephant was sitting on her over the past 2 hours. She was also sweating, even though her temperature in the ED was about 96°F. She stated that she felt nauseous and dizzy and had intermittent feelings of heartburn more than usual.

What could be causing the women's symptoms?

Answer: Acute cardiopulmonary disease, including possible myocardial infarction (MI), must be considered.

What additional information should be gathered in the ED?

Answer: Vital signs and electrocardiogram (ECG) should be assessed and laboratory testing should be performed to include complete blood count (CBC), blood glucose, C-reactive protein, cardiac troponin, and chest x-ray. CBC may be helpful in identifying possible anemia or increased white blood cell (WBC) count associated with infection. C-reactive protein is an inflammatory marker; higher levels are associated with development of heart failure, diabetes, and adverse cardiovascular events. Blood glucose should be monitored in patients with diabetes mellitus and for management of plasma glucose. Cardiac troponins T and I are the preferred biomarkers to assess for acute MI.

   Upon physical examination, it was noted that the woman's heart rate was increased and irregular. Her respiratory rate was increased, as was her blood pressure. Laboratory tests and results at admission were as follows:

- ECG showed ST-segment elevation with increased heart rate.
- CBC monitor was normal for WBCs (count and differential) as well as red blood cells (RBCs) and platelets.

- C-reactive protein was increased.
- Blood glucose (nonfasting) was 210 mg/dL.
- Cardiac troponin at admission was above normal reference range levels.
- Arterial blood gas showed decreased Pao_2, decreased $Paco_2$, and slightly elevated pH.

Laboratory tests and results 3 hours after admission were as follows:

- Cardiac troponin increased above admission levels.
- CBC showed increased WBCs with an increase in polymorphonuclear cells, normal RBCs, and decreased platelets.

What could be causing this woman's symptoms?

Answer: The woman's presentation and results of her physical examination, ECG monitor, and laboratory tests strongly suggest that she is having a myocardial infarction.

What additional diagnostic tests would be needed?

Answer: An ECG should be performed to assess heart function. Chest x-ray may help rule out pneumonia. B-type natriuretic peptide can be measured to further confirm a diagnosis of heart failure. CK and CKMb (cardiac muscle enzymes) support the diagnosis of myocardial infarction.

References

1. Tefferi A, Hanson C, Inwards DJ. How to interpret and pursue an abnormal complete blood cell count in adults: concise review for clinicians. *Mayo Clin Proc.* 2006;80:923–936.
2. Harmening D. *Clinical Hematology and Fundamentals of Hemostasis,* 5th ed. Philadelphia: F. A. Davis; 2008.
3. Lichtman, MA, Beutler E, Kipps, TJ, Seligsohn U, Kaushansky K, Prchal JT. *Williams Hematology,* 7th ed. New York: McGraw Hill; 2006.
4. Rodak B, Fritsma G, Doig K. *Hematology: Clinical Principal and Applications,* 3rd ed. St. Louis, MO: Elsevier; 2008.
5. Rodak B, Carr J (2008). *Clinical Hematology Atlas,* 3rd ed. St. Louis, MO: Elsevier; 2008.
6. Turgeon ML. *Clinical Hematology Theory and Procedures,* 3rd ed. Philadelphia: Lippincott Williams & Wilkins; 2005.
7. Deutsch VR, Tomer A. Megakaryocyte development and platelet production. *Br J Haematol.* 2006;134(5):453–466.
8. Tanaka K, Key N, Levy J. Blood coagulation: hemostasis and thrombin regulation. *Anesth Analg.* 2009;108(5):1433–1446.
9. Burtis CA, Ashwood ER, Bruns DE (eds.). *Tietz Fundamentals of Clinical Chemistry,* 6th ed. St. Louis, MO: Saunders; 2008.
10. Comprehensive metabolic panel. Lab Tests Online. August 30, 2012. http://labtestsonline.org/understanding/analytes/cmp/tab/test. Accessed December 13, 2013.
11. Dufour DR. Sources and control of preanalytical variation. In: Kaplan LA, Pesce AJ (eds.). *Clinical Chemistry: Theory, Analysis, Correlation.* St. Louis, MO: Mosby; 2010: 322–341.
12. American Diabetes Association. Standards of medical care in diabetes—2013. *Diabetes Care.* 2013;36(suppl 1):S11–S66.
13. Kaplan JM, First MR. Renal Function. In: Kaplan LA, Pesce AJ (eds.). *Clinical Chemistry: Theory, Analysis, Correlation.* St. Louis, MO: Mosby; 2010: 567–585.
14. Sunheimer RL, Graves L. Amino acids and proteins. In: Sunheimer RL, Graves L. *Clinical Laboratory Chemistry.* Upper Saddle River, NJ: Pearson; 2011: 179–199.
15. *ATP III Guidelines At-A-Glance Quick Desk Reference.* NIH Publication No. 01-3305, May 2001. Washington, DC: U.S. Department of Health and Human Services. http://www.nhlbi.nih.gov/guidelines/cholesterol/dskref.htm. Accessed December 19, 2013.
16. Sunheimer RL, Graves L. Cardiac function. In: Sunheimer RL, Graves L. *Clinical Laboratory Chemistry.* Upper Saddle River, NJ: Pearson; 2011: 390–412.
17. Dufour DR. The liver: function and chemical pathology. In: Kaplan LA, Pesce AJ (eds.). *Clinical Chemistry: Theory, Analysis, Correlation.* St. Louis, MO: Mosby; 2010: 586–600.
18. Lorenz JM. Physiology and pathophysiology of body water and electrolytes. In: Kaplan LA, Pesce AJ (eds.). *Clinical Chemistry: Theory, Analysis, Correlation.* St. Louis, MO: Mosby; 2010: 527–549.
19. Dufour RD. The pancreas: function and chemical pathology. In: Kaplan LA, Pesce AJ (eds.). *Clinical Chemistry: Theory, Analysis, Correlation.* St. Louis, MO: Mosby; 2010: 651–676.
20. Sunheimer RL, Graves L. Body water and electrolyte homeostasis. In: Sunheimer RL, Graves L. *Clinical Laboratory Chemistry.* Upper Saddle River, NJ: Pearson; 2011: 265–282.
21. Sherwin JE. Acid-base control and acid-base disorders. In: Kaplan LA, Pesce AJ (eds.). *Clinical Chemistry: Theory, Analysis, Correlation.* St. Louis, MO: Mosby; 2010: 550–566.
22. Oussama I, Tsang RC. Bone disease. In: Kaplan LA, Pesce AJ (eds.). *Clinical Chemistry: Theory, Analysis, Correlation.* St. Louis, MO: Mosby; 2010: 550–566.
23. Baron EJ, Miller JM, Weinstein MP, et al. A guide to utilization of the microbiology laboratory for diagnosis of infectious diseases: 2013 recommendations by the Infectious Diseases Society of America (IDSA) and the American Society for Microbiology (ASM). *Clin Infect Dis.* 2013;57(4):e22–e121.
24. Carroll KC. 2002. Laboratory diagnosis of lower respiratory tract infections: controversy and conundrums. *J Clin Microbiol.* 40(9):3115–3120.
25. Baron EJ, Thomson Jr, RB. Specimen collection, transport, and processing: bacteriology. In: Versalovic J, Carroll KC, Funke G, Jorgensen JH, Landry ML, Warnock DW (eds.). *Manual of Clinical Microbiology,* 10th ed. Washington, DC: ASM Press; 2009: 228–272.

26. Anevlavis S, Petroglou N, Tzavaras A, et al. A prospective study of the diagnostic utility of sputum Gram stain in pneumonia. *J Infect.* 2009;59(2):83–89.

27. Wieser A, Schneider L, Jung J, Schubert S. MALDI-TOF MS in microbiological diagnostics—identification of microorganisms and beyond. *Appl Microbiol Biotechnol.* 2012;93(3):965–974.

28. Muthukumar A, Zitterkopf NL, Payne D. Molecular tools for the detection and characterization of bacterial infections: a review. *Lab Med.* 2008;39(7):430–436.

29. Kuper KM, Boles DM, Mohr JF, Wanger A. Antimicrobial susceptibility testing: a primer for clinicians. *Pharmacotherapy.* 2009;29(11):1326–1343.

30. Simmerville JA, Maxted WC, Pahira JJ. Urinalysis: a comprehensive review. *Am Fam Physician.* 2005;71(6):1153–1162.

31. Ringsrud KM, Linne JJ. *Urinalysis and Body Fluids. A Colortext and Atlas.* St. Louis, MO: Mosby; 1995.

32. Wever PC, Yzerman EPF, Kuijper EJ, Speelman P, Dankert J. Rapid diagnosis of Legionnaires' disease using an immunochromatographic assay for *Legionella pneumophila* serogroup 1 antigen in urine during an outbreak in the Netherlands. *J Clin Microbiol.* 2000;38:2738–2739.

33. Murdoch DR, Laing RTR, Mills GD, et al. Evaluation of a rapid immunochromatographic test for the detection of *Streptococcus pneumoniae* antigen in urine samples from adults with community-acquired pneumonia. *J Clin Microbiol.* 2001;39(10):3495–3498.

34. Kohler RB, Winn Jr, WC, Wheat LJ. Onset and duration of urinary antigen excretion in Legionnaires disease. *J Clin Microbiol.* 1984;20(4):605–607.

35. Dionne M, Hatchette T, Forward K. Clinical utility of a *Legionella pneumophila* urinary antigen test in a large university teaching hospital. *Can J Infect Dis.* 2003;14(2):85–88.

36. Yang H, Kruh-Garcia NA, Dobos KM. Purified protein derivatives of tuberculin—past, present, and future. *FEMS Immunol Med Microbiol.* 2012;66(3):273–280.

37. Nayak S, Acharjya B. Mantoux test and its interpretation. *Indian Dermatol Online J.* 2012;3(1): 2–6.

38. Pal M, Zwerling A, Menzles D. Systematic review: T-cell-based assays for the diagnosis of latent tuberculosis infection: an update. *Ann Intern Med.* 2008;149:177–184.

39. Abubakar I, Staff HR, Whitworth H, Lalvani A. How should I interpret an interferon gamma release assay result for tuberculosis infection? *Thorax.* 2013;68(3):298–301.

40. Li JT. Allergy testing. *Am Fam Physician.* 2002;66(4):621–624.

41. Saiki R, Scharf S, Faloona F, Mullis K, Horn G, Erlich H. Enzymatic amplification of beta-globin genomic sequences and restriction site analysis for diagnosis of sickle cell anemia. *Science.* 1985;230:1350–1354.

42. Saiki RK, Gelfand DH, Stoffel S, et al. Primer-directed enzymatic amplification of DNA with a thermostable DNA polymerase. *Science.* 1988;239(4839):487–491.

43. U.S. Food and Drug Administration. Nucleic acid based tests. http://www.fda.gov/MedicalDevices/ProductsandMedicalProcedures/InVitroDiagnostics/ucm330711.htm. Accessed December 17, 2013.

44. Muldrew KL. Molecular diagnostics of infectious diseases. *Curr Opin Pediatr.* 2009;21(1):102–111.

45. Murdoch DR. Molecular genetic methods in the diagnosis of lower respiratory tract infections. *APMIS.* 2004;112(11–12):713–727.

46. Mermin J, Ekwaru JP, Were W, et al. Utility of routine viral load, CD4 count, and clinical monitoring among adults with HIV receiving antiretroviral therapy in Uganda: randomized trial. *BMJ.* 2011;9:343:d6792.

47. Terrault NA, Pawlotsky JM, McHutchison J, et al. Clinical utility of viral load measurements in individuals with chronic hepatitis C infection on antiviral therapy. *J Viral Hepat.* 2005;12(5):465–472.

48. Razonable RR, Hayden RT. Clinical utility of viral load management of Cytomegalovirus infection after solid organ transplantation. *Clin Microbiol Rev.* 2013;26(4):703–727.

49. Valsamakis A. Molecular testing in the diagnosis and management of chronic Hepatitis B. *Clin Microbiol Rev.* 2007;20(3):426–439.

50. Khanna M, Fan J, Pehler-Harrington K, et al. The pneumoplex assays, a multiplex PCR-enzyme hybridization assay that allows simultaneous detection of five organisms, *Mycoplasma pneumoniae, Chlamydia (Chlamydophila) pneumoniae, Legionella pneumophila, Legionella micdadei and Bordetella pertussis,* and it real-time counterpart. *J Clin Microbiol.* 2005;43:565–571.

51. Mahoney JB. Detection of respiratory viruses by molecular methods. *Clin Microbiol Rev.* 2008;21(4):716–747.

52. Centers for Disease Control and Prevention. 2009 H1N1 flu. http://www.cdc.gov/h1n1flu/. Accessed December 18, 2013.

53. H5N1 Avian Flu (H5N1 Bird Flu). FLU.gov. http://www.flu.gov/about_the_flu/h5n1/. Accessed December 18, 2013.

54. Centers for Disease Control and Prevention. Avian Influenza Virus (H7N9). http://www.cdc.gov/flu/avianflu/h7n9-virus.htm. Accessed December 18, 2013.

55. Centers for Disease Control and Prevention. Severe Acute Respiratory Syndrome (SARS). http://www.cdc.gov/sars/. Accessed December 18, 2013.

56. Centers for Disease Control and Prevention. Middle East Respiratory Syndrome (MERS). http://www.cdc.gov/coronavirus/mers/. Accessed December 18, 2013.

57. Mahoney J, Chong S, Merante F, et al. Development of a respiratory virus panel test for detection of twenty human respiratory viruses by use of multiplex PCR and a fluid microbead-based assay. *J Clin Microbiol.* 2007;45(9):2965–2970.

58. Popowitch EB, O'Neill SS, Miller MB. Comparison of the Biofire FilmArray RP, Genmark eSensor RVP, Luminex xTAG RVPv1, and Luminex xTAG RVP fast multiplex assays for detection of respiratory viruses. *J Clin Microbiol.* 2013;51(5):1528–1533.

59. Nolte FS. Molecular diagnostics for detection of bacterial and viral pathogens in community-acquired pneumonia. *Clin Infec Dis.* 2008;47(S3):S123–S126.

60. Balasingham SV, Davidsen T, Szpinda I, Frye SA, Tonjum T. Molecular diagnostics in tuberculosis: basis and implications for therapy. *Mol Diagn Ther.* 2009;13(3):137–151.

61. Kalokhe AS, Shafiq M, Lee JC, et al. Multidrug-resistant tuberculosis drug susceptibility and molecular diagnostic testing. *Am J Med Sci.* 2013;345(2):143–148.

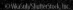

CHAPTER

10

Cardiac Assessment and the Electrocardiogram

Viva Jo Siddall and David C. Shelledy

CHAPTER OUTLINE

Introduction to the Electrocardiogram
Components of the ECG Tracing
Rhythm Strip Interpretation
Myocardial Infarction
Congestive Heart Failure
Management of Cardiac Arrhythmias
12-Lead ECG Interpretation
ECG for Diagnostic Purposes

CHAPTER OBJECTIVES

1. Provide an overview of the anatomy and function of the heart.
2. Describe the flow of an electrical impulse resulting in depolarization and repolarization of the atria and ventricles.
3. Describe electrocardiogram (ECG) lead placement.
4. Contrast different cardiac leads and "views" of the heart.
5. Recognize the components of an ECG tracing.
6. Recognize abnormal waves, segments, and intervals on an ECG tracing and describe the pathologies associated with each.
7. Interpret various cardiac rhythms.
8. Explain the application of Einthoven's triangle and estimation of the cardiac axis.
9. Describe the components of a 12-lead ECG.
10. Interpret a 12-lead ECG.
11. Explain the causes, diagnosis, and treatment of myocardial infarction.
12. Explain the causes, diagnosis, and treatment of congestive heart failure.
13. Review other cardiac diagnostic testing methods.

KEY TERMS

acute myocardial infarction
arrhythmia/dysrhythmia
atrial flutter
atrioventricular (AV) block
atrioventricular (AV) junction
axis deviation
Bachmann's bundle
bundle of His
bradycardia
congestive heart failure (CHF)
cor pulmonale
depolarization
Einthoven's triangle
electrocardiogram (ECG)
endocardium
epicardium
Holter monitoring
intervals
myocardium
non-ST segment elevation MI (NSTEMI)
P wave
pacemaker cells
pericardium
premature atrial contractions (PACs)
premature junctional contractions (PJCs)
premature ventricular contractions (PVCs)
PR segment
Purkinje fibers
QRS complex
repolarization
sinoatrial (SA) node
ST segment elevation MI (STEMI)
ST segment
T wave
tachycardia
U wave
unstable angina
ventricular flutter
ventricular fibrillation

Overview

Cardiac assessment should include review of the patient's medical record, history and physical examination, vital signs, laboratory and imaging studies, and the electrocardiogram (ECG, also known as EKG). The ECG is an essential tool for cardiac assessment. Prior to discussing the assessment of the ECG, we will briefly review cardiac anatomy and physiology. Next, the components of an ECG will be described and the causes and identification of various dysrhythmias will be discussed. Finally, other cardiac diagnostic testing will be reviewed.

Introduction to the Electrocardiogram

A primary purpose of the heart is to rhythmically pump blood rich in oxygen and nutrients to the tissues of the body and to return deoxygenated, CO_2^- laden blood to the lungs for gas exchange. Therefore, the heart could be considered to function as an electrically timed pump.[1] The electrical activity of this pump can be captured beat by beat on graph paper or displayed on a monitor, and this graphic display is the **electrocardiogram (ECG)**. The ECG remains an essential tool for assessment of patients with known or suspected cardiac disease. The ECG also provides an important method of monitoring cardiac function in the acute and intensive care settings. The respiratory care clinician must be able to monitor and interpret the basic ECG and to identify and treat harmful dysrhythmias. The ECG is useful to evaluate cardiac rate and rhythm, conduction abnormalities, myocardial ischemia, and other heart abnormalities.[2–6] **Box 10-1** summarizes the uses of the ECG.

Overview of Cardiac Function

The heart is a hollow organ not much bigger than a fist located in the center of the chest (**Figure 10-1**). It rests

BOX 10-1

ECG Assessment of the Heart

The ECG is useful for assessing:
- Cardiac rate
- Cardiac rhythm
- Cardiac conduction abnormalities
- Myocardial ischemia
- Myocardial infarction
- Other cardiac/cardiovascular disease:
  - Valvular heart disease (e.g., aortic, mitral, tricuspid, or pulmonary valve stenosis; valve insufficiency; valve regurgitation)
  - Cardiomyopathy (i.e., myocardial disease leading to heart failure)
  - Pericarditis (i.e., inflammation of the pericardium due to infection)
  - Hypertension
- Monitoring in the intensive care unit or acute care setting
- Evaluation of response to therapy (e.g., drugs, ventilation, oxygenation)

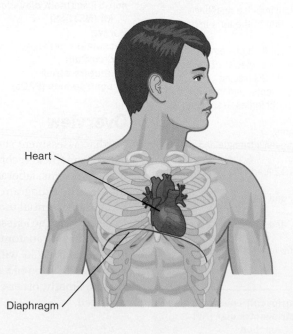

FIGURE 10-1 The heart in the thorax.

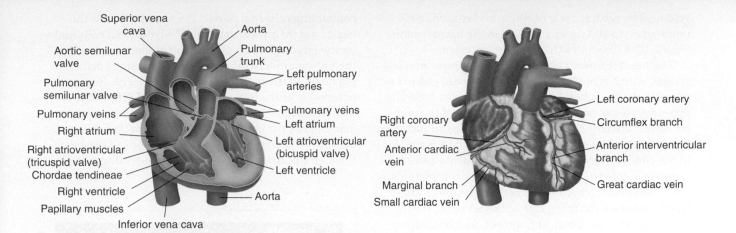

FIGURE 10-2 Anatomy of the heart.

on the diaphragm and is almost entirely surrounded by the lungs. It has four chambers and its own blood supply (**Figure 10-2**). The heart itself has three walls: the **epicardium** (outer layer), the **myocardium** (cardiac muscle), and the **endocardium**, which lines the inside of the heart chambers (**Figure 10-3**). The heart is contained within the **pericardium**, which reduces friction as the heart moves. The heart receives deoxygenated blood from the entire body by way of the superior and inferior vena cavae. The blood next enters the right atrium, passing across the tricuspid valve into the right ventricle, where it is pumped across the pulmonic valve into the pulmonary artery for delivery to the lungs for oxygenation and removal of CO_2. The oxygenated blood is returned to the left atrium, where it then moves across the mitral valve to the left ventricle, which pumps the blood across the aortic valve and out to the aorta. The first branches of the aorta are the left and right coronary arteries, and they supply oxygenated blood to the myocardium and endocardium. The

arterial system then delivers the oxygenated blood throughout the body via the systemic circulation.

The heart moves blood through the circulatory system using a rhythmic motion produced by ventricular relaxation (diastole) and contraction (systole). During ventricular diastole, the aortic and pulmonic valves close and the atria fill with blood. As the ventricles relax, the mitral and tricuspid valves open, allowing the ventricles to begin to fill. Next, the atria contract, expelling blood into the ventricles, allowing them to fill completely. This atrial contraction adds about 10% to 30% to the total cardiac output under normal conditions.[4-6] The blood volume added by the atria during end-ventricular diastole is sometimes referred to as the "atrial kick." Ventricular systole begins when the mitral and tricuspid valves close and the atria relax. The ventricles then contact, expelling blood across the now open aortic and pulmonic valves, pumping blood to the lungs via the pulmonary circulation and out to the tissues of the body through the systemic circulatory

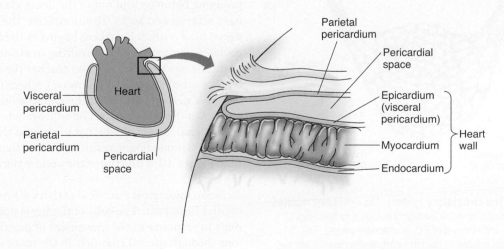

FIGURE 10-3 The layers of the heart.

system. The cardiac cycle of filling and emptying is repeated 60 to 100 times a minute in the normal adult.[6] **Figure 10-4** illustrates the circulatory system.

The heart is under control of the autonomic nervous system, which is made up of the sympathetic and parasympathetic branches. Each branch produces generally opposing effects on the heart. Stimulation of the sympathetic (adrenergic) nervous system causes an increase in the firing of the sinoatrial (SA) node, an increase in the conductivity of the electrical impulses, and an increase in force of atrial and ventricular contractions. Parasympathetic (cholinergic) nervous system stimulation decreases the firing rate of the SA node, slowing conduction of electrical impulses, which results in a decrease in heart rate, cardiac output, and blood pressure.

The heart is composed of three unique cardiac cell types: (1) **pacemaker cells** that serve as the power and timing source for electrical activity, (2) electrical conducting cells that moved the impulse across the heart, and (3) myocardial cells.[7,8] Myocardial cells make up the largest portion of the heart tissue and provide the muscular force for repeated contractions delivering blood to the body (see Figure 10-3). The dominant pacemaker of the heart is the **sinoatrial (SA) node**, which is located in the right atrium; however, every cardiac cell has the ability to act as a pacemaker. The conducting cells carry impulses to all regions of the heart through the atrial and ventricular conducting systems.

> ### RC Insights
>
> The dominant pacemaker of the heart is the sinoatrial (SA) node, which maintains a normal heart rate of 60 to 100 beats per minute.

The atrial conducting system includes the interatrial conduction tract (**Bachmann's bundle**) and internodal atrial conduction tracts. Normally, the heartbeat begins when the SA node "fires." The electrical signal spreads across the right and then left atrium with corresponding atrial depolarization and contraction. Following atrial depolarization, the electrical signal arrives at the atrioventricuar (AV) junction and is then transmitted to the ventricles. The ventricular conducting system consists of three parts: (1) the **atrioventricular (AV) junction**; (2) the **bundle of His**, branching to the right and left bundle branches; and (3) the terminal **Purkinje fibers** and myocardium. When the atrial signal reaches the AV node, it is delayed briefly (about one-tenth of a second) to allow the ventricles to completely fill before being relayed to the bundle of His, the right and left bundle branches, the Purkinje fibers, and the myocardium.

Ventricular depolarization and contraction occurs from the apex of the heart in an upward direction, pumping blood up and out of the heart via the pulmonary arteries and aorta. To summarize, the electrical signal for a normal heartbeat begins at the SA node and proceeds across the atria, resulting in atrial contraction. The electrical signal then reaches the AV node (via the atrial internodal pathways), where it is delayed briefly, and then conducted through the bundle of His and down the right and left bundle branches. The electrical signal is next conducted out across the ventricles via the Purkinje fibers, resulting in ventricular contraction. **Figure 10-5** illustrates the conduction system of the heart.

Innate biological electrical activity allows for the regular heartbeat. The cells of the heart contract and relax in response to the movement of positively charged ions through special channels in the myocardial cell membrane, resulting in electric impulses that are

Capillary beds of lungs

Pulmonary circuit

Pulmonary arteries

Pulmonary veins (4)

Superior and inferior vena cavae

Aorta and branches

Right ventricle

Left ventricle

Systemic circuit

Arterioles

Capillary beds of all body tissues

Venules

Oxygen-poor, CO2-rich blood

Oxygen-rich, CO2-poor blood

Pulmonary circuit

Systemic circuit

FIGURE 10-4 The circulatory system. The right heart receives deoxygenated blood from the body and pumps it to the lungs for oxygenation and removal of CO2 (pulmonary circuit). The oxygenated blood returns to the left heart, which then pumps the blood to the body (systemic circuit).

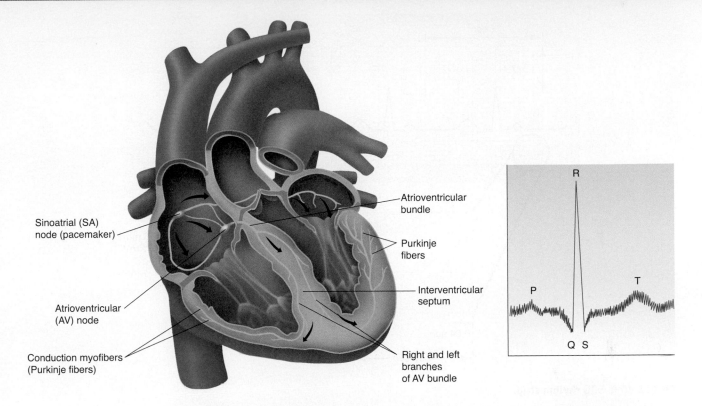

FIGURE 10-5 The electrical conduction system of the heart and the ECG tracing. The normal heartbeat originates in the SA node. Conduction proceeds across the atria, resulting in atrial contraction (P wave on ECG). The electrical signal then arrives at the AV node and is transmitted to the ventricles, and ventricular contraction occurs. The QRS complex corresponds to ventricular deoplarization, and the T wave to ventricular repolarization.

measured in millivolts (mV).[7,8] The positive ions are sodium, potassium, and calcium. Cardiac cells in a resting, or *polarized*, state have positive ions surrounding the cell and negative ions inside the cell. When pacemaker cells **depolarize**, they lose their internal negative charge, resulting in a wave of electrical current that moves through the heart. The cells **repolarize** by restoring ions to the cells through the use of membrane pumps.

The Electrocardiogram

The direction and strength of the electric current generated during depolarization and repolarization of the cells of the heart can be detected through the use of surface electrodes and recorded or displayed using a cardiac monitor or ECG machine. An ECG tracing is made up of waves, segments, and **intervals**. The ECG may be printed using graph paper that has vertical and horizontal lines. The light lines make up small 1×1 mm squares, or blocks, and the dark lines define large 5×5 mm squares.[2] The horizontal axis measures time in seconds, with one small square representing 0.04 seconds and a large square representing 0.2 seconds. Voltage is measured on the vertical axis, with one small square representing 0.1 mV and one large square 0.5 mV. **Figure 10-6** provides an example of a standard

ECG rhythm strip with units of measure indicated. **Table 10-1** provides the specifications for ECG recording paper.

Lead Placement

The electrical activity of the heart is captured by electrodes (leads) placed on the limbs and/or chest. These

TABLE 10-1
Description of ECG Paper

ECG Attribute	Equivalent
1 small block (or square)	0.04 sec
5 small blocks	One big box
1 big box	0.20 sec
25 small blocks	1 second
5 big boxes	1 second
1500 small blocks	1 minute
300 big boxes	1 minute
1 small block	1 millimeter

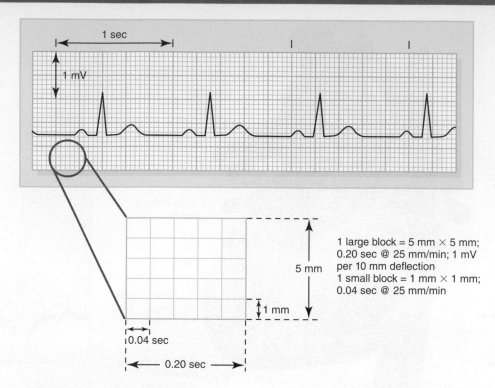

1 large block = 5 mm × 5 mm; 0.20 sec @ 25 mm/min; 1 mV per 10 mm deflection
1 small block = 1 mm × 1 mm; 0.04 sec @ 25 mm/min

5 mm

1 mm

0.04 sec

0.20 sec

FIGURE 10-6 ECG rhythm strip.

electrodes measure the difference in electrical potential between two different points on the body (*bipolar*) or one point and a virtual reference point (*unipolar*). Depolarization waves that move toward a positive lead will produce an upright inflection or tracing, whereas depolarization waves that move toward a negative lead produce an inverted deflection or tracing. An isoelectric (flat) line is produced when no net current is generated.

A simple three-lead ECG system uses electrodes placed on the right arm (RA), left arm (LA), and left leg (LL). Using these three electrodes, three different bipolar electrical views of the heart can be obtained by changing the relationship of the positive, negative, and ground leads:

- *Lead I*: LA = positive (+); RA = negative (−); LL = ground; provides information about the left lateral wall of the heart muscle (myocardium).
- *Lead II*: LA = ground; RA = negative (−); LL = positive (+); provides information about the inferior wall of the heart muscle.
- *Lead III*: LA = negative (−); RA = ground; LL = positive (+); provides information about the inferior wall of the heart muscle.

This lead placement forms **Einthoven's triangle**. Einthoven's law states that lead I + lead III = lead II, which means that the height of the QRS of leads I and III added together should equal the height of the QRS in lead II. This will help differentiate between an abnormal ECG or just improper lead placement.[2] Normal

ECG tracings for leads I, II, and III are illustrated in **Figure 10-7**. Einthoven's triangle is illustrated in **Figure 10-8**.

Chest Monitoring Leads

In the acute or critical care setting, it is common to place monitoring leads directly on the patient's chest. Placement of the electrodes on the chest can mimic limb leads I, II, and III, as illustrated in **Figure 10-9**. Lead II is commonly used in the acute care setting and provides a good monitoring lead for most patients (see Figure 10-9). A modified chest lead, known as MCL_1, is also sometimes used in the acute care setting because it allows for the better assessment of the width of the QRS complex (see Figure 10-9). **Table 10-2** summarizes the three bipolar limb leads. **Box 10-2** describes each of the standard monitoring leads.

> **RC Insights**
>
> The most common monitoring lead is lead II.

Standard 12-Lead ECG

In addition to the three bipolar limb leads described above, three unipolar *augmented limb leads* are measured as a part of the standard 12-lead ECG: aV_R, aV_L, and aV_F. These amplified unipolar leads are measured with one positive lead and all of the others negative.

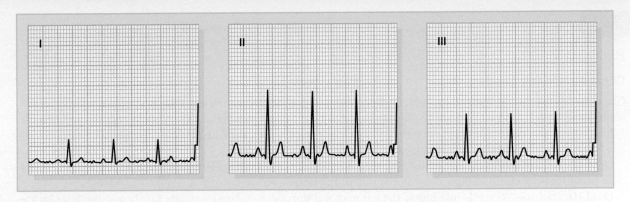

FIGURE 10-7 Normal ECG tracings for leads I, II, III.

Reproduced from: Ajay Bharadwaj and Umanath Kamath, Cypress Semiconductor Corp. Techniques for accurate ECG signal processing. EE Times. February 14, 2011. http://www.eetimes.com/document.asp?doc_id=1278571

TABLE 10-2
Bipolar Limb Leads

Lead	Measures Current Traveling	Negative Pole	Positive Pole
I	Right arm (–) to left arm (+)	Right arm	Left arm
II	Right arm (–) to left leg (+)	Right arm	Left leg
III	Left arm (–) to left leg (+)	Left arm	Left leg

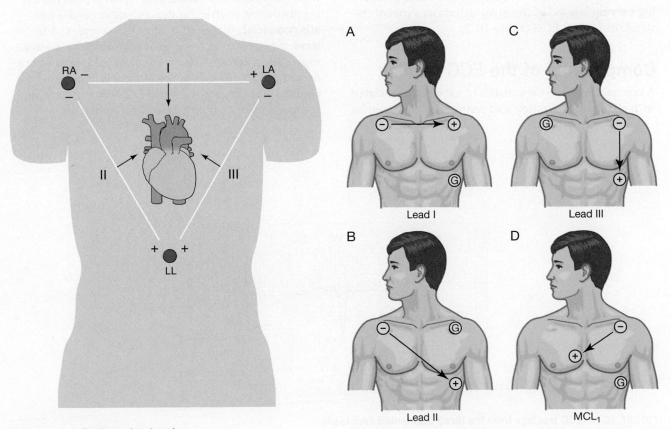

FIGURE 10-8 Einthoven's triangle.

Courtesy of Tomas B. Garcia, MD.

FIGURE 10-9 Monitoring leads.

BOX 10-2

Chest Monitoring Leads

Chest leads are often employed for patient monitoring in the acute care setting. Chest leads can mimic limb leads for leads I, II, and III. Electrode placement for the commonly used monitoring leads is described below.

Lead I: Positive electrode just below the left clavicle; negative electrode just below the right clavicle; provides information about the left lateral wall of the heart.

Lead II: Positive electrode just below the left pectoral muscle; negative electrode just below the right clavicle; provides information about the inferior wall of the heart.

Lead III: Positive electrode just below the left pectoral muscle; negative electrode just below the left clavicle; provides information about the inferior wall of the heart; P waves seen in this lead usually of lower amplitude than in leads I and II and are more likely to be biphasic (partly positive and partly negative).

MCL_1 **(modified chest lead):** Negative electrode just below the left clavicle; positive electrode to the right of the sternum (fourth intercostal space); provides information about the anterior wall of the heart; can be used for assessment of the width of the QRS complex to differentiate supraventricular tachycardia (SVT) from ventricular tachycardia (VT).

Figure 10-10 provides an example of ECG tracings obtained from these augmented leads. The addition of six chest leads to the six limb leads allows for obtaining varying "views" of the myocardium as a part of the standard 12-lead ECG (**Table 10-3**).

Components of the ECG Tracing

A normal cardiac cycle consists of a **P wave** (associated with atrial depolarization and contraction) followed by a **QRS complex** (associated with ventricular depolarization and contraction) followed by a **T wave** (associated with ventricular repolarization). Atrial repolarization occurs during ventricular depolarization and is usually completely obscured by the QRS complex. A **U wave** may be seen in some leads following the T wave, especially in certain cases, such as hypokalemia or bradycardia, but the cause of the U wave is uncertain.[4–6] **Figure 10-11** displays a normal ECG tracing showing waves, complexes, intervals, and segments.

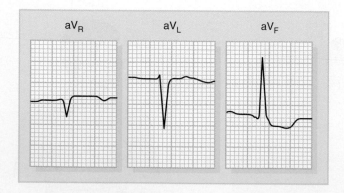

FIGURE 10-10 ECG tracings from the three augmented limb leads.

Reproduced from: Ajay Bharadwaj and Umanath Kamath, Cypress Semiconductor Corp. Techniques for accurate ECG signal processing. EE Times. February 14, 2011. http://www.eetimes.com/document.asp?doc_id=1278571

TABLE 10-3
Leads and Corresponding View of Myocardial Wall

Lead	Myocardial Wall "View"
Limb lead	
I	Lateral
II	Inferior
III	Inferior
aV$_R$	Endocardial wall to surface of right atrium
aV$_L$	Lateral
aV$_F$	Inferior
Chest lead	
V$_1$	Septal
V$_2$	Septal
V$_3$	Anterior
V$_4$	Anterior
V$_5$	Lateral
V$_6$	Lateral

RC Insights

A normal ECG tracing has the following waveform sequence:
P–QRS–T.

The P Wave

The P wave is initiated by the SA node and begins the normal cardiac cycle. The P wave is typically a smooth, rounded, upright deflection (leads I and II) from baseline and represents the electrical activity associated with the depolarization (and contraction) of the right and left atria (see Figure 10-11). Usually the P wave has a duration ≤ 0.10 seconds (this corresponds to 2–5 small boxes on standard ECG paper) and has an amplitude of 0.5 to 2.5 mm.[2]. With a normal sinus rhythm, a QRS complex follows a P wave and corresponds with the depolarization (and contraction) of the ventricles. It must be noted that although the P wave and QRS complex are associated with atrial and ventricular contraction, electromechanical dissociation (i.e., electrical activity without mechanical contractions) may occur under certain conditions. This condition is also known as *pulseless electrical activity*.

The P wave is normally positive (upright) in leads I, II, aV$_F$, and V$_3$ through V$_6$ and negative (inverted) in aV$_R$. The P wave may be positive, negative, or biphasic (positive and negative) in leads III and aV$_L$; in leads V$_1$ and V$_2$ the P wave may be upright or biphasic.[5] An abnormal P wave can mean atrial disease. For example, in lead II the P wave may be widened (> 120 msec) due to left atrial enlargement, and the P waves may appear to be tall (> 2 mm) with right atrial enlargement.[9] Causes of increased right atrial pressure and right atrial enlargement include increased pulmonary vascular resistance (e.g., chronic obstructive pulmonary disease [COPD], chronic hypoxia, severe asthma, or pulmonary embolism).[9–11] Causes of increased left atrial pressure (and enlargement) include systemic hypertension, congestive heart failure (CHF), mitral or aortic valvular disease, and acute myocardial infarction (MI).[9–11]

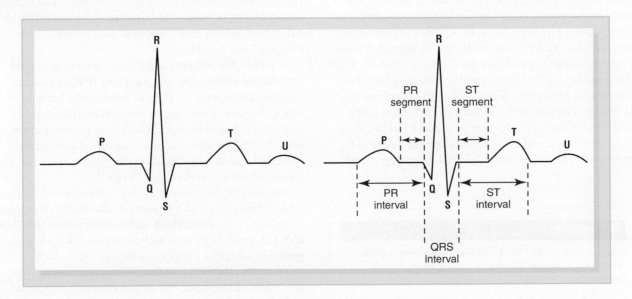

FIGURE 10-11 The normal ECG tracing showing waves, complexes, intervals, and segments.

The PR Segment and Interval

A horizontal isoelectric **PR segment** connects the P wave to the QRS complex (see Figure 10-11). The PR segment is measured from the end of atrial depolarization (i.e., the end of the P wave) to the beginning of ventricular depolarization (i.e., the beginning of the QRS complex). The *PR interval* (also seen in Figure 10-11) is measured from the start of atrial depolarization (i.e., beginning of the P wave) to the start of ventricular depolarization (i.e., the beginning of the QRS complex). The PR interval may be normal (0.12 to 0.20 seconds) or abnormal (> 0.20 seconds or < 0.12 seconds).[2] The PR interval is decreased with a rapid heart rate and increased with a slowed heart rate. The PR interval provides information about the conduction of the electrical signal across the atria through the AV junction. PR intervals < 0.12 seconds can be caused by an ectopic pacemaker in the atria or at the AV junction, whereas intervals > 0.20 seconds (> 5 small boxes) indicate a slowing of the electric impulse through the AV node, bundle of His, or the bundle branches.[4] Normally, the P wave is followed by a QRS complex, and the PR interval is < 0.20 seconds. A PR interval > 0.20 is a *first-degree AV heart block*.[4–6] With a first-degree AV heart block, there is still a 1:1 relationship between P waves and QRS complexes. A *second-degree AV heart block* occurs when there is an abnormal relationship between P waves and QRS complexes.[4–6] There are two types of second-degree heart block. A progressive increase in the length of the PR interval followed by a blocked signal to the ventricles is a *second-degree AV block type I* (aka Mobitz I or Wenckebach). A series of conducted P waves followed by a nonconducted (dropped) P wave is a *second-degree AV block type II* (aka Mobitz II). With a second-degree AV block type II, there may be a fixed relationship between P waves and QRS complexes (e.g., 2:1 or 3:1). *Third-degree AV block* occurs when there is no conduction of the electrical signal from the atria to the ventricles, and thus no relationship between P waves and QRS complexes.[4–6] Third-degree AV heart

blocks occur below the AV node. Heart blocks will be further discussed further later in this chapter.

The QRS Complex

The QRS complex represents the depolarization of the ventricles and is composed of three waves (see Figure 10-11). The Q wave is the first negative deflection of the QRS complex. Q waves are associated with depolarization of the interventricular septum; they are not prominent in most leads in normal patients. Pathologic Q waves (Q waves > 0.04 seconds and ≥ 25% of QRS height) may be due to tissue damage seen with MI.[6] Pathologic Q wave development may be part of the progression of ECG changes seen with an acute MI or may be present due to an MI that occurred sometime in the past. Prominent Q waves are also sometimes seen with ventricular enlargement, altered conduction, and other conditions.[12]

The first positive deflection (leads I, II, and III) of the QRS complex is the R wave, which represents depolarization of the left ventricle. The R-R interval is the time between two successive ventricular depolarizations and normally represents one complete cardiac cycle. The interval will be regular or irregular depending on the underlying rhythm. The interval will be short if the heart rate is fast and long if the heart rate is slow.

Following the R wave, the S wave is a negative deflection representing terminal ventricular depolarization. The QRS starts where the first wave deviates from baseline and ends where the last wave begins to flatten out at, above, or below the baseline. A normal QRS has a duration of 0.06 to 0.10 seconds and an amplitude ranging from 1 to 15 mm.[4]

A wide QRS complex (≥ 0.12 seconds) is seen with **premature ventricular contractions (PVCs)**; conduction disturbances (e.g., right or left bundle branch block, Purkinje fiber block); electrolyte disturbances (e.g., severe hypokalemia); ventricular pre-excitation (e.g., Wolff-Parkinson-White syndrome, a congenital disorder); use of a ventricular pacemaker; and toxic levels of certain antiarrhythmic drugs.[13]

Myocardial ischemia or infarction can result in irritable ectopic foci that can serve as the origin of ectopic heartbeats (e.g., **premature atrial contraction [PAC]** or PVC). A rapid heart rate with a narrow QRS complex generally suggests a supraventricular tachycardia.[13] A rapid heart rate with a wide QRS usually means that the origin of the rapid rate is ventricular (ventricular tachycardia).[14,15]

QRS Axis

The electrical axis of the heart normally ranges from about −30° to +90° in adults and can be determined by examining the QRS complex as viewed by the frontal plane limb leads (i.e., leads I, II, III, aV$_R$, aV$_L$, aV$_F$).[4,5,14] Each lead has a positive and negative pole. The electrical axes of these leads are shown in **Figure 10-12**. For example, the positive pole of lead II is +60°, whereas the negative pole of lead II is −120°. If the net QRS is positive in leads I and II, the QRS axis is normal.

A *left axis deviation* is < −30° (i.e., −30° to −90°) and is associated with a net positive QRS deflection in lead I and a net negative deflection in lead II.[6] Left axis deviation may be caused by left ventricular hypertrophy (e.g., left-sided CHF), inferior wall MI, and left anterior hemiblock (aka left anterior fascicular block, which is a partial block of the anterior half of the left bundle branch).[4,14] **Box 10-3** summarizes the assessment of the mean QRS axis.

A *right axis deviation* is > 90° (i.e., 90° to 180°) and is associated with a net negative QRS deflection in lead I and a net positive deflection in lead II.[4,14] A right axis deviation may be caused by right ventricular hypertrophy (e.g., cor pulmonale) or left posterior hemiblock and may also be seen in thin, healthy individuals.[4,14] An extreme axis deviation (extreme right or extreme left) is between −90° and −180°.

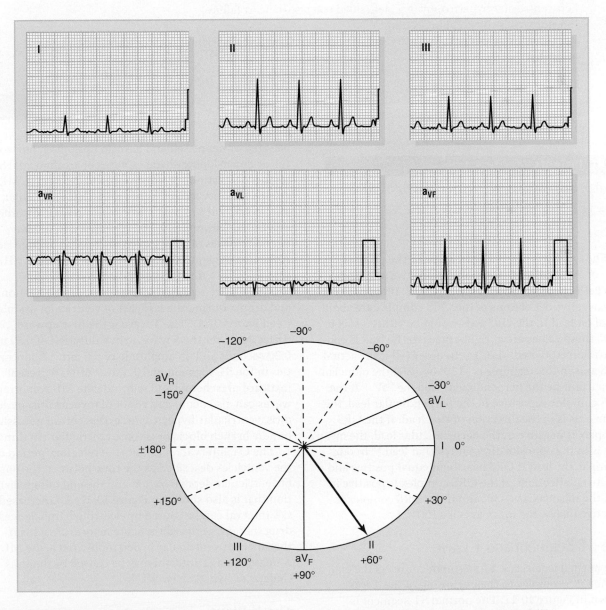

FIGURE 10-12 **The electrical axis of the heart as viewed by the frontal plane limb leads (I, II, III, aV$_R$, aV$_L$ and aV$_F$).**

This article was published in *Clinical Assessment in Respiratory Care*. 6th ed., Wilkins RL, Dexter JR, Heuer AJ, eds., Interpretation of electrocardiogram tracings, Pages 211-238, Copyright Mosby 2010.

BOX 10-3

Mean QRS Axis Deviation

Normal QRS axis: −30° to +90° ➜ Net QRS is positive in leads I and II.

Right axis deviation: > 90° ➜ Net negative QRS deflection in lead I and a net positive deflection in lead II. Possible causes include:

- Right ventricular hypertrophy (e.g., cor pulmonale)
- Left posterior hemiblock (partial block of the posterior half of the left bundle branch)
- Certain types of left ventricular myocardial infarction (e.g., left ventricular apicolateral wall infarction)
- Dextrocardia
- Left-side pneumothorax
- May be seen in normal children, young adults, and thin, otherwise healthy individuals

Left axis deviation: < −30° ➜ Net positive QRS deflection in lead I and a net negative deflection in lead II. Possible causes include:

- Left ventricular hypertrophy (e.g., left-sided congestive heart failure)
- Inferior wall myocardial infarction
- Left anterior hemiblock (left anterior fascicular block, which is a partial block of the anterior half of the left bundle branch)
- May be seen in normal patients

RC Insights

A right axis deviation (> 90°) may be caused by cor pulmonale.

The QRS axis lies at a right angle to the positive pole of any limb lead in which the positive and negative deflections are about equal.[4,5] Thus, if the positive and negative deflections of the QRS complex are about equal on lead II, the QRS axis would be either +150° *or* −30°; these values are at right angles to the lead II configuration (+60° and −120°).[4,5] In order tell if the actual QRS axis in this example is +150° or −30°, the clinician must examine the perpendicular lead (i.e., aV$_L$). If the QRS complex is positive in the perpendicular lead, the mean axis is in the direction of that lead. If the QRS complex is negative in the perpendicular lead, the mean axis is in the opposite direction of that lead.[4,5] In our example, the lead II QRS has about equal positive and negative deflections; if the QRS complex is positive in aV$_L$, the mean axis is −30° and if the QRS complex is negative in aV$_L$, the mean axis is +150°.[4,14]

The ST Segment and T Wave

The normal isoelectric **ST segment** connects the end of the QRS complex to the beginning of the T wave shown in Figure 10-11. The normal ST segment is ≤ 0.20 seconds and represents the time from the end of ventricular depolarization to the start of ventricular repolarization.[4] An abnormal ST segment can be elevated or depressed and have an upsloping, horizontal, or downsloping shape.[5] Causes of an abnormal ST segment elevation include myocardial ischemia, MI, coronary artery spasm, pericarditis, left ventricular aneurysm, and Brugada syndrome (a genetic disorder associated with specific ECG changes and sudden death).[6] Causes of ST segment depression include ischemia, nontransmural MI (partial wall thickness MI), digitalis effect, and left ventricular hypertrophy.[6]

The T wave represents ventricular repolarization and occurs during the last part of ventricular systole (see Figure 10-11). The T wave is the first upward deflection after the S wave, with a duration of 0.10 to 0.20 seconds and an amplitude of ≤ 5 mm.[4] Abnormalities in the ST segment and T waves often represent myocardial ischemia and may indicate MI. Abnormal T waves can also occur as a result of myocarditis, pericarditis, ventricular hypertrophy, excess serum potassium, bundle branch block, or ectopic ventricular rhythms.

The QT interval represents the refectory period of the ventricles described as the time between the onset of ventricular depolarization and the end of repolarization that is also shown in Figure 10-11. An increased QT interval can be caused by electrolyte imbalances, drug therapy, pericarditis, acute myocarditis, hypothermia, left ventricular hypertrophy, and acute MI.[4,5,12] A decreased QT interval may be caused by digitalis therapy or hypercalcemia.[4,5,12]

The U Wave

The U wave is thought to represents the final stage of ventricular repolarization (see Figure 10-11).[4,5] The

TABLE 10-4
Normal and Abnormal Components of Waves, Segments, and Complexes

Component	Normal Duration	Abnormal Duration	Amplitude	Lead II Morphology
P wave	0.12–0.20 sec	< 0.12 or > 0.20 sec	0.5–2.5 mm	Positive (upright), smooth, rounded
QRS complex	0.06–0.10 sec	> 0.10 sec	1–15 mm	Positive (upright), negative (inverted), equiphasic (both), narrow, sharp-pointed
T wave	0.10–0.25 sec		< 5 mm	Positive (upright), slightly asymmetrical, rounded
U wave	Undetermined		< 2 mm, > 2 mm abnormal	Positive (upright), symmetrical, rounded
PR interval	0.12–0.20 sec	< 0.12 or > 0.20 sec		
QT interval	Depends on rate			
R-R interval	Depends on rate			
S-T segment	≤ 0.20 sec		< 1.0 mm abnormal	Slightly elevated flat, concave, or arched Slightly depressed flat, down-sloping
P-R segment	0.02–0.10 sec		Isoelectric	

normal U follows the T wave and is small, rounded, and upright in lead II. An abnormally large U wave may be present in patients receiving certain medications or due to hypokalemia. **Table 10-4** summarizes the components of ECG waves, segments, and complexes.

Rhythm Strip Interpretation

The components of an ECG wave have been described. The next step in evaluating the ECG is the basic interpretation of the ECG rhythm strip, or monitoring lead.[5,8] A systematic approach is helpful, and we suggest the following steps in assessing the ECG strip:

1. Calculate and evaluate the heart rate.
2. Evaluate the cardiac rhythm.
3. Assess the P waves, PR interval, and relationship of P waves to QRS complexes.
4. Assess the QRS complex.
5. Inspect the ST segment.
6. Determine the QRS axis.
7. Assess the overall ECG.

Each of these steps and related ECG findings will be discussed below.

Step 1: Calculate and Evaluate the Heart Rate

The first step in ECG rhythm strip interpretation is estimation of the patient's heart rate (HR). Normal HR in adults is 60 to 100 beats per minute (bpm); HR < 60 bpm is **bradycardia** and HR > 100 bpm is **tachycardia**.[8,15] Often clinicians will monitor heart rate by observing the HR display on a cardiac monitor or pulse oximeter. These numbers, however, can be inaccurate

in the presence of arrhythmia (e.g., irregular rhythm, hypotension). The clinician should verify monitored rates by taking the patient's pulse, as described in Chapter 5. There are also several methods that can be used to calculate the heart rate based on the ECG rhythm strip. The ECG can be recorded on paper strips that operate at a speed of 25 mm per second and contain:

- 5 large blocks (or squares) per second on the x-axis; each large block is 0.20 seconds and 5.0 mm in length:
  - 1 large block = 0.20 seconds
  - 5 large blocks = 1 second
  - 15 large blocks = 3 seconds
  - 30 large blocks = 6 seconds
- 5 small blocks per large block; each small block is 0.04 seconds and 1.0 mm in length:
  - 1 small block = 0.04 seconds
  - 5 small blocks = 1 large block = 0.20 seconds
- Hash marks at the top of the paper denote 1- or 3-second intervals.

Figure 10-6 illustrates a typical ECG rhythm strip layout.

The *6-second method* to estimate heart rate is simple, fast, and fairly accurate if the cardiac rhythm is regular. To estimate the heart rate, count the number of QRS complexes in a 6-second interval (30 large blocks) and multiply the number by 10.[4,8] Thus, if there are 8 QRS complexes in a 6-second interval (30 large blocks) the heart rate would be:

HR = 8 QRS complexes per 6-second interval × 10
    = 80 bpm

When a 6-second interval is not available, a 3-second interval (15 large blocks) may be used where:

HR = Number of QRS complexes in 3 seconds × 20

Another method used to estimate HR is to *measure the R-R interval*. To use this method, measure the time in seconds between the R waves of two consecutive QRS complexes and divide the number into 60. For example, if there are 20 small blocks (or 4 large blocks) between the R waves, the time in seconds would be 20 small blocks × 0.04 seconds per block = 0.80 seconds:

HR = 60 ÷ R-R interval (seconds) = 60 ÷ 0.80 seconds = 75 bpm

An alternative to calculating the length of the R-R interval in seconds is to simply count the number of small blocks between the R waves (i.e., the R-R interval) and divide the number into 1500.[4] This rule is based on the fact that ECG strips operate at 25 mm/sec or 1500 mm/min (25 mm/sec × 60 sec/min = 1500 mm/min). If there are 20 small blocks between R waves, the rate would be:

HR = 1500 ÷ number of small blocks between R waves = 1500 ÷ 20 = 75 bpm

---

RC Insights

Heart rate (HR) = 1500 ÷ number of small blocks in the R-R interval.

Figure 10-13 illustrates heart rate estimation using this method.

Last, the *triplicate method* is fast and commonly used. ECG strips operate at a rate of 25 mm per second (i.e., 5 large blocks per second), which is equal to 300 large boxes per minute. To employ the triplicate method, count the number of large blocks between R waves and divide by 300, as follows:

R-R Interval (large blocks)	Heart Rate (bpm)
1	300 (300 ÷ 1)
2	150 (300 ÷ 2)
3	100 (300 ÷ 3)
4	75 (300 ÷ 4)
5	60 (300 ÷ 5)
6	50 (300 ÷ 6)
7	43 (300 ÷ 7)
8	38 (300 ÷ 8)

Figure 10-14 provides an example of calculation of HR based on R-R interval using the triplicate method. It should be noted that this method only provides an approximate estimate of cardiac rate and is not accurate if the heart rate is irregular. **Figure 10-15** provides an example of a normal sinus rhythm (NSR) and rate. Evaluation of alterations in the cardiac rate is described following.

Tachycardia

Tachycardia is defined as a heart rate > 100 bpm. Causes of tachycardia include hypoxia, anemia, blood

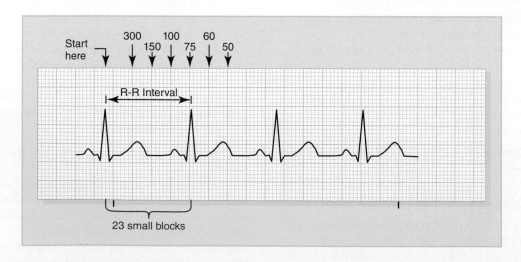

FIGURE 10-13 Calculation of cardiac rate based on R-R interval. To estimate heart rate (HR), count the number of small blocks in the R-R interval and divide into 1500. In this example, the number of small blocks in the R-R interval is approximately 23, so the heart rate (HR) would be: HR = 1500 ÷ 23 = 65 beats per minute.

From *Arrhythmia Recognition: The Art of Interpretation*, courtesy of Tomas B. Garcia, MD.

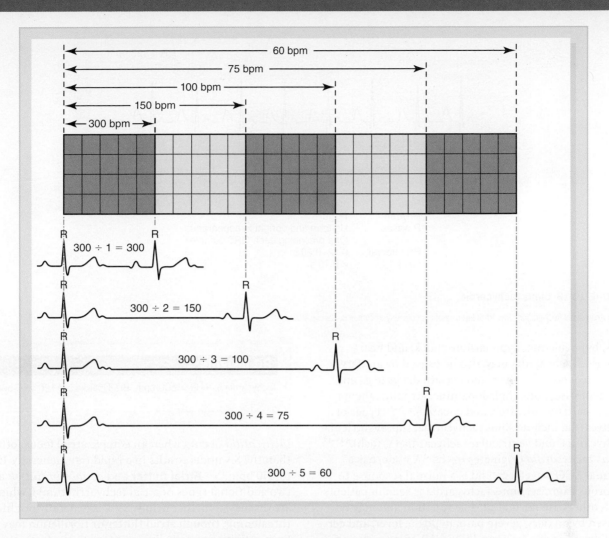

FIGURE 10-14 Heart rate calculation based on R-R interval using triplicate method. Count the large blocks in the R-R interval and divide into 300 to estimate heart rate.

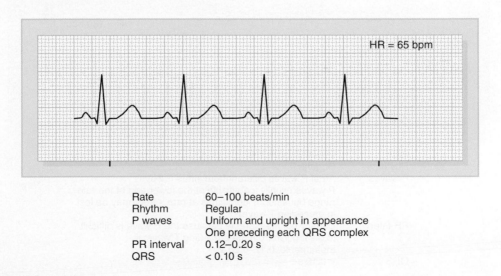

Rate	60–100 beats/min
Rhythm	Regular
P waves	Uniform and upright in appearance
	One preceding each QRS complex
PR interval	0.12–0.20 s
QRS	< 0.10 s

FIGURE 10-15 Normal sinus rhythm (NSR).

From *Arrhythmia Recognition: The Art of Interpretation*, courtesy of Tomas B. Garcia, MD.

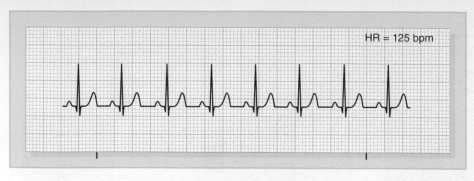

Rate	100–160 beats/min
Rhythm	Regular
P waves	Uniform and upright in appearance
	One preceding each QRS complex
PR interval	0.12–0.20 s
QRS	< 0.10 s

FIGURE 10-16 Sinus tachycardia.

From *Arrhythmia Recognition: The Art of Interpretation*, courtesy of Tomas B. Garcia, MD.

loss, hypovolemia, hypotension, shock, and heart disease. Tachycardia may also be caused by anxiety, uncontrolled pain, fever, and certain drugs (e.g., epinephrine, isoproterenol, dopamine, atropine, theophylline, caffeine, nicotine, and cocaine).[8,15–17] Types of tachycardia include sinus tachycardia, supraventricular tachycardia, and ventricular tachycardia (V-tach).[8,15–17] *Sinus tachycardia* originates in the SA node, has a normal ECG waveform, and is a normal response to vigorous exercise. Sinus tachycardia is seen in patients with otherwise normal cardiac function and may be caused by anxiety, severe pain, hypoxia, fever, and certain drugs or medications. **Figure 10-16** provides an example of a sinus tachycardia.

Supraventricular tachycardia (SVT) is a rapid heart rate that originates at or above the SA node. *Atrial*

tachycardia occurs when an ectopic atrial focus (other than the SA node) results in a rapid rate, generally 100 to 250 bpm.[15–16] **Atrial flutter** and *atrial fibrillation* are two additional types of atrial tachyarrhythmia, which are discussed further below. SVT is generally not life threatening, though atrial flutter or fibrillation may limit activities of daily living or lead to the formation of blood clots along the walls of the atria, which can dislodge and result in a stroke. **Figure 10-17** provides an example of SVT. **Figure 10-18** provides an example of

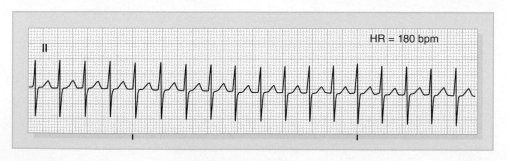

Rate	150–250 beats/min
Rhythm	Regular
P waves	Atrial P waves different from sinus P waves
	P waves usually identifiable at the lower end of the rate range but seldom identifiable at rate > 200 (may be lost in preceding T wave)
PR interval	Usually not measurable because the P wave is difficult to distinguish from the preceding T wave; if measurable, 0.12–0.20 s
QRS	< 0.10 s

FIGURE 10-17 Supraventricular tachycardia.

From *Arrhythmia Recognition: The Art of Interpretation*, courtesy of Tomas B. Garcia, MD.

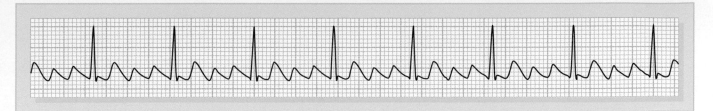

Rate	Usually 60–100 beats/min but may be faster or slower
Rhythm	Irregular
P waves	Uniform and upright in appearance
	One preceding each QRS complex
PR interval	0.12–0.20 s
QRS	< 0.10 s

FIGURE 10-18 Atrial flutter.

From *Arrhythmia Recognition: The Art of Interpretation*, courtesy of Tomas B. Garcia, MD.

atrial flutter, whereas **Figure 10-19** provides an example of atrial fibrillation.

Ventricular tachycardia (V-tach) appears as a series of ventricular depolarizations at a rate above normal (i.e., HR > 100 bpm).[11,16] The QRS complex is wide (> 0.12 seconds), and each complex looks like a PVC. V-tach may occur in runs of three or more consecutive depolarizations.

Causes of V-tach include acute myocardial ischemia, MI, CHF, hypoxia, hyperkalemia, and with use of certain medications (e.g., digoxin or antiarrhythmic agents).[11,16] Ventricular tachycardia is associated with increased cardiac mortality, and sustained V-tach may cause heart failure, angina, and hemodynamic instability.

Treatment of ventricular tachycardia depends on the patient's condition and whether the V-tach is sustained or nonsustained. For asymptomatic nonsustained

V-tach, no treatment may be necessary. For symptomatic nonsustained V-tach, antiarrhythmic drugs may be prescribed. For example, stable, symptomatic patients with V-tach associated with ventricular dysfunction may be managed with β-blockers (e.g., propranolol) or amiodarone, a class III antiarrhythic agent.

Synchronized cardioversion should be considered for unstable patients and those with hemodynamic instability; automatic implantable cardioverter-defibrillator (ICD) insertion should be considered in patients with V-tach and moderately severe to severe left ventricular dysfunction (generally an ejection fraction < 30–35%).[11,16] Catheter ablation therapy may also be considered in certain patients with V-tach.[11,16] MI patients with V-tach will often improve once myocardial ischemia is reversed. **Figure 10-20** provides an example of V-tach as seen on ECG.

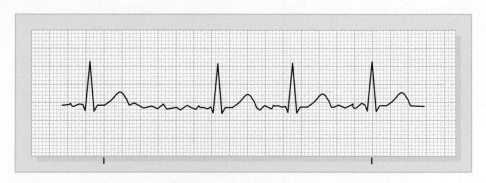

Rate	Atrial rate usually > 400 beats/min
	Ventricular rate variable
Rhythm	Atrial and ventricular very irregular (regular, bradycardic ventricular rhythm may occur as a result of digitalis toxicity)
P waves	No identifiable P waves
	Erratic, wavy baseline
PR interval	None
QRS	Usually < 0.10 s

FIGURE 10-19 Atrial fibrillation.

From *Arrhythmia Recognition: The Art of Interpretation*, courtesy of Tomas B. Garcia, MD.

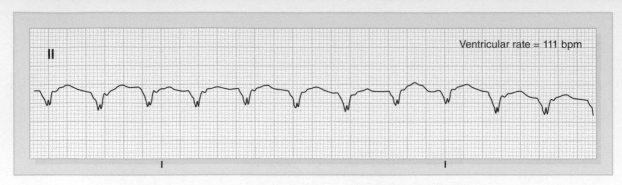

Ventricular rate = 111 bpm

Rate	Atrial rate not discernible; ventricular rate 100–250 beats/min
Rhythm	Atrial not discernible; ventricular essentially regular
P waves	May be present or absent; if present, they have no set relationship to the QRS complexes, appearing between the QRSs at a rate different from that of the VT
PR interval	None
QRS	Usually < 0.12 s
	Often difficult to differentiate between the QRS and the T wave

Note: Three or more PVCs occurring sequentially are referred to as a "run" of VT

FIGURE 10-20 Ventricular tachycardia (monomorphic VT).

From *Arrhythmia Recognition: The Art of Interpretation*, courtesy of Tomas B. Garcia, MD.

Bradycardia

Bradycardia (HR < 60 bpm) can be caused by severe hypoxia, vagal stimulation, severe acidosis, cardiac disease, arrhythmia (e.g., heart block), and the administration of certain medications (e.g., β-blockers).[6,8] Well-trained athletes may have a resting HR of 40 to 50 bpm. **Figure 10-21** provides an example of a patient with sinus bradycardia.

Step 2: Evaluate the Cardiac Rhythm

The next task is to determine if the rhythm is regular, regular but interrupted, or irregular. Atrial regularity is determined by the spacing of the P waves. The regularity of the ventricular rhythm can be assessed by determining if the distances between QRS complexes (i.e., R-R intervals) are equal. If the R-R intervals are equal across time, the ventricular rhythm is regular. If the length of the R-R interval varies more than 0.04 seconds, the rhythm is irregular. An irregular rhythm may vary in a set pattern, and this is known as a *regularly irregular* rhythm. In contrast, an irregular rhythm may be random, and this is known as an *irregularly irregular* rhythm. Examples of types of cardiac rhythms include:

- Regular rhythm and rate
- Regular rhythm and abnormal rate (i.e., bradycardia or tachycardia)

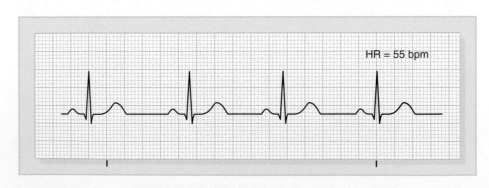

HR = 55 bpm

Rate	< 60 beats/min
Rhythm	Regular
P waves	Uniform and upright in appearance
	One preceding each QRS complex
PR interval	0.12–0.20 s
QRS	0.10 s

FIGURE 10-21 Sinus bradycardia.

From *Arrhythmia Recognition: The Art of Interpretation*, courtesy of Tomas B. Garcia, MD.

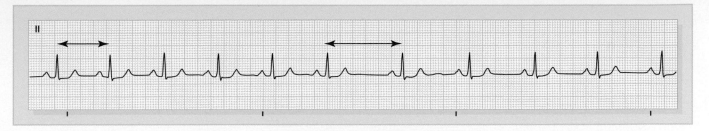

Rate	Variable; usually 60–100 beats/min but may be faster or slower
Rhythm	Irregular. Note the varying time in the R-R interval
P waves	Uniform and upright in appearance
	One preceding each QRS complex
PR interval	0.12–0.20 s
QRS	0.10 s

FIGURE 10-22 Irregular sinus rhythm.

From *Arrhythmia Recognition: The Art of Interpretation*, courtesy of Tomas B. Garcia, MD.

- Irregular rhythm
  - Regular except for an occasional early beat or late beat
  - Regularly irregular pattern with normal or abnormal rate
  - Irregularly irregular rhythm with normal or abnormal rate

Figure 10-22 provides an example of an irregular sinus rhythm.

Types of Premature Beats

Premature atrial contractions (PACs; aka *atrial premature complexes*, or *APCs*) are due to premature activation of the atria by an atrial site other than the sinus node. The PAC is an early beat on ECG that may appear similar to a normal sinus rhythm, though the shape of the P wave may be different. With PACs, the PR interval may be normal, increased, or decreased, and the QRS complex may be normal or wide.[6,11] The frequency of PACs increases with age, and PACs are also associated with alcohol and caffeine consumption. They are also associated with structural heart disease (e.g., chronic renal or pulmonary disease), early-state MI, and pericarditis.[6,11] Symptoms include palpitations, noticeably skipped beats, and, in some cases, dizziness.[6,11] The PR interval may be normal, increased, or decreased, and the QRS complex may be normal or wide. Treatment includes addressing the underlying cause and elimination of caffeine and alcohol from the diet.[6,11] β-blockers may be helpful in symptomatic patients; calcium channel blockers and class IC antiarrhythmic sodium channel antagonists (e.g., flecainide and propafenone) may be considered.[6,11] **Figure 10-23** provides an example of premature atrial complexes.

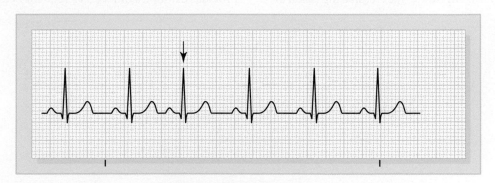

Rate	Usually normal, but depends on the underlying rhythm
Rhythm	Irregular because of PACs
P waves	P wave of the early beat differs from sinus P waves and is premature (arrow)
	May be flattened or notched
	May be lost in the preceding T wave
PR interval	Varies from 0.12–0.20 s when the pacemaker site is near the SA node to 0.12 s
QRS	Usually 0.10 s but may be prolonged

FIGURE 10-23 Premature atrial complexes (PACs).

From *Arrhythmia Recognition: The Art of Interpretation*, courtesy of Tomas B. Garcia, MD.

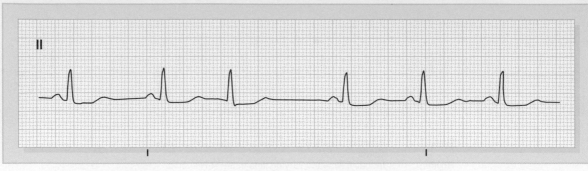

Rate	Atrial and ventricular rate depend on underlying rhythm
Rhythm	Irregular because of premature complex
P waves	May occur before, during, or after the QRS; if seen, will be inverted (retrograde)
PR interval	If the P wave occurs before the QRS, the PR interval will usually be ≤ 0.12 s
QRS	< 0.10 s

FIGURE 10-24 Premature junctional complexes (PJCs).

From *Arrhythmia Recognition: The Art of Interpretation,* courtesy of Tomas B. Garcia, MD.

Premature junctional complexes (PJCs) are premature beats that originate in the AV node, the area around the AV node, or the bundle of His.[6,11] Possible causes of PJC include digitalis toxicity, hypokalemia, and MI.[6,11] Symptoms may include palpitations, skipped beats, dizziness, and fainting; most patients with PJCs do not have symptoms.[6,11] **Figure 10-24** provides an example of PJCs as seen on ECG.

Premature ventricular contractions (PVCs) are ectopic beats caused by early depolarization of the ventricles. PVCs originate in one of the ventricles, often due to irritable myocardial tissue (e.g., irritable myocardial foci) and enhanced automaticity. Automaticity is an intrinsic property of all myocardial cells that enables them to act as pacemakers for the heart. PVCs can be caused by anxiety; excessive ingestion of

alcohol, tobacco, or caffeine; and use of certain medications (e.g., catecholamines, theophylline). Myocardial ischemia, MI, hypoxia, severe acidosis, and electrolyte disturbances may also cause PVCs. Symptoms include skipped beats, palpitations, dizziness, and fainting. Generally, infrequent, single PVCs are innocuous and do not pose a threat to the patient's well-being.[8,11] Frequent PVCs (e.g., multiple PVCs in 1 minute), however, can lower the effective heart rate and reduce cardiac output.[8,11] *Bigeminy* refers to PVCs alternating with sinus beats, whereas *couplets* are two PVCs in a row and *salvos* are three or more PVCs in a row. PVCs that have more than one configuration (i.e., multifocal PVCs) indicate more than one area of myocardial irritation (i.e., multiple irritable myocardial foci).[8,11] **Figure 10-25** provides examples of PVCs as seen on ECG.

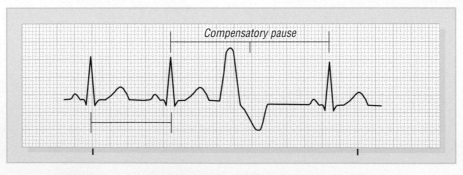

Rate	Atrial and ventricular rate depend on underlying rhythm
Rhythm	Irregular because of PVC
	If the PVC is interpolated (sandwiched between two normal beats), the rhythm will be regular
P waves	No P wave is associated with the PVC
PR interval	None with the PVC because the ectopic originate in the ventricles
QRS	< 0.12 s
	Wide and bizarre
	T wave frequently in opposite direction of the QRS complex

FIGURE 10-25 Premature ventricular complexes (PVCs).

From *Arrhythmia Recognition: The Art of Interpretation,* courtesy of Tomas B. Garcia, MD.

With heart disease, PVCs are associated with poorer outcomes, and MI patients with PVCs are at greater risk for death.[8,11] Multiple PVCs (couplets, salvos, or bigeminy) and multifocal PVCs are ominous findings, and the patient should be monitored closely. Treatment of symptomatic PVCs should include the use of a β-blocker.[11] Alternatives include amiodarone (an antiarrhythmic medication) or catheter ablation. With catheter ablation, radiofrequency energy (i.e., heat) is used to destroy the offending heart tissue.[11]

Step 3: Assess the Strip for P Waves, PR Interval, and the Relationship of the P Waves to the QRS Complexes

For this step, assess the P waves and the relationship between P waves and QRS complexes, and then measure the PR interval. A normal sinus rhythm is initiated in the SA node, and the P wave should appear as smooth and upright in lead II. The P wave represents both right atrial and left atrial depolarization, and amplitude and duration may be affected by a right- or left-side atrial enlargement. For example, a P wave > 2.5 mm in lead II may be associated with right atrial hypertrophy, whereas a biphasic P wave in V_1 may be caused by left atrial hypertrophy.[6] P waves should be followed by a QRS complex, and the PR interval should be 0.12 to 0.20 seconds in length. A PR interval > 0.20 seconds is a first-degree heart block when each P wave is followed by a QRS complex. An abnormal relationship between the P wave and QRS complex is a second-degree heart block. No relationship between the P wave and QRS interval is a third-degree heart block. **Figure 10-26** provides an example of a first-degree heart block as seen on ECG. **Figures 10-27, 10-28**, and **10-29** provide examples of second-degree heart blocks type I and II. **Figure 10-30** provides an example of a third-degree heart block.

Step 4: Describe the QRS Complexes, Noting Their Duration, Shape, and Regularity

If the QRS complexes differ, this may indicate an ectopy or aberrancy. Are the QRS complexes normal in duration (i.e., 0.06 to 0.10 seconds)? If the answer is yes, the QRS complex probably represents the normal pathway from the SA node to the Purkinje fibers and normal ventricular depolarization. If the answer is no (i.e., QRS ≥ 0.12 seconds), the complex is widened and suggests that ventricular depolarization is taking place in the ventricles themselves instead of the conduction system. A QRS > 0.10 seconds but < 0.12 seconds is generally considered abnormal; however, a QRS ≥ 0.12 seconds has a higher specificity for structural heart disease. Q waves may suggest infarction, whereas a wide QRS may be caused by premature beats (e.g., PVC), bundle branch blocks, toxic levels of certain drugs, or severe hypokalemia. Ventricular hypertrophy may be suggested by increased QRS voltage.[4–6,11]

Step 5: Inspect the ST Segment

Note the presence of ST segment elevation or depression and whether the T waves are abnormal. ST elevation may be caused by acute MI, pericarditis, or ischemia (e.g., blockage or spasm). ST depression may be caused by digitalis intoxication or increased myocardial work (e.g., ventricular hypertrophy, ischemia, or nontransmural MI).[4–6,11] Tall, peaked T waves may be

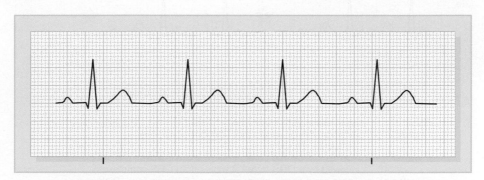

Rate	Atrial and ventricular within normal limits and the same
Rhythm	Atrial and ventricular regular
P waves	Normal in size and configuration; one P wave for each QRS
PR interval	Prolonged (> 0.20 s) but constant
QRS	< 0.10 s

FIGURE 10-26 First-degree AV block.

From *Arrhythmia Recognition: The Art of Interpretation*, courtesy of Tomas B. Garcia, MD.

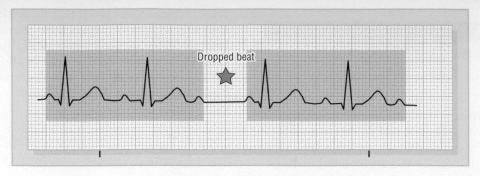

Rate	Atrial rate > ventricular rate; both are usually within normal limits
Rhythm	Atrial regular (P waves plot through) Ventricular irregular
P waves	Normal in size and configuration; some P waves are not followed by a QRS (more P waves than QRS complexes)
PR interval	There is a progressive increase in the PR interval with each cycle (although lengthening may be slight) until a P wave appears without a QRS (e.g., dropped or blocked QRS)
QRS	< 0.10 s but is dropped periodically

FIGURE 10-27 Second-degree AV block, type I (Wenckebach, Mobitz I).

From *Arrhythmia Recognition: The Art of Interpretation*, courtesy of Tomas B. Garcia, MD.

seen with hyperkalemia and acute MI.[4–6,11] The height of the T wave represents K+ and thus hyperkalemia induces tall T waves.

Inverted T waves may be seen with digitalis electrolyte disturbances, non-Q-wave MI, and increased intracranial pressure.[4–6,11]

Step 6: Determine the QRS Axis

The mean QRS axis can be determined by examining the QRS complex in leads I and II. A normal QRS axis is primarily positive in these leads (I and II).[4–6,11] Figure 10-12 describes the electrical axis of the heart, as described earlier in this chapter.

Step 7: Overall Assessment

Review the heart rate, rhythm, P waves, PR interval, QRS complex, ST segment and T waves, QRS axis, and waveform morphology. Common abnormal findings on ECG include abnormal heart rate (i.e., tachycardia or bradycardia), abnormal cardiac rhythm (e.g., PAC),

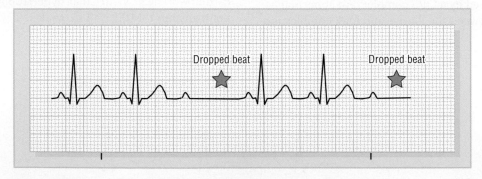

Rate	Atrial rate > ventricular rate
Rhythm	Atrial regular (P waves plot through) Ventricular irregular
P waves	Normal in size and configuration; some P waves are not followed by a QRS (more P waves than QRS complexes)
PR interval	There are a series of nonconducted P waves (e.g., P wave without QRS) followed by a conducted P wave. PR interval may be normal or prolonged but is constant for each conducted QRS.
QRS	< 0.10 s but is dropped periodically

FIGURE 10-28 Second-degree AV block, type II (Mobitz II).

From *Arrhythmia Recognition: The Art of Interpretation*, courtesy of Tomas B. Garcia, MD.

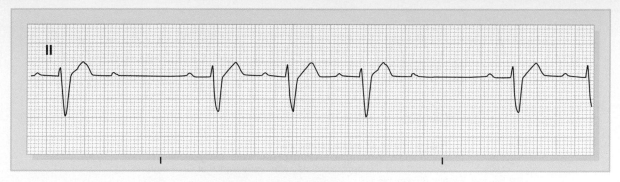

Rate	Atrial rate > ventricular rate
Rhythm	Atrial regular (P waves plot through)
	Ventricular regular
P waves	Normal in size and configuration
	Every other P wave is followed by a QRS (more P waves than QRS complexes)
PR interval	Constant
QRS	Within normal limits if the block occurs above the bundle of His (probably type I)
	Wide if the block occurs at or below the bundle of His (probably type II)
	Absent after every other P wave

FIGURE 10-29 Second-degree AV block, 2:1 conduction.

From *Arrhythmia Recognition: The Art of Interpretation*, courtesy of Tomas B. Garcia, MD.

heart blocks (first-, second-, or third-degree), alteration in the QRS complex (e.g., PVC, ventricular tachycardia, bundle branch blocks), pathologic Q wave development (e.g., MI), ST segment changes (e.g., acute MI, ischemia), QRS axis deviation (e.g., right ventricular hypertrophy), and T wave changes (e.g., ischemia, electrolyte imbalance).[4–6,11–13]

Ventricular flutter, fibrillation, and asystole represent medical emergencies that require the immediate application of advanced cardiac life support (ACLS).

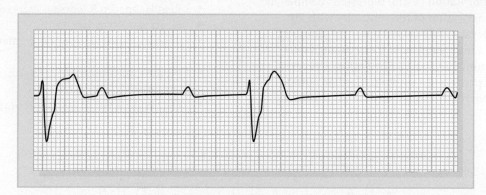

Rate	Atrial rate > ventricular rate; ventricular rate determined by the origin of the escape rhythm
Rhythm	Atrial rhythm regular and ventricular rhythm regular through atrial and ventricular rhythms are disconnected
P waves	Normal in size and configuration
	P waves are "disconnected from QRS (more P waves than QRS complexes)
PR interval	None—the atria and ventricles beat independently of each other; no relationship between the P waves an QRS complexes
QRS	Narrow or wide depending on the location of the escape pacemaker and the condition of the interventricular conduction system.
	Narrow QRS → junctional pacemaker
	Wide QRS → ventricular pacemaker

FIGURE 10-30 Third-degree heart block.

From *Arrhythmia Recognition: The Art of Interpretation*, courtesy of Tomas B. Garcia, MD.

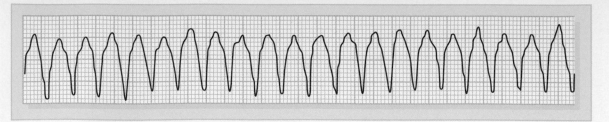

Rate	Rate is 280 to 300 beats per minute
Rhythm	Rapid and monomorphic – a form of ventricular tachycardia
P waves	Generally not discernible but may alter appearance of QRS morphology
PR interval	Not discernible
QRS	A monomorphic form of ventricular tachycardia with wide QRS complexes

FIGURE 10-31 **Ventricular flutter (rapid ventricular tachycardia).**

Copyright 2007 Munther Hamoud, MD. Ventricular flutter. From Hamoud MK. Cardiovascular Pathophysiology. "Figure 10-31: Ventricular Flutter". Published in Tufts OpenCourseWare (2005–2014). http://ocw.tufts.edu/Content/50/lecturenotes/634401/634452. [Retrieved date 08/19/2014]. Reproduced with permission of the author and publisher. Licensed under the Creative Commons Attribution-Noncommercial-Share Alike 3.0 Unported License.

Ventricular flutter is a form of ventricular tachycardia in which the rate is usually about 300 bpm and each QRS is approximately the same in appearance (i.e., monomorphic).[4–6,11] Torsades de pointes is a form of ventricular tachycardia in which the QRS complexes vary in appearance (i.e., polymorphic). **Figure 10-31** provides an example of ventricular flutter; **Figure 10-32** provides an example of torsades de pointes. Cardioversion should be applied as soon as possible in patients who are hemodynamically unstable.

Ventricular fibrillation (V-fib) represents completely uncoordinated activation of the ventricles with an irregular and elevated rate (> 300 bpm).[4–6,11] Initially, V-fib often has a high amplitude (i.e., coarse fibrillation), which diminishes to fine fibrillation. Untreated V-fib will often progress to asystole. Cardiac output during V-fib is virtually absent, and treatment should

begin immediately using ACLS protocols (i.e., chest compressions and rapid performance of defibrillation). **Figure 10-33** provides an example of fine and coarse fibrillation as seen on ECG, whereas **Figure 10-34** shows asystole.

To summarize, for overall assessment of normal sinus rhythm and common arrthymias observe for:

- Normal sinus rhythm
  - Narrow QRS, width < 0.10 seconds, uniform shape
  - Regular spaced R waves
  - Heart rate 60 to 100 bpm
  - P waves upright, rounded, "married" to QRS complexes in lead II
  - PR interval constant 0.12 to 0.20 seconds
- Arrhythmias
  - Heart rate is fast (> 100 bpm) or slow (< 60 bpm)

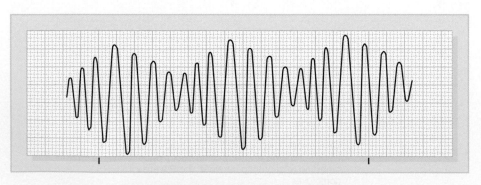

Rate	Atrial not discernible; ventricular 150–250 beats/min
Rhythm	Atrial not discernible; ventricular may be regular or irregular
PR interval	None
QRS	Gradual alteration in the amplitude and direction of the QRS

FIGURE 10-32 **Torsades de pointes.**

From *Arrhythmia Recognition: The Art of Interpretation,* courtesy of Tomas B. Garcia, MD.

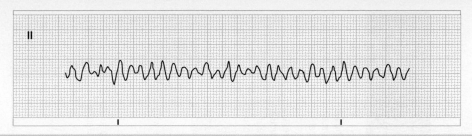

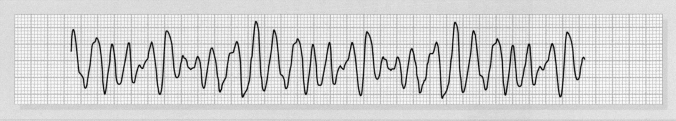

Rate	Cannot be determined because waves or complexes are not discernible to measure
Rhythm	Rapid and chaotic with no pattern or regularity
P waves	Not discernible
PR interval	Not discernible
QRS	Not discernible

FIGURE 10-33 Ventricular fibrillation.

From *Arrhythmia Recognition: The Art of Interpretation*, courtesy of Tomas B. Garcia, MD.

- Irregular or interrupted rhythm
- Premature beats present (e.g., PACs, PVCs)
- Abnormal PR interval
- Abnormal relationship between P waves and QRS complexes (e.g., heart blocks)
- Abnormal ST segment
- Pathologic Q waves
- Abnormal QRS axis
- Major arrhythmia (e.g., V-fib, V-flutter, asystole)

Table 10-5 provides a summary of the major cardiac arrhythmias.

Myocardial Infarction

Acute myocardial infarction (acute MI) occurs when part of the heart muscle is damaged or dies due to lack of blood flow. The most common cause of acute MI is blockage of one of the coronary arteries by a blood clot. Coronary artery disease with plaque buildup (i.e., atherosclerotic heart disease) may lead to MI. The site of blockage of myocardial blood supply will determine which parts of the heart are affected. For example, occlusion of the left anterior descending coronary artery may cause an anterior wall MI.[18] Occlusion of the

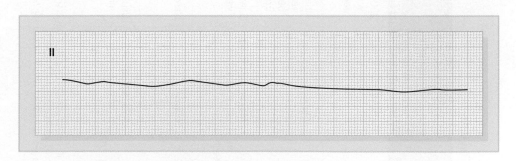

Rate	Ventricular usually indiscernible, but may see some atrial activity
Rhythm	Atrial may be discernible; ventricular indiscernible
P waves	Usually not discernible
PR interval	Not measurable
QRS	Absent

FIGURE 10-34 Asystole (ventricular asystole, ventricular standstill).

From *Arrhythmia Recognition: The Art of Interpretation*, courtesy of Tomas B. Garcia, MD.

TABLE 10-5
Summary of Cardiac Rhythms

	Normal Sinus[1]	Paroxysmal Supraventricular Tachycardia	Atrial Flutter	Atrial Fibrillation	Ventricular Tachycardia	Ventricular Fibrillation	First-Degree AV Block	Second-Degree AV Block, Type I	Second-Degree AV Block, Type II	Complete AV Block (Type III)
Rate (beats per minute)	60–100	150–250	250–350 atrial; ventricular rate varies	Atrial rate > 400; ventricular rate varies	100–250 ventricular	Difficult to discern	Normal	Atrial > ventricular; both usually normal	Atrial > ventricular; both usually normal	Atrial > ventricular; both usually normal
Rhythm	Regular	Regular	Atrial is regular; ventricular can be regular or irregular	Irregular	Regular ventricular	Rapid and chaotic	Regular	Atrial regular; ventricular pauses	Atrial regular; ventricular irregular with pauses	Regular
P waves	Uniform, upright, one before each QRS	May be hard to see	Sawtooth P waves	No P waves identifiable	Usually not discernible	Not discernible	Prolonged, constant PR interval	Progressive widening, then dropped	Some P waves not followed by QRS	No relationship between P and QRS
QRS[2]	Narrow	Narrow	Narrow	Narrow	Wide	Not discernible	Narrow	Narrow; sometimes dropped	Can be wide	Narrow or wide
Clinical severity[3]	Normal	Mild to moderate	Usually mild to moderate	Mild to severe, depending on context	Severe to life threatening	Life threatening	Mild	Mild to moderate, depending on context	Severe to life threatening	Life threatening

[1]If rate is < 60 beats per minute, it is called sinus bradycardia. If rate is > 100 beats per minute, it is sinus tachycardia.

[2]Narrow is defined as ≤ 0.12 second and wide as > 0.12 second.

[3]This clinical severity is used as a general guide for clinicians in training, but the actual severity takes into account numerous factors of a patient's illness and the clinical context and thus should be interpreted accordingly.

right coronary artery or left circumflex coronary artery may cause an inferior wall MI.[18]

Acute MI is often identified based on symptoms (e.g., chest pain not fully relieved by rest or nitroglycerin, anxiety, nausea) and physical findings (e.g., pallor, diaphoresis, and tachycardia) and confirmed by ECG changes and elevation of cardiac biomarkers (e.g., elevated troponins T and I; CKMB).[6] It is important to note, however, that up to 25% of patients with MI may be asymptomatic.[6]

STEMI and NSTEMI

There are two broad categories of acute MI based on ECG findings. **ST segment elevation MI (STEMI)** typically shows ST segment elevation followed by T wave inversion and then Q wave development over a period of several hours if the heart muscle is not reperfused.[6,18-21] **Non-ST segment elevation MI (NSTEMI)**; (aka non-Q-wave MI), in contrast, manifests with ST segment depression and/or T wave inversion in two or more leads *without Q wave development*.[16,18-21] Thus, abnormalities in the ST segment and T waves with MI may be followed by formation of pathologic Q waves (STEMI) or without Q wave development (NSTEMI).[6,18-21]

RC Insights

ST segment elevation may be caused by acute MI.

The location of ischemic or infarcted myocardial tissue can sometimes be determined by the nature of the ECG changes as viewed via different leads. For example, ST segment elevation or Q waves in leads I and aV_L and one (or more) of leads V_1 through V_6 is associated with anterior and apical heart wall ischemia or infarction.[6,18-21] ST segment shifts or Q waves in leads II, III, and aVF are associated with inferior wall ischemia.[6,18-21] ST segment depression with a large R wave in V_1 or V_2 or ST elevation as seen in leads V_6 through V_9 (the posterior ECG leads) may suggest acute posterior wall MI.[6,18-21] Echocardiography may also be useful in clarifying the location of myocardial wall infarction.[20] **Box 10-4** lists Q wave ECG changes associated with specific sites of infarction. **Figure 10-35** provides an example of ST segment elevation. **Figure 10-36** provides an example of a pathologic Q wave.

The treatment of STEMI and NSTEMI are similar, but not the same. Initial treatment of STEMI may include:[20,21]

- Initial assessment (clinical manifestations of MI, vital signs).
- Immediate administration of aspirin (162 to 325 mg, chewed).
- Oxygen therapy if SpO_2 < 90%; establish IV access, begin cardiac monitoring, and implement ACLS protocols if indicated (e.g., ventricular arrhythmia present).
- An ECG to identify STEMI is performed within 10 minutes of arrival in the healthcare facility.

BOX 10-4

Site of Myocardial Infarction and Q Wave ECG Findings

Site of Myocardial Infarction	ECG Changes
Apical wall	Pathologic Q waves* leads V_3–V_4
Anterioseptal wall	Pathologic Q waves in leads V_1–V_2
Anterolateral wall	Pathologic Q waves in leads I, aV_L, V_5–V_6
Inferior wall	Pathologic Q waves in leads II, III, and aV_F or ST segment shifts or Q waves in leads II, III, and aV_F
True posterior	Pathologic Q waves in leads V_1–V_2 (tall R, not deep Q)

*Pathologic Q waves are > 0.04 seconds and ≥ 25% of QRS height.

Modified from: Longo DL, Fauci AS, Kasper DL, Hauser SL, Jameson JL, Loscalzo J, eds. *Harrison's Manual of Medicine*. 18th ed., p. 804. Copyright © 2013 by McGraw-Hill Education. Reprinted by permission.

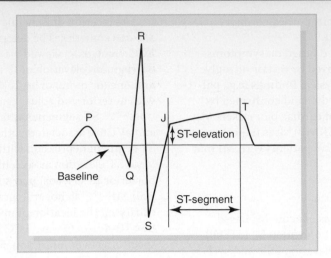

FIGURE 10-35 ST segment elevation characteristic of myocardial injury.

Courtesy of AMC/R.C.B. Kreuger.

ST segment elevation (> 1 mm) in two contiguous limb leads *or* > 2 mm in two continuous precordial leads *or* new left bundle branch block (LBBB) indicates STEMI. Contiguous leads "view" adjacent areas of the heart muscle and are listed below:

- Septal leads (V_1, V_2)
- Inferior leads (II, III, aV_F)
- Lateral leads (I, aV_L, V_5, V_6)
- Anterior leads (V_3, V_4)

■ Measure cardiac biomarkers, electrolytes, and hemoglobin/hematocrit and obtain coagulation studies.
- Measurement of cardiac troponins is preferred (e.g., troponins T and I); these remain elevated 7 to 10 days following acute MI.
- Alternative cardiac biomarkers include creatine phosphokinase (CK), myoglobin, and creatine kinase isoenzyme MB mass (CK-MB$_{mass}$).
- Biomarkers may be normal early in MI.

■ Evaluate and arrange for percutaneous coronary intervention (PCI; aka coronary angioplasty) or IV fibrinolytic agent for myocardial reperfusion.
- If available, PCI should be performed within a specific window of time (i.e., ≤ 90 minutes from first medical contact and transport to a PCI-capable hospital or ≤ 120 minutes if transfer to a PCI capable hospital is required).[20,21]
- Provide fibrinolytic agents to patients with symptom onset of ≤ 12 hours who cannot receive rapid PCI (i.e., within 120 minutes).

- Thrombolytic agents include alteplase, tenecteplase, reteplase, and streptokinase.
- Patients should receive therapy in < 30 minutes after arrival in hospital.[20,21]
- Contraindications must be considered and include history of intracranial hemorrhage or ischemic stroke, internal bleeding, etc.

■ Treat angina (e.g., sublingual nitroglycerin tablets) and persistent anxiety and/or discomfort (e.g., morphine sulfate).[20,21]

■ Manage arrhythmia.

■ Provide β-blocker to prevent recurrent ischemia and ventricular arrhythmias.[20,21]

NSTEMI and **unstable angina** are similar conditions. Elevated biomarkers in combination with unstable angina and ECG changes that do not include ST-segment elevation indicate NSTEMI.[22,23] Unstable angina can be acute, severe, new-onset angina; angina at rest or with minimal activity; or a recent increase in intensity and frequency of chronic angina.[22,23] Initial treatment of unstable angina and NSTEMI is similar to STEMI with the exception of fibrinolysis (tPA), which should *not* be done in cases of NSTEMI.[22,23] Initial treatment of NSTEMI should include providing relief of ischemic pain (e.g., nitroglycerin, morphine), oxygen therapy, assessment and support of hemodynamic status, antithrombotic therapy (e.g., antiplatelet and anticoagulant therapy), and β-blocker therapy to prevent recurrent ischemia and prevent life-threatening arrhythmias.[22,23] Consideration of possible cardiac

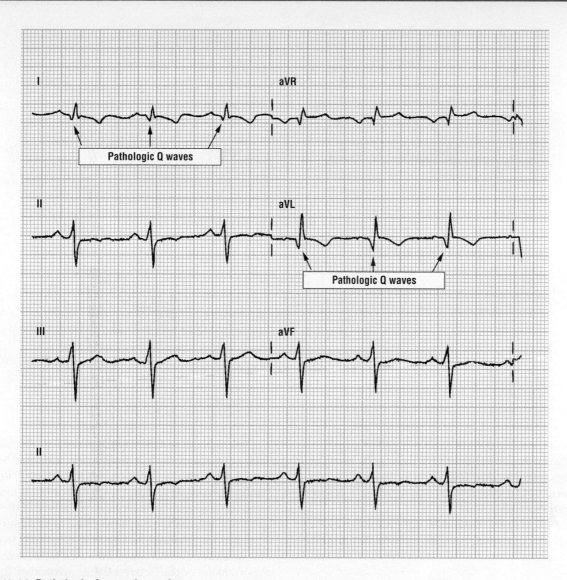

FIGURE 10-36 Pathologic Q wave formation.

From *Arrhythmia Recognition: The Art of Interpretation*, courtesy of Tomas B. Garcia, MD.

catheterization (PCI), coronary artery bypass graft (CABG), or a conservative medical strategy will depend on the patient's condition and estimation of risk. Risk scores using instruments such as the TIMI (Thrombolysis in Myocardial Infarction), GRACE (Global Registry of Acute Coronary Events), and PURSUIT (Platelet glycoprotein IIb/IIIa in Unstable angina: Receptor Suppression Using Integrilin) have been developed for patients with acute cardiac syndrome.[22,23] These risk scores are useful in identifying high-risk patients who may benefit most from myocardial revascularization (e.g., PCI or CABG) and are accurate predictors of mortality.[22,23]

Evolution of Myocardial Infarction

ECG findings typically change as an MI evolves. With very early MI, the ECG may be normal.[18,19] Early tall T waves may be followed by ST segment changes.[18,19] In some cases, elevation of the ST segment is the earliest sign of an acute MI, often followed by T wave inversion (with or without Q wave formation) in a few hours to days following the MI.[18,19] T wave inversions may persist indefinitely or resolve in a few days.[18,19] Most patients continue to show ECG changes (e.g., Q waves with or without inverted, flat, or upright T waves) with a chronic or "old" MI. To summarize, the following are common changes with evolving STEMI:

- Preinfarction is characterized by T wave inversion. Myocardium is ischemic.
- Very early/acute MI is characterized by marked elevation of the ST segment and upright T wave. Acute MI has begun with myocardial injury.
- Acute phase is characterized by significant Q wave formation (may take several hours to appear); ST segment elevation; and upright T wave. Partial myocardial tissue death occurs.

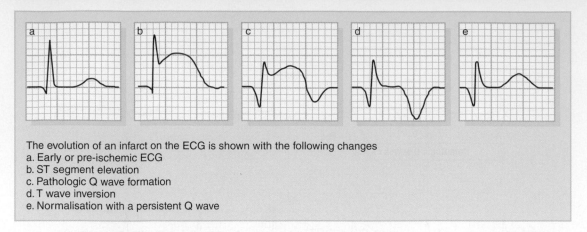

The evolution of an infarct on the ECG is shown with the following changes
a. Early or pre-ischemic ECG
b. ST segment elevation
c. Pathologic Q wave formation
d. T wave inversion
e. Normalisation with a persistent Q wave

FIGURE 10-37 ECG changes with evolution of MI.

- Acute, evolving MI is characterized by significant Q wave and then inverted T wave a few hours to days following MI. Infarction is almost complete.
- Recent MI is characterized by significant Q wave with inverted T wave.
- Old MI is characterized by significant Q wave and ST segment at baseline with flat or upright T wave.

With some patients, the ECG changes are such that the age of the MI cannot be determined. A STEMI of indeterminate age may show a significant Q wave with the ST segment back to baseline (or nearly back to baseline) and an inverted T wave. **Figure 10-37** provides an example of ECG changes sometimes seen with evolution of MI. It must be emphasized, however, that the ECG pattern of evolution in MI is variable.

Congestive Heart Failure

Congestive heart failure (CHF), or "pump failure," can be simply defined as a disease state or condition in which the heart fails to maintain adequate blood circulation. Heart failure can be left-sided, right-sided, or both. *Left ventricular failure* refers specifically to failure of the left side of the heart to adequately pump blood out to the body, whereas *right-sided heart failure* refers to failure of the right side of the heart to adequately pump blood to the lungs. In fact, when the left ventricle fails, blood will "back up" in the pulmonary system, pulmonary vascular pressures will rise, and eventually the right heart may fail.

Development of CHF is associated with coronary artery disease, chronic hypertension, enlarged heart (cardiomegaly), and cardiac valvular disease.[10] Reduction in ventricular ejection fraction is sometimes referred to as *systolic heart failure*. Failure of the heart to fill during diastole may also cause heart failure (e.g., diastolic heart failure in which the heart fails to relax during diastole, which may be caused by untreated hypertension or restrictive cardiac myopathy). Episodes of CHF may be triggered by excessive salt intake, worsening hypertension, acute MI, development of arrhythmias, pulmonary embolus, infection, anemia, and certain drugs.[10]

Patients with CHF often experience dyspnea (e.g., orthopnea, paroxysmal nocturnal dyspnea), fatigue, and peripheral edema (e.g., swelling of the ankles). CHF patients may suffer repeated hospitalizations and often have a reduced health-related quality of life and increased mortality.[10] Increased heart rate and respiratory rate, peripheral edema, jugular venous distension, enlarged liver, and ascites are seen on physical examination.[10] Chest exam may reveal dullness to percussion over areas of pleural effusion due to CHF and rales or crackles upon auscultation of the chest, which are associated with development of pulmonary edema.[10] The chest radiograph may show an enlarged heart, pleural effusion, and Kerley B lines associated with increased pulmonary vascular fluid (see Chapter 11) and the development of interstitial or pulmonary edema. Echocardiography may reveal left ventricular dysfunction.

As noted above, left ventricular failure may lead to right-sided heart failure due to fluid backup and increased pulmonary vascular pressures. **Cor pulmonale** is right-sided heart failure caused by lung disease. For example, chronic hypoxia due to chronic lung disease often causes an increase in pulmonary vascular resistance (i.e., hypoxemic vasoconstriction), chronic pulmonary hypertension, and right ventricular hypertrophy.[10] COPD, bronchiectasis, cystic fibrosis, and interstitial lung disease (ILD) are all associated with chronic hypoxemia and the development of cor pulmonale.[10] Other causes include chronic restrictive pulmonary disease, sickle cell anemia, and diseases that occlude the pulmonary vasculature.[10]

ECG with Heart Failure

The ECG should be obtained in patients with suspected CHF to help identify the cause and to detect any arrhythmias that may be present. For example, CHF patients may exhibit PVCs, episodes of V-tach, or atrial fibrillation, all of which may worsen CHF.[4,5,24] The ECG may also help identify AV heart block, bundle branch block, or other conduction abnormalities.[4,5,24] The ECG is also essential in identifying myocardial ischemia or acute MI.[24] ECG changes may also help identify the presence of left ventricular hypertrophy secondary to chronic hypertension.[4,5,24] For example, the following ECG changes are associated with left ventricular hypertrophy:[6]

- S wave in V_1 + R wave in V_5 or $V_6 \geq 35$ mm

  OR

- R wave in $aV_L > 11$ mm

Right ventricular hypertrophy may result in right axis deviation (> 90°), and the R wave may be greater than the S wave in the V_1 lead.

Treatment of Heart Failure

Treatment of CHF may include diuretics for fluid retention and use of an ACE inhibitor and β-blocker for patients with left ventricular systolic disease.[24] General measures may include salt restriction, avoidance of nonsteroidal anti-inflammatory drugs (NSAIDs), and preventive immunizations (e.g., influenza and pneumococcal pneumonia vaccines).[24]

Management of Cardiac Arrhythmias

Arrhythmias are abnormal rhythms (cardiac dysrhythmias) associated with abnormal electrical activity of the heart. As we have seen, there are a large number of types and causes of cardiac arrhythmia, and these may be described in terms of the source of the abnormal heartbeat. For example, an abnormal cardiac rhythm may originate in the SA node, the atria, the AV junction, or the ventricles.

Management of cardiac arrhythmias will depend on the type of arrhythmia and the patient's clinical condition. Certain arrhythmias are associated with sudden cardiac death, whereas others may cause hemodynamic instability. Treatment of sudden cardiac death requires immediate application of cardiopulmonary resuscitation (CPR), which usually includes electrical defibrillation. Treatment of arrhythmias often includes use of antiarrhythmia medications. Nonpharmacologic treatment of arrhythmias may include use of cardiac pacemakers to treat bradyarrhythmia and electrical cardioversion or radiofrequency ablation to treat certain tachyarrhythmias. Cardiac defibrillation in combination with ACLS protocols are used to treat asystole and ventricular fibrillation.

Pharmacologic Treatment

Arrhythmia management in cases where clinical symptoms are present, hemodynamic instability has occurred, or the patient is at risk for sudden cardiac death often includes pharmacologic therapy. Antiarrhythmic drugs are categorized by class. Class I medications include moderate sodium channel blockers (Class IA) and weak sodium channel blockers (Class IB). Examples of Class IA agents include quinidine, procainamide, and disopyramide.[11] These agents are sometimes useful in treatment of supraventricular and ventricular arrhythmias.[11] Class IB medications include lidocaine, tocainide, mexiletine, and phenytoin.[11] Class IB agents are sometimes useful for treating ventricular tachyarrhythmias.[11] Class IC antiarrhythmic agents are the most potent sodium channel blockers. Class IC agents include flecainide, propafenone, and moricizine.[11] Like Class IA drugs, Class IC agents may be effective in treating both supraventricular and ventricular arrhythmias. Unfortunately, the use of flecainide or moricizine following MI has been shown to increase mortality, and thus both agents are contradicted in these patients.[11]

Class II antiarrhythmic agents are the β-blockers and include propranolol, metoprolol, and atenolol.[11] The β-blockers are useful to control the rate with atrial flutter and atrial fibrillation and some forms of supraventricular tachycardia. β-blockers are also used to prevent recurrent ischemia and ventricular arrhythmia in patients with acute MI.

Class III antiarrhythmic agents are potassium channel blockers; amiodarone is an example of a drug that is mainly Class III.[11] Amiodarone is useful in treating a wide range of supraventricular and ventricular tachyarrhythmias.[11] Amiodarone may be especially useful in the treatment of patients with atrial fibrillation with heart failure, and it can sometimes help prevent recurrence of ventricular tachycardia or ventricular fibrillation.[11] Other Class III drugs include sotalol, bretylium, ibutilide, and dofetilide.[11]

Class IV antiarrhythmic drugs include verapamil and diltiazem.[11] These medications are calcium channel blockers that are sometimes effective for controlling the heart rate with atrial fibrillation and atrial flutter.[11]

Nonpharmacologic Treatment

Cardiac pacemakers are sometimes useful in treatment of bradyarrhythmias. Examples where cardiac pacing is indicated include certain forms of atrioventricular block (e.g., third-degree block).[11] Pacing can be applied transcutaneously to treat transient bradyarrhythmia until reversed or implanted permanently. Cardiac pacemakers are available that pace the atrium, the ventricle, or both. Newer pacemakers may be responsive to the patient's level of activity in that they have a rate-responsive mode.

Cardioversion techniques involve the application of a synchronized electrical shock to treat tachyarrhythmias such as atrial flutter, atrial fibrillation, and ventricular tachycardia. The electrical shock is typically less than 50 to 100 joules (biphasic) for atrial flutter, whereas atrial fibrillation may require 120 to 200 joules (biphasic).[11] Risks of cardioversion include of precipitation of ventricular fibrillation and embolization of an atrial thrombus.[11]

Ventricular defibrillation applies a high-energy, unsynchronized shock in the range of 200 to 250 joules (biphasic) or 300 to 360 joules (monophasic). Ventricular defibrillation is indicated in all patients with ventricular fibrillation as a part of ACLS. Automatic, implantable cardioverter defibrillators are available for use in certain patients at high risk of sudden cardiac death. Radiofrequency catheter ablation may be indicated in certain patients with tachyarrhythmias in whom drug therapy is not effective. With radiofrequency ablation, electrical energy is applied using radio waves to cause a lesion to a specific site in the endocardium. Radiofrequency ablation is sometimes effective in controlling atrial flutter and certain types of supraventricular tachycardia.[11] Radiofrequency ablation therapy is also sometimes useful in treating atrial fibrillation and, to a lesser extent, ventricular tachycardia.

Rhythms Initiated in the Sinus Node

The sinus node (SA) is the kingpin of the conduction system, and rhythms that start in the SA node are predictable. A normal sinus rhythm (NSR) originates in the SA node with an identical normal P wave before every QRS complex at a regular rate of 60 to 100 beats per minute. The PR interval is 0.12 to 0.20 seconds. Sinus rhythms have waves that are upright in lead II, a married QRS complex, and constant PR intervals.[2] When a dysrhythmia is present, the goal is to return the heart back to a sinus rhythm, if possible.

Sinus Tachycardia

When the SA node is the pacemaker for a rate of greater than 100 beats per minute, sinus tachycardia is present.[8,16,17] With sinus tachycardia, there is a P wave for every QRS complex, the rhythm is regular, and the rate can be anywhere from 100 to 150 beats per minute. The PR intervals are constant but short due to the rapid rate. Sinus tachycardia is a normal response to the body's demand for more blood flow (e.g., exercise) or it may be caused by hypoxemia, the ingestion of stimulants, smoking, increased catecholamines or sympathetic tone, fever, anemia, hypoxia, hypervolemia, CHF, pulmonary embolism, acute MI, or hypotension. Other causes include use of certain medications, such as epinephrine, isoproterenol, norepinephrine, and excessive amounts of atropine. Treatment should target the underlying cause. Sinus tachycardia is generally not life threatening; however, it may signal an underlying condition that can be life threatening (e.g., severe hypoxemia). Tachycardia also increases myocardial oxygen consumption and may lead to inadequate filling during diastole and myocardial ischemia (see Figure 10-16 for an example of sinus tachycardia). Causes of sinus tachycardia are listed in **Box 10-5**.

Sinus Bradycardia

Sinus bradycardia is a normal rhythm initiated in the SA node resulting in a rate of less than 60 beats per minute.[8,17,25] Sinus bradycardia can be caused by increased vagal tone, drugs and medications, hyperkalemia, hypothyroidism, and hypothermia (see also Box 10-5).[25] Well-conditioned athletes often have a resting HR < 60 bpm.[17] Thus, it is the change in HR compared to the patient's baseline that should be considered when evaluating patients with sinus bradycardia. Bradycardia in patients may result in hypotension and symptoms such as dizziness, syncope, and fatigue. Figure 10-21 provides an example of sinus bradycardia. **Clinical Focus 10-1** provides an example of a patient with bradycardia.

Sinus Rate Fluctuation

An abnormal increase or decrease in the firing rate of the SA node during breathing provides another example of a sinus dysrhythmia. In this case, there is a P wave for every QRS complex; however, the rate may increase with inspiration and decrease during expiration. This type of dysrthymia is common in children, young adults, and the elderly and may be caused by changes in intrathoracic pressure or vagal parasympathetic effect on the SA node during breathing. This dysrhythmia is also sometimes seen in adults with heart disease and those taking certain medications, such as digitalis or morphine.

Sinus Arrest or Pause

A sinus pause or arrest is caused by failure of the SA node to fire.[6,11,25] No P wave is seen, and if the duration of SA node inactivity is prolonged (i.e., sinus arrest) the pause may be followed by an atrial, a junctional, or a ventricular escape beat or by asystole. The intrinsic resting HR of the SA node is 60 to 100 bpm. If the SA node fails to fire, the initiation of the heartbeat may be taken over by the atria (other than the SA node), the AV junction, or the ventricles in hierarchical order and with a characteristic heart rate:

- Atrial escape rate of 60 to 80 bpm
- Junctional escape rate of 40 to 60 bpm
- Ventricular escape rate of 20 to 40 bpm

Sinus pause or arrest is not the same as a sinoatrial exit block (abnormal conduction from the SA node to the atrium) or nonconducted atrial premature complexes.[6,11,25] Sinus arrest or pause can be a result of increased vagal parasympathetic tone, hypoxia, hyperkalemia, or medications such as digitalis, propranolol, and quinidine. It may also be seen with acute inferior MI, acute myocarditis, or forms of fibrosis.[6,11,12] If the sinus arrest is transient or asymptomatic, then no treatment is necessary. If lightheadedness, syncope, or other symptoms occur, treatment may include correcting

BOX 10-5

Causes of Sinus Tachycardia and Sinus Bradycardia

Sinus tachycardia (HR > 100 bpm)
- Normal response to exercise
- Hypoxia
- Cardiac and circulatory problems:
  - Heart disease
  - Anemia
  - Blood loss
  - Hypovolemia
  - Hypotension
  - Shock
- Anxiety
- Uncontrolled pain
- Fever
- Drugs and medications:
  - Catecholamines: Epinephrine, isoproterenol, dopamine, β_1-agonist bronchodilators
  - Atropine
  - Xanthines: Theophylline, caffeine, nicotine
  - Cocaine, methamphetamines
- Medical procedures (e.g., endotracheal suctioning, manipulation of tracheostomy tubes, or tracheostomy tube ties)

Sinus bradycardia (HR < 60 bpm)
- Increased vagal tone:
  - Healthy young athletes
  - Carotid sinus massage
  - Valsalva maneuver
  - Vomiting
  - Increased intracranial pressure (ICP)
  - Vasovagal syncope (e.g., fainting due to emotional distress)
- Drugs and medications:
  - Digitalis
  - β-blockers (e.g., propranolol, metoprolol)
  - Calcium channel blockers (e.g., diltiazem, verapamil)
  - Antiarrhythmic agents (e.g., sotalol, amiodarone)
- Hyperkalemia
- Hypothyroidism
- Hypothermia

CLINICAL FOCUS 10-1

Bradycardia

Problem

A 28-year-old male with the diagnosis of asthma starting at age 6 was admitted to the hospital for initiation of propafenone, an antiarrhythmic for atrial and ventricular dysrhythmia. Propafenone slows the influx of Na^+ into the cardiac muscle cells, and it is metabolized rapidly in the liver. The patient was placed on telemetry, and titration of the medication was started at 900 mg/dL. The patient became lightheaded, complained of increasing shortness of breath, and his heart rate dropped from 40 to 30 beats per minute with a blood pressure of 50/30 mm Hg. Breath sounds on auscultation revealed bilateral wheeze. The ECG showed sinus bradycardia with a first-degree block followed by a wide-complex tachycardia. What treatment should be administered? What existing morbidities put this patient at risk?

Solution

Cardiopulmonary resuscitation should be administered to help with perfusion of the vital organs until temporary heart pacing can be applied. Medical treatment should include epinephrine and catecholamines. Side effects of propafenone include dizziness, gastrointestinal upset, and bronchospasm. The patient has a history of asthma, which may be exacerbated by propafenone. Quick administration of supportive measures, both circulatory and respiratory, will allow this patient time to recover.

Data from: Wozakowska-Kaplon B, Stepien-Walek A. Propafenone overdose: Cardiac arrest and full recovery. *Cardiol J.* 2009;17:619–622.

---

the underlying cause, stopping medications that suppress the SA node, and, in some cases, inserting a pacemaker.[6,11,25]

Rhythms that start in the atria but outside of the SA node are considered ectopic rhythms and usually result in a rapid rate. When the patient is symptomatic, the goal is to return the heart to a normal sinus rhythm. Atrial rhythms will have varied P waves depending on the site of the ectopic pacemaker. Examples include premature atrial contractions, atrial flutter, and atrial fibrillation.

Rhythms Initiated in the Atria

Premature Atrial Contraction

Premature atrial contractions (PACs) are due to premature activation of the atria by an atrial site other than the sinus node. The PAC is an early beat on ECG that may appear similar to a normal sinus rhythm, though the shape of the P wave may be different. With PACs the PR interval may be normal, increased, or decreased, and the QRS complex may be normal or wide.[6,11] PACs are more common in older patients and are also associated with alcohol and caffeine consumption. PACs are also associated with structural heart disease, early, state MI, and pericarditis.[6,11] Symptoms include palpitations, noticeably skipped beats, and, in some cases, dizziness.[6,11] Treatment includes addressing the underlying cause and eliminating caffeine and alcohol from the diet.[6,11] β-blockers may be helpful in symptomatic patients; calcium channel blockers and class IC antiarrhythmic sodium channel antagonists (e.g., flecainide and propafenone) may be considered.[25]

Atrial Flutter

A rapid sawtooth or flutter appearance on the ECG is indicative of an arrhythmia known as atrial flutter. The abnormal direction of the depolarization of the atria results in atrial waves that have an undetermined onset and end, an amplitude of 1 to 5 mm, and that precede, are buried in, and follow a normal QRS complex.[2] The sawtoothed appearance results from a common conduction ratio of two waves for every QRS complex (2:1; rhythm 120 bpm and regular), but it can also be 3:1, 4:1, or more when a physiologic AV block is present.[2] The atrial flutter rate is between 240 and 360 bpm, whereas the ventricular rate is about one-half the atrial rate.[2] The rhythm is regular if the AV conduction ratio is constant. Because the atria do not regularly contract, the ventricles cannot completely fill, resulting in a decreased cardiac output. Atrial flutter is commonly seen in middle-aged and elderly persons with valve disease, coronary heart disease, advanced rheumatic heart disease, acute hypoxia, CHF, cardiomyopathy, pericarditis, or myocarditis. A person with atrial flutter may feel palpitations, anxiety, weakness, shortness of breath, chest pain, and even syncope. The goal of treatment is to restore a normal sinus rhythm. A vagal maneuver such as carotid sinus massage or Valsalva maneuver may slow the ventricular rate. The patient should avoid stimulants and may be given medications such as warfarin or heparin to decrease the possibility of blood clots. In some cases, radiofrequency catheter ablation may be required. This technique destroys abnormal conduction pathways in the atria. Figure 10-18 provides an example of atrial flutter.

Atrial Fibrillation

A dysrhythmia originating from multiple ectopic pacemakers or sites of rapid reentry in the atria is called atrial fibrillation. The atrial waves represent incomplete depolarizations and are chaotic, lacking definition as to their onset or end. The amplitude of the waves varies from 1 millimeter to several millimeters. The QRS complexes are normal but have no relationship to the P waves, and only one-half to one-third of the electrical impulses make it through to the AV junction. The rate is irregular, with an atrial rate at 350 to 600 waves per minute and a ventricular rate at 160 to 180 beats per minute.[2] Advanced rheumatic heart disease, coronary heart disease, and thyrotoxicosis are all associated with atrial fibrillation. In some individuals, atrial fibrillation may appear with excessive ingestion of alcohol or caffeine, metabolic imbalances, lung disease, sleep apnea, heart surgery, viral infections, or during periods of great emotional stress. The goal for treatment is to reset the rhythm and to prevent blood clots by maintaining anticoagulation therapy. Resetting the rhythm (which increases cardiac output) may be accomplished through the use of medications, electrical cardioversion, radiofrequency catheter ablation, or by performing a surgical maze during open heart surgery. See Figure 10-19 for an example of atrial fibrillation. It is interesting to note that there is some evidence that resetting cardiac rhythm may not reduce the rate of stroke.

Rhythms Initiated at the AV Junction

Rhythms that start in the AV junction will send electrical impulses in both directions antegrade toward the ventricles and retrograde toward the atria, resulting in varied P wave formations. These rates are usually slower than atrial rhythms.

A **premature junctional complex (PJC)** stems from irritable tissue in the AV junction in the form of an ectopic pacemaker. This ventricular beat may yield a normal or an abnormal QRS complex and may or may not have a P wave preceding or buried within the QRS complex. The P waves will appear abnormal, varying in size, shape, and direction. The rhythm is irregular, as seen in the R-R intervals, and the inherent rate is 40 to 60 beats per minute.[2] PJC may appear as isolated beats or in couplets or in a pattern of bigeminy, trigeminy, or quadrigeminy. The most common cause is digitalis toxicity; however, other causes include hypoxia;

stimulants; increased parasympathetic tone; cardiac medications such as procainamide and quinidine or sympathomimetic drugs, such as epinephrine, isoproterenol, and norepinephrine; CHF; or AV junction damage. Treatment may be necessary if symptoms are present, usually with slow rates. See **Figure 10-24** for an example of a premature junctional complex.

A *junctional* or *escape rhythm* originates from an escape pacemaker in the AV junction. P waves may or may not be present and will not be married to the QRS complexes. The rate is regular but only 40 to 60 beats per minute.[2] This type of rhythm can be caused by vagal simulation, hypoxia, heart disease, or sinus node ischemia. Cardiac output may decrease with slower rate and should be treated with transcutaneous pacing, atropine, dopamine, or epinephrine.

Irritable tissue at the level of the AV junction may result in a tachycardia or an accelerated *junctional tachycardia*. P waves may or may not be present, and they may not have any relationship with the normal-looking QRS complexes. The rhythm is regular at a rate of 60 to 150 beats per minute.[2] This rhythm is most often caused by digitalis toxicity but can also occur in people with heart disease, sympathetic stimulation, electrolyte imbalance, or hyperventilation. It can also occur during stress or with the use of stimulants. If symptoms appear as a result of decreased output, medications such as β-blockers, calcium channel blockers, or adenosine may be prescribed and carotid massage can be used to slow the heart rate. If the patient is unstable, cardioversion is an option (see **Figure 10-38**).

Rhythms Initiated in the Ventricles

With the exception of ventricular tachycardia, ventricular rhythms are often slow and have wide QRS complexes with or without remarkable P waves. The treatment for these rhythms includes medications or electric shock. Note that ventricular rhythms can be fatal despite treatment.

A *premature ventricular contraction* (PVC) is an early beat stemming from irritable ventricular tissue. The QRS complexes are wide and bizarre in shape, usually greater than 0.12 seconds in width, and P waves are usually not seen. The rhythm is irregular when PVCs are present, and the rate is determined by the underlying rhythm. A compensatory pause usually follows a PVC, which allows the regular underlying rhythm to resume right on time. The T wave will slope in the opposite direction of the QRS complex. Unifocal PVCs can have a single focus and all look alike, whereas multifocal PVCs differ from each other because they stem from different irritable tissue sites in the ventricles. Occasional PVCs are not a problem unless they cause symptoms such as palpitations, weakness, dizziness, and syncope. Heart disease, hypokalemia, and hypoxia are the main causes of PVCs; however, stimulant use,

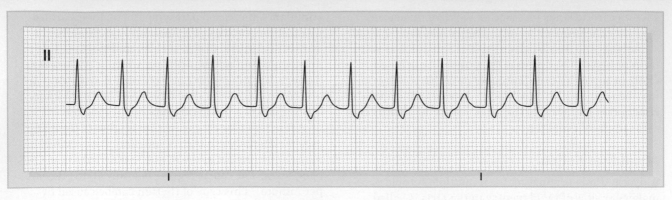

Rate	100–180 beats/min
Rhythm	Atrial and ventricular very regular
P waves	May occur before, during, or after the QRS; if seen, will be inverted (retrograde)
PR interval	If the P wave occurs before the QRS, the PR interval will usually be ≤ 0.12 s
QRS	< 0.10 s

FIGURE 10-38 Junctional tachycardia.

From *Arrhythmia Recognition: The Art of Interpretation*, courtesy of Tomas B. Garcia, MD.

hypomagnesium, stress, and anxiety can also trigger PVCs. If PVCs are frequent (i.e., more than six per minute) or fall too close to the T wave, an R-on-T phenomenon can cause the progression to a lethal dysrhythmia.[4] Treatment for symptomatic PVCs should be focused on the cause. Oxygen should be administered, and medications such as atropine may be given to increase the heart rate. See Figure 10-25 for an example of PVCs. **Clinical Focus 10-2** provides an example of a patient with PVCs.

An *idioventricular rhythm* (IVR) is a ventricular regular escape beat at a rate of 20 to 40 per minute. The QRS is wide and bizarre with no P waves or PR interval. The T waves slopes in the opposite direction of the QRS complexes. The individual will have decreased output and vascular collapse, and each beat may or may not result in a palpable pulse due to massive damage to the heart and/or body or hypoxia. Treatment includes epinephrine, oxygen, and pacemaker insertion. If the blood pressure is not adequate to perfuse the brain, then CPR should be initiated. See **Figure 10-39** for an example of accelerated idioventricular rhythm.

Ventricular tachycardia (V-tach) originates from irritable ventricular tissue that is rapidly firing. Wide and bizarre QRS complexes are present with no P waves. The rate is regular and greater than 100 beats per minute.[2,16,18] Ventricular tachycardia is often lethal unless treated with medications, cardioversion, or initiation of CPR. Symptoms may include palpitations, weakness, dizziness, angina, and syncope caused by cardiomyopathy, heart failure, myocarditis, valvular heart disease, electrolyte imbalance, hypoxia, acid-based imbalance, or use of certain medications. See Figure 10-20 for an example of ventricular tachycardia.[8,16]

A polymorphic ventricular tachycardia known as *torsades de pointes* (a French term meaning "twisting of the points") is sometimes seen in certain patients. With torsades de pointes, the QRS complexes start by pointing up and then become smaller, oscillating around an axis until they point down. Torsades de pointes is not tolerated well and will often deteriorate into ventricular fibrillation. The QRS complexes are wide and bizarre. The QT interval is prolonged, and the T wave, if present, is opposite of the QRS complexes. Torsades de pointes may be inherited (e.g., long QT syndrome) or caused by amiodarone, procainamide, and quinidine, as well as by cardiomyopathy, heart failure, myocarditis, valvular heart disease, electrolyte imbalance, hypoxia, and acid-based imbalance. Treatment consists of magnesium administration, electrical cardioversion, or defibrillation, depending on the individual's symptoms. See Figure 10-32 for an example of torsades de pointes.

Ventricular fibrillation occurs when the heart has multiple ectopic pacemaker sites all firing at different times in different areas. With ventricular fibrillation, the rhythm is chaotic; distinct QRS complexes, P waves, or T waves are absent; and there is no detectable rate. Cardiac output is zero, and the patient exhibits no palpable pulse. Causes include cardiomyopathy, heart failure, myocarditis, hypovolemic shock, blunt or penetrating trauma, valvular heart disease, electrolyte imbalance, hypoxia, and acid-based imbalance, as well as drowning, drug overdose, and accidental electric shock. Emergent treatment is required, including electrical defibrillation, CPR, ventilatory support, and medications. See Figure 10-33 for an example of ventricular fibrillation.

CLINICAL FOCUS 10-2

Premature Ventricular Contractions

Problem

A 58-year-old female is seeking medical advice from her pulmonary physician concerning a chronic cough associated with palpations and syncope. Having recently quit smoking and no recent history of respiratory infection, the persistent cough was affecting her quality of life. The patient denies any shortness of breath. Upon examination, her blood pressure is 90/60 mm Hg. The ECG was normal except during coughing, when a sinus rhythm with unifocal premature ventricular contractions (PVCs) was noted. What diagnostic tests should be ordered? What is the mechanism for cough-induced PVCs? What treatment should be considered?

Solution

The patient underwent an echocardiography that showed mild mitral valve prolapse with regurgitation. An external event monitor captured multiple episodes of bigeminy that coincided with coughing episodes. Medications were ineffective. Spirometry, chest radiograph, and histamine challenge were all negative. GERD was ruled out along with other possible abnormalities following a thorough physical examination.

The patient was referred to a specialist for possible radiofrequency (RF) ablation. An isoproterenol infusion was administered to induce PVC activity. The PVCs disappeared after the fifth pulse of RF energy focused on the posterior area of the right ventricle below the pulmonary valve.

Dysrhythmias caused by cough are not common. A possible cause is the distension of the pulmonary trunk, which stimulates sympathetic innervation in the pulmonary artery.

Data from: Stec S, Dabrowska, M, Bielicki P, et al. Premature ventricular complex-induced chronic cough and cough syncope. *Eur Resp J.* 2007;30:391–394.

Asystole is the absence of any electrical activity in the heart (i.e., cardiac death). The ECG tracing will be a flat line because the heart rate is zero; no QRS complexes are present, and waves of any kind are absent. Asystole is caused by profound states such as complete cardiac collapse, severe hypoxia, or other catastrophic body system damage or failure. Treatment includes immediate application of CPR, chest compressions, epinephrine, oxygen, ventilatory support, and attention to causative factors. Figure 10-34 provides an example of asystole as seen on ECG.

Rhythms Initiated by Atrioventricular Blocks

With an **atrioventricular (AV) block**, the SA node fires normally but there is a problem in the downstream

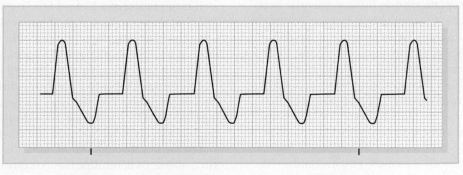

Rate	Atrial not discernible; ventricular 40–100 beat/min
Rhythm	Atrial not discernible; ventricular essentially regular
P waves	Absent
PR interval	None
QRS	> 0.12 s

FIGURE 10-39 **Accelerated idioventricular rhythm (AIVR).**

From *Arrhythmia Recognition: The Art of Interpretation,* courtesy of Tomas B. Garcia, MD.

conduction of the electrical impulse to the ventricles. There are three types, or degrees, of blocks, with varying heart rates, P waves, and symptoms. Treatment is focused on normalizing the heart rate and rhythm.

First-degree AV block manifests in a rhythm with a normal P wave married to a normal QRS complex; however, the PR interval is prolonged—greater than 0.20 seconds. This dysrhythmia can be caused by ischemia or medications such as digitalis, β-blockers, or calcium channel blockers. There should be no symptoms, and treatment is targeted at the cause. See Figure 10-26 for a sinus rhythm with first-degree block.

Second-degree Mobitz I (Wenckebach) AV block is usually a temporary dysrhythmia. Normal P waves are followed by normal QRS complexes; however, the PR interval becomes increasingly longer until the AV node is unable to pass along the impulse to the ventricles and the ensuing QRS complex is dropped. The P-P intervals are of equal distance. The rate is irregular, usually between 60 to 100 beats per minute.[2,8] The atrial rate is faster than the ventricular rate due to the dropped beats. Second-degree Mobitz I can be caused by MI, digitalis toxicity, or side effects from medications. If signs and symptoms occur, a transcutaneous pacemaker may be required to support cardiac output and observation for worsening blocks. See Figure 10-27 for an example of second-degree Mobitz I AV block.

Second-degree Mobitz II AV block is a result of a problem with conduction through the AV node or bundle branches. There are normal P waves with normal QRS complexes, except for the blocked P waves. The P-P interval is regular, but the overall rhythm may be regular or irregular at a rate of 60 to 100 beats per minute.[2,8] The PR intervals will be constant with conducted beats. The QRS complex will be < 0.12 seconds when the AV node is blocked and > 0.12 seconds if the block occurs in the bundle branches.[2] The heart rate may be slow, resulting in a decreased cardiac output. Causes include MI, medication side effects, hypoxia, ethanol poisoning, obstructive sleep apnea, cardiac tumors, valvular heart disease, or lesions in the conduction system. Treatment calls for immediate transcutaneous pacing, oxygen, atropine, epinephrine, or dopamine. See Figure 10-28 for an example of second-degree Mobitz II AV block.

A *2:1 AV block* is a second-degree block defined by having two P waves for every QRS complex. The first P wave of the pair is the blocked beat. The QRS complexes are normal and < 0.12 seconds with a block in the AV node and > 0.12 seconds with a bundle branch block. The PR intervals are constant with conducted beats, and the rate is 60 to 100 beats per minute and regular. The causes and treatments are the same for a Mobitz II block. See Figure 10-29 for an example of second-degree 2:1 AV block. **Clinical Focus 10-3** describes a patient with a heart block.

Third-degree or *complete heart block* occurs when the SA node sends out impulses but none of them get through to the ventricles. The ventricles are controlled by their own pacemaker site, resulting in P waves and QRS complexes that have no relationship (i.e., they are not married). The term for this phenomenon is *AV dissociation*. The rhythm is regular with an atrial rate of 60 to 100 beats per minute and a ventricular rate of 20 to 60 beats per minute.[4] The QRS complexes may be narrow or wide, depending on where the block is located. A complete heart block can be caused by MI, medication side effects, hypoxia, or conduction system lesions. Treatment is focused on resolving the underlying cause. When treating symptoms of low cardiac output as a result of the slow rate, a transcutaneous pacer, oxygen, atropine, epinephrine, or dopamine should be considered. See Figure 10-30 for an example of third-degree block.

12-Lead ECG Interpretation

A 12-lead ECG is obtained to identify cardiac waveform morphology and determine if there are abnormalities caused by arrhythmias, electrolyte imbalance, toxicities, or disease. The individual being tested is at rest and in the supine position. This is a noninvasive procedure that measures the electrical impulses emitted through cardiac tissue from different angles and records the rate and rhythm of the heart.

Placement for the leads when obtaining a 12-lead ECG requires that the limb leads be positioned as follows: right arm (RA) on the right forearm or wrist, left arm (LA) on the left forearm or wrist, left leg (LL) on the left lower leg, and the right leg (RL) or ground lead on the lower right leg. The precordial leads are placed in the following positions:[2,8]

V_1	Fourth intercostal space, right sternal border
V_2	Fourth intercostal space, left sternal border
V_3	Between V_2 and V_4
V_4	Fifth intercostal space, midclavicular line
V_5	Anterior axillary line, straight in line with V_4
V_6	Midaxillary line, straight in line with V_4 and V_5

Interpretation of a 12-lead ECG involves six steps.[2] The first step is to look at the basic rhythm by examining the heart rate; heart rhythm; PR, QRS, and QT intervals; QRS complex; and ST segments, and then deciding if they are normal or abnormal.

The second step is to identify the direction of the electrical impulse flow through the heart by determining the axis. The normal electrical impulse flow through the heart starts at the SA node and travels downward and to the left through the AV junction into the Purkinje fibers. To determine the axis quadrant, a compass is used to depict north, south, east, and west, with lines depicting the frontal leads, I, II, III, aV_R, aV_L, and aV_F. Lead I runs from right to left, whereas the aV_F lead runs north to south. All the other leads are separated by 30° increments around the axis circle. The current in a normal heart flows on an axis of 60°. The circle forms four quadrants: normal, 0 to +90°; left axis deviation 0 to

CLINICAL FOCUS 10-3

Heart Block

Problem

A 65-year-old female presented to the hospital with an exacerbation of end-stage COPD. Her chief complaint was faintness and shortness of breath. She received β-adrenergic inhalers and oxygen via 4 L nasal cannula. ECG on admission revealed a sinus rate of 126 beats per minute and a 2:1 AV block resulting in a ventricular rate of 63 beats per minute. The patient was placed on telemetry, which showed numerous episodes of Mobitz type II blocks. What is the mechanism for this type of block? What treatment is contraindicated? What type of management should the patient undergo?

Solution

Patients' with heart block localized to a site distal to the bundle of His and Purkinje system will not respond to the same sympathetic and parasympathetic stimulus as those that result from the sinus atrial (SA) or atrioventricular (AV) nodes. Treatments such as carotid massage and intravenous β-blockers may slow the sinus rate and paradoxically improve the AV conduction; however, atropine administration could increase the sinus rate, resulting in worsening AV conduction. The treatment of choice is a permanent pacemaker, according to the 2008 ACC/AHA/HRS Guidelines. Patients who present with 2:1 AV block are at risk for developing complete heart block, which may progress to cardiac arrest.

Data from: Littman L, Holshouser JW. Not so fast: Acceleration-dependent or Mobitz type II second-degree AV block. *Am J Med.* 2012;125(10). Accessed http//dx.doi.org/10.1016/J.amjmed.2012.06.011; ACC/AHA/HRS 2008 guidelines for device-based therapy of cardiac rhythm abnormalities: A report of the American College of Cardiology/American Heart Association Task Force on Practice Guidelines. *J Am Coll Cardiol.* 2008;51(21):e1–e62. doi:10.1016/j.jacc.2008.02.032.

−90 °; right axis deviation +90 to ±180°; and indeterminate −90 to 180 ° (see **Figure 10-40**).[2]

The third step is to determine if bundle branch blocks (BBBs) are present. A BBB occurs when either of the branches become blocked and will not allow impulses to pass. A right or left BBB will have an abnormally wide (> 0.12 seconds) QRS complex and a T wave that is inverted opposite the QRS complex. BBBs are a symptom of the impaired conduction system and do not cause symptoms. A right bundle branch block (RBBB) can be seen in normal healthy people, whereas a left bundle branch block (LBBB) is seen in people with extensive heart disease. Because a new onset of BBB is a sign of a dysfunctional conduction system, immediate treatment should be sought.

The fourth step involves checking for ventricular hypertrophy through the use of the V_1 and V_5–V_6 leads to examine the QRS complexes for signs of abnormality. Ventricular hypertrophy is usually a result of disease that causes thickening of the heart muscle. If the heart muscle is thick, it will require more current to depolarize the tissue, which is indicated by a QRS complex with greater-than-normal amplitude. The most common cause of right ventricular hypertrophy (RVH) is chronic lung disease. It can be identified by a tall R wave in lead V_1 along with a right **axis deviation** with a possible inverted T wave. Left ventricular hypertrophy (LVH) is most often the result of hypertension. It can be seen on a 12-lead ECG as a taller-than-normal R wave with a deeper-than-normal S wave in leads V_1 and V_2. A formula can be used to assess for the possibility of LVH: R wave in V_5 or V_6 (whichever is taller) + S wave in $V_1 \geq 35$ mm.

The fifth step involves scanning all of the leads for disturbances caused by electrolyte imbalances or medications. Hyperkalemia with levels of 6 could cause tall, pointy, narrow T waves, and levels of 8 cause wide QRS complexes and are a sign that cardiac arrest may be imminent. Hypokalemia will result in a prominent U wave and flattened T waves. Hypercalcemia causes shortened T segments, making the T wave look as if it is on top of the QRS complex. Hypocalcaemia will reveal itself with prolonged ST segments. The digitalis effect causes scooping ST segments along with prolonged PR intervals.

The final step is to check for signs of an infarction or ischemia. This can be seen with ST depression or elevation, inverted T waves, and significant Q waves. An infarction will cause tissue to die and turn black, resulting in significant Q waves. Ischemia decreases blood flow to the muscle, turning the tissue a pale white and inverting the T waves on an ECG. See Figure 10-35 for an example of ST segment elevation and Figure 10-36 for a pathologic Q wave.

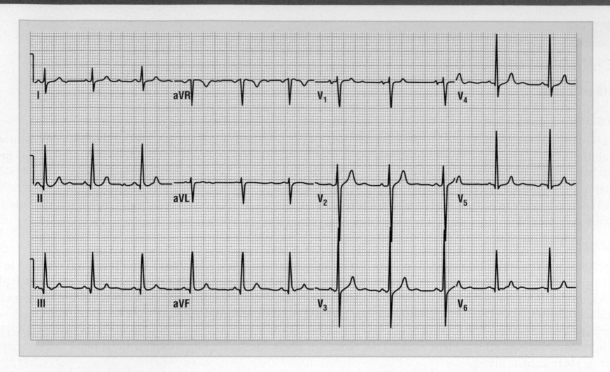

FIGURE 10-40 Twelve-(12-) lead ECG.

ECG for Diagnostic Purposes

To rule out various disease processes, a diagnostic ECG is acquired. Three types of diagnostic tests are available: stress testing, resting ECG, and ambulatory monitoring. The resting ECG is most commonly performed in a clinic, physician's office, emergency department or hospital. The ambulatory ECG allows for monitoring of patients' ECG pattern as they go about their normal activities in order to detect any abnormal rhythms which occur with activity.

Stress Testing

In determining the diagnosis of coronary artery disease, **stress testing** or exercise tolerance testing is employed.[3,26] The goal is to increase the heart rate through the use of physical exertion or the administration of medication. During a stress test, an ECG is recorded, as well as any symptoms the patient may have, to generate information concerning the patency of the coronary arteries. Stress testing is done with patients who have recently undergone cardiac bypass surgery or angioplasty or have a history of heart disease. It is also performed to diagnose exercise-induced arrhythmias or as a follow up to cardiac rehabilitation. Absolute contraindications to stress testing include an acute MI < 48 hours old, unstable angina, uncontrolled arrhythmia with decreased cardiac output, acute pulmonary embolism, and symptomatic aortic stenosis.

Normal changes to an ECG during a stress test include shortened PR intervals, tall T waves, lower-voltage QRS complexes, and an increased heart rate. Normal signs and symptoms may include increased cardiac output, blood pressure, respiratory rate, sweating, fatigue, muscle cramping, and J point depression. The J point is found at the junction of the QRS complex and the ST segment.

A positive stress test is revealed with a depressed ST segment of ≥ 1.0 to 1.5 mm that does not return to baseline within 0.08 seconds, with the onset of inverted U waves, and ST elevation.[3]

Ambulatory Monitoring

Ambulatory, or Holter, monitoring allows the patient to be ambulatory in order to rule out arrhythmias or ischemia that might not be present during a routine ECG.[3] This type of test is indicated for patients with syncope, intermittent chest pain, shortness of breath, or suspected arrhythmias. It may also be performed to determine the effectiveness of a treatment. Abnormalities that may be revealed with **Holter monitoring** include tachycardia, bradycardia, presence of pauses, and ST segment depression.

Other Diagnostic Test and Procedures

The chest radiograph is often useful in assessing cardiovascular disease and may be used to evaluate cardiac enlargement, dilation of the aorta or pulmonary arteries, and pulmonary venous congestion. Echocardiography may be used to assess cardiac size, structure, and function. Blood flow in the heart and major vessels can be assessed using Doppler echocardiography. Transesophageal echocardiography (TEE) allows for high-resolution imaging that can sometimes be useful in evaluating conditions such as aortic dissection, infective endocarditis, and intracardiac sources of embolism. TEE is also sometimes used in the intensive care unit (ICU) for rapid evaluation of unexplained hypotension or hypoxemia and complications following MI. Nuclear cardiology may sometimes be used for myocardial perfusion imaging with exercise or pharmacologic stress testing. Cardiac catheterization allows for measurement of the intracardiac pressures and visualization of the heart chambers, coronary arteries, and major vessels.

Key Points

▶ Cardiac assessment should include review of the patient's medical record, history and physical examination, vital signs, laboratory testing, imaging studies, and the ECG.

▶ An increased PR interval indicates a delay (or block) of the electrical signal from the atria to the ventricles.

▶ Wide QRS complexes are associated with premature ventricular beats, bundle branch blocks, severe hypokalemia, and toxic levels of certain antiarrhythmic drugs (e.g., quinidine, flecainide, propafenone).

▶ Excessive amounts of antiarrhythmic agents may result in a prolonged QT interval and result in a "twisting of the points" known as torsades de pointes. Torsades de pointes looks like ordinary ventricular tachycardia except that the QRS complexes change their axis and amplitude. The two dysthymias are treated differently.

▶ The presence of an abnormal ST segment is common in patients with acute myocardial infarction.

▶ If the heart rate appears to be slow or grossly irregular, a 12-second strip should be used and the resulting count should be multiplied by 5 to establish approximate beats per minute.

▶ Sinus bradycardia is common in patients with an acute inferior myocardial infarction.

▶ Premature atrial contraction (PAC) may be a warning for more serious dysrhythmias, such as atrial tachycardia, atrial flutter, atrial fibrillation, or paroxysmal supraventricular tachycardia.

▶ Cardiac output can be reduced by as much as 25% due to the loss of the atrial kick.

▶ Multifocal atrial tachycardia is found in patients with respiratory failure.

▶ Atrial fibrillation is commonly associated with congestive heart failure (CHF).

▶ Supraventricular tachycardia (SVT) is a rapid heart rate that originates at or above the SA node.

▶ Ventricular rhythms are the most lethal of all dysrhythmias, requiring due diligence on the part of the healthcare provider.

▶ Premature ventricular contractions (PVCs) can be classified as couplets, bigeminy, trigeminy, or quadrigeminy beats, just like PACs.

▶ Sometimes the SA node will still fire even though the ventricles are too damaged to depolarize. As a result, there will be P waves and nothing else on the ECG strip. These P waves will eventually stop because there is no perfusion to or from the heart.

▶ If there is no QRS complex, there is no cardiac output.

▶ Normal QRS complexes are less than 13 mm, or 13 small boxes, high in any lead.

▶ In determining the age of a myocardial infarction, ST elevation reveals an acute injury; significant Q waves, ST at baseline, and inverted T waves point to an age-indeterminate injury; and significant Q waves, ST at baseline, and an upright T wave indicate an old injury.

▶ Absolute contraindications to stress testing include an acute MI < 48 hours old, unstable angina, uncontrolled arrhythmia with decreased cardiac output, acute pulmonary embolism, and symptomatic aortic stenosis.

References

1. Goldberger AL, Goldberger ZD, Shvilkin A. *Clinical Electrocardiography: A Simplified Approach*, 8th ed. Philadelphia: Elsevier Saunders; 2013.

2. Ellis KM. *EKG Plain and Simple*, 3rd ed. Boston: Pearson; 2012.

3. Thaler MS. *The Only EKG Book You'll Ever Need*, 6th ed. Philadelphia: Lippincott Williams & Wilkins; 2010.

4. Goldberger AL. Basic principles of electrocardiographic interpretation. In: *UpToDate*, Basow, DS (ed.), UpToDate, Waltham, MA, 2013.

5. Prutkin JM. ECG tutorial: Basic principles of ECG analysis. In: *UpToDate*, Basow, DS (ed.), UpToDate, Waltham, MA, 2013.

6. Longo DL, Fauci AS, Kasper DL, Hauser SL, Jameson JL, Loscalzo J. Electrocardiography. In: Longo DL, Fauci AS, Kasper DL, Hauser SL, Jameson JL, Loscalzo J, eds. *Harrison's Manual of Medicine*, 18th ed. New York: McGraw-Hill; 2013: 800–804.

7. Beachey W. Functional anatomy of the cardiovascular system. In: Beachey W, ed. *Respiratory Care Anatomy and Physiology*, 2nd ed. St. Louis, MO: Elsevier-Mosby; 2007: 274–299.

8. Beachey W. The electrocardiogram and cardiac arrhythmias. In: Beachey W, ed. *Respiratory Care Anatomy and Physiology*. 2nd ed. St. Louis, MO: Elsevier-Mosby; 2007: 314–334.

9. Longo DL, Fauci AS, Kasper DL, Hauser SL, Jameson JL, Loscalzo J. Pulmonary hypertension. In: Longo DL, Fauci AS, Kasper DL, Hauser SL, Jameson JL, Loscalzo J, eds. *Harrison's Manual of Medicine*, 18th ed. New York: McGraw-Hill; 2013: 895–898.

10. Longo DL, Fauci AS, Kasper DL, Hauser SL, Jameson JL, Loscalzo J. Heart failure and cor pulmonale. In: Longo DL, Fauci AS, Kasper DL, Hauser SL, Jameson JL, Loscalzo J, eds. *Harrison's Manual of Medicine*, 18th ed. New York: McGraw-Hill; 2013: 879–886.

11. Hamdan MH. Cardiac arrhythmias. In: Andreoli TE, Benjamin IJ, Griggs RC, Wing EJ, eds. *Andreoli and Carpenter's Cecil Essentials of Medicine*, 8th ed. Philadelphia: Saunders Elsevier; 2010: 118–144.

12. Goldberger AL. Pathogenesis and diagnosis of Q waves on the electrocardiogram. In: *UpToDate*, Basow, DS (ed.), UpToDate, Waltham, MA, 2013.

13. Podrid PJ, Ganz LI. Aproach to the diagnosis and treatment of wide QRS complex tachycardias. In: *UpToDate*, Basow, DS (ed.), UpToDate, Waltham, MA, 2013.

14. Beachey W. Cardiac electrophysiology. In: Beachey W, ed. *Respiratory Care Anatomy and Physiology*, 2nd ed. St. Louis, MO: Elsevier-Mosby; 2007: 300–313.

15. Sauer WH. Normal sinus rhythm and sinus arrhythmia. In: *UpToDate*, Basow, DS (ed.), UpToDate, Waltham, MA, 2013.

16. Longo DL, Fauci AS, Kasper DL, Hauser SL, Jameson JL, Loscalzo J. Tachyarrhythmias. In: Longo DL, Fauci AS, Kasper DL, Hauser SL, Jameson JL, Loscalzo J, eds. *Harrison's Manual of Medicine*, 18th ed. New York: McGraw-Hill; 2013: 867–878.

17. LeBlond RF, Brown DD, DeGowin RL. Vital signs, anthropometric data, and pain. In: LeBlond RF, Brown DD, DeGowin RL, eds. *DeGowin's Diagnostic Examination*, 9th ed. New York: McGraw-Hill; 2009: 51–87.

18. Prutkin JM. ECG tutorial: Myocardial infarction. In: *UpToDate*, Basow, DS (ed.), UpToDate, Waltham, MA, 2013.

19. Goldberger AL. Electrocardiogram in the diagnosis of myocardial ischemia and infarction. In: *UpToDate*, Basow, DS (ed.), UpToDate, Waltham, MA, 2013.

20. Longo DL, Fauci AS, Kasper DL, Hauser SL, Jameson JL, Loscalzo J. ST-segment elevation myocardial infarction (STEMI). In: Longo DL, Fauci AS, Kasper DL, Hauser SL, Jameson JL, Loscalzo J, eds. *Harrison's Manual of Medicine*, 18th ed. New York: McGraw-Hill; 2013; 844–854.

21. Reeder GS, Kennedy HL, Rosenson RS. Overview of the acute management of ST elevation myocardial infarction. In: *UpToDate*, Basow, DS (ed.), UpToDate, Waltham, MA, 2013.

22. Longo DL, Fauci AS, Kasper DL, Hauser SL, Jameson JL, Loscalzo J. Unstable angina and non-ST-elevation myocardial infarction. In: Longo DL, Fauci AS, Kasper DL, Hauser SL, Jameson JL, Loscalzo J, eds. *Harrison's Manual of Medicine*, 18th ed. New York: McGraw-Hill; 2013: 855–858.

23. Breall JA, Aroesty JM, Simons M. Overview of the acute management of unstable angina and non-ST elevation myocardial infarction. In: *UpToDate*, Basow DS (ed.), UpToDate, Waltham, MA, 2013.

24. Colucci WS, Evaluation of the Patient with Heart Failure or Cardiomyopathy. In: UpToDate, Basow, DS (ed.), UpToDate, Waltham, MA, 2013.

25. Longo DL, Fauci AS, Kasper DL, Hauser SL, Jameson JL, Loscalzo J. Bradyarrhythmias. In: Longo DL, Fauci AS, Kasper DL, Hauser SL, Jameson JL, Loscalzo J, eds. *Harrison's Manual of Medicine*, 18th ed. New York: McGraw-Hill; 2013: 864–867.

26. Singh J. Cardiac Assessment. In: Hess DR, MacIntyre NR, Mishoe SC, Galvin WF, Adams AB, eds. *Respiratory Care: Principles and Practice*, 2nd ed. Sudbury, MA: Jones & Bartlett Learning; 2012: 113.

CHAPTER

11
Cardiopulmonary Imaging

Laura P. Vasquez, David C. Shelledy, and Jay I. Peters

CHAPTER OUTLINE

CHAPTER OBJECTIVES

1. Explain how x-ray images are produced.
2. Define the terms *radiolucent* and *radiopaque*.
3. Contrast x-ray penetration depending on object density for metal, bone, fluid, soft tissue, and air.
4. Explain how the distance between the x-ray source, patient, and film or detector affects the radiographic appearance of anatomic structures on the film.
5. Describe the technique, indications, and advantages and disadvantages of the various chest radiographic techniques to include the posteroanterior (PA), anteroposterior (AP), left lateral, and lateral decubitus views.
6. Describe a standard approach to chest radiograph interpretation.
7. Identify normal anatomic structures on the chest radiograph.
8. Identify placement of endotracheal tubes, lines and catheters (e.g., central venous pressure (CVP) lines, pulmonary artery catheters, nasogastric tubes), and chest tube placement on the chest radiograph.
9. Identify major abnormalities as seen on the chest radiograph to include pneumothorax, bronchial intubation, pleural effusion, atelectasis, interstitial and alveolar fluid, tumor or abscess, and consolidative processes.
10. Explain the significance of the silhouette sign and air bronchogram.
11. Describe the technique, indications, and advantages and disadvantages for computerized tomography (CT scan) for evaluation of cardiopulmonary disease.
12. Describe the technique, indications, and advantages and disadvantages of magnetic resonance imaging (MRI) for evaluation of cardiopulmonary disease.
13. Explain the technique and indications for ventilation–perfusion scans and how specific conditions (e.g., embolism, atelectasis, pneumonia) affect lung scans.
14. Describe the techniques and indications for pulmonary angiography, cardiac-interventional radiography, and vascular-interventional radiography.
15. Describe the technique, indications, and advantages and disadvantages of diagnostic medical sonography (ultrasound imaging) for evaluation of cardiopulmonary disease.
16. Recognize clinical and imaging findings for specific cardiopulmonary diseases.

KEY TERMS

angiography
asthma
atelectasis
blebs
bronchiectasis
bronchitis
bullae
calcification
cardiomegaly
chest x-ray (CXR)
chronic obstructive pulmonary disease (COPD)
consolidation
contrast agent
computed tomography (CT)
edema
emphysema
fissures
fluoroscopy

ground-glass opacification
hilum
honeycombing
idiopathic pulmonary fibrosis (IPF)
infarction
infiltrate
lymphadenopathy
magnetic resonance imaging (MRI)
mass
nodular pattern
nuclear medicine (NM)
opacity
parenchyma
pneumomediastinum
pneumonia
pneumothorax
positron emission tomography (PET)

pulmonary edema	reticulonodular pattern
radiolucent	silhouette sign
radiopaque	tension pneumothorax
reticular pattern	ultrasonography

Overview

Imaging studies are often needed for the accurate diagnosis, treatment, and monitoring of patients with cardiopulmonary disease. The respiratory care clinician must be able to evaluate medical radiographs such as the chest x-ray and upper airway/neck radiograph. Other imaging studies of special interest include reports of computed tomography (CT) scans, magnetic resonance imaging (MRI) scans, diagnostic ultrasound studies, positron emission tomography (PET) studies, and ventilation–perfusion ($\dot{V}/\dot{Q}$) scans. Results of angiography (coronary, pulmonary, and bronchial) can also be very helpful in identifying conditions such as coronary artery disease or pulmonary embolus. This chapter will describe the basic principles, indications, and clinical use of imaging studies for the assessment of the cardiopulmonary patient. Assessment of the chest radiograph, CT scan, and MRI will be discussed. Next, the chapter will review the principles of nuclear medicine imaging, cardiac and cardiovascular interventional radiography, and ultrasonography (diagnostic medical sonography). Last, this chapter will describe common imaging findings with the major cardiopulmonary diseases.

Introduction to Medical Imaging

Medical imaging techniques play an important role in the assessment of patients with cardiopulmonary disease. In the acute care setting, imaging studies are needed to verify the presence of pneumonia, atelectasis, pulmonary edema, and acute respiratory distress syndrome (ARDS) and are part of the diagnostic evaluation of patients with thoracic trauma. Imaging studies are also often needed to evaluate patients with interstitial lung disease, pleural effusion, lung cancer, and heart disease. Review of imaging studies may allow for recognition and treatment of abnormalities that may be life threatening, as in the case of tension pneumothorax. In the intensive care unit, imaging studies are used to monitor and evaluate line and tube placement. Imaging devices may also be used as an aid to the performance of specific procedures at the bedside. For example, small portable ultrasound imaging devices are now available that can be used to help guide insertion of central venous catheters or arterial lines. On the more mundane side, selection of chest physiotherapy procedures and postural drainage positions should be based, if possible, on chest x-ray findings.

Many medical imaging techniques are dependent on the application of the electromagnetic spectrum to generate images. Electromagnetic waves include radio

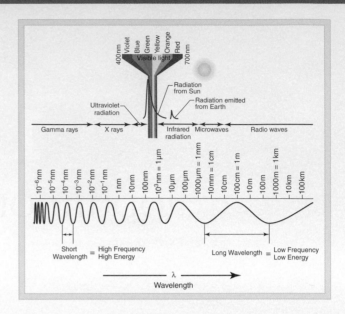

FIGURE 11-1 **Electromagnetic radiation.**

waves, infrared light, visible light, x-rays, and gamma rays. The energy of these waves is determined by the frequency of the waves and the wavelength; as frequency increases, wavelength decreases. **Figure 11-1** illustrates the relationship between wavelength and wave frequency and the relative frequencies for radio waves, visible light, x-rays, and gamma rays.

Many imaging studies, such as conventional radiographs and CT scans, involve the use of x-rays. X-rays were first discovered by Wilhelm Roentgen in 1895, who found that shadow images of his wife's hand bones could be produced by passing mysterious rays through the hand onto a photographic plate. X-rays are generated using a cathode ray tube to produce an electron stream that is directed to a tungsten target, as shown in **Figure 11-2**. The interaction of the electron stream and tungsten target results in the production of

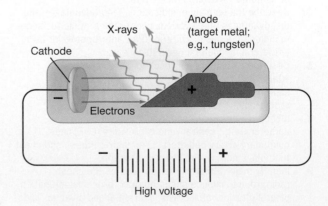

FIGURE 11-2 **X-ray generation.**

x-rays, which are a form of electromagnetic radiation, as shown in Figure 11-1. X-rays have sufficient energy to penetrate gas and air, which are of low density (i.e., **radiolucent**), resulting in dark or black images on x-ray film. X-rays do not generally penetrate high-density (i.e., **radiopaque**) objects such as bone, metal, or contrast media, and the resulting image appears white. Liquid, body fluids, and blood are relatively radiopaque, and appear grayish-white on the radiograph, whereas soft tissue (e.g., muscle, fat) is denser than air but less dense than bone, and appears as shades of gray. Box 11-1 compares x-ray absorbance by tissue type.

Computed tomography (CT) uses x-rays and computer processing to produce tomographic images of cross sections of the body. The thoracic CT scan provides cross-sectional images of the chest and upper abdomen and is especially useful in the detection of pulmonary embolus, aortic aneurysm or dissection, and pulmonary abnormalities (nodules and pleural disease) and for the staging of bronchogenic carcinoma. High-resolution CT (HRCT) scans may detect lung disease in patients with normal chest radiographs. HRCT is also useful in the evaluation of patients with emphysema or interstitial lung disease and in detection or verification of bronchiectasis.

Bronchography and **angiography** use contrast media and conventional x-ray technology to provide images of the tracheobronchial tree (bronchogram) or pulmonary vasculature (pulmonary angiogram), though CT has diminished the need for these techniques.

Magnetic resonance imaging (MRI) uses a strong magnetic field and pulses of radio waves to produce digital images of body structures with good contrast between soft tissues (e.g., joints, muscle, fat). MRIs are especially useful in evaluation of soft tissue injuries, as well as the brain (e.g., stroke, tumor) and heart (e.g., cardiac sarcoidosis, ischemic heart disease). MRIs do not produce ionizing radiation, allowing for more frequent imaging procedures as compared to conventional x-rays or CT scans. The MRI of the chest provides information not available using conventional x-rays or CT scans and may be used to evaluate chest wall problems, such as chest wall tumors, chest wall infection, or pleural disease. The thoracic MRI is of more

---

BOX 11-1

X-Ray Absorbance and Penetration

The energy of x-rays determines the degree of x-ray penetration:

$$E = P \times f$$

where E = energy; P = Planck's constant; and f = frequency. Thus, as frequency increases, penetration of specific substances also increases.

Density of materials also affects x-ray absorption and penetration. More dense materials absorb more x-rays (i.e., less penetration) and less dense materials absorb fewer x-rays (i.e., more penetration). In summary:

- Dense materials (e.g., bone, metal, or water) absorb more x-rays.
  - If a dense material is placed between an x-ray source and an x-ray detector (e.g., x-ray film) few x-rays will pass completely through the material and the film (or x-ray detector) will be unexposed or less exposed.
  - The resulting image will be white or grey-white.
- Less dense materials (e.g., normal lung tissue, air) absorb fewer x-rays.
  - If a less dense material is placed between an x-ray source and an x-ray detector (e.g., x-ray film), many x-rays will pass through the material and the film (or x-ray detector) will be more exposed.
  - The resulting image will be black or dark grey.
- The relative order of radiographic densities (least dense to most dense) is:
  - Gas: Present in lungs, stomach, intestines
  - Fat: Surrounds kidney; present along the abdominal wall and other organs
  - Water: Same density as heart and blood vessels
  - Bone: More dense than other tissues
  - Metal: Foreign objects, prostheses, contrast media.

Ionizing radiation can cause biological damage; exposure should be limited.

This article was published in *Merrill's atlas of radiographic positions and radiologic procedures*, vols. 1–3, 10th ed., Ballinger, P. W., & Frank, E. D., Copyright Mosby 2003.

limited value in evaluation of the lung **parenchyma**. MRIs are contraindicated in patients with certain medical implants, such as cardiac pacemakers or other implanted electronic devices.

Diagnostic medical sonography, also known as **ultrasonography**, uses sound waves to produce images of body structures. One form of diagnostic medical sonography is the echocardiogram, which allows for assessment of the size of the atria and ventricles (e.g., hypertrophy), heart wall movement (which may be compromised with myocardial infarction), heart valves, pericardium (e.g., effusion, tamponade), and intracardiac shunts. Critical care ultrasound is becoming the standard of care to detect pneumothorax, pericardial effusion, cardiogenic shock, and deep venous thrombosis by intensivists in the ICU setting.

Positron emission tomography (PET) is a nuclear medicine technique that provides physiologic information about tissue function that is especially useful in evaluation of possible malignancies (e.g., lung cancer) and identifying occult infections (e.g., workup of fever of unknown origin). Other nuclear medicine techniques allow for the production of ventilation and perfusion scans using radioactive substances to assess pulmonary blood flow and the distribution of ventilation. Single-photon emission computed tomography (SPECT, or tomographic radionuclide scintigraphy) allows for visualization of slices of the chest that can be manipulated by computer.

To summarize, medical imaging techniques can be broadly grouped into those that use ionizing radiation and those that do not. Images generated using ionizing radiation use x-rays or gamma rays. Nonionizing techniques include those that use acoustic pulses (e.g., ultrasound) or high-field magnets (e.g., MRI). Newer "fusion" imaging techniques may combine the use of two forms of ionizing radiation (e.g., PET-CT), ionizing and nonionizing radiation (e.g., CT and ultrasound or CT and MRI), or two forms on nonionizing radiation (e.g., MRI and ultrasound). We will discuss each of these techniques in the following sections.

Conventional Radiography

Despite the many advances in medical imagery, conventional chest radiography remains the imaging technique of choice for initial evaluation of the lung.[1] The conventional **chest x-ray (CXR)** is fast and easy to obtain, relatively inexpensive, and administers a relatively low dose of radiation.[2] Every respiratory care clinician should be able to examine a routine chest radiograph and recognize:

- Normal anatomic structures
- Tube, catheter, and line placement (e.g., endotracheal tubes, nasogastric tubes, chest tubes, central venous lines, pulmonary artery catheter placement)

- Gross abnormalities to include:
  - Improper endotracheal tube placement
  - Pneumothorax
  - Rib fractures
  - Pleural effusion
  - Atelectasis
  - Interstitial or alveolar fluid (e.g., ARDS, pulmonary edema, interstitial edema)
  - Tumor or abscess
  - Consolidative processes (pneumonia)
  - Hyperinflation (e.g., emphysema, acute asthma)
  - Enlarged heart

Conventional radiography offers lower contrast resolution than CT and MRI. However, conventional radiology offers greater spatial resolution when compared to MRI and CT. Conventional radiography equipment is also relatively easy to operate and much less expensive than CT, MRI, or PET.[2] If done correctly and read by well-trained personnel, conventional radiology can be a powerful diagnostic tool.

How It Works

Conventional radiography (i.e., projectional, analog, or plain-film radiography) refers to images produced on special liquid silver–processed film using traditional x-ray machines.[3] The resulting images are often called *chest films, chest x-rays,* or *CXRs.* In practice, the rather messy film processing of the past has largely been replaced by quicker, easier-to-produce alternatives that usually involve digital technology.[4]

To obtain an x-ray image on film, patients are bombarded with electromagnetic radiation, more specifically x-ray photons. The x-ray photons either collide with or pass through the patient's body. The processes of attenuation and absorption are responsible for the resulting image on the radiograph.[3] Contrast-enhancement media may be used to compensate for biologic structures of comparable density that would otherwise be indistinguishable from one another.[5]

To obtain a conventional chest x-ray image, the patient is placed between an x-ray tube and a flat panel detector or film. When the patient is standing (or sitting) facing the detector/film and the x-ray machine is activated from behind the patient, a posteroanterior (PA) x-ray is obtained. Note: the patient reaches around the cassette and the scapula are rotated outside the lung fields in a PA film.[3] **Figure 11-3A** is an example of a PA projection. For a PA chest x-ray, the film or flat panel detector is placed directly in front of the sternum and anterior chest wall. This is the most common type of chest x-ray done in the radiology department; it usually results in a better image with fewer distortions than other views.[6]

If the x-rays are delivered from the front of the body to the back, it is called an anteroposterior (AP) chest x-ray. **Figure 11-3B** is an example of an AP projection.[3]

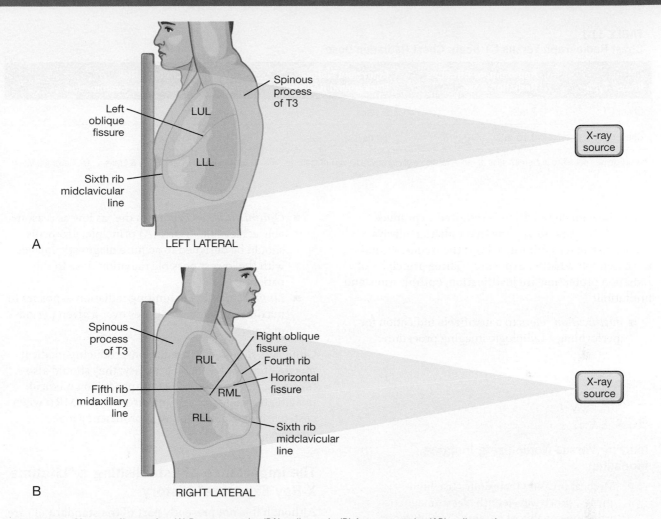

FIGURE 11-3 Chest radiographs. (A) Posteroanterior (PA) radiograph. (B) Anteroposterior (AP) radiograph.

For an AP chest x-ray, the film or flat panel detector is placed directly behind the patient, often with the patient laying on the film canister or flat panel detector.[3] This type of chest x-ray is commonly performed on bedridden patients and patients in the emergency department (ED) or intensive care unit (ICU). Because the patient is supine or reclining with the film or detector panel against the back, and because the distance between the x-ray source and film or detector may vary, AP images need to be interpreted differently than those produced with PA x-rays.[7] For example, because the film or detector is farther from the heart in an AP film, the heart generally appears larger in AP views, sometimes prompting a misdiagnosis of cardiomegaly.[8] Figure 11-3 also demonstrates AP versus PA projection. Note: in the AP view, the patient is lying on the flat panel and the scapula are seen within the lung fields.

In addition to PA and AP chest films, lateral chest x-rays are sometimes obtained to better view structures behind the heart and can provide unique views of the lungs, pleura, thoracic cage, pericardium, heart, upper abdomen, and mediastinum.[3] When no specific side is specified, a left lateral view is the default choice.

Radiation Exposure

Medical imaging is responsible for only a portion of the radiation exposure that occurs, and natural sources of radiation are ubiquitous.[3] In fact, the average person in the United States is exposed to about 3 mSv (milliSievert) per year from natural sources, although actual counts vary by location.[3] In physics, this is known as *background radiation*, to distinguish it from human-produced radiation. As a point of reference, one chest x-ray delivers the equivalent of 10 days of natural background radiation exposure.[3] **Table 11-1** compares the radiation dose for a chest x-ray versus a chest CT scan. CT imaging procedures account for the majority of medical radiation exposure.[9] One chest CT is equal to approximately 48 chest x-rays in terms of exposure, and one abdominal CT is equal in radiation exposure to approximately 200 chest x-rays.[9,10] The risk of radiation injuries linked to use of CT scans continues to be a topic of concern. **Box 11-2** describes the ionizing versus nonionizing imaging modalities.[3]

Although the medical imaging–related radiation exposure of patients is thought to be safe, no one really

TABLE 11-1
Chest Radiograph Versus CT Scan: Chest Radiation Dose

Image Type	Approximate Effective Radiation Dose	Equivalent Natural Background Radiation	Additional Lifetime Risk of Fatal Cancer from Examination
Chest CT	7 mSv	2 years	Low
Chest x-ray	0.15 mSv	10 days	Minimal

This article was published in *Merrill's atlas of radiographic positions and radiologic procedures*, vols. 1–3, 10th ed., Ballinger, P. W., & Frank, E. D., Copyright Mosby 2003.

knows how much radiation is required to produce disease.[11] It is best to assume that radiation always carries risk and to minimize both the frequency and the extent of radiation exposure.[3] Three principles of radiation protection are justification, optimization, and limitation:

- *Justification* refers to a justifiable indication for performing a radiologic imaging procedure.[3]

- *Optimization* incorporates the "as low as reasonably achievable" (ALARA) principle; protocols should be designed to acquire diagnostic images with the lowest possible radiation dose to the patient.[3]
- *Limitation* refers to limiting radiation exposure to maximum cumulative doses over a given period of time.[3]

Clinicians should order radiation-producing medical imaging tests only when necessary; they should also take advantage of non-radiation-producing medical imaging technologies (e.g., ultrasound and MRI) when cost, feasibility, and diagnostic proficiency make it possible.

The Importance of Establishing a "Lifetime X-Ray Exposure" History

Although it is not presently part of the standard of care, every patient should be provided with a "lifetime x-ray exposure" record. With the advent of standardized electronic records, it may become easier for healthcare providers to determine potential risks and employ exposure-minimization strategies. This is of particular importance for people with compromised health status, those with a genetic predisposition to cancer, pregnant women, children, and those older than age 60.[8,12] Monitoring lifetime exposure is also important for those who have been exposed to dangerously high levels of radiation, either from repeated radiographic testing or occupational exposure. Such individuals may be advised to avoid ionizing-radiation imaging except in life-threatening situations. These patients may, for example, have such a limitation noted on their medical ID bracelets. The availability of newer imaging techniques that do not use ionizing radiation may allow for limiting radiation exposure in some circumstances. Ultrasound, for example, is considered especially safe for developing fetuses.[13] As a general rule, x-rays pose a special risk to reproductive anatomy, so limiting exposure should be a goal for anyone of reproductive age, whether pregnant or not.[14]

In addition to x-rays, it is important to consider radiation exposure from the radioactive tracers used

BOX 11-2

Ionizing Versus Nonionizing Imaging Modalities

- Medical imaging techniques use high-energy, short-wavelength electromagnetic radiation capable of passing through most body tissues.
- Medical imaging techniques can be broadly grouped into those that use ionizing radiation versus those that do not.
  - Ionizing radiation techniques provide medial images using either:
    - X-rays (e.g., radiography, computed tomography)
    - Gamma rays (e.g., nuclear scintigraphy, positron emission tomography)
  - Nonionizing radiation techniques provide medical images using either:
    - Acoustic pulses (ultrasound) imaging (e.g., diagnostic medical sonography [DMS], including echocardiography, vascular ultrasonography)
    - Radio waves combined with high-field magnets (e.g., magnetic resonance imaging)

Data from: Ballinger PW, Frank ED. *Merrill's Atlas of Radiographic Positions and Radiologic Procedures*, vols. 1–3, 10th ed. St. Louis, MO: Mosby; 2003.

in nuclear medicine (NM) contexts, such as PET scans. The radioactive tracers used with PET usually have a short life span and are only in the body for a limited time.[15] Nevertheless, radiation exposure has a cumulative effect, and nuclear medicine scans, like x-rays, pose a risk.[15] Another group of patients requiring special consideration is breast-feeding mothers. The special radiopharmaceutical agents used in some nuclear medicine examinations can be passed on to babies through the mother's breast milk.[12] Consequently, breast-feeding mothers are advised to avoid such tests, if possible, or to forego nursing for some time before and after such procedures.[12]

Radiation Exposure Measurement

Radiation cannot be seen, heard, smelled, or even felt, except in the case of high, skin-warming doses. Radiation is usually only detectable using special devices such as dosimeters and Geiger counters. Several units of measurement are used for radiation; they include grays, Sieverts, roentgens, rems, and rads.[9,11] Calculation of the *effective dose* provides an estimate of cancer risk due to radiation exposure. Defined as the entire-body-averaged-exposure radiation dose risk, effective dose is usually expressed in milliSieverts (mSv).[9,11] The concept of effective dose was developed because different parts of the body have different cellular damage thresholds; that is, some areas are more susceptible than others to cancer.[3] For example, the thyroid, lung tissue, breast tissue, stomach, colon, and bone marrow are highly sensitive to high doses of radiation, whereas the skin, spleen, and kidneys have low sensitivity.[3] Effective dose is useful in quantifying risk and as a tool for comparison using well-known sources of radiation such as medical imaging and background radiation.[3]

The Normal Chest X-Ray

The ability to recognize a normal chest x-ray is a prerequisite for recognizing abnormalities. In evaluating the routine chest x-ray, the clinician first must ensure that the image being viewed is for the correct patient. Next, the clinician should consider the gender and age of the patient, the type of x-ray (i.e., AP, PA, lateral), and the image quality.[3] Technical factors that affect image quality include degree of x-ray penetration and patient position.[3]

Posteroanterior Chest Film

The posteroanterior chest film is taken with the patient standing upright following a full inspiration. The patient's shoulders should be rotated forward to move the scapulae up and out of lung fields as much as possible. The x-ray source is behind the patient with the film or detector against the patient's sternum. The x-ray source should be 72 inches from the film or detector.[3]

Advantages of the PA view include:

- Very good visualization of anatomic structures and specific abnormalities.
- The scapulae are rotated out of the lung fields (as compared to an AP view).
- The film (or flat panel detector) is against the sternum, so the heart does not appear enlarged (as with an AP view).
- The diaphragm is lower than in a film taken with the patient supine.
- Fluid moves caudally due to the upright patient position, allowing for observation of a meniscus sign in the presence of pleural effusion or an air-fluid level with abscess or hydropneumothorax.

The major disadvantage to the PA film is that it requires the patient be transported to the radiology department or a dedicated imaging room with the appropriate equipment installed. This takes time and may be difficult to accomplish with critically ill patients, especially those receiving mechanical ventilation.

Anteroposterior Chest Film

The anteroposterior chest film is often taken with the patient in bed using a portable x-ray machine. As noted, most films taken in the ICU or ED are "portables" with the film (or flat panel detector) placed against the patient's back. AP films can often be identified by the scapula appearing within the lung fields. The x-ray source for a portable is often 36 to 40 inches from the film, though a distance of 72 inches is preferred if space in the room permits.[3]

The following are some of the advantages of the AP film:

- It is relatively fast and easy to obtain.
- It does not require patient transport to the radiology department.
- It enables for verification of endotracheal tube placement.
- It is useful for identification of major abnormalities (e.g., pneumothorax, bronchial intubation, atelectasis, pneumonia, ARDS).

The following are some of the disadvantages of the AP view:

- The image is not as clear as the PA film and is often somewhat distorted, coarse, and of lower resolution.
- The patient may be twisted, and patient position may result in distortion of anatomic structures.
- A good inspiratory effort is often lacking.
- The scapulae obscure more of the lung tissue.
- The heart appears larger than on a PA view.
- Often there are many artifacts present (e.g., ECG monitoring leads, catheters, tubes, lines).

- Visualization of anatomic structures and specific abnormalities may be poor.
- Diaphragm is often higher than as seen in a film taken with the patient standing.
- Pleural fluid may be spread out, depending on patient position.

In spite of the disadvantages, the portable chest film remains an essential tool for evaluation of very sick patients seen in the ED or ICU. Often, the time and effort required to transport the very sick patient to the radiology department for a PA film makes AP film a good alternative. This is especially true of patients receiving mechanical ventilatory support. **Figure 11-4** provides examples of normal PA and AP chest radiographs.

Lateral Films

The lateral chest film complements the PA view and is normally taken with the film (or flat panel detector) against the left side of the chest (i.e., left lateral view) with the patient's arms raised.[3] The lateral view allows the clinician to visualize structures behind the heart that would be otherwise obscured by the heart shadow.

The left lateral film reduces magnification of the heart. A right lateral film may be obtained to better evaluate a right-side density or lesion. On a lateral film, the right hemidiaphragm is usually higher than the left.[8] A lateral view is especially useful to evaluate flattening of the diaphragm as seen with lung overinflation (e.g., COPD, emphysema). A lateral decubitus view refers to lateral films taken with the patient lying flat, on the right or left side. The lateral decubitus view is sometimes useful in evaluation of suspected or known pleural effusion.[2] Thoracentesis can be safely accomplished if there is 10 mm of fluid observed on the decubitus film. With pleural effusion, the pleural fluid will tend to collect in the dependent part of the pleural space due to gravity. **Figure 11-5** provides an example of a normal lateral chest radiograph.

Lateral films may be used to:

- Visualize structures behind the heart.
- Clarify a lobar collapse or consolidation.
- Explore a retrocardiac or retrosternal "shadow."
- Localize lesions spotted on frontal chest x-rays.
- Establish whether trapped fluid is present in an oblique fissure.

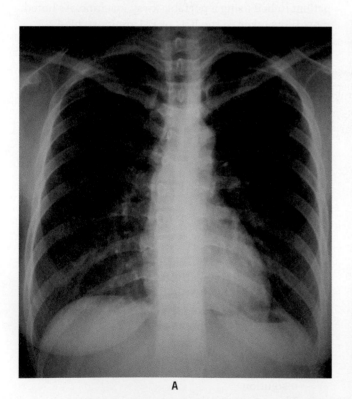

A

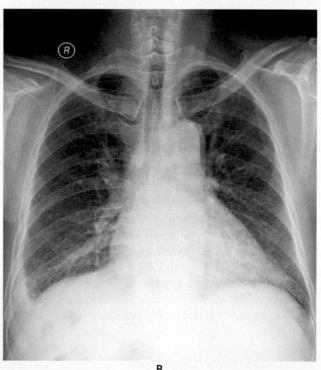

B

FIGURE 11-4 Normal chest radiographs on posteroanterior (PA) and anteroposterior (AP) views. (A) Normal PA chest radiograph of a female patient. Good position. Ten posterior ribs visible, which is an excellent inspiration. In many patients, nine posterior ribs is an adequate inspiration. Good visualization of anatomic structures. The scapulae are rotated out of the lung fields, as compared to an AP view. (B) Normal AP chest radiograph for a male patient. Patient position is good with adequate inspiration. Good visualization of trachea, carina, right and left mainstream bronchi, heart and major vessels, diaphragm, and costophrenic and cardiophrenic angles.

(A) © sinngern/iStock/Thinkstock; (B) © windcatcher/iStock/Thinkstock.

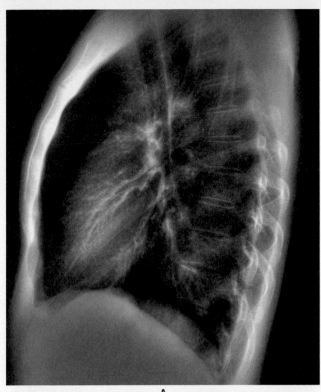

A

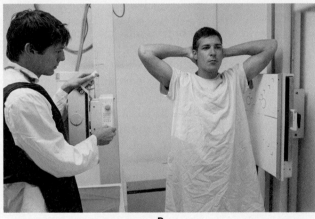

B

FIGURE 11-5 Normal left lateral chest radiograph. Note that the film detector is against the left side of the chest. The image is normally viewed with the vertebral column on the viewer's right.

(A) © Lukasz Panek/iStock/Thinkstock; (B) © Wavebreakmedia Ltd/Wavebreak Media/Thinkstock.

- View the dome of the diaphragm and observe for pulmonary overinflation (flattening of the hemidiaphragms).
- Evaluate pleural fluid (lateral decubitus view).

Lateral airway (i.e., neck) x-rays are sometimes obtained in children. For example, with epiglottitis (inflammation of the epiglottis) the resultant swelling may result in visualization of the "thumb sign" in which

the epiglottis looks like a thumb on the lateral neck x-ray view.[13] Epiglottitis is usually caused by a bacterial infection (e.g., *Haemophilus influenzae, Streptococcus,* other) and may lead to complete airway obstruction if not promptly identified and treated.[13] Subglottic edema may be a result of larygnotracheobronchitis, or croup, which is a viral infection of the upper respiratory tract. It may sometimes be seen as the "pencil sign" or "steeple sign" in which the trachea narrows in the subglottic area as viewed on neck films.[14] Children are also prone to aspiration of foreign bodies (e.g., candy, peanuts, small toys), and these may sometimes be visualized on a lateral upper airway radiograph. **Figure 11-6** provides examples of the neck x-ray findings sometimes seen with croup (pencil sign or steeple sign) and epiglottis (thumb sign).

Technical Factors Affecting the Chest X-Ray

Following identification of the chest x-ray view (i.e., PA, AP, lateral), the clinician should consider technical aspects of the image relating to penetration, rotation, inspiration, and angulation. It is also important to ensure that the proper distance between the x-ray source and the patient was used in obtaining the chest x-ray.[3] This is particularly important for radiographs taken at the bedside, such as in the ICU or ED, and when patients are supine.[7] If the x-ray source is too close or too far from the patient, quality issues arise. If the patient was rotated or twisted when the image was obtained, this will affect the image and may lead to an incorrect interpretation. Issues related to rotation or position are more common with AP films taken while the patient is in bed. It should also be noted that older, film-based x-rays may be degraded and images hard to discern.[3]

Penetration

Penetration refers to whether the film (or digital image) is overexposed, underexposed, or properly exposed. As noted earlier, on x-ray film less dense material, such as air, appears dark or black. More dense material (e.g., bone or fluid) appears white or gray.[3] Overexposed x-ray film tends to result in very dark images, whereas underexposure results in very white images. In an overexposed chest radiograph, the lung fields appear very dark. If the film is properly exposed (i.e., good penetration), clinicians should be able to barely see the thoracic spine through the heart. In addition, a good-quality chest x-ray image should allow 8 to 11 ribs to be clearly seen, as well as the clavicles, sternum, trachea, heart, and lungs.[3]

If the chest film is underpenetrated, the left hemidiaphragm (and left lung base) may not be visible and the pulmonary vascular markings will appear abnormally prominent.[3]

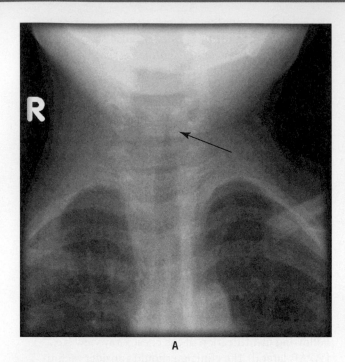

A

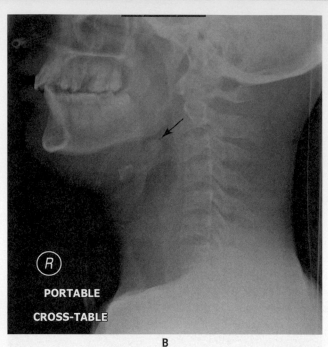

B

FIGURE 11-6 Neck x-ray findings. (A) Croup (the "pencil" or "steeple" sign). (B) Epiglottitis (the "thumb sign").

(A) Courtesy of Dr. Michael Sergant/Radiopaedia; (B) Courtesy of Dr. Andrew Ho/Radiopaedia.

Inspiration Versus Expiration

A good-quality chest x-ray is taken on inspiration, ideally after the patient takes a deep breath. A poor inspiratory effort or chest x-ray taken at end expiration will crowd lung markings and may lead to the incorrect conclusion that the patient has airspace disease. The degree of inspiration can be assessed by counting the number of visible posterior ribs. Ten visible posterior ribs indicate an excellent inspiration; nine visible posterior ribs is an adequate inspiration.[3] The respiratory care clinician should be able to identify anterior and posterior ribs on the standard chest x-ray. Posterior ribs are those that are most apparent on the chest x-ray. Posterior ribs run more or less horizontally. Anterior ribs will be visible but are harder to see and run more or less at a 45-degree angle down and toward the feet.[3]

Density and Image Appearance

As noted, the densest objects on a chest x-ray, including bones (e.g., ribs, vertebrae), metal (e.g., artifacts such as pacemaker wires or metal jewelry on the surface of the chest), and calcium will appear bright white; these materials are radiopaque.[3] Fluid and fluid-filled vessels appear as white, whereas soft tissue will appear grayish white, not as bright as bone. Scar tissue (fibrotic tissue) is also relatively radiopaque.[3] Abnormal findings on a chest x-ray that are white or gray are often referred to as *areas of opacity* or **opacities**. Low-density materials, such as air, are radiolucent and will appear as pitch black [3]

The normal lung contains air-filled lung tissue, airways, and vessels and is relatively radiolucent. The lung tissue is visualized between the ribs and should appear mostly dark with vascular markings.[3] Pitch-black areas inside the rib cage without vascular markings suggests free air, such as may be present with pneumothorax. Vessels and the heart are filled with fluid and appear white. Fluid in the alveoli (e.g., pneumonia, pulmonary edema, ARDS), pleural fluid (e.g., pleural effusion), and interstitial fluid (e.g., interstitial edema) result in areas of increased opacity on the conventional chest x-ray.[3]

An **infiltrate** is simply an abnormal substance (e.g., water, pus, or blood) that has penetrated the interstitial and/or alveolar space in the lung and is visualized on chest x-ray as an area of increased opacity. The term *interstitium* refers to the space between the air sacs and represents the supporting structures of the lungs. Interstitial lung disease (ILD) is a very large group of diseases affecting the interstitial space, with fluid and/or scar tissue accumulation (e.g., fibrosis). Interstitial opacities as seen on chest x-ray may be classified as *linear*, **reticular**, **nodular**, or **reticulonodular patterns**.[14] A linear interstitial pattern on chest x-ray may be characterized by branching linear streaks or opacities (e.g., white lines) with multiple thin strands radiating to the periphery of the lung.[14] Linear patterns are sometimes referred to as *Kerley lines*, which represent thickening of the interlobular septa. Kerley A lines are longer linear opacities that are oriented radially to the hila. Kerley B lines (also called septal lines or septal thickening) are shorter and run at right angles to the lateral pleural surface.[14] A common cause of a linear interstitial pattern on chest x-ray is hydrostatic pulmonary edema (e.g., cardiogenic pulmonary edema) in which fluid leaks into the interstitial space due to high vascular pressures. A linear pattern may also be caused by atypical interstitial pneumonias (e.g., *Chlamydophila*, cytomegalovirus, or respiratory synctial virus [RSV]) or cancer (e.g., metastatic tumor obstruction of the lymphatics).

Reticular interstitial patterns are lines that produce a mesh or lacelike appearance on chest x-ray. A classic cause of a reticular pattern is pulmonary fibrosis, which is sometimes described as a "honeycomb lung" because of the reticular appearance of the opacities on chest x-ray.[15] For example, **idiopathic pulmonary fibrosis (IPF)** typically shows a reticular interstitial pattern with **honeycombing** (peripheral cystic scarring of the lung at least two layers thick with cysts measuring 3 to 5 mm in diameter) on chest x-ray. The tissue histology associated with IPF is known as usual interstitial pneumonia (UIP).[15]

A nodular interstitial pattern is one of discrete opacities (small dots). Pulmonary nodules are seen on chest x-ray as well-defined areas of opacity and may be caused by alveolar or interstitial disease.[16] Causes of a nodular pattern include lung metastases, pneumoconiosis (dust-caused disease), and granulomatous diseases (e.g., tuberculosis, histoplasmosis, cryptococcosis, sarcoidosis).[16] For example, multiple fibrotic nodules may be seen on chest x-ray with silicosis (caused by silica dust inhalation, a type of pneumoconiosis). A reticulonodular pattern (the most common pattern in ILD)

combines the appearance of a nodular and reticular pattern, and causes of both reticular and nodular disease should be considered.[17] **Figure 11-7** provides examples of linear, reticular, nodular, and reticulonodular patterns seen with ILD.

An *alveolar filling pattern* refers to the pattern seen on chest x-ray due to filling of the alveoli with fluid.[18] For example, infectious pneumonia may cause focal or diffuse airspace opacities due to alveolar filling with exudative fluid (e.g., pus, white blood cells, plasma proteins, fluid).[1] A typical alveolar filling pattern results in fluffy, poorly demarcated infiltrates that obscure vascular markings. The term **ground-glass opacification** is sometimes used to describe the appearance on chest x-ray of hazy areas with preservation of bronchial and lung markings.[18] This ground-glass appearance is thought to be due to partial filling of the alveoli and may be caused by infectious disease, ILD, or pulmonary edema (e.g., cardiogenic or ARDS). Air-filled bronchi adjacent to fluid-filled alveoli (e.g., consolidative lobar pneumonia) may result in an *air bronchogram* seen on chest x-ray.[19]

Artifacts such as endotracheal and tracheostomy tubes, central venous catheters, chest tubes, pulmonary artery catheters, and nasogastric tubes are also relatively radiopaque and easily visualized on the chest x-ray. Imaging findings with various pulmonary diseases are discussed later in this chapter.

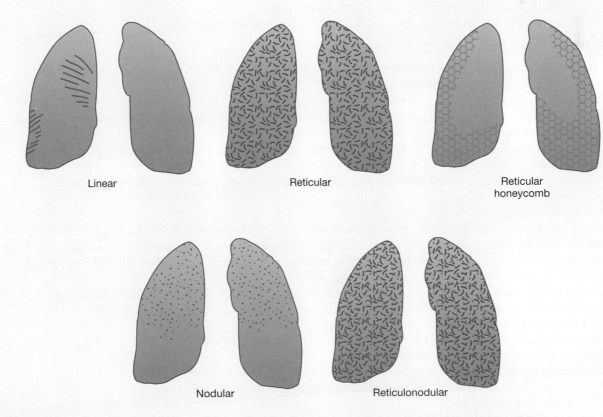

Linear

Reticular

Reticular honeycomb

Nodular

Reticulonodular

FIGURE 11-7 **Linear, reticular, nodular and reticulonodular patterns seen with interstitial lung disease (ILD).**

Data from: Collins J, Stern EJ. *Chest Radiology: The Essentials.* 2nd ed. Philadelphia, PA: Lippincott Williams and Wilkins; 2007.

Approach to the Chest Radiograph

Inspection of the chest x-ray should be done in a systematic way beginning with assessment of the image quality, type of view (i.e., AP, PA, lateral, other), patient position, and whether a full inspiration was achieved. Next, the respiratory care clinician should inspect the trachea for patency, position, narrowing, and the presence of endotracheal or tracheostomy tubes. Any tracheal deviation to right or left should be noted.[3] For example, unilateral atelectasis may pull the trachea towards the affected side, whereas a tension pneumothorax or a large pleural effusion will tend to push the trachea towards the opposite side. The carina should be identified, and the right and left main stem bronchi visualized.

The aorta and right and left **hilum** should then be inspected. The hila contain the major bronchi and vessels, including the pulmonary arteries and veins. Heart size, shape, borders, and cardiophrenic angles should be noted. The cardiothoracic (CT) ratio should also be determined. The hemidiaphragms should be inspected and costophrenic angles reviewed.[3] The ribs should be inspected and rib position and intercostal spaces assessed. For example, a difference between right- and left-side rib spacing may indicate a unilateral lung problem, whereas an increase in space bilaterally may be caused by lung overinflation (e.g., COPD, acute asthma).[14] Next, the lung parenchyma should be inspected followed by inspection of the soft tissues of the neck and chest wall.[3] **Box 11-3** provides a check list for inspection of the AP or PA chest film.

BOX 11-3

Checklist for Chest Radiograph Evaluation

A checklist for evaluation of the chest x-ray should include:

Quality of the Film

- ☐ Is the image PA, AP, or lateral?
- ☐ Is the film overpenetrated, underpenetrated or good exposure?
- ☐ Is the patient upright and flat or twisted in position?
- ☐ Is there anything outside of the chest such as jewelry, etc., that might be misinterpreted?
- ☐ Verify right as opposed to left side as follows: observe stomach bubble and shape and position of left border and aorta; note identifying differences in ribs and parenchyma; note marker on film.
- ☐ Was film taken at full inspiration, or is it a full or partial expiration film?

Review of the Chest Film

- ☐ Trachea: Position, patency, normal narrowing at larynx and normal slight deviation to right at aorta.
- ☐ Carina: Note endotracheal tube position, if present.
- ☐ Aorta: Size, shape, calcification, tortuosity.
- ☐ Hila: Pulmonary arteries, main and branches; enlarged nodes; calcium; eggshells; relationship right versus left; left hilum normally slightly above right.
- ☐ Heart: Size, shape, straight left border, calcified valves, prostheses, mediastinal air, cardiophrenic angles, double contour, enlarged atrium, CT ratio.
- ☐ Hemidiaphragms: Right hemidiaphragm normally slightly above left, scalloping, "adhesions," calcific plaques.
- ☐ Costophrenic angles.
- ☐ Obliques: Posterior ribs can be identified as horizontal; anterior ribs run diagonally; abnormal shadows can be located as anterior or posterior by tendency to remain in relationship to one or the other in two different views.
- ☐ Bones and joints: Old or recent fractures, degree of calcification, notching of upper and under margin of ribs, moth-eaten areas, cervical ribs, deformities.
- ☐ Parenchyma: Character of abnormal shadows, that is mottling; stringy, homogeneous, clear, or vague margins; calcific, spicular radiations; air bronchogram; silhouette sign; interstitial as opposed to alveolar infiltrates; vascularity or bronchovascular markings.
- ☐ Soft tissues of neck and chest wall: Air, foreign objects, calcifications, sinus tracts.
- ☐ Specific abnormalities on CXR include:
    - ☐ Tracheostomy and endotracheal tube position with respect to the carina.
    - ☐ Position of a central lines (CVP) or pulmonary artery (Swan-Ganz) catheter.
    - ☐ Chest tube placement
    - ☐ Interstitial or alveolar infiltrates
    - ☐ Pleural effusion

☐ Pneumothorax
☐ Rib fractures and chest trauma
☐ ARDS and pulmonary edema
☐ Hyperinflation and COPD
☐ Fibrotic lung disease
☐ Deviated trachea
☐ Enlarged heart
☐ Pulmonary arteries

*Most modern x-ray departments today use digital imaging; however, we will use the term "film" loosely to mean the digital image or film image.

Data from: Radiology Masterclass 2007–2013. Available at: http://radiologymasterclass.co.uk/tutorials/chest/chest_pathology/chest_pathology_page2.html.

Normal Anatomy

Recognition of normal thoracic and lung anatomy is a prerequisite for identification of abnormalities.[2] The respiratory care clinician should be familiar with normal anatomy, as viewed via the conventional radiograph. Many structures of the chest are readily visible on a chest x-ray, but others are difficult to see. In fact, some important structures, such as the phrenic nerve, are not visible at all, and other anatomic structures, such as the pleura, only become clearly visible when abnormal. The key structures that are generally visible on a chest x-ray include bones, soft tissue, the mediastinum, the heart, the diaphragm, the trachea and bronchi, the costophrenic angles, the lung lobes and fissures, the pleura, the lung zones, and the hilar structures.[20] **Box 11-4** lists key points regarding normal anatomy as viewed in the chest x-ray. **Figure 11-8** provides normal thoracic anatomy as viewed on the chest film and suggests an "inside out" approach to reviewing the chest radiograph. **Figure 11-9** illustrates normal anatomy as seen on the PA and lateral chest radiograph.

Trachea and Carina

The trachea extends from the cricoid cartilage (at the level of C6 [sixth cervical vertebra]) to the carina, a distance of approximately 10 to 12 cm. At the carina,

the trachea splits into the right and left main bronchi. As a reference point, the carina lies approximately in line with the sternal angle, which is the junction of the manubrium and body of the sternum (angle of Louis).[2] This usually corresponds with the level of the fifth thoracic vertebra (T5). If an endotracheal tube is present, it should be at least 2 cm above the carina, preferably in the middle third of the trachea. The trachea and larger conducting airways contain supportive cartilage and are known as the *cartilaginous airways*.[2]

Mediastinum

The mediastinum is the central cavity within the thorax and is divided into compartments along a horizontal plane at the level of the sternal angle to the T4–T5 disk.[2] Located above this plane is the superior compartment and located below the plane is the inferior compartment.

Major structures of the superior mediastinum include the esophagus; the trachea; the aorta, carotid, and subclavian arteries; the superior vena cava; the innominate veins; one of the intercostal veins; the thymus; the left recurrent, phrenic, and vagus nerves; the lymph nodes; and the thoracic duct.[2] Important anatomic landmarks often visualized on chest x-ray include the aortopulmonary window, the aortic knob, the

BOX 11-4

Normal Anatomy on Chest Imaging

Large Airways

- The trachea should be clearly visible and extend from the larynx (cricoid cartilage) to the carina, where it bifurcates into the right and left main bronchi.
- The trachea begins about the level of sixth cervical vertebra (C6) and extends to about the level of the fifth thoracic vertebra (the carina is about the level of the fifth thoracic vertebra [T5]).

The Hila (Lung Roots)

- The hilum is the "lung root" where the large airways and vessels enter the lung.
- Each hilum contains the major bronchi and pulmonary vessels.
- There are also lymph nodes on each side (not visible unless abnormal).
- The left hilum is often higher than the right.
- If a hilum is out of position, ask yourself if it has been pushed or pulled.
- In addition to position, also check the size and density of the hila.

Heart Size and Contours

- The heart size is assessed as the cardiothoracic (CT) ratio.
- A CT ratio > 50% is abnormal (PA view only).
- The cardiophrenic angles on the right and left are formed by the intersection of the heart and diaphragm.
- The left hemidiaphragm should be visible behind the heart.
- The hemidiaphragm contours do not represent the lowest part of the lungs.

Lung Lobes and Fissures

- The left lung has two lobes and the right has three.
- Each lobe has its own pleural covering.
- The horizontal fissure (right) is often seen on a normal frontal view.
- The oblique fissures are often seen on a normal lateral view.

Diaphragm

- The hemidiaphragms are domed structures.
- Each hemidiaphragm should be well defined.
- The left hemidiaphragm should be visible behind the heart.
- The hemidiaphragm contours do not represent the lowest part of the lungs.
- The costophrenic angles (right and left) are the angles between the diaphragm and chest wall.

Bones and Joints

- There are 12 ribs on each side (1–12) corresponding to the 12 thoracic vertebrae (T1 to T12).
- The first rib is attached to the first thoracic vertebra (T1).
- Each rib then attaches to the adjacent thoracic vertebrae; the head of each rib typically attaches to the bodies of two adjacent vertebrae.
- The ribs slope slant downward as they move anteriorly, making their vertebral attachment higher than their sternal attachment.
- The sternum is made up of three parts from top to bottom: the manubrium, body, and xiphoid process.
- The "angle of Louis," or the sternal angle, is the anterior angle formed by the junction of the manubrium and body of the sternum and is at about the level of T4 or T5 and adjacent to the second costal cartilage.
- The angle of Louis generally corresponds with the level of the carina.
- The first seven ribs (the vertebrosternal ribs), attach to the sternum directly, and thus are often called the "true" ribs.
- Ribs 8–10 (the vertebrochondral ribs) attach to the sternum indirectly via a common cartilage.
- Ribs 11–12 do not attach to the sternum, and thus are referred to as the "floating" ribs.

Soft Tissues

- Soft tissues of the thorax include muscle, fat, and connective tissue.
- Thick soft tissue may obscure underlying structures.
- Black within soft tissue may represent gas.

Data from: Radiology Masterclass 2007–2013. Available at: http://radiologymasterclass.co.uk/tutorials/chest/chest_pathology/chest_pathology_page2.html.

aortic knuckle, and the right paratracheal stripe. These landmarks are important to clinicians, in part, because disease often changes their appearance. **Figure 11-10** outlines the trachea, carina, mainstem bronchi, hilar areas, heart, and major vessels as seen on a normal PA chest radiograph. On chest x-ray, the mediastinum is assessed for growth or invasion of tumor **masses** and the presence of free air (pneumomediastinum) or blood. The mediastinum can appear as widened due to a vascular abnormality or mediastinal mass.[2]

Aortic Knob and Aortic Knuckle

The aortic knob or knuckle is the prominent shadow of the aortic arch as viewed on a frontal chest radiograph. Specifically, the aortic knuckle is the left lateral border of the aorta seen arching posteriorly over the left main pulmonary vessels and bronchus. It is the portion of

1. Mediastinum (trachea, heart, lymph vessels, blood vessels)
   a. Trachea position, patency
   b. Carina; endotracheal tube position, if present
   c. Aorta
   d. Heart size, borders (cardiophrenic angles, cardio-thoracic (C/T) ratio)
2. Hilum – pulmonary arteries, veins, bronchi
3. Lung fields (vascular marking, infiltrates, air bronchograms, and silhouette sign [if present])
4. Dome of diaphragm (shape, flattening)
5. Pleural surface
5a. Costophrenic angles
6. Bones (humerus, clavicles, scapulae, vertebrae, ribs [position, fractures, intercostalspaces, deformities])
7. Skin and soft tissue (neck and chest wall)
8. Sub-diaphragm (observe for stomach bubble on left)

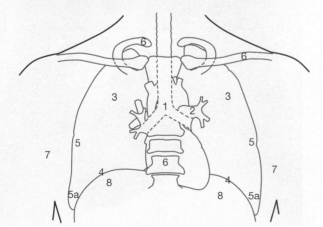

FIGURE 11-8 Normal anatomy as seen on the chest radiograph.

Data from: Ballinger PW, Frank ED. *Merrill's Atlas of Radiographic Positions and Radiologic Procedures*, vols. 1–3, 10th ed. St. Louis, MO: Mosby; 2003.

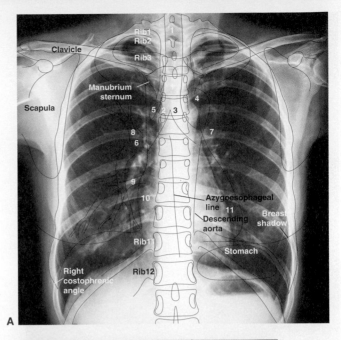

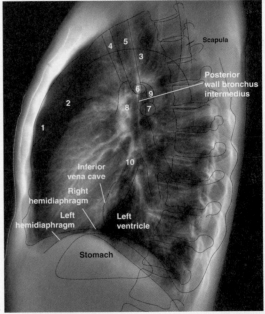

A. Structures include:
   1. Trachea
   2. Right main stem bronchus
   3. Left main stem bronchus
   4. Aortic "knob" or arch
   5. Azygos vein emptying into superior vena cava
   6. Right interlobar pulmonary artery
   7. Left pulmonary artery
   8. Right upper lobe pulmonary artery (truncus anterior)
   9. Right inferior pulmonary vein
   10. Right atrium
   11. Left ventricle
   12. Labeled structures (clavicle, scapulae, sternum, right costophrenic angle, breast shadow, ribs 11 and 12, stomach)

B. Structures include:
   1. Retrosternal airspace
   2. Ascending aorta
   3. Aortic arch
   4. Brachiocephalic vessels
   5. Trachea
   6. Right upper lobe bronchus
   7. Left upper lobe bronchus
   8. Right pulmonary artery
   9. Left pulmonary artery
   10. Confluence of pulmonary veins
   11. Labeled structures

FIGURE 11-9 Normal chest radiograph. (A) Posteroanterior (PA) view. (B) Lateral view.

(A) © stockdevil/iStock/Thinkstock; (B) © Lukasz Panek/iStock/Thinkstock.

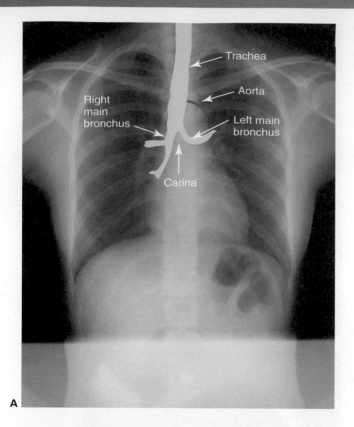

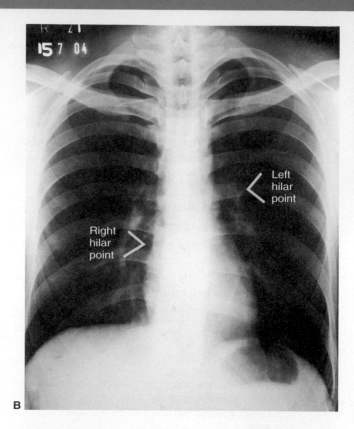

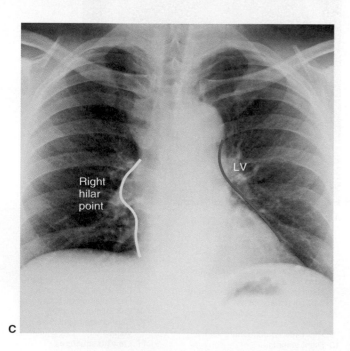

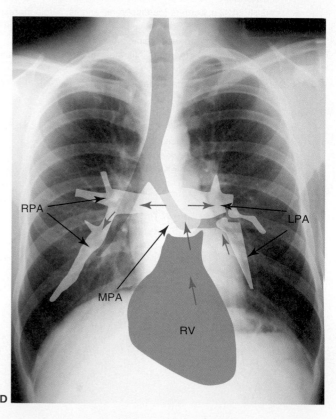

FIGURE 11-10 The large airways, mediastinum, and hila. The major airways, hila, heart, aorta and pulmonary arteries are shown as seen on normal PA views. The right ventricle is normally obscured on CXR by the left ventricle. RA, right atrium; LV, left ventricle; RV, right ventricle position; MPA, main pulmonary artery; LPA, left pulmonary artery; RPA, right pulmonary artery

(A) © Chen Wei Seng/ShutterStock, Inc.; (B) © hald3r/ShutterStock, Inc.; (C) © Susan Law Cain/Dreamstime.com; (D) © Van Hart/ShutterStock, Inc.

the aortic arch where the aorta turns downward and becomes the descending aorta.[2] Shifting of normal position or unclearly demarcated organ borders suggests pathology, such as adjacent lung consolidation, an aneurysm, or a tumor.[3]

Aorto-Pulmonary Window

The aorto-pulmonary window is located between the arch of the pulmonary arteries and the aorta. Abnormally large lymph nodes can sometimes be seen on x-rays near this structure. The aorto-pulmonary window should be visible between the left pulmonary artery and the aortic knuckle. Its posterior boundary is delineated by the descending aorta. Nearby is the ascending aorta.[2]

Right Paratracheal Stripe

The trachea's right edge looks like a thin white stripe extending from the clavicles to the azygous vein because of the lower air density on either side of the denser tracheal wall. The lower density areas display darker, whereas the denser structures appear white on medical images. If this stripe measures more than 3 mm, it could be an indication of disease, such as enlarged lymph nodes or a paratracheal growth. The trachea's left side is not as well-defined because of the location of the great vessels and the aortic arch.[2]

Heart

The heart occupies most of the left side of the mediastinum. The heart should be clearly visible, and the clinician should be able to identify the right atrium, left ventricle, and the right and left cardiophrenic angles.[21] The appearance of the heart can be a helpful diagnostic tool. **Figure 11-11A** provides an example of normal cardiac contours. If the contours of the heart are obscured or blurred, it can mean there is increased density in the tissue adjacent the heart; this is known as the **silhouette sign**.[2] For example, right middle-lobe pneumonia may obscure the right heart margin. In contrast, right lower-lobe pneumonia may blur the diaphragm on the right side. When the left contours of the heart (e.g., left ventricle) are obscured, the cause may be disease of the lingula.[2]

Examining the size of the heart is an important step in the review of any chest radiograph. This is done simply by calculating the ratio of cardiac width to thoracic width. Specifically, the cardiothoracic (CT) ratio is the maximum width of the heart compared to the maximum total width of the thoracic cage at the level of the diaphragm.[3] The width of the thorax is measured from the inner edge of the ribs or pleura. A normal CT ratio on a PA chest film is less than 50% (i.e., CT ratio < 0.50). In adults, if the width of the heart is greater than 50% of the total width of the thoracic cage at the level of the diaphragm in the PA view, then the heart may be enlarged (**cardiomegaly**).[8] Clinicians should remember, however, that the heart may appear to be enlarged on AP radiographs or if the patient's body was rotated even slightly to the right or the left. The standard (preferred) chest x-ray is a PA film. With a PA film, the heart is closer to the film (or flat panel detector) and heart size

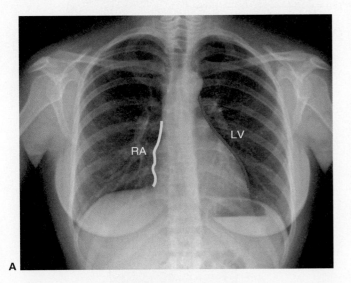
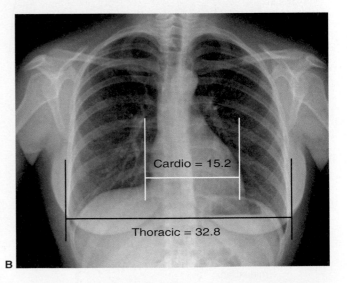

FIGURE 11-11 Normal heart as viewed on PA radiograph. (A) The left heart contour (red line) consists of the left lateral border of the left ventricle (LV). The right heart contour is the right lateral border of the right atrium (RA). (B) Cardiac size is measured by drawing parallel lines at the most lateral point on each side of the heart and measuring the distance across the heart. Thoracic width is determined by drawing parallel lines down the inner aspect of the widest points of the rib cage, and measuring the distanced across the thorax. In (B), the cardiothoracic ratio (CTR) is approximately 15.2:32.8 (arbitrary units) or about 0.46 or 46%. This is less than 50%, which is normal. A CT ratio > 50% suggests an enlarged heart.

is not artificially magnified.[3] In an AP image, the heart is farther away from the film (or detector) and is more magnified. Portable chest x-rays are almost always done AP. **Figure 11-11B** provides an example of a normal CT ratio and heart size on chest x-ray.

> **RC Insights**
>
> On a PA chest radiograph, the width of the heart should be less than half of the overall width of the thorax.

Lungs

The right lung (appearing on the viewer's left when facing the chest x-ray) has three lobes with three corresponding lobar bronchi. The right upper lobe and right middle lobe are separated by the *horizontal fissure* (aka the minor fissure), whereas the right lower lobe is separated from the right upper and middle lobes by the *oblique fissure* (aka the major fissure).[2] The left lung has only two lobes with corresponding lobar bronchi. The left upper lobe and the left lower lobe are separated by the oblique or major fissure on the left. The *lingula* is part of the left upper lobe and roughly corresponds to the right middle lobe, although the lingula is not considered a separate lobe and the left lung has no minor fissure.[2] On the conventional PA chest x-ray, the minor fissure on the right can often be seen; however, the major fissures cannot be seen unless there is fluid in the fissure.[2] The major fissures can often be seen on the lateral chest x-ray. **Figure 11-12** illustrates lung lobes and fissures.

There are 10 *lung segments* on the right and eight on the left, although several of the segments on the left are sometimes "double counted" to arrive at a total of 10 segments on each side.[2] The three lobar bronchi on the right branch into a total of 10 *segmental bronchi*, one for each lung segment. The two lobar bronchi on the left branch into a total of eight distinct segmental bronchi. Segmental bronchi then branch to *subsegmental* bronchi and continue to branch into smaller and smaller conducting airways. The trachea is considered

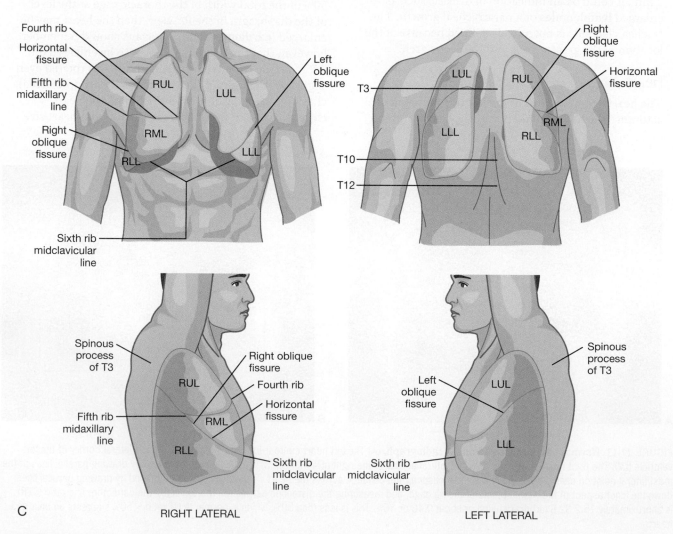

FIGURE 11-12 Lung anatomy.

generation zero, whereas the right and left main bronchi are generation one and the lobar and segmental bronchi are generations two and three, respectively. At each level, beginning with the trachea, the airways branch into two smaller airways (i.e., dichotomous branching).[2] After 10 to 15 generations, cartilage is no longer present and the airways are very small, approximately 1 mm in diameter (i.e., bronchioles). The last conducting airway is the terminal bronchiole, which appears at the 16th to 19th generation. Beyond the terminal bronchioles lie the gas exchange units of the lung (i.e., respiratory bronchioles, alveoli).[2]

As noted, the dichotomous branching of conducting airways of the lung occurs from trachea to main bronchi to lobar bronchi to segmental bronchi to subsegmental bronchi to bronchioles. The conventional chest film usually allows only for visualization of the trachea and mainstem bronchi; lobar, segmental, and subsegmental bronchi can be routinely identified using thin-section CT.[2] Use of contrast media (e.g., bronchograms) with conventional radiography also allows for visualization of the small airways. Bronchograms were used in the past to verify a diagnosis of **bronchiectasis**, which is characterized by cough, mucopurulent sputum production, and thickening and dilation of the small airways.[22] Today, CT or HRCT are the preferred imaging technique for evaluation of bronchiectasis.

Lung Hila

The two hila (right hilum and left hilum) are the point at which the major bronchi and vessels enter the lung and can be considered the lung's root.[2] The hila are complex structures consisting of the major bronchi and the pulmonary veins and arteries. These structures pass through the narrow hila on each side and then branch as they widen out into the lungs. There are also hilar lymph nodes on each side; these are not visible on chest x-ray unless there is an abnormality present.[2] Figure 11-10 provides a view of the pulmonary arteries as seen on chest x-ray.

The hila are not symmetrical but contain the same basic structures on each side. Usually, the left hilum is higher than the right.[2] If the hila are out of position, it may be due to a disease state or condition that pushes or pulls in one direction, such as tension pneumothorax or massive atelectasis on one side (e.g., bronchial intubation). Figure 11-10 also demonstrates normal hilar position.

Fissures

The lung **fissures** are sometimes helpful in pinpointing or identifying disease because diseases are sometimes restricted to specific lobes, each of which has its own pleural covering.[2] The pleural space is only visible when there is an abnormality (e.g., pleural effusion), and normally lung markings should extend to the thoracic

wall on chest x-ray. On a PA view, the right horizontal or minor fissure may be visualized.[3] With lateral chest x-rays, the oblique or major fissures can be seen. Beginning posteriorly at T4–T5, the oblique fissures traverse the hilum. Whereas the right fissure ends up behind the costophrenic angle, the left fissure ends 5 cm posterior to the same angle and has a steeper incline.[2] Separating the right upper lobe from the middle lobe, the horizontal fissure proceeds anteriorly from the hilum. The left lung lacks a horizontal fissure.

Costophrenic Angles

Disease identification is sometimes further aided by the use of the costophrenic angles and costophrenic recesses as anatomic landmarks.[2] The *costophrenic recesses* are formed by the hemidiaphragms and the chest wall. They contain the rim of the lung bases that lie over the dome of each hemidiaphragm.[2] On a frontal chest x-ray, the recess is seen in only one place on each side, where an angle is formed by the lateral chest wall and the dome of each hemidiaphragm. These sharp angles are the *costophrenic angles* and are partial views of costophrenic recesses. Costophrenic angles should appear sharp in frontal chest x-rays, forming acute angles and ending in a sharp point. The *cardiophrenic angles* are the medial angles formed by the heart and the diaphragm on each side.[2] The cardiophrenic angles are more likely to look smooth rather than sharp. **Figure 11-13** provides an example of a normal costophrenic and cardiophrenic angles as seen on a PA chest radiograph.

The left and right hemidiaphragms are almost superimposed on a lateral view. Anteriorly, the left hemidiaphragm blends with the heart and becomes indistinct, as shown in Figure 11-13. When viewing lateral x-rays, costophrenic recesses are visible where the posterior and anterior costophrenic angles are formed by the hemidiaphragms' domes and the chest wall.[2] This costophrenic angle–blunting phenomenon is sometimes confused with a pathologic aberration such as pleural effusion. Costophrenic angle blunting can be related to other pleural disease or to underlying lung disease. Lung hyperexpansion can also lead to blunting of the costophrenic angles. This is because the domes of the diaphragm are pushed downward, and the angle formed is no longer acute.[3]

When reading chest x-rays, one must be keenly aware of possible "pseudo-blunting" of the costophrenic angle. The left costophrenic angle may appear blunt at first sight.[2] This false impression can be produced if the patient was rotated, causing the appearance of thicker breast tissue on the left in comparison to the right, superimposed over the left costophrenic angle. As mentioned earlier, costophrenic angle–blunting phenomenon is sometimes confused with a pathologic aberration such as pleural effusion.[2]

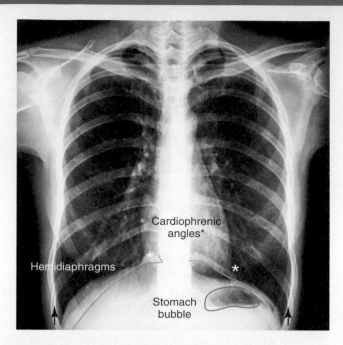

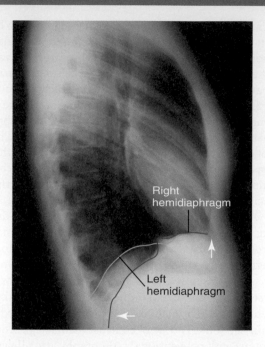

FIGURE 11-13 Diaphragm, costophrenic, and cardiophrenic angles. The costophrenic angles are indicated by the arrows. The cardiophrenic angles are indicated by the white asterisks.

(A) © stockdevil/iStock/Thinkstock; (B) Courtesy of Dr. Thomas Hooten/CDC.

Pleura

The visceral pleura line the surface of the lung, whereas the parietal pleura line the surface of the interior chest wall.[2] Normally, the visceral and parietal pleura are separated only by a thin, serous fluid that reduces friction as the lungs inflate and deflate within the thorax. The pleura only become visible on chest x-ray with abnormalities such as pleural thickening (seen, for example with asbestosis), pleural effusion, or pneumothorax.[2] With pleural effusion, the pleural space fills will fluid, whereas pneumothorax is air in the pleural space; both conditions separate the visceral and parietal pleural surfaces. Anteriorly, the left hemidiaphragm blends with the heart and becomes indistinct. Junctional lines are normal lines that consist of four layers of pleura (two visceral and two parietal) not always seen on chest x-ray. **Figure 11-14** illustrates the location of the pleura as seen on the PA chest radiograph.

Diaphragm and Hemidiaphragms

The diaphragm provides an important demarcation line between the lower-density, darker pulmonary tissue and the denser, white-appearing abdominal structures. Having a sharp, white edge contrasted by the nearby dark lungs, the "domed" oval appearance of the hemidiaphragms should be clearly visible.[2] The right hemidiaphragm is slightly more elevated than the left, which should be clearly visible behind the heart. Although this is sometimes explained by the dome of the liver on the right, it is more likely due to the fact that the large (and heavy) left ventricle sits over the left diaphragm.[3]

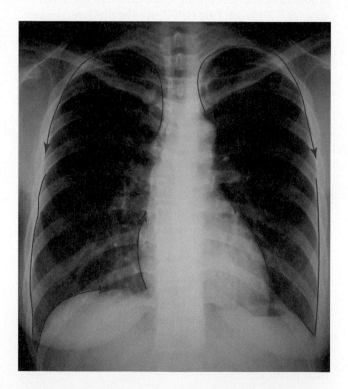

FIGURE 11-14 Normal pleura and pleural spaces. The pleura are outlined in red. When assessing the pleurae, the clinician should begin at the hilum and trace round the entire edge of the lung where pleural abnormalities are more readily seen. The clinician should be on the alert for pleural thickening, pneumothorax (lung markings should be visible to the chest wall) or effusion. The costophrenic angles and hemidiaphragms should be well defined.

© sinngern/iStock/Thinkstock.

Appearing as a lower-density, dark, hanging bubble, air is generally seen beneath the left hemidiaphragm within the stomach. Interestingly, this bubble sometimes serves as a transparent aperture for the most caudal parts of the lungs; in other words, normal lung tissue should be visible through it.[2] Though tricky, it is possible to distinguish between the two diaphragms; spotting gastric air is one way to do so. As noted, Figure 11-13 shows the hemidiaphragms on frontal and lateral views. Lying beneath the contours of the hemidiaphragms are the lowest sections of the lungs; they also reside within the posterior costophrenic recesses. The contours of the hemidiaphragms should be distinguishable from the most caudal parts of the lungs.[2]

The liver is just below the right hemidiaphragm. Below both hemidiaphragms one can see lung markings. The hemidiaphragms' contours should be visible traversing medially all the way to the spine.[2]

In a lateral chest x-ray, the hemidiaphragms should both be visibility enhanced by the nearby darkness of lung air and the softer grayish shade of fluid-filled soft tissue in the abdomen. The heart obscures the left hemidiaphragm's anterior end.[3]

Bone

The densest living tissue visible on a chest x-ray is bone. Bones display as bright white, in comparison with the air inside the lungs, which appears black.[3] Despite the fact that x-rays are ideal for displaying bones, mistakes are sometimes made in identifying single, perhaps small, abnormalities, such as small fractures or dislocations, and diffuse bone disease. This problem is especially important when it comes to less-visible bones such as the ribs, the spine, and the scapulae.[3] The respiratory care clinician should assess the bones of the chest on every chest x-ray, checking for single-bone abnormalities (e.g., fractures) and diffuse bone disease. Review of the appearance of the bone on the chest x-ray is also helpful in assessing the quality of the image. For example, overpenetrated chest x-rays will tend to wash out bones. The position of the vertebral column and ribs can also indicate if the patient is twisted or turned to one side.[2]

The identifiable bones on a chest x-ray include the ribs, the scapulae, the clavicles, some of the spine and the spinous processes, and the upper parts of the humeri. The clavicles are the only bones that are completely visible.[2] Technically, the sternum is also visible, but only as a superimposed structure and, therefore, not clearly delineated. The bones can be used as first-step radiograph quality referential markers. How well the bones can be seen and where they appear on the radiograph are indicators of x-ray penetration, patient rotation, and inspiration. **Figure 11-15** illustrates the appearance of the clavicles, scapulae, and ribs on the conventional PA x-ray.[3]

The clavicles and the vertebral spinous processes between the clavicular medial ends should be clearly demarcated.[2] Should such centrality of the spinous processes not be seen, rotation of the patient may have occurred (note: paratracheal masses or upper lobe fibrosis may also cause shifting of the appearance the spinous processes). The scapulae and humeri are also usually visible on a chest x-ray. In addition to revealing fractures and dislocations, the appearance of all these bones can help pinpoint disease, such as tumors, including those that may have metastasized.[3]

Soft Tissue

The soft tissues of the thorax are made up of the chest and neck muscles and fatty tissue (e.g., breasts). Although the examination of soft tissue is often not emphasized when teaching basic chest x-ray interpretation (probably because x-rays are not ideal for studying it), the appearance of the soft tissue on images can be helpful in rendering diagnoses. A careful review of the chest x-ray should include a close look at the soft tissue of the thoracic wall, the neck, and the breasts.[23] Soft tissue can either impair or assist in diagnosis; in obese patients, for example, some areas may be obscured by fat. Similarly, oversized breasts can hide the costophrenic angles and falsely give the impression that pleural effusion is present. Another important point is that black areas within soft tissue indicate the presence of gas.[24]

When examining the pectoral area, it is also important to pay close attention to possible breast asymmetry, which is fairly common. This can cause lung markings on one side to appear denser when compared to the opposite side. Generally, with breast asymmetry the fine lung markings are denser on the left than on the right. One must avoid mistaking this for a sign of lung disease. In fact, sometimes breast tissue is not visible on one side, but one should not automatically conclude the patient has had a mastectomy unless that fact is known. Yet another set of soft-tissue anatomic landmarks are the nipple markings.[3] Care must be taken not to confuse the nipples for lung masses or nodules. Metallic markers may be used to mark the exact nipple placement on the chest if a second x-ray is taken to evaluate unclear findings.

Fat is less dense than muscle and appears darker on a radiograph.[3] In addition to sometimes being confused with diseased tissue, fat can sometimes obscure other abnormalities. The edges of fat tissue should be smooth. Black areas with irregular edges in soft tissue may be a sign of subcutaneous air tracking, also called *surgical emphysema* or, more commonly, *subcutaneous emphysema*.[14] Following a pneumothorax, subcutaneous emphysema may develop and can be seen in the soft tissues of the neck and face. Subcutaneous emphysema appears as radiolucent streaks in the subcutaneous and muscle tissue.

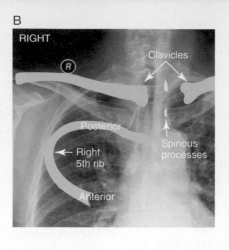

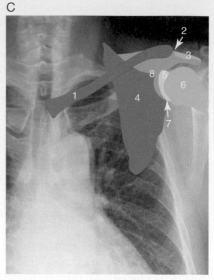

Structures include:
1. Clavicle
2. Acromioclavicular joint
3. Acromion process of scapula
4. Body of scapula
5. Glenoid fossa of scapula
6. Head of left humerus
7. Glenohumeral joint
8. Coracoid process of scapula

FIGURE 11-15 Bones of the thorax. This figure illustrates the major bones seen on the chest radiograph (clavicles, ribs, scapula, and vertebrae). The posterior ribs tend to be more horizontal in position, while the anterior ribs slope down and toward the feet. The scapulae should be rotated up and out of the lung fields in a good PA image, while the clavicles should be even, suggesting the patient is not twisted or rotated. Posterior ribs are more or less horizontal, while anterior ribs run at about a 45-degree angle downward toward the feet and are harder to see.

(A) © windcatcher/iStock/Thinkstock; (B) © windcatcher/iStock/Thinkstock; (C) © windcatcher/iStock/Thinkstock.

Computed Tomography

Computed tomography, also referred to as *computed axial tomography, CT, CAT,* or *CT scan,* was invented in 1972, and since then it has undergone technologic advances that have been truly extraordinary.[3] Modern CT imaging is fast, readily available, and highly detailed. CT scanners can be used to study any part of the human body, including bone and soft tissue.[25] CT can also be used to obtain images of moving organs, as in cardiac studies, as well as the vasculature studies of the circulatory system.[26]

How It Works

Whereas regular x-ray machines concentrate on one angle, or "view," of the human body, CT produces images of the human body in sections. This is known as cross-sectional imaging.[27] In fact, the word *tomography* comes from the Greek words *tomos,* which means "slice" or "section," and *graphe,* which means "drawing."[3] Thus, CT scans provide a "slice" view of the inside of the human body.[28] The clinician can then study each slice from the outer edge to the center. Stacking these slices together creates a multidimensional image,

providing a more realistic view than seen in a flat x-ray image.[28] **Figure 11-16** illustrates a cross-sectional medical image. **Clinical Focus 11-1** describes the cross-sectional anatomy that must be understood to evaluate the thoracic CT. **Figure 11-17** illustrates the various body planes.

CT imaging is based on the same physical principles as conventional radiography: the differential absorption of x-rays by tissues and other substances of differing atomic number (i.e., different density).[3] CT scanners incorporate an x-ray tube source and an array of x-ray detectors; a computer reconstructs the signal from the x-ray detectors.[3] The speed at which the CT scanner captures a single sectional image depends on the period of time the x-ray source takes to rotate around the patient.[3] Each slice is very detailed, accurate, and less susceptible to image-disrupting factors such as patient movement during the scan.[28]

Volumetric CT (aka spiral or helical CT) has greatly influenced clinical CT imaging protocols.[29] The fundamental principle of volumetric CT involves continuous acquirement of data as the patient is moving at a constant rate through the CT scanner.[29] Today, high-speed scanners are capable of producing very thin sections

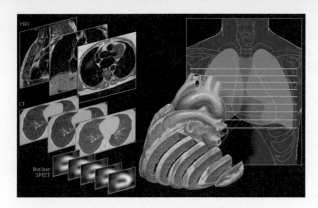

FIGURE 11-16 Cross-sectional medical imaging.

Courtesy of Dr. Patrick Lynch.

with exquisite detail in one or two breath holds, resulting in a significant increase in the speed of examination. Multislice helical CT provides a technical advance over helical CT scanning and allows for improved detection of aortic dissection or aneurysm, pulmonary emboli, or diffuse lung disease.[30]

Current multidetector CT scanners have a 256-slice capacity per rotation.[19] A very large number of slices can be acquired with high spatial and contrast resolution, resulting in detailed multidimensional images.[19] CT scans provide much more information than traditional single-view, monodimensional radiographs. The images produced allow for assessment of organ and tissue morphology and dimensions, current biological condition, defects, and aberrations (**Figure 11-18**).[3] The two-, three-, and four-dimensional images produced can be manipulated, corrected, or enhanced.[22] Because the images are usually digitized, they can easily be saved or transmitted to other locations. This makes it possible for facilities to obtain outside help in interpreting the images as well as providing opportunities to use images for consultative or educational purposes.[27] Instantaneous output to high-resolution printers or to computer systems with 3-D displays can also be performed.

In recent years, CT scanners have improved in multipurpose capacity, speed, number of images possible per rotation, and visual quality of the resulting images.[26] For example, CT scanners are now capable of spiral or helical scanning in addition to axial mode.[27] These new scanners provide more images, with greater detail and in less time, while also limiting the patient's exposure to ionizing radiation.[27] Electron-beam CTs (EBCTs) do not require moving components to create anatomic snapshots and are also faster than conventional CTs.[3] HRCT scanners are being used to accurately identify inflammation and scarring in the lungs.[27] Thin-section CT (1.5 to 3 mm) slices allows for better detection and assessment of solitary pulmonary nodules, metastatic lesions, emphysema (e.g., bullae), bronchiectasis, and CT pulmonary angiograms. HRCT (1 to

CLINICAL FOCUS 11-1

Cross-Sectional Anatomy

In order to study sectional anatomy, the clinician must understand the planes of the body and orientation of anatomic structures within each plane. Sectional images may be obtained in numerous body planes, including axial, or transverse; sagittal; oblique; and coronal. Sagittal planes pass vertically through the body, dividing it into right and left portions. Sagittal images allow for identification of structures from the anterior to posterior, as well as proximal or distal and superior or inferior. Sagittal images slice the body from lateral to medial. It is sometimes difficult to localize anatomy without an entire series of images.

Coronal planes are vertical planes that pass through the body, dividing it into anterior and posterior portions. Anatomy is seen as being closer to midline (deep) or closer to surface (lateral). Closer to the surface may also be described as *superficial*. Proximal and distal structures are demonstrated on coronal images.

The axial (transverse) plane passes horizontally though body, dividing it into superior and inferior portions. Axial images show anterior from posterior, as well as medial to lateral structures. Structures that are closer to surface, as compared to those located deeper in the body, can also be distinguished. Because the part or body is imaged in transverse sections from top to bottom, it is difficult to distinguish which structures are more proximal or distal without an entire series of axial images.

Sectional imaging can demonstrate a variety of diseases of the lungs, bronchi, and pleura, including infections, traumatic injuries, and neoplasms.

Data from: Kelley LL, Petersen C. *Sectional Anatomy for Imaging Professionals*, 3rd ed. St. Louis, MO: Mosby Elsevier; 2007.

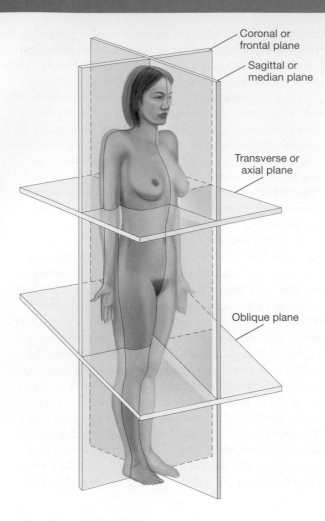

Coronal or frontal plane

Sagittal or median plane

Transverse or axial plane

Oblique plane

FIGURE 11-17 Body planes.

1.5 mm) may be especially useful in evaluation of ILD and can be used to identify linear, reticular, or nodular patterns of opacity. It should be noted that HRCT often takes cuts every 10 mm and thus can miss some nodules. Thin-section CT cuts are generally every 2 to 3 mm.

To enhance images or produce images that would not otherwise be visible, CT scans may employ the use of radio-contrast agents. **Contrast agents** may be introduced into the body by intravenous injection, through a catheter, or via a natural aperture, such as the rectum or esophagus. These agents make an area more visible or help identify abnormalities within bone, tissue, or vessels by making the area temporarily denser and easier to distinguish from other nearby structures. CT pulmonary angiography incorporates spiral (helical) CT scans using intravenous contrast media for diagnosis of pulmonary emboli. CT scans can be merged with PET scans (PET-CT) to provide precise anatomic locations for cancer tumors or other metabolic abnormalities.

Indications for CT Scans

Thoracic CT scans are used to explore problems related to the heart, lungs, esophagus, trachea, major blood vessels, and soft-tissue organs in the chest.[24] Some of the abnormalities that may be found by a CT scan include interstitial or alveolar disease, lung cancer, pulmonary emboli, and aneurysm.[3] CT scans may also reveal evidence of metastasized cancer, which is

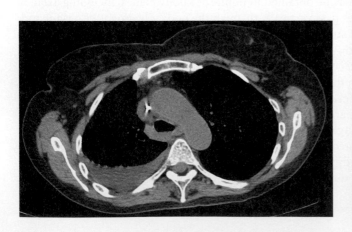

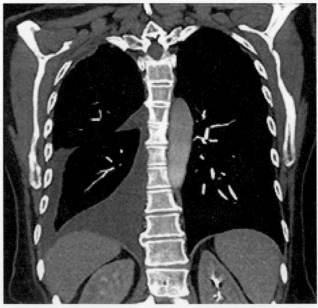

FIGURE 11-18 71-year-old female with right pleural malignant effusion. (A) Axial CT showing right pleural effusion. (B) Coronal CT and right pleural effusion.

cancer that has spread from its original site.[23] CT of the chest may be especially useful for detection and/or evaluation of:

- Interstitial lung disease
- Pulmonary embolus
- Aortic aneurysm or aortic dissection
- Chest pain (e.g., to rule out pulmonary embolus or aortic dissection)
- Lung nodules
- Lymph nodes (e.g., lymphadenopathy, mediastinal lymph nodes)
- Pleural fluid
- Pericardial fluid
- Lung abscess
- Lung cancer (e.g., staging of bronchogenic carcinoma)
- Cortical bone masses

CT for Lung Cancer Screening

Lung cancer currently has a 5-year survival rate of about 16%, and it is the leading cause of cancer deaths.[31] New evidence suggests that low-dose CT lung cancer screening can reduce lung cancer deaths by 20% compared to conventional chest radiographs.[31,32] Based on these findings, low-dose CT (LDCT) scans may be considered for current or former tobacco smokers who meet the following criteria:[31]

- Currently smoke or who have quit smoking within the past 15 years
- Age 55 to 74 years
- Smoking history ≥ 30 packs a year
- No prior history of lung cancer

Further, chest radiographs should not be used for routine lung cancer screening.

CT scans are also used to guide or help correctly plot minimally invasive interventional procedures. Examples include using CT scans to guide needle insertion for tissue biopsy or abscess drainage. CT scans are also used for staging procedures to determine the extent or severity of cancer. As noted, CT angiography is being increasingly used to diagnose pulmonary emboli. **Box 11-5** contrasts CT scans with conventional radiography. **Box 11-6** lists factors that can limit or adversely affect CT scan results.

Procedures for the Exam

To perform a CT scan, the patient is asked to lie flat in the scanner. The table is drawn through a doughnut-shaped gantry containing the x-ray source, which rotates around the patient as the patient moves through the gantry. A rotating fan-shaped beam of x-rays is projected onto (and through) the patient, and sensitive detectors record the results. The constantly changing viewpoints or angles result in extensive data that are collected and sent to a computer. The computer uses sophisticated algorithms to organize and manipulate the data and construct multidimensional images of the organs, bone, or tissue being studied. Although the

---

BOX 11-5

Advantages of CT Imaging

Advantages of CT Imaging include:

- Better differentiation between types of soft tissue disease (e.g., differentiating tumors from cysts).
- Superior bone imaging.
- Superior contrast as compared to conventional radiography.
- Reduced acquisition time as compared to other cross sectional imaging techniques.

CT, computed tomography

BOX 11-6

Factors Impacting Use of CT Scans

Factors that may adversely affect patients or limit the application of CT imaging include:

- Allergies to contract agents, such as iodine
- Certain medications, such as those containing bismuth
- Claustrophobia
- Gastroesophageal reflux disease (GERD)
- Heart disease
- Jewelry or removable prostheses
- Kidney problems; contrast agents can adversely affect the kidneys
- Myeloma
- Neurological or mental health issues that make it difficult for the person to remain still or follow directions
- Pregnancy or breast-feeding
- Respiratory disease or distress, especially dyspnea when lying supine in an enclosed place

CT, computed tomography

actual scanning takes only a few seconds, the entire procedure may take between 15 and 30 minutes. Most of the time is spent on preparatory procedures.[3] More time may be devoted if multiple scanning sessions are planned or if interventional procedures, such as biopsies, have been scheduled in addition to the diagnostic exams.[3]

What Patients Can Expect

Although the procedure is essentially painless, there are aspects that may be inconvenient, uncomfortable, or intolerable for certain patients. Some patients may find it difficult to lie still for extended periods of time.

In some cases, patients will have an IV catheter inserted for the administration of sedatives or contrast agents, such as iodine. Contrast is used to identify pulmonary emboli, to distinguish mediastinal lymph nodes from vessels, and to better outline the pleural space. The IV is usually placed in the arm, wrist, or hand area. Some people report feeling a slight burning, warm, or flushed sensation when the contrast agent is introduced into their system, followed by a metallic taste in their mouths. These sensations are considered normal and are usually short-lived. The radiology technologist should make sure that the patient is comfortable and should deal with any complications or mishaps expeditiously and supportively.

Magnetic Resonance Imaging

Edward Purcell and Felix Bloch discovered the concept of magnetic resonance in 1946. In 1952, they won the Nobel Prize for Physics for this discovery.[33] Before it was used for medical imaging, magnetic resonance was used for physical and chemical molecular analyses. In 1971, Raymond Damadian determined that the specific nuclear magnetic relaxation periods of normal tissue cells and tumor cells differed.[33] This motivated scientists to consider the use of magnetic resonance for disease identification. Two years later, Godfrey Hounsfield introduced x-ray–powered computerized tomography.[33] It was around this time that hospitals adopted the idea of investing in medical imaging machinery and technology, opening the door for further development.

How It Works

Magnetic resonance imaging (MRI), originally known as nuclear magnetic resonance imaging (NMR), is a minimally invasive technique that uses nonionizing radiation produced by large, powerful magnets and radio waves to create accurate, detailed images of the human body.

As with CT scans, the images produced are called *slices.* Sectional images may be obtained across various body planes, including axial, or transverse; sagittal; coronal; and oblique views.

The human body contains a very large quantity of hydrogen atoms, and each hydrogen atom produces a nuclear magnetic resonance signal that can be used to generate images. The signal is created by the spin of the hydrogen atom's single proton.[33] The MRI scanner incorporates a strong, circular magnet that generates a powerful magnetic field. This magnetic field is used to align the hydrogen protons within the body. When exposed to radio waves, the hydrogen atoms absorb kinetic energy, changing the energy state of the protons.[33] The energy imparted is then released, producing distinct signals for different tissues. The signals produced by abnormal tissue are different from those produced by healthy cells. Thus, the cellular mapping created by MRI is very detailed.[33] The MRI is especially useful for visualization of body soft tissues, which contain water and thus an abundance of hydrogen atoms.

Patients undergoing MRI are prohibited from wearing anything containing metal, including clothing, jewelry, and certain internal or external medical devices. Metal objects can lead to metal artifacts on the images.[2,33] More important, they pose a danger to the patient because of the strong magnets in use. Metal objects are also not allowed in the MRI imaging suite, because the magnetic field produced can cause a metal object to become a dangerous projectile missile.[33]

For an MRI scan, the patient lies on a flat table that then moves the patient's body inside a gantry. The confined, narrow structure of the MRI scanner can be troublesome for people with even mild claustrophobia. Thus, "open" MRI scanners have been specifically developed for claustrophobic or morbidly obese patients. Coils are placed around, under, or over the areas to be studied to assist in the reception and transmission of radio waves and help enhance the images. Electrocardiogram (ECG) leads are placed on the patient's chest when synchronizing the image acquisition with the patient's heartbeat and respiration is required, such as in cardiac and vasculature imaging.[33]

Indications for MRI

MRI is an excellent tool for identifying vascular diseases and abnormalities, soft tissue injuries, abnormal fluid deposits, signs of **calcification** and stenosis, internal bleeding, and infection.[2,3] It can also clarify the findings of other imaging tests. The thoracic MRI is often used to evaluate certain thoracic or cardiovascular problems and can pinpoint problems in the heart's atria, ventricles, and valves; lung lobes, bronchioles, capillaries, and thoracic blood vessels; thymus; trachea; thoracic spine, and esophagus.[2,33,34] **Figure 11-19** demonstrates a normal chest MRI. The MRI is often used to evaluate chest wall problems, such as chest wall

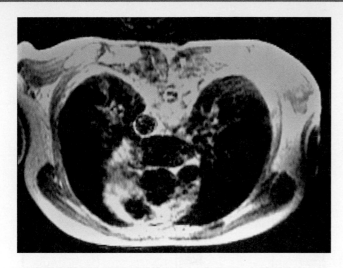

FIGURE 11-19 Normal chest MRI.

© Mediscan/Visuals Unlimited, Inc.

tumors, chest wall infection, or pleural disease. The thoracic MRI is of more limited value in evaluation of the lung parenchyma.[21]

MRI is also used to detect difficult-to-spot blood circulation abnormalities, especially when the problem is minor; these include aneurysms, pulmonary embolus, and blockages in arteries and veins caused by calcification, plaque, or foreign objects. Contrast agents are particularly important in these types of vascular assessments.[34]

MRI is very useful for the detection of bone pathology and imperfections and provides useful information about bone integrity. MRI may confirm a bone fracture not clearly visible on x-ray, as well help evaluate the condition of joints, bone marrow, tendons, cartilage, and ligaments. MRI can also help diagnose arthritis, malignancies, and infections and may be useful for assessing fetal development.[2,12] The MRI is also the most specific test in identifying brain or spinal cord abnormalities that may be missed on CT scans.

Like CT, MRI is increasingly being combined with other imaging techniques, such as radionuclide scintigraphy or ultrasound, though initial costs are high. In summary, MRI of the thorax may be especially useful for assessment of:[35]

- Lung apices
- Diaphragm
- Spinal column (e.g., paraspinal masses)
- Pleural disease (e.g., lesions, effusions)
- Mediastinum and hila (e.g., tumor, lymphoma staging)
- Chest wall (e.g., tumors, infection, masses)
- Bone (e.g., metastatic bone marrow invasion)

MRI Risks

MRI is considered to be one of the safest imaging procedures, though there are a number of important safety issues. For example, MRI-related accidents in the United States have risen over 500% from 2000 to 2009.[36] Reported hazards include burns, tinnitus, near-field effects, and projectile accidents.[36] As scanners become more powerful, the likelihood of a projectile missile increases. The physical design of the MRI suite can diminish risks inherent in the MRI environment. However, the increasing use of MRI for older and more acutely ill patients increases the hazards associated with medical devices.[37] Interventional applications for MRI also bring more people and more equipment into the MRI suite and increase risk.[36, 37]

Adverse reactions to contrast agents pose a risk, and persons with kidney disease may develop postprocedure renal complications.[3] For example, use of gadolinium-containing contrast agents has been associated with the development of nephrogenic systemic fibrosis in patients with severe kidney failure.

The powerful magnet used during MRI can disrupt or damage implanted medical devices. Patients with pacemakers, defibrillators, insulin pumps, and similar devices should be informed regarding this hazard and the risks of MRI for such patients must be carefully considered.[3] Also, any metallic material in the body can shift during MRI; this can result in damage to implants or, worse, a metal piece breaking off and inflicting damage to vital organs, tissue, vessels, nerves, or bones.[3] **Box 11-7** lists factors that may interfere with MRI.

Considerations in Transporting Critically Ill Patients

Nursing personnel and a respiratory therapist may be required to transport critically ill patients to and from the imaging department for MRI; a qualified healthcare professional must also remain with unstable or critically ill patients during the procedure.[33] Certain instances, such as procedural sedation, require a clinician to remain with the patient during the procedure to manage sedation.

In patients requiring mechanical ventilation, an MRI-compatible ventilator is available and is usually housed in MRI zone 4, which is the scanning room. **Figure 11-20** is an example of the MRI suite safety zones.[33] The respiratory therapist should determine if the MRI-compatible ventilator will be used or if the patient will need to be ventilated manually.

All MRI facilities are required to have clear signage that indicates the hazards present and access restrictions. Equipment, instruments, and devices should be clearly labeled to indicate their safety in the MRI environment.[33]

BOX 11-7

Factors that Impact MRI Procedures

Factors that may adversely affect MRI procedures include:

- Dialysis
- Embedded metal fragments (e.g., bullet fragments, shrapnel)
- Implants or medical prosthesis
  - Artificial heart valves
  - Artificial joints or limbs
  - Cardiac pacemakers
  - Cardioversion (defibrillator) implants
  - Cerebral aneurysm clips
  - Cochlear implants
  - Dental implants, bridges, braces, or fillings
  - Insulin pumps or medication infusion devices
  - Intrauterine devices
  - Metal clips, pins, screws, or plates
  - Vascular stents, filters, or coils
- Issues related to the use of contrast agents
  - Allergy
  - Diabetes mellitus
  - Kidney disease
  - Sickle cell anemia
- Medication—delivery patches, which may overheat during MRI
- Metal dust in cosmetics, tattoos, body paints, tattooed eyeliner (e.g., iron pigment)
- Occupational exposure to metal dust or debris (e.g., metal dust in the eyes)
- Pregnancy

MRI, magnetic resonance imaging

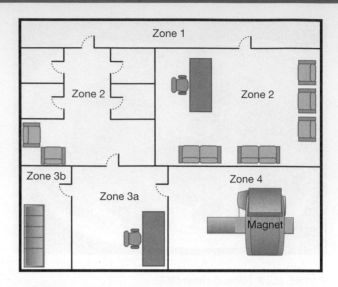

FIGURE 11-20 MRI suite safety zones.

perfusion, neuroendocrine tumors, adrenocortical adenomas, and disseminated thyroid cancer.[38] Ventilation–perfusion ($\dot{V}/\dot{Q}$) scans can be used to assess the distribution of ventilation and pulmonary blood flow. For example, areas of the lung that are ventilated but not perfused may suggest pulmonary emboli, and $\dot{V}/\dot{Q}$ scans are considered the gold standard for evaluating chronic pulmonary emboli resulting in pulmonary hypertension.

Positron emission tomography (PET) is a nuclear medicine technique that provides physiologic information about metabolically active tissue (e.g., O_2 consumption and glucose metabolism).[38] PET is very useful for evaluation of cancers and cancer metastases. Single-photon emission computed tomography (SPECT), also known as tomographic radionuclide scintigraphy, is a newer technique that allows for visualization of slices of the chest that can be manipulated by computer.[38] We will discuss each of these techniques below.

Nuclear Medicine

Nuclear medicine (NM) imaging techniques use radioactive materials to diagnose disease, assess disease progression, and treat certain medical conditions. Because nuclear medicine techniques can identify physiologic and pathophysiologic processes, they may identify problems that are not apparent using other imaging techniques, allowing for earlier treatment.[38] Nuclear medicine technology can also be used to plan and assess the effectiveness of treatment. Radionuclide scanning is frequently ordered to identify metastatic disease (e.g., bone scan), and specialized radionuclide scans can be performed to assess for myocardial

How It Works

Nuclear medicine imaging is minimally invasive, generally painless, and low risk. The scans conducted make use of energy-emitting radiotracers (i.e., radiopharmaceuticals). Although radioactive, these substances usually have a short life span, minimizing the amount of radiation exposure.[38] The radiation imparted by these radiotracers is relatively small; however, the short life span also helps ensure that any substance remaining in the body does not continue to emit potentially harmful radiation.[3]

Radiotracers may be delivered orally, by injection, or by inhalation; they then follow a particular path, depending on what is being targeted, and are then usually concentrated in specific organs or parts of the body.[20] The medical image produced is created from the emitted energy of the radiotracer and the chemical reactions occurring at the sites through which (or into which) the tracers travel; the gamma rays thus produced may be monitored and recorded using gamma cameras, PET scanners, and special probes.[20]

Radiotracers tend to concentrate in the more active areas of the body, such as tumor cells. These cells often consume large amounts of glucose and force the body to supply additional blood flow through newly created blood vessels, a process known as *angiogenesis*.[21] These "hot spots," help identify diseased tissue.[21] So-called "cold spots"—areas where little or no activity is detectable, particularly in contrast to the surrounding areas—can also be signs of pathology, as in the case of dead or diseased tissue, such as might be found in certain parts of the heart following a myocardial infarction (MI).[3]

Lung Ventilation and Perfusion Imaging

A lung ventilation–perfusion scan, also known as a $\dot{V}/\dot{Q}$ scan, is an imaging test that evaluates air and blood flow in the lungs.[39] $\dot{V}/\dot{Q}$ scans may be used to rule out or diagnose pulmonary embolism and are commonly used in patients with renal disease where contrast media may further injure the kidneys. The $\dot{V}/\dot{Q}$ scan actually involves two separate imaging exams: one for ventilation and one for lung perfusion. The ventilation scan demonstrates the distribution of air in the lung; the perfusion scan accesses pulmonary blood flow.[39] Both scans utilize radioisotopes that emit ionizing radiation but have a short life span.[3] For the ventilation portion of the exam, the patient inhales a small amount gas containing the radioactive tracer; for the perfusion portion of the scan, the radioisotopes are introduced

directly into a vein.[3] One of the few side effects sometimes experienced by patients undergoing these tests is an allergic reaction to the tracer.[40] The ventilation scan generally requires that patients lie on a moving table while the scanner is manipulated over them.[3] Wearing a special mask, the patient inhales a gas mixture that is composed primarily of oxygen with a small amount of radioisotope tracer.[40] As the patient breathes, the scanner takes pictures showing air flowing into the lungs.[40] The scan is quick and painless; one of its few disadvantages is the small amount of radiation exposure that patients receive.[40]

In the perfusion test, a tiny amount of radioisotope (radioactive microaggregated albumin) is injected into a vein.[41] The scanner then obtains images of vascular sections and processes within and near the lungs.[41] Although it is a relatively safe procedure, the radioisotope injection can cause some discomfort. As with any test involving radiation exposure, women who are breast-feeding or pregnant should exercise caution and consider the relative risks and benefits of the test, because fetuses and infants are much more sensitive to radiation than adults.[33]

The test is performed for three main reasons: (1) to help find or diagnose a pulmonary embolus, (2) to look for shunts, and (3) to test pulmonary function (e.g., distribution of ventilation and perfusion) in patients with COPD and other similar diseases.[3] For example, $\dot{V}/\dot{Q}$ scans are sometimes useful to assess air trapping in patients with obstructive lung disease (e.g., COPD, smoke injury, or rejection after lung transplantation). When combined with clinical findings, the $\dot{V}/\dot{Q}$ test is highly accurate in correctly identifying patients with pulmonary embolus, whereas a normal $\dot{V}/\dot{Q}$ test virtually excludes pulmonary embolus.[3] **Figure 11-21**

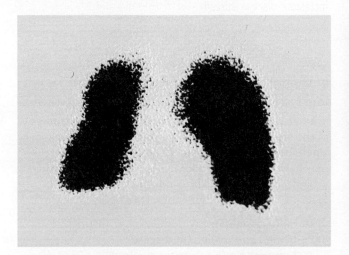
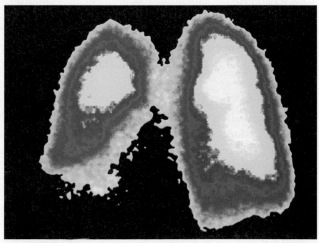

FIGURE 11-21 (A) A lung perfusion scan. (B) Scintigram with perfusion of technetium 99m (Tc 99m) showing a pulmonary embolism, posterior view and a thrombosis of the right lower pulmonary vein.

(A) © Z070/Custom Medical Stock Photo, Inc.; (B) © Sovereign/ISM /Phototake.

provides an example of a ventilation perfusion scan of a patient with pulmonary embolus using SPECT.

PET Scans and Fusion Imaging

PET scans can assess important chemical and metabolic activities and reactions occurring deep inside the body, such as oxygen utilization, circulation of blood and other essential fluids, and glucose metabolism.[3] Observing how well these functions are proceeding can help physicians determine the health status of organs, tissue, and bones. PET scans can also help point out the existence of pathology, even at very early stages, when treatment can do the most good.[3] When the biologically active molecule used for PET is the glucose analog fluorodeoxyglucose (18-fluoro-2-deoxyglucose, or FDG), the resultant images are able to depict metabolic activity in tissue based on where the tracer is absorbed.[42] This type of tracer is especially useful in identifying cancer metastases, because cancer cells tend to readily absorb glucose.[42] Taking advantage of this characteristic of cancer cells, F-18 FDG-PET can help reveal whether and where cancer is present in the body. Using different radiotracers, PET can help detect and diagnose other disorders.[42,43]

Image fusion/coregistration combines nuclear medicine techniques with other imaging techniques (e.g., CT or MRI). For example, superimposition of images from nuclear medicine techniques and CT scans can create a comprehensive, very detailed image. One example of this "fusion" technology is the popular trend of combining SPECT with CT in a single medical imaging scanner.[44] These combined techniques make it possible to have the anatomic detail of CT and the chemical/metabolic information provided by SPECT or PET exams, all done the same day during the same medical-imaging exam session.[44,45] **Figure 11-22** provides an example of combined PET and CT imaging of lung cancer. Image fusion can provide much more detailed images and may lead to better health outcomes. Currently, PET/CT is probably more popular than SPECT/CT. Another promising device expected to be available for use in the near future is a combination PET/MRI scanner.

What Patients Can Expect

The time required for PET scans can vary widely. First, the patient is prepped. Then, the patient must lie quietly still for approximately 60 minutes to allow the radiotracer to spread through the body.[45] The time needed for the exam itself depends on whether the patient is having a PET scan or a combined PET-CT scan, the parts of the body being radiographed, the number of tests being performed, and whether any interventional procedures have also been scheduled. For a combined test, the CT scan is generally done first, followed by the PET scan.

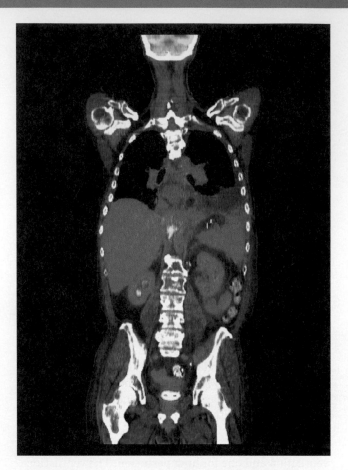

FIGURE 11-22 A color-enhanced image obtained from a combined positron emission tomography (PET) computerized tomography (CT) scan. This is a frontal (coronal) image with the data from the PET scan combined with the anatomic/spatial data from a CT scan. PET images look at the metabolic activity of the tissues. The CT scan is used for precise structural/anatomic information. The fusion of the data from the PET scan and the CT scan provides imaging information from the PET scan with spatial anatomic information from the CT scan. This patient has lung cancer and underwent PET/CT to look for metastatic disease (spread).

© Living Art Enterprises, LLC/Science Source.

Indications for PET and Fusion Imaging

F-18 FDG-PET and PET-CT are especially useful for evaluation of malignant disease (i.e., cancer). Cancers of the oral cavity, pharynx, larynx, esophagus, stomach, small intestine, colon, liver, gallbladder, and pancreas may be evaluated using PET. The following conditions provide some of the indications for the use of F-18 FDG-PET or PET-CT for thoracic imaging:[46]

- Solitary pulmonary nodules (e.g., distinguishing benign and malignant disease)
- Lung cancer (e.g., cancer staging)
- Monitoring for recurrence of lung cancer
- Metastatic esophageal cancer

Limitations of Nuclear Medicine Scans

The resolution obtained with nuclear medicine imaging is not as anatomically sophisticated as that obtained from MRI or CT, though this drawback may be less important in light of the physiologic information provided by nuclear medicine techniques.[47] It should be noted that PET scans can provide erroneous results, especially if the patient has chemical imbalances that are not related to the disease or injury being studied.[48] For example, patients who eat or drink certain substances prior to the exam, despite instructions to fast, may trigger confusing test results.[3] Diabetes mellitus, implanted devices, and impaired kidney function, among other conditions, can limit findings. **Box 11-8** provides a summary of the limitations of nuclear medicine procedures that should be considered.

Nuclear Medicine Cardiac Imaging

Radionuclide cardiac imaging utilizes a gamma camera to create an image of the cardiac blood vessels after the injection of a radioactive substance into the bloodstream.[49] This exam is performed to assess coronary artery disease, cardiomyopathy, valvular or congenital cardiac diseases, and other cardiac disorders.[49] SPECT utilizes rotating cameras and computer-managed tomographic reconstruction to produce detailed 3-D images of imaged areas. With multihead SPECT systems, imaging may be completed in less than 10 minutes.[48] Using SPECT, posterior and inferior abnormalities and otherwise imperceptible areas of **infarction**, as well as the vessels responsible for infarction, may be pinpointed. The sections of viable and infarcted myocardium can be quantified, which may aid in rendering a prognosis.[49]

BOX 11-8

Risks and Hazards of Nuclear Medicine Imaging Procedures

Nuclear medicine scans are not suitable for certain people or in certain situations. Examples include:

- *Pregnant women.* In general, fetuses should not be subjected to radioactive medical imaging; breast-feeding women should exercise caution regarding such tests because traces of radiation may be imparted through the milk if breast-feeding takes place too soon after the test, and even small amounts of radiation may constitute significant exposure for a baby.
- *Patients who use certain medications or nutritional supplements, such as herbs, vitamins, and minerals.* Because nuclear medicine scans measure chemical reactions, patients need to report all medications and supplements they are taking before undergoing an exam. Patients may be advised to forego certain substances that may interfere with or cloud the PET results.
- *Patients with specific known allergies or previous reactions to contrast agents used in nuclear medicine tests.* In particular, nuclear medicine tests may be contraindicated in patients with allergies to seafood or iodine.
- *Patients with diagnosed medical problems or conditions that may interfere with, hinder, or complicate the exam, such as nephrologic disorders and diabetes mellitus.* Patients who have recently had a kidney transplant or who are receiving radiation therapy for cancer may also not be good candidates for nuclear medicine tests.
- *Patients who ignore instructions regarding eating and drinking before the test.* Failure to follow these instructions may require the test to be redone.
- *Obese patients.* Like CT and MRI equipment, PET scanning equipment has weight and size limits. Scanning facilities should provide this information to healthcare providers.
- *Patients undergoing radiation therapy or with an extensive history of radiation-conferring tests.* Although the amount of radiation exposure from nuclear medicine tests is small, it still contributes to the patient's lifetime radiation exposure. Care should be exercised to ensure that these tests are done only when necessary and with even more caution when dealing with patients who are currently receiving radiation therapy, have had extensive radiation-conferring tests in the past 5 years, or have been exposed to unusually large doses of radiation over their lifetimes.

This article was published in *Essentials of Nuclear Medicine Imaging*, Fred A. Mettler, Jr, and Milton J. Guiberteau, Copyright Saunders 2005.

Myocardial perfusion imaging is utilized in conjunction with cardiac stress tests to assess patients with chest pain of unknown etiology, to assess the functional ramifications of coronary artery stenosis or collateral vessels previously examined through angiography, or to assess the efficacy of perfusion interventions, such as percutaneous intervention, thrombolysis, and coronary artery bypass grafting (CABG).[49] Following acute myocardial infarction, myocardial perfusion imaging may identify perfusion abnormalities, extent of scarring due to former infarcts and residual peri-infarct, or additional areas of reversible ischemia.[49] *Radionuclide ventriculography* is utilized to assess ventricular functionality.[50] It is most applicable for the measurement of exercise and resting ejection fraction in valvular cardiac disease, coronary artery disease, and congenital cardiac disease.[50] Some physicians prefer this test for repeated evaluations of ventricular functionality in patients who have been prescribed cardiotoxic cancer chemotherapy. The multiple-gated acquisition (MUGA) aspect of this technology, which helps provide better imaging, is still useful, despite the fact that radionuclide ventriculography has largely been replaced by echocardiography.[51]

Diagnostic Arteriography

Arteriography is an invasive exam that seeks to create an arteriogram, which is essentially a map of arteries that need to be examined.[52] The procedure is similar to an x-ray and is utilized both for diagnosis and to plot a course for treatment.[52] Arteriography may be used to diagnose blockages, stenosis, and vessel degradation ailments, or it may help determine whether additional procedures, such as angioplasty, surgery, or stent placement, are necessary.[53] Diagnostic arteriograms are the most commonly conducted vascular procedures for gastrointestinal disorders.[52] Using angioplasty and thrombolysis, interventional radiologists can sometimes treat blocked, narrowed, or damaged arteries on the same day that arteriography is performed (see below).[53]

After injecting the patient with a contrast agent, the radiologist inserts a catheter into the femoral artery, most often from the groin area. Using medical imaging for guidance, the radiologist then threads the catheter to the desired part of the body, such as the heart or the lungs.[52,53] X-ray images are taken for further study of the arteries in question; the contrast agent increases the density of the vessels being studied so that they are more visible on radiographs. The procedure is performed under local anesthesia and IV sedation. In addition to its diagnostic uses, the catheter can also directly deliver medications, such as blood clot dissolvers, or other treatment, such as radioactive seeds to kill cancerous cells.[52] The catheter may also be used to inject medicines directly into a diseased organ through one of its main arteries.[52] Diagnostic arteriography may also

be used for stent placement, to guide angioplasty, and to determine whether to conduct a surgical procedure, such as a heart bypass, and the best approach for doing so.[43] Some other uses of arteriography fall into the category of endovascular treatments. Revascularization and embolization to treat of blood vessel pathologies, such as malformations, aneurysms, fistulae, and stenoses, may be done using smaller catheters or microcatheters and other instruments suitable for the particular situation.[52]

The same type of catheter used for diagnostic angiography can be utilized for deliberate vessel occlusion or *embolization*.[52] This might be done to stem, prevent, or help reduce bleeding anticipated after or during a surgical procedure or following some form of trauma.[53] Bronchial embolization is now one of the primary therapies for patients with significant hemoptysis secondary to bronchiectasis, lung cancer, or cavitary lung disease. With *scintigraphy*, a radiographic tracer with a short half-life is deposited into the bloodstream to check for circulatory problems.[52,53] This procedure is used primarily to diagnose diseases that disrupt the blood–brain barrier, such as abscesses, tumors, and hemorrhages. Scintigraphy is useful when trying to differentiate between different aberrations with similar pathophysiologic signs and clinical symptoms.[52]

Pulmonary angiography is an imaging procedure that utilizes a contrast agent and x-rays to determine how well blood is flowing through vessels in the lungs.[52] After numbing the area with a local anesthetic, a radiologist inserts a catheter into a vein, usually in the arm or the groin. The catheter is guided into the right side of the heart and into the pulmonary artery.[52] The physician then injects a contrast agent, which enhances the appearance of the vessels being studied.[52] In addition to showing blood flow through the lungs, this procedure may also help spot damaged, clogged, or diseased vascular tissue.[53] Pulmonary angiography may also be used to deliver anticoagulant medications if a pulmonary embolus is seen or suspected.[53] Pulmonary angiography may also be ordered to diagnose pulmonary hypertension, pulmonary artery aneurysms, congenital pulmonary vascular stenosis, and arteriovenous malformation of the lungs.[53] The test may discover a variety of abnormal findings, including lung tumors, primary pulmonary hypertension, aneurysm of pulmonary vessels, pulmonary embolism, and pulmonary vascular stenosis.[53]

Interventional Radiology

Historically, radiology has been primarily concerned with the diagnosis of disease. Modern technology and training, however, have allowed for the development of the field of interventional radiology. Simply put, interventional radiology is the use of medical imaging techniques and procedures for treatment.[52] Modern imaging techniques allow for minimally invasive procedures that are often less risky, less expensive, less painful, less time-consuming, and more convenient than the methods they are replacing, such as exploratory surgery.[52]

Interventional radiologists use imaging devices to guide small tools such as needles, catheters, probes, and ablation-purposed radioactive substances through veins, arteries, organs, and other structures to conduct therapeutic procedures.[52] Disease states or conditions sometimes treated using *vascular-interventional radiology* procedures include pulmonary embolus, carotid artery disease, peripheral arterial disease, gastrointestinal bleeding, and lung tumors.[3,53] Vascular-interventional radiology procedures include balloon angioplasty and stent placement to hold open occluded vessels, catheter-directed thrombolysis (e.g., blood clot dissolution), radiofrequency ablation (e.g., tumors, cardiac arrhythmias, pain management), and embolization to selectively occlude vessels to treat bleeding (e.g., hemoptysis) or certain tumors by blocking blood flow.[3,53] Interventional radiologists also provide specific cancer treatments, including transarterial chemoembolization, with or without drug-eluting beads, and transarterial radioembolization.

Cardiac-interventional radiology procedures include cardiac catheterization, cardiac angiography, cardiac angioplasty, and catheter-directed thrombolysis. Cardiac catheterization is used to assess the condition of the coronary arteries and determine how well the heart is working, primarily by examining the pressures in the heart's chambers.[52,53] To accomplish this, a catheter is threaded through an artery in the arm, groin, or other part of the body; the catheter is then advanced slowly and methodically into the aorta and heart using medical imaging to guide the procedure.[52] Patients receive local anesthesia and usually remain awake during the procedure, which is often performed on an outpatient basis. During cardiac catheterization, a dye contrast agent may be injected into the coronary arteries to check for blockages caused by calcification or plaque, fatty tissue, or blood clots.[53] With coronary artery disease (CAD), plaque may narrow the coronary arteries, leading to partial or complete occlusion. This may cause myocardial ischemia and the development of irritable ectopic foci and arrhythmia.[53] Blood clots may also form on the surface of ruptured plaque leading to complete occlusion and MI. Indications for coronary angiography include new onset angina, unstable angina, a history of previous or recent MI, possible aortic stenosis, atypical chest pain, or abnormal cardiac stress test.[52] **Figure 11-23** provides an example of the images seen using cardiac angiography.

Percutaneous transluminal coronary angioplasty (PTCA) is a procedure used to dilate narrow or blocked coronary arteries and restore blood flow to the heart using a catheter with an inflatable balloon at the tip.[52] By restoring blood flow, the procedure relieves myocardial ischemia and may prevent infarction, or the worsening of infarction. PTCA is normally completed immediately following coronary angiography to identify blocked vessels. The catheter is guided to the blocked coronary artery, where it is positioned and the balloon inflated using a standardized protocol.[52] Inflation of the balloon compresses the plaque and opens the artery. Fluoroscopy is used to guide catheter placement, and a newer technique, intravascular ultrasound (IVUS), may also be used to provide images of the coronary vessels.[52]

In some cases, it may necessary perform an atherectomy to remove plaque using tiny blades or a rotating tip at the end of the catheter. As an alternative, laser atherectomy may be performed to vaporize the plaque. Once the vessel is open, a small, expandable metal coil, or *stent*, may be inserted to ensure the vessel stays open. Over time, scar tissue may form inside the stent and obstruct blood flow.[53] Drug-eluting stents (DES) are coated with medication to prevent formation of scar tissue inside the stent.

As discussed in Chapter 10, there are two broad categories of acute MI, based on ECG findings: ST segment elevation MI (STEMI) and non-ST segment elevation MI (NSTEMI). The preferred treatment of STEMI is the PTCA (aka percutaneous coronary intervention, or PCI). If available, PTCA should be performed within a specific time frame (e.g., ≤ 90 minutes from first medical contact and transport to a PTCA lab [door to balloon time]; ≤ 120 minutes if transfer to a PCI-capable hospital is required). If PTCA is not possible within the suggested time frame, administration of thrombolytic agents should be considered. Initial treatment of NSTEMI should include providing relief of ischemic pain, oxygen therapy, hemodynamic support, antiplatelet and anticoagulant therapy (but not thrombolytics), and β-blocker therapy. With NSTEMI, the approach will depend on the patient's condition and estimation of risk. Options include cardiac catheterization, coronary artery bypass graft (CABG), or a conservative medical strategy.

Catheter-Directed Thrombolysis

One of several powerful, minimally invasive treatments in the arsenal of interventional radiologists, catheter-directed thrombolysis is used to dissolve clotted blood in narrowed or obstructed blood vessels.[52] When blood does not flow well through the blood vessels, it begins to coagulate into a partially solidified gel called a *thrombus*. As a thrombus increases in size, it may cut off the blood supply to a particular area of the body, which may lead to damage at the cellular level.[52] Thrombi can also dislodge and move through the blood vessels, eventually blocking smaller vessels in a process known as *embolization*. Thrombosis or embolization

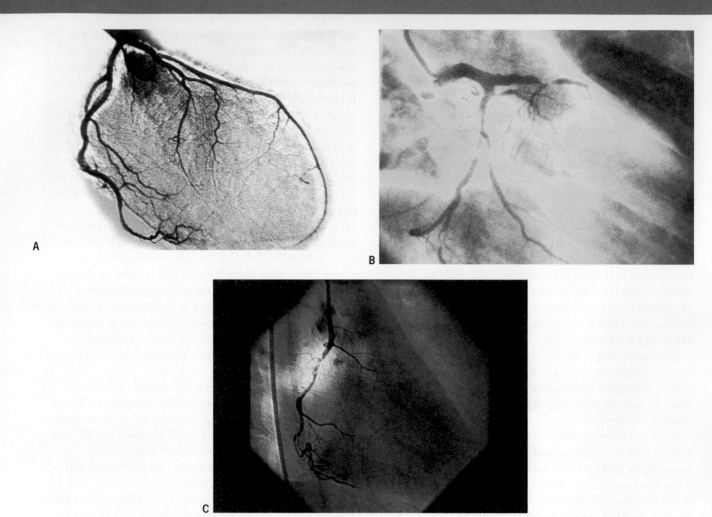

FIGURE 11-23 Coronary angiograms. (A) Normal heart angiogram visualizing the morphology of the right and left coronary arteries. (B) Coronary artery stenosis. Colored angiogram x-ray of the heart of a 60-year-old man showing stenosis (narrowing) in the left anterior descending coronary artery. The coronary arteries (red) run on the surface of the heart, feeding blood to the heart muscle. Here, a pinched section of the coronary artery (top center in artery arc) is due to an obstruction of blood flow. This is caused by atherosclerosis, in which the artery has become narrowed due to deposits of fatty plaque on the artery walls. Chest pain may occur, while complete artery blockage may cause a heart attack. An x-ray opaque dye was injected into the coronary arteries to obtain this image. (C) Coronary artery disease. A false-color coronary artery angiogram showing stenosis of the right coronary artery, an obstruction of blood flow in one of the arteries that supply the heart. In digital angiography, the arterial supply to the heart is outlined by means of a radio-opaque contrast medium injected via a catheter, and visualized using digital x-ray equipment. Here, the heart is roughly outlined in red; the right coronary artery appears as a black ribbon, and the obstruction appears as a pinched, narrowed section (yellow highlight). This lesion is complicated by the presence of a smaller artery (running to the left) and (just below) a "bubble" (possibly a clot).

can lead to tissue and organ damage and, in the worst case, death.[52] Using catheter-directed thrombolysis, interventional radiologists can help unblock obstructed vessels and prevent further damage.[52]

Catheter-directed thrombolysis is used to treat arm or leg arterial thrombosis, deep vein thrombosis (DVT), compromised circulation (e.g., lower leg ischemia), thrombosis of dialysis fistulas or grafts, and occasionally for thrombosis of the portal vein or other mesenteric veins and pulmonary embolus.[53] As with other modalities that may employ contrast media, it is

important to screen patients for potential allergies (e.g., iodine). In some cases, thrombolysis is not technically feasible. Moreover, clot removal cannot address tissue damage that has already occurred. Such damage may or may not heal on its own after the procedure. Finally, the underlying condition that led to the formation of blood clots may continue to cause problems unless it is resolved.[53] A newer technique for breaking up clots is ultrasound-accelerated, catheter-directed thrombolysis, which may be useful in the treatment of massive pulmonary embolus.

Percutaneous Abscess Drainage

Abscesses are pockets of infected fluid that collect in certain parts of the body.[53] They are generally accompanied by pain, chills, and fever; these symptoms may also be related to the underlying condition that brought about the abscesses.[52] Medical imaging is often used to diagnose the existence and determine the cause of these abnormalities. Percutaneous abscess drainage (PAD) is one tool that interventional radiologists may use to remove infected fluid, most commonly from the abdomen or pelvis, though the procedure may be useful to drain lung abscesses or mediastinal abscesses. In this procedure, the interventional radiologist uses medical-imaging guidance to introduce a very small needle that can drain the infected fluid from the area in question.[53] In some cases, the procedure involves leaving a drainage tube in place for a while. Surgery is often necessary when percutaneous abscess drainage is not possible.

Radiation Exposure Considerations

Interventional radiology procedures may expose patients to more radiation than simple medical-imaging procedures.[20] Exposure risk must be weighed against the potential benefits of treatment and does not necessarily disqualify patients from interventional radiology procedures.[20]

Ultrasound

How It Works

Ultrasound medical imaging transmits high-frequency, inaudible sound waves through the body and then measures the echo, or reflection, of those waves after they encounter organs, vessels, bones, and other structures, allowing for image generation.[54] The sound waves are sent and received by a transducer.[54] The received signals are digitally analyzed and stored in a computer, which then creates an image of the area in question.[54]

Ultrasound does not use ionizing radiation, has a low risk profile, and is a good tool for fetal imaging.[54] Ultrasound imaging is also a good alternative for patients who have previously acquired significant radiation exposure and for those who may not be able to tolerate or who are poor candidates for nuclear medicine or CT procedures. Ultrasound imaging is also a good choice for patients with metal implants in the body.[54]

The quality of information generated by ultrasound is determined by the ultrasound frequency, amplitude, and time parameters involved in the exam.[54] Other key factors that affect image quality include the skill of the ultrasound technologist (sonographer) and the body tissue examined.[54] For example, it may be difficult to acquire diagnostic quality ultrasound images when examining a very obese patient or when scanning a nonfasting patient with excessive bowel gas.

Ultrasound is often used as a guide to specific procedures, such as arterial or central line placement or chest tube placement. Another example would be a percutaneous abscess drainage guided by ultrasound. Assessment and drainage of pleural fluid and evaluation and treatment of pneumothorax may also be guided by ultrasound imaging.[54]

Real-time imaging using ultrasound allows clinicians to assess functional processes as they occur, such as blood flow (e.g., Doppler ultrasound) or cardiac wall motion (e.g., echocardiogram).[54] Vascular ultrasound techniques are used to assess arteries, veins, and capillaries. In addition, ultrasound can help determine patient candidacy for certain procedures, such as angioplasty, and can be used to evaluate the efficacy of past vascular bypass or grafting procedures.[54] Other uses of ultrasound imaging include evaluation of patients for gallstone disease, kidney size, presence of peritoneal fluid, or enlarged lymph nodes in the neck.[54] **Figure 11-24** provides examples of the images seen using vascular ultrasound techniques.

Doppler Ultrasound

Doppler ultrasound is a special type of ultrasound that can help identify problems such as vascular stenosis, blood clots, congenital vascular aberrations, and tumors by measuring the speed and direction of blood cells in veins and arteries.[54] Doppler ultrasound may also be used in the evaluation of patients with arterial atherosclerotic disease or suspected DVT. The motion of blood cells creates a detectable alteration in the pitch of the sounds being reflected, which is known as the *Doppler effect*. The process is captured by computer and represented using graphs and/or colored images.[54]

Echocardiograms

An echocardiogram is completed in a similar fashion to other ultrasound tests, but is restricted to the heart and the immediate area surrounding it.[54] The transducer transmits sound waves to the chest which, when echoed back, are converted to electrical impulses. These impulses are used by the computer to create real-time still or video images of the heart that can be stored, retrieved, and studied. Heart size (atria, ventricles), the heart valves, the pericardium (e.g., effusion, tamponade), and the intracardiac shunts all can be assessed using the echocardiogram.[3] Heart wall motion can be evaluated, which is especially useful in assessment of the myocardium following MI. **Box 11-9** lists indications for the echocardiogram. **Box 11-10** provides examples of specialized echocardiograms.[54] **Figure 11-25** provides an example of the images seen using echocardiography.

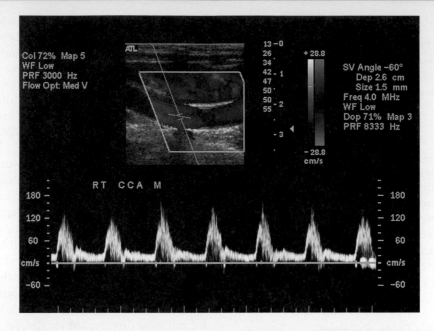

FIGURE 11-24 A composite from a noninvasive duplex ultrasound exam of the carotid arteries in the neck. Data of the blood flow velocities in addition to a color-enhanced 2-D ultrasound image of the blood vessel.

© Living Art Enterprises, LLC/Science Source.

BOX 11-9

Indications for Echocardiogram

Indications for an echocardiogram include:

- Evaluating heart valve malfunctions
- Determining the etiology of a heart murmur
- Assessing heart structure changes
- Determining damage to the heart after a myocardial infarction
- Studying heart functionality in patients with chronic heart disease
- Locating edema in or near the heart
- Confirming masses in or near the heart
- Diagnosing congenital defects
- Examining blood flow efficacy
- Determining the extent of vascular damage after trauma
- Assessing cardiovascular capacity and status in critically ill patients
- Assisting in the diagnosis of angina
- Diagnosing thrombus in heart chambers

Data from: American Institute of Ultrasound in Medicine. AIUM practice guideline for the performance of fetal echocardiography. *J Ultrasound Med.* 2011;30(1):127–136. Fetal Echocardiography Task Force; American Institute of Ultrasound in Medicine Clinical Standards Committee; American College of Obstetricians and Gynecologists; Society for Maternal-Fetal Medicine.

BOX 11-10

Types of Specialized Echocardiograms

Specialized types of echocardiograms include:

- *Stress echocardiogram*: Logs heart activity during cardiac stress-testing exams.
- *Contrast echocardiogram*: Employs contrast agents to help enhance captured heart images.
- *Echocardiogram with Doppler ultrasound*: Helps diagnose blood flow conditions.
- *Transesophageal echocardiogram*: Visualizes the heart from a closer distance by positioning a small transducer into the esophagus; useful for obese patients and in patients with pulmonary disease.

Data from: American Institute of Ultrasound in Medicine. AIUM practice guideline for the performance of fetal echocardiography. *J Ultrasound Med.* 2011;30(1):127–136. Fetal Echocardiography Task Force; American Institute of Ultrasound in Medicine Clinical Standards Committee; American College of Obstetricians and Gynecologists; Society for Maternal-Fetal Medicine.

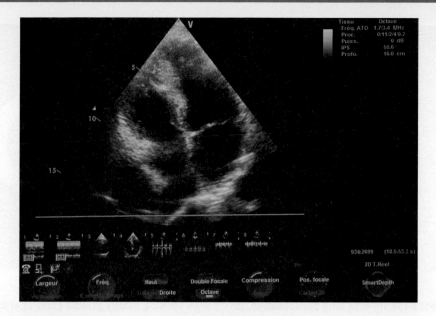

FIGURE 11-25 Echocardiography display screen. Middle-aged patient undergoing a heart ultrasound scan. A transducer (held against his chest) emits ultrasonic waves and detects the reflected echoes. The change in frequency is used to build images of the heart structures and to assess the velocity and direction of blood flow.

© AJ Photo/Custom Medical Stock Photo, Inc.

Cardiopulmonary Disease

The respiratory care clinician will often rely on the radiologist or other imaging specialist to provide assessment and interpretation of thoracic, pulmonary, cardiac, and cardiovascular imaging studies. However, the respiratory care clinician should understand the imaging findings associated with specific cardiopulmonary diseases. These include atelectasis, pneumonia, ARDS, pleural effusion, asthma, chronic obstructive pulmonary disease (COPD), interstitial lung disease, pulmonary vascular disease, pneumothorax, and neoplastic disorders of the lung. In addition, the respiratory care clinician must be able to recognize placement of chest tubes and lines as well as endotracheal tubes.

Alveolar Lung Disease

The term *alveolar lung disease* is sometimes used to describe disease characterized by exudates and **edema** in the pulmonary airspaces, more specifically, the alveoli and acini.[18,19] It may be classified as either chronic or acute. If the alveoli and small airways fill with dense material, the lung is said to be **consolidated**. It is important to be aware that consolidation does not always mean there is infection, and the small airways may fill with material other than pus (as in pneumonia), such as fluid (pulmonary edema), blood (pulmonary hemorrhage), or cancer cells. An air bronchogram is seen when an air-filled small airway is surrounded by consolidated lung tissue.[18] **Figure 11-26** provides

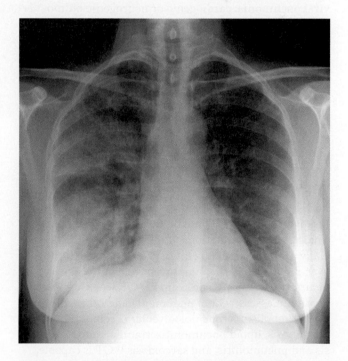

FIGURE 11-26 Pneumonia. This is an x-ray of the chest of a 49-year-old female patient with pneumonia affecting the right lung (viewer's left).

© Du Cane Medical Imaging Ltd./Science Source.

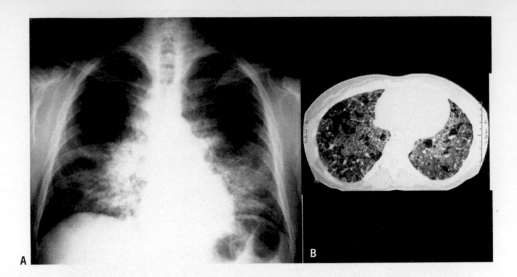

FIGURE 11-27 (A) Chest x-ray showing lung consolidation. (B) CT scan showing mostly ground glass opacity.

(A) Courtesy of Laura Vasquez; (B) Courtesy of Laura Vasquez.

an example of an x-ray of the chest of a 49-year-old female patient with pneumonia affecting the right lung. **Figure 11-27** provides an example of areas of consolidation as seen on chest radiograph and CT scan.

Etiology

Acute airspace disease is brought about by bacterial or viral pneumonia, cardiogenic or neurogenic pulmonary edema, systemic lupus erythematosus, pulmonary embolism, pulmonary hemorrhage (as in Goodpasture syndrome), granulomatosis with polyangiitis (GPA), or idiopathic pulmonary hemosiderosis.[19] Chronic airspace disease may be brought about by alveolar cell carcinoma, pulmonary alveolar proteinosis, the alveolar form of sarcoidosis, mineral oil pneumonia, tuberculosis, lymphoma, desquamative interstitial pneumonia, and metastases.[19]

Important Radiologic Concepts

Portable chest x-rays are often obtained in the ICU; however, clinicians should be cautious regarding the findings due to limitations of the procedure. CT is especially useful in assessing interstitial lung disease; however, it can also play an important role in the assessment of airspace disease.[55] For example, CT scans are often helpful in assessment of pneumonia and other infections, embolism, bronchioloalveolar carcinoma, alveolar proteinosis, lipoid pneumonitis, trauma, radiation fibrosis and pneumonitis, and sarcoidosis.[19] CT is capable, for example, of discovering early, opportunistic pneumonia before it is observable on simple radiographs.[56] Location and disease severity are also better delineated by CT, as are concomitant aberrations such as lymphadenopathy, abscesses, and pleural effusion.[19] Specific alveolar airspace diseases will be discussed next.

Pneumonia

Pneumonia is an infection of the lung parenchyma, usually caused by bacterial or viral infection. It can run the gamut from mild cases that are usually treatable at home and are sometimes termed *walking pneumonia* to very severe, potentially fatal cases.[19,56] Community-acquired pneumonia (CAP) is acquired at home, work, or school; nosocomial pneumonia may occur after 48 to 72 hours of hospitalization (hospital-acquired pneumonia [HAP]).[56] Ventilator-associated pneumonia (VAP) occurs following intubation and institution of mechanical ventilatory support, whereas healthcare-associated pneumonia (HCAP) refers to a pneumonia acquired in other healthcare facilities, such as nursing homes, long-term care units, or clinics (e.g., hemodialysis or intravenous infusion centers).[55,56] Common bacterial causes of pneumonia include *Streptococcus pneumoniae*, *Haemophilus influenzae*, *Legionella* sp., *Staphylococcus aureus*, and, occasionally, gram-negative bacilli.[57] Viral pneumonia may be caused by influenza, parainfluenza, RSV, adenovirus, and human metapneumovirus. Atypical pneumonias include those caused by *Mycoplasma pneumoniae*, *Chlamydia psittaci*, and *Coxiella burnetii*.[57,58]

Diagnosis of Pneumonia

Diagnosis of pneumonia is based on clinical signs and symptoms, imaging studies, and laboratory data. Productive cough, shortness of breath, chest pain, fever, chills, and malaise are common symptoms. Many, but not all, patients with CAP have fever, though elderly patients often do not develop fever.[58] Physical examination often reveals crackles (historically referred to as *rales*) upon auscultation, and signs of consolidation may be noted (e.g., E-a egophony, tactile vocal fremitus;

see Chapter 5). Mucopurulent sputum production is common with bacterial pneumonia, whereas patients with atypical pneumonias may have watery sputum.[58] Sputum characteristics, however, are of limited value in directing clinical decision making.[58]

Initial diagnostic tests for CAP should include a chest x-ray and complete blood count (CBC). A single conventional chest x-ray may be sufficient to diagnose pneumonia; the presence of an infiltrate and corresponding clinical and microbiologic features provide diagnostic confirmation.[58] The role of sputum and blood cultures remains controversial, though cultures are suggested for certain patients (see below). Bronchoscopy, bronchoalveolar lavage, and/or thoracentesis may be useful in assessment of patients with pneumonia (see Chapter 13). The diagnosis of HAP, VAP, and HCAP are based on the findings of a new or progressive infiltrate on chest x-ray, worsening hypoxemia, fever, and/or elevated white blood cell count.[59] Recently, procalcitonin (a peptide precursor of calcitonin) has been shown to rise with bacterial infection but decline with viral disease. It has become an evolving test in supporting the diagnosis of pneumonia and reducing the duration of antibiotic therapy. **Figures 11-27** and **11-28** provide examples of imaging studies showing lung consolidation associated with pneumonia.

Ideally, laboratory identification of specific pathogens will direct antibiotic therapy, though microbiology testing is considered optional in outpatients. Sputum Gram stains and cultures are indicated in patients who fail outpatient antibiotic therapy and for those with pleural effusion, cavitary infiltrates, severe COPD or other chronic respiratory disease, and current alcohol abusers. Urinary antigen tests (UATs) are available for *Legionella* and *Streptococcus pneumoniae*, and patients with a positive UAT should have a sputum culture performed.[58] ICU patients should have both sputum and blood cultures performed, and intubated patients should have their tracheal aspirate tested.[58]

Blood cultures should also be obtained for patients with pleural effusion, cavitary infiltrates, active alcohol abuse, chronic severe liver disease, leukopenia, absence of normal spleen function (asplenia), or a positive pneumococcal UAT.[58]

Treatment

Initial treatment for CAP is usually empiric based on severity of illness, comorbid factors, and the likelihood of infection with a drug-resistant pathogen.[60] For uncomplicated CAP managed outside the hospital, a macrolide antibiotic (e.g., azithromycin, clarithromycin, or clarithromycin XL) or doxycycline (a tetracycline antibiotic) may be prescribed.[1,60] A typical treatment course of antibiotic therapy is 7 to 10 days.[1] COPD patients and those with other comorbid conditions (e.g., renal disease, cancer, diabetes, and heart disease) may receive a respiratory fluoroquinolone (e.g., gemifloxacin

or levofloxacin) or combination therapy (e.g., amoxicillin or amoxicillin plus cefuroxime and azithromycin or clarithromycin).[60]

For hospitalized patients with CAP, combination therapy with a β-lactam antibiotic (e.g., ceftriaxone, cefotaxime, ceftaroline, ertapenem, or ampicillin-sulbactam) and a macrolide antibiotic (e.g., azithromycin or clarithromycin XL) have been suggested.[60] ICU patients may require a β-lactam antibiotic (e.g., ceftriaxone, cefotaxime, or ampicillin-sulbactam), often in combination with a macrolide or quinolone (e.g., azithromycin, levofloxacin, or moxifloxacin).[60] Vancomycin may be added if methicillin-resistant *Staphylococcus aureas* (MRSA) is suspected.[60]

Vaccines may help prevent the development of certain types of pneumonia. These may be especially important to older patients and persons with asthma, emphysema, COPD, diabetes, cancer, HIV/AIDS, and other chronic ailments. **Box 11-11** lists the key points about pneumonia.[60]

Nosocomial Pneumonia

Nosocomial pneumonia is the most common cause of infection in the ICU and the second most common cause of infection in hospitalized patients.[1] Critically ill patients, ventilator patients, and those with compromised immune systems are especially vulnerable for development of nosocomial pneumonia. Nosocomial pneumonia is caused by the introduction of contaminated material into the lower respiratory tract. The most common source of infection is aspiration of contaminated secretions from the oropharynx or GI tract.

Aspiration occurs when foreign material such as food, liquid, gastric contents, or oral secretions are introduced into the lung. About 45% of all normal people routinely aspirate small amounts of oropharyngeal secretions during sleep (microaspiration).[59] Critically ill patients with depressed levels of consciousness or altered respiratory tract anatomy are at special risk for aspiration. Alcohol or drug intoxication, neurologic illness, seizures, head trauma, administration of sedative or narcotic medications, and the presence of nasogastric tubes, endotracheal tubes, and tracheostomy tubes predispose patients to aspiration. Individuals with conditions that interfere with proper swallowing, such as stroke, Parkinson disease, and amyotrophic lateral sclerosis (ALS) are also at risk for development of aspiration pneumonia.

Colonization of the oropharynx and gastric contents with gram-negative bacteria may be facilitated by the administration of medications to reduce gastric acidity in acutely ill patients. Aspiration of these contaminated oral or gastric secretions may then cause nosocomial pneumonia. Ventilator patients may also be infected due to contact with environmental reservoirs such as humidifiers, nebulizers, or ventilator circuits. Common gram-positive microorganisms associated with

BOX 11-11

Key Points about Pneumonia

Definition: Inflammation of the lung parenchyma usually caused by bacterial or viral infection, although other pathogenic organisms (e.g., fungi, amoebae, parasites) may cause pneumonia.

- Pneumonia may be community-acquired (CAP) or nosocomial.
- Nosocomial infections include hospital-acquired pneumonia (HAP), ventilator-associated pneumonia (VAP), or healthcare-associated pneumonia (HCAP).
- Pneumonia may be characterized by cause (e.g., bacterial, viral) and/or anatomic site of infection (e.g., lobar, interstitial, diffuse). For example, lobar pneumonia affects an entire lobe, whereas bronchopneumonia may involve several lobes and atypical pneumonia may be diffuse.

Causes may be bacterial, viral, fungal or due to other pathogens.

- Bacterial causes include gram-positive bacteria (e.g. *Streptococcus pneumoniae, Staphylococcus aureus*) and gram-negative bacteria (e.g., *Haemophilus influenzae, Legionella pneumophila, Pseudomonas aeruginosa, Klebsiella pneumoniae*).
- *Mycobacterium tuberculosis* is an acid-fast rod that causes tuberculosis (TB).
- Viral causes include influenza virus and hantavirus.
- Causes of atypical pneumonia include *Mycoplasma pneumoniae, Chlamydia psittaci*, and *Coxiella burnetii*.
- Fungal lung infections include *Pneumocystis jiroveci* (aka *Pneumocystis carinii* [PCP]). Coccidiodomycosis, histoplasmosis, and blastomycosis are forms of fungal lung disease.

Diagnosis of pneumonia is typically based on the clinical picture, complete blood count (CBC), and chest x-ray.

- Clinical findings include productive cough, shortness of breath, chest pain, fever, chills, and malaise.
  - Many, but not all, patients have fever.
  - Tachypnea, tachycardia, and other signs of respiratory failure may be present.
  - Crackles upon auscultation and signs of consolidation (dullness to percussion, increased fremitus, bronchial breath sounds).
- CBC will often (but not always) show increased WBC; a left shift with immature cells may be present.
- A lung infiltrate on imaging is the gold standard for diagnosis of pneumonia.
  - The chest x-ray will show parenchymal opacity, which may be diffuse or focal.
  - Alveolar consolidation is a hallmark although other causes must be ruled out.
  - Air bronchograms indicate opacities are parenchymal.
  - CAP may show lobar consolidation, interstitial infiltrates, and/or cavitation.
- The diagnosis of HAP, VAP, and HCAP are based on the findings of a new or progressive infiltrate on chest x-ray, worsening hypoxemia, fever, and/or elevated WBC.
- Sputum may be obtained for Gram stain, culture, and sensitivity to guide patient management.
- Blood cultures should be done in patients with pleural effusion, cavitary infiltrates, active alcohol abuse, chronic severe liver disease, leukopenia, absence of normal spleen function (e.g., asplenia), or a positive pneumococcal UAT.
- Serum procalcitonin (PCT) may be helpful to evaluate bacterial infection severity and response to treatment.
- Urinary antigen tests (UATs) are available for *Legionella* and *Staphylococcus pneumoniae*.

Treatment is based on the causative agent, although empirical antibiotic treatment without laboratory examination of sputum has been suggested for uncomplicated CAP. Some suggest pretreatment examination of sputum when possible to help guide therapy, especially in hospitalized patients.

nosocomial pneumonia include *S. pneumoniae* and *S. aureus*. Common gram-negative pathogens include *H. influenzae, Escherichia coli, Klebsiella pneumoniae, Pseudomonas aeruginosa,* and *Acinetobacter baumannii*.[1,59] Nosocomial pneumonias caused by antibiotic-resistant pathogens, such as MRSA or drug-resistant *Streptococcus pneumoniae* (DRSP), can be especially problematic. Fungal, viral, and parasitic pneumonias often affect people with compromised immune systems. Pathogens that may be harmless to most people may cause pneumonia in patients who have had an organ transplant or have AIDS. Some pharmaceuticals, such as chemotherapeutic agents and corticosteroids, can also suppress the immune system, increasing an individual's vulnerability.

Empiric antimicrobial therapy should be started in patients with suspected nosocomial pneumonia who have a new or progressive infiltrate on chest x-ray and at least two of the following: fever (> 38° C), abnormal white blood cell count (e.g., leukocytosis or leukopenia) and purulent secretions.[59] Antibiotic therapy may include combined therapy with a β-lactam antipseudomonal penicillin or cephalosporin in combination with an aminoglycoside or quinolone. Cultures of endotracheal tube or bronchoscopic secretion samples may be helpful in identifying the causative organism.

Radiologic Considerations with Pneumonia

A lung infiltrate on imaging is the gold standard for diagnosis of pneumonia. The chest x-ray will show parenchymal opacity, which may be diffuse or focal. Diffuse opacities may be found across the lung, whereas focal opacities are limited to a specific area of the lung. Infectious, especially bacterial, pneumonias are the most common cause of focal opacities, whereas fungal, mycobacterial, and viral pneumonias may be focal or diffuse. Alveolar consolidation is a hallmark of pneumonia, although other causes must be ruled out. Other causes of an abnormal chest x-ray that should be considered include pneumonitis, cancer, bleeding, pulmonary edema, and pulmonary embolism.[58]

The presence of an air bronchogram indicates that an opacity is parenchymal in nature and is classically seen with *pneumococcal* or *Klebsiella* pneumonia (see Figure 11-26). CAP may show lobar consolidation, interstitial infiltrates, and/or cavitation.[58] **Figure 11-28** shows a patient with a lobar consolidation due to right middle-lobe pneumonia. The diagnosis of HAP, VAP,

and HCAP are based on the findings of a new or progressive infiltrate on chest x-ray, worsening hypoxemia, fever, and/or elevated white blood cell count.[59]

The anatomic location of a lung infiltrate following aspiration is related to where the aspirate deposited. Aspiration tends to affect the dependent portions of the lung, and this is determined by the patient's position at the time of aspiration. For example, aspiration will tend to affect the right lower lobe (superior segment) or right upper lobe (posterior segment) in patients who are supine.[59]

Following diagnosis and initiation of treatment, repeated chest x-rays are not generally needed for patients responding to therapy.[60] A follow-up chest x-ray in older patients after 7 to 12 weeks to document resolution of the pneumonia has been suggested.[60]

In some hospitalized patients with suspected pneumonia, a false-negative chest x-ray may be obtained. In these cases, empiric antibiotic therapy may be started and the chest x-ray repeated in 24 to 48 hours.[58] The HRCT scan is more sensitive and has higher resolution than the chest x-ray; CT may be useful in patients with suspected pneumonia with a negative chest film.[58] CT scans may detect specific lesions or define anatomic changes.[58] It should be noted that following treatment, symptoms often improve before the chest x-ray clears.[60]

Pulmonary Edema

Pulmonary edema is an abnormal accumulation of fluid in the alveolar and interstitial spaces. Pulmonary edema may be caused by (1) high pressures in the pulmonary capillaries (pulmonary capillary wedge pressure > 18 mm Hg) causing a fluid leak, as seen with left-sided congestive heart failure, or (2) increased permeability of the pulmonary capillaries due to disease (e.g., leaky capillaries) with low or normal pulmonary

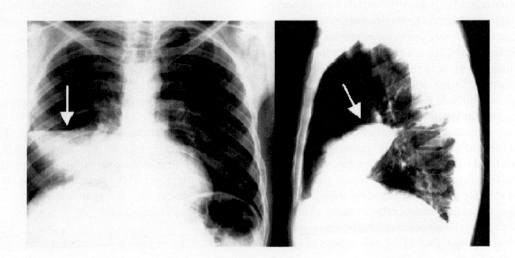

FIGURE 11-28 PA and lateral chest x-ray showing lobar consolidation and a right middle-lobe pneumonia.

Courtesy of Laura Vasquez.

capillary pressures (pulmonary capillary wedge pressure ≤ 18 mm Hg). ARDS provides the best example of low-pressure pulmonary edema. Often it is difficult to distinguish between high-pressure and low-pressure pulmonary edema, and some conditions appear as mixed states.

Cardiogenic pulmonary edema is the most common type of high-pressure pulmonary edema. Cardiogenic pulmonary edema is usually caused by congestive heart failure (CHF) in which the left heart fails (left-sided CHF) and fluid backs up into the lungs. The resultant high pulmonary vascular pressures cause a fluid leak, first into the interstitial space and then into the alveoli.[19] Causes of left-sided CHF include coronary heart disease (atherosclerotic heart disease), chronic hypertension, cardiac ischemia or infarction, valvular heart disease (e.g., aortic or mitral valve regurgitation), certain toxins and medications, and myocarditis.[61] Cigarette smoking, hypertension, obesity, and diabetes predispose patients to the development of CHF. Factors that may lead specifically to the development of cardiogenic pulmonary edema include myocardial ischemia and/or infarction, volume overload, valvular heart disease, and renal disease.[61]

Noncardiogenic pulmonary edema is generally due to damaged or leaky pulmonary capillaries, though elevated pulmonary capillary pressures may be present in some forms of noncardiac pulmonary edema. The most common causes of noncardiogenic pulmonary edema include shock, sepsis, severe trauma, and overwhelming pneumonia. Other potential causes of noncardiogenic pulmonary edema include head trauma or cerebral hemorrhage (e.g., neurogenic pulmonary edema), altitude (e.g., high-altitude pulmonary edema [HAPE]), opiate overdose (e.g., methadone or heroin), salicylate toxicity, viral infection, and multiple or massive pulmonary emboli.[19] Re-expansion pulmonary edema may occur following rapid expansion of a collapsed lung (e.g., following pneumothorax). Another potential cause of noncardiogenic edema is obstruction of the upper airways, known as negative-pressure pulmonary edema. Pulmonary veno-occlusive disease is a rare disorder involving vascular occlusion with scar tissue that may also cause pulmonary edema.[51] Other, less common causes of pulmonary edema include hantavirus pulmonary syndrome, arteriovenous malformation, and venom injection (e.g., *Atrax robustus*, an Australian spider).[51]

ARDS is a form of noncardiogenic pulmonary edema defined by bilateral infiltrates on chest x-ray, severe hypoxemia, with pulmonary capillary wedge pressures (PCWP) ≤ 18 mm Hg. ARDS is caused by alveolar injury resulting in release of proinflammatory cytokines and damage to the alveolar epithelial and capillary endothelial damage. **Box 11-12** lists causes of acute pulmonary edema.

BOX 11-12

Causes of Acute Pulmonary Edema

Acute pulmonary edema is generally characterized as cardiogenic or noncardiogenic. Cardiogenic pulmonary edema is due to increased pressures in the pulmonary capillaries resulting in a fluid leak into the interstitial and then alveolar spaces. The most common cause is *left ventricular failure* resulting in increased left-side pressures (e.g., elevated left atrial and pulmonary capillary wedge pressures). Noncardiogenic pulmonary edema is generally due to leaky pulmonary capillaries *without* elevated pulmonary capillary wedge pressures as seen with ARDS. Possible causes of acute pulmonary edema are listed below.

Cardiogenic Pulmonary Edema

- Myocardial ischemia (e.g., coronary artery disease)
- Myocardial infarction
- Acute, severe hypertension
- Chronic hypertension resulting in left ventricular hypertrophy
- Mitral or aortic valve disease (e.g., mitral stenosis, aortic stenosis, aortic or mitral regurgitation)
- Arrhythmias
- Volume overload (e.g., blood transfusion, IV fluid adminstration)
- Renal disease (e.g., severe kidney disease, renal artery stenosis resulting in chronic hypertension)

Noncardiogenic Pulmonary Edema

- ARDS
- High altitude pulmonary edema (HAPE)
- Neurogenic pulmonary edema (e.g., head trauma, surgery or hemorrhage)
- Heroin or methadone overdose
- Aspiration
- Pulmonary embolus
- Rapid re-expansion of collapsed lung (e.g., treatment of pneumothorax)
- Transfusion related lung injury
- Viral infection (e.g., hantavirus infection)
- Pulmonary contusions (e.g., chest trauma)
- Upper airway obstruction (e.g., negative pressure pulmonary edema)
- Aspirin toxicity

Pulmonary edema associated with CHF and ARDS is discussed in the following sections.

Congestive Heart Failure

Disease, trauma, or constant high level of work required may damage or weaken the left ventricle, reducing cardiac output and causing fluid to back up in the system, raising left ventricular end-diastolic pressures and left atrial pressures.[19] The increase in left atrial pressure results in increased pulmonary vascular pressures that are transmitted to the pulmonary capillaries.[19] When the pressure increases sufficiently, fluid begins to seep from capillaries into the interstitial and then alveolar space—a condition known as *cardiogenic pulmonary edema*.[19] PCWP is sometimes used as a surrogate for left atrial pressure. As a rough guide, when PCWP exceeds 18 mm Hg, fluid begins to leak into the interstitial space. A PCWP > 20 mm Hg is associated with interstitial edema, whereas a PCWP > 25 mm Hg is associated with alveolar filling. A PCWP > 30 mm Hg is associated with frank pulmonary edema. It should be noted that pulmonary edema may occur at lower pressures if albumin and the resulting colloid oncotic pressures are low. As noted, causes of left-sided CHF include coronary artery disease, volume overload, hypertension, certain toxins (e.g., ethanol, cocaine, methamphetamine), aortic valve disease, and mitral valve disease and viral myocarditis.[19] There are also a number of less common causes of CHF and cardiomyopathy, including idiopathic cardiomyopathy and metabolic/endocrine-related CHF. Right-sided CHF may occur if the right ventricle is overwhelmed by an increased pulmonary artery pressure due to left heart failure, pulmonary hypertension, or chronic pulmonary disease.[19]

Pulmonary edema in patients with CHF may be triggered by events such as a myocardial infarction that results in an arrhythmia or an overload of fluid in the lungs due to renal failure. A myocardial infarction will weaken the heart wall and may involve rupture of the papillary muscles or damage to the ventricular septum.[19] The mechanics of these disruptions can induce volume overload in the cardiovascular system and promote pulmonary edema.[19]

Aggressive intravenous therapy may bring about pulmonary edema even in the absence of heart failure (e.g., iatrogenic fluid overload). When shortness of breath manifests as orthopnea and paroxysmal nocturnal dyspnea, this may be an indication of chronic pulmonary edema associated with CHF. Patients with chronic CHF are prone to fluid overload, often accompanied by pitting skin, peripheral edema, hepatomegaly, and increased jugular venous pressure.[55] Treatment of acute pulmonary edema should be aimed at maintaining oxygenation and hemodynamic stability.

Lymphatic Considerations

The lymph nodes help to maintain a suitable fluid balance within the lungs by getting rid of colloids, solutes, and liquids within interstitial spaces.[55] As long as the pressures and fluid exchanges remain normal, the lymphatic system helps protect the lungs from pulmonary edema.[55] However, a sudden increase in pulmonary arterial capillary pressure can increase fluid filtration into the interstitium to the point where the lymphatic drainage is not be able to keep up with the changes. Obstruction of lymph nodes may also contribute to the development of pulmonary edema.[19]

Renal Disorders and Sodium Retention

Sodium retention brought about by disease, such as left ventricle systolic dysfunction, can play a role in the development of pulmonary edema.[49] Some renal disorders, for example, can induce both volume overload and sodium retention, which may be particularly severe in the case of patients with hemodialysis-dependent renal failure who fail to comply with their dietary restrictions and miss hemodialysis sessions.[49]

Imaging Considerations with Pulmonary Edema

The chest x-ray, which is a primary tool in the diagnosis of pulmonary edema, will show both lungs appearing whiter than usual. The chest x-ray may show the development of pulmonary edema even before clinical signs are present.[62] Severe cases of pulmonary edema will display significant opacification, often resulting in minimum visualization of the lungs' normal fields. Heart size should be assessed on every chest radiograph, and cardiogenic pulmonary edema will often include enlargement of the cardiac silhouette. Pulmonary vascular congestion and redistribution and interstitial and alveolar opacities are common findings. Although interstitial and alveolar opacities are typical, interstitial edema may appear prior to alveolar filling. Interstitial edema may result in blurring of the margins of blood vessels, hazy thickening of the bronchial walls, subpleural edema, and visualization of Kerley A and B lines.[62] Alveolar filling usually results in the development of widespread patchy, bilateral opacities.[62] Accumulation of fluid in the perihilar area may result in a "bat wing" or "butterfly" appearance to the shadow.[62]

In contrast to pneumonia, pulmonary edema tends to develop quickly and clear rapidly. Pleural effusion is also a common finding. **Figure 11-29** provides examples of findings seen with congestive heart failure and pulmonary edema. Note the enlarged heart, as evidenced by a CT ratio > 50% in Figure 11-29A; Figure 11-29B shows septal lines (Kerley B Lines) on chest x-ray.[62]

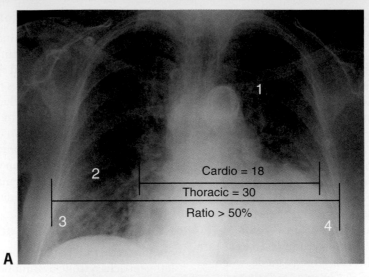

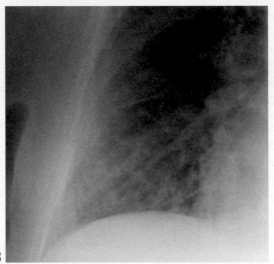

FIGURE 11-29 Cardiogenic pulmonary edema.

© Kallista Images/Custom Medical Stock Photo.

Echocardiography, a cardiac diagnostic ultrasound exam, may be used to confirm the existence of cardiogenic pulmonary edema by displaying evidence of high central vein pressure, left ventricle impairment, and high lung artery pressure; other heart disorders this test may reveal include abnormal motion of a ventricle's walls, valve malfunctions, congenital defects, and pericardial effusion.[54] Echocardiography can also help measure cardiac ejection fraction (EF), which is the quantity of blood ejected by the left ventricle with each heartbeat, as well as whether there is abnormally high pressure in the right atrium or ventricle.[54] A low ejection fraction indicates that a heart abnormality may be responsible for the pulmonary edema; nevertheless, a normal ejection fraction can be obtained despite the presence of pulmonary edema.[54] Echocardiography can also detect diastolic dysfunction (the inability of the ventricle to relax), which is another common cause of heart failure. Another testing option is transesophageal echocardiography (TEE). This involves introducing an ultrasound transducer through the esophagus to obtain closer imaging of the heart. This test provides more accurate imaging than a standard ultrasound.

Information from a Swan-Ganz catheter may also aid in diagnosis. A PCWP > 18 mm Hg is suggestive of cardiogenic etiology.[53] This procedure may be done by an intensivist and usually takes place in an ICU setting.

If other tests fail to determine the cause for pulmonary edema, cardiac catheterization may be performed.[53] In this test, a catheter is threaded into a vein or artery and then into the patient's heart.[53] If a contrast agent is used, then the procedure is called a coronary angiogram.[54] Typically, this procedure is performed by an interventional cardiologist, and it may be used to unblock an artery.[54] Cardiac catheterization may also be employed to evaluate heart valves, measure heart chamber pressures, and discover possible hidden causes of pulmonary edema.[54]

Acute Respiratory Distress Syndrome

ARDS is a type of hypoxemic respiratory failure often described as noncardiogenic pulmonary edema. The recent Berlin definition of ARDS includes the presence of new or worsening respiratory symptoms following a known clinical insult with bilateral infiltrates on chest imaging and marked hypoxemia (see **Table 11-2**). Chest x-ray findings must *not* be due to effusions, lobar or lung collapse, or pulmonary nodules. The associated pulmonary edema must *not* be of cardiac origin or due to fluid overload. The severity of the patient's oxygenation problem is determined by the Pao_2 to Fio_2 ratio, which must be ≤ 300 mm Hg while the patient is receiving at least 5 cm H_2O of positive end-expiratory pressure (PEEP) or continuous positive airway pressure (CPAP). Severity of ARDS is then based on the Pao_2 to Fio_2 ratio (see Chapter 6).

ARDS is a serious, potentially fatal pulmonary disorder that interferes with oxygen getting from the alveoli into the pulmonary capillaries and being distributed throughout the body. The cause usually involves damage to the lungs from injury or disease, such as pneumonia, inhalation of toxic chemicals, aspiration of gastric contents, lung transplantation, septicemia, septic shock, or severe trauma. Massive transfusion and hematopoietic stem cell transplant are also risk factors for development of ARDS. Drug overdose (e.g., aspirin, cocaine, opioids, tricyclic antidepressants) and alcohol abuse have been associated with the development of ARDS.[63]

ARDS generally culminates in the abnormal accumulation of fluid, protein, and fibrin in the alveoli. This misplaced fluid can then block absorption of sufficient oxygen. Another consequence is that the lungs become stiff, heavy, and unable to fully expand. Oxygen levels for patients with ARDS can remain precariously low, even with the assistance of mechanical ventilators using endotracheal tubes and PEEP. This disorder can accompany the failure of vital organs, including the kidneys and the liver. Other risk factors include alcohol and tobacco use, acute pancreatitis, obesity, near drowning, and cardiopulmonary bypass.[63]

Medical Imaging Considerations with ARDS

The chest radiograph with ARDS typically shows diffuse, widespread, bilateral pulmonary infiltrates that are not due to effusions, lobar or lung collapse, or pulmonary nodules. Radiologic findings may at first be normal or may initially show minimal interstitial edema or decreased lung volume.[64] The chest x-ray then typically progresses to demonstrate symmetrical and bilateral infiltrates that may start out as patchy and ill-defined but then coalesce or grow together.[64] Late in ARDS, the patient may develop alveolar cell proliferation with collagen deposition.[68] The chest x-ray may then show an interstitial pattern that may include honeycombing.[64]

Care must be exercised to rule out cardiogenic pulmonary edema. The x-ray findings with cardiogenic pulmonary edema and ARDS are very similar; however, ARDS does not typically include cardiomegaly, vascular redistribution, or pleural effusion.[64] An echocardiogram can help evaluate the heart and recognize hypertrophy, assess ventricular function, and identify valve disorders. **Figure 11-30** provides an example of noncardiogenic pulmonary edema (i.e., ARDS) as seen on an AP chest radiograph.

Other Alveolar Airspace Disease

Sarcoidosis is a granulomatous disease of unknown origin that affects multiple body systems and primarily strikes young adults.[65] Chest x-rays reveal bilateral hilar

---

TABLE 11-2
Imaging Finding with ARDS

ARDS is defined based on imaging findings, timing (e.g., worsening symptoms with 1 week of a known clinical insult), origin of the observed pulmonary edema, and degree of oxygenation defect based on Pao_2/Fio_2 ratio ≤ 300 mm Hg* while receiving 5 cm H_2O or more of PEEP/CPAP. Imaging findings with ARDS include:

- Bilateral chest opacities on chest radiograph or CT scan not explained by lobar or lung collapse or lung nodules.
- Pulmonary edema that is not due to increased hydrostatic pressure (e.g., not due to CHF) as verified by:
  - Echocardiography or
  - PCWP < 18 mm Hg.

CPAP, continuous positive airway pressure; Fio_2, fraction of inspired oxygen; Pao_2, partial pressure of arterial oxygen; PEEP, positive end-expiratory pressure.

*If altitude is higher than 1000 m, then correction factor should be calculated as follow: Pao_2/Fio_2 × (barometric pressure/760).

Data from: ARDS Definition Task Force, Ranieri VM, Rubenfeld GD, et al. Acute respiratory distress syndrome: the Berlin Definition. *JAMA.* 2012;307(23):2526–2533. doi: 10.1001/jama.2012.5669.

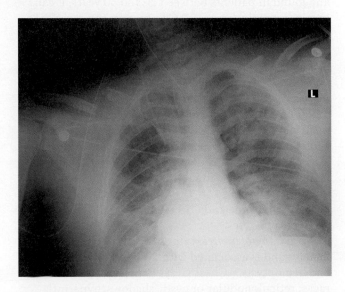

FIGURE 11-30 AP chest radiograph showing ARDS in a 17-year-old male patient.

© PhotoStock-Israel/Science Source.

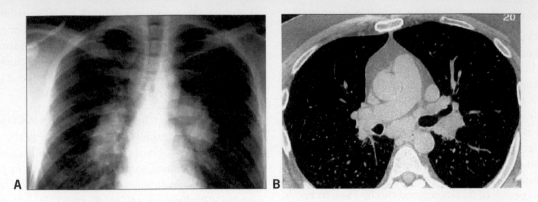

FIGURE 11-31 Sarcoidosis, thoracic. (A) Sarcoidosis as seen on a standard PA chest radiograph in a 28-year-old man. Note the extensive bilateral hilar and mediastinal lymph node enlargement, which was not associated with a pulmonary abnormality. (B) High-resolution CT scan in the same patient shows uniformly small, bilateral nodules in a miliary pattern with mediastinal and hilar adenopathy.

(A) Courtesy of Laura Vasquez; (B) Courtesy of Laura Vasquez.

adenopathy in the first stages, parenchymal infiltrates and hilar adenopathy in the second stages, only parenchymal infiltrates in the third stages, and significant lung damage and fibrosis in later stages.[65] **Figure 11-31** provides an example of sarcoidosis as seen on chest x-ray and CT scan.

Hypersensitivity pneumonitis is an allergy or hypersensitivity reaction disorder triggered by animal proteins, microbial spores, and certain chemicals.[66] Farmer's lung falls under this category. In chronic cases, chest x-rays reveal honeycombing and worsening fibrosis; for acute cases, it can reveal reticulonodular patterns.[66] *Eosinophilic granuloma* (now called pulmonary langerhan cell histiocytosis [PLCH]) is a chronic or subacute regenerative disease of unknown etiology that features granulomatous infiltration of bone and lung tissue.[66] Usually associated with smoking and found in patients between 20 and 50 years, it can involve pneumothoraces.[66] Chest x-rays can reveal honeycomb cysts and reticular or nodular densities in the upper or middle lungs.[66]

Pulmonary vasculitis can refer to granulomatosis and pulmonary angiitis (GPA or *Wegener's granulomatosis*); which involves vasculitis and necrotizing granulomas), *Goodpasture syndrome* (a pulmonary/renal syndrome), or *Churg-Strauss syndrome* (CSS; which involves necrotizing vasculitis, eosinophilia, and asthma).[67] Chest x-rays for GPA may reveal alveolar hemorrhage, diffuse interstitial disease, and bilateral nodules measuring 1 to 9 cm.[67] Chest x-rays for Goodpasture syndrome and CSS often reveal diffuse or focal alveolar infiltrates.[67]

Lymphangioleiomyomatosis (LAM) occurs in females and is associated with dyspnea, chylothorax, and hemoptysis.[68] Chest x-rays may reveal pneumothoraces, reticulonodular or cystic shadows, hyperinflation, and pleural effusions.[68] Lung biopsy may show hamartomatous regeneration of smooth muscle interstitium and numerous thin-walled parenchymal cysts.[68]

Chronic alveolar filling diseases are another special group of airspace diseases.[19] Chest x-ray findings common to these diseases include lobar, butterfly, or segmental patterns; puffy cloud margins; air alveologram or bronchogram; and early coalescence.[19] Some of the diseases under this heading are pulmonary alveolar proteinosis, alveolar hemorrhage syndrome, and idiopathic pulmonary hemosiderosis.[19]

Drug-induced pulmonary diseases are yet another special group of airspace diseases.[69] Illnesses related to drug side effects occur in 18% of hospital patients; some factors, including being older than age 70, increase a patient's risk.[69] The underlying chest x-ray findings include well-defined nodular changes, upper lobe predilection, diffuse interstitial changes, visible interstitial fibrosis, and pneumonitis.[69] Some of the offending drugs include amiodarone, methotrexate, sulfasalazine, nitrofurantoin, narcotics, salicylates, and thiazides; radiation therapy may also be a culprit.[69]

Bronchiolitis obliterans is a lung disease involving fibrosis that primarily affects the smaller airways and largely spares the interstitium.[70] Chest x-rays reveal significant interstitial or airspace changes but usually reflect air trapping (emphysema-like) and a mosaic pattern on CT scans. This condition may be caused by toxic fumes or an infectious pathogen.[70]

Atelectasis

Atelectasis involves the loss of lung volume with partial or complete collapse of alveoli. Unlike alveolar lung disease, atelectasis does not involve substantial filling of the alveoli with fluid or other material.[71] A common cause of atelectasis is obstruction of bronchioles or bronchi resulting in absorption of the gas distal to the obstruction and collapse of the alveoli (*obstructive atelectasis*). Sources of obstruction include secretions, mucous plugs, tumor (e.g., bronchogenic carcinoma, other neoplasms), or aspirated foreign bodies.[71] A malpositioned endotracheal tube (e.g., right main bronchus intubation) is an important hazard in the ICU, especially among ventilated patients, that may cause significant atelectasis on the opposite side (e.g., complete left lung collapse).[72] Postoperative atelectasis is a major cause for concern in patients following thoracic or abdominal surgery, which can lead to postoperative respiratory failure and significantly increased morbidity and mortality.[14]

Nonobstructive and Obstructive Atelectasis

Atelectasis may broadly be categorized as either nonobstructive or obstructive.[14] The most common type of atelectasis is obstructive. In this form of atelectasis, gas is reabsorbed from the alveoli if the obstruction occurs between the trachea and the alveoli.[14] The seriousness of atelectasis hinges on the inspired gas composition, levels of collateral ventilation, and other such mechanisms.[39] Indications of an infection of the respiratory system, such as pneumonia, on a child's chest x-ray may in fact be due to a foreign body aspiration; for children, this is the most common cause of obstructive atelectasis.

Nonobstructive atelectasis can occur due to lack of contact between the visceral and parietal pleura, loss of surfactant, parenchymal tissue replacement by infiltrative or scarring diseases, and by compression.[14] Types of nonobstructive atelectasis include *passive atelectasis* (caused by pleural effusion or pneumothorax), *compression atelectasis* (caused by compression by a space-occupying lesion), *adhesive atelectasis* (due to surfactant deficiency), *cicatrization atelectasis* (associated with fibrosis), and *replacement atelectasis* (caused by replacement of lung tissue, e.g., bronchioloalveolar cell carcinoma).[14] Absorptive atelectasis sometimes occurs with administration of high F_{IO_2} combined with low tidal volumes.

With atelectasis, gas exchange in the alveoli is reduced or eliminated; in the worst case scenario, respiratory failure may result.[14] Acute atelectasis can occur after chest or abdominal surgery or following a traumatic injury.[14] A surfactant deficiency may cause atelectasis, such as what occurs in respiratory distress syndrome (RDS) of the premature neonate. Chronic atelectasis may feature a complex mix of infection, airlessness, bronchiectasis (overextended bronchi), fibrosis, and tissue destruction.[14]

Radiologic Considerations in Atelectasis

Atelectasis is one of the most frequently encountered chest imaging abnormalities and can generally be diagnosed with a chest x-ray. Classic findings on the chest x-ray with atelectasis include:[71]

- Abnormal lung opacification (may require significant loss of lung volume)
- Diaphragm elevated due to volume loss

- Crowding of pulmonary vessels and/or crowded air bronchograms
- Displacement of anatomic features due to partial or complete collapse of lung tissue
  - Interlobular fissures displaced
  - Mediastinal structures displaced
  - Hilum displaced
- Obscured heart borders
- Obscured diaphragm borders
- Compensatory expansion of lung tissue adjacent to area of atelectasis
- Ribs may appear closer together on the affected side with unilateral atelectasis

Atelectasis may affect an entire lung lobe (lobar atelectasis) or more than one lobe. For example, combined right lower lobe and right middle lobe atelectasis is not uncommon with bronchial obstruction.[71] *Nonlobar atelectasis* can be round, discoid, or subsegmental.[71] *Round atelectasis* is a type of chronic atelectasis seen with pleural disease (e.g., asbestos-related pleural disease).[71] *Discoid atelectasis* is also known as platelike or linear atelectasis and is associated with peripheral volume loss and is *not* due to obstruction.[71] Discoid atelectasis is commonly seen in hospitalized and bedridden patients or following abdominal or thoracic surgery or multiple trauma. Shallow breathing and an inadequate cough following surgery may predispose patients to the development of discoid atelectasis. Incentive spirometry is often ordered for postoperative patients to promote deep breathing and prevent discoid atelectasis

Figure 11-32 provides an example of a right lower lobe obstructive atelectasis as seen on chest radiograph. CT scans are more revealing than x-rays because they can help determine lung volume. CT can also determine if a tumor is to blame for atelectasis; chest x-rays may not reveal tumors, especially when they are small.[3] Ultrasound can be used to identify pleural effusion. In addition, ultrasound can help guide fluid-removal procedures.[20] A bronchoscopy to remove obstructions such as foreign bodies, mucus plugs, and blood clots from airways may be needed in some cases.[20]

Other Infectious Pulmonary Diseases

Infectious pulmonary diseases include upper respiratory tract infections, acute bronchitis, pneumonia (bacterial, viral, atypical, fungal), and *Mycobacterium tuberculosis* (TB). Pneumonia has been discussed as a form of alveolar lung disease. We will now briefly review TB, acute bronchitis, croup, and epiglottitis.

Pulmonary Tuberculosis

Pulmonary tuberculosis (TB) is a lung infection of bacterial etiology; it can also spread to other organs (disseminated TB). Caused by the *Mycobacterium*

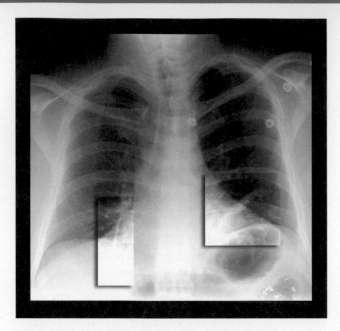

FIGURE 11-32 A color enhanced frontal chest x-ray shows the typical appearance of linear and discoid atelectasis of the lung. These regions are highlighted by the smaller boxes. Atelectasis is where there are areas of collapse of regions of the lung. These can be small, as in this case, or they can involve large regions of the lungs.

© Living Art Enterprises/Science Source.

tuberculosis bacillus, TB infection is spread by the inhalation of aerosolized droplets expelled from infected individuals. These inhaled droplets (droplet nuclei) may reach the alveoli, where they most often cause a latent infection. If this latent infection is not eliminated by host defenses, it may cause active disease that includes infection of alveolar macrophages, proliferation of the bacilli, and the formation of a granulomatous tubercle. Those who inhale these droplets and become infected are said to have *primary tuberculosis.* Unchecked infection leads to a caseating necrosis of the lung tissue (necrotizing granuloma).[1] The bacteria also enter adjacent lymph nodes; **lymphadenopathy** is a feature of primary TB.[1] The formation of a Ghon complex occurs when the tubercle results in calcification of the lung parenchyma and regional lymph node.[1] Reactivation of previously dormant TB may occur (reactivation TB) with fibrocavitary lesions in the upper lobes.

Clinical manifestations of TB include cough, fever, night sweats, weight loss, and/or hemoptysis. Patients infected with TB often have tender or swollen lymph nodes (lymphadenopathy). A positive tuberculin skin test and/or interferon-gamma release assay (IGRA) confirms TB exposure (latent TB), but not necessarily active disease. Patients with a cough of more than 2 to 3 weeks and at least one additional symptom should have a chest x-ray performed followed by three sputum samples for acid-fast bacilli (AFB) and culture if the chest

x-ray is suggestive of TB.[73] The interval between each sputum sample should be at least 8 hours, and at least one sample should be obtained early in the morning, before breakfast.[73] A nucleic acid amplification (NAA) test may be performed on one sputum sample in at-risk patients.[73] NAA testing can reliably detect *M. tuberculosis* bacteria in specimens 1 or more weeks earlier than culture. The AFB stain is a fast and inexpensive tool; however, sputum cultures require at least 3 weeks for the results and in some cases may take 4 to 8 weeks. Cultures are necessary to determine drug sensitivity, and newer techniques that are faster are now available. These include the microscopic-observation drug-susceptibility (MODS) and thin-layer agar (TLA) assays and use of molecular beacons for drug resistance.[73] An automated NAA test, the Xpert MTB/RIF assay, is also now available that can rapidly identify *M. tuberculosis* and assess for rifampin resistance.[73]

Patients at special risk for the development of TB include those who have had a recent exposure to an infected individual, a prior positive test for TB by skin test or IGRA, HIV infection, drug abuse, or who live in low-income, underserved communities or are recent immigrants. Other risk factors include chronic disease (e.g., renal failure, diabetes), immunosuppression (e.g., corticosteroids, organ transplant), silicosis, gastrectomy, and certain carcinomas.[73]

Other tests sometimes performed to diagnose TB include CT scans, bronchoscopy, and thoracentesis for pleural effusion. Rarely, pleural biopsies are performed, and gastric aspiration is sometimes performed in children when a sputum specimen cannot be obtained.

Treatment of Tuberculosis
Treatment of active TB includes a combination of four or more drugs: rifampin, isoniazid, pyrazinamide, and ethambutol (called RIPE therapy).[1] Typically, these medications are continued for 2 months, after which therapy is modified based on drug-sensitivity studies and continued for an additional 4 months; therapy for the last 4 months typically consists of isoniazid and rifampin.[1]

Because TB patients need to take a number of different medications for several months to be cured, some patients fail to follow recommended procedures. This may result in the development of difficult to treat, drug-resistant strains of TB. Drug-resistant TB may be treated with a combination of at least three drugs that the patient has not received in the past and guided by drug-sensitivity studies.[1] Complications of TB include hemoptysis, pneumothorax, and bronchiectasis. TB patients may also be at risk for development of lung cancer and chronic pulmonary aspergillosis.[73] TB cases generally must be reported to the health department.

Radiologic Manifestations of TB
A chest x-ray should be obtained in symptomatic patients with suspected TB. *Infiltrates (usually*

fibronodular) with or without cavitation in the upper lobes or the superior segments of the lower lobes are suggestive of TB.[73] It should be noted, however, that the chest x-ray alone cannot distinguish between active and inactive TB.[73]

The pulmonary foci of primary TB (also known as TB pneumonia) may be distributed randomly throughout the lungs and may range from small parenchymal opacities to segmental or lobar opacification.[64] An important radiographic feature of primary TB is lymphadenopathy (hilar and/or mediastinal), usually on one side.[64] Hilar lymph node calcification is seen in about one-third of cases and unilateral pleural effusions are not uncommon.[64] Alveolar infiltrates are common, whereas cavitation is rare. Lobar pneumonia has a strong association with lymphadenopathy. Atelectasis often affects the anterior upper lobes or medial segments of the right middle lobe. Pleural effusion is more likely to be seen in adults than in children. Because the fluid collects painlessly and slowly, TB patients are rarely seen with pleural fluid in small quantities. Parenchymal pathology will very rarely accompany pleural effusion; lymphadenopathy is more common. If apical pleural scarring is present, it is likely due to causes other than TB.

Focal infiltration of the upper lobes or lower lobes is a common finding with reactivation TB.[73] Often, the earliest chest x-ray finding with reactivation disease is one or more ill-defined opacities in the posterior segments of the upper lobes or the superior segment of the lower lobes.[64] Cavitation with reactivation TB tends to indicate active infection.[64] Other patterns sometimes seen with reactivation include lobar pneumonia, diffuse bronchopneumonia, and miliary TB.[64]

Transbronchial spread may be seen, usually from the upper lobes of one lung to the lower lobes of the opposite lung. Asymptomatic bronchiectasis may also be present. In addition, stricture and fibrosis may cause bronchostenosis. Years after the infection, evidence of middle lobe syndrome may be present—bronchus distortion and atelectasis due to fibrosis. Tuberculoma, or solitary pulmonary nodules, may be present just as in primary TB; these present as oval or round lesions with discrete, tiny shadows near the lesion. If pleural effusion is found, then spread of the disease into the pleural cavity can be assumed, as well as the presence of an empyema, which is a very rare but rather serious development.

CT scans are more sensitive than conventional chest x-rays, though they are not generally needed for management of TB.[73] CT scans may be helpful for discriminating active processes (e.g., infectious disease or neoplasms) from fibrosis.[73] It must also be noted that mycobacteria other than *M. tuberculosis* may cause lung disease. **Figure 11-33** provides an example of a cavitary TB as seen in an HIV patient.

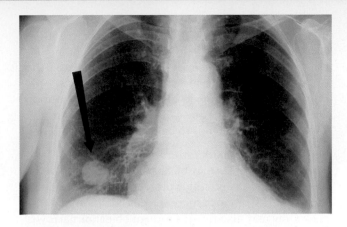

FIGURE 11-33 Cavitary pulmonary tuberculosis as seen on chest radiograph. Note cavitation in right lower lung field.

Acute Bronchitis

Acute **bronchitis** is upper respiratory tract inflammation, usually due to viral infection (e.g., influenza, parainfluenza, coronavirus, rhinovirus, RSV, or metpneumovirus).[74] *Mycoplasma pneumoniae* is a fairly common cause acute bronchitis in young adults, and other bacteria may also cause acute bronchitis (e.g., *Chlamydophila pneumoniae, Bordetella pertussis*). Acute bronchitis cannot be distinguished from a simple upper respiratory tract infection (i.e., common cold) in the first few days. Initial diagnosis of acute bronchitis is based, in part, on acute cough with or without sputum production that lasts for more than 5 days.[74]

Chest radiographs are not typically useful in the diagnosis of acute bronchitis, other than to exclude other causes of acute cough (e.g., pneumonia, interstitial lung disease, pleural effusion). Chest x-ray is specifically indicated in cases where vital signs are elevated (e.g., increased respiratory rate, increased heart rate, fever) or in the very elderly where pneumonia is suspected.[19,20,74] Thickening of the bronchial walls in chest x-ray is sometimes reported with acute bronchitis. In addition to pneumonia, diseases that should be ruled out in cases of suspected acute bronchitis include postnasal drip, gastroesophageal reflux disease (GERD), asthma, and chronic bronchitis. Treatment of acute bronchitis may include aspirin, acetaminophen, a nonsteroidal anti-inflammatory medication (e.g., ibuprofen), and/or ipratropium by inhalation.[74]

Croup

Croup, or laryngotracheobronchitis, is a disease that produces breathing difficulty and a classic "barking" cough.[19,20,74] Most common in children and infants, the condition is caused by swelling around the vocal cords.[12,13,74]

Causes of croup include bacterial infection, viral infection, allergies, GERD, and inhalation of irritating gases and substances.[12,13,74] One of the most common causes is the parainfluenza virus.[14,74] Other viruses that can case croup include measles, RSV, adenovirus, and influenza. When croup develops quickly in association with a mild cold it may be called *spasmodic croup*.[74] This type of croup tends to be recurrent.[74]

Radiographic Considerations

An x-ray of the neck may be obtained in order to determine if there is a noticeable obstruction and to assess for epiglottitis, a much more serious condition.[13,14,74] A neck x-ray may also reveal a foreign object or narrowing of the trachea. Children with croup ordinarily have a noticeable upper airway narrowing, which can be observed on x-rays.[13,14,74]

The subglottic edema due to larygnotracheobronchitis may sometimes be seen on imaging as the "pencil sign" or "steeple sign" in which the trachea narrows in the subglottic area (see Figure 11-6). An AP radiograph of the neck's soft tissues classically shows a steeple sign in croup, which indicates subglottic narrowing; a lateral neck view may show a distended, ballooning pharynx during inspiration.[12-14] However, these signs may be absent in as many as half of all croup cases involving children. Furthermore, a steeple sign may be seen in patients not suffering from croup, requiring consideration of other differential options for this radiologic finding, such as epiglottitis, angioneurotic edema, thermal injury, or bacterial tracheitis.[12-14] Patients undergoing imaging in these circumstances should be monitored closely because airway obstruction can rapidly become life threatening.[14] An ordinary chest x-ray can help confirm a diagnosis of croup or help exclude other conditions that may mimic croup by causing stridor, such as an esophageal foreign body, an aspirated foreign body, congenital subglottic stenosis, epiglottitis, and retropharyngeal abscess. Croup requires a clinical diagnosis. A chest x-ray can help confirm the diagnosis but is not required except in complicated cases.

Epiglottitis

Epiglottitis is caused by a bacterial infection such as *Haemophilus influenzae* or *Streptococcus* sp. Epiglottitis can be life threatening and may lead to complete airway obstruction if not promptly identified and treated. Lateral upper airway (neck) x-rays are sometimes obtained in children to evaluate upper airway inflammation.[12-14] With epiglottitis, swelling may result in the "thumb sign," in which the epiglottis looks like a thumb on the lateral neck x-ray view (see also Figure 11-6).

Pulmonary Vascular Diseases

Pulmonary vascular diseases range from idiopathic (primary) pulmonary arterial hypertension (IPAH) to pulmonary hypertension caused by hypoxemia, left ventricular failure, or thromboembolic disease (e.g., pulmonary embolus).[20] The pulmonary artery arises from the right ventricle's base. It moves upwards to the left side of the ascending aorta, and then it bifurcates beneath the aortic arch into the left and right pulmonary arteries.[20] The separation is situated anteriorly, inferiorly, and left-wise to the tracheal division. Pulmonary hypertension may be defined as a mean pulmonary artery pressure > 25 mm Hg.[20]

Pulmonary Hypertension

Pulmonary hypertension occurs as the result of changes in pre- or postcapillary pulmonary circulation.[75] Precapillary (vascular) pulmonary hypertension may be due to primary pulmonary hypertension (e.g., IPAH); acute or chronic pulmonary thromboembolic disease; widespread pulmonary embolisms caused by foreign materials, parasites, or intravascular malignant cells; pulmonary vasculitis; or peripheral pulmonary artery stenosis. Other causes include chronic interstitial lung disease, emphysema and COPD, bronchiectasis, and other diseases associated with chronic hypoxemia.[75] Postcapillary (cardiac or venous) pulmonary hypertension may occur due to left-sided atrial or ventricular heart disease, valvular heart disease (e.g., mitral stenosis), or constrictive pericarditis or secondary to focalized venous constriction or restricted venous drainage because of left atrium neoplasia. With pulmonary veno-occlusive disease (a very rare form of postcapillary pulmonary hypertension), the cause is unknown.

Classic radiologic characteristics of pulmonary hypertension (both pre- and postcapillary) include enlargement of the central pulmonary arteries and sharply pruned peripheral pulmonary artery branches.[7] CT scans better depict the size of the heart chambers and pulmonary arteries.

Right ventricular enlargement is often viable on the lateral chest film and small to moderate pericardial effusions are not uncommon.[7] The radiologic findings associated with postcapillary pulmonary hypertension may also include small pleural effusions, prominent septal lines, and sometimes airspace opacities.

Pulmonary Thromboembolic Disease

Pulmonary embolus refers to obstruction of the pulmonary artery or one of its branches by a blood clot (thromboembolus), fat, air, or tumor. Of these, thromboembolus is the most common. Pulmonary thromboembolus is usually due to thrombosis of the deep veins of the lower extremities, though other sources of clots are possible.[1,19] Factors associated with development of pulmonary embolus include venous stasis, venous thrombosis, hypercoagulability, and endothelial damage.[1,14] Massive pulmonary embolus is a life-threatening event that causes hypotension and may result in acute right ventricular failure and death within a few hours.

Although blood clots are the usual cause of pulmonary emboli, they may also be caused by fat from the marrow of a broken bone, air bubbles introduced through an IV line or a syringe, or part of a dislodged tumor.[27] Solitary emboli are rare; usually, numerous clots are involved.[1] Arterial blockage can lead to tissue damage and may interfere with oxygenation, depending on how severely the damage compromises gas exchange.[27]

Clinical manifestations of acute pulmonary embolus include dyspnea, chest pain, hemoptysis, severe hypoxemia, and hypotension. Calf or thigh pain may be present due to deep vein thrombosis. Breath sounds may include crackles and/or wheezing, and blood gases often show hypoxemia, with or without hypercapnea and acidemia. Pulmonary embolus increases ventilatory dead space, and patients may exhibit an increased rate and depth of breathing, but normal $Paco_2$. There may or may not be electrocardiogram (ECG) changes associated with right heart strain; other laboratory studies tend to be nonspecific. The three main diagnostic tests for pulmonary embolus are imaging techniques. These are the $\dot{V}/\dot{Q}$ scan, spiral CT, and pulmonary angiogram. A lower extremity Doppler study or venogram may also be ordered to identify lower extremity venous thrombosis.

Imaging Considerations with Pulmonary Embolus

Pulmonary embolism is difficult to diagnose; this is especially true for patients already suffering from other lung or heart disease. A chest x-ray is not an accurate tool for detecting pulmonary embolism. The chest x-ray can, however, help identify problems that may mimic pulmonary embolism and evaluate conditions that may be present along with (or without) pulmonary embolus, such as enlarged heart, atelectasis, pleural effusion, or parenchymal lung disease.[27]

The pulmonary angiogram has been considered the definitive test for pulmonary embolus. To obtain a pulmonary angiogram, a catheter is inserted through a large vein and threaded to the right side of the heart and into the pulmonary artery. A contrast agent is then injected to provide an image of pulmonary blood flow.[19,55] A negative pulmonary angiogram rules out pulmonary embolus. This test must be performed by highly trained interventional radiologists and should only be used if other tests are not sufficient to make a diagnosis. Across many medical centers, CT angiograms have largely replaced the need for conventional pulmonary angiography. Pulmonary angiography should be reserved for patients in whom other tests are inconclusive.[19,55]

Spiral (helical) CT with intravenous contrast media (e.g., CTPA or CT pulmonary angiogram) is now considered to be an excellent alternative to conventional angiography in those institutions experienced in its application.[26,27] The spiral CT scan provides a sensitive test for pulmonary embolus that is noninvasive. Using an injected intravenous contrast agent, a spiral CT scan can provide an accurate picture of arterial and venous blood flow in the lungs. In a patient with acute pulmonary embolism, a CT angiogram may show an intraluminal filling defect occluding the front basal segmental artery of the right lower lobe.[26] Another sign that may be visible is an infarction of the affected lung, indicated by a triangle-shaped, pleural-based consolidation (sometimes referred to as a Hampton hump). **Figure 11-34** provides an example of a pulmonary embolus as seen on CTPA.

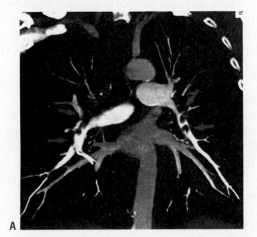
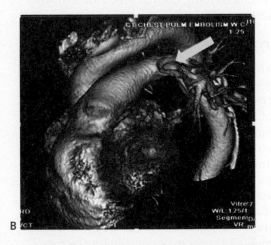

FIGURE 11-34 **(A) Computerized tomography pulmonary angiogram (CTPA) of pulmonary embolism.** Images show coronal maximum intensity projections reconstruction of a CTPA in a patient with multiple, bilateral pulmonary embolisms (arrows). **(B) 3D reconstruction image of a left pulmonary artery with embolus (yellow arrow).**

(A) Courtesy of Laura Vasquez; (B) Courtesy of Laura Vasquez.

The $\dot{V}/\dot{Q}$ scan is a nuclear medicine technique that compares ventilation to pulmonary perfusion. The $\dot{V}/\dot{Q}$ scan uses mildly radioactive tracers to provide images that are used to evaluate the distribution of air flow and blood flow in the lungs and can help to detect blockages.[76] Areas of ventilation without perfusion are suggestive of pulmonary embolus. Patients with a combination of a high probability of embolus based on the clinical picture and a high-probability $\dot{V}/\dot{Q}$ scan are very likely to actually have pulmonary embolus. A normal $\dot{V}/\dot{Q}$ scan virtually rules out pulmonary embolus.[76]

Duplex venous ultrasonography, also known as a duplex scan or compression ultrasonography, may be used to check for thrombosis in the veins of the upper and lower extremities (deep vein thrombosis), though the usefulness and quality of this test is dependent on the technician performing the exam.[3] An echocardiogram can estimate right ventricular size and blood pressure in the right side of the heart. These may be elevated with pulmonary embolus. MRI is of limited value in diagnosing pulmonary embolism, though this may change with advances in the technology.[3]

Treatment of Pulmonary Embolus

Treatment of pulmonary thromboembolus may include support of oxygenation and hemodynamic status, thrombolytic medications (e.g., tissue plasminogen activator [TPA] for massive emboli) to dissolve existing clots, and anticoagulants (e.g., low-molecular-weight heparin, subcutaneous fondaparinux, intravenous or subcutaneous unfractionated heparin) to prevent additional clot formation. Contraindications and risks of thrombolytic and anticoagulant drugs must be considered. Other treatments include insertion of vena caval filters to screen new clots and catheter or surgical thromboembolectomy, both of which are high-risk procedures.[20]

Chronic Obstructive Pulmonary Disease

Patients with pulmonary **emphysema** (a form of COPD) may exhibit significant changes in pulmonary vessel structure and function.[77,78] Impairment of gas exchange, obliteration of pulmonary capillaries (e.g., vascular remodeling), and chronic hypoxemia resulting in intense pulmonary vasoconstriction cause development of pulmonary hypertension. This is known as *secondary pulmonary hypertension,* which is one of the chief reasons COPD patients often die prematurely.[77, 78] Hypoxemia, endothelial cellular dysfunction, and damage caused by inflammation-inducing toxins and cigarette smoking appear to be contributing factors.[77,78] *Cor pulmonale* (right ventricular hypertrophy and heart failure) is sometimes seen with COPD patients, other patients with chronic lung disease/hypoxemia, and in patients with IPAH.

The Role of MRI for Pulmonary Vasculature Disease

MRI is playing an increasingly important role in imaging of pulmonary vasculature diseases, primarily because it is noninvasive and uses no ionizing radiation. Some of the specific clinical applications of MRI in this area include evaluating vascular involvement by intrinsic and extrinsic tumors, diagnosing vascular lung lesions, identifying central thromboembolic disease, and performing pre- and postoperative assessments of congenital abnormalities.[79]

Pneumothorax, Pneumomediastinum, and Hemothorax

Pneumothorax

A **pneumothorax** is the abnormal collection of air in the pleural space.[5] Symptoms are variable but may include sudden-onset dyspnea and sharp pleuritic chest pain, especially during inspiration or coughing.[26] Types of pneumothorax include simple pneumothorax, tension pneumothorax, and open or traumatic pneumothorax. A simple pneumothorax is not usually life threatening, whereas a tension pneumothorax in a mechanically ventilated patient represents a medical emergency.[26] An iatrogenic pneumothorax is one resulting as a complication of a surgical or medical intervention. Transthoracic needle biopsy, thoracentesis, transbronchial biopsy, and subclavian central venous catheter placement are common causes. Bilateral pneumothoraxes have occurred in patients following heart–lung transplant.

Types of trauma that may cause a pneumothorax include stab wounds, gunshot wounds, collision with a hard surface (as in a car accident), and surgical procedures involving the opening of the thoracic cavity; a rib fracture may also puncture a lung.[29] In cases involving rib fractures, the first rib is often broken posteriorly. In the case of numerous fractured ribs down the anterior or midlateral chest wall, the result may be a flail chest, potentially leading to a pneumothorax.[29]

Blunt trauma incidents, auto accidents in which the passengers are unrestrained, falls, and pugilistic blows to the chest can also trigger a pneumothorax. Air bag deployment in car accidents has been known to cause traumatic pneumothorax, as has participation in high-risk activities such as skydiving, skiing, and flying.

An occult traumatic pneumothorax is a special type of pneumothorax that usually cannot be seen on chest x-rays despite being discernible on CT scan. Studies have shown that some asymptomatic victims of chest stab wounds later develop a delayed hemothorax or pneumothorax.[29]

A *primary spontaneous pneumothorax* (PSP) may occur without a precipitating event or known pulmonary disease due to the rupture of a pleural bleb.

Apical pleural **blebs**, or air blisters, seem to be more common in tall, thin people.[19] Blebs can rupture at any time; they are more likely to rupture, though, in people who travel by airplane, scuba dive, or who climb mountains at high altitudes.[19] PSP has been associated with smoking, Marfan syndrome, and a family history of PSP; patients are often young men in their early 20s.[19]

Pneumothorax may also occur as a complication of lung disease (*secondary pneumothorax*). Lung diseases in which a secondary pneumothorax may occur include COPD, cystic fibrosis, necrotizing pneumonia, and lung malignancy. Bullous emphysema is a form of COPD in which blebs or bullae form; these may rupture causing pneumothorax.[19] *Birt-Hogg-Dubé syndrome* is a genetic disorder whose symptomatology includes, among other things, pulmonary cysts and an increased risk for development of spontaneous pneumothorax.[19] About 22% of patients with Birt-Hogg-Dubé syndrome develop pneumothorax.[19] A genetic test is available to detect the syndrome. Occurring rarely and striking 1 to 3 days after menstrual cycle onset, *catamenial pneumothorax* usually afflicts women between 30 and 50 years old and may be attributable to thoracic endometriosis. Women between 30 and 40 years who manifest a right-sided and recurrent pneumothorax within 2 days of menstruation should be suspected of having a catamenial pneumothorax.[19]

A **tension pneumothorax** is present when pleural gas is pressurized. Damage to the parietal pleura, visceral pleura, and/or the tracheobronchial tree resulting in the creation of a one-way valve can lead to tension pneumothorax in a spontaneously breathing patient.[19] The ICU sees many instances of tension pneumothorax in patients receiving positive pressure ventilation; the respiratory care clinician must always consider this possibility in the event of changes in hemodynamic and/or respiratory status in ventilated patients.[19] Aspirated meconium can act as a one-way air valve in infants, potentially inducing a tension pneumothorax.[12] Infants who require ventilatory assistance are also at higher risk for tension pneumothorax.[12] Without treatment, tension pneumothorax can be rapidly fatal. Learning the signs of this condition, as well as emergency thoracic decompression techniques, can save lives.[19] Immediate treatment is so urgent that waiting for chest x-ray results should not forestall aggressive treatment in patients with hemodynamic compromise.[19]

Tension and traumatic pneumothorax occur more frequently than spontaneous pneumothoraces.[19] As noted, iatrogenic pneumothorax has been associated with the placement of central venous catheters, thoracentesis, positive pressure ventilation, and other interventions.[19] For example, thoracentesis leads to pneumothorax only 4% of the time when performed by experienced healthcare providers, but when performed by inexperienced medical professionals pneumothorax

rates may be as high as 30%.[19] In summary, procedures that may cause pneumothorax include:[19]

- Thoracentesis
- Pleural or transbronchial biopsy
- Transthoracic needle aspiration or pulmonary nodule biopsy (32% to 37% of reported cases)
- Intercostal nerve block
- Central venous catheterization (internal jugular or subclavian)
- Tracheostomy
- Positive pressure ventilation
- Cardiopulmonary resuscitation (CPR; the chance of a pneumothorax increases in proportion to ventilation/support difficulty)
- Placement of nasogastric feeding tube

Clinical Manifestations of Pneumothorax

The clinical manifestations of pneumothorax vary with the type and severity of the disease. A small, simple pneumothorax may be asymptomatic. With a larger pneumothorax, dyspnea and pleuritic chest pain may occur. Tachypnea and changes in blood pressure may occur and oximetry may demonstrate hypoxemia. Chest wall movement may be reduced on the affected side, breath sounds may be absent or diminished on the affected side, and the affected side of the chest may be hyperresonant to percussion. With tension, the trachea and point of maximal impulse (PMI; the point where the apical pulse is strongest) of the heart may be shifted to the opposite side. Untreated tension pneumothorax may rapidly lead to profound alterations in ventilatory and hemodynamic status (e.g., hypotension that may be followed by cardiac arrest and death).

Imaging Findings with Pneumothorax

The chest radiograph and CT scan are the preferred imaging techniques for identifying pneumothorax. The CT scan is the most accurate method to identify and assess a pneumothorax; however, CT is generally needed only in complex cases.[80] A portable chest radiograph is often preferred in very sick patients where time is of the essence (e.g., ICU or emergency department). The chest x-ray may be taken with the patient in the upright, lateral decubitus, or supine positions. Of these, the upright or lateral decubitus positions are preferred; the supine view is least sensitive.[80]

The main finding on chest x-ray with pneumothorax is free air in the pleural space (i.e., black with no vascular markings). A separation of the visceral and parietal pleura can be seen as a white visceral pleural line. Pneumothorax is often accompanied by a visible loss of lung volume; with a large pneumothorax there may be complete lung collapse on one side. In the upright chest radiograph, free air in the pleural space tends to collect in the apex. Supine chest radiography may show a "deep sulcus" sign where the costophrenic sulcus is outlined by anterior and basal pleural gas. The costophrenic sulcus is between the ribs and the most lateral part of the diaphragm (i.e., costophrenic angle); the deep sulcus sign refers to a unilateral increase in the size of the costophrenic angle.[81] Formulas are available that can be used to estimate the size of a pneumothorax as a percentage based on imaging studies, though some clinicians prefer to simply classify pneumothorax as large or small.

Radiologic manifestations of tension pneumothorax include air in the pleural space and loss of lung volume. In addition, with tension there is often a tracheal and mediastinal shift away from the affected side. The chest on the affected side may appear to be hyperexpanded, and the hemidiaphragm may be depressed.[3] Ventilatory and hemodynamic compromise are also often present. Rapid identification and decompression of a tension pneumothorax can be lifesaving. Pneumomediastinum (free air in the mediastinum) often occurs with tension pneumothorax. The development of subcutaneous emphysema (air in the subcutaneous tissue) and/or pneumoperitoneum (air in the peritoneum) may also occur.

Bedside ultrasound of the chest is sometimes used to assess patients with suspected pneumothorax in the critical care setting. Ultrasound may be more effective in identifying pneumothorax than the supine chest radiograph, though the supine view is the least preferred chest x-ray for evaluation of pneumothorax. Findings on ultrasonography that may rule out the presence of a pneumothorax are the "sliding lung" and B lines or "comet tail."[80] Lung sliding refers to the normal motion or sliding of the visceral and parietal pleura against each other as the lung expands and contracts during normal breathing as seen during ultrasonography. B lines (the comet tail) refer to characteristic lines perpendicular to the pleura seen in the ultrasound image during normal breathing. The absence of lung sliding and B lines suggest pneumothorax.[80]

Because a large variety of malignancies, including sarcomas and primary lung cancer, have been associated with pneumothoraces, patients with a history of, predisposition to, or other indications of cancer should be examined or closely monitored with appropriate medical imaging for metastasized malignancies. In addition, some chemotherapeutic medicines are suspected of inducing secondary spontaneous pneumothoraces. There are several conditions that may look similar to a pneumothorax on imaging studies. These include large lung bullae, skin folds, and traumatic rupture of the diaphragm with stomach herniation into the chest.[80]

Figure 11-35 demonstrates a right-side pneumothorax with the beginning of tension. **Figure 11-36** clearly shows a left-side tension pneumothorax, whereas **Figure 11-37** provides an example of a pneumothorax as seen on CT scan. **Figure 11-38** provides an example of an iatrogenic pneumothorax that developed

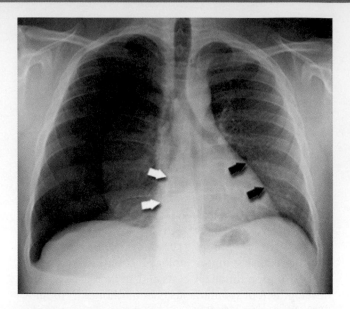

FIGURE 11-35 Large right side pneumothorax—early tension. This image demonstrates a large pneumothorax in the right. The right lung is largely collapsed and the right heart border (white arrows) and left heart border (black arrows) are shifted to the left, indicating the development of tension on the right side. The right hemidiaphragm is also slightly depressed—it should be higher than the left hemidiaphragm.

Courtesy of Laura Vasquez.

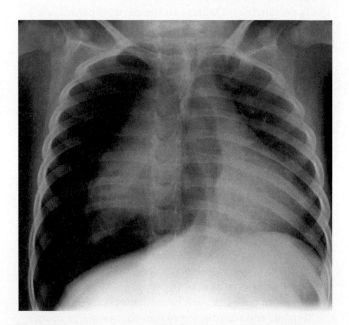

FIGURE 11-36 Tension pneumothorax. The right hemithorax is black with no vascular markings due to air in the pleural cavity. The right lung is completely collapsed. The trachea is pushed to the opposite side due to the pressure that has built up on the right side (e.g., tension) and the heart is shifted to the contralateral side. Note the right heart border is pushed to the left. The right hemidiaphragm is depressed.

© Mediscan/Visuals Unlimited, Inc.

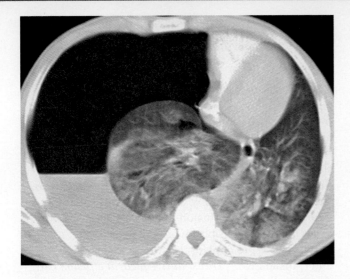

FIGURE 11-37 Traumatic hemopneumothorax. A chest CT scan, axial section.

© Pr. Michel Brauner/ISM/Phototake.

following a thoracentesis to evaluate a pleural effusion. **Figure 11-39** shows a traumatic pneumothorax.

Treatment of Pneumothorax

Treatment of simple pneumothorax may include administration of supplemental oxygen, needle aspiration (if the pneumothorax is large), and possible placement of chest tubes. Tension pneumothorax may be life threatening, and management includes rapid decompression via thoracostomy.[19,52] Ideally, tension pneumothorax should be confirmed by chest x-ray prior to thoracostomy, though this may not always be possible.[20] In the presence of worsening dyspnea, diminished breath sounds on one side, tracheal shift, distended neck veins, and hypotension, immediate thoracostomy for chest decompression should be performed. If a standard chest tube is not immediately available, a needle thoracostomy should be performed to decompress the chest followed by chest tube insertion. For needle decompression, a 14- to 16-gauge needle with intravenous catheter is attached to a syringe (5 to 10 mL). The needle is then inserted along the superior (top) margin of the second or third rib at the midclavicular line on the affected side. The needle is inserted until the trapped air is aspirated through the needle syringe; the rush of escaping air is proof that a tension pneumothorax was present. The needle is then removed, leaving

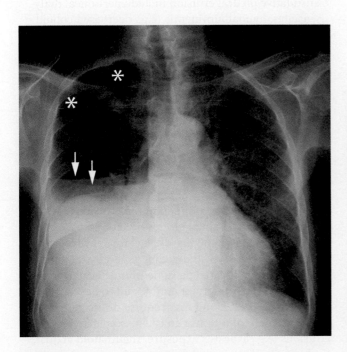

FIGURE 11-38 Iatrogenic pneumothorax. A pneumothorax can be the consequence of instrumentation of the chest. In this case, a thoracocentesis (pleural aspiration) was performed to evaluate a pleural effusion. After invasive procedures such as this, a chest x-ray should be requested, specifically to check for pneumothorax. This x-ray shows dense opacification of the right lower zone due to consolidation and a residual effusion (arrows) and a large pneumothorax (*). The direct contact between air and water results in a flat interface (arrows) rather than the classical meniscus shape of a simple pleural effusion.

Modified from: Radiology Masterclass 2007–2013. Available at http:// radiologymasterclass.co.uk/.

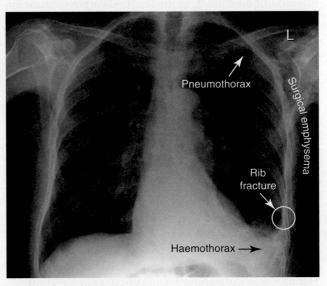

FIGURE 11-39 Traumatic pneumothorax. A minimally displaced rib fracture is visible on the left. This fracture is complicated by blood obscuring the left costophrenic angle (e.g., hemothorax) and free air seen in the upper portion of the right hemithorax (e.g., pneumothorax). Subcutaneous air (e.g., subcutaneous emphysema) is also seen on the right due to the trauma. This represents air in the soft tissue and is sometimes referred to as "surgical" emphysema as it can be caused by surgery or traumatic injury.

Modified from: Radiology Masterclass 2007–2013. Available at http:// radiologymasterclass.co.uk/.

the catheter in place.[52,53] This procedure turns a tension pneumothorax into a simple pneumothorax, and chest tube placement should follow as soon as possible. Possible complications of needle thoracostomy include lung laceration and air embolism. Rapid re-expansion of a large pneumothorax may cause pulmonary edema. As noted, if no hemodynamic compromise exists, it is best to wait for confirmation from an emergency chest x-ray prior to intervention.[53] However, needle thoracentesis can be a life-saving procedure and should not be withheld when indicated.[52,53]

Pneumothorax in Infants

Respiratory distress syndrome (RDS) is the most common cause of pneumothorax among infants, especially those born prematurely.[12] Because their still-developing lungs lack sufficient surfactant, premature infants' alveoli have difficulty functioning properly.[12] Use of a mechanical ventilator to address the problem can expose the already fragile alveoli to too much pressure and pneumothorax may occur.[20] Another cause of pneumothorax in newborns is meconium aspiration syndrome. More common in boys than in girls, this condition occurs when, during the birth process, infants inhale traces of their first bowel movements, known as meconium. The ensuing breathing difficulties may call for assisted ventilation.

Pneumomediastinum

Pneumomediastinum, or mediastinal emphysema, is air in the mediastinum.[52] This condition, which may occur spontaneously, after trauma, or following a medical procedure, often results from increased intrathoracic pressure.[20,53] It may also be instigated by seizures, the Valsalva maneuver, a slight esophageal perforation, or endoscopy.[19] If the infiltrating air enters the membrane surrounding the heart, the condition is called a *pneumopericardium*. On a chest x-ray, a pneumomediastinum may appear as a radiolucent area around the border of the left side of the heart.[3] As noted, tension pneumothorax often causes pneumomediastinum.

Hemothorax

The abnormal presence of blood in the pleural space is called a hemothorax.[19] In short, a hemothorax is a bloody pleural effusion (see pleural effusion, below). Hemothorax is diagnosed using chest x-rays, pleural fluid analysis, thoracentesis, or a CT scan.[3] MRI is able to image pleural blood and distinguish between fresh blood and older blood.[82] Causes of hemothorax include trauma, administration of anticoagulants, metastatic disease, and leak from an aortic aneurysm.[82] To treat the condition, it is necessary to address the cause and remove accumulated air and blood from the pleural space. In serious, uncontrollable cases of bleeding, a thoracotomy may be required. Trauma

and rib fractures may cause pneumothorax and/or hemothorax.

Pleural Effusion

The surfaces of the pleurae are kept moist by small amounts of fluid (≤ 10 mL) that act as a lubricant between the visceral and parietal pleura as they move as the lung expands and contracts during normal ventilation.[20] Pleural effusion is the accumulation of excess fluid in the pleural space.[83] Pleural effusion may be diagnosed using chest x-rays, CT scans, thoracentesis, thoracic ultrasonography, and pleural fluid analysis. Typically, a pleural effusion must exceed 250 mL in order to be easily visible on chest x-ray.[83]

The two types of pleural effusion are exudative and transudative.[83] *Transudative pleural effusion* can develop when changes in osmotic and hydrostatic pressures within vessels cause fluid to leak into the pleural space.[83] Transudative pleural effusions may be bilateral or occur on one side. Congestive heart failure often results in elevated osmotic pressures and is the most common cause of a transudative pleural effusion that is usually bilateral. Other conditions that can cause a transudative pleural effusion include peritoneal dialysis, ascites, hypoalbuminemia (e.g., decreased colloid osmotic pressure), malnutrition, nephrotic syndrome (a form of kidney disease), and liver cirrhosis.[83] Transudates due to cirrhosis are often unilateral on the right side. Transudates may be relatively small and may not require drainage.

Exudative pleural effusion occurs when there are changes to vascular permeability resulting in fluid leaks in the pleura. This most commonly occurs due to infection, such as bacterial pneumonia (e.g., parapneumonic effusion). Thoracentesis can also be used to examine the chemical and biological makeup of a pleural effusion. Uncomplicated parapneumonic effusions are associated with certain pleural fluid lab values (e.g., pH > 7.1 to 7.2; glucose > 60 mg/dL; lactate dehydrogenase [LDH] < 1000 units/L) and do not generally require drainage.[83] Complicated parapneumonic effusions do not respond to antibiotic therapy, tend to have a pleural fluid pH < 7.1 to 7.2, and may require drainage.[83] Other inflammatory conditions can cause exudative pleural effusions (e.g., asbestos exposure, rheumatoid arthritis, lupus erythematosus); however, the second most common cause of exudative effusion is malignancy. Findings of a specific organism (i.e., infective agent) or malignant cells in the pleural fluid can identify the cause of pleural effusion in about 25% of cases.[84]

Exudative effusions can be sometimes be distinguished from transudative effusions based on measurement of pleural fluid protein, pleural fluid LDH, serum protein LDH, and serum LDH. Exudates are associated with one or more of the following: pleural fluid protein to serum protein ratio > 0.50; pleural fluid LDH to serum LDH ratio ≥ 0.60; or pleural fluid LDH ≥ two-thirds of the upper limit of normal.[84]

Imaging Findings with Pleural Effusion

Although analysis of pleural fluid can help in the differential diagnosis of pleural effusion, the initial identification of an effusion is often dependent on imaging studies. A conventional chest x-ray may be the first tool used to discover or confirm the presence of pleural fluid.[83,84] Pleural effusions are often easily seen on frontal (PA), lateral, and decubitus radiographs.

Pleural effusions will usually accumulate in the most dependent part of the thorax due to gravity. Pleural fluid volume can be estimated using standard upright frontal (PA) and lateral views. Pleural fluid typically forms an arc or meniscus that obscures the costophrenic angle and increasing portions of the diaphragm as the volume of fluid increases. On a frontal (PA) radiograph, the costophrenic angle will often be obviously obscured when pleural fluid volume exceeds 250 mL.[83] In the upright PA view, pleural fluid > 75 mL may obscure the posterior costophrenic sulcus, and fluid > 175 mL may obscure the lateral costophrenic sulcus.[82] A pleural fluid volume of > 500 mL usually obscures the entire diaphragm on one side. The costophrenic sulcus is the recess between the lateral-most portion of the diaphragm and the ribs, seen on chest x-ray as the costophrenic angle.[82]

A lateral decubitus view with the patient lying on the affected sided can be used to verify the presence of a small pleural effusion (vs. pleural thickening), quantify the volume of fluid present, and clarify if the fluid is free flowing. Loculated pleural effusions are those that are not free flowing and are confined to one or more fixed pockets in the pleural space. Loculated pleural effusions are often associated with empyema (or complicated parapneumonic effusions).[82] Other causes include hemothorax, chylothorax (due to lymph fluid or chyle), and pleuritis caused by tuberculosis.[82] Loculated pleural effusions must be distinguished from masses or abscesses, and this may be best accomplished by CT scan. CT scans can detect very small pleural effusions (< 10 mL) and are helpful in assessing empyema, pleural masses, and pleural thickening. Subpulmonic pleural effusions are those that appear to be below the lung and may be confused with an elevated hemidiaphragm.[82]

Thoracic ultrasound can also be used to identify pleural effusion and to guide thoracentesis.[82] MRI can identify pleural effusion, pleural tumors, and other chest wall soft tissue abnormities. **Figure 11-40** provides examples of pleural effusion as seen on imaging studies.

Interstitial Lung Disease

The category of interstitial lung disease (ILD) involves a very large group of disorders characterized by diffuse,

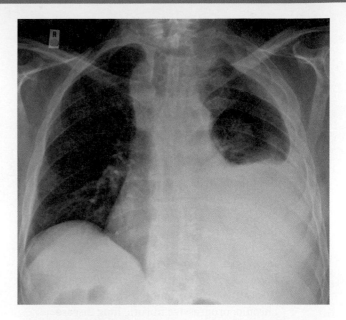

FIGURE 11-40 Pleural effusion. This image provides an example of a large, left-side pleural effusion as seen on conventional chest x-ray. Note the trachea and mediastinum are shifted to the right.

Modified from: Radiology Masterclass 2007–2013. Available at http://radiologymasterclass.co.uk/.

often chronic, lung injury. ILD typically involves varying degrees of lung inflammation resulting in the formation of scar tissue (e.g., pulmonary fibrosis). Dyspnea on exertion and a dry cough are often the main symptoms, though symptoms vary greatly with different forms of ILD.[85] Pulmonary function testing will often show a restrictive pattern with gas exchange abnormalities. The chief characteristic of imaging studies is diffuse lung disease. HRCT scans can be useful to identify imaging patterns associated with specific types of ILD. Most ILDs present with chronic, progressive symptoms, though some may present as acute disease (e.g., acute pneumonitis).[85]

ILD is sometimes grouped into categories that may include idiopathic interstitial pneumonitis (IIP), granulomatous disorders, connective tissue ILDs, drug-induced ILDs, and pulmonary vaculitis/diffuse alveolar hemorrhage–related ILD. Sometimes, the term *interstitial pneumonia* is used to refer to a number of interstitial diseases, but the term *pneumonia* is more accurately applied to lung tissue inflammation due to infection. Because there are a number of causes for ILD, most of which are not related to infection, the label *interstitial pneumonitis* may be more appropriate when referring to inflammation not caused by infection.[85] Specific ILDs include:[85]

- *Pneumoconiosis*: Dust-caused lung disease, including coal workers' pneumoconiosis (CWP), asbestosis, silicosis, and berylliosis.

- *Idiopathic interstitial pneumonias (IIP)*: These are ILDs of unknown origin. IIPs may be grouped by common clinical course, though IIPs can be sub-acute or chronic.
  - *Acute clinical course*: Acute interstitial pneumonia (AIP).
  - *Subacute clinical course*: Nonspecific interstitial pneumonia (NSIP—may be chronic in some patients); cryptogenic organizing pneumonia (COP), respiratory bronchiolitis ILD (RB-ILD), desquamative interstitial pneumonia (DIP), and lymphoid interstitial pneumonia (LIP).
  - *Subacute or chronic clinical course*: Usual interstitial pneumonia (UIP; may be fairly aggressive in some patients).
  - *Interstitial pulmonary fibrosis (IPF)*: Also known as cryptogenic fibrosing alveolitis, this is the most common form of IIP. IPF is a chronic, progressive fibrotic lung disease.
  - *Bronchiolitis obliterans with organizing pneumonia (BOOP)*: This is an older term that was used to refer to diffuse ILD that caused inflammation of the bronchioles, alveolar ducts, and alveolar wall. The term BOOP has been replaced by the term *cryptogenic organizing pneumonia* (COP).
- *Hypersensitivity pneumonitis:* Also referred to as *extrinsic allergic alveolitis*, hypersensitivity pneumonitis occurs in response to environmental exposure to specific agents such as birds (e.g., pigeon breeders' lung), moldy hay (e.g., farmers' lung), sugar cane (e.g., bagassosis), chemicals (e.g., epoxy resin lung), fungi (e.g., maple bark-strippers' disease), or bacteria (e.g., hot tub lung).
- *Connective tissue–related ILD*: Examples include systemic lupus erythematosus, rheumatoid arthritis, scleroderma, polymyositis, and Sjögren syndrome.
- *Drug-induced ILD*: Many drugs may induce ILD. Examples include chemotherapeutics (e.g., bleomycin, busulfan, gefitinib), antimicrobials (e.g., nitrofurantoin), cardiovascular agents (e.g., amiodarone), and illicit drugs (e.g., opiates, cocaine).
- *Sarcoidosis*: This is the most common type of granulomatous lung disease. Sarcoidosis is a multisystem disease characterized by formation non-caseating granulomas in the lung.
- *Radiation-exposure ILD*: ILD associated with radiation therapy for cancer.
- *Other ILDs*: Pulmonary Langerhans cell histiocytosis and lymphangioleiomyomatosis.

Imaging Considerations with ILD

An abnormal chest x-ray showing diffuse lung disease suggests the possibility of ILD. The most common imaging finding with ILD is a reticular pattern on the chest radiograph. Reticular interstitial patterns are lines that produce a mesh or lacelike appearance on the chest x-ray.[3] Nodular or mixed patterns are also not unusual with ILD. A nodular interstitial pattern is one of discrete opacities or nodules. A mixed pattern is one in which increased interstitial markings and alveolar filling are present. It must also be noted that a normal chest x-ray is sometimes seen in about 10% of patients with ILD.[86] As described earlier, Figure 11-7 contrasts the appearance of linear, reticular, nodular, and reticulonodular patterns as seen on imaging studies.

HRCT scans may be obtained in patients with diffuse ILD to help narrow the specific diagnosis. For example, the HRCT may discriminate between peripheral disease, central disease, and disease that is predominately in the upper lung zones.[86] ILDs that tend to have a peripheral lung zone distribution include asbestosis, connective tissue disease, COP/BOOP, and eosinophilic pneumonia. Lymphangitic carcinoma is an ILD associated with central disease and bronchovascular thickening.[86] ILDs associated with upper zone predominance include granulomatous disease (e.g., pulmonary histiocytosis X [eosinophilic granuloma], chronic hypersensitivity pneumonia, tuberculosis, histoplasmosis) and pneumoconiosis (silicosis, berylliosis, CWP).[86] IPF and asbestosis may have a peripheral or lower lung zone pattern; sarcoidosis may show upper zone predominance or a central pattern.[86] It must also be noted that ILD may be present even though chest x-ray and HRCT show a normal pattern.

HRCT may be alveolar (e.g., airspace opacities), reticular, or nodular. The following summarizes typical findings with some of the more important ILDs when viewed using HRCT:[86]

- *IPF*: Reticular pattern with peripheral lung zone or lower lung zone predominance. **Figure 11-41** provides an example of a reticular pattern as seen with IPF.
- *Sarcoidosis*: Nodular pattern with central or upper zone predominance (HRCT may also be normal). Bilateral hilar adenopathy further suggests sarcoidosis or other granulomatous disease. Figure 11-31 provides an example of the nodular pattern as seen with sarcoidosis.
- *Pneumoconiosis* (silicosis, CWP): nodular pattern with upper lung zone predominance (see **Figure 11-42**). Pneumoconiosis represents an immune response to inorganic antigens, such as silica.
- *Asbestosis*: Reticular with a peripheral or lower lung zone predominance (HRCT may also be normal). Pleural plaques with linear calcification may be present.
- *Hypersensitivity pneumonitis*: Hazy or ground-glass airspace opacities and/or nodules with upper lung zone predominance (HRCT may also be normal). Hypersensitivity pneumonitis represents an immune response to organic antigens. **Figure 11-43** provides an example of a patient with hypersensitivity pneumonitis.

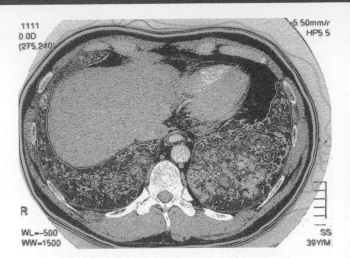

FIGURE 11-41 Reticular patterns as seen with interstitial pulmonary fibrosis (IPF).

© James Cavallini/Science Photo Library

■ *Chronic infectious disease*: Diseases such as TB or histoplasmosis show granulomatous inflammation with upper lung zone predominance. **Figure 11-44** provides an example of a patient with histoplasmosis.

Lung consolidation may also be seen with eosinophilic pneumonia, COP/BOOP, alveolar proteinosis, and alveolar cell carcinoma, whereas metastatic cancer may show as nodules.[86]

An echocardiogram may be used to assess the condition of the right side of the heart, which is

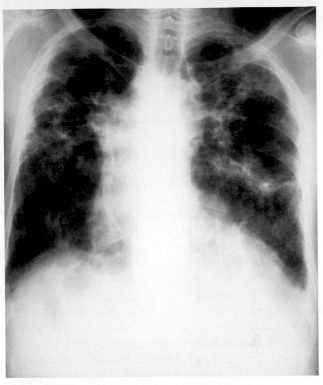

FIGURE 11-43 A chest x-ray showing a patient with hypersensitivity pneumonitis, also referred to a farmer's lung.

© Biophoto Associates/Science Source.

sometimes affected because of the chronic hypoxemia and increased pulmonary vascular resistance seen with chronic ILD. Treatment of ILD varies by underlying cause, but may include avoidance of precipitating

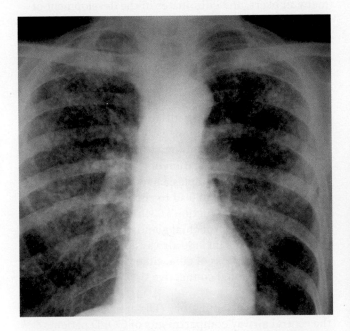

FIGURE 11-42 X-ray of silicosis from sandstone dust. Silicosis is an occupational respiratory disease caused by inhaling silica dust and is marked by inflammation and scarring in the form of nodular lesions in the upper lobes of the lungs.

© Biophoto Associates/Science Source.

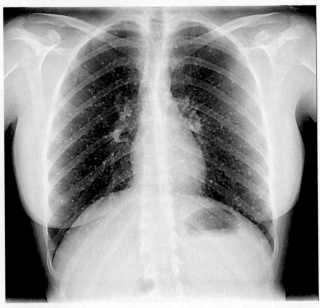

FIGURE 11-44 Histoplasmosis. A chest x-ray of a 23-year-old female with disseminated histoplasmosis.

© Z070/Custom Medical Stock Photo.

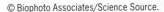

factors, use of immunosuppressants, supplemental oxygen therapy, and pulmonary rehabilitation.

Asthma

Asthma is characterized by airway inflammation, airway hyperreactivity, and reversible airflow obstruction.[87] Diagnosis is based on clinical manifestations, which typically include chronic cough, wheezing, and episodes of dyspnea.[87] Wheezing is not always present and, when present, may be caused by other diseases. Symptoms often get worse at night and early morning. Cough may be productive, and chest pain or chest tightness may occur. Diagnostic evaluation often includes pulmonary function testing before and after bronchodilator administration to document reversibility of airway obstruction. Bronchoprovocation testing by methacholine/mannitol challenge may be needed in cases in which airway obstruction is difficult to document due to its intermittent nature or in cases where cough may be the only symptom of obstruction. Other tests that are sometimes useful include skin tests to identify household and other antigens and blood tests for increased levels of IgE or eosinophilia. The management of asthma may include patient education, avoidance of triggers, use of rescue bronchodilators for acute episodes, and regular use of anti-inflammatory medications for control of moderate to severe asthma.

Radiological Considerations in Asthma

The chest x-ray is almost always normal in the asthma patient.[88] The primary value of a chest x-ray for the asthma patient is in cases where pulmonary infection may be present, such as pneumonia. The chest x-ray may also be used to help rule out other causes of the observed symptoms, especially in new-onset disease. Chest x-rays may be useful in difficult to manage asthma and when comorbid conditions are suspected.[88] For example, infiltrates in the difficult manage asthma patient may be due to allergic bronchopulmonary aspergillosis. In the case of allergic bronchopulmonary aspergillosis, eosinophilia, increased IgE, and *Aspergillus* precipitins may be found in the blood.

Specific conditions for which a chest x-ray should probably be obtained in the asthma patient include fever, chronic purulent sputum, hemoptysis, unexplained weight loss, clubbing, or inspiratory crackles.[88] Severe hypoxemia or moderate to severe airflow obstruction that does not reverse following bronchodilator administration should also prompt obtaining a chest x-ray in the asthma patient.[88] CT scans should be considered when the chest x-ray is abnormal and there is a need to further clarify the cause. For example, thin cut CT or HRCT may be obtained if bronchiectasis or ILD are suspected.[88]

During an asthma exacerbation, a chest x-ray may be obtained when infection or other comorbid conditions are suspected. During asthma exacerbation, the findings on chest x-ray are often consistent with air trapping and lung overinflation (pulmonary hyperinflation). Acute, severe asthma exacerbation represents a medical emergency. In addition to administration of inhaled β-agonists, with or without inhaled anticholinergics; oxygen therapy; and systemic glucocorticoids, support of ventilation is sometimes required. The respiratory care clinician must be on guard for the development of pneumothorax, pneumomediastinum, pneumonia, and atelectasis, though these complications are relatively rare.[88]

Chronic Obstructive Pulmonary Disease

Chronic obstructive pulmonary disease (COPD) includes chronic bronchitis, emphysema, and small airways disease. Often these conditions are present in the same patient. Specifically, emphysema is defined as a permanent enlargement of the air spaces distal to the terminal bronchiole.[87] Chronic bronchitis is defined as a chronic cough with sputum production for more than 3 months of each of the last 2 years.[87] Often, COPD patients exhibit both emphysema and chronic bronchitis. Small airways disease refers to inflammation of the airways less than 2 mm in diameter (respiratory bronchiolitis).

Characteristics of COPD include irreversible airflow disease. Tobacco smoking is the primary risk factor for COPD, though inhalation of other toxic gases and particles may also be at fault.[93] The disease begins with inflammation of the lungs, already the case for many smokers, and culminates in the development of pathological lesions specific to COPD.[78] An imbalance of antiproteinases and proteinases may also be at play; along with inflammation, oxidative stress is also part of the classical pathogenesis.[78] The pattern of pathogenic mechanisms in COPD induces pathologic changes that, in turn, induce physiologic abnormalities, including air flow limitations and hyperinflation, mucus hypersecretion and ciliary dysfunction, gas exchange aberrations, systemic effects, and pulmonary hypertension.[19]

One clinical manifestation of COPD is the occurrence of goblet cell metaplasia and bronchial gland hypertrophy, which can lead to chronic bronchitis and excessive mucus production.[1] Cellular infiltrates may also be seen in the bronchial glands.[78] Changes visible in the airway walls include airway epithelium squamous metaplasia, loss of cilia, ciliary dysfunction, and growth of additional connective tissue and smooth muscle.[19,78]

A variety of inflammatory cells are predominant in the central airway compartments of COPD patients.[78,87] These include lymphocytes (mostly the CD8+ types) and, as the ailment progresses, neutrophils.[78] Neutrophils, lymphocytes, and macrophages may also be seen in the airspaces.[78] The radiograph of a person with chronic bronchitis may show a thick muscle bundle and gland enlargement.[3] If the enlarged glands are more closely observed, evidence of chronic inflammation involving mononuclear, polymorphonuclear, and plasma cells may be seen.[55]

In peripheral airway manifestations of COPD, bronchiolitis may be present early on in the disease, along with an abnormal extension of squamous metaplasia and goblet cells.[19] The inflammatory cells in the airspaces and airway walls are similar to those seen in the larger airways. Increased collagen deposition and fibrosis appear as the condition progressively worsens.[19]

Emphysema, defined as pathologic air space enlargement distal to the terminal bronchioles, frequently occurs in the pulmonary parenchyma of patients with COPD.[87] Emphysema often results in the loss of alveolar attachments, which contributes to peripheral airway collapse.[87]

The two primary types of emphysema are distinguished based on the distribution of damage in the acinus.[87] *Centrilobular emphysema* is primarily characterized by destruction and dilatation of the respiratory bronchioles, whereas *panlobular emphysema* is characterized by destruction of the entire acinus.[19] The former is the most commonly seen type of COPD emphysema and primarily affects the upper zones of the lungs; the latter is most prevalent in individuals who have a deficiency of α-1 antitrypsin and primarily affects the lower zones of the lungs.[62]

Early in its course, COPD is marked by microscopic lesions.[3] Eventually these may evolve into macroscopic lesions known as **bullae**, which are categorized as emphysematous spaces > 1 cm in diameter.[62] Bullous disorder can occur even in the absence of COPD.

Persisting throughout the duration of the disease, the alveolar wall inflammatory cell pattern is identical to that seen within the airways. Some studies suggest that inflammation in the distal and proximal airspaces persists even after COPD patients quit smoking.[62]

Pulmonary vascular changes start soon after development of the disease. At first, these changes involve endothelial dysfunction and thickening of vessel walls.[83] What follows is an increase in the amount of vascular smooth muscle tissue and inflammatory cell infiltration of vessel walls, including CD8+ T lymphocytes and macrophages.[83] In the more advanced stages of the disease, emphysematous capillary bed destruction and collagen deposition occur.[83] These mechanical changes invariably induce pulmonary hypertension and cor pulmonale.[83]

The pathophysiology behind the inflammation that accompanies COPD is marked by an increase in macrophages, neutrophils, and T lymphocytes throughout the lung—a factor that affects the degree of airflow limitation.[83] Some patients also exhibit an increase in eosinophils; this is most notable in exacerbated cases of the disease.[83]

The inflammatory cells at work can release various inflammatory mediators and cytokines; however, the inflammatory mechanisms of COPD differ from those seen in bronchial asthma patients.[83] Inflammatory changes can persist even after patients quit smoking, though why this is so is not known.[83]

COPD brings about a proteinase and antiprotease imbalance.[83] Cigarette smoking and other risk factors for COPD, in addition to causing inflammation, can also induce oxidative stress.[83] This oxidative stress motivates inflammatory cells, such as neutrophils and macrophages, to emit proteinases but also helps deactivate various antiproteinases through oxidation.[83] Neutrophil elastase is a powerful inducer of mucus secretion and mucous gland hyperplasia; neutrophils are also responsible for parenchymal destruction in COPD.[83]

Oxidative stress contributes to the pathology of COPD by oxidizing biological molecules capable of cell disruption, destroying the extracellular matrix, deactivating important antioxidant defense mechanisms, and altering gene expression.[83] Some markers of oxidative stress in the lungs include exhaled condensates, urine, hydrogen peroxide, lipid peroxidation products, and nitric oxide.[83]

The pathologic mechanisms thus far described create the abnormal architecture leading to COPD: ciliary dysfunction, mucus hypersecretion, airflow hyperinflation and limitation, gas exchange abnormalities, systemic effects, and pulmonary hypertension.[83] Expiratory airflow limitation is the pathologic hallmark of COPD; unfortunately, it is usually incurable.[78]

Pathologic ventilation–perfusion distribution ratios are the primary abnormal gas exchange mechanisms in COPD.[93] Pulmonary hypertension (often caused by untreated hypoxemia) occurs later in the course of the disease, well after serious gas exchange abnormalities are established.[19] Finally, COPD also involves extrapulmonary effects, including skeletal muscle wasting and systemic inflammation.[78] These systemic breakdowns limit the amount of exercise COPD patients can engage in, thus worsening their prognosis, regardless of pulmonary capacity.[19]

Pulmonary Emphysema

Pulmonary emphysema can be described as an irregular, inalterable enlargement of the airspaces farthest from the terminal bronchioles, including damage to the alveolar wall, although without the clear presence of fibrosis.[19] The disease is one of a heterogeneous collection of abnormalities within the framework of COPD and encompasses four distinctive, yet connected, morphologic subtypes: paracicatricial emphysema, paraseptal emphysema, panlobular emphysema, and centrilobular emphysema. The panlobular and centrilobular subtypes are described above. Other types of pulmonary emphysema are idiopathic giant bullous emphysema (also called vanishing lung syndrome), congenital lobar emphysema, and pulmonary interstitial emphysema.[19]

It is important to distinguish the clinical manifestations of emphysema from the symptoms of chronic bronchitis.[1] Those afflicted with emphysema tend to be hypocapnic and are sometimes unkindly referred to as "pink puffers."[19] In contrast, chronic bronchitis is characterized by hypercapnea and cyanosis, which has led to victims being described as "blue bloaters." Medically speaking, the two conditions both fall under the heading of COPD.[19]

Radiologic Manifestations of COPD

The conventional chest radiograph is useful primarily to evaluate the COPD patient for comorbidities or to rule out alternative diagnoses. Comorbidities that must be considered include lung cancer, bronchiectasis, ILD, congestive heart failure, and pleural disease. The chest x-ray should also be employed when pneumonia or pneumothorax is suspected.

Typical chest x-ray findings with COPD include lung hyperinflation as indicated by an increased retrosternal air space and flattened diaphragms (especially on lateral view). The space between the ribs may appear to be increased, and the lungs may appear large and hyperlucent. The heart shadow may appear long and narrow.[87] With advanced COPD, there may be signs of cardiac enlargement, pulmonary hypertension, and cor pulmonale. For example, the hilar vascular shadows may be increased.[87] CT scans are helpful for the detection of emphysema, but not asthma or chronic bronchitis.

Except in advanced cases of emphysema accompanied by bullous formations, the chest x-ray is not a reliable method of diagnosing emphysema. CT is the modality most often chosen for diagnosing emphysema, and often HRCT is preferred.[87] HRCT, however, is not needed for the diagnosis of COPD. At present,

however, a diagnosis of emphysema in patients is never completely reliable because of the difficulty of confirming the pathology.[3] For example, approximately 20% of patients with emphysema do not exhibit signs of disease on CT scan; by the same token, some 40% of patients with abnormal CT findings have normal pulmonary function tests.[87] In many cases, however, CT is able to differentiate between panacinar (panlobular), centriacinar (centrilobular), and paraseptal emphysema.[87] **Figure 11-45** provides an example of typical imaging findings seen with COPD.

MRI is still under investigation as a means of diagnosing emphysema and, for that matter, all pulmonary parenchymal pathologies.[35] Dynamic-breathing MRI, however, may someday play a key role in evaluating pulmonary emphysema.

Treatment of COPD includes smoking cessation, avoidance of complications, bronchodilator therapy, oxygen therapy in hypoxemic patients, and pulmonary rehabilitation. Inhaled corticosteroids may improve symptoms and reduce exacerbations.

Neoplastic Disorders of the Lung

Solitary Pulmonary Nodules

Solitary lung nodules are seen in 1 to 2 out of every 1000 chest x-rays.[89] **Figure 11-46** shows a solitary pulmonary nodule. Roughly 30% to 50% of these nodules in adults are malignant and 10% to 15% are benign tumors.[89] The remaining nodules tend to be infectious. These types of tumors comprise a heterogeneous class of neoplastic lesions with pulmonary structure origin. They include hamartomas, bronchial adenomas, and a class of uncommon neoplasms that includes fibromas, chondromas, lipomas, leiomyomas, teratomas,

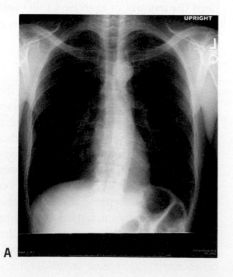
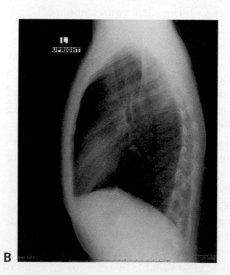

A   B

FIGURE 11-45 COPD. Note flattened diagrams, blunting of costophrenic angles, increased AP diameter, increased retrosternal air space, and lung overinflation as demonstrated by dark, hyperlucent lung fields.

(A) Courtesy of Laura Vasquez; (B) Courtesy of Laura Vasquez

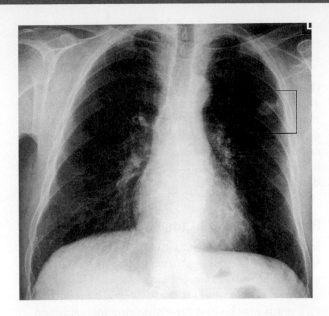

FIGURE 11-46 Solitary pulmonary nodule. Note solitary pulmonary nodule within bracket.

Courtesy of Laura Vasquez.

hemangiomas, endometriomas, pseudolymphomas, and bronchial glomus growths. Risk of a pulmonary nodule being cancer is age related; it occurs in 40% to 60% of smokers aged 40 to 60 years.

Although benign pulmonary masses are generally treatable and not as dangerous as malignant tumors, they can nevertheless lead to serious disease, especially if the lesions are obstructive. Diseases attributable to benign pulmonary masses include atelectasis, pneumonia, and hemoptysis. Additionally, benign tumors have the potential to become malignant. Fewer women than men succumb to benign tumors; the average age of those afflicted is 56 years old.

Solitary pulmonary nodules (SPNs) may be found incidentally on chest x-rays or CT scans. Defined as round lesions < 3 cm in diameter that are enveloped by pulmonary parenchyma and lack other abnormal classifications, SPNs are found at a rate of 1 to 2 per 1000 routine chest x-rays.[89] They are discovered with even more frequency on CT scans.[89] The discovery of an SPN is cause for concern because it may be an indication of primary lung cancer or solitary metastasis from an area outside the lungs. Patients are usually asymptomatic and have undergone a chest x-ray for an unrelated reason.[89] Granulomas and hamartomas account for the majority of SPNs.[89] Statistically, 30% prove to be malignant, but because CT scans now routinely pick up smaller nodules, the malignancy rate may decline.[89]

Lung Carcinoma

Lung carcinoma (i.e., lung cancer) is the most prevalent cause of mortality from neoplasia in developed nations.[90] Formerly restricted mostly to males, lung carcinoma now also affects many women between the ages of 40 and 70.[90] These growths are divided into two groups: *non-small-cell lung cancers* (NSCLC) and *small-cell lung carcinoma* (SCLC).[48] Most of these develop in the main bronchi, whereas others develop within the peripheral airways or alveoli.[48]

Lung cancer originates in the cells that line the bronchi, bronchioles, or alveoli.[48] As noted, there are two primary types of lung cancer: NSCLC, which is the most prevalent type, and SCLC, which accounts for approximately 20% of cases.[48] Mixed small-cell and non-small-cell lung cancer is a combination of both categories. Cancer that spreads to the lungs from elsewhere in the body is classified as *metastatic lung cancer.*[90]

Lung cancer is one of the deadliest types of cancer for both men and women.[90] It is estimated that more people die from lung cancer than from prostate, breast, ovarian, and colon cancer combined. The disease is more commonly found in older adults; rarely it is be found in patients younger than 45.[91] The prognosis is generally not good, especially in advanced cases when the cancer has spread.[91] Cigarette smoking is a leading risk factor for the disease, but lung cancer can also strike nonsmokers.[48]

Clinical Manifestations

Lung cancer is often found when performing a chest x-ray or CT scan for other medical concerns.[92] Unfortunately, signs and symptoms of lung cancer typically occur only when the disease is advanced.[89] Symptoms include coughing that does not abate, coughing of mucus with blood, weight loss, hoarseness, and pain that does not go away.[89]

SCLC occurs almost exclusively in heavy smokers and those with consistent and extensive exposure to a known carcinogen.[48] NSCLC is actually a group of lung cancers with similar characteristics.[48] The three main types of NSCLC are adenocarcinoma, large-cell carcinoma, and squamous cell carcinoma. Adenocarcinomas are sometimes seen in the peripheral or outer areas of the lungs, whereas squamous cell carcinomas are often centrally located in the bronchi.[48]

The classifications of SCLC and NSCLC are based on the appearance of tumor cells under the microscope.[48] These cells grow and spread differently.[91] SCLC is the most predatory and most quickly growing type of lung cancer. Generally associated with cigarette smoking, only 1% of SCLC masses occur in nonsmokers.[48] SCLC spreads rapidly, leading to its eventual discovery. SCLC cells are sometimes called "oat cell" carcinomas.[48]

Lung cancer often leads to pleural effusion, which is one reason to check for cancer when pleural effusion is diagnosed.[48] When looking for cancer, clinicians need to consider the possibility of metastasis even if only one cancerous mass is found on an x-ray.[93] Metastasized cancer spread to other parts of the body may include vital organs, bones, and the brain.[93]

Chest x-rays may reveal abnormal nodules or masses, but CT scans may pick up smaller or less-noticeable malignancies.[94] A physician may perform a biopsy using bronchoscopy, mediastinoscopy, or needle biopsy, often using medical imaging to guide needle placement for tissue sampling.[95]

The progression of lung cancer is broken down into stages.[48] Medical imaging may be used to ascertain the stage of a cancer once it has been detected.[95] A stage 1 cancer is still within the lungs and has not spread to the lymph nodes; the mass is usually < 5 cm. In stage 2, the mass may be > 5 cm or it may be smaller but also involve lymph nodes or other nearby structures, such as the pleura, chest wall, or diaphragm.[83] In stage 3, the tumor often has grown rather large and has spread to the mediastinal lymph nodes or other organs near the lungs; alternatively, stage 3 may involve a relatively small mass but include malignancy in lymph nodes outside the lungs.[3] Stage 4 cancer has metastasized to both lungs and to other parts of the body.[83]

SCLC is sometimes classified as being either limited or extensive, meaning it is either limited to one lung or has spread beyond the initially affected lung.[48] Radiation therapy is sometimes used to treat lung cancer. The patient can be subjected to x-rays, or radioactive substances can be introduced into the body through needles, catheters, or seeds and placed near the cancer, as in brachytherapy.[91] This may be combined with other treatments. If the cancer is very small, stereotactic body therapy may be utilized.[91] In this procedure, a concentrated beam of radiation is aimed from different angles at the specific lung cancer.[91] The treatment may be repeated as needed.

Medical imaging can also detect benign masses in the lungs.[91] Such masses do not spread and can usually be removed, thus preventing them from becoming malignant.[91] In contrast, malignant tumors are always destructive and usually pose the threat of spreading to other parts of the body, or metastasizing. The liver, brain, adrenal glands, and bones are the most likely destinations for cancer metastasis.[91]

Radiography and Lung Cancer

Masses revealed by chest x-rays may include calcified nodules and benign tumors, such as hamartomas, which may be mistaken for lung cancer.[56] CT scans are often a better tool for spotting lung cancer, and PET scans may be best for identifying metastasized masses.[94] MRI may be used to better identify the location of tumors as well as to map out treatment strategies; it may also be used to ascertain the effect of treatment.[94] Other techniques for diagnosis include bronchoscopy, needle biopsy, and thoracentesis. **Figure 11-47** provides an example of lung cancer as seen on conventional chest radiograph and CT scan.

It should be noted that PET and CT scans can sometimes lead to a misdiagnosis of lung cancer when inflammation of the lungs is misinterpreted as a malignant lesion.[94] For inflammatory lesions, diffusion-weighted MRI can be more accurate and spare individuals without malignant pathology from undergoing additional procedures.[94]

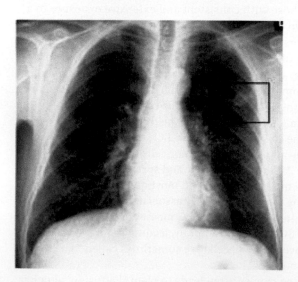
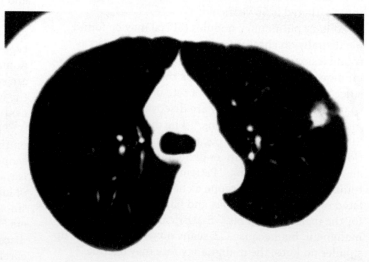

FIGURE 11-47 Lung cancer as seen on chest x-ray and CT. Note the well-defined area of increased density in the left lung on chest x-ray (box), which corresponds to the area of opacity in CT scan.

Courtesy of Laura Vasquez.

Miscellaneous Chest Conditions

When reviewing medical imaging tests that have been requested to further explore symptoms, the results of a physical exam, or blood work findings, radiologists often make discoveries that are unrelated to the reasons for ordering the imaging but nevertheless demand immediate attention. In fact, many diagnoses are rendered based on findings that are totally unrelated or only tangentially related to the condition that caused the patient to seek medical attention in the first place. Such findings may be loosely labeled as miscellaneous chest conditions or incidental lesions.

For example, chest CT is often used to assess disorders involving the mediastinum, the lung, the pleura, the diaphragm, or the chest wall.[26] It is common to incidentally find both malignant and benign breast lesions on these chest CT scans.[26] Radiologists using chest CT scans should be fully aware of the manifestations of various breast diseases so that they do not overlook or dismiss such findings.[3]

Placement of Chest Tubes and Lines and Endotracheal Tubes

ICU patients require advanced care and monitoring involving many types of technology, some of which are utilized for extended time periods.[20] It is the responsibility of those who monitor patients in intensive care units to make sure that tubes, lines, and other medical devices are correctly placed, functioning properly, and benefiting the patient. Portable chest x-rays are extremely useful in monitoring the patient's condition and assessing the position of lines, tubes, and other supportive devices.[20] It is recommended that a chest x-ray be taken immediately following the placement of tubes, catheters, and lines to ensure that no damage has been caused during their insertion and to verify that they are properly positioned.[20]

Nasogastric Tubes

Nasogastric (NG) tubes and orogastric (OG) tubes are used to feed patients and to aspirate gastric contents; in either case, the tip of the device should rest within the stomach.[20] NG tubes come with multiple side holes and terminal lead balls that can help identify the tip of the device. Ideally, the tip of the NG tube rests with its side holes within the gastric antrum.[20] The recommended procedure to ascertain proper placement is to push air into the NG tube while simultaneously auscultating with a stethoscope laid flat over the stomach. If the side holes remain within the esophagus, there is a chance of aspiration. Consequently, the tip of the NG tube should be located at least 10 cm inferiorly to the gastroesophageal junction.[20] The tip of a nasoduodenal feeding tube should be positioned at least 10 to 12 cm into the small bowel. Mistakenly inserting an NG tube into the bronchus or trachea can cause pneumonia, pulmonary laceration, or pulmonary contusion. Esophageal and pharyngeal perforations are also possibilities, although rare.[20]

Endotracheal Tubes

Endotracheal (ET) tubes are used to ventilate the lungs and to prevent aspiration.[7,20] Each ET tube has a cuff and a terminal hole. The appropriate positioning of an ET tube is with the distal tip at least 2 cm superior to the carina in the adult patient (range of 2 to 6 cm above the carina).[7] If the carina is not visible, the tip of the ET tube should be approximately at the level of the medial clavicular ends.[7,20] Ideally, the tip of the tube should rest midway between the carina and the larynx (i.e., middle one-third of the trachea) to avoid trauma to these structures and to prevent complications such as inadvertent extubation or unintentional mainstem bronchus intubation. ET tubes have distance markers, and the insertion depth of for an oral tube is about 21 cm in adult females and about 23 cm in adult males. Following insertion, placement in the trachea should immediately be verified using an end-tidal carbon dioxide (CO_2) detector and assessment of adequate bilateral breath sounds during spontaneous or mechanically supported (e.g., ventilator or manual resuscitator bag) breathing.[7] ET tube placement is then verified using a portable chest x-ray, and the tube position is adjusted as indicated.

Typically, if the ET tube is advanced too far, it will enter and reside in the right mainstem bronchus. An unintentional bronchial intubation may cause collapse of the contralateral lung, a pneumothorax, or hyperinflation of the ipsilateral lung. Inadvertent esophageal intubation is another possible complication; this condition can be diagnosed clinically. As noted, lung placement is confirmed by breath sounds and expired CO_2. Esophageal intubation is suggested by the absence of breath sounds and expired CO_2 and rapid decline in the patient's clinical condition. With accidental esophageal intubation, air movement can also sometimes be heard over the stomach when positive pressure is applied to the ET tube. Radiographically, esophageal intubation may be detected by seeing an overdistended stomach. **Figure 11-48** contrasts proper ET tube placement versus placement in the right mainstem bronchus (bronchial intubation).

Tracheostomy

The tip of a tracheostomy tube should rest approximately halfway between the carina and the tracheal stoma. The position of this type of tube, unlike the endotracheal tube, should be maintained with neck extension and flexion.[96] The tube's width should be two-thirds of the tracheal width; the tracheal wall should not be distended by the cuff.[96] The tube should rest parallel to the trachea. Potential complications of tube misplacement are pneumomediastinum, subcutaneous emphysema, pneumothorax, hemorrhage, and

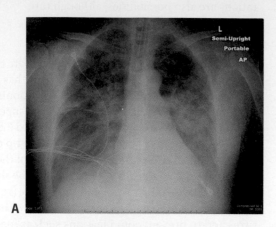
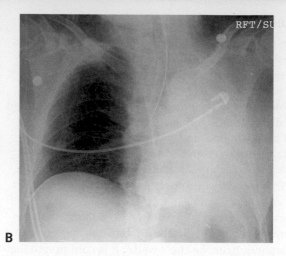

FIGURE 11-48 Tracheal and right mainstem intubation. (A) Endotracheal tube properly positioned with tip in the middle third of the trachea 2–6 cm above the carina. (B) A 25-year-old female with an endotracheal tube in the right mainstem bronchus with total left lung atelectasis.

(A) Courtesy of Laura Vasquez; (B) Courtesy of Laura Vasquez.

tracheal stenosis. Hematoma can cause widening of the superior mediastinum.[3]

Chest Drainage Tubes

An intercostal chest drainage tube, also known as a pleural tube or thoracostomy tube, is sometimes inserted in the treatment of pneumothorax, hemothorax, or pleural effusion. The chest tube insertion site varies with the indication. For a pneumothorax, the chest tube is generally inserted through the fourth or fifth intercostal space at the midaxillary or anterior axillary anterior line.[52] It is then guided posterior-inferiorly to address effusion and anterior-superiorly to address a pneumothorax.[53] The chest tube has a terminal hole and side holes. The side holes can be distinguished on a chest x-ray.[3] No side holes should rest outside of the pleural cavity, and the tube should not appear to float above the effusion.[53] Misplacement of these tubes occurs in about 10% of cases, making them ineffective or only marginally effective. At times, the tip of the tube may rest in a fissure or even within the lung parenchyma. Lateral and frontal chest x-rays are sometimes necessary to verify properly position these tubes, though recently bedside ultrasound techniques have been used to aid in chest tube placement.

Central Venous Lines

Central venous lines are catheters that provide long-term venous access. They can be used for a number of reasons, including hemodialysis, hemodynamic pressure monitoring, and administration of nutrition and medications.[52] Central venous lines are inserted via a major vein (internal jugular, subclavian, or femoral vein) into the superior vena cava. The tip of the line should be distally located to the farthest venous valve, at the junction of the internal jugular and the subclavian veins.[52] Viewed on a chest x-ray, the valve's position corresponds to the inner border of the first rib. Central venous lines, in general, have two or three lumens. If the tip of the line is located in the lower portion of the superior vena cava, all these orifices will be distal to the farthest venous valve. Proper central venous line position is then verified using medical imaging techniques.[52] Portable chest radiography or **fluoroscopy** are commonly used, though ultrasound is being increasingly employed. In the operating room setting, transesophageal echocardiography may be employed. **Figure 11-49** provides examples of proper and improper central venous line position, as seen on chest x-ray.[53]

Swan-Ganz Catheter

A Swan-Ganz catheter is a balloon-tipped, flow-directing pulmonary artery catheter. The balloon inflates so that it can measure capillary wedge pressure.[52] This device is often used to monitor circulation hemodynamics as part of the management a variety of critical pathologies.[52] To determine capillary wedge pressure and pulmonary artery pressure, the catheter's tip must be in the left or right pulmonary artery. Complications are avoided by making sure that the tip of the catheter is not more than 1 cm lateral to the margin of the mediastinum.[53]

As a general rule, when viewed on a chest x-ray, the Swan-Ganz catheter should not go past the pulmonary hilum; if it does, it must be retracted.[52] To diminish the possibility of pulmonary infarction, the balloon is inflated only during insertion and for PCWP

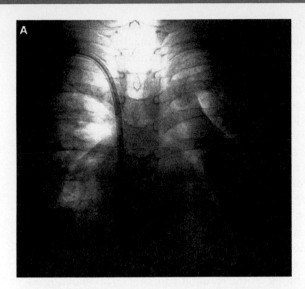 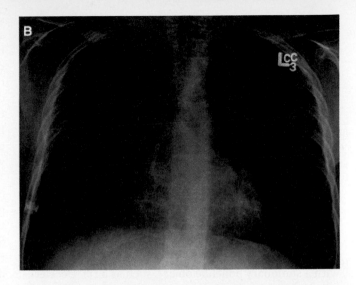

FIGURE 11-49 Central venous catheter placement. (A) Improper placement of a central venous catheter with the tip at the inferior vena cava–right atrial junction. (B) Corrected central line placement following repositioning. Note the upright PA chest radiograph confirms that the tip is optimally positioned within the superior aspect of the right atrium.

(A) Courtesy of Laura Vasquez; (B) Courtesy of Laura Vasquez.

measurement.[53] Other possible complications include intracardial knotting, pulmonary artery perforation, cardiac perforation, arrhythmias, and misplaced insertion into the inferior vena cava.

Other Medical Devices

Medical imaging is an indispensable tool in monitoring the placement and functionality of many devices inserted in patients. Medical imaging may help guide the placement of a device, determine its correct position, or ascertain if a misplacement has occurred.[52] Medical imaging is often used in conjunction with insertion of implantable cardiac pacemakers, mechanical circulatory assistance devices, and other implantable devices. Medical imaging makes it possible to ensure that these devices are properly positioned and function when and how they should, thus reducing injury and mortality from device misplacement. Additional examples of medical devices sometimes assessed using imaging techniques include enteric drainage and feeding tubes, implantable cardiac defibrillators, ventricular assist devices, and intraesophageal monitoring devices (e.g., temperature probe, pressure monitor, pH monitor).

Inferior vena cava filters (IVC filters) are sometimes inserted at the bedside of critically ill patients (e.g., DVT or pulmonary embolus).[52] Their insertion is guided using portable radiographic equipment or with the use of an intravascular ultrasonographic scanning machine.[52] Filters can be deployed in the superior vena cava to help prevent fatal or symptomatic pulmonary embolisms in patients with upper extremity DVT.[53]

Pulmonary embolisms are seen in approximately 12% of patients with upper extremity DVT.[52] Treatment can include elevation of the affected arm, rest, thrombolysis, and anticoagulation therapy. Central venous catheters play a role in 17% to 47% of upper extremity DVTs.[53] The placement of a superior vena cava filter calls for the utilization of a modified technique.[53] A filter made for jugular access is implanted using a femoral approach to maintain the correct filter orientation; alternatively, a filter made for femoral access may be implanted using a jugular approach.[53] The Gunther Tulip filter was approved by the FDA in 2003. Because this filter is constructed from nonferromagnetic conichrome, it may be useful for patients who may subsequently require MRI scans.[53] Although it can only be inserted and retrieved via a jugular approach, this device may nevertheless be useful for a number of patients.[5] Many IVC filters are now removable and may be placed in patients that cannot be anticoagulated due to acute bleeding but removed weeks to months later.

Imaging the Trauma Patient

Properly conducted imaging of trauma patients is invaluable in guiding appropriate treatment and diagnosis for patients whose lives may depend on the steps taken by medical personnel.[3] For example, CT scanning immediately upon admission to a trauma center can make a big difference in outcome, especially if head or chest trauma is involved.[26] Multidetector computed tomography (MDCT) can be very effective in the assessment of complicated, multifaceted, internal injuries of trauma patients; most experts say that MDCT sets the standard in diagnostic potential.[26]

Although all trauma is serious, chest trauma is of particular concern. Blunt thoracic trauma accounts for 20% to 25% of trauma fatalities and is a primary complicating factor in another 50% of trauma-associated fatalities.[25] The two most common causes of chest trauma are falls and motor vehicle accidents (MVAs).[25] Other causes include assaults, stabbings, gunshot wounds, and sports injuries.[25] Blunt-force trauma is the most common type of chest trauma; the three primary mechanisms by which it may occur are direct impact, thoracic compression, and deceleration injuries.[26] Direct impact is most likely to occur in a motor vehicle accident, from a direct blow to the chest, or a fall.[26] Thoracic compression occurs when soft tissue collides with a stationary bonelike object, such as a rib. Deceleration injuries occur when a person keeps moving while the vehicle in which the person is riding stops suddenly, as when a car hits a tree.[25]

The entire bony thorax, including the clavicles, the ribs, the scapulae, and the vertebrae, should be carefully examined and assessed for fractures.[26] Particular attention should be paid to *rib fractures*, which are among the most frequently seen fractures in trauma cases; fractured ribs can puncture vital organs and vessels.[3] Portable x-ray imaging of supine patients is not particularly sensitive and may reveal only about 20% of all rib fractures. Fractures of the first rib may indicate severe blunt chest trauma and may be associated with aortic tears, bronchial tears, and subclavian vessel injuries. If a fractured rib punctures a lung, it may cause a pneumothorax.[26]

Flail chest is said to be present if five or more ribs in a row are fractured or if three or more ribs have segmental fractures, meaning they are broken in two places (thus the flail portion of the chest moves inward on inspiration and outward on expiration in a spontaneously breathing patient).[26] It is important to recognize a flail chest because respiratory failure may develop from paradoxical motion of the flail segment.[87] In cases of flail chest, soft tissue should be evaluated for opacification and subcutaneous emphysema.[87] The lung fields may reveal pneumothorax, consolidation suggesting lung contusion, and/or hemothorax.[26] Radiographic aberrations of the mediastinum, especially widening of the mediastinum, pneumomediastinum, or shift of the mediastinum, may indicate airway rupture, tension pneumothorax, and aortic disruptions.[3] Additionally, evaluation of the cardiac silhouette can assist in the diagnosis of blunt myocardial injury, including *pericardial tamponade*.[26] Pericardial tamponade as a result of blunt trauma is very rare. **Figure 11-50** provides an example of flail chest as viewed on conventional radiograph.

Subclavian vascular injury should be suspected if the patient has fractures of the first three ribs, the scapula, and the clavicle, especially if accompanied by significant extrapleural hematoma, fracture displacement, or radiologic evidence of mediastinal hemorrhage.[25] Sternal fractures are rare; if one is suspected, oblique and lateral thoracic views may be required for diagnosis. If a fracture of the sternum is present and the chest x-ray shows an abnormal mediastinal contour, injury to the great vessels is also a possibility. As noted, pericardial tamponade as a result of blunt trauma is very rare.

Pulmonary contusion following traumatic injury may be identified by airspace opacification on chest radiograph or CT. Air bronchograms may be absent because the smaller airways are likely to be filled with blood.[3] Shadowing may be extensive, patchy, or confluent; diffuse, multifocal, or solitary; and bilateral or unilateral, depending on the traumatic force.[25] Focal hematomas may exhibit cavitation as they are forming.[26] Consolidation distribution is nonsegmental and usually progresses quickly in the first day or two following injury.[26] Pulmonary contusion may be associated with nearby rib fractures and homogeneous infiltrates, which tend to be nonsegmental and peripheral.[26] Such injuries often resolve rapidly; in fact, the lungs may return to normal within a week.[26] When the injury does not resolve promptly, there is a possibility of superimposed atelectasis, infection, aspiration, or a laceration-associated blood clot.[25] Contusions are usually associated with the maximum impact area, although countercoup injuries are also possible.[25] Additional fractures may overlay the area of impact.[25] Pulmonary lacerations are often associated with pulmonary contusion, but are generally not detectable on a chest x-ray.[25] CT scans are more sensitive for this purpose than standard x-rays.[3]

Diaphragmatic rupture occurs in 8.8% of blunt thoracic trauma cases.[25] The chest x-ray is abnormal in 77% of patients, but the results are usually nonspecific and the diagnosis is often missed.[25] Signs of a diaphragmatic rupture on chest x-rays include a raised irregular or asymmetric diaphragm, loss of the diaphragmatic contour, the presence of a nasogastric or bowel tube in the chest, a mediastinal shift to the opposite side, and elevation of the hemidiaphragm.[26] Diaphragmatic injuries should be suspected in situations involving a left-sided, penetrating thoracic wound inferior to the fourth intercostal space anteriorly, the sixth intercostal space laterally, or the eighth intercostal space posteriorly.[3] Consecutive chest images can display the progressive changes indicative of a diaphragmatic rupture.[8] Pleural effusions, atelectasis, lung contusions, or paralysis of the phrenic nerve can mimic or mask traumatic diaphragmatic tears.[3] Ruptured hemidiaphragms are more commonly seen on the left side than on the right. Nonspecific signs can include apparently elevated hemidiaphragms, distortion or obliteration of the contours of the hemidiaphragm, pleural effusion, and contralateral mediastinal displacement.[8] The appearance of gas-filled

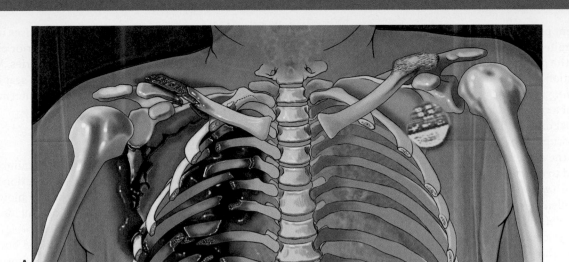

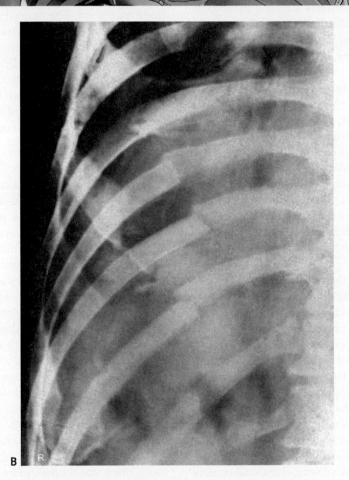

FIGURE 11-50 Flail chest. Flail chest is defined as multiple adjacent rib fractures each broken in two or more places. The result is an unstable chest wall that tends to sink in upon inspiration. A common complication of flail chest is pneumothorax and patients may also require ventilator support.

(A) © Nucleus Medical Media/Visuals Unlimited, Inc.; (B) © BSIP/Science Source.

viscera in the thorax, especially if accompanied by a focal constriction traversing a gas-filled bowel section, is pathognomonic.[8]

Tracheobronchial tears are seen in approximately 1.5% of blunt chest trauma cases.[97] These injuries often go unnoticed on initial exams, leading to delayed diagnoses.[97] In 80% of patients with bronchial fractures, the fracture is located within 2 to 0.5 cm of the carina.[97] A bronchial tear should be considered when radiographs display worsening subcutaneous emphysema, a persistent pneumothorax despite proper placement of chest drains, the presence of a pneumomediastinum, and/or the presence of a pneumothorax.[97] Tracheal transection may occur in cases of neck trauma. A *fallen-lung sign* is the unexpected or unusual manifestation of a collapsed lobe or lung in connection with a bronchial injury.[97] This peculiarity is believed to derive from disruption of the normal hilar lung attachments, forcing the collapsed lung to droop peripherally, as opposed to centrally.[97]

Aortic injury should be considered when chest x-rays show widening of the mediastinum by more than 8 cm, a loss of definition of the aortic knuckle, nasogastric tube displacement to the right of the T4 spinous process, and the presence of left apical pleural caps.[98] Additional suggestive evidence includes widened paraspinal lines, disappearance of the descending aorta line, and a right paratracheal stripe that has widened by more than 5 mm.[107] A normal chest x-ray has a negative predictive value of 98%.[3]

Esophageal rupture may occur due to trauma and should be considered when chest x-rays showing an extensive left pneumothorax, subcutaneous emphysema, expansive pneumomediastinum, left lower-lobe atelectasis, left pleural effusion, and V-shaped air lucency in the left lower mediastinal area (Naclerio's V sign) are present.[3] CT manifestations of esophageal rupture may include focal extraluminal air pockets at the tear site and a hematoma of the esophageal wall or the mediastinum.[3] The diagnosis of an esophageal rupture is often affirmed with a swallowing test using nonionic contrast agents.[4]

In cases of *impalement injury* or *projectile injury*, a chest x-ray can reveal the intrathoracic foreign body, especially if it is made of metal.[3] Visualization of the foreign body is easier in the presence of pleural effusion, pneumothorax, and lung lacerations.[98] A chest x-ray can also indicate the proximity of the foreign body to vital intrathoracic structures.[3] CT scans can more clearly show vascular injuries. Aortography can also be of use if there are hematomas near the aorta or if a major artery leak is strongly suspected.[98] *Penetrating cardiac trauma* (e.g., stabbing injury or bullet wound) is the leading causes of mortality in urban environments.

Other pathologies associated with chest wall trauma include contusions and soft tissue hematomas; lacerations of chest wall arteries can lead to extensive chest wall hematomas.[25] These injuries can be diagnosed with chest CT scans, which can also be used to ascertain the region of primary impact.[3] The appearance of hematomas or overlying soft tissue edema on CT scan generally points to injury of a rib or another bony structure.[25] The potential existence of these injuries should be investigated by reviewing the images utilizing bone window settings reformatted with the aid of an edge-enhancing algorithm. Using the cine-paging mode can simplify bone image review. Seat belt trauma resulting from a three-point restraint may lead to bruises in the subcutaneous tissues and fat of the anterior chest wall.[25] CT scans can help identify these injuries. When severe enough to produce dermal abrasions, seat belt trauma may be associated with distinctive internal injuries in 30% of trauma patients.[25]

Foreign Body Aspiration

Acute choking accompanied by respiratory failure due to laryngeal or tracheal foreign body obstruction can sometimes be successfully treated with back blows and abdominal thrusts. Even in nonemergency incidents, the quick removal of tracheal or bronchial foreign bodies is essential. Bronchoscopy may be utilized both therapeutically and diagnostically in cases of foreign body aspiration. The majority of foreign bodies are radiolucent. Before attempting to extract a foreign body, it is necessary to confirm its existence as well as its anatomic location, condition, shape, position, composition, and entrapment parameters, as indicated by granulation tissue or edema. Fortunately, once they are identified and found, almost all aspirated foreign bodies can be extracted bronchoscopically.

Key Points

▶ Medical imaging techniques use electromagnetic radiation to generate images.

▶ Imaging techniques may use ionizing radiation (x-rays or gamma rays) or nonionizing radiation (e.g., ultrasound or magnetic resonance imaging).

▶ X-rays easily penetrate low-density, radiolucent materials (e.g., air). Radiolucent materials appear dark or black with x-ray imaging.

▶ X-rays do not easily penetrate high-density materials (e.g., bone or fluid). These materials appear as white or gray with x-ray imaging and are considered radiopaque.

▶ Conventional radiography remains the imaging technique of choice for initial evaluation of the lungs.

▶ Artifacts that are often seen and evaluated using conventional radiography include endotracheal and tracheostomy tubes, central venous catheters, chest tubes, pulmonary artery catheters, and nasogastric tubes.

▶ Conventional chest radiographs are especially useful for evaluation of patients with pneumonia, atelectasis, pleural effusion, pulmonary edema, tumor or abscess, an enlarged heart, chest trauma, or pneumothorax and for determining the position of an endotrachial tube.

▶ Conventional chest radiographs may provide anteroposterior (AP), posteroanterior (PA), or lateral views. Each has advantages and disadvantages.

▶ Radiation exposure has risks; thus the dose should be "as low as reasonably achievable," or ALARA.

▶ An infiltrate is caused by accumulation of fluid, protein, or cells that fill the interstitial and/or alveolar space.

▶ Interstitial opacities can be classified as linear, reticular, nodular, or reticulonodular.

▶ An alveolar filling pattern (i.e., bronchopneumonia pattern) results in fluffy, poorly demarcated infiltrates that obscure vascular markings. A lobar pattern results in homogeneous opacity with air bronchograms.

▶ Ground-glass opacification describes hazy areas with preserved bronchial and lung markings.

▶ Air bronchograms are seen with alveolar filling adjacent to air-filled bronchi.

▶ Inspection of the chest radiograph should include assessment of image quality, type of view (i.e., AP, PA, lateral, other), patient position, and volume of air within the lung.

▶ A systemic approach to review of the chest radiograph should include inspection of the large airways, hila, heart, lung parenchyma, diaphragm, bones and joints, and soft tissues.

▶ Computed tomography (CT) may be especially useful for evaluation of shortness of breath and chest pain to rule out embolus or aortic dissection, lung nodules, lymph nodes, interstitial lung disease, pleural fluid, pericardial fluid, lung abscess, and lung cancer.

▶ Low-dose CT scans (LDCT) have been recommended by some for screening current or former smokers who meet certain guidelines.

▶ Magnetic resonance imaging (MRI) uses nonionizing radiation and is especially useful for evaluation of soft tissue injuries and pleural disease.

▶ MRI of the thorax may be especially useful for assessment and evaluation of the chest wall and diaphragm, pleura, paravertebral masses, and the mediastinum and hila.

▶ Positron emission tomography (PET) is a nuclear medicine technique that provides physiologic information about metabolically active tissue, such as cancer or infection.

▶ Thoracic PET or PET-CT scans are useful for evaluating solitary pulmonary nodules, staging lung cancer, and monitoring for lung cancer recurrence.

▶ Imaging tests useful for the diagnosis of pulmonary embolus include ventilation–perfusion scans, spiral CT, and pulmonary angiograms.

▶ A normal ventilation–perfusion scan virtually excludes the presence of pulmonary embolus.

▶ Pulmonary angiography is the definitive diagnostic test for pulmonary emboli but is being replaced by high-quality CT angiograms (the CT PE protocol).

▶ Interventional radiography techniques include cardiac catherization, percutaneous transluminal coronary angioplasty (PTCA), catheter-directed thrombolysis, and percutaneous abscess drainage.

▶ Bedside ultrasound imaging may be used to guide arterial or central line placement, chest tube insertion, rapid assessment of pneumothorax, and assessment of pleural fluid.

▶ Doppler ultrasound techniques are sometimes useful to evaluate deep vein thrombosis (DVT) or heart valve function (e.g., Doppler echocardiogram).

▶ Abnormal findings on chest radiograph associated with increased tissue density most commonly due to fluid are sometimes called *areas of opacity* or *opacities*.

▶ The silhouette sign is caused by increased density in the lung tissue adjacent to the heart resulting in obscured or blurred heart contours.

▶ Pneumonia is an infection of the lung parenchyma usually caused by bacterial or viral infection.

▶ Diagnosis of pneumonia is based on clinical signs and symptoms, imaging studies, and laboratory data. Initial diagnostic tests often include a chest x-ray and a complete blood count.

▶ Alveolar consolidation is a hallmark of pneumonia, although other causes must be ruled out.

▶ An air bronchogram is seen when air-filled airways are surrounded by consolidated lung tissue.

▶ Pulmonary edema is an abnormal accumulation of fluid in the alveolar and interstitial spaces.

▶ Pulmonary edema may be caused by either high pressures in the pulmonary capillaries or increased permeability of the pulmonary capillaries due to disease (e.g., leaky capillaries).

▶ Pulmonary edema on chest x-ray will show both lungs appearing whiter than usual, with interstitial and then alveolar filling.

▶ Acute respiratory distress syndrome (ARDS) is a form of noncardiogenic pulmonary edema defined by bilateral infiltrates on chest x-ray, severe hypoxemia, and normal left ventricular function (pulmonary capillary wedge pressures ≤ 18 mm Hg or normal function by echocardiography).

▶ Atelectasis involves the loss of lung volume with partial or complete collapse of alveoli. Atelectasis does not involve substantial filling of the alveoli with fluid or other material.

▶ Radiologic findings with atelectasis may include abnormal lung opacification, elevated diaphragm, crowding of pulmonary vessels, displacement of anatomic features due to partial or complete collapse of lung tissue, and obscured diaphragm and/or heart borders. If the atelectasis is unilateral, the ribs may appear closer together on the affected side.

▶ Fibronodular infiltrates with or without cavitation in the upper lobes and/or the superior segments of the lower lobes are suggestive of tuberculosis (TB).

- Lateral upper airway (neck) x-rays are sometimes obtained in children to evaluate epiglottitis (thumb sign) or croup (pencil sign).
- Types of pneumothorax are spontaneous, traumatic, and tension; each has characteristic findings on chest radiograph, which includes free air in the pleural space.
- Pleural effusion may be exudative or transudative. Exudates are due to inflammation of the pleura (commonly caused by infection, malignancy, or connective tissue disease).
- Transudative pleural effusions may be caused by elevated vascular pressures as may be seen with congestive heart failure (CHF), cirrhosis (liver failure), renal failure, or decreased colloid osmotic pressure (e.g., hypoalbuminemia).
- Pleural effusions usually accumulate in the dependent parts of the thorax and often obscure the costophrenic angle on the affected side.
- Interstitial lung disease (ILD) includes a very large group of disorders characterized by diffuse, often chronic, lung injury.
- ILD typically involves varying degrees of lung inflammation resulting in the formation of scar tissue (pulmonary fibrosis).
- Dyspnea on exertion and a dry cough are often the main symptoms of ILD, though symptoms vary greatly with different forms of ILD.
- Interstitial opacities as seen on chest x-ray may be classified as linear, reticular, nodular, or reticulonodular.
- ILD is sometimes grouped into categories that may include idiopathic interstitial pneumonitis (IIP), granulomatous disorders, connective tissue ILDs, drug-induced ILDs, and pulmonary vasculitis/diffuse alveolar hemorrhage–related ILD.
- Pneumoconiosis is dust-caused lung disease; examples include coal workers' pneumoconiosis (CWP), asbestosis, silicosis, and berylliosis.
- Idiopathic interstitial pneumonias (IIP) are ILDs of unknown origin and may be grouped by clinical course.
- Hypersensitivity pneumonitis (extrinsic allergic alveolitis) is caused by environmental exposure to specific organic proteins (e.g., molds).
- Connective tissue–related ILDs include systemic lupus erythematosus, rheumatoid arthritis, scleroderma, polymyositis, and Sjögren syndrome.
- ILD may be induced by certain chemotherapeutic, antimicrobial, and cardiovascular agents and certain illicit drugs (e.g., opiates, cocaine).
- Sarcoidosis is the most common type of noninfectious granulomatous lung disease.
- Asthma is characterized by airway inflammation, airway hyperreactivity, and reversible airflow obstruction.

- Chest imaging with asthma is usually normal, though conventional imaging may be useful for identification of comorbid conditions (e.g., pneumonia) in asthma patients.
- COPD includes chronic bronchitis, emphysema, and small airway disease.
- Conventional chest radiography of COPD patients may demonstrate lung hyperinflation, increased AP diameter, increased retrosternal airspace, and a flattened diaphragm. The lungs may appear hyperlucent.
- The chest radiograph for COPD patients is used primarily to identify or rule out comorbid conditions (e.g., pneumonia, congestive heart failure, lung cancer, pleural disease).
- High-resolution CT (HRCT) scans can sometimes differentiate between types of emphysema (i.e., panlobular, centrilobular, paraseptal) and some types of IIPs.
- Lung cancer originates in the cells that line the bronchi, bronchioles, or alveoli.
- The two primary types of lung cancer are non-small cell lung cancer (NSCLC) and small-cell lung cancer (SCLC).
- Cancer that spreads to the lungs from elsewhere in the body is classified as metastatic lung cancer (vs. primary lung cancer).
- Solitary pulmonary nodules (SPNs) are small round lesions enveloped by pulmonary parenchyma that may be caused by a primary lung cancer or solitary metastasis from an area outside the lungs; however, the majority of SPNs are not malignant.
- Imaging the trauma patient is essential to identify rib fractures, flail chest, pneumothorax, hemothorax, lung contusions, and other thoracic injuries.
- In many cases, foreign body aspiration may be confirmed by chest radiography.

References

1. Collins J, Stern EJ. Mediastinal masses. In: Collins J, Stern EJ (eds.). *Chest Radiology: The Essentials*, 2nd ed. Philadelphia: Wolters Kluwer Health, Lippincott Williams & Wilkins; 2008: 78–100.
2. Kelley LL, Petersen C. *Sectional Anatomy for Imaging Professionals*, 3rd ed. St. Louis, MO: Mosby Elsevier; 2012.
3. Ballinger PW, Frank ED. *Merrill's Atlas of Radiographic Positions and Radiologic Procedures*, vols. 1–3, 10th ed. St. Louis, MO: Mosby; 2003.
4. Collins J, Stern EJ. Peripheral lung disease. In: Collins J, Stern EJ (eds.). *Chest Radiology: The Essentials*, 2nd ed. Philadelphia: Wolters Kluwer Health, Lippincott Williams & Wilkins; 2008: 206–214.
5. Swenson SJ, Morin RL, Schueler BA, et al. Solitary pulmonary nodule: CT evaluation of enhancement with iodinated contrast material. *Radiology*. 1992;182(2):343–347.
6. Raghu G, Mageto YN, Lockhart D, Schmidt RA, Wood DE, Godwin JD. The accuracy of the clinical diagnosis of new-onset

idiopathic pulmonary fibrosis and other interstitial lung disease. A prospective study. *Chest*. 1999;116(5):1168–1174.

7. Collins J, Stern EJ. Airways. In: Collins J, Stern EJ (eds.). *Chest Radiology: The Essentials*, 2nd ed. Philadelphia: Wolters Kluwer Health, Lippincott Williams & Wilkins; 2008: 215–237.

8. Celli BR. Diseases of the diaphragm, chest wall, pleura, and mediastinum. In: Goldman L, Schafer AI (eds.). *Goldman's Cecil Medicine*, 24th ed. Philadelphia, PA: Elsevier Saunders; 2011: chap 99.

9. Collins J, Stern EJ. Chest trauma. In: Collins J, Stern EJ (eds.). *Chest Radiology: The Essentials*, 2nd ed. Philadelphia: Wolters Kluwer Health, Lippincott Williams & Wilkins; 2008: 119–137.

10. Sun JK, LeMay DR. Imaging of facial trauma. *Neuroimaging Clin N Am*. 2002;12(2):295–309.

11. Collins J, Stern EJ. Pleura, chest wall, and diaphragm. In: Collins J, Stern EJ (eds.). *Chest Radiology: The Essentials*, 2nd ed. Philadelphia: Wolters Kluwer Health, Lippincott Williams & Wilkins; 2008: 138–163.

12. Carlo WA. The fetus. In: Kliegman RM, Stanton BF, Gemell JW, Schor NF, Behrman RE, *Nelson Textbook of Pediatrics*, 19th ed. Philadelphia: Saunders Elsevier; 2011: chap 90.

13. Roosevelt GE. Acute inflammatory upper airway obstruction (croup, epiglottitis, laryngitis, and bacterial tracheitis). In: Kliegman RM, Stanton BF, Gemell JW, Schor NF, Behrman RE, eds. *Nelson Textbook of Pediatrics*, 19th ed. Philadelphia: Saunders Elsevier; 2011: chap 377.

14. Elfenbein DS, Felice ME. Adolescent pregnancy. In: Kliegman RM, Stanton BF, Gemell JW, Schor NF, Behrman RE, eds. *Nelson Textbook of Pediatrics*, 19th ed. Philadelphia: Saunders Elsevier; 2011: chap 112.

15. Selman M. Hypersensitivity pneumonitis. In: Schwarz MI, King TE (eds.). *Interstitial Lung Disease*, 4th ed. Hamilton, Ontario, BC: Decker; 2003.

16. Mukhopadhyay S, Gal AA. Granulomatous lung disease: an approach to the differential diagnosis. *Arch Pathol Lab Med*. 2010;134(5):667–690.

17. Cantin L, Chartrand LC, Lepanto L, et al. Chest tube drainage under radiological guidance for pleural effusion and pneumothorax in a tertiary care university teaching hospital: review of 51 cases. *Can Respir J*. 2005;12(1):29–33.

18. Ely EW, Johnson MM, Chiles C, et al. Chest X-ray changes in air space disease are associated with parameters of mechanical ventilation in ICU patients. *Am J Respir Crit Care Med*. 1996;154(5):1543–1550.

19. Torres A, Menendez R, Wunderink. Pyogenic bacterial pneumonia and lung abscess. In: Mason RJ, Broaddus VC, Martin TR, et al. (eds.). *Murray & Nadel's Textbook of Respiratory Medicine*, 5th ed. Philadelphia: Saunders Elsevier; 2010: 741–753.

20. Chernecky CC, Berger BJ. *Laboratory Tests and Diagnostic Procedures*, 5th ed. St. Louis, MO: Saunders; 2008.

21. Gupta NC, Maloof J, Gunel E. Probability of malignancy in solitary pulmonary nodules using fluorine-18-FDG and PET. *J Nucl Med*. 1996;37(6):943–948.

22. Limper AH. Overview of pneumonia In: Goldman L, Schafer AI, (eds.). *Goldman's Cecil Medicine*, 24th ed. Philadelphia, PA: Elsevier Saunders; 2011: chap 97.

23. Yi JG, Kim SJ, Marom EM, et al. Chest CT of incidental breast lesions. *J Thorac Imaging*. 2008;23(2):148–155.

24. Alfaro V, Roca-Acin J, Palacios L, Guitart R. Multiple inert gas elimination technique for determining ventilation/perfusion distributions in rat during normoxia, hypoxia and hyperoxia. *Clin Exp Pharmacol Physiol*. 2001;28(5–6):419–424.

25. Barboza R, Fox JH, Shaffer LE, Opalek JM, Farooki S. Incidental findings in the cervical spine at CT for trauma evaluation. *Am J Radiol*. 2009;192(3):725–729.

26. Tanaka N, Newell JD, Brown KK, Cool CD, Lynch DA. High-resolution computed tomography findings based on the pathologic classification. *J Comput Assist Tomogr*. 2004;28(3):351–360.

27. Shaw AS, Dixon AK. Multidetector computed tomography. In: Adam A, Dixon AK (eds.). *Grainger & Allison's Diagnostic Radiology: A Textbook of Medical Imaging*, 5th ed. New York: Churchill Livingstone; 2008: chap 4.

28. Elliot TL, Lynch DA, Newell JD Jr, et al. High-resolution computed tomography features of nonspecific interstitial pneumonia and usual interstitial pneumonia. *J Comput Assist Tomogr*. 2005;29(3):339–345

29. Novelline RA, Rhea JT, Rao PM, Stuk JL. Helical CT in emergency radiology. *Radiology*. 1999;213(2):321–339.

30. Gilk T. MRI safety: accidents are not inevitable. MedicalPhysicsWeb, January 10, 2012. Available at: http://medicalphysicsweb.org/cws/article/opinion/48264. Accessed June 13, 2013.

31. American Lung Association. Providing guidance on lung cancer screening to patients and physicians. Available at: http://www.lung.org/lung-disease/lung-cancer/lung-cancer-screening-guidelines/lung-cancer-screening.pdf. Accessed June 22, 2013.

32. Jacklitsch MT, Jacobson FL, Austin JHM, et al. The American Association for Thoracic Surgery guidelines for lung cancer screening using low-dose computed tomography scans for lung cancer survivors and other high-risk groups. *J Thorac Cardiovasc Surg*. 2012;144(1):33–38.

33. Wilkinson ID, Paley MNJ. Magnetic resonance imaging: basic principles. In: Adam A, Dixon AK (eds.). *Grainger & Allison's Diagnostic Radiology: A Textbook of Medical Imaging*, 5th ed. New York: Churchill Livingstone; 2008: chap 5.

34. Garter WB, Hatabu H. Evaluation of pulmonary vascular anatomy and blood flow by magnetic resonance. *J Thorac Imaging*. 1993;8(2):122–136.

35. Chernoff, D, Stark, P. Magnetic resonance imaging of the thorax. In: UpToDate, Basow, DS (ed.), UpToDate, Waltham, MA, 2013.

36. Gilk T. MRI safety: accidents are not inevitable. Medical PhysicsWeb. January 10, 2012. Available at: http://medicalphysicsweb.org/cws/article/opinion/48264. Accessed June 13, 2013.

37. Kodali S, Baher A, Shah D. Safety of MRIs in patients with pacemakers and defibrillators. *Methodist Debakey Cardiovasc J*. 2013;9(3):137–141

38. Levin DC, Intenzo CM, Rao VM, et al. Comparison of recent utilization trends in radionuclide myocardial perfusion imaging among radiologists and cardiologists. *J Am Coll Radiol*. 2005; 2(10):821–824.

39. Marsh S, Barnden L, O'Keeffe D. Validation of co-registration of clinical lung ventilation and perfusion SPECT. *Australas Phys Eng Sci Med*. 2011;34(1):63–68.

40. Dolovich M, Labiris R. Imaging drug delivery and drug responses in the lung. *Proc Am Thorac Soc*. 2004;1:329–337.

41. Collins J, Stern EJ. Interstitial lung disease. In: Collins J, Stern EJ (eds.). *Chest Radiology: The Essentials*, 2nd ed. Philadelphia: Wolters Kluwer Health. Lippincott Williams & Wilkins; 2008: 34–50.

42. Collins J, Stern EJ. Alveolar lung disease. In: Collins J, Stern EJ (eds.). *Chest Radiology: The Essentials*, 2nd ed. Philadelphia: Wolters Kluwer Health. Lippincott Williams & Wilkins; 2008: 51–62.

43. Casserly B, Rounds S. Essentials in critical care medicine. In: Andreoli TE, Benjamin IJ, Griggs RC, Wing EJ (eds.). *Andreoli and Carpenter's Medical Essentials of Medicine*, 8th ed. Philadelphia: Elsevier Saunders; 2012: 259–265.

44. Rounds S, Jankowich MD. Disorders of respiratory control. In: Andreoli TE, Benjamin IJ, Griggs RC, Wing EJ (eds.). *Andreoli and Carpenter's Medical Essentials of Medicine*, 8th ed. Philadelphia: Elsevier Saunders; 2012: 245–247.

45. Collins J, Stern EJ. Pulmonary vasculature disease. In: Collins J, Stern EJ, eds. *Chest Radiology: The Essentials*, 2nd ed. Philadelphia: Wolters Kluwer Health, Lippincott Williams & Wilkins; 2008: 271–286.

46. Stark P. Thoracic positron emission tomography. In: *UpToDate*, Basow DS (ed.), UpToDate, Waltham, MA, 2013.

47. Rounds S. Pulmonary vascular disease. In: Andreoli TE, Benjamin IJ, Griggs RC, Wing EJ (eds.). *Andreoli and Carpenter's Medical Essentials of Medicine*, 8th ed. Philadelphia: Elsevier Saunders; 2012: 241–244.

48. Johnson DH, Blot WJ, Carbone DP, et al. Cancer of the lung: non-small cell lung cancer and small cell lung cancer. In: Abeloff MD, Armitage JO, Niederhuber JE, Kasten MB, McKenna WG (eds.). *Abeloff's Clinical Oncology*, 4th ed. Philadelphia: Churchill Livingstone Elsevier; 2008. 1307–1366.

49. Rounds S, Jankowich MD. The lung in health and diseases. In: Andreoli TE, Benjamin IJ, Griggs RC, Wing EJ (eds.). *Andreoli and Carpenter's Medical Essentials of Medicine*. 8th ed. Philadelphia: Elsevier Saunders; 2012: 188–191.

50. Van Heertum RL. Infarct avid imaging study in the radionuclide diagnosis of acute myocardial infarction. *Bull NY Acad Med.* 1981;57(9):747–754.

51. McCool DF. Evaluating lung structure and function. In: Andreoli TE, Benjamin IJ, Griggs RC, Wing EJ (eds.). *Andreoli and Carpenter's Medical Essentials of Medicine*. 8th ed. Philadelphia: Elsevier Saunders; 2012: 198–212.

52. Kandarpa K, Machan L. *Handbook of Interventional Radiologic Procedures*, 4th ed. Philadelphia: Lippincott Williams & Wilkins; 2011.

53. Snopek AM. *Fundamentals of Special Radiographic Procedures*, 5th ed. Philadelphia: WB Saunders; 2006.

54. Rumack CM, Wilson SR, Charboneau WJ, Levine D. *Diagnostic Ultrasound*, 4th ed. Philadelphia: Mosby; 2011.

55. Raghu G, Brown KK. Interstitial lung disease: clinical evaluation and keys to an accurate diagnosis. *Clin Chest Med.* 2004;25(3):409–419, v.

56. Collins J, Stern EJ. Upper lung disease, infection, and immunity. In: Collins J, Stern EJ (eds.). *Chest Radiology: The Essentials*, 2nd ed. Philadelphia: Wolters Kluwer Health, Lippincott Williams & Wilkins; 2008: 164–194.

57. Niewoehner D. COPD. In: Goldman L, Schafer AI (eds.). *Goldman's Cecil Medicine*, 24th ed. Philadelphia, PA: Elsevier Saunders; 2011: chap 88.

58. Bartlett, JG. Diagnostic approach to community-acquired pneumonia in adults. In: *UpToDate*, Basow DS (ed.), UpToDate, Waltham, MA, 2012.

59. File TM. Epidemiology, pathogenesis, microbiology, and diagnosis of hospital-acquired, ventilator-associated, and healthcare-associated pneumonia in adults. In: *UpToDate*, Basow, DS (ed.), UpToDate, Waltham, MA, 2013.

60. File TM. Treatment of community-acquired pneumonia in adults who require hospitalization. In: *UpToDate*, Basow, DS (ed.), UpToDate, Waltham, MA, 2012.

61. Frazier AA, Galvin JR, Franks TJ, et al. From the archives of the AFIP: pulmonary vasculature: hypertension and infarction. *Radiographics.* 2000;20(2):491–524.

62. Collins J, Stern EJ. Signs and patterns of lung disease. In: Collins J, Stern EJ (eds.). *Chest Radiology: The Essentials*, 2nd ed. Philadelphia: Wolters Kluwer Health Lippincott Williams & Wilkins; 2008: 16–33.

63. Siegel, MD. Acute respiratory distress syndrome: epidemiology; pathophysiology; pathology; and etiology. In: *UpToDate*, Basow DS (ed.), UpToDate, Waltham, MA, 2012.

64. Collins J, Stern EJ. Normal anatomy of the chest. In: Collins J, Stern EJ (eds.). *Chest Radiology: The Essentials*, 2nd ed. Philadelphia: Wolters Kluwer Health, Lippincott Williams & Wilkins; 2008: 52.

65. Fishbach FT, Dunning MB III (eds.). *Manual of Laboratory and Diagnostic Tests*, 8th ed. Philadelphia: Lippincott Williams and Wilkins; 2009.

66. Selman M. Hypersensitivity pneumonitis. In Schwarz MI, King TE (eds.). *Interstitial Lung Disease*, 4th ed. Hamilton, Ontario, BC: Decker; 2003.

67. Kliegman RM, Behrman RE, Jenson HB, et al. *Nelson Textbook of Pediatrics*, 19th ed. Philadelphia, PA: Saunders Elsevier; 2011.

68. Casserly B, Rounds S. Infectious diseases of the lung. In: Andreoli TE, Benjamin IJ, Griggs RC, Wing EJ (eds.). *Andreoli and Carpenter's Medical Essentials of Medicine*, 8th ed. Philadelphia: Elsevier Saunders; 2012: 254–258.

69. Schwartz MI. CCNU, 1-(2-chloroethyl)-3-(4-methylcyclohexyl)-1-nitrosourea. Data from Camus P: Drug-induced infiltrative lung diseases. In Schwarz MI, King TE (eds.). *Interstitial Lung Disease*, 4th ed. Hamilton, Ontario, BC: Decker; 2003: 485–534.

70. Cohen A, King TE, Jr, Downey, GP. Rapidly progressive bronchiolitis obliterans with organizing pneumonia. *Am J Respir Crit Med.* 1994;149(6):1670–1675.

71. Collins J, Stern EJ. Atelectasis. In: Collins J, Stern EJ, eds. *Chest Radiology: The Essentials*, 2nd ed. Philadelphia: Wolters Kluwer Health, Lippincott Williams & Wilkins; 2008: 195–205.

72. Hudson LD, Slutsky AS. Acute respiratory failure. In: Goldman L, Schafer AI (eds.). *Goldman's Cecil Medicine*, 24th ed. Philadelphia, PA: Elsevier Saunders; 2011: chap 104.

73. Bernardo J. Diagnosis of pulmonary tuberculosis in HIV-negative patients. In *UpToDate*, Basow DS (ed.), UpToDate, Waltham, MA, 2012.

74. Everard ML. Acute bronchiolitis and croup. *Pediatr Clin North Am.* 2009;56(1):119–133.

75. Casserly B, Rounds S. General approach to patients with respiratory disorders. In: Andreoli TE, Benjamin IJ, Griggs RC, Wing EJ (eds.). *Andreoli and Carpenter's Medical Essentials of Medicine*, 8th ed. Philadelphia: Elsevier Saunders; 2012: 192–197.

76. Nagata Y, Kumada K, Yamada R, et al. Pulmonary thromboembolism following angioplasty for membranous occlusion of the vena cava: case report. *Cardiovasc Intervent Radiol.* 1989;12(6):304–306.

77. Jogi J, Ekberg M, Jonson B, Bozovic G, Bajc M. Ventilation/perfusion SPECT in chronic obstructive pulmonary disease: an evaluation by reference to symptoms, spirometric lung function and emphysema, as assessed with HRCT. *Eur J Nucl Med Mol Imaging.* 2011;38:1344–1352.

78. Jones PW, Agusti AG. Outcomes and markers in the assessment of chronic obstructive pulmonary disease. *Eur Respir J.* 2006;27(4):822–832.

79. Garter WB, Hatabu H. Evaluation of pulmonary vascular anatomy and blood flow by magnetic resonance. *J Thorac Imaging.* 1993;8(2):122–136.

80. Stark P. Imaging of pneumothorax. In *UpToDate*, Basow DS (ed.), UpToDate, Waltham, MA, 2012.

81. Hyzy RC. Pulmonary barotrauma during mechanical ventilation. In *UpToDate*, Basow DS (ed.), UpToDate, Waltham, MA, 2012.

82. Stark P. Imaging of pleural effusions in adults. In *UpToDate*, Basow DS (ed.), UpToDate, Waltham, MA, 2012.

83. McCool DF. Disorders of the pleura, mediastinum, and chest wall. In: Andreoli TE, Benjamin IJ, Griggs RC, Wing EJ, eds. *Andreoli and Carpenter's Medical Essentials of Medicine*, 8th ed. Philadelphia: Elsevier Saunders; 2012: 248–253.

84. Heffner JE. Diagnostic evaluation of a pleural effusion in adults: initial testing. In *UpToDate*, Basow DS, (ed.), UpToDate, Waltham, MA, 2012.

85. Aliotta JM, Jankowich MD. Interstitial lung diseases. In: Andreoli TE, Benjamin IJ, Griggs RC, Wing EJ (eds.). *Andreoli and Carpenter's Medical Essentials of Medicine*, 8th ed. Philadelphia: Elsevier Saunders; 2012:225–240.

86. Talmadge E.K. Approach to the adult with interstitial lung disease: diagnostic testing. In *UpToDate*, Basow DS (ed.), UpToDate, Waltham, MA, 2012.

87. Jankowich MD. Obstructive lung diseases. In: Andreoli TE, Benjamin IJ, Griggs RC, Wing EJ (eds.). *Andreoli and Carpenter's Medical Essentials of Medicine*, 8th ed. Philadelphia: Elsevier Saunders; 2012: 213–224.

88. Fanta CH. Diagnosis of asthma in adolescents and adults. In *UpToDate*, Basow DS (ed.), UpToDate, Waltham, MA, 2012.

89. Swenson SJ, Silverstein MD, Ilstrup DM, et al. The probability of malignancy in solitary nodules: application to small radiologically indeterminate nodules. *Arch Intern Med.* 1997;157(8):849–855.

90. Jankowich MD, Aliotta JM. Neoplastic disorders of the lung. In: Andreoli, TE, Benjamin, IJ, Grigg, RC, Wing EJ, (eds.). *Andreoli and Carpenter's Medical Essentials of Medicine*, 8th ed. Philadelphia: Elsevier Saunders; 2012: 266–271.

91. McCool FD. Diseases of the diaphragm, chest wall, pleura, and mediastinum. In: Goldman L, Schafer AI (eds.). *Goldman's Cecil Medicine*, 24th ed. Philadelphia, PA: Elsevier Saunders; 2011: chap 99.

92. Collins J, Stern EJ. Solitary and multiple pulmonary nodules. In: Collins J, Stern EJ, eds. *Chest Radiology: The Essentials*, 2nd ed. Philadelphia: Wolters Kluwer Health, Lippincott Williams & Wilkins; 2008: 101–118.

93. Cummings SR, Lillington GA, Richard RJ. Estimating the probability of malignancy in solitary pulmonary nodules. *Am Rev Respir Dis.* 1986;134(3):449–452.

94. Henschke CI, Yankelevitz DF, Naidich DP, et al. CT screening for lung cancer: suspiciousness of nodules according to size on baseline scans. *Radiology.* 2004;231(1):164–168.

95. Libby DM, Smith JP, Altorki NK, et al. Managing the small pulmonary nodule discovered by CT. *Chest.* 2004;125(4):1522–1529.

96. Collins J, Stern EJ. Monitoring and support devices-tubes and lines. In: Collins J, Stern EJ, eds. *Chest Radiology: The Essentials*, 2nd ed. Philadelphia: Wolters Kluwer Health, Lippincott Williams & Wilkins; 2008: 63–77.

97. Grimm LJ. Tracheobronchial tear imaging. Medscape. Updated May 1, 2014. http://emedicine.medscape.com/article/362315-overview.

98. Bilello JF, Davis JW, Cagle KM, Kaups KL. Predicting extubation failure in blunt trauma patients with pulmonary contusion. *J Trauma Acute Care Surg.* 2013;75(2):229–233.

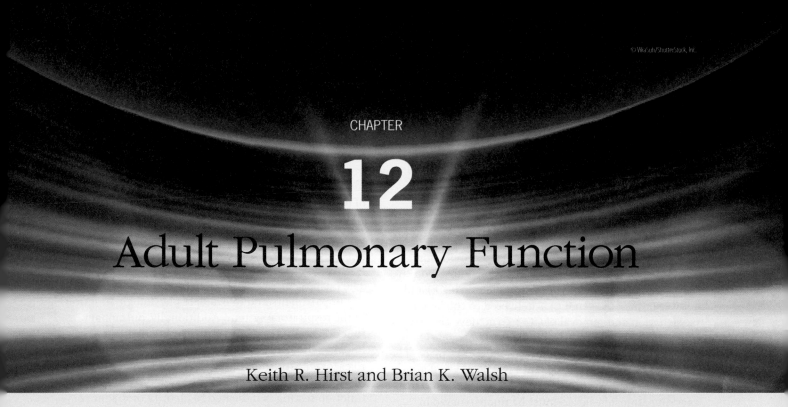

CHAPTER OUTLINE

CHAPTER OBJECTIVES

1. Explain the purpose for performing pulmonary function tests (PFTs).
2. Summarize the steps required to perform pulmonary function testing.
3. Explain the methods that are used to calculate lung volumes.
4. Describe the four methods of determining total lung capacity.
5. Understand the differences among spirometry, flow-volume loops, diffusion capacity, and respiratory system forced conductance oscillation.
6. Determine when blood gases, pulse oximetry, and exhaled gas measures such as end-tidal CO_2 or fraction of exhaled nitric oxide may provide valuable information.
7. Categorize obstructive and restrictive disease based on pulmonary function testing.

8. Describe the appropriate use of bronchoprovocation testing and what constitutes a response.
9. Describe common causes of restrictive and obstructive lung disease.
10. List the major indications for pulmonary exercise testing.
11. Explain the clinical use of exercise tests such as the 6-minute walk.
12. Explain the concepts of oxygen consumption and carbon dioxide elimination.
13. Explain the anaerobic threshold and how it pertains to exercise testing.
14. Describe the indications and contraindications for exercise testing.
15. Identify the major components of a pulmonary function testing laboratory.
16. Describe how height, weight, age, gender, and patient effort affect pulmonary function test measurements.
17. Define and list approximate normal values, factors affecting, and the significance of the following: tidal volume, minute volume, total lung capacity, vital capacity, residual volume, expiratory reserve volume, functional residual capacity, inspiratory reserve volume, inspiratory capacity, and maximal voluntary ventilation.
18. Define the normal values and factors affecting the following: FEV_1, FEV_3, $FEF_{25-75\%}$, PEF.
19. Describe the purpose and interpretation of pre- and postbronchodilator pulmonary function testing.
20. Describe the purpose of quality control of pulmonary function testing equipment.
21. Interpret the results of pulmonary function testing.
22. Assess the need for and application of pulmonary function testing in specific patients.

KEY TERMS

airway resistance (R_{aw})
American Thoracic Society (ATS)
body plethysmograph
body temperature, pressure, and saturation (BTPS)

Boyle's law
diffusing capacity (D_{LCO})
European Respiratory Society (ERS)
expiratory reserve volume (ERV)

forced oscillation technique (FOT)
forced vital capacity (FVC)
functional residual capacity (FRC)
inspiratory capacity (IC)
maximal expiratory pressure (MEP)
maximal inspiratory pressure (MIP)

maximal voluntary ventilation (MVV)
peak expiratory flow (PEFR or PEF)
residual volume (RV)
RV/TLC ratio
slow vital capacity (SVC)
total lung capacity (TLC)
vital capacity (VC)

Overview

The primary function of the lungs is to provide for gas exchange (i.e., respiration). Mixed venous blood containing a higher level of carbon dioxide (CO_2) and a lower level of oxygen (O_2) is delivered to the lung for oxygenation and removal of CO_2. To achieve the goal of respiration (i.e., to eliminate CO_2 and provide O_2 to cells) several physiologic processes must take place. The respiratory muscles must expand the thorax and lung, creating a negative pressure gradient. Second, airways carrying atmospheric gas must be unobstructed in order for alveolar ventilation to occur. Third, CO_2 and O_2 must be able to diffuse across the alveolar–capillary membrane. Fourth, blood must circulate through ventilated regions of the lung. A full range of pulmonary function testing can provide insight into each of these areas. This chapter will review pulmonary function testing that can provide a valuable and objective assessment of the chest wall, lung, airway, respiratory muscle strength, and gas exchange.

Introduction to Pulmonary Function Testing

The lungs contain a number of branching and tapering airways that originate at the nose and mouth and terminate at the alveolus. Surrounding the alveoli is a complex network of capillaries that provide a rich supply of blood that starts at the pulmonary arteries and ends at the pulmonary veins. The pulmonary system is the only organ that receives 100% of the cardiac output and is exposed to atmospheric air. Pulmonary function tests (PFTs) help us identify abnormalities through a series of measurements that either directly or indirectly assess lung function. These studies include spirometry, pre- and postbronchodilator administration, flow-volume loops (FVL), lung volume and diffusion capacity (D_L) studies, and gas exchange measurements. It may also include airway resistance (R_{aw}), respiratory system forced conductance oscillation, arterial blood gas (ABG) measurements, and the patient's response to exercise and bronchial provocation. Other studies may include a 6-minute walk test, metabolic testing, and oxygen-saturation testing for use of home oxygen.

These tests may be done in either an outpatient or inpatient setting and are usually performed by a qualified technologist (usually a respiratory therapist with PFT credentials) under the direction of a physician who has been trained in interpretation of PFTs. The technologist's role is to assist with selection of the appropriate test, execute the ordered test according to lab and national guidelines, and maintain the equipment. This chapter will describe proper pulmonary function testing to include indications and assessment of results.

Purpose of Pulmonary Function Testing

The purpose of pulmonary function testing is to identify impairments and to evaluate physiologic function of the respiratory system. Additionally, pulmonary function testing is designed to classify the degree of impairment. These classifications have two primary roles: diagnostic and therapeutic.

According to Crapo[1] and Miller et al.,[2] pulmonary function testing is indicated to identify or diagnose pulmonary disease, to monitor therapeutic interventions such as medications or surgery, to determine degree of disability or impairment to qualify for programs, or to determine pulmonary function for epidemiologic surveys or research. The most common use of pulmonary function testing is to evaluate the absence or presence of abnormal pulmonary function.

Predicted Values

The results of a pulmonary function test are only useful if an individual patient's results are compared to an appropriate normal range for healthy people of the same age, gender, and race. This normal range is often referred to as *predicted values* or *predicteds*. If the measured results deviate from the predicted values, clinicians can determine impairment. The predicted values are based on height, gender, age, and race. Several large epidemiologic studies have been conducted from which these reference ranges have been developed. A number of reference equations are available, and the specific equations used are often determined by the personal preference of the interpreter or specific PFT laboratory. Previously used reference equations should be used for trending purposes. Some national and international references may not be a good representative of the specific study patient at hand; therefore, the clinician should choose the reference range most representative of the population the PFT laboratory is most likely to see.

Reference Ranges

The most recent set of predicted normal values is the Third National Health and Nutrition Examination Survey (NHANES III). The values in this study were derived from healthy, lifelong nonsmoking individuals aged 8 to 80 years from the following racial categories: Caucasian, African American, and Mexican American.[3] However, a new study (Global Lung Initiative 2012 [GLI 2012]) looked at Caucasians, African Americans, and Northeast and Southeast Asians between the ages of 3 and 95.[4] The data are starting to be compared with the NHANES III data to see if these values can be used.[5] To date, there are only small differences when using the GLI 2012 compared to the NHANES III values.[6,7]

RC Insights

A good pulmonary history should be completed along with a physical assessment. This helps with PFT interpretation.

Factors That Influence Predicted Values

Height

Height is probably the most important factor influencing lung size. Taller people typically have a larger thoracic compartment. In most cases, a taller person will have larger predicted lung volumes, higher flow rates, and a greater uptake for both oxygen (O_2) and carbon monoxide (CO), which will be reflected in their **DLCO (diffusing capacity)**.

RC Insights

Know the question(s) being asked before the PFT begins.

Weight

Weight typically does not affect lung volumes and flow rates unless a person is obese (body mass index [BMI] > 30).[8] Truncal obesity may restrict expansion of the thorax.[9] In obese subjects, the expiratory reserve volume (ERV) is found to be out of proportion to the total lung capacity (TLC). Serial tests are sometimes required to determine if obese patients have underlying restrictive disease. Low body weight may suggest malnutrition, which can reduce the diaphragm's strength and thereby limit the patient's ability to take a deep breath. As TLC is reduced, the patient's ability to produce maximal flows, such as the forced expiratory volume in 1 second (FEV_1) are proportionately reduced. Although weight may affect lung function, this variable is not typically incorporated into the equations used to determine a patient's normal range; it is left to the interpreting clinician to determine if any lung function abnormalities are attributable to patient weight.[9] One way to help determine if weight may play a role is to calculate the patient's BMI. If a patient is found to be obese based on BMI, this should be considered when reviewing PFT results. If abnormal PFT results are thought to reflect obesity, then serial studies are required to document stability, which then suggests an absence of active pulmonary disease.

Gender

Males typically have larger lungs than females, and females will achieve their maximum lung volumes at a younger age than males. Additional gender-related factors, such as muscle composition, might influence lung volumes and flow rates.[9] Young people who regularly perform aerobic exercise tend to develop larger lung volumes then those who do not. Children taking glucocorticoids on a regular basis may have slower or slightly lower lung volume increases as they get older.

Age

Most individuals reach their maximum lung function in their 20s to early 30s.[8,10] In children and adolescents, the FEV_1/FVC ratio has been shown to increase during adolescence rather than decreasing from childhood to adulthood as previously thought.[7] This is explained by the FVC "outgrowing" the total lung capacity and FEV_1.[7] This leads to a decline in the FEV_1/FVC ratio that reverses during adolescence.[7] Lung function begins to decline in the late 30s to early 40s, even among those who are healthy nonsmokers with no exposure to air pollution. This decline is at a rate of approximately 30 mL per year.[7] Those smoking at an early age may see a decline sooner than those who do not smoke.[8] Patients who are nonsmokers will see a decrease in their vital capacity (VC) while their residual volume (RV) increases, which leaves their TLC intact. Diffusing capacity declines linearly with age as well. FEV_1 will decline slowly at first, but as the patient ages the FEV_1 decrease will accelerate.[10]

Race

Race plays a role in PFT results. If at all possible, equations that are race specific should be used.[11] African Americans, Asians, and East Indians generally have a 12% lower lung volume when compared to Caucasians of the same age, height, and gender.[3,4,11] It should be noted that adjustment of PFT values for Asians and East Indians raised in the U.S. remains controversial. This is thought to be due to the fact that they have greater lower extremity length and a smaller thoracic cavity than their Caucasian counterparts. Hispanics and Native Americans have lung volumes that typically do not need correction if using the NHANES III predicted values.

Other Considerations

Pulmonary function testing is effort-dependent and requires patient cooperation. It is up to the technologist performing the test to ensure that the test is performed correctly and meets established standards. This may take several tests with proper coaching to ensure repeatability.

Pulmonary Function Laboratory Equipment

Spirometer

The word *spirometer* in respiratory care is commonly used to describe a system that measures flow or volume. Within the pulmonary function lab the spirometer is the primary instrument employed. The first spirometers were volume-displacement systems. These water, bellows, or dry rolling-seal systems would directly measure volume by displacing a column of air in which a pen would plot the volume over a timed paper feed. The change in volume over time would later be used to calculate flow rate. Since the development of the first spirometers, advancements have been made to determine flow rates and therefore calculate volumes (flow over time) in a more efficient manner.

Pneumotachometer

The spirometer that is most often utilized in the modern PFT lab is a pneumotachometer. These devices measure flow in several different ways, including by pressure differences (e.g., pressure differential pneumotachometer), the effect of gas flow on temperature (e.g., thermistor pneumotachometer), and by rotating fan blade (e.g., turbinometer). Measuring flow allows the calculation of volume. The pneumotachometer is popular because of its low resistance to flow, ease of use, portability, ease of disinfection, and low maintenance cost.

Pressure Differential Pneumotachometer

The Fleisch-type pneumotachometer measures the change in pressure as gas flows through a resistor. Manufactures have developed different versions of the pressure differential pneumotachometer by adding different resistors or heating the sensor to improve durability and accuracy.

Thermistor Pneumotachometer

A pneumotachometer that measures flow by the change in temperature is known as a thermistor. More specifically, highly accurate thermistors used in the PFT lab are constant-temperature anemometers. Utilizing the Wheatstone Bridge hotwire or hot film anemometer system, the element within the sensor is warmed. As flow passes over the wire or film, it is cooled. This decreases the electrical resistance, and additional energy (i.e., an increase in electrical flow) is required to keep the sensor at a constant temperature. This cooling and subsequent increase in electrical flow enable the calculation of gas flow.

Turbinometer

Spirometers that utilize the rotation of fan blades are called turbinometers. The number of rotations determines the volume, and the speed of rotation determines the flow rate. The most popular turbinometer is the Wright respirometer. Due to the small size of this spirometer, it is often used in the acute care setting for bedside monitoring.

Forced Oscillation

Small-amplitude pressure oscillations at different frequencies have been applied to determine respiratory mechanics. Random-frequency noise-called **forced oscillation technique (FOT)** can be used to determine airway resistance and conductance. The FOT system uses a loudspeaker to generate a FOT signal in spontaneously breathing patients. FOT signals are filtered to eliminate the influence of high- or low-frequency artifacts. The signals are sampled at a rate of 128 Hz and fed into a computer for analysis.[12]

Today, most PFT equipment is computerized and designed to measure or calculate flow rates, lung volumes, and capacities with very little effort on the technologist's part. These highly sophisticated computer systems often offer visual incentives that help patients perform the test. These systems also often offer technical assistance in determining the patient's best effort and quality of the test performed. Many are connected electronically to the medical record, allowing the interpreting physician to review results remotely, which may increase the efficiency of these tests.

Preparing the Patient

Prior to patient testing, a past medical history needs to be obtained. The following patient information should to be obtained and documented:

- Age
- Height
- Weight
- Race/ethnic origin
- Sex (M/F)
- Pulmonary history
- Personal history
  - Smoking history
  - Family history
  - Occupational/environmental history

- Symptoms (e.g., dyspnea, cough, chest pain, sputum production)
- Current medications

Contraindications

The pretest interview is used to identify contraindications. There are very few absolute contraindications to PFT. The **American Thoracic Society (ATS)** and the **European Respiratory Society (ERS)** list a myocardial infarction (MI) within 1 month of testing to be an absolute contraindication due to the physical demands that are placed on the patient during testing.[9] The following are also considered absolute contraindications:[13] acute MI or angina, ascending aortic aneurysm, pulmonary embolism, and severe or uncontrolled hypertension. The following are relative contraindications:[13] recent thoracic/abdominal surgery; recent brain, eye, ear, airway, or throat surgery; pneumothorax; hemoptysis; acute diarrhea; and confusion or dementia. Other factors, according to Miller et al., which may adversely affect PFT results include patients' inability to follow instructions, claustrophobia (e.g., body plethysmography), pain (e.g., oral, facial, chest or abdominal), and missing teeth.[9] All contraindications should be discussed with the patient prior to performing a pulmonary function test.

Positioning

The patient needs to be either sitting upright or standing during the testing.[9] The preference is sitting, because the exertion needed during the testing may, on rare occasions, cause the subject to have a syncopal episode. The chair should be secured from moving and have arms. For subjects who wish to stand, a chair should be right behind them in case they need to sit. The position of the subject should be noted, and the same position should ideally be used for all subsequent testing. This is important because certain patient populations, such as obese patients, may have different results from sitting to standing.[2]

The ATS/ERS guidelines have developed a list of activities that are to be avoided prior to testing. These activities may skew the results and result in an invalid test. The following activities should be avoided:[9]

- Smoking for at least 1 hour prior to the test
- Consuming alcohol or caffeine-containing products for at least 4 hours prior to the test
- Performing vigorous exercise within 30 minutes of testing

- Wearing clothes that restrict the chest or abdominal cavities
- Eating a large meal within 2 hours of the test

Measurements and Documentation

The patient's age, height, weight, and race should be recorded prior to the test beginning and entered into the computer. If the patient has loose-fitting dentures, they should be removed prior to the start of the testing. However, dentures—loose or tight—may help reduce mouthpiece leaks. Height may be calculated from the arm span of patients in whom height may be difficult to obtain or may be inaccurate, such as patients with significant kyphoscoliosis, lower extremity amputation, or inability to stand. A nose clip is recommended to ensure that no gas volume is lost through the nares.

Medications

The decision to prohibit bronchodilator use prior to testing is determined by the ordering clinician. This decision is usually based on the clinical questions being addressed and an assessment as to whether the patient can tolerate stopping a particular medication. If the test is to determine the underlying disease or diagnosis, then it is recommended to withhold bronchodilator medications prior to testing. However, if the test is to assess a patient's response to treatment, inhaled medications should not be withheld.[9] Whatever decision is made should be consistent to allow comparisons over time.

During the Test

Pulmonary function testing usually follows a prescribed order and generally begins with dynamic studies, such as spirometry (e.g., FVC, FEV_1). Spirometry tends to be more demanding, and beginning with spirometry allows for the opportunity to repeat spirometry later in the session if initial testing results are not adequate or useable. Static lung volume measurement often follows the dynamic studies, followed by diffusing capacity and bronchodilator or provocation studies, if ordered. The technologist needs to ensure that any of the following have not occurred in order for the test to meet acceptability criteria: slow start, cough, early termination, Valsalva maneuver, glottic closure, poor effort throughout the maneuver, leak, obstructed mouth piece, or evidence of an extra breath.[2] **Figure 12-1** demonstrates some of the common conditions that will disqualify the test during a FVC maneuver.

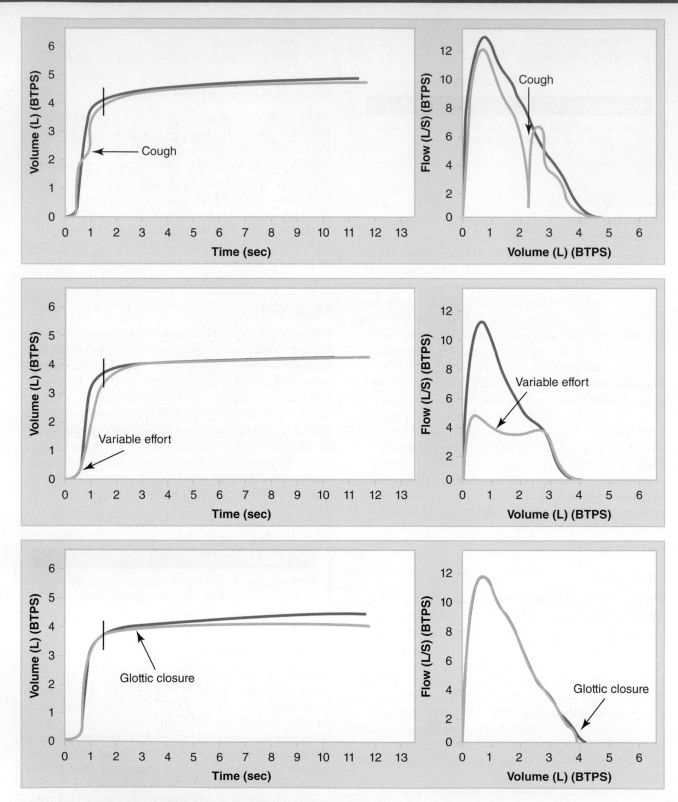

FIGURE 12-1 **Invalid pulmonary function tests.**

Modified from: Spirometry Quality Assurance: Common Errors and Their Impact on Test Results, 2012. CDC. NIOSH.

Reproducibility

Reproducibility is a hallmark of a high-quality test. The technologist should verify test reproducibility between testing maneuvers. Once reproducibility is established, the technologist can proceed to the next test or conclude the study if no additional testing has been ordered. For spirometry, a minimum of three acceptable maneuvers is required. The following ATS/

ERS criteria have to be met in order for the test to be acceptable: (1) the two largest FVC values must be within 0.150 L of each other and (2) the two largest FEV_1 values must be within 0.150 L of each other.[11] If both of these criteria are met, the test is acceptable. If both of these criteria are not satisfied, testing should be repeated until both of the criteria are met. A maximum of eight tests may be performed.[2] Testing may be halted if the patient cannot continue due to exhaustion or distress.[2] If the technologist is having difficulty obtaining an acceptable test, a brief break or moving on to the next test with the intent on coming back may be warranted.

It should be noted that even under ideal conditions, each pulmonary function maneuver is highly patient dependent (e.g., adequate effort and cooperation). It is up to the technologist overseeing the testing to ensure that the patient makes a maximal effort for each maneuver. To ensure this, coaching and demonstrations are needed, along with lots of encouragement. Because each maneuver can be tiresome to the patient, the technologist should ensure that the patient has enough time to recover between maneuvers. Modern spirometers will indicate if the patient effort is adequate, but it is up to the technologist to ensure that each maneuver is done properly and meets current guidelines and recommendations.

Lung Volumes

Prior to describing the interpretation of the tests, it is worthwhile to discuss the lung volumes and capacities that are measured clinically. **Figure 12-2** illustrates how lung volumes and capacities relate to each other. With the exception of residual volume (RV), lung volumes can be measured directly via spirometry. This section will briefly define these volumes.

Tidal Volume

Tidal volume (V_T) is the amount of air that is moved during quiet breathing. The average is approximately 500 mL for both men and women. The range is 400 to 700 mL.

Minute Ventilation

Minute ventilation ($\dot{V}_E$) is the volume of gas that is exhaled over 1 minute. A normal range is 5 to 10 L/min while at rest. $\dot{V}_E$ is the product of the patient's respiratory rate (normal 12 to 18 or 20 breaths/min) and tidal volume (400 to 700 mL). Minute ventilation may increase in response to exercise, fever, pain, hypoxemia, or acidosis. It may be diminished due to neurologic conditions or the presence of pharmacologic suppressive agents.

Inspiratory Reserve Volume

Inspiratory reserve volume (IRV) is the volume of air that can be inspired above and beyond the normal inspired tidal volume when a person inspires with full force. It is approximately 3000 mL for men and 2000 mL for women.

Expiratory Reserve Volume

Expiratory reserve volume (ERV) is the maximum volume of air the can be expired by forceful expiration after the end of a normal tidal expiration. It is

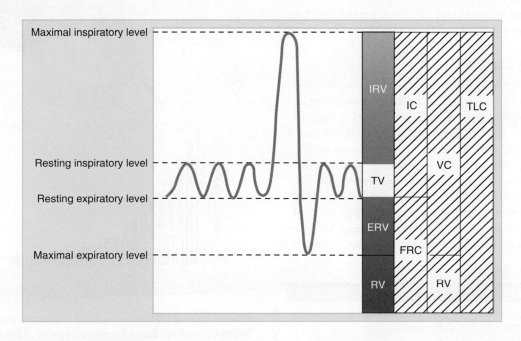

FIGURE 12-2 Lung volumes and capacities.

approximately 1200 mL in a healthy young adult. Obesity, poor effort, and restrictive lung disease may reduce ERV.

Residual Volume

Residual volume (RV) is the volume of air remaining in the lungs following a forced expiration. This volume of air cannot be exhaled. It is approximately 1200 mL for both men and women. It may be abnormally high in obstructive diseases. Residual volume cannot be measured directly via spirometry. Methods for indirect measurement of RV include helium equilibration, nitrogen washout, and use of body plethysmograph.

X-ray Planimetry

Lung volume can also be estimated based on radiographic images; however, this method is not widely used and typically is only considered when the patient will be receiving radiation for other diagnostic purposes. Using posteroanterior (PA) and lateral chest x-rays, chest computed tomography (CT) scan, or magnetic resonance imaging (MRI) images, lung volume can be calculated by subtracting the volume occupied by the heart and great vessels from the total volume within the thoracic cavity. This method is useful for patients when traditional methods of obtaining lung volumes are not feasible.[14] Although imaging software is commercially available for this purpose, one major concern with this technique is the ability for correct interpretation because determination of lung values requires maximum inspiration and expiration that are often difficult to obtain during clinical studies.[14]

Lung Capacities

Whereas lung volumes can be directly measured, lung capacities are extrapolated from two or more volumes.

Inspiratory Capacity

Inspiratory capacity (IC) is the sum of V_T plus IRV. It is the amount of air a person can breathe in beginning at the normal expiratory level and distending the lungs to the maximum amount. A normal IC is about 3600 mL in a healthy young adult or 50 mL/kg of ideal body weight (IBW). An IC-like maneuver is performed during incentive spirometry, a technique used to prevent atelectasis in postoperative patients and others at risk for the development of atelectasis in the acute care setting. An ideal volume goal for incentive spirometry is at least 33% of predicted IC. Incentive spirometry should be accompanied by

> **RC Insights**
>
> Inspiratory capacity is 75% of vital capacity, and expiratory residual capacity is 25% of vital capacity.

additional deep-breathing exercises, directed coughing, early mobilization, and avoidance of excessive sedation.

Functional Residual Capacity

Functional residual capacity (FRC) is the sum of ERV plus RV. A normal FRC is about 2400 mL in a normal healthy young adult. It is the amount of air that remains in the lungs at the end of a passive expiration. It represents the balance between the chest wall's tendency to expand and the lung's elasticity (i.e., tendency to collapse). A loss of lung elastic tissue (as in patients with chronic obstructive lung disease [COPD]) will increase FRC as lung recoil is reduced. Elevated FRCs in a patients with COPD may be caused by air trapping or hyperinflation related to their obstructive disease. Often, this will cause a corresponding decrease in VC, although TLC is within normal range. Conversely, in patients with pulmonary fibrosis (in whom the lung tissue is more elastic), FRC is decreased due to an increase in lung recoil.

Nitrogen Washout Method

The method for performing the nitrogen washout (**Figure 12-3**) is fairly simple. The patient breathes 100% oxygen for about 7 minutes until all the nitrogen

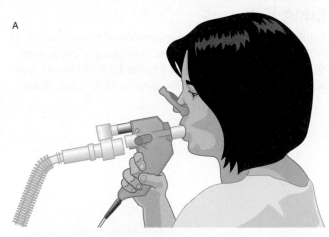

A

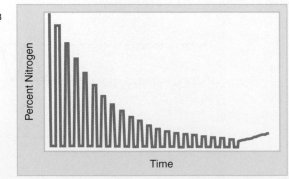

B

FIGURE 12-3 **(A) Nitrogen washout procedure and (B) Nitrogen washout curve for measurement of functional residual capacity (FRC).**

is washed out from the patient's lungs.[15] The exhaled gas volume is collected, and the initial and final alveolar N_2 concentration levels are used to calculate FRC:

$$FRC = \frac{(\text{Volume } N_2 \text{ washed out}) - (\text{Volume } N_2 \text{ tissue excreted})}{\text{Initial} - \text{final alveolar } N_2 \text{ concentration}}$$

The N_2 tissue excreted is based on tables that use the patient's height and weight. The patient breathes until there are three continuous measurements of < 1.5% nitrogen.[14] For interpretation, only one acceptable result is required.

Helium Dilution Method

Another method for indirect measurement of FRC is the closed-circuit helium dilution method (**Figure 12-4**). Helium, which is an inert gas, is not readily absorbed by the blood. This method is based on the principle that if a patient breathes a known volume and concentration of helium (10%), the helium will dilute in proportion to the lung volume to which the gas was added. This equilibration takes approximately 7 minutes. Oxygen must be added and carbon dioxide (CO_2) removed from the system during the test to match O_2 consumption and to ensure that CO_2 does not build up. At the end of the test, the helium concentration in the system (i.e., lungs plus spirometer) is used to calculate FRC, using the following formula:

$$FRC = \frac{(\text{Initial helium} - \text{Final helium}) \times V \times BTPS}{\text{Final helium}}$$

where V is the volume in the spirometer and **BTPS** is a correction factor for **body temperature, pressure, and saturation** (of air with water).

Vital Capacity

Vital capacity (VC) is the sum of the IRV, V_T, and ERV. VC is about 4800 mL in a healthy young adult. It is the maximum amount of air a person can expel from the lungs after first filling the lungs to their maximum extent and then expiring to the maximum extent. If the patient gently exhales all the volume, it is referred to as a **slow vital capacity (SVC)** maneuver. If the patient exhales the volume forcefully, it is called a **forced vital capacity (FVC)** maneuver. SVC is usually slightly greater than FVC and may be significantly higher in patients with air trapping. When differences between the FVC and SVC are significant, the SVC should be used in calculation of the FEV_1 to vital capacity ratio (FEV_1/VC).

Vital capacity measurement has several clinical uses, particularly in patients with restrictive disease. Vital capacity measurement may be used to assess for disease progression or response to treatment in patients with

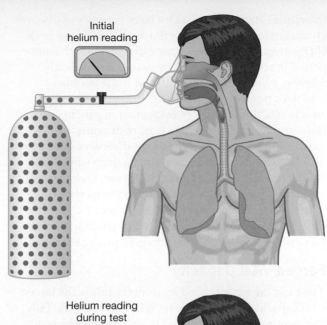

Initial helium reading

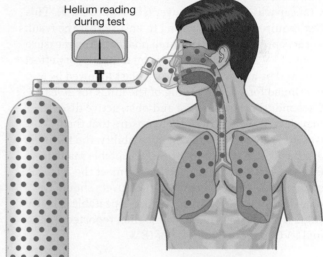

Helium reading during test

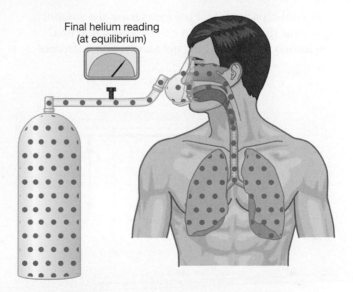

Final helium reading (at equilibrium)

FIGURE 12-4 Helium equilibration for measurement of functional residual capacity (FRC).

interstitial lung disease (ILD; a large category of diseases characterized by pulmonary fibrosis). A decrease in an ILD patient's VC of 10% or more over a 6-month time period is associated with an increased risk of death, whereas an improvement of 10% or more is associated with improved survival. VC measurement plays an important role in the management of patients with respiratory muscle weakness (e.g., neuromuscular disease). Patients with neuromuscular disorders should be evaluated for hypoventilation during sleep when their VC decreases to 40% or less of predicted. Endotracheal intubation should be considered in patients with Guillain-Barré syndrome when VC decreases to ≤ 20 mL/kg (or < 1.0 L), because this can signal impending respiratory failure. A normal VC is about 70 mL/kg of IBW.

Forced Vital Capacity

The most commonly used spirometry test is the forced vital capacity (FVC) maneuver (see **Figure 12-5**). This test requires proper coaching to ensure that the results are acceptable. There are three phases to the measurement of FVC. The first is a maximal inspiratory effort followed by an initial expiratory blast followed by a continued forceful emptying of the lungs for at least 6 seconds. Both restrictive and obstructive diseases may decrease FVC. In order to ensure that the FVC was done correctly and has repeatability, the technologist needs to have at least three acceptable maneuvers (see section "During the Test") that meet the ATS/ERS standards.[16] Three acceptable maneuvers should be obtained, of which at least two are repeatable. The FVC value from the best maneuver is then reported. A normal FVC is about 70 mL/kg of IBW.

Slow Vital Capacity

Slow vital capacity (SVC) is a measure of the amount of volume that a patient can exhale after a maximal inspiration while breathing out slowly. The difference

between a SVC and the FVC is that the FVC is a forced maximal effort and is done in about 6 seconds; the SVC may take up to 30 seconds for the patient to completely exhale. The patient may produce a larger VC during the SVC maneuver due to less air trapping.[16]

Total Lung Capacity

Total lung capacity (TLC) is the sum of SVC plus RV. It is the amount of air contained in the lungs following a maximal inspiratory effort. A normal TLC in a healthy young adult is about 6 L. Normal values ranges from 80% to 120% of predicted, but more specific predicted ranges are commonly used by each laboratory. Similar to other PFT parameters, the TLC is a function of the patient's height, age, race, and gender. Patients with obstructive lung disease may have an increase in TLC due to hyperinflation (e.g., TLC > 120% predicted). Patients with restrictive disease will have a lower TLC value (e.g., TLC < 80% predicted). Because the RV cannot be directly measured by simple spirometry, it needs to be measured in one of four ways: body plethysmography, open-circuit nitrogen washout, closed-system helium dilution, or x-ray planimetry. Only body plethysmography will be described below, as the others were described earlier. Restrictive lung disease causes a decrease in TLC, typically to < 80% of predicted values. TLC > 120% predicted is defined as lung hyperinflation.

Body Plethysmography

Body plethysmography (also called a "body box," see **Figure 12-6**) uses **Boyle's law**, which states that the pressure and volume of a gas vary inversely if the temperature remains constant. This test measures all the gas within the chest. When the patient is positioned in the body box, two volumes are considered: the volume of the box that is known and the volume of compressible gas (largely within the chest/lungs) that is unknown. The formula is as follows:

$$V_1 = \frac{V_2 \times P_2}{P_1}$$

where:

V_1 = Lung volume
P_1 = Gas pressure of the lung
V_2 = Body box volume
P_2 = Gas pressure of the box

Body plethysmography is more accurate for measurement of FRC than gas dilution or washout methods because it measures trapped as well as exhaled gas. Gas dilution or washout methods cannot measure the trapped gas and thus may underestimate TLC in patients with COPD (e.g., air trapping) or in patients with bullae (air-filled pockets that do not communicate with the airways). Body boxes are large and expensive

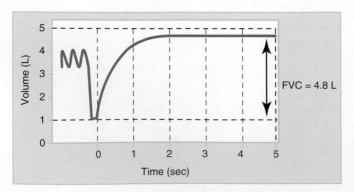

FIGURE 12-5 Forced vital capacity maneuver.

Data from: Ruppel GL. *Manual of Pulmonary Function Testing.* St. Louis, MO: Mosby Elsevier; 2009:58.

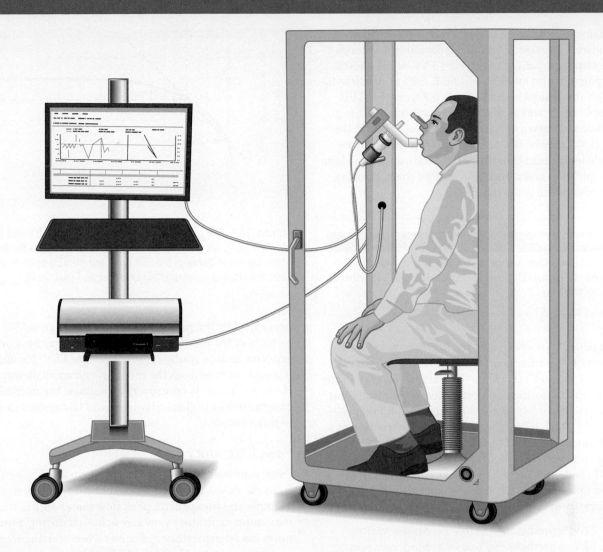

FIGURE 12-6 Body plethysmography.

and may be limited to high-volume pulmonary function labs. Body plethysmography is considered the gold standard when TLC must be accurately measured.[17] According to Wanger et al., when air trapping is present, most (but not all) patients will have a greater FRC when measured by plethysmography as compared to measurement by gas dilution. [14]

Flow Determination

Measurement of Airflow

Several different measures are used clinically to assess gas flow out of the lung. These parameters are useful for diagnosing, trending, and tracking obstructive lung diseases, such as asthma and COPD, and assessing disease progression and/or response to treatment. The three most commonly used measures are:

- Forced expiratory volume in 1 second (FEV_1)
- Forced expiratory flow, midexpiratory phase ($FEF_{25-75\%}$)
- Peak expiratory flow (PEF; peak flow)

Improvements in technology allow any of these three flow measures to be performed outside of the PFT lab. The small portable units that can be used to obtain these measures are ideal for outpatient use, as well as for testing hospitalized patients, eliminating the need to transport the patient to the pulmonary function laboratory. Data capturing is available with most devices that enables graphical displays to be generated for self-management as well as use by the primary care provider.

Forced Expiratory Volume in 1 Second

The forced expiratory volume in 1 second, or FEV_1, is the volume of air that is exhaled during the first second of a forced expiration. Normal subjects are able to exhale 83% of their total FVC in 1 second. In other words, a normal FEV_1/FVC ratio is 0.83. The normal value for FEV_1 is 80% to 100% of predicted. Predicted values are commonly based on 95% confidence intervals; therefore, some patients will have results that exceed 100%. FEV_1 may be reduced in both obstructive and restrictive disease, but not for the reasons one would think. Patients suffering from a restrictive disease may not have a large enough FVC to exhale the normal amount of volume expected in 1 second. For example, a patient may have a FVC of 2.0 L (50% of predicted) and an FEV_1 of 1.65 L (50% of predicted), though the patient's FEV_1/FVC is 0.83, or 83%. This example illustrates that with a reduction in FVC (e.g., restrictive disease), the FEV_1 will be reduced, but the FEV_1/FVC may be normal. Patients with respiratory muscle weakness often cannot generate enough volume on inspiration and cannot forcefully exhale, limiting their results and reducing FEV_1.

> ### RC Insights
> For FVC maneuvers, remember the following: the two largest values of FVC and FEV_1 must be within 0.150 L of each other to be acceptable.

In patients in whom an obstructive component is suspected, it is important to examine the calculated ratio of FEV_1 to FVC. When this ratio is lower than the lower limit of normal, an obstructive defect is present.[11] The current guidelines for the diagnosis and management of COPD define the presence of obstruction as a postbronchodilator FEV_1/FVC < 0.70 (or 70%).

Once obstruction has been identified (e.g., FEV_1/FVC < 0.70), Pellegrino et al.[11] have suggested that the FEV_1 percent predicted (FEV_1% predicted) be used to classify the severity of lung function impairment as follows:

- FEV_1% predicted 70% to 79%: Mild severity
- FEV_1% predicted 60% to 69%: Moderate severity
- FEV_1% predicted 50% to 59%: Moderately severe
- FEV_1% predicted 35% to 49%: Severe
- FEV_1% predicted < 35%: Very severe

The Global Institute for Chronic Obstructive Lung Disease (GOLD) standards suggest a similar approach for classification for airflow limitation in COPD in patients, where:

- FEV_1% predicted ≥ 80% and FEV_1/FVC < 0.70: Mild airflow limitation
- FEV_1% predicted 50% to 79% and FEV_1/FVC < 0.70: Moderate airflow limitation
- FEV_1% predicted 30% to 49% and FEV_1/FVC < 0.70: Severe airflow limitation
- FEV_1% predicted < 30% and FEV_1/FVC < 0.70: Very severe airflow limitation

Forced Expiratory Flow, Midexpiratory Phase

The forced expiratory flow, midexpiratory phase ($FEF_{25-75\%}$) measures the mean expiratory flow between 25% and 75% of the FVC (see **Figure 12-7**). The value is taken from the test with the largest sum of the FEV_1 and FVC of the existing acceptable FVC maneuvers

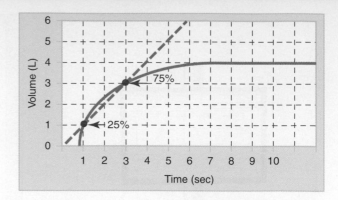

FIGURE 12-7 **$FEF_{25-75\%}$.** In this example, the FVC is 4.0 L and 25% of FVC is 1.0 L, while 75% of FVC is 3.0 L. The $FEF_{25-75\%}$ is the slope of the line drawn between the 25% point and the 75% point. In this case, the slope is approximately 1.0 L/sec and thus the $FEF_{25-75\%}$ is 1.0 L/sec.

performed by the patient.[2] The normal range is 65% to 100% of the predicted value. $FEF_{25-75\%}$ may be more sensitive to airway obstruction than the FEV_1 because it measures flow from the medium and small airways. However, its use is controversial, because the normal ranges are less well standardized and test results can be highly variable.

Peak Expiratory Flow

Peak expiratory flow (**PEF** or **PEFR**) can be obtained from the flow-volume curve data or through the use a simple and inexpensive peak flow meter. PEF is the maximum expiratory flow rate achieved during a maximum forced expiratory maneuver when starting from a point of maximal inflation.[2] The patient performs three maneuvers, and the best flow is reported. PEF is highly dependent on patient effort, but it can be useful in assessing airflow limitation in patients with asthma, thereby helping to assess how well a patient's disease is controlled on the current medical regimen or to detect an asthma exacerbation. A normal PEF in a healthy young adult is about 7.5 to 10 L/sec.

> ### RC Insights
> PEF has to be within 0.67 L/sec. The highest, or best, PEF is used.

Choice of Best Test

As has been noted, FVC maneuvers have to meet certain criteria. For forced spirometry maneuvers, at least three acceptable maneuvers should be obtained in which at least two are repeatable. For reporting, the technologist then chooses the largest FVC and largest FEV_1, even if these values are taken from separate curves. For $FEF_{25-75\%}$ and PEF, the "best test curve" is used, which is the curve with the largest sum of FVC plus FEV_1. For example, the following three tests all meet criteria for an acceptable test:

Parameter	Trial 1	Trial 2	Trial 3	Reported Value
FVC (L)	5.20	5.30	5.35	5.35
FEV_1 (L)	4.41	4.35	4.36	4.41
FEV_1 + FVC (L)	9.61	9.65	9.71	NA
FEV_1/FVC	0.85	0.82	0.82	0.82
$FEF_{25-75\%}$ (L/sec)	3.87	3.92	3.94	3.94
PEF (L/sec)	8.39	9.44	9.89	9.89

The sum of FEV_1 + FVC is used to determine the "best curve." In this example, the best FVC was obtained in trial 3, the best FEV_1 was obtained in trial 1, and the best curve was obtained in trial 3. The best curve is utilized to report $FEF_{25-75\%}$ and PEF. The best FVC occurred during trial 3, whereas the best FEV_1 occurred during trial 1, and those values are reported (i.e., FVC = 5.35 L and FEV_1 = 4.41 L).

RC Insights

After three FVC maneuvers are performed, the largest values are reported. The FEV_1 and FVC ratio is made up from the two best FEV_1 and FVC maneuvers.

Flow-Volume Loops

The flow-volume loop (FVL) is the graphic representation of the flows generated during an FVC maneuver versus the volume change (see **Figure 12-8**). The patient performs a FVC maneuver by inspiring fully and then exhaling as rapidly as possible. To complete the loop, the patient inspires as rapidly as possible from the maximal expiratory level back to maximal inspiration. The single best test maneuver (highest sum of FEV_1 and FVC) is used for reporting purposes.

Graphical inspection of the FVL can be diagnostic. There are several distinct patterns of flow limitation that can assist the clinician in diagnosing, or pursuing additional testing for, specific diseases. During normal respiration, elastic fibers within the lung tissue help keep the small airways open. During exhalation, these elastic fibers shorten and decrease their tethering on the airways, which eventually (at low lung volumes) cause the airways to collapse. Smooth muscle in the walls of the small airways can constrict (bronchospasm) decreasing the airway diameter and decreasing expiratory flow. The administration of a fast-acting β-agonist aerosol (such as albuterol) can cause bronchial smooth muscle relaxation and can rapidly improve expiratory flow rates.

The ATS/ERS has a list of standards that must be met in order for the FVL test to be acceptable. The four standards are: (1) rapid rise from maximal inspiration to PEF, (2) maximal effort until flow returns to zero with no glottic closure or abrupt end of flow, (3)

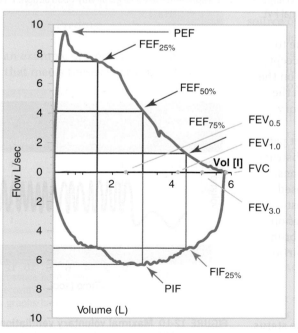

PEF-peak expiratory flow rate
PIF-peak inspiratory flow rate
FVC-forced vital capacity
FEF-forced expiratory flow rate at 25%, 50%, and 75% of FVC
FEV-forced expiratory volume at 0.5, 1.0, and 3.0 sec

FIGURE 12-8 Normal flow-volume loop.

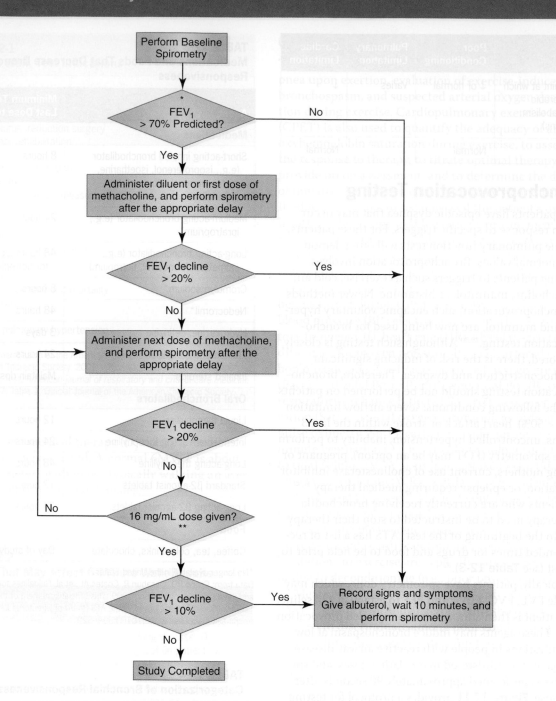

FIGURE 12-11 Flow chart for a methacholine challenge testing sequence.

Reprinted with permission of the American Thoracic Society. Copyright © 2014 American Thoracic Society. 1999 *Am J Respir Crit Care Med* 2000;161:309-329, Figure 2. Official Journal of the American Thoracic Society.

Pulmonary Function Test Interpretation

Quality Control

One of the most important aspects of pulmonary function testing is ensuring the quality of the test results, which includes the accuracy of the instruments within the laboratory. The technologist must understand the equipment's capacity, accuracy, error, resolution, precision, linearity, and output. Many of the computerized systems currently in use will step the technologist through warm-up, calibration, and quality-control procedures; however, it is the responsibility of the lab manager and medical director to ensure that manufacturer and international recommendations and standards are followed.

The ATS and ERS have developed a set of standards that must be met in order for testing to be considered valid.[9] Equipment used in the lab should meet ATS/ERS guidelines and be calibrated on a daily basis.[16] This ensures accurate and validated test results from that laboratory. Most well-equipped PFT laboratories have the following equipment:

- Spirometer for measuring flows and volumes
- Body plethysmograph for measuring total lung capacity, thoracic gas volume (e.g., FRC) and airway resistance
- Gas analysis systems
  - Diffusion testing (CO, CO_2, O_2)
  - Metabolic testing ($\dot{V}CO_2$, $\dot{V}O_2$,)
  - Blood gas and co-oximetry analysis
- Nebulizer equipment for delivering both bronchodilators and bronchoprovocation agents
- Treadmill or bicycle for exercise testing
- A defibrillator (e.g., AED), oxygen, and resuscitation equipment

Before any interpretation can proceed, it is important that the test meets all ATS standards for quality, acceptable test results, and reproducibility. All tests should be recorded at BTPS. Finally, the test results need to be compared to reference values or ranges for normal subjects of the same age, height, gender, and race (e.g., NHANES III). Guidelines are available for using such published references values or ranges.

Pattern Recognition

For spirometry, there are three basic abnormal pulmonary function patterns: obstructive, restrictive, and mixed. ATS recommends initially focusing on the FEV_1, FVC, FEV_1/FVC, and TLC for interpreting PFT results.[16] According to Pellegrino et al., limiting the number of PFT parameters examined for interpretation purposes will help avoid reporting an inordinate number of "abnormal" test results.[11] It may be helpful to use an algorithm such as provided in **Figure 12-12** to interpret PFT results. This allows most clinicians to come up with a diagnosis. The ATS recommends starting with FEV_1/FVC ratio and FVC.[11] Abnormal values are those below the 5th percentile of the predicted value.[11]

Spirometry values for FEV_1, FVC, FEV_1/FVC, and TLC that are below the 5th percentile of the predicted values are consistent with a pulmonary defect.[16] However, if the values lay close to the lower limits of normal, then further investigation is suggested, because these numbers may not separate subjects with early lung disease from normal subjects. It is probably safer to interpret lung testing results on the conservative side and recommend serial studies until a confirmed diagnosis can be made. Many diseases have additional symptoms, and PFTs are often used to confirm and quantify the disease state. Borderline results warrant additional testing or retesting, especially in the absence of any physical symptoms.

For a patient with a suspected obstructive component, the FEV_1/FVC ratio is the best parameter to review. Specifically, an FEV_1/FVC (or FEV_1/VC) below the 5th percentile of the predicted value defines airway obstruction.[11] As an alternative, a FEV_1/FVC ratio < 0.70 may be used to identify obstruction. Once the

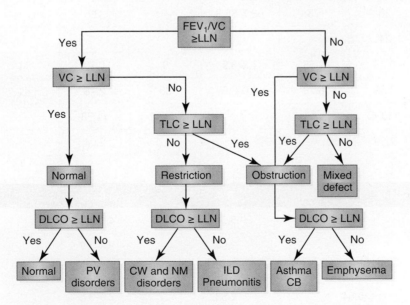

VC, vital capacity; LLN, lower limit of normal; TLC, total lung capacity;
D$_{LCO}$, diffusing capacity; PV, pulmonary vascular disorder; CW, chest wall disorders;
NM, neuromuscular disorders; ILD, interstitial lung disease; CB, chronic bronchitis.

FIGURE 12-12 Lung function interpretation algorithm.

R. Pellegrino, G. Viegi, V. Brusasco, R. O. Crapo, F. Burgos, R. Casaburi, A. Coates, C. P. M. van der Grinten, P. Gustafsson, J. Hankinson, R. Jensen, D. C. Johnson, N. MacIntyre, R. McKay, M. R. Miller, D. Navajas, O. F. Pedersen, and J. Wanger, Interpretative strategies for lung function tests, *Eur Respir J November 2005 26:948-968; doi:1 0.1183/09031936.05.00035205.*

FEV_1/FVC ratio (or FEV_1/VC ratio) determines the presence of obstruction, $FEV_1\%$ predicted is used to classify the degree of severity of obstruction (e.g., mild, moderate, or severe). Different cut values may be used for different disorders when reviewing $FEV_1\%$ predicted (e.g., asthma vs. COPD). **Clinical Focus 12-1** describes the evaluation of a patient with dyspnea and a long history of smoking. **Clinical Focus 12-2** describes the evaluation of an apparently healthy subject.

> **RC Insights**
>
> An increase in TLC, RV, or the RV/TLC ratio above the upper limits may suggest the presence of emphysema, bronchial asthma, or other obstructive diseases, as well as lung hyperinflation.

CLINICAL FOCUS 12-1

Evaluation of Dyspnea in a Smoker

Mrs. Smith is a 55-year-old female who works in a bakery and has a 70-pack-year smoking (2 packs/day for 35 years) history. She is seen by her primary care physician with a complaint of dyspnea. She is referred to a respiratory care clinician, who obtains a complete set of pulmonary function tests.

Personal Data

Sex: Female
Age: 55 years
Height: 66 inches
Weight: 172 lbs
Race: Caucasian

Spirometry

	Pre	Ref	CI Range	%Ref	Post	%Ref	%Chg
FVC (L)	2.27	3.62	2.9–4.4	63	2.79	77 + 0.52	23
FEV₁ (L)	0.63	2.82	2.2–3.4	22	0.81	29	29 + 0.18
FEV₁/FVC (%)	28	78	68.7–88.3		29		
FEV₁/SVC (%)	24						
FEF₂₅₋₇₅% (L/sec)	0.23	2.56	1.2–3.9	9	0.29	11	24
PEF (L/sec)	2.39	6.73	4.9–8.6	35	2.78	41	16
FET 100% (sec)	11.04				11.78		7
FIF 50% (L/sec)	2.69				2.04		−24

Lung Volumes

	Pre	Ref	CI Range	%Ref
TLC (L)	7.07	5.30	4.3–6.3	133
VC (L)	2.59	3.04	2.4–3.7	85
IC (L)	1.43			
FRC PL (L)	5.64	2.83	2.0–3.6	200
ERV (L)	1.05			
RV (L)	4.48	1.97	1.4–2.5	228
RV/TLC (%)	63	38	28.8–48.0	

Diffusing Capacity

	Pre	Ref	CI Range	%Ref
D$_{LCO}$ (mL/mm Hg/min)	11.3	22.6	16.1–29.1	50
D$_L$ Adj (mL/mm Hg/min)	11.3	22.6	16.1–29.1	50
D$_{LCO}$/V$_A$ (mL/mm Hg/min/L)	2.87	4.38	3.1–5.7	65
D$_L$/V$_A$ Adj (mL/mm Hg/min/L)	2.87			
V$_A$ (L)	3.94	5.17	4.1–6.2	76
IVC (L)	2.66			

Resistance

	Pre	Ref	%Ref
R$_{aw}$ (cm H$_2$O/L/sec)	3.00	1.34	224
G$_{aw}$ (L/sec/cm H$_2$O)	0.333	0.683	49
sR$_{aw}$ (cm H$_2$O/L/s/L)	18.90	3.81	496
sG$_{aw}$ (L/s/cm H$_2$O/L)	0.053	0.262	20

Technologist's Comments

Good patient cooperation and effort. After three acceptable curves were obtained, FVC and FEV$_1$ met ATS reproducibility standards. Albuterol (PROVENTIL HFA) 360 mcg given via spacer. Tolerated treatment well. Room air Spo$_2$ was 97%.

Flow-Volume Loop

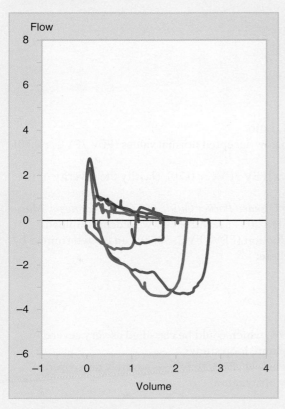

(*continues*)

Forced Vital Capacity

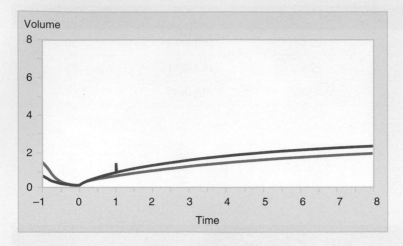

Lung Volumes

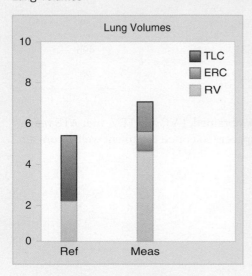

Clinical Assessment Questions

1. Reviewing Mrs. Smith's PFT results, describe the FEV_1/FVC ratio.
   The prebronchodilator FEV_1/FVC ratio is 0.28 (28%), well below accepted normal values ($FEV_1/FVC \geq 0.70$), which indicates obstruction.

2. Given that the patient has a demonstrated obstructive defect ($FEV_1/FVC < 0.70$), classify the severity of the patient's airflow limitation.
   Based on the *Global Initiative for Chronic Obstructive Lung Disease Pocket Guide to COPD Diagnosis, Management, and Prevention for Healthcare Professionals* (updated 2014 see: http://www.goldcopd/upload), severity of airflow limitation in patients with FEV_1/FVC reduction ($FEV_1/FVC < 0.70$) can be determined by examination of the postbronchodilator $FEV_1\%$ predicted, where:

   Mild: $FEV_1 \geq 80\%$ predicted
   Moderate: FEV_1 50% to 79% predicted
   Severe: FEV_1 30% to 49% predicted
   Very severe: $FEV_1 < 30\%$ predicted

   Mrs. Smith has a postbronchodilator $FEV_1\%$ predicted of 29%, which could be classified as very severe.

3. What is the interpretation of the prebronchodilator flow-volume loop study?
   Obstructive ventilatory defect is present (FEV_1/FVC max is below 95% CI). FEV_1 is severely decreased (< 30%). The flow-volume loop is consistent with expiratory obstruction.

4. Did Mrs. Smith demonstrate a response to the bronchodilator?

   Following bronchodilator administration, Mrs. Smith's FVC increased 23%, and her FEV_1 increased 29%. To be considered significant, improvement following bronchodilator administration must be at least 12% *and* at least 200 mL. For Mrs. Smith, the percent improvement was greater than 12% and greater than 200 mL.

5. What is your interpretation of the lung volumes?

   TLC is elevated at 133% predicted. Also elevated are the RV (at 228% predicted), RV/TLC ratio (at 0.63, or 63%), and FRC (at 200% predicted). With airflow obstruction, TLC may be normal or increased. A normal TLC is 80% to 120% predicted, and a normal RV/TLC ratio is about 0.40 (or 40%). The term *air trapping* (as seen in asthma and COPD) is sometimes used when there is an increase in RV and FRC, but no increase in TLC.

6. Provide your interpretation of Mrs. Smith's diffusion capacity results.

   Diffusion capacity is decreased: D_{LCO} was 11.3 mL/mm Hg/min, or 50% of predicted. This indicates a diffusion defect, which could be classified as a moderate decrease (see section on diffusion defect).

7. Describe Mrs. Smith's airway resistance (R_{aw}).

   Normal R_{aw} is about 1 to 2 cm H_2O/L/sec. Mrs. Smith's R_{aw} is increased at 3.0 cm H_2O/L/sec.

8. What is the cause of the patient's symptoms?

   Smoking, and perhaps flour/dust inhalation (she works at a bakery).

9. What other tests might be indicated?

   Arterial blood gases (ABGs) may be helpful.

10. What treatment might be recommended based on these findings.

    Initiate bronchodilator and inhaled steroids. Refer to smoking cessation program.

CLINICAL FOCUS 12-2

Apparently Healthy Individual

Mr. Williams is an apparently healthy 22-year-old male who participates in triathlons. He wants to join the Navy as a pilot. He has a history of taking albuterol in the past for a slight cough and chest tightness, but has not taken it in years. The Navy recruiter sent him for a PFT workup to see if he has any lung condition. The patient does not have a smoking history.

Personal Data

Sex: Male
Age: 23 years
Height: 72 inches

Weight: 191 lbs
Race: Caucasian

Spirometry

	Pre	Ref	CI Range	%Ref	Post	%Ref	%Chg
FVC (L)	6.79	5.82	4.9–6.9	115	6.87	116	1
FEV₁ (L)	4.86	4.88	4.0–5.7	100	5.51	113	13
FEV₁/FVC (%)	72	83	73.6–93.0		80		
FEV₁/SVC (%)	71						
FEF₂₅₋₇₅% (L/sec)	3.54	5.02	3.3–6.7	71	5.03	100	42
PEF (L/sec)	12.60	10.63	8.2–13.1	119	12.62	119	0
FET 100% (sec)	7.81				7.68		–2
FIF 50% (L/sec)	6.53				5.03		–23

(continues)

Lung Volumes

	Pre	Ref	CI Range	%Ref
TLC (L)	8.44	7.54	6.4–8.7	112
VC (L)	6.81	5.87	4.9–6.8	116
IC (L)	4.53			
FRC PL (L)	3.91	3.41	2.4–4.4	115
ERV (L)	2.25			
RV (L)	1.63	1.67	1.0–2.3	98
RV/TLC (%)	19	23	13.9–31.8	

Diffusing Capacity

	Pre	Ref	CI Range	%Ref
D_{Lco} (mL/mm Hg/min)	46.9	37.7	29.8–45.7	124
D_L Adj (mL/mm Hg/min)	46.9	37.7	29.8–45.7	124
D_{Lco}/V_A (mL/mm Hg/min/L)	5.48	5.27	4.1–6.5	104
D_L/V_A Adj (mL/mm Hg/min/L)	5.48			
V_A (L)	8.56	7.16	5.7–8.6	120
IVC (L)	6.89			

Resistance

	Pre	Ref	%Ref
R_{aw} (cm H_2O/L/sec)	1.33	1.10	121
G_{aw} (L/sec/cm H_2O)	0.755	0.954	79
sR_{aw} (cm H_2O/L/s/L)	6.22	4.37	142
sG_{aw} (L/s/cm H_2O/L)	0.161	0.229	70

Technologist's Comments

Good patient cooperation and effort. After three acceptable curves were obtained, FVC and FEV_1 met ATS reproducibility standards. Room air SpO_2 was 99%. Proventila HFA 360 mcg given via spacer. Tolerated treatment well.

Forced Vital Capacity

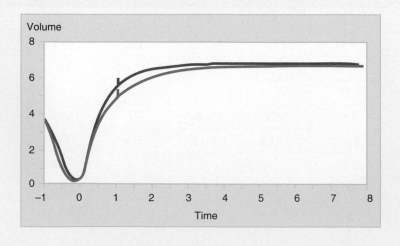

(continues)

Flow-Volume Loop

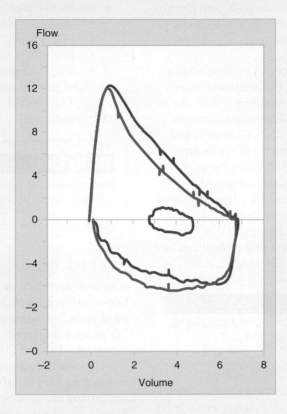

Patient Assessment Questions

1. **What is your interpretation of the prebronchodilator study?**
    Very slight obstructive ventilatory defect may be present (FEV_1/FVC_{max} is < 95% CI); however, the FEV_1/FVC ratio prebronchodilator is 0.72. FEV_1 is normal (80% or greater). Flow-volume loop is normal.

2. **What is your interpretation of the patient's response to bronchodilators?**
    There is a significant improvement in the FEV_1 (> 12% and > 200 mL).

3. **What is your the interpretation of the patient's lung volume results?**
    TLC is normal.

4. **What is your interpretation of the airway resistance and conductance?**
    Normal.

5. **What is the cause of the patient's symptoms?**
    The patient has some response to bronchodilator therapy, and exercise-induced bronchospasm is a possibility.

6. **What other tests might be indicated?**
    Patient might benefit from a bronchoprovocation study; however, because he has no symptoms and is in good condition, this might not be warranted.

7. **What treatment might be recommended based on these findings?**
    Albuterol MDI as needed.

Occasionally, a patient may have a decreased FEV_1/FVC ratio (e.g., $FEV_1/FVC < 0.70$) and a normal FEV_1.[11] In otherwise healthy patients, the interpretation is not clear cut, and the patient may require additional testing.[11] Where respiratory disease has been established, a decreased FEV_1/FVC ratio and normal FEV_1 may signal early disease and may be predictive of future morbidity and mortality.[11]

Although the severity of obstructive lung disease is generally based on $FEV_1\%$ predicted, this does not apply to upper airway obstruction. It should also be noted that although $FEV_1\%$ predicted correlates better than other PFT parameters with symptoms, it is not by itself a strong prognostic predictor. For example, other parameters (VC and DLCO) are better predictors of mortality in patients with ILD. Additionally, exercise tolerance often does not correlate well with FEV_1, so assessing both lung function and exercise capacity (typically with the 6-minute walk test) permits a more accurate evaluation of the individual patient. **Table 12-5** summarizes typical patterns of pulmonary function by disease state.

A restrictive ventilatory defect can be defined as a TLC below the 5th percentile of the predicted value with a normal FEV_1/FVC (or normal FEV_1/VC).[11] As an alternative, a reduced FVC (or VC) with a normal (or increased) FEV_1/FVC (or FEV_1/VC) is consistent with a restrictive defect. In cases where there is a reduced FVC (or VC) and normal FEV_1/FVC ratio, the presence of restrictive disease should be confirmed by measurement of TLC, as a reduced VC often does not predict low TLC. For example, poor patient effort may result in a low FVC or VC, even though TLC is normal. **Clinical Focus 12-3** describes the evaluation of a patient with dyspnea for possible restrictive lung disease.

RC Insights

Restrictive abnormalities have a reduction in TLC below the 5th percentile of predicted and a normal FEV_1/FVC.

To summarize, pulmonary function abnormalities may be classified as an obstructive pattern, a restrictive pattern, or mixed:

- Obstructive pattern
  - FVC normal or decreased
  - FEV_1 decreased
  - FEV_1/FVC decreased
  - TLC normal or increased
- Restrictive pattern
  - FVC decreased
  - FEV_1 normal or decreased
  - FEV_1/FVC decreased
  - TLC decreased

A mixed pattern is suggested when there is obstruction (e.g., $FEV_1/FVC < 0.70$) and restriction (e.g., TLC < 0.80% predicted).

RC Insights

Mixed abnormalities are identified when both FEV_1/FVC and TLC are below the 5th percentile.

Approach to Interpretation of Results

A general approach to interpretation of PFT results is to begin with review of the FEV_1/FVC ratio to determine if an obstructive defect is present. If $FEV_1/FVC < 0.70$ (or 5th percentile of predicted value), then the FEV_1 % predicted may be used to classify the severity of the defect. If an obstructive defect is present, the clinician may then assess for a significant bronchodilator response by comparing pre- and postbronchodilator FEV_1 and FVC. Finally, the clinician should determine if a gas transfer (diffusing capacity) defect is present using DLco. This is especially important in separating asthma (normal DLco) from COPD (usually a reduced DLco) and for identifying early ILD (often with a reduced DLco

TABLE 12-5
Typical Patterns of Abnormal Pulmonary Function

	Restrictive Disease		Obstructive Disease	
	Lung Tissue	**Mechanical Factors**	**Asthma**	**COPD**
FVC	↓	↓	N or ↓	N or ↓
FEV_1	↓	↓	↓	↓
FEV_1/FVC	N	N	< 0.70	< 0.70
TLC	↓	↓	N or ↑	N or ↑
RV/TLC	N	↑	N or ↑	N or ↑
R_{aw}	N	N	↑	↑
DLco	↓	N	N	↓ (emphysema)

N, normal; R_{aw}, airway resistance capacity; DLco, diffusion capacity (typical single-breath carbon monoxide).

With obstructive disease (e.g., COPD or asthma), there is a decrease in FEV_1 and a decrease in the FEV_1/FVC ratio. With COPD, there also may be a decrease in FVC. Airway resistance (R_{aw}) is increased with obstructive disease. With emphysema, diffusion capacity is reduced, whereas with asthma and "pure" chronic bronchitis (i.e., no alveolar destruction) DLco may be normal. Restrictive disease may be due to lung tissue disease (e.g., parenchymal disease, such as fibrotic lung disease) or mechanical problem (e.g., neuromuscular disease, chest wall deformity). In both cases, FVC and TLC are reduced. With parenchymal disease, DLco may be reduced, whereas with mechanical disease DLco may be normal.

Data from: Section 3- Respiratory Disorders, Chapter 23 - Pulmonary Function Testing – By Dr Jay I. Peters, MD and Dr David Shelledy, PhD

CLINICAL FOCUS 12-3

Dyspnea Evaluation

Mrs. Trevia is a 43-year-old female who has been complaining of shortness of breath for several months. The patient has been referred to the PFT lab for further workup by her physician. The patient is a stay-at-home mom.

Personal Data

Sex: Female
Age: 45 years
Height: 66 inches
Weight: 185 lbs
Race: African American

Spirometry

	Pre	Ref	CI Range	%Ref	Post	%Ref	%Chg
FVC (L)	2.03	3.31	2.6–4.1	61			
FEV$_1$ (L)	1.66	2.72	2.1–3.4	61			
FEV$_1$/FVC (%)	82	83	72.6–94.0				
FEV$_1$/SVC (%)	79						
FEF$_{25-75\%}$ (L/sec)	1.68	2.95	1.5–4.4	57			
PEF (L/sec)	6.11	6.93	4.8–9.1				
FET 100% (sec)	7.38						
FIF 50% (L/sec)	2.11						

Lung Volumes

	Pre	Ref	CI Range	%Ref
TLC (L)	2.93	5.3	4.3–6.3	55
VC (L)	2.09	3.49	2.8–4.2	60
IC (L)	1.77			
FRC PL (L)	1.16	2.81	2.0–3.6	41
ERV (L)	0.31			
RV (L)	0.84	1.70	1.1–2.3	49
RV/TLC (%)	29	33	23.1–42.3	

Diffusing Capacity

	Pre	Ref	CI Range	%Ref
D$_{LCO}$ (mL/mm Hg/min)	15.2	24.5	18.0–31.0	62
D$_L$ Adj (mL/mm Hg/min)	15.2	24.5	18.0–31.0	62
D$_{LCO}$/V$_A$ (mL/mm Hg/min/L)	5.59	4.65	3.3–6.0	120
D$_L$/V$_A$ Adj (mL/mm Hg/min/L)	5.59			

(continues)

	Pre	Ref	CI Range	%Ref
V$_A$ (L)	2.73	5.28	4.2–6.3	52
IVC (L)	1.95			

Resistance

	Pre	Ref	%Ref
R$_{aw}$ (cm H$_2$O/L/sec)	3.85	2.02	190
G$_{aw}$ (L/sec/cm H$_2$O)	0.260	0.473	55
sR$_{aw}$ (cm H$_2$O/L/sec/L)	7.30	4.0	183
sG$_{aw}$ (L/sec/cm H$_2$O/L)	0.137	0.250	55

Technologist's Comments

Good patient cooperation and effort. After three acceptable curves were obtained, FVC and FEV$_1$ met ATS reproducibility standards. Room air SpO$_2$ was 98% at rest.

Forced Vital Capacity

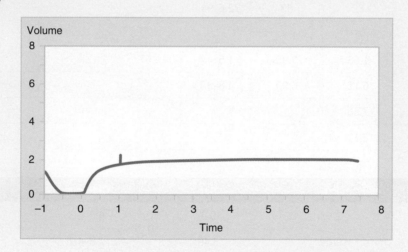

Lung Volumes

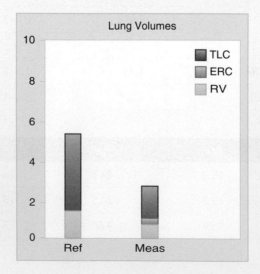

Flow-Volume Loop

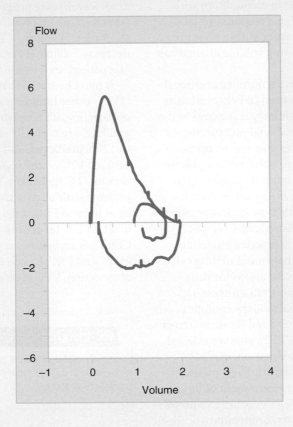

Patient Assessment Questions

1. What is your interpretation of the PFT study?

   FEV_1/FVC is 0.82, which is normal (i.e., no obstruction). Reduced FVC (below 95% CI). FEV_1 is moderately decreased. FVL contour is normal but with reduced volume. A normal FEV_1/FVC ratio with reduced FVC is consistent with restrictive lung disease.

2. Why were pre- and postbronchodilators not given?

   This patient appears to have no airway obstruction.

3. What is your interpretation of the lung volumes?

   TLC indicates a severe restrictive defect.

4. What is your interpretation of airway resistance and conductance?

   Normal.

5. What is the interpretation of the DLCO?

   Moderate decrease in diffusion capacity for CO.

6. What other tests might be indicated?

   Further workup (CT scan and bronchoalveolar lavage [BAL]) led to a diagnosis of interstitial lung disease (sarcoidosis).

7. What treatment might be recommended based on these findings?

   Pulmonary rehabilitation and steroid therapy should be recommended.

with normal lung volumes). In cases where the FEV_1/FVC ratio is normal (or increased), the FVC should be reviewed. A reduced FVC (or VC) in the absence of obstruction suggests a restrictive defect, which may be confirmed by measurement of TLC.

From this information, a combination of defects may be reported. A number of specific diseases (lung and otherwise) are suggested by these combinations. For example, a COPD patient may exhibit an obstructive defect with a gas transfer defect, suggestive of emphysema. It must be recognized that multiple conditions can coexist in an individual patient and that a given disease may have several different patterns, so PFT results must always be used in conjunction with a patient's clinical and radiographic presentation to arrive at the correct diagnosis. Lung volumes should be measured and tracked over time in conjunction with an intervention to best determine a response or lack thereof.[11] A change of 15% or greater within a year is an indication that a significant lung volume change has occurred.

Pulmonary function tests have a number of clinical applications. As noted, they are used to help clinicians diagnose specific diseases. Spirometry is integral to the diagnosis of COPD, for example. Serial measurements are used to assess disease progression and response to treatment. PFTs are often used in preoperative pulmonary evaluation, particularly in patients preparing to undergo lung resection (e.g., for lung cancer). Guidelines exist to aid clinicians in this type of preoperative workup. Examples include the American College of Chest Physicians (ACCP) clinical practice guidelines (CPG) for the diagnosis and management of lung cancer.[33] Likewise, PFTs can be used to assess for drug toxicity (e.g., amiodarone or bleomycin pulmonary toxicity) and to stratify risk of pulmonary complications following hematopoietic stem cell (bone marrow) and solid organ transplantation. PFTs also are utilized to select patients for lung transplantation; cardiopulmonary exercise testing is used similarly in heart transplantation. In addition to measurement of forced spirometry (e.g., FVC, FEV_1, FEV_1/FVC), lung volumes (TLC and FRC), diffusion capacity, bronchoprovocation testing, measurement of airway resistance, MIP and MEP, and exercise testing may be considered, depending on the patient's presentation.

Obstructive Defects

Pulmonary obstructive defects can occur in the upper airway, bronchi, or bronchioles. Lung diseases that are included in (but are not limited to) this category are α1-antitrypsin deficiency, asthma, acute and chronic bronchitis, bronchiectasis, cystic fibrosis, and emphysema. According to Pellegrino et al., an obstructive ventilatory defect is present when there is a disproportionate reduction in maximal expiratory airflow with respect to the the maximal volume (i.e., VC) that can be exhaled.[11] Obstructive diseases are generally signaled by a reduction in measures of expiratory airflow below the lower limit of normal. This reduction in airflow may be caused by bronchospasm, airway inflammation, increased secretions in the airway, and/or due to loss of lung elastic recoil. More specifically, airflow obstruction can be identified by a reduction in the ratio of the FEV_1 to FVC. Expiratory airflow limitation (i.e., obstruction) is generally defined as an FEV_1/FVC ratio below the 5th percentile of the predicted value. Some guidelines utilize a fixed percent, typically FEV_1/FVC < 0.70, but it must be recognized that this strategy risks classifying some "normal" individuals (particularly older adults) as "abnormal." A concave shape that may

be seen on the flow-volume curve indicates the slowing of the expiratory flow. According to Pellegrino et al., as airway disease progresses and/or more central airways become involved, FEV_1 will decrease more than VC (or FVC) and the FEV_1/FVC (or FEV_1/VC) ratio will decrease.[11] **Clinical Focus 12-4** describes the evaluation of a patient with cystic fibrosis.

It must be noted that obstructive lung disease often affects other lung volumes and capacities. With airflow obstruction, TLC maybe normal or increased and RV and FRC are typically elevated. A normal TLC is 80% to 120% predicted, and a normal **RV/TLC ratio** is about 0.40 (or 40%). *Lung hyperinflation* refers to an elevation in TLC (generally TLC > 120% predicted). Some patients with obstructive disease may have an increase in in RV and FRC, a decrease in VC, and no increase in TLC. The term *air trapping* (as seen in asthma and COPD) is sometimes used when there is an increase in RV and FRC, but no increase in TLC. With severe obstruction, FVC is often decreased.

> ### RC Insights
>
> Bronchodilator response is positive when there is both an increase of 12% or more in the FEV_1 or FVC and an increase of 200 mL or more.

Upper and Large Airway Obstruction

Obstruction in the upper or large airway (e.g., larynx, trachea) will cause changes in the FVL that are characteristic depending on the location and type of the obstruction. A fixed large airway obstruction will result in flattened expiratory and inspiratory FVL limbs, whereas variable large airway obstruction (occurring during only one phase of the respiratory cycle) will impair predominantly either inspiratory or expiratory flow. Specifically, extrathoracic obstruction (e.g., vocal cord paralysis) will reduce inspiratory flow, whereas intrathoracic obstruction (e.g., tracheal tumor) may reduce expiratory flow. However, FVL has a low sensitivity for detecting upper or large airway obstructions, and if upper or large airway obstruction is suspected, further investigation is warranted.[34] Examples of variable intrathoracic obstruction include localized tumors of the lower trachea or mainstem bronchus and tracheomalacia. Unilateral and bilateral vocal cord paralysis, vocal cord adhesions, vocal cord constriction, laryngeal edema, and upper airway narrowing associated with obstructive sleep apnea are all examples of variable extrathoracic obstructions. The following may cause fixed airway obstruction: goiters, endotracheal neoplasms, stenosis of both main bronchi, and post-intubation tracheal stenosis. Sorting out if there is intrathoracic or extrathoracic obstruction

CLINICAL FOCUS 12-4

Adult with Cystic Fibrosis

Mrs. Gonzalez is a 40-year-old female who has a long-standing diagnosis of cystic fibrosis (CF). Patient is in for follow-up spirometry.

Personal Data

Sex: Female
Age: 40 years
Height: 63 inches
Weight: 132 lbs
Race: Caucasian

Spirometry

	Pre	Ref	CI Range	%Ref	Post	%Ref	%Chg
FVC (L)	1.89	3.45	2.8–4.1	55			
FEV_1 (L)	0.90	2.76	2.2–3.3	33			
FEV_1/FVC (%)	48	81	70.8–90.4				
FEV_1/SVC (%)							
$FEF_{25-75\%}$ (L/sec)	0.31	2.78	1.6–4.0				
PEF (L/sec)	3.11	6.64	5.0–8.3				
FET 100% (sec)	9.46						
FIVC (L)	1.61						
PIF (L/sec)	3.81						

Technologist's Comments

Good patient cooperation and effort. After three acceptable curves were obtained, FVC and FEV_1 met ATS reproducibility standards. Room air SpO_2 was 98% at rest.

Forced Vital Capacity

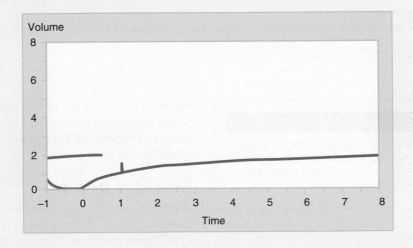

(*continues*)

Flow-Volume Loop

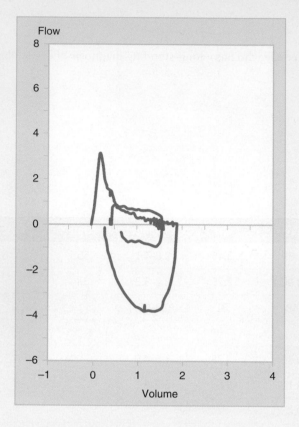

Clinical Assessment Questions

1. What is your interpretation of the PFT results?
    Obstructive defect present (FEV_1/VC max is below the 95% CI). The FEV_1/FVC ratio is 0.48, which indicates obstruction. The FEV_1% predicted is consistent with severe obstruction. Contour of the FVL is concave, consistent with diffuse expiratory airway obstruction.
2. What other information would you like to have?
    Indices from previous tests, which would allow for evaluation of any decline of > 10% in FEV_1 or FVC over time.
3. What is your impression of the study?
    Very severe obstructive ventilatory defect is present that is consistent with known cystic fibrosis.

can be difficult. Figure 12-9 provides examples of FVLs with variable and fixed airway obstruction. **Table 12-6** compares specific PFT measures for extrathoracic and intrathoracic obstruction.

Restrictive Defects

A patient with restrictive disease will typically have a decrease in lung volumes to less than 80% of predicted (TLC below the lower limit of normal) and a normal FEV_1/FVC. Restrictive defects may be caused by chest wall dysfunction, neurologic disease, diaphragm dysfunction, lung resection, ILD, atelectasis, and obesity. According to Pellegrino et al., a reduction in TLC below the 5th percentile of the predicted value with a normal

TABLE 12-6
Lung Function Parameters Capable of Differentiating Extrathoracic and Intrathoracic Obstruction

	Extrathoracic Obstruction		Intrathoracic Obstruction
	Fixed	**Variable**	
PEF	Decreased	Normal or decreased	Decreased
MIF_{50}	Decreased	Decreased	Normal or decreased
MIF_{50}/MEF_{50}	~ 1	< 1	> 1

PEF, peak expiratory flow; MIF_{50}, maximum inspiratory flow at 50% of forced vital capacity (FVC); MEF_{50}, maximum expiratory flow at 50% of FVC.
R. Pellegrino, G. Viegi, V. Brusasco, R. O. Crapo, F. Burgos, R. Casaburi, A. Coates, C. P. M. van der Grinten, P. Gustafsson, J. Hankinson, R. Jensen, D. C. Johnson, N. MacIntyre, R. McKay, M. R. Miller, D. Navajas, O. F. Pedersen, and J. Wanger, Interpretative strategies for lung function tests, *Eur Respir J November 2005* 26:948-968; doi:10.1183/09031936.05.00035205

FEV_1/VC (or normal FEV_1/FVC) suggests restrictive disease.[11] A restrictive ventilatory defect is suspected when VC (or FVC) is reduced, the FEV_1/VC (or FEV_1/FVC) is normal or increased and the flow-volume curve shows a convex shape.[11]

In the setting of obstructive lung disease (e.g. COPD), any significant decrease in TLC over time should be investigated to assess for combined restrictive and obstructive disease (see also below). About 5% of COPD patients develop ILD, a restrictive lung disease. These patients may have an increased TLC (e.g., TLC = 120% predicted) due to obstructive disease. If the COPD patient then develops ILD and TLC begins

to decline, the TLC may never reach the LLN. Thus, a decline in TLC in these patients should be evaluated, even of the TLC is > LLN.

To summarize, spirometry, though helpful, may not be able to accurately identify a restrictive defect, and TLC measurement should be performed if restrictive disease is suspected.[35] It also must be noted that with severe obstruction, TLC can be greatly underestimated by gas dilution or washout techniques, and this significantly increases the risk of misclassifying any PFT abnormality in these patients.[11] **Clinical Focus 12-5** describes the evaluation of an obese patient with dyspnea and possible restrictive disease.

CLINICAL FOCUS 12-5

Dyspnea and Obesity

Mrs. Treveno is a 70-year-old female who has a history of dyspnea. Patient is in for follow-up and spirometry. Known previous smoking history (60-pack-year history). Mrs. Treveno is retired; she used to work as a secretary.

Personal Data

Sex: Female
Age: 70 years
Height: 62 inches
Weight: 360 lbs
Race: African American

Spirometry

	Pre	Ref	CI Range	%Ref	Post	%Ref	%Chg
FVC (L)	1.25	2.25	1.6–2.9	56	1.22	54	−2
FEV_1 (L)	0.89	1.75	1.2–2.3	51	0.96	55	8
FEV_1/FVC (%)	71	78	67.5–88.9		79		
FEV_1/SVC (%)	62						
$FEF_{25-75\%}$ (L/sec)	0.56	1.69	0.4–3.0	33	0.86	51	54

(continues)

	Pre	Ref	CI Range	%Ref	Post	%Ref	%Chg
PEF (L/sec)	3.84	4.82	2.9–6.7	80	5.0	1.4	30
FET 100% (sec)	9.26				7.39		−20
FIF 50% (L/sec)	2.59				1.98		−24

Lung Volumes

	Pre	Ref	CI Range	%Ref
TLC (L)	2.84	4.57	3.6–5.6	62
VC (L)	1.43	2.32	1.6–3.0	62
IC (L)	1.4			
FRC PL (L)	1.44	2.59	1.8–3.4	56
ERV (L)	0.03			
RV (L)	1.41	1.9	1.3–2.5	74
RV/TLC (%)	50	41	31.5–50.6	

CI range: 95% Confidence Interval

Diffusing Capacity

	Pre	Ref	CI Range	%Ref
D$_{LCO}$ (mL/mm Hg/min)	9.1	20.1	13.6–26.6	45
D$_L$ Adj (mL/mm Hg/min)	9.1	20.1	13.6–26.6	45
D$_{LCO}$/V$_A$ (mL/mm Hg/min/L)	3.68	4.44	3.1–5.8	83
D$_L$/V$_A$ Adj (mL/mm Hg/min/L)	3.68			
V$_A$ (L)	2.48	4.53	3.6–5.4	55
IVC (L)	1.36			

Technologist's Comments

Good patient cooperation and effort. After three acceptable curves were obtained, FVC and FEV$_1$ met ATS reproducibility standards. After multiple attempts, patient was unable to reproduce PEF on pre- and postspirometry.

Forced Vital Capacity

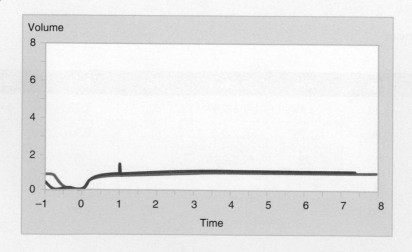

Flow-Volume Loop

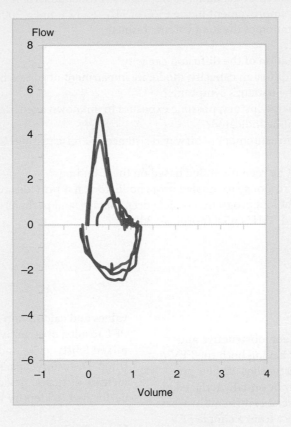

Lung Volumes

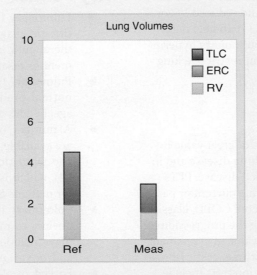

Clinical Assessment Questions

1. What is your interpretation of the prebronchodilator study?

   The prebronchodilator FEV_1/FVC is 0.71 (71%), which is within the 95% CI. For COPD, the GOLD standards for airflow limitation are a postbronchodilator $FEV_1/FVC < 0.70$. This patient's postbronchodilator FEV_1/FVC is 0.79. Although the FEV_1 is reduced (51% of predicted), a large portion of this reduction is due to the reduction in available volume (FVC = 1.25 L). When $FEV_1/FVC > 0.70$ and FVC (and VC) are reduced, a restrictive defect should be considered (and confirmed by measurement of TLC).

(continues)

2. What is your interpretation of the patient's response to bronchodilators?
   There is no significant improvement in the FVC or FEV_1 (> 12% and > 200 mL).
3. What is your interpretation of the lung volume results?
   Mild restrictive defect.
4. What is your interpretation of the diffusion capacity?
   Moderate decrease in diffusion capacity, moderate impairment of gas exchange.
5. What is the cause of the patient's symptoms?
   Obesity, previous smoking history, possible exposure to unknown agent causing restrictive disease.
6. What other tests might be indicated?
   Arterial blood gases, measurement of airway resistance, exercise testing, CT scan, and/or bronchoscopy may be considered.
7. What treatment might be recommended based on these findings?
   Despite no significant response to inhaled bronchodilators, if it provides relief then it should be continued. Consultation for weight loss program, possible drug therapy, and perhaps evaluation for bariatric surgery. The patient's calculated BMI is 65.8 (normal < 30).

Mixed Abnormalities

A patient may have a mixed defect (obstructive and restrictive), which is defined by having both the FEV_1/FVC and TLC below the 5th percentiles of their predicted values.[11] Because VC may be equally reduced by restrictive or obstructive disease, it is difficult to assess if a patient has a combined defect from a simple FEV_1 and VC measurement. Patients with COPD often have reduced FEV_1/FVC (obstruction) and reduced VC or FVC. Measurement of FRC and TLC can help determine if VC reductions are due to pulmonary hyperinflation, air trapping, or concomitant restrictive lung disease.

Summary

Pulmonary function testing can be of great value in assessing patients with suspected lung disease and in monitoring patients with established disease. PFTs may be especially helpful in assessing current or past cigarette smokers, verifying suspected COPD, classifying COPD severity, and monitoring the progression of the disease. PFTs are also of great value in assessment and monitoring of patients with asthma, cystic fibrosis, and ILD. Routine pulmonary function tests include measurement of forced spirometry (FVC, FEV_1, FEV_1/FVC, $FEF_{25-75\%}$), lung volumes (TLC, FRC, RV, VC), and diffusion capacity (DLCO). Additional tests commonly employed include pre- and postbronchodilator tests, bronchoprovocation testing, measurement of MIP and MEP, and exercise testing. Successful pulmonary function testing requires accurate and reliable equipment, proper testing technique, and adequate patient effort. Interpretation of pulmonary function tests often involves comparison of patient values to predicted values and calculation of percent predicted. Based on PFT results, obstructive defects, restrictive defects, or mixed (obstructive and restrictive) defects may be identified. Diffusion capacity (DLCO) may be measured to identify diffusion defects, and exercise testing may be performed to identify limitations to exercise.

Key Points

▶ Pulmonary function testing is intended to identify or diagnose pulmonary disease, monitor therapeutic interventions, and quantify impairment or disability.

▶ Pulmonary function test results are compared to normal predicted values based on the patient's age, height, gender, and race.

▶ A number of predicted datasets and equations are available, including the Third National Health and Nutrition Examination Survey (NHANES III), which is recommended for reference values for patients 8 to 80 years of age.

▶ Pulmonary function testing equipment includes devices to measure gas flow and volume. These may include volume-displacement spirometers and/or various types of pneumotachometers.

▶ Forced oscillation technique (FOT) uses small-amplitude pressure oscillation to measure respiratory mechanics.

▶ Pulmonary function testing should be preceded by a thorough pulmonary history, review of past medical records, and physical assessment.

▶ The results of the pulmonary function test must be reproducible. For spirometry, the two largest values (out of three acceptable tests) must be within 0.15 L of one another; the two largest FEV_1 values must also be within 0.15 L.

- For forced expiratory volume spirometry, a maximum of eight tests may be done; testing should be terminated if the patient becomes exhausted or distressed.
- The four lung volumes are tidal volume (V_T), inspiratory reserve volume (IRV), expiratory reserve volume (ERV), and residual volume (RV).
- Lung capacities are made up of two or more lung volumes.
- Lung capacities include vital capacity (VC), inspiratory capacity (IC), functional residual capacity (FRC), and total lung capacity (TLC).
- A normal IC is about 50 mL/kg of ideal body weight (IBW).
- A normal VC is about 70 mL/kg of IBW.
- RV, FRC, and TLC cannot be directly measured because RV cannot be exhaled.
- Methods to indirectly measure FRC, RV, and TLC include helium dilution, nitrogen washout, and body plethysmography.
- Basic spirometry includes measurement of FVC, FEV_1, $FEF_{25-75\%}$, and PEF.
- The best indicator of obstruction is the FEV_1/FVC ratio < 0.70.
- Once obstruction is identified (e.g., FEV_1/FVC < 0.70), the degree of airflow impairment can be classified based on FEV_1.
- The flow-volume loop allows for observing the characteristics of the expiratory and inspiratory curves to identify various types of obstruction (e.g., small airway obstruction, upper or large airway obstruction).
- Maximal voluntary ventilation (MVV) can be reduced with decreased respiratory muscle strength, decreased compliance, increased resistance, or presence of obstructive disease.
- DLCO measures diffusion capacity; DLCO is decreased when there is a loss of alveolar–capillary surface area (e.g., emphysema).
- The 6-minute walk can be used to assess exercise tolerance.
- Bronchoprovocation testing may identify patients with hypersensitive airways.
- Pulmonary function abnormalities include obstructive, restrictive, and mixed disorders.
- Obstruction is best identified by a reduced FEV_1/FVC ratio; restriction is indicated by a reduced TLC.
- A normal FEV_1/FVC ratio with a reduced VC and FVC suggests restriction, which should be confirmed by TLC measurement.
- A decreased FEV_1/FVC and a decreased TLC suggest a mixed, obstructive/restrictive disorder.
- An increased FRC is associated with pulmonary hyperinflation or air trapping.
- Upper airway obstruction (UAO) can sometimes be identified via flow-volume loop.
- Types of UAO include fixed versus variable and extrathoracic versus intrathoracic obstruction.
- Cardiopulmonary exercise testing can help discriminate among poor conditioning, pulmonary limitation, and cardiac limitation to exercise.

References

1. Crapo RO. Pulmonary-function testing. *N Eng J Med.* 1994; 331(1):25–30.
2. Miller MR, Hankinson J, Brusasco V, et al. Standardisation of spirometry. *Eur Respir J.* 2005;26(2):319–338.
3. Hankinson JL, Odencrantz JR, Fedan KB. Spirometric reference values from a sample of the general U.S. population. *Am J Respir Crit Care Med.* 1999;159(1):179–187.
4. Quanjer PH, Stanojevic S, Cole TJ, et al. Multi-ethnic reference values for spirometry for the 3-95-yr age range: The global lung function 2012 equations. *Eur Respir J.* 2012;40(6):1324–1343.
5. Quanjer PH, Brazzale DJ, Boros PW, Pretto JJ. Implications of adopting the Global Lungs Initiative 2012 all-age reference equations for spirometry. *Eur Respir J.* 2013;42(4):1046–1054.
6. Brazzale DJ, Hall GL, Pretto JJ. Effects of adopting the new global lung function initiative 2012 reference equations on the interpretation of spirometry. *Respiration.* 2013;86(3):183–189.
7. Quanjer PH, Hall GL, Stanojevic S, Cole TJ, Stocks J, Global Lungs Initiative. Age- and height-based prediction bias in spirometry reference equations. *Eur Respir J.* 2012;40(1):190–197.
8. Robbins DR, Enright PL, Sherrill DL. Lung function development in young adults: Is there a plateau phase? *Eur Respir J.* 1995; 8(5):768–772.
9. Miller MR, Crapo R, Hankinson J, et al. General considerations for lung function testing. *Eur Respir J.* 2005;26(1):153–161.
10. Knudson RJ, Lebowitz MD, Holberg CJ, Burrows B. Changes in the normal maximal expiratory flow-volume curve with growth and aging. *Am Rev Respir Dis.* 1983;127(6):725–734.
11. Pellegrino R, Viegi G, Brusasco V, et al. Interpretative strategies for lung function tests. *Eur Respir J.* 2005;26(5):948–968.
12. Oostveen E, MacLeod D, Lorino H, et al. The forced oscillation technique in clinical practice: Methodology, recommendations and future developments. *Eur Respir J.* 2003;22(6):1026–1041.
13. Cooper BG. An update on contraindications for lung function testing. *Thorax.* 2011;66(8):714–723.
14. Wanger J, Clausen JL, Coates A, et al. Standardisation of the measurement of lung volumes. *Eur Respir J.* 2005;26(3):511–522.
15. Newth CJ, Enright P, Johnson RL. Multiple-breath nitrogen washout techniques: including measurements with patients on ventilators. *Eur Respir J.* 1997;10(9):2174–2185.
16. Brusasco V, Crapo R, Viegi G. Coming together: the ATS/ERS consensus on clinical pulmonary function testing. *Eur Respir J.* 2005;26(1):1–2.
17. AARC (American Association for Respiratory Care) clinical practice guideline. Spirometry. *Respir Care.* 1991;36(12):1414–1417.
18. Cavalheri V, Hill K, Donaria L, Camillo CA, Pitta F. Maximum voluntary ventilation is more strongly associated with energy expenditure during simple activities of daily living than measures of airflow obstruction or respiratory muscle strength in patients with COPD. *Chron Respir Dis.* 2012;9(4):239–240.
19. AARC (American Association for Respiratory Care) clinical practice guideline. Assessing response to bronchodilator therapy at point of care. *Respir Care.* 1995;40(12):1300–1307.
20. Macintyre N, Crapo RO, Viegi G, et al. Standardisation of the single-breath determination of carbon monoxide uptake in the lung. *Eur Respir J.* 2005;26(4):720–735.
21. McCormack M. Diffusing capacity for carbon monoxide. In: UpToDate, Stoller JK (ed.), UpToDate, Waltham, MA.
22. Ruppel G. *Manual of Pulmonary Function Testing.* St. Louis, MO: Elsevier; 2009.

23. AARC clinical practice guideline. Metabolic measurement using indirect calorimetry during mechanical ventilation. American Association for Respiratory Care. *Respir Care.* 1994;39(12):1170–1175.

24. Casanova C, Celli BR, Barria P, et al. The 6-min walk distance in healthy subjects: Reference standards from seven countries. *Eur Respir J.* 2011;37(1):150–156.

25. Enright PL. The six-minute walk test. *Respir Care.* 2003;48(8):783–785.

26. American Thoracic Society. ATS statement: guidelines for the six-minute walk test. *Am J Respir Crit Care Med.* 2002;166(1):111–117.

27. Ross RM. ATS/ACCP statement on cardiopulmonary exercise testing. *Am J Respir Crit Care Med.* 2003;167(10):1451; author reply 1451.

28. Feiner JR, Severinghaus JW, Bickler PE. Dark skin decreases the accuracy of pulse oximeters at low oxygen saturation: The effects of oximeter probe type and gender. *Anesth Analg.* 2007;105(6 Suppl):S18–23, tables of contents.

29. Davis BE, Cockcroft DW. Past, present and future uses of methacholine testing. *Expert Rev Respir Med.* 2012;6(3):321–329.

30. Stickland MK, Rowe BH, Spooner CH, Vandermeer B, Dryden DM. Accuracy of eucapnic hyperpnea or mannitol to diagnose exercise-induced bronchoconstriction: A systematic review. *Ann Allergy Asthma Immunol.* 2011;107(3):229–234 e228.

31. Borges Mde C, Ferraz E, Vianna EO. Bronchial provocation tests in clinical practice. *Sao Paulo Med J.* 2011;129(4):243–249.

32. Crapo RO, Casaburi R, Coates AL, et al. Guidelines for methacholine and exercise challenge testing–1999. This official statement of the American Thoracic Society was adopted by the ATS Board of Directors, July 1999. *Am J Respir Crit Care Med.* 2000;161(1):309–329.

33. Rivera MP, Mehta AC, Wahadi MM. Establishing the diagnosis of lung cancer: Diagnosis and management of lung cancer, 3rd ed: American College of Chest Physicians evidence-based clinical practice guidelines. *Chest.* 2013;143(5 Suppl:e142S–65S).

34. Modrykamien AM, Gudavalli R, McCarthy K, Liu X, Stoller JK. Detection of upper airway obstruction with spirometry results and the flow-volume loop: a comparison of quantitative and visual inspection criteria. *Respir Care.* 2009;54(4):474–479.

35. Aaron SD, Dales RE, Cardinal P. How accurate is spirometry at predicting restrictive pulmonary impairment? *Chest* 1999;115(3):869–873.

CHAPTER

13

Bronchoscopy and Other Diagnostic Studies

Anisha Arora, Karla Diaz, Jay I. Peters, and Adriel Malavé

CHAPTER OUTLINE

History
Clinical Indications for Bronchoscopy
Diagnostic Bronchoscopy
Thoracentesis
Surgical Lung Biopsy

CHAPTER OBJECTIVES

1. Describe the indications and contraindications to bronchoscopy.
2. Explain the use of bronchoscopy in patients with hemoptysis, pneumonia, masses of the lung, solitary pulmonary nodules, foreign bodies, and interstitial lung disease.
3. Compare and contrast flexible and rigid bronchoscopy in terms of indications, contraindications, and hazards.
4. Explain the steps in performing a flexible bronchoscopy.
5. Describe the indications and technique for obtaining a sterile brush sample, cytologic brush sample, transbronchial biopsy (TBBx), and bronchoalveolar lavage (BAL).
6. Discuss the significance of a bronchoalveolar lavage.
7. Explain the purpose of the endobronchial ultrasound (EBUS).
8. Describe the use of bronchoscopy in the intensive care unit.
9. Describe the indications and procedure for thoracentesis.
10. Discuss the role of a surgical lung biopsy in evaluating pulmonary patients.
11. Contrast the use of video-assisted thoracoscopic surgery (VATS) and open lung biopsy (OLBx).

KEY TERMS

bronchoalveolar lavage
  (BAL)
bronchoscopy
computed tomography (CT)
endobronchial
endobronchial ultrasound
  (EBUS)
endotracheal tube (ETT)
flexible bronchoscopy
foreign body aspiration
hemoptysis
immunocompromised
interstitial lung disease
  (ILD)
mediastinoscopy
opacification
open lung biopsy (OLBx)
parenchyma
pneumocystis pneumonia
  (PCP)
pneumothorax
rigid bronchoscopy
solitary pulmonary nodule
  (SPN)
surgical lung biopsy (SLB)
thoracentesis
thoracotomy
transbronchial biopsy
  (TBBx)
video-assisted thorascopic
  surgery (VATS)

Overview

When to subject a patient to an invasive pulmonary procedure is often a difficult decision. Advances in technology have provided respiratory care clinicians with a diverse array of tools that can help in the diagnosis and management of patients with cardiopulmonary disease. The bronchoscope allows the clinician to visualize the patient's airway and obtain samples that can aid in the diagnosis of infection, malignancy, and other diseases. **Bronchoscopy** can be used for therapeutic purposes to remove foreign bodies or to clear mucus plugs directly from the airway. Thoracentesis allows for removal of pleural fluid for both diagnostic and therapeutic benefit. Ultrasound technology can be used to locate even a small pocket of fluid in the pleural space for diagnostic purposes. This chapter will provide the respiratory care clinician with a more comprehensive understanding of the various tools and special procedures available to assist in the diagnosis and treatment of patients with cardiopulmonary disease.

History

Historically, more than half of accidental aspirations of a foreign body or particulate matter caused either death or chronic illness from purulent infection, abscess formation, fistulas, or malnutrition. As far back as 460–370 BC, Hippocrates advised the insertion of a hollow reed or tube into the airway of a suffocating patient. Others described intubation as a means to explore the trachea and suggested use of instrumentation to remove foreign bodies. Early obstacles to developing bronchoscopy as a medical procedure included the need to find a safe way of inserting an instrument into a patient's trachea while maintaining oxygenation and ventilation. Other obstacles included the need to sedate the patient and the need to develop an instrument with a light source to navigate the airway. Interestingly, one of the first anesthetics used for endoscopy was cocaine. It was first described as a new "miracle drug" and aid to endoscopy by an ophthalmologist named Koller. Initially tested in rabbits and then patients, Koller presented his findings at a lecture on September 15, 1884, to the Annual Congress of German Ophthalmologists in Heidelberg.

The first successful modern bronchoscopy was performed by Gustav Killian in 1897, when he introduced an early bronchoscope into the trachea of a patient with the assistance of a light source. Killian would introduce the bronchoscope and advance it to the point where the diameter of the trachea was no longer greater than that of the scope. Later, in 1897, he went on to remove two foreign bodies from patients using this instrument. Killian described his use of "direct bronchoscopy" at the sixth meeting of the Society of South German Laryngologists in Heidelberg on May 29, 1898.[1]

Shigeto Ikeda introduced glass-fiber illumination for the rigid bronchoscope in 1962 and later went on to develop the first flexible bronchoscope. Further advancements in science and technology have led to the modern day bronchoscope. Respiratory therapists are key in assisting physicians with bronchoscopies. They often are the primary personnel responsible for the maintenance of the scope and assist during the procedure with providing technical support to the physician.[1]

Clinical Indications for Bronchoscopy

Clinical indications for bronchoscopy include assessment of hemoptysis to include determination of the site of bleeding, removal of foreign bodies from the airway, and assessment of various pulmonary problems (e.g., interstitial lung disease, cancer, hemoptysis, pneumonia). These conditions are discussed in the following sections.

Hemoptysis

Hemoptysis, or coughing up of blood, is usually not life threatening, and patients with lung disease often cough up small amounts of blood. However, massive hemoptysis can be present. *Massive hemoptysis* is defined as massive blood loss from the pulmonary tree of approximately 200 to 600 mL of blood within a 12- to 24-hour time frame. Hemoptysis has many causes, and an exact etiology can be difficult to discern based on chest radiographs. A complete blood count (CBC) and assessment of coagulation parameters (prothrombin time and international normalized ratio [PT/INR], partial thromboplastin time [PTT], and a platelet count) are frequently obtained in patients with hemoptysis. Arterial blood gases (ABGs) may be useful in assessing the patient's oxygenation and ventilatory status, but are of little or no value in determining the cause of hemoptysis. When the cause is unclear, flexible bronchoscopy can be useful to identify the source and location of bleeding. Generally, it is beneficial to perform a bronchoscopy earlier rather than waiting 48 hours after the bleeding has stopped in most patients. A rigid bronchoscopy may provide for superior visualization of the airways and ability for intervention in cases of massive hemoptysis, but if time is of the essence, waiting for an operating room in which to perform a rigid bronchoscopy may not be a good option.[2] **Table 13-1** lists various causes of hemoptysis.

Pneumonia

The value of bronchoscopy in assessing patients with pulmonary infection may not be readily apparent, and clinicians may simply ask, "Why not just give antibiotics?" For most patients with pneumonia, an invasive procedure such as bronchoscopy is not necessary. However, certain patients (e.g., immunosuppressed patients or those with subacute or chronic symptoms) may not be able to cough up sputum for testing, and bronchoscopy will allow for obtaining a suitable sample. It also may be important to obtain sputum samples to identify difficult-to-grow organisms such as mycobacteria or to obtain cytology to diagnose **pneumocystis pneumonia (PCP)**, especially in **immunocompromised** patients. Knowing which organisms are the causative agents for pulmonary infection will allow the clinician to select antibiotics for those organisms. Also, pneumonia may overwhelm the patient, resulting in respiratory failure that requires intubation and mechanical ventilatory support. In these cases, a bronchoscopy may be needed to identify the causative agent leading to the overwhelming infection and can be easily obtained in intubated patients.

Masses and Solitary Pulmonary Nodules

Pulmonologists often are asked to perform a bronchoscopy in order to obtain **transbronchial biopsies (TBBx)** for tissue sampling when a **solitary pulmonary nodule (SPN)** or lung mass is seen on chest radiograph or **computed tomography (CT)** scan. Although radiologists can

TABLE 13-1
Causes of Hemoptysis

Airway	Pulmonary Parenchyma	Pulmonary Vasculature	Miscellaneous

Acute bronchitis
Trauma
Bronchiectasis
Bronchopleural fistula
Dieulafoy's disease
Foreign bodies
Neoplasms
	Genetic defect in connective
	  tissues
	Infection (tuberculosis, abscess)
	Inflammatory/autoimmune
		Left atrial hypertension
		Pulmonary arteriovenous
		  malformation
		Pulmonary thromboembolism
			Bevacizumab (chemotherapeutic
			  agent)
			Catamenial hemoptysis
			Coagulopathy
			Cocaine use
			Cryptogenic
			Iatrogenic
			Nitrogen dioxide

sometimes perform successful percutaneous biopsies if the lesions are peripheral, oftentimes central SPNs or masses cannot be safely reached via percutaneous biopsy. In these cases, flexible bronchoscopy is a valuable tool in assisting in diagnosis. A central mass often will extrinsically compress the airways, and this is visible upon bronchoscopic evaluation of the airway. TBBx via a flexible bronchoscopy is an important means of diagnosing both central lesions as well as peripheral lesions.[3]

Foreign Bodies

Foreign bodies (FB) are commonly aspirated into the tracheobronchial tree. FBs may consist of food (e.g., popcorn, vegetables, corn, chicken bones, beans/legumes) or other items, such as lost teeth, coins, or nails, that have been placed in the mouth and then inhaled. **Foreign body aspiration** can cause serious problems, including pneumonias that do not resolve and symptoms such as significant shortness of breath. A flexible bronchoscopic examination can evaluate the airways but also offers a means of removing the FB with forceps or snares that can be passed through the working channel of the bronchoscope. In cases of FB aspiration, it is a good idea to have a rigid bronchoscope on hand in case the foreign body cannot be successfully removed using flexible bronchoscopy. It should be noted that flexible bronchoscopy for FB removal has certain risks. For example, the FB can move further down the tracheobronchial tree as removal is attempted, and this illustrates the importance of having rigid bronchoscopy available as an alternative. In a recent study, 57 of 60 patients had a successful removal of the FB either through flexible or rigid bronchoscopy.[4]

Interstitial Lung Disease

Interstitial lung disease (ILD) is an abnormality of the lung **parenchyma** involving the space between alveoli. There are many different types of ILD, and it is often necessary to have an interdisciplinary team of clinicians, radiologists, and pathologists working together to correctly diagnose the specific type. Frequently, a high-resolution computed tomography (HRCT) scan

will show a particular pattern of inflammation or fibrosis. For example, usual interstitial pneumonia (UIP) is associated with a subpleural reticular pattern of fibrosis and honeycombing (3- to 5-mm cysts) affecting the lower lobes, with or without traction bronchiectasis.

An ILD diagnosis, however, cannot always be made based solely upon the CT scan imaging results. Blood studies such as an autoimmune panel (e.g., assessing for diseases such as systemic lupus) and specific antibodies (e.g., assessing for fungal diseases or other infectious agents) are usually ordered.

TBBx can be useful to sample random areas of lung tissue to help obtain tissue for diagnosis. Often, the bronchoscopist will obtain **bronchoalveolar lavage (BAL)** samples from various lobes of the lung to look for cancer, alveolar bleeding, or infection.[5]

> **RC Insights**
>
> Bronchoscopy is mainly used to obtain tissue for diagnosis or to assist in the direct visualization of an area of concern.

Diagnostic Bronchoscopy

A diagnostic bronchoscopy is a procedure that involves using a bronchoscope to visualize the major airways and to obtain tissue, secretions, or fluid samples. The fiber-optic bronchoscope is a device composed of a long tube (about 2 feet in length) with a light source at its tip and an inner channel or passageway through which tools, such as forceps, can be passed. There are two types of commonly used bronchoscopes: rigid and flexible. The bronchoscope is typically inserted through the nose (for flexible scopes) or the mouth (for rigid or flexible scopes) past the epiglottis and through the vocal cords into the trachea. Flexible scopes may also be inserted through an endotracheal or tracheostomy tube or a tracheostomy stoma.

Diagnostic bronchoscopy may be used to investigate otherwise unexplained pulmonary symptoms, such as persistent cough, wheezing, dyspnea, or hemoptysis. Bronchoscopy may also be used to investigate unresolved atelectasis, which may be caused by obstruction due to mucus, tumor, or foreign body. Imaging studies, such as chest x-ray or CT scan, may reveal a mass or infiltrate that requires further evaluation by bronchoscopy to appraise for infection, cancer, or ILD.

Flexible Bronchoscopy

Flexible bronchoscopy is more commonly performed than rigid bronchoscopy. The flexible bronchoscope is less than 0.5 inches wide and is about 2 feet long. The flexible bronchoscope is composed of a flexible sheath containing the necessary cables to allow flexion and extension of the tip of the scope (ranging from 130 degrees in one direction and 160 degrees in the opposite direction[6]) while harboring encapsulated fibers that transmit the **endobronchial** images from a small camera at the tip onto a video screen or to a camera. The bronchoscope also contains a light source and a working channel to facilitate the use of forceps, sterile brush, cytology brush, fine-needle aspiration, and suctioning of bronchoalveolar samples.[7] Flexible bronchoscopes allow for visualization of the vocal cords, larynx, trachea, and tracheobronchial tree down to the segmental airways (the fourth or fifth generation in most patients). See **Figures 13-1** and **13-2**.

Flexible bronchoscopy is used for sampling of parenchymal masses and nodules suspicious for cancer; obtaining bronchoalveolar samples to diagnose infection, such as bacterial, fungal, viral, or atypical infections; and evaluating hemoptysis, cough, and infiltrates in the immunocompromised host.[7] Flexible bronchoscopy can also be used for diagnostic sampling of mediastinal lymphadenopathy, assessing endobronchial tissue for an obstructing lesion, and sampling of both endobronchial and parenchymal tissue to assess for conditions such as sarcoid, ILD, and cancer.[7–9] Flexible bronchoscopy is useful for removal of foreign bodies and suctioning of the airway to clear an obstruction secondary to mucus impaction.

Flexible bronchoscopy should not be performed without formal patient consent or when the operator is inexperienced, though less experienced personnel may practice under the careful supervision of an experienced clinician. Bronchoscopy should also not be performed without adequate support should a complication arise. Relative contraindications to bronchoscopy include a recent history of myocardial infarction (within the last 6 weeks), unstable arrhythmias, poorly controlled bronchial asthma, respiratory insufficiency with hypoxia or hypercarbia (as this may necessitate intubation), coagulopathy, uremia, and/or significant hypo/hypertension.[10]

Procedure for Flexible Bronchoscopy

Before the procedure is initiated, the patient must undergo a prebronchoscopy assessment. A careful history includes evaluating the patient's airway (see also Figure 15-8). A careful history should be taken to include smoking history; active alcohol or drug use; reactions to medications; allergy; and history of pulmonary, cardiac, or renal disease. The use of dentures or

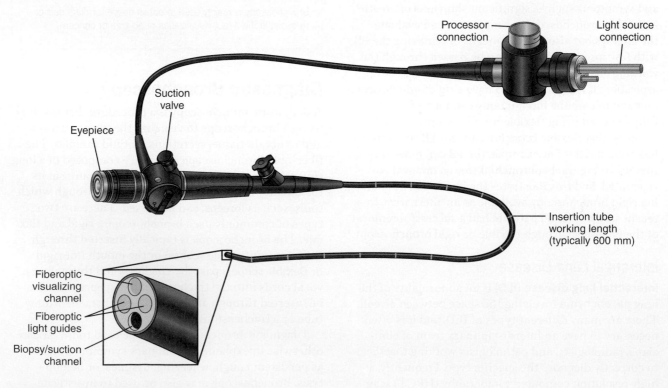

FIGURE 13-1 Flexible bronchoscope components.

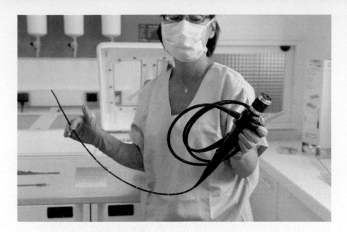

FIGURE 13-2 **The flexible bronchoscope.**

© BSIP SA/Alamy

TABLE 13-2
Indications and Contraindications to Bronchoscopy

Indications	Contraindications	Relative Contraindications
Evaluation of airways	Patient or surrogate does not consent	Recent myocardial infarction (6 weeks)
Infection	Bronchoscopist is inexperienced	Unstable arrhythmias
Lung mass or nodule	Facilities are inadequate to provide support should a complication arise	Unstable bronchial asthma
Hemoptysis		Respiratory insufficiency with hypoxia or hypercarbia
Unexplained cough		Coagulopathy
Removal of foreign body		Uremia
		Hypo- or hypertension

other oral appliances should be noted, and these should be removed prior to performance of the procedure. Flexible bronchoscopy does not require general anesthesia; most clinicians use conscious sedation to ensure that the patient is comfortable but can be aroused easily after the procedure.[11] Patients are provided supplemental oxygen during the procedure via nasal cannula at 2 to 6 L/min in order to prevent hypoxemia. Should the need arise, patients can be given higher concentrations of oxygen by mask. Occasionally, patients may require intubation (often over the bronchoscope) to protect the airway and provide 100% oxygen. During the procedure, the patient's vital signs are continuously monitored to note heart rate, blood pressure, and ability to oxygenate and ventilate (oximetry with or without capnography). Vital signs guide the administration of analgesics and sedatives and provide a measure of overall ability of the patient to tolerate the procedure. Each patient is unique, and adjustments are made accordingly. For example, a patient may be too hypertensive to tolerate the procedure; others may have problems with oxygenation or ventilation. Complications such as bleeding may prevent the clinician from completing the procedure as planned. Care to optimize the patient's comorbidities prior to bronchoscopy should be provided in order to ensure that he or she is able to tolerate the procedure while experiencing minimal complications.[12] **Table 13-2** lists the indications and contraindications for bronchoscopy.

Once the patient has been appropriately assessed and sedated, the bronchoscope is introduced either through the nares and nasal passage or the mouth and oropharynx. Oral insertion requires prior placement of a bite block to prevent the patient from biting down and damaging the scope.[12] A well-trained assistant (respiratory therapist or nurse) is critical to the procedure's success. The assistant must actively participate with the bronchoscopist to ensure that the procedure is safe and effective. The bronchoscope is advanced through the oropharynx and passed anterior to the epiglottis. Next, the vocal cords are visualized. At this point, lidocaine solution is inserted through the side port of the scope to anesthetize the vocal cords.[12] This helps ensure patient comfort and decreases cough. Once adequate analgesia has been provided, the scope is advanced through the vocal cords into the trachea (**Figure 13-3**). The trachea is again anesthetized with lidocaine as to minimize the sensation of a foreign body (the scope) in the airway. Once the patient is comfortable, the bronchoscopist will proceed with a visual exam of the airway anatomy, making sure to assess the right upper lobe, the right middle lobe, and the right lower lobe with all of their subsegmental bronchi. Next, the left upper and left lower lobes are viewed to include their subsegmental bronchi. The bronchoscope can enter

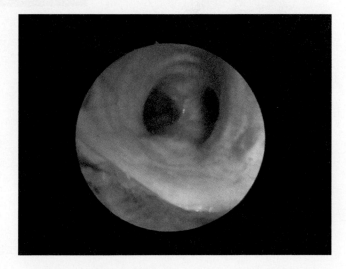

FIGURE 13-3 **Bronchoscopic view of the trachea and carina.**

© CNRI/Science Photo Library

most fourth-order bronchi and one-third of all fifth-order bronchi. After an endobronchial exam has been performed, samples of tissue, secretions, or fluid are obtained based on the indications for the procedure. For example, if a nodule in one of the subsegments of the lung is visualized via fluoroscopic guidance during the procedure, the bronchoscopist may take samples in this order:[12]

1. Sterile brush sample for microbiology
2. Cytologic brush sample to assess for malignant cells
3. TBBx of tissue sample to assess for infection and malignancy
4. Bronchoalveolar lavage (BAL) samples to look for malignant cells

The instrumentation used for sampling includes forceps (smooth or serrated), a sterile brush to collect microbiology samples, and a cytology brush to collect cytology specimens. All of these instruments can be passed through the hollow working channel of the standard bronchoscope. Larger-diameter scopes (therapeutic bronchoscopes) are typically used when the clinician believes additional tools may be needed. Smaller-diameter scopes may be used to perform a visual survey of the airways without obtaining biopsy samples.

The smooth-edged forceps are typically used to sample lung parenchyma with random biopsy samples. Serrated forceps may be used when a mass is visualized and a larger piece of tissue is required for sampling. Serrated forceps are capable of cutting tissue and are preferred if a larger sample is needed. Forceps are metallic and can be seen on fluoroscopy in real time. Fluoroscopy during bronchoscopy can help guide the clinician to the site of interest in the lungs and ensure that the procedure is performed safely. Care should be taken to not extend the forceps to the periphery of the lung where they can damage the pleura and cause a **pneumothorax**. During fluoroscopy, lead aprons are worn by all the members of the team to protect them from radiation exposure.

In this discussion of instrumentation, it is important to mention shielded versus unshielded brushes. Unshielded brushes are not protected by a sterile outer plastic sheath. Unshielded brushes are primarily used to obtain samples of masses or suspicious parenchymal tissue to send for cytologic analysis. The shielded sterile brush has an inner layer that is protected by a plastic outer layer. This is to protect the sterile inner brush from contamination because the scope is passed through the nose or mouth where respiratory flora live. Contamination of the brush with oral or nasal flora can lead the clinician to falsely conclude that those microbes were found in the lower airway. When the shielded brush has been passed through the scope and is visualized on fluoroscopy in the lower airway, the bronchoscopist will then instruct the assistant to "push the brush out." This maneuver pushes out a sterile

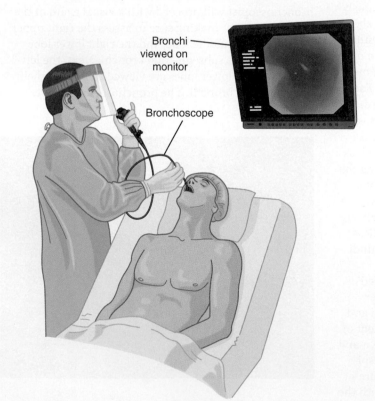

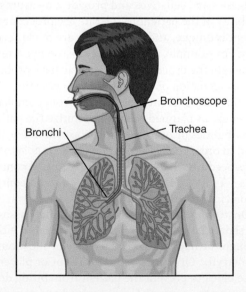

FIGURE 13-4 Flexible bronchoscopy.

wax plug that protects the inner layer of the brush and readies the brush for sampling. The inner brush is then advanced, and uncontaminated samples are taken from the area of interest. The clinician then asks the assistant to "pull the brush in" to ensure that the lower airway sample is not contaminated as the brush is removed. Once the entire brush is removed from the scope, the tip of the brush is cut by the assistant and inserted into a sterile container containing sterile normal saline.[6]

Bronchoalveolar Lavage

The BAL requires the assistance of the respiratory therapist or nurse (see **Figure 13-5**). First, the bronchoscopist locates the subsegment of the lung of interest. The tip of the scope is then wedged into that subsegment of the airway.[13,14] Next, the respiratory therapist or nurse inserts approximately 20 to 40 mL of saline into the side port of the scope and out into the small airway. The bronchoscopist then suctions this fluid back into a collection container or trap that the assistant attaches to the outside of the scope.[13,14] The fluid obtained by performing a BAL provides a sample of material from bronchial subsegments that cannot otherwise be visualized or assessed by bronchoscopy because these airways are smaller than the diameter of the scope. The BAL sample is then sent to the laboratory to run tests to diagnose infection, determine total and differential cell counts, assess cytology (e.g., cancer), or perform immunologic studies.

As with any procedure, possible complications must be disclosed to the patient and anticipated by those performing and assisting with the procedure. Risks associated with bronchoscopy include infection, bleeding due to trauma from the scope and/or biopsy samples taken, and pneumothorax (usually seen in the setting of TBBx should the biopsies be taken too peripherally and biopsy of the pleura is taken instead of the desired lung parenchyma).[7] Other complications include difficulty with oxygenation and ventilation, hypertension and tachycardia due to pain or underlying cardiac conditions, and rarely, death. The experience and skill of the bronchoscopist helps minimize the risk of adverse outcomes; however, even the most skilled clinician must be alert to the possible hazards and complications of the procedure.

Endobronchial Ultrasound

Endobronchial ultrasound (EBUS) is a variation of flexible bronchoscopy. The EBUS is very similar to the flexible bronchoscope, except that the EBUS has a curvilinear ultrasound probe at the end with Doppler capability to better assess vascular structures and lymph nodes. It utilizes a transducer to produce the sound waves and receive the reflected sound waves. A processor integrates the signal reflected by tissues

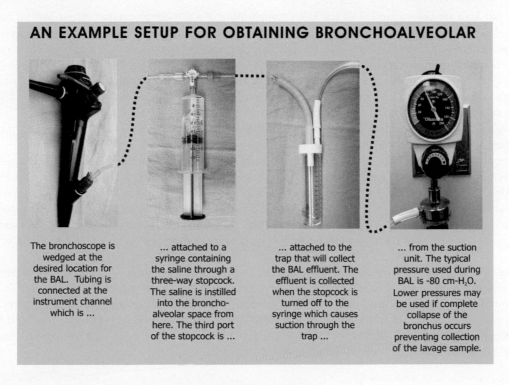

AN EXAMPLE SETUP FOR OBTAINING BRONCHOALVEOLAR

The bronchoscope is wedged at the desired location for the BAL. Tubing is connected at the instrument channel which is ...

... attached to a syringe containing the saline through a three-way stopcock. The saline is instilled into the bronchoalveolar space from here. The third port of the stopcock is ...

... attached to the trap that will collect the BAL effluent. The effluent is collected when the stopcock is turned off to the syringe which causes suction through the trap ...

... from the suction unit. The typical pressure used during BAL is -80 cm-H_2O. Lower pressures may be used if complete collapse of the bronchus occurs preventing collection of the lavage sample.

FIGURE 13-5 Setup for obtaining a bronchoalveolar lavage (BAL) specimen.

Courtesy of Augustine Lee

and generates the two-dimensional ultrasound image. Because water is an excellent conductor of sound waves, the device is designed with a balloon that can be filled with water in order to improve the image.[15] The image quality can also be adjusted for gain, brightness, and contrast. The field of view is 90 degrees, and the direction of view is 35 degrees forward oblique.[15] This mode of bronchoscopy has become more popular with clinicians recently due to its utility in sampling mediastinal and hilar lymph nodes. EBUS sampling of mediastinal lymph nodes is a safer, less invasive, and more cost-effective than a surgical biopsy technique such as **mediastinoscopy**.[5] Once the lymph nodes have been visualized with EBUS, transbronchial needle aspiration can be performed through the working channel of the scope to obtain tissue for histopathologic analysis.[15] This can be especially helpful as a quick and efficient alternative to surgical mediastinoscopy when hilar and mediastinal lymphadenopathy is present.

Complications and contraindications are similar to that of flexible bronchoscopy; a recent meta-analysis noted only two serious complications in 1299 patients.[1,16] **Clinical Focus 13-1** provides an example of bronchoscopy for the evaluation of a patient with interstitial lung disease.

Bronchoscopy in the Intensive Care Unit

Normally, bronchoscopy is performed in the bronchoscopy suite; however, there are several clinical situations in which bronchoscopy performed in the intensive care unit (ICU) is indicated and potentially lifesaving. For example, a patient receiving invasive mechanical ventilation may experience a sudden oxygen desaturation with a chest radiograph showing complete **opacification** (or "white out" that obscures the regular lung tissue on a chest radiograph) on the one side. A bedside bronchoscopic evaluation may demonstrate a mucus plug obstructing a large airway. The plug may be then suctioned out, allowing for immediate improvement in oxygenation and re-expansion of the lung.[12] As another example, a patient in the ICU may be experiencing hemoptysis that is not clarified by imaging studies, sputum, blood cultures, or hematology. A bedside bronchoscopy may differentiate possible causes of the hemoptysis, such as an obstructing lesion, trauma,

CLINICAL FOCUS 13-1

Interstitial Lung Disease

A 56-year-old African American female has been complaining of a dry cough on and off for several months. She has also had raised, red, painful spots on her legs for the about same amount of time. She complains of generalized fatigue, shortness of breath, and joint pain. Her primary care doctor performed a routine chest radiograph that suggests hilar lymphadenopathy.

The patient is referred for further evaluation. A CT scan confirms hilar lymphadenopathy, but not lung parenchymal abnormalities. The clinician wants to schedule the patient for a procedure to obtain a tissue sample to help establish a diagnosis.

Which of the following procedures will enable obtaining endobronchial biopsies using conscious sedation: flexible bronchoscopy, rigid bronchoscopy, endobronchial ultrasound (EBUS), or open lung biopsy?

The patient will likely be scheduled for a flexible bronchoscopy as the first line of testing. The patient's presentation is consistent with a diagnosis of sarcoidosis. Sarcoidosis causes interstitial lung disease (ILD) and inflammation of various body systems (e.g., lymph nodes, lungs, liver, eyes, skin, other). Sarcoidosis may be caused by an immune response to infection, hypersensitivity to environmental agents, or genetic factors. Symptoms include dry cough, dyspnea, chest pain, fatigue, joint pain, hair loss, rash, and erythema nodosum (raised, red skin sores on the front of the lower legs). Sarcoidosis is more common among African Americans than other groups.

As a clinician, you may suggest an EBUS to evaluate the patient's lymph nodes and hilar lymphadenopathy. An EBUS would definitely be of value in patients with sarcoidosis. However, patients with sarcoidosis can have involvement of airway mucosa, and this can be evaluated during flexible bronchoscopy by tissue sampling using forceps biopsies of endobronchial tissue. Diagnostic fine-needle aspiration (FNA) of mediastinal and hilar lymph nodes during EBUS can also be useful; however, flexible bronchoscopy probably should be done first, and EBUS may not be needed.

abscess, infection, or an autoimmune condition. Bedside bronchoscopic evaluation with BAL sampling may help guide appropriate treatment.

A bronchoscopy on a patient receiving mechanical ventilation with an **endotracheal tube (ETT)** in place is performed differently than a bronchoscopy on a nonventilated patient. A bronchoscopic adapter must be connected between the ETT and the mechanical ventilator circuit to allow passage of the bronchoscope into the airway without interrupting the ventilator circuit. Typically, the ventilated patient is already sedated with intravenous medication drips such as fentanyl (a narcotic analgesic that will reduce coughing) and midazolam (a sedative that induces short-term amnesia). The dose of these medications may be increased, as needed, for the bronchoscopy procedure to be well tolerated by the patient. The bronchoscopist stands on one side of the patient while the respiratory therapist adjusts the alarms on the ventilator. In particular, the peak pressure alarm must be adjusted prior to bronchoscopy because as the scope is advanced through the ETT, partial occlusion of the airway lumen by the scope will increase airflow resistance, raising peak pressures and often reducing delivered tidal volume.[12] The fractional concentration of oxygen (F_{IO_2}) delivered must also be increased (often to 100%) to avoid hypoxemia while the scope partially obstructs the ETT. The bronchoscopic evaluation of the ICU patient is performed in the same general manner as described previously, though it usually cannot be as comprehensive. For example, TBBx are often obtained in the bronchoscopy suite, but infrequently done in the ICU on ventilated patients due to the risk of a tension pneumothorax in patients receiving positive pressure ventilation. It is also difficult to obtain fluoroscopic bedside guidance during bronchoscopy in the ICU. As mentioned earlier, complications of the procedure can occur, and patients who are critically ill in the ICU may be more likely to experience complications than patients receiving a more routine bronchoscopy. The complications were listed in the flexible bronchoscopy section. It is important to optimize the patient's condition prior to the procedure, especially in the ICU, because these patients tend to be severely ill. As with any procedure, the respiratory care clinician should always attempt to anticipate potential adverse outcomes and be equipped to handle them should they arise.

Clinical Focus 13-2 provides an example of bedside bronchoscopy for the evaluation of a patient in the ICU.

Rigid Bronchoscopy

Rigid bronchoscopy is a specialized procedure that may be performed when flexible bronchoscopy will not suffice. The rigid bronchoscope is a long, hollow, straight metal tube with a light source, telescope, and viewing monitor. Rigid bronchoscopy allows for access to the trachea and proximal airways to remove large foreign bodies, to insert metal stents into airways that are stenotic, to manage massive hemoptysis or very thick secretions, or to debulk large tracheal or endobronchial tumors.[17] Rigid bronchoscopy is typically performed in a controlled setting, usually the operating room. Patients undergo general anesthesia, because complete muscle relaxation is desired while manipulating the rigid bronchoscope. Should the need arise, patients can be intubated through the larger diameter of the rigid bronchoscope once it is inserted into the airway.

Clinicians may elect to introduce a flexible bronchoscope through the larger diameter rigid scope for a light source, though newer rigid scopes typically have light sources included. With advances in technology, rigid bronchoscopes are now equipped with technology allowing for sharp, real-time images that can be seen directly on a viewing screen during the procedure. This enables those with more advanced skills to teach others during the procedure.

Rigid bronchoscopy requires an advanced skill set given potential complications such as damaging the oropharynx, breaking/chipping of teeth, cutting of patients, lips with the scope, or harming the vocal cords. Airway perforation during the procedure is a serious risk, particularly the posterior membranous portion of the trachea. This procedure shares the same contraindications as that for flexible bronchoscopy; in addition, spinal cord injury is a contraindication to this procedure. **Figure 13-6** illustrates the rigid bronchoscope.

> ### RC Insights
>
> Flexible bronchoscopy is the most commonly used means of bronchoscopic evaluation.

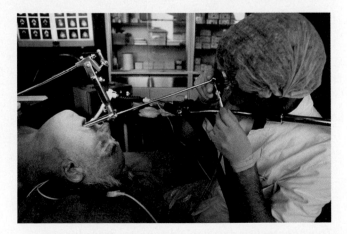

FIGURE 13-6 Rigid bronchoscopy. Rigid bronchoscopy may be used to visualize the trachea and bronchi, obtain tissue samples or remove foreign bodies.

© Philippe Plailly/Science Photo Library

CLINICAL FOCUS 13-2

Bronchoscopy in the ICU

A 33-year-old male who is HIV positive is admitted to the medical intensive care unit for acute hypoxemic respiratory failure. The patient is being supported with mechanical ventilation via endotracheal tube requiring an FIO_2 of 0.60 (60%) and a PEEP of 8 cm H_2O in the volume-control mode. The patient's chest radiograph shows bilateral alveolar airspace opacities that are consistent with acute respiratory distress syndrome (ARDS), pulmonary edema, or multifocal pneumonia. The physician taking care of this patient would like to perform a bedside flexible bronchoscopy for the purpose of clarifying the diagnosis.

1. *What actions should the respiratory care clinician take to ensure that the procedure is safe and effective?*

    The patient has hypoxemic respiratory failure requiring PEEP and an increased FIO_2. This patient may have a pneumonia related to the HIV infection and resulting immunocompromised state. The respiratory care clinician should be prepared to make ventilator adjustments during the bronchoscopy procedure to ensure adequate oxygenation and ventilation. The peak pressure will increase when the bronchoscope is introduced into the airway, so the peak airway pressure alarm and limit will need to be increased. If the alarm and pressure limit are not increased, the alarm will sound every time the machine volume cycles and the delivered tidal volume will decrease. The FIO_2 will also need to be increased during the procedure, probably to 100%, and the patient's oximetry values (SpO_2), vital signs (heart rate, blood pressure), and electrocardiogram (ECG) should be also monitored carefully. A manual resuscitator bag, endotracheal tube adapter, and PEEP valve must be available in case the patient needs to be bagged during the procedure. Suctioning and airway equipment should also be kept nearby in case of a problem; the code crash cart should also be readily available.

2. *Which of the following tests might the clinician expect to be completed during the procedure: forceps biopsy, FNA of lymph node(s), bronchoalveolar lavage (BAL) and microbiology brush, or BAL and cytology brush?*

    Immunocompromised patients are at risk for opportunistic infections (e.g., pneumocystis pneumonia [PCP]) and community-acquired pneumonia. Sterile microbiology brush is the ideal test for these possible infections, given the high diagnostic value. Ideally, the clinician would also perform a BAL to send for culture, stains, and cytology. The respiratory care clinician should be prepared for serial BAL samples to evaluate for alveolar hemorrhage, because the patient's chest x-ray findings could also be caused by alveolar hemorrhage. At least three consecutive and separate BAL samples in each lung segment will be needed, using a new collection container with each BAL specimen. If alveolar hemorrhage is present, the last BAL should be a darker red than the initial sample. BAL cytology will also confirm hemorrhage (if present) or PCP (if present), though the laboratory diagnosis will take several days. Forceps biopsies and FNA are rarely done in the ICU and are not useful to evaluate infection. Cytology brush also has no utility in the evaluation of infection.

RC Insights

Always be overprepared for possible procedure risks and complications. There is no harm in having more equipment and supplies and personnel at your disposal; if you have less than needed in an emergency, it can put the patient's life in danger.

Thoracentesis

Thoracentesis is a valuable diagnostic procedure in patients with pleural effusions of unknown origin. Pleural fluid analysis can determine if the fluid is a transudate (a product of unbalanced hydrostatic forces) or an exudate (a product of increased capillary permeability from inflammation or lymphatic obstruction).[18]

Examples of conditions associated with transudative pleural effusion include left ventricular failure (e.g., congestive heart failure), renal failure, liver failure, or cirrhosis. Exudative effusions can be caused by infection (e.g., bacterial or viral pneumonia), cancer, or pulmonary embolus. Thoracentesis can also be performed to remove pleural fluid and reduce respiratory distress in patients with large pleural effusions. If the effusion has an obvious cause, such as congestive heart failure, treatment of the underlying process is recommended and thoracentesis is not indicated.[18]

Although there are no absolute contraindications to thoracentesis, the clinician must consider conditions such as a bleeding diathesis (predisposition to bleeding), coagulopathy, and poorly defined anatomic landmarks that would make the procedure more challenging to perform. Other considerations include the degree of respiratory impairment of the contralateral lung, size of the effusion (small vs. large), and the presence of loculations that would make drainage more difficult. The clinician must also consider whether the patient can tolerate the procedure with respect to required positioning, analgesia, and ability to follow commands needed to successfully complete the procedure.[10]

The procedure is typically performed while the patient is in a sitting position on the edge of the bed, leaning forward, with his or her arms resting on a bedside table. If the patient is unable to sit upright, the lateral recumbent or supine position may be used. **Figure 13-7** illustrates the proper patient positioning for a thoracentesis.

The location and extent of the effusion should be estimated on the basis of diminished or absent breath sounds on auscultation, dullness to percussion, and decreased or absent fremitus.[18] With the advent of newer technology, ultrasound-guided thoracentesis is being performed with more regularity. In the hands of a skilled practitioner, ultrasound imaging can be used to locate deep pockets of pleural fluid located away from structures, such as the diaphragm and lung tissue, so as to avoid damaging complications.[19] Once the anatomic site has been located using ultrasound guidance, the area is marked and cleansed with an antiseptic. The clinician should wear sterile gloves and gown, face mask, and head cover, and a sterile drape should be placed over the patient's back. The skin is anesthetized using lidocaine and a small-bore needle and syringe. Lidocaine is also used to anesthetize the deeper tissues. A larger needle and aspirating syringe are then employed. The needle is inserted over the superior surface of the rib and then advanced into the pleural space. It is important to ensure that the needle goes over the superior margin of the rib to avoid the intercostal nerves and arteries that are located in the inferior margin.[18] Once pleural fluid is aspirated into the syringe, the needle is no longer advanced. The depth of penetration is noted prior to withdrawing the needle. An 18-gauge over-the-needle catheter is next attached to a syringe and advanced along the superior surface of the rib to the predetermined depth while continuously pulling back on the plunger. Once pleural fluid is obtained, the plastic catheter is guided over the needle and the needle is removed. A large syringe is connected to the catheter and fluid is aspirated into a collection bag or vacuum bottle. Caution should be taken to note the volume of fluid removed during thoracentesis, because patients can experience re-expansion pulmonary edema. Re-expansion pulmonary edema is rare and can probably be avoided by limiting therapeutic aspirations to less than 1500 mL.[18]

Pneumothorax is a rare but possible complication of thoracentesis. A postprocedure chest radiograph can confirm the presence and size of pneumothorax. Pneumothorax caused by thoracentesis may not require the placement of a chest tube if the visceral pleura has not been injured.[18] The patient's symptoms, degree of underlying lung disease, and the size of a pneumothorax should guide the decision to place chest tubes. Other complications of thoracentesis include pain, coughing, and localized infection. More serious complications include hemothorax, injury to an intra-abdominal organ, air embolism, and postexpansion pulmonary edema.

> **RC Insights**
>
> Ultrasound should *always* be used when available for performing a thoracentesis. It is a safer way to perform this procedure.

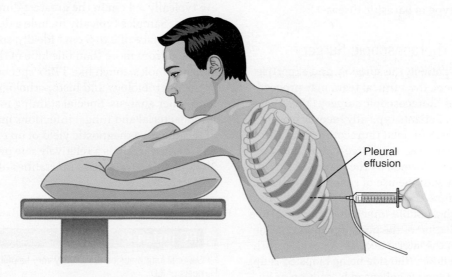

FIGURE 13-7 Proper patient position for thoracentesis.

Surgical Lung Biopsy

A **surgical lung biopsy (SLB)** is indicated in a subset of patients who have clinical findings suggestive of ILD. With ILD, the lung parenchyma is affected by a recurrent insult, such as autoimmune or collagen vascular disease, leading to a specific radiographic pattern (dots and lines referred to as a reticulonodular pattern) within the lung. Idiopathic pulmonary fibrosis (IPF) is a specific type of ILD that can typically be diagnosed by symptoms, history, physical examination, and chest imaging (e.g., CT scan).[20] However, when radiographic findings are atypical for IPF or other types of ILD are suspected, a tissue sample is needed. Tissue samples can be obtained by flexible bronchoscopy (e.g., TBBx); however, most samples obtained by flexible bronchoscopy tend to be small and are often nondiagnostic.[20] With suspected ILD of unknown etiology, specific causes must be identified. A surgical lung biopsy may then be performed, either via **video-assisted thoracoscopic surgery (VATS)** or **open lung biopsy (OLBx)**.

Indications for SLB include ILD with atypical features for IPF and chest imaging suggestive of ILD not consistent with IPF. SLB may also be used to exclude infectious processes and rule out neoplastic disease. SLB may be indicated to evaluate unexplained hypoxia, hemoptysis, or signs of an inflammatory lung process.[20] SLB is not indicated in cases of ILD if the risk of complications outweighs the benefits. SLB may also be avoided by careful integration of clinical, radiologic, and BAL/TBBx findings resulting in a confident diagnosis.

Patients with an elevated pulmonary artery pressure (> 25 to 35 mm Hg) and those with coagulopathies may not be good candidates for either nonsurgical or surgical lung biopsy because they can be at higher risk of bleeding. Caution should also be taken with patients who have vascular tumors, end-stage interstitial fibrosis, arteriovenous aneurysms, and hydatid cysts (cysts associated with a type of parasitic disease).[10]

Video-Assisted Thoracoscopic Surgery

Depending on the patient, the surgeon, and expertise of the team members, the surgical team may proceed with video-assisted thoracoscopic surgery (VATS) or open **thoracotomy**. Patients typically recover from VATS more quickly than open thoracotomy, but the underlying disease process may force a more invasive approach. VATS is performed by the surgical team in an operating room with the use of general anesthesia. During the procedure, the patient receives mechanical ventilation through a double-lumen endotracheal tube (allowing for ventilation of the nonsurgical lung). The patient is placed in the lateral decubitus position with the ventilated side down (the side being biopsied is up). The nondependent lung is collapsed by suction or by positive pressure introduced into the pleural cavity.

Most therapeutic procedures require three incision sites, each ≤ 2 cm in diameter. Incision length may need to be increased depending on the patient, the surgeons, and the procedure requirements. The incision must be sufficient to allow the endoscopic tools to pass through the skin and for manipulation to view and obtain tissue samples. Once the procedure has been completed, one or more chest tubes may be placed to allow for drainage of air and/or fluid from the pleural space. The chest tubes are connected to suction until the lung is completely reinflated and the fluid volume is < 100 mL per day. Chest tubes are typically managed by the pulmonary or the cardiothoracic surgery services.

Open Lung Biopsy

If other procedures have been nondiagnostic or the clinician feels that BAL/TBBx and/or VATS will not be useful, then open lung biopsy (OLBx) may be performed. OLBx is the gold standard for obtaining tissue samples. OLBx is also performed by a surgical team in an operating room with the use of general anesthesia. During the procedure, the patient receives mechanical ventilation through an endotracheal tube. The site for the biopsy is chosen by the surgeon using radiographic imaging to help guide where the greatest yield of tissue can be obtained to aid in diagnosis. Usually at least two specimens are obtained. During OLBx, the surgeons have the advantage of touching and visualizing the anatomic structures, which aid in diagnostic yield.

Complications of both OLBx and VATS include infection, bleeding, creation of a bronchopleural fistula, postprocedure pneumonia, and postprocedure atelectasis. With OLBx, surgeons can visualize the pleural space and anatomic structures and repair any damaged structures. There is always the chance of damaging adjacent anatomic structures during surgery, though this is usually a rare complication.

Surgical lung tissue specimens obtained by SLB are typically > 4 cm in the greatest dimension when inflated. Samples typically include a depth from the pleural surface of 3 to 5 cm.[4] Ideally, specimens are obtained from more than one lobe of the lung. These biopsy samples, much like TBBx specimens, are sent to the microbiology and histopathology laboratories for further analysis. Special staining to assess for mycobacterial and fungal infections may be employed. SLB can have a diagnostic yield of up to 81% for specific diseases. SLB is a relatively safe procedure with 30- and 90-day operative mortalities of 2.7% and 4.1%, respectively.[21]

> **RC Insights**
>
> Surgical lung biopsies are usually very helpful to aid in the diagnosis of ILD.

Key Points

▶ Bronchoscopy can be done to diagnose infection, tumor, or interstitial lung disease. It can also be used to evaluate the location and cause of hemoptysis.

▶ Bronchoscopy can have complications such as pneumothorax, infection, bleeding, and hypoxemia.

▶ The most common type of bronchoscopy is flexible bronchoscopy using a fiber-optic bronchoscope.

▶ Alternative forms of bronchoscopy include rigid bronchoscopy (to assess and treat tracheal lesions) and endobronchial ultrasound (EBUS; to sample mediastinal lymph nodes).

▶ Local anesthesia using lidocaine and sedation with a short-acting benzodiazepine and narcotic are used for bronchoscopy.

▶ Thoracentesis is helpful in the evaluation of a pleural effusion or removal of fluid for symptomatic relief.

▶ Proper patient positioning is important when performing a thoracentesis.

▶ Thoracentesis using ultrasound guidance is becoming the standard of care for this procedure.

▶ Surgical lung biopsy may be needed if bronchoscopic biopsies are nondiagnostic.

▶ A successful bronchoscopy requires the teamwork of a physician to operate the bronchoscope, a respiratory therapist to assist in the handling of samples and tools, and a nurse who can carefully monitor the patient and administer medications.

▶ It is important to know the indications and contraindications to bronchoscopy. Not every patient is low risk for such a procedure.

▶ A variety of instruments are available for use with either the flexible or rigid bronchoscope that aid in diagnosis, some of the most common being forceps and sterile brushes that can be passed through the scope.

▶ Bronchoscopy can be helpful in the intensive care setting when critically ill patients need a diagnosis (in regards to pneumonia) or have a mucus plug that needs to be cleared.

▶ EBUS is a newer modality used to visualize and sample lymph nodes using ultrasound to assess for malignancy.

References

1. Ernst A (ed.). *Introduction to Bronchoscopy*. Cambridge, UK: Cambridge University Press; 2009.

2. Differential diagnosis of hemoptysis. In: UpToDate, Waltham, MA. (Accessed June 20, 2014).

3. Gasparini S, Ferretti M, Secchi EB, Beldelli S, Zuccatosta L, Gusella P. Integration of transbronchial and percutaneous approach in the diagnosis of peripheral pulmonary nodules or masses. Experience with 1,027 consecutive cases. *Chest*. 1995;108(1):131–137.

4. Limper AH, Prakash UB. Tracheobronchial foreign bodies in adults. *Ann Intern Med*. 1990;112(8):604–609.

5. Spruit MA, Chavannes NH, Herth FJ, Poletti V, Ley S, Burghuber OC, Clini E, Cottin V. Clinical highlights from the 2011 ERS Congress in Amsterdam. *Eur Respir J*. 2012;39(6):1501–1510.

6. Dexter J. Flexible fiberoptic bronchoscopy. In: Wilkins RL, Dexter JF, Heuer A, (eds.). *Clinical Assessment in Respiratory Care*. Philadelphia: Elsevier Health Sciences; 2009: 366–376.

7. British Thoracic Society guidelines on diagnostic flexible bronchoscopy. *Thorax*. 2001;56(Suppl 1):i1–i21.

8. Kawaraya M, Gemba K, Ueoka H, et al. Evaluation of various cytological examinations by bronchoscopy in the diagnosis of peripheral lung cancer. *Br J Cancer*. 2003;89(10):1885–1888.

9. Mazzone P, Jain P, Arroliga, Matthay RA. Bronchoscopy and needle biopsy techniques for diagnosis and staging of lung cancer. *Clin Chest Med*. 2002;23(1):137–158, ix.

10. Crossno JT Jr. Procedures in pulmonary medicine. In: Hanley M, Welsh C (eds.). *CURRENT Diagnosis and Treatment in Pulmonary Medicine*. New York: McGraw-Hill; 2003; 57–65.

11. Wahidi MM, Jain P, Jantz M, et al. American College of Chest Physicians consensus statement on the use of topical anesthesia, analgesia, and sedation during flexible bronchoscopy in adult patients. *Chest*. 2011;140(5):1342–1350.

12. Wang, KP, Mehta, CA, and Turner, Jr. JF (eds). *Flexible Bronchoscopy*. Oxford, UK: Wiley-Blackwell; 2011, p. 53–70; 317–324.

13. Anzueto A, Levine SM, Jenkinson SG. The technique of bronchoalveolar lavage. A guide to sampling the terminal airways and alveolar space. *J Crit Illn*. 1992;7(11):1817–1824.

14. Baughman RP. Technical aspects of bronchoalveolar lavage: recommendations for a standard procedure. *Semin Respir Crit Care Med*. 2007;28(5):475–485.

15. Sheski FD, Mathur PN. Endobronchial ultrasound. *Chest*. 2008;133(1):264–270.

16. Du Rand IA, Barber PV, Goldring J, et al. British Thoracic Society guideline for advanced diagnostic and therapeutic flexible bronchoscopy in adults. *Thorax*. 2011;66(Suppl 3):iii1–iii21.

17. Ayers ML, Beamis JF Jr. Rigid bronchoscopy in the twenty-first century. *Clin Chest Med*. 2001;22(2):355–364.

18. Thomsen TW, DeLaPena J, Setnik GS. Videos in clinical medicine. Thoracentesis. *N Engl J Med*. 2006;355(15):e16.

19. Feller-Kopman D. Ultrasound-guided thoracentesis. *Chest*. 2006;129(6):1709–1714.

20. Bradley B, Branley HM, Egan JJ, et al. Interstitial lung disease guideline: The British Thoracic Society in collaboration with the Thoracic Society of Australia and New Zealand and the Irish Thoracic Society. *Thorax*. 2008;63(Suppl 5):v1–58.

21. Sigurdsson MI, Isaksson HJ, Gudmundsson G, Gudbjartsson T. Diagnostic surgical lung biopsies for suspected interstitial lung diseases: a retrospective study. *Ann Thorac Surg*. 2009;88(1):227–232.

14

Acute and Critical Care Monitoring and Assessment

David L. Vines, Kyle Jendral, Joshua Wilson, and Ramandeep Kaur

CHAPTER OUTLINE

Overview
Introduction to Acute and Critical Care Monitoring and Assessment
Ventilatory Parameters
Noninvasive Monitoring
Cardiac Monitoring
Hemodynamic Monitoring
Summary

CHAPTER OBJECTIVES

1. Discuss commonly monitored ventilatory parameters in critically ill patients.
2. Differentiate between normal and abnormal ventilatory parameters.
3. Discuss the effect of spontaneous breathing efforts on the inspiratory-to-expiratory ratio (I:E) using assist-control or synchronized intermittent mandatory ventilation (SIMV) modes.
4. Explain how peak inspiratory pressure and plateau pressure will be affected by changes in compliance or airway resistance.
5. Distinguish between normal and abnormal bedside spirometry findings.
6. Identify indicators of poor respiratory muscle strength.
7. Recognize common abnormalities on ventilator graphics.
8. Discuss how various ventilator dyssynchronies identified on ventilator graphics are corrected.
9. Explain how total-PEEP is measured and how auto-PEEP is calculated.
10. State the appropriate depth of an endotracheal tube.
11. State the appropriate artificial airway cuff pressure.
12. Describe the technologic principles behind pulse oximetry, capnography, transcutaneous monitoring, and exhaled nitric oxide monitoring.
13. Recognize the clinical relevance for pulse oximetry, capnography, transcutaneous monitoring, and exhaled nitric oxide monitoring.
14. Discuss the role of hemodynamic monitoring in critically ill patients.
15. Discuss the effects of preload, contractility, and afterload on cardiac output.
16. Differentiate between cardiopulmonary disorders based on measured and calculated hemodynamic variables.
17. Calculate compliance, airway resistance, cardiac output, systemic vascular resistance, pulmonary vascular resistance, and oxygen delivery.
18. Discuss the use of $S\bar{v}_{O_2}$ in monitoring critically ill patients.

KEY TERMS

afterload
airway resistance (R_{aw})
auto-PEEP
capnometry
contractility
exhaled nitric oxide (FeNO)
forced expiratory volume in 1 second (FEV_1)
forced vital capacity (FVC)
inspiratory-to-expiratory ratio (I:E)
maximal expiratory pressure (MEP)
maximal inspiratory pressure (MIP)
minute ventilation ($\dot{V}_E$)
negative inspiratory force (NIF)
oxygen delivery ($\dot{D}_{O_2}$)
peak expiratory flow (PEF)
peak inspiratory pressure (PIP)
plateau pressure ($P_{plateau}$)
preload
pressure control ventilation (PCV)
pressure support ventilation (PSV)
pulse oximetry
respiratory rate (f)
slow vital capacity (SVC)
spirometer
tidal volume (V_T)
total-PEEP
transcutaneous monitoring (TCM)
vital capacity (VC)
volume control ventilation
work of breathing (WOB)

Overview

This chapter will provide an overview of the assessment and monitoring of critically ill patients with a focus on patients receiving mechanical ventilatory support. Common ventilator parameters, ventilator graphics, lung mechanics, noninvasive monitoring, and hemodynamic monitoring will be discussed. The respiratory care clinician should be able to interpret information from the patient, the ventilator, and surrounding monitors to reach sound clinical decisions when caring for critically ill patients.

Introduction to Acute and Critical Care Monitoring and Assessment

Chapters 3, 4, and 5 provide the foundational information needed to complete a thorough patient assessment, including review of the medical record, history, and physical examination. Many patients seen in the critical care unit have disturbances of oxygenation and/or ventilation, and these topics are covered in detail in Chapters 6 and 7. Arterial blood gases, electrocardiogram (ECG), and laboratory and imaging studies are discussed in Chapters 8 through 11. This chapter will review these assessment fundamentals in light of the additional information that may be gathered from various monitoring systems employed in the acute and critical care setting. The goal is to provide the respiratory care clinician with the tools needed to monitor patient safety and determine when changes in the care of the acutely or critically ill patient are needed.

An important difference between a general hospital bed and an intensive care unit (ICU) bed is the amount of patient monitoring and bedside care that is provided. Regardless of the location, the respiratory care clinician must decide on the amount of monitoring and frequency of assessments needed to ensure patient safety. Increased monitoring and/or frequency of assessments directly increases healthcare costs. Lack of adequate monitoring or inappropriate frequency of assessment places patients at unnecessary risk. The clinician must weigh the cost-benefit relationship with respect to the level of monitoring desired and frequency of assessments. Some monitoring systems, especially noninvasive systems, pose little risk to the patient and provide valuable clinical data. A pulse oximeter is an example of a noninvasive monitoring device that provides valuable data at a relatively low cost. Pulse oximeters can be used to continuously monitor heart rate and oxygen saturation (Spo_2) with little or no risk. Spo_2 monitoring is part of routine vital sign assessment in today's ICU. Invasive monitoring systems may provide information that cannot be obtained noninvasively or through physical assessment but usually increase the patient's risk for complications or harm. A pulmonary artery catheter is an example of an invasive monitoring technique that can provide the clinician with continuous hemodynamic data, including pulmonary artery pressures and cardiac output. The placement of this catheter and associated increased risk of infection put the patient at a higher risk of complications and increases healthcare costs.[1] Technological advances in ultrasound allow for the periodic noninvasive assessment of cardiac function, identification of pneumothorax and pleural effusion, as well as assessment of volume status (e.g., inferior vena cava [IVC] size changes via ultrasound imaging). Minimally invasive monitoring may shift the risk-benefit ratio in favor of patient safety.[2]

Regardless of the type of monitoring used, the respiratory care clinician must be able to interpret the information provided. Are the data accurate? Are the findings important? Does the patient's respiratory care plan need to be changed, or should monitoring be continued? These are just a few of the questions that clinicians must be able to answer when assessing critically ill patients. Respiratory care clinicians use physical assessment techniques, critical care monitoring devices, and laboratory and imaging studies to identify and evaluate changes in the patient's condition. For this reason, the respiratory care clinician may be the most valuable monitoring system available. **Clinical Focus 14-1** provides an example of a patient requiring an assessment by a respiratory care clinician.

Ventilatory Parameters

A number of ventilatory parameters need to be assessed by the respiratory care clinician when monitoring a critically ill patient. One of the most important vital signs to monitor is the patient's respiratory rate. The **respiratory rate (f)** is the total number of breaths taken every minute. The respiratory rate can be counted by the clinician during the physical assessment or can be visualized on a monitoring device. An abnormal respiratory rate can be caused by a number of different physiologic changes that may be occurring. A fast respiratory rate, tachypnea (f > 20 breaths/min), is often the body's response to hypoxia, hypercapnea, increased **work of breathing (WOB)**, fever, pain, and/or anxiety. A slow respiratory rate, bradypnea (f < 12 breaths/min), can indicate a decrease in consciousness due to sedation or severe hypercapnia, which may occur when patients with chronic obstructive pulmonary disease (COPD) and chronic hypercapnia receive high oxygen concentrations. The clinician must also assess the patient's **tidal volume (V_T)**, which is the amount of air passively exhaled after a normal inspiration from functional residual capacity. Tidal volume will often increase when temperature, metabolic demands, and/or dead space increase. Tidal volume may decrease with heavy sedation, neuromuscular disease, and increased WOB. A decreasing tidal volume and increasing respiratory rate (e.g., rapid, shallow breathing) may be signs of impending respiratory failure. The patient's respiratory rate multiplied by the tidal volume is the patient's **minute ventilation ($\dot{V}_E$)**, which provides an assessment of the patient's overall ventilatory status. It is usually recorded in liters per minute (L/min). Generally, a minute volume of 80 to 100 mL/kg/min is needed to maintain a normal $Paco_2$ and acid-base balance. Without

CLINICAL FOCUS 14-1

Hypercapnic Respiratory Failure Secondary to Drug Overdose

A 21-year-old male found unresponsive at a public transportation bus stop was bought to the emergency room. On arrival, his vitals were: heart rate 123 bpm, blood pressure 142/80 mm Hg, respiratory rate 8 breaths/min, Spo_2 94%. Urine toxicology was performed and was positive for both cocaine and opiates. Initial arterial blood gases on room air showed pH of 7.15, $Paco_2$ 72 mm Hg, Pao_2 87 mm Hg, HCO_3^- 23.2 mEq/L, and Sao_2 93.5%.

Clinical Assessment Questions

1. What is your initial impression of this clinical scenario?
    This patient was in acute ventilatory failure (hypercapnic respiratory failure) secondary to a narcotic drug overdose.

2. What are the clinical, laboratory, or radiologic features associated with this condition?
    Blood gases typically show elevated $Paco_2$ and normal serum bicarbonate (no renal compensation) consistent with uncompensated respiratory acidosis (i.e., acute ventilatory failure). In acute ventilatory failure, pH drops 0.08 for every 10 mm Hg rise in $Paco_2$. For this patient, the $Paco_2$ has elevated by 32 mm Hg (72 − 40 = 32) with a pH decrease of 0.24 (7.40 − 7.16 = 0.24), which correlates with a decrease in pH of about 0.08 for every 10 mm Hg rise in $Paco_2$. The hypercapnia and respiratory acidosis present confirm acute ventilatory failure. The positive drug screen suggests narcotic drug overdose.

3. How would you manage this situation?
    The initial approach would be to intubate the patient, secure the airway, and initiate mechanical ventilation. Ventilator strategies should be aimed to achieve a minute ventilation of about 100 mL/kg/min to correct the respiratory acidosis and bring pH to the normal range (7.35 to 7.45). Opioid overdose has impaired the ventilatory drive for this patient, which is reversible by administration of an opioid antagonist such as naloxone (Narcan).

an adequate minute volume, oxygenation and carbon dioxide removal may be insufficient and hypoxia and acidosis may occur. Determining the underlying cause and correction of a low minute ventilation is critical to preventing ventilatory failure and the associated adverse patient outcomes.

> ### RC Insights
>
> Decreasing tidal volume and increasing respiratory rate (f > 30 breaths/min, V_T < 300 mL) are signs of an increased WOB and fatiguing respiratory muscles that may require mechanical ventilatory support.

Monitoring Volume and Rate During Mechanical Ventilation

Respiratory rate, tidal volume, and minute ventilation must also be assessed during mechanical ventilatory support of patients. During mechanical ventilation the respiratory care clinician can set the ventilator rate, tidal volume (or pressure), inspiratory time (or flow), and mode (e.g., assist-control [A/C; aka continuous mandatory ventilation or CMV], synchronized intermittent mandatory ventilation [SIMV], pressure support ventilation [PSV], or pressure control ventilation [PCV]). During mechanical ventilation there is also typically a measured total rate, tidal volume, and minute volume. The set rate is the minimum number of mandatory breaths that will be delivered by the ventilator every minute. The total rate is the total number of breaths the patient receives per minute, which includes both the set "machine" rate and any spontaneous breaths initiated by the patient.

Assist-Control Mode or Continuous Mandatory Ventilation

Assist-control mode (aka A/C or CMV) refers to a mode of mechanical ventilation in which the patient receives a preset tidal volume (or pressure) with each machine-delivered breath. If the patient makes no inspiratory effort, the breaths are delivered at a preset rate. If the patient makes an inspiratory effort, the ventilator is triggered, and a mechanical breath is delivered. In other words, patients' inspiratory efforts will result in mechanically supported breaths being delivered, typically with a preset tidal volume or pressure. These "machine" breaths provide the same tidal volume or pressure each breath. Typically, in the assist-control mode the clinician will also set the inspiratory time

(I-time), or inspiratory flow rate for each breath. If the patient breathes at a faster rate than set, the ventilator will trigger at that increased rate, and the minute volume will increase.

Assuming a constant inspiratory time or flow rate, as the patient increases his or her rate the expiratory time (E-time) will decrease and the **inspiratory-to-expiratory ratio (I:E)** will increase. Specifically, the I:E ratio increases because E-time decreases when the rate increases and the I-time remains the same. For example, in the assist-control mode if the ventilator rate (f) is set at 12 with a tidal volume (V_T) of 500 mL and I-time of 1 second and there is no patient effort, the minute volume ($\dot{V}_E$) will be 6 L/min:

$$\dot{V}_E = V_T \times f = 500 \text{ mL} \times 12 \text{ breaths / min}$$
$$= 6000 \text{ mL / min} = 6 \text{ L / min}$$

In this case, the patient's respiratory cycle time is 5 seconds (60 sec/min ÷ 12 breaths/min = 5 sec). If the I-time is 1 second, then the E-time is 4 seconds and the I:E ratio is 1:4.

If the patient begins to trigger the ventilator 20 times per minute by making inspiratory efforts, the patient's actual minute volume will increase to 10 L/min (instead of 6 L/min):

$$\dot{V}_E = V_T \times f = 500 \text{ mL} \times 20 \text{ breaths / min}$$
$$= 10,000 \text{ mL / min} = 10 \text{ L / min}$$

In this case the respiratory cycle time will decrease to 3 seconds (60 sec/min ÷ 20 breaths/min = 3 sec). If the I-time remains 1 second, the E-time will decrease to 2 seconds and the I:E ratio will increase to 1:2 (instead of 1:4). If this patient continues to increase his spontaneous efforts and rate, the E-time will continue to decrease, and at some point significant air trapping may occur because enough time to exhale has not been provided.

Synchronized Intermittent Mandatory Ventilation

Synchronized intermittent mandatory ventilation (SIMV) refers to a mode of providing mechanical ventilatory support that combines aspects of assist-control ventilation and spontaneous breathing. In the SIMV mode, mandatory breaths provided by the ventilator at a set rate are interspersed with spontaneous breaths. The mandatory breaths are delivered using a preset tidal volume (or pressure). The tidal volumes during spontaneous breaths vary and are usually less than the mandatory breath tidal volumes. Spontaneous breaths may be supported (e.g., PSV). PSV levels are usually much less than the pressures used during mandatory breaths.

If the patient described above is receiving ventilation in the SIMV mode and the ventilator rate is set at 12 breaths/min, then the total rate will be determined by the sum of the "machine" set rate and the spontaneous

rate. If the total rate is 20 breaths/min, the patient will get 12 mandatory breaths at 500 mL (as an example) and the "machine" minute volume will be 6 L/min (machine $\dot{V}_E$ = 500 mL × 12 breaths/min = 6000 mL = 6 L/min). However, the patient in this example is breathing spontaneously at a total respiratory rate of 20 breaths/min. This means that the 12 mandatory "machine" breaths are interspersed with 8 spontaneous breaths, for a total rate of 20 breaths/min. If each of these spontaneous breaths averaged 250 mL, the "spontaneous" minute volume would be 2 L/min (spontaneous $\dot{V}_E$ = 250 mL × 8 breaths/min = 2000 mL = 2 L/min.). The patient's total minute volume would then be 8 L/min (total $\dot{V}_E$ = machine $\dot{V}_E$ + spontaneous $\dot{V}_E$ = 6 + 2 = 8 L/min).

For spontaneous breaths in SIMV, the tidal volume, inspiratory time, and spontaneous respiratory rate are determined by the patient's ventilatory drive, lung mechanics, and respiratory muscle strength. If the spontaneous tidal volumes are less than normal or the patient is tachypneic, PSV can be added to increase the "spontaneous" tidal volume by assisting the patient's inspiratory efforts. This inspiratory assist provided by PSV can normalize tidal volume, lower WOB, and lessen the tachypnea.

Other Modes of Ventilation

Many newer modes of ventilation have been introduced with varying degrees of success. These include adaptive pressure control, adaptive support ventilation (ASV), airway pressure release ventilation (APRV), and proportional assist ventilation (PAV). Each of these modes are reported to have specific advantages and disadvantages, but none have been clearly shown to improve patient outcomes when compared to more traditional modes of ventilation (e.g., assist-control, SIMV, PCV, PSV). Regardless of the mode chosen, it is essential that the patient's actual ventilatory rates and volumes be carefully monitored.

Bedside Measures of Ventilation

A **spirometer** can be used to measure a patient's tidal volume and/or minute ventilation at the bedside. These two ventilatory parameters are rarely measured in nonintubated patients except for certain patients with neuromuscular disorders (e.g., Guillain-Barré, myasthenia gravis). Clinicians often categorize spontaneous ventilation as either sufficient or insufficient based on their clinical assessment. If the clinician visualizes good chest excursion, auscultates bilateral breath sounds, and counts a normal respiratory rate, then the patient's minute ventilation should be sufficient to maintain adequate oxygenation and CO_2 removal. Unless they are critically ill, most patients can adjust their spontaneous respiratory rate and/or tidal volume to maintain sufficient minute ventilation.

Minute volume alone may not ensure adequate alveolar ventilation. For example, a patient with a normal tidal volume of 0.5 L and respiratory rate of 16 breaths/min would have a normal minute volume of 8 L (8 L = 0.5 L × 16 breaths/min). If this patient's tidal volume decreased to 0.25 L due to pulmonary disease, and in compensation he increased his respiratory rate to 32 breaths/min, the minute volume would remain constant at 8 L (8 L= 0.25 L × 32 breaths/min). Unfortunately, although the minute volume in this example is maintained, the rapid, shallow breathing pattern that has developed is such that the patient's dead space volume represents a much larger portion of each breath, and alveolar ventilation declines. Rapid, shallow breathing is a troubling breathing pattern that clinicians should recognize. Rapid, shallow breathing often occurs in patients with acute reductions in pulmonary compliance (e.g., pneumonia, acute respiratory distress syndrome [ARDS]) and is associated with an elevated WOB that the patient may not be able to sustain for an extended period. The end result may be ventilatory failure in which the patient is unable to maintain adequate oxygenation and ventilation. Thus, small tidal volumes with an elevated respiratory rate may be inadequate to maintain alveolar ventilation and oxygenation even if minute volume is maintained. The clinician can confirm the sufficiency of ventilation and oxygenation by performing an arterial blood gas (ABG) study. Chapter 7 provides an in depth discussion of assessment of ventilation, to include the effects of dead space on alveolar ventilation.

Assessment of Ventilation During Mechanical Ventilatory Support

During mechanical ventilation it is essential to assess tidal volume, respiratory rate, minute volume, and airway pressures. With volume ventilation, the tidal volume is generally set at 6 to 8 mL/kg of ideal body weight (IBW) and the respiratory rate is set to achieve a minute volume of 80 to 100 mL/kg/min. Slightly larger tidal volumes (e.g., 10 mL/kg IBW) may be used in patients with normal lung compliance (e.g., neuromuscular disease) in order to prevent atelectasis. An adequate tidal volume, respiratory rate, and minute volume are essential to maintain good gas exchange. Inspired and expired tidal volume should be monitored on the ventilator to ensure that the desired tidal volume is being delivered (± 5% to 10%) in volume control mode or targeted volumes are achieved in pressure limited modes (PCV or PSV). The airway pressures required to achieve a given tidal volume will vary depending on the patient's lung mechanics (i.e., lung compliance and airway resistance).

Peak inspiratory pressure (PIP) is the maximum pressure that results from the flow of gas into the lungs during ventilatory support with positive pressure. In the volume control mode, the PIP is usually reached at the end of the dynamic portion of inspiration and reflects both **airway resistance (R_{aw})** and respiratory system compliance (C_{rs}). As C_{rs} decreases or R_{aw} increases, PIP will increase. **Plateau pressure ($P_{plateau}$)** is a static measurement when flow has ceased at end inspiration and reflects alveolar pressure. This pressure is measured by creating an inspiratory hold, or plateau, after the tidal volume has been delivered. As C_{rs} decreases, the plateau or static pressure increases. The difference between the PIP and plateau pressure is due to the resistance that is present; PIP is > plateau pressure in the volume control mode.

When low flow rates (e.g., < 30 to 40 L/min) and/or very small tidal volumes (e.g., 4 to 5 mL/kg) are used, the patient's inspiratory effort may exceed the flow and/or tidal volume provided by the ventilator. If this occurs, the PIP will decrease, WOB will increase, and the patient may "fight" the ventilator. Ventilator inspiratory gas flow should be adjusted to ensure that it exceeds the patient's inspiratory demand to avoid dyssynchrony between patient effort and the ventilator settings.

Respiratory Mechanics

PIP, $P_{plateau}$, tidal volume, and inspiratory flow are used to calculate respiratory mechanics during mechanical ventilation. Typically, total compliance (respiratory system compliance [C_{rs}]) and R_{aw} are calculated and monitored for change during mechanical ventilation. Compliance is calculated as the change in volume over the change in pressure (mL/cm H_2O) during a mechanically supported breath. Total compliance (C_{total}) includes both thoracic (aka chest wall) and lung compliance. C_{rs} is a measure of C_{total} and is calculated based on the volume delivered to the lungs and change in alveolar pressure associated with this volume.

In older ventilators, a portion of the tidal volume is "lost" during inspiration due to expansion of the ventilator circuit when pressurized due to the compliance of the tubing (tubing compliance, or TC). In these cases, volume lost due to TC must be subtracted from the values measured at the expired gas port of the ventilator. To adjust for TC, tidal volume is corrected by multiplying the difference between PIP and positive end-expiratory pressure (PEEP) by the tubing compliance (TC) factor and then subtracting that volume from the exhaled tidal volume measured at the expiratory port of the ventilator:

$$\text{Corrected } V_T = V_T \text{ exhaled} - [(\text{PIP} - \text{PEEP}) \times \text{TC factor}]$$

The TC factor is simply the volume loss due to tubing compliance expressed as mL/cm H_2O. For example, if the TC factor were 3 mL/cm H_2O, the V_T exhaled was

600 mL with PIP = 30 cm H_2O and PEEP = 5 cm H_2O, the corrected V_T would be:

$$Corrected\ V_T = 600\ mL - [(30 - 5) \times 3]$$
$$= 600\ mL - 75\ mL = 525\ mL$$

The volume of gas lost to tubing compliance in the example would be 75 mL.

The TC factor is calculated for a ventilator circuit before connection to the patient by setting the tidal volume at 100 mL and dividing it by the change in pressure that occurs while the ventilator circuit "Y" is occluded. Today's ventilators usually automatically correct for this volume lost to the circuit, and the exhaled tidal volume is reported as corrected for TC. More sophisticated ventilators actually adjust the delivered tidal volume to make up for the loss due to TC. In either case, once the corrected tidal volume is measured, total compliance is calculated by dividing this volume by the difference between plateau pressure and PEEP (C_{total} = $V_T/P_{plateau}$ – PEEP). Normal total compliance is 60 to 100 mL/cm H_2O.

Airway resistance (R_{aw}) is typically calculated in the volume control mode using a square flow waveform. An inspiratory hold is set to obtain plateau pressure. The difference between the PIP and plateau pressure is divided by the inspiratory flow in L/sec to calculate airway resistance:

$$R_{aw} = (PIP - P_{plateau}) \div Inspiratory\ flow\ (L/sec)$$

This calculation can be simplified by using a constant (square wave) inspiratory flow of 60 L/min, which is 1 L/sec. With this flow rate, the difference between PIP and plateau pressure is the airway resistance. Airway resistance in an intubated patient is normally less than 10 cm H_2O/L/sec. Chapter 7 provides additional discussion of factors that may affect patients' compliance and resistance.

RC Insights

Increases in both PIP and plateau pressure are caused by a decrease in compliance. If PIP increases but the plateau pressure remains the same, it is the result of an increase in airway resistance.

Inspiratory-to-Expiratory Ratio

Another aspect of the patient's ventilation during mechanical ventilatory support that deserves more discussion is the I:E ratio. This ratio is normally maintained at 1:2 or 1:3. An I:E ratio that changes from 1:2 to 1:4 is said to have *decreased*; inspiratory time would have to decrease or expiratory time increase for this change to occur. If the ratio changes from 1:2 to 1:1, the I:E ratio is said to have *increased*, which means inspiratory time increased or expiratory time decreased. If the

ratio changes, for example, from 1:1 to 1.5:1 or 2:1, then it is referred to as an inverse ratio.

The I:E ratio can provide useful information to the clinician regarding pulmonary mechanics. A prolonged expiratory time during spontaneous breathing may indicate obstruction or increased airway resistance. Patients with severe asthma exacerbation routinely recruit expiratory muscles to help force air out of their lungs due to bronchospasm and the resultant obstruction. COPD patients typically have prolonged expiratory times due to airway obstruction or decreased lung elastic recoil, as seen with emphysema.[3] Pursed-lip breathing is sometimes used by these patients in an attempt to prevent airway collapse and allow the lungs to empty and prevent air trapping. Prolonged expiratory times may occur as a result of pursed-lip breathing. Fixed obstructions (e.g., tumor, foreign body) can also cause prolonged inspiratory times. A depressed respiratory drive or short gasps due to fatigue may result in short inspiratory times and small tidal volumes.

Although assessing a patient's I:E ratio during spontaneous breathing can provide insight into the underlying pathophysiology, the I:E ratio should be monitored carefully in patients receiving mechanical ventilatory support. Specifically, inappropriate ventilator settings can result in harmful effects related to the resultant inspiratory or expiratory times or I:E ratios. For example, inadequate expiratory times can result in air trapping, lung overinflation, and elevations in mean airway pressures that reduce venous return and cardiac output. Note, however, that increasing inspiratory time can sometimes be useful to improve the distribution of inspired gas and oxygenation in certain types of patients.

In certain ventilators (e.g., Puritan Bennett 840, Puritan Bennett 980, Covidien) in the volume control mode, inspiratory time (I-time) is determined by the set tidal volume, the inspiratory flow rate, and the inspiratory waveform (e.g., square wave, descending ramp). An increase in flow rate, a change from descending ramp to square wave, or a decrease in tidal volume will *decrease* inspiratory time. A decrease in flow rate, a change from square wave to descending ramp, or an increase in tidal volume will *increase* I-time. E-time is determined by respiratory rate, and an increase in rate will *decrease* E-time, whereas a decrease in rate will *increase* E-time.

Other ventilators (e.g., Servo-s, MAQUET, Hamilton S1, Hamilton Medical AG) in the volume control mode have controls to set I-time (instead of inspiratory flow rate) and inspiratory pause time. For ventilators in this family of devices, inspiratory time is set directly in seconds. An inspiratory pause or plateau may also be set, usually as a percent of the total respiratory cycle time. The expiratory time is determined by the respiratory rate.

For **pressure control ventilation (PCV)**, typically I-time and rate are set, and these determine E-time and the I:E ratio. With **pressure support ventilation (PSV)**,

I-time is determined by the pressure support level and the patient's interaction with the ventilator. The inspiratory phase is terminated when the inspiratory flow decreases to a certain level. The use of other modes of ventilation (e.g., SIMV, pressure regulated volume control [PRVC], proportional assist ventilation [PAV]) further complicate the interaction of the ventilator and patient and the resultant I-time, E-time, and I:E ratio. Regardless of the mode of ventilation employed, the respiratory care clinician must always be aware of the effects of specific ventilator settings on I-time, E-time, and I:E ratio, because inappropriate settings can cause serious harm to patients.

Bedside Spirometry

Many devices are available that a clinician can use to assess a patient's lung function at the bedside. One of the simplest devices is the bedside spirometer. These devices are used to measure a patient's vital capacity (or the exhaled volume over approximately 6 seconds; FEV_6). Recall from Chapter 12 that **vital capacity (VC)** is the maximum amount of air one can exhale from the lungs after a maximum inspiratory effort. Measuring vital capacity and how fast an individual can exhale that volume are helpful in identifying underlying lung pathology. A normal vital capacity is about 70 mL/kg IBW, and normally at least 70% of VC can be exhaled in 1 second with a maximal patient effort. A VC < 70 mL/kg may represent a restrictive lung defect (e.g., neuromuscular or interstitial lung disease). A VC < 30 mL/kg IBW is associated with a weak cough and increased potential for development of atelectasis.[4] Vital capacity can be measured either by a **slow vital capacity (SVC)** technique or a **forced vital capacity (FVC)** technique (see Chapter 12). The main difference between these two is the speed at which the patient is instructed to exhale. SVC is primarily performed in patients with obstructive lung disease to avoid air trapping associated with a forceful exhalation. SVC is often greater than FVC in patients with emphysema, tracheal malacia (tracheal cartilage softening or weakness), or tracheal collapse. SVC is also routinely measured at the bedside using a simple respirometer (e.g., Wright respirometer) as a gross measure of pulmonary function.

FVC is performed to determine the total volume and how fast the patient can exhale. The patient's **forced expiratory volume in 1 second (FEV_1)** can then be compared to the total FVC to assess for airway obstruction. Remember, a normal FEV_1 is 70% (or more) of vital capacity. Thus, an FEV_1/FVC ratio of less than 0.70 (or 70%) suggests airway obstruction.* Measurement of FEV_1 can then be repeated after administering a bronchodilator to determine if the obstruction is reversible. An improvement in $FEV_1 \geq 12\%$ and at least 200 mL (or improvement in $FVC \geq 12\%$ and at least 200 mL) is generally considered indicative of reversibility (see also Chapter 12).

In the critical care setting, SVC < 15 mL/kg IBW or 1.0 L is widely accepted as an indicator of impending ventilatory failure[4] and often indicates poor respiratory muscle strength in patients with neuromuscular disease. A number of factors can contribute to a decreased VC. Sedation may reduce a patient's drive to breathe and ability to follow commands. Pain can influence a patient's ability to breathe deeply, especially following abdominal or thoracic surgery. A pneumonectomy or multiple lobectomies can result in a reduced VC. COPD patients with severe obstruction and significant air trapping often have a reduced VC. The diaphragm accounts for about 70% of the inspiratory tidal volume in a healthy patient.[5] Diaphragmatic injury or weakness may reduce VC. If VC decreases by more than 15% to 20% when a patient is placed in the supine position, diaphragmatic weakness may be present.[5] Monitoring of vital capacity is important in patients at risk of developing atelectasis and respiratory failure.

Peak expiratory flow (PEF) is another measurement that can be made at the bedside to determine the severity of obstruction and assess patients' response to therapy. Peak flow meters measure the maximum speed at which patients can force airflow out of their lungs, usually recorded in liters per second (L/sec) or liters per minute (L/min). PEF can be measured in the pulmonary function laboratory using sophisticated equipment or at the bedside using simple, inexpensive, and highly portable peak flow meters. Simple peak flow meters are also often provided to asthmatic patients for home self-monitoring. Bronchial constriction can cause PEF to decline depending on the severity of the obstruction. In asthma, a PEF of less than 50% of the patient's predicted (or personal best) generally represents severe obstruction. Monitoring PEF over time can be useful for trending, especially for asthma patients. An increase in PEF would suggest improvement, possibly in response to therapy. PEF measurement can also be performed before and after bronchodilator treatments. A significant improvement in PEF following bronchodilator therapy provides evidence of effectiveness. Other factors that may influence PEF include patient cooperation, patient effort, quality of the clinician's instruction of the patient, and patient understanding of the procedure. The measurement of PEF during acute asthma exacerbations is somewhat controversial and may not provide a good way to classify severity of illness under

---

* The GOLD criteria for COPD suggest that $FEV_1/FVC < 0.70$ represents obstruction. In the pulmonary function laboratory, the criterion for obstruction is FEV_1/FVC below the 95% confidence interval based on the NHANES III data (see Chapter 12). $FEV_1/FVC < 0.70$ generally represents obstruction, whereas FEV_1 alone can be reduced with obstruction *or* restriction.

these conditions. The clinician should to take all these factors into consideration when evaluating the results of PEF measurement.

Pressure manometers can be used at the bedside to measure a patient's ability to generate a negative (i.e., subatmospheric) or positive pressure during inspiration or expiration as measures of ventilatory muscle strength. The maximum negative pressure a patient can generate during an inspiratory effort is referred to as **maximal inspiratory pressure (MIP)** or **negative inspiratory force (NIF)**, and the two terms can be used interchangeably. MIP measurement is achieved by instructing the patient to breathe out completely (to residual volume) and then attempt to inhale in as hard as possible against a closed-valve system, thus allowing the pressure manometer to register the negative pressure generated. This can be explained to patients by comparing the maneuver to trying to suck a thick milkshake through a small straw. MIP provides information about the patient's inspiratory muscle strength and ability to take a deep breath. Depending on age and gender, a normal MIP is between −75 and −100 cm H_2O.[6] An MIP of at least −20 cm H_2O (or more negative) is suggested when considering weaning from mechanical ventilation (see also Chapter 7).

Pressure manometers can also be used to measure a patient's **maximal expiratory pressure (MEP)**. MEP is the maximum amount of force that the patient can generate during exhalation (after taking a deep breath) when exhaling against a closed-valve system connected to a pressure manometer. MEP measurement is helpful to assess whether a patient can generate an effective cough. An MEP < 40 cm H_2O is considered abnormal.[4]

Clinicians can perform spot or routine checks for MIP and MEP to monitor a patient's ventilatory muscle strength. These measures along with VC are often helpful in the evaluation of patients with neuromuscular disease. Analyzing trends in these parameters may allow for interventions prior to the development of ventilatory failure. Some suggest review of VC, MIP, and MEP and applying the "20/30/40 rule" to evaluate ventilatory muscle strength and possible need for mechanical ventilatory support. If VC, MIP, and MEP values are suboptimal (i.e., VC < 20 mL/kg, MIP > −30 cm H_2O, and MEP < 40 cm H_2O), the patient may have difficulty maintaining adequate spontaneous breathing and may require mechanical ventilatory support. If VC > 20 mL/kg IBW, MIP < −30 cm H_2O, and MEP > 40 cm H_2O, then ventilator weaning may be

successful. **Clinical Focus 14-2** reviews the indications for mechanical ventilation.

Assessment of the Intubated Patient Receiving Mechanical Ventilation

Assessing the intubated patient receiving mechanical ventilation can be one of the most challenging and complex procedures that the respiratory care clinician performs. The entire clinical picture has to be reviewed in order to reach sound decisions. The assessment of the patient begins with a review of the medical record. The patient's diagnosis, problem list, physician's orders, history, physical examination, results of any imaging or laboratory studies, and progress notes should be reviewed. Chapter 3 provides a detailed discussion of items that should be reviewed in the medical record and the significance of specific findings. A sufficient review of the patient's record will provide the clinician with an expectation of the patient's condition prior to entering the patient area or room.

Following a review of the medical record, the respiratory care clinician will then complete a patient assessment at the bedside. Upon entering a critically ill patient's room, it is important to pay attention to the surroundings. Scanning the room for things like a "crash cart," IV pumps, cardiac monitor, type of ventilator equipment, chest drainage systems, cooling blankets, urinary catheters, and collection chambers or bags provides valuable information about the patient's condition. Monitoring equipment may allow for quick assessment of the patient's vital signs (including SpO_2), and the ECG monitor can be checked for arrhythmias. The patient's overall appearance, sensorium, and color can help the clinician rapidly decide if the patient is stable or unstable.

Physical assessment is a vital part of the evaluation and monitoring of the critically ill patient. This should include assessment of the patient's general appearance (resting, anxious, signs of distress), skin (color, temperature, diaphoresis, edema), mental status (awake and alert, oriented, responsive, comatose), head and neck (eyes, nose, and mouth; jugular venous distension [JVD]; accessory muscle use), thorax (inspection, auscultation, palpation, percussion), heart (heart sounds, point of maximal impulse [PMI]), abdomen (swelling, ascites), and extremities (edema). Vital signs should be reviewed to include heart rate, blood pressure, temperature, and SpO_2. Chapter 5 provides a detailed discussion of physical assessment findings and their significance.

After the physical assessment is completed the respiratory care clinician can begin to assess the mechanical ventilator and patient–ventilator interaction. This generally includes review of the ventilator settings (mode, rate, tidal volume, inspiratory pressure, oxygen concentration, PEEP or CPAP). Most ventilators also allow for setting I-time (or inspiratory flow),

---

RC Insights

The clinician can use the "20/30/40 rule" as an indicator of poor muscle strength and possible impending ventilatory failure: VC < 20 mL/kg IBW; MIP > −30 cm H_2O; MEP < 40 cm H_2O.

CLINICAL FOCUS 14-2

Indications for Mechanical Ventilation

A 48-year-old woman with no significant past medical history presented to the emergency department complaining of shortness of breath, cough with yellow-colored sputum, and fever with chills for 2 weeks. She was alert and oriented but spoke in short sentences due to difficulty breathing. On physical examination, she was using her inspiratory accessory muscles for breathing, was diaphoretic, and had nasal flaring. Auscultation revealed coarse crackles on the right. Chest x-ray demonstrated bilateral infiltrates with air bronchograms in the right middle and lower lobes. Vital signs were: heart rate 124 bpm, respirations 33 breaths/min, blood pressure 158/90 mm Hg, oral temperature 101.5° F, and SpO_2 85% on room air. Arterial blood gas values on a nonrebreathing oxygen mask were: pH 7.45, $PaCO_2$ 36 mm Hg, PaO_2 54 mm Hg, HCO_3^- 22.4 mEq/L, SaO_2 88%.

Clinical Assessment Questions

1. What is your initial impression of this clinical scenario?
   The patient's initial presentation with fever, cough, yellow-colored sputum, and acute distress are suggestive of pneumonia with hypoxemic respiratory failure.
2. What is your assessment of this patient's condition?
   Based on the clinical findings, the patient was in acute respiratory distress, as indicated by accessory muscle use, diaphoresis, nasal flaring, tachypnea, tachycardia, and hypoxia.
3. What oxygenation indices can be calculated on this patient?
   The $P(A - a)O_2$ and PaO_2/FIO_2 ratio are sometimes calculated for assessment of the severity of hypoxemia.
   The arterial blood gas values are reflective of an oxygenation defect, confirmed by the low PaO_2/FIO_2 ratio and widened $P(A - a)O_2$ gradient. Assuming that the patient is receiving close to 100% O_2 via the nonrebreathing mask, the calculations are:

$$P_AO_2 = 1.0(713) - 36/0.8 = 668 \text{ mm Hg}$$

$$P(A - a)O_2 = 668 - 54 = 614 \text{ mm Hg}$$

and

$$PaO_2/FIO_2 = 54$$

   A normal $P(A - a)O_2$ while breathing 100% O_2 is about 100 to 150 mm Hg, and a normal PaO_2/FIO_2 ratio is > 300. The presence of bilateral infiltrates and air bronchograms throughout the lung fields further suggest the presence of an infective etiology like pneumonia. A complete blood count should be obtained to confirm the diagnosis.
4. How would you now describe this patient's condition?
   The low PaO_2/FIO_2 ratio (normal > 300) and high $P(A - a)O_2$ (normal on 100% O_2 is 100 to 150 mm Hg) indicates the presence of severe hypoxemia due to intrapulmonary shunting. Shunting is further confirmed because the PaO_2 was low while receiving high concentrations of oxygen via nonrebreathing mask (FIO_2 of 0.60 to 1.0).
5. What are the indications for mechanical ventilation?
   The four main indications for mechanical ventilation are:
   a. Apnea
   b. Acute ventilatory failure
   c. Impending ventilatory failure
   d. Severe oxygenation problems (e.g., refractory hypoxemia)
   This patient has refractory hypoxemia and possible impending ventilatory failure. Treatment of refractory hypoxemia seen with ARDS may require the application of positive end-expiratory pressure (PEEP) or continuous positive airway pressure (CPAP), typically provided by invasive mechanical ventilation. PEEP or CPAP may be indicated in this patient to improve oxygenation by increasing functional residual capacity (FRC) and decreasing shunting. In this scenario, invasive mechanical ventilation with PEEP was considered to be appropriate because of the profound oxygenation deficit and severe respiratory distress.

flow waveform, trigger sensitivity, pressure support, and various alarms. Monitored values will include measured airway pressures (PIP, $P_{plateau}$, mean airway pressure [$\bar{P}_{aw}$]), PEEP/CPAP), analyzed F_{IO_2}, measured ventilatory volumes (V_T, $\dot{V}_E$), respiratory rate (machine rate, patient spontaneous rate, total rate), I:E ratio, and airway temperature.

Mechanically ventilated patients who are making spontaneous breathing efforts should be assessed for ventilator–patient synchrony. Ventilator dyssynchrony is associated with poor outcomes and may reduce weaning success and prolong the time required for mechanical ventilation.[7] The first aspect of ensuring adequate ventilator–patient synchrony is maintaining proper ventilator trigger sensitivity. Trigger sensitivity should be set at the most sensitive setting possible without causing automatic triggering. Flow triggering is associated with less trigger work than pressure triggering[8] and is usually preferred. In patients well synchronized with the ventilator, diaphragmatic efforts will correspond to the initiation of gas flow from the ventilator, and a "smooth" inspiratory phase will follow with no signs of respiratory distress. Signs of dyssynchrony include failure to trigger despite a patient effort, patient agitation, paradoxical breathing, severe tachypnea, tachycardia, retractions, diaphoresis, hypertension, hypoxemia, and head bobbing in infants. Ventilator graphics are useful in identifying and correcting patient–ventilator dyssynchrony.

Ventilator Graphics

Ventilator graphics packages are commonly available on modern ventilators. The three most common graphic displays are pressure, flow, and volume waveforms. Pressure, flow, and volume curves are typically displayed versus time. These signals can also be used to create pressure–volume curves and flow-volume "loops."

Pressure Waveforms

Pressure waveforms allow for the visualization of the pressure curves generated during mechanical ventilation displayed in real time as pressure (*y*-axis) versus time (*x*-axis). Most patients receive mechanical ventilatory support in the assist-control or control mode of ventilation. In the assist-control mode, inspiration is initiated by time or patient effort (whichever occurs first). For example, the machine rate may be set at 12 breaths/min, and if the patient makes no effort to breathe she will still receive 12 breaths per minute in the control mode. In this case, each breath is time triggered and breaths occur every 5 seconds. If the patient begins to trigger the ventilator by making spontaneous breathing efforts at a rate of 14 breaths/min, the total rate would increase to 14 "assisted" breaths per minute. Every "assist" breath would be patient triggered.

If the patient was then heavily sedated and spontaneous breathing efforts ceased, she would still receive 12 time-triggered breaths per minute (i.e., control mode). In the assist or assist-control mode of ventilation, a negative deflection in the pressure waveform caused by a patient inspiratory effort should trigger the start of the inspiratory phase and gas flow from the ventilator. In the time-triggered mode (i.e., control mode), there will be no negative deflection in the pressure waveform prior to initiation of the inspiratory phase. In the assist or assist-control modes, if the ventilator is not triggered immediately following a patient inspiratory effort, then patient–ventilator dyssynchrony has occurred, and the ventilator trigger sensitivity should be adjusted.

Peak Inspiratory Pressure

Following initiation of inspiration by time or patient trigger, pressure at the airway rises and a peak inspiratory pressure (PIP) can be observed. The inspiratory phase can be provided by a constant flow of gas (e.g., square wave flow pattern) or variable flow of gas (e.g., descending flow waveform) depending on the ventilator mode chosen and ventilator settings. For example, some ventilators in the volume control (volume limited) mode have controls for the operator to choose the inspiratory flow waveform, and this choice affects the inspiratory pressures generated. In other modes (e.g., PSV, PCV), the flow waveform is determined by the characteristics of that mode. Both PSV and PCV generate a descending (i.e., decelerating) flow waveform.

As noted, during inspiration the pressure at the patient airway rises. PIP usually occurs near or at the end of a volume-limited inspiration. PIP may occur early during inspiration with PSV or PCV, and that pressure may then be sustained throughout the remainder of the inspiratory phase. The rate of rise in inspiratory pressure is related to the gas flow rate, delivered volume, patient lung mechanics (R_{aw}, C_{rs}), patient spontaneous effort, and the resistance of the ventilator circuit and artificial airway. During **volume control ventilation**, PIP represents the maximum pressure that results from overcoming these factors during a "mechanical" breath. PIP is a dynamic measurement that occurs while gas is flowing into the lungs. PIP increases with decreases in lung compliance, decreases in chest wall (thoracic) compliance, or with increases in airway resistance (volume control mode). Improvements in any of these will tend to decrease PIP (volume control mode). It should also be noted that changes in ventilator settings can increase or decrease PIP. For example, if the ventilator's inspiratory flow rate is increased or I-time decreased, PIP will increase (volume control mode). A change from a descending expiratory flow waveform to a square waveform will tend to increase PIP. A decrease in inspiratory flow rate or a change from a square waveform to a descending flow waveform will often decrease PIP. **Clinical Focus 14-3**

CLINICAL FOCUS 14-3

Recognizing Tension Pneumothorax

The alarm system of a mechanical ventilator being used for support of an intubated patient with acute respiratory distress syndrome (ARDS) suddenly begins signaling high peak inspiratory pressures. The patient develops tachycardia, tachypnea, hypoxemia, and hypotension.

Clinical Assessment Questions

1. **What are possible causes of a sudden increase in peak inspiratory pressures during mechanical ventilation?**
   High peak inspiratory pressures (PIP) can develop for several reasons. Any condition leading to elevated airway resistance or decreased compliance can cause high PIP. In assessing this patient, the first step is to ensure that the patient is being adequately ventilated. Secretions or plugs in the artificial airway may result in partial or complete occlusion, which will result in high PIP. Ensuring endotracheal tube (ETT) patency by attempting to pass a suction catheter can establish if the tube is patent. Suctioning the patient may also remove any secretions in the tube.

   Once ETT patency has been confirmed, the respiratory care clinician should focus on other factors that may cause increased airway resistance, such as bronchospasm or secretions in a larger airway. If there are no signs of bronchospasm or airway secretions, the clinician should consider factors that may reduce lung compliance. In patients with ARDS, decreases in lung compliance may be due to worsening of the disease process over hours to days. In this case, the *sudden* increase in PIP and decrease in blood pressure should prompt the clinician to access the patient's breath sounds and inspect the chest wall for equal bilateral chest wall movement. One possible cause of a sudden increase in PIP with hypoxemia, tachycardia, and hypotension is the development of a tension pneumothorax. A tension pneumothorax is a life-threatening event requiring rapid identification and treatment.

2. **What are the clinical, laboratory, and radiologic features associated with tension pneumothorax?**
   Physical examination findings associated with tension pneumothorax include absent (or markedly decreased) breath sounds on the affected side, a hyperresonant percussion note on the affected side, and a contralateral tracheal shift indicating that the mediastinum is being pushed towards the unaffected side. A chest radiograph should be ordered immediately to rule out (or confirm) tension pneumothorax. Radiologic features of a tension pneumothorax include mediastinal shift towards the unaffected side, absence of pulmonary vascular markings on the affected side (i.e., free air in the thorax), and lung collapse. The affected side will often also show increased space between the ribs and the thorax will tend to be expanded on the affected side. SpO_2 and arterial blood gases will generally show hypoxemia and possibly acute hypercapnea.

3. **How would you manage a tension pneumothorax in a patient receiving mechanical ventilation?**
   Tension pneumothorax with severe hypotension represents is a life-threatening situation that must be resolved immediately. As pressure in the thorax increases, venous return to the right heart decreases, which decreases cardiac output, causing hypotension and tachycardia. A life-saving measure in this situation is emergent decompression of the chest. This may be accomplished using an 18-gauge intravenous catheter inserted in the second or third intercostal space on the anterior chest at the midclavicular line of the affected side. This is a temporary solution for decompression that should be followed with conventional chest tube placement.

describes a patient receiving mechanical ventilation with an increasing PIP.

Inspiratory Plateau

Many mechanical ventilators allow the operator to set a inspiratory hold, or plateau in the volume-control mode. Plateau pressures can then be graphically identified, typically using a 1-second inspiratory hold. Plateau pressures are measured at the end of inspiration when there is no gas flow. To obtain an accurate plateau, the patient must *not* be actively breathing during the inspiratory hold nor can a leak be present in the system. With an inspiratory hold of approximately 1 second, plateau pressures should reflect alveolar pressures. Plateau pressures increase with decreases in lung compliance or decreases in thoracic compliance. Plateau pressures decrease with improvements in compliance. **Figure 14-1** provides a graphic display of PIP and plateau pressure.

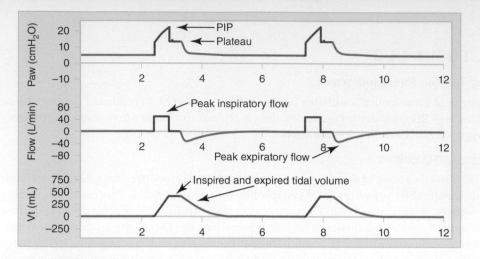

FIGURE 14-1 Pressure, flow, and volume versus time graphics during VCV: square flow waveform with an inspiratory plateau. Note: There is a noticeable difference between PIP and Plateau pressures due to an elevated airway resistance.

Changes in airway resistance tend to have little effect on plateau pressures. When PIP increases but plateau pressure remains the same, an increase in R_{aw} has occurred. This change could be due to factors such as water in the circuit, secretions in the airway, bronchospasm, partial occlusion of the endotracheal tube, or other causes of increased airway resistance. When both PIP and plateau pressure increase, lung and/or chest wall compliance have decreased.

In the volume control mode, PIP is always higher than the plateau pressure unless the patient's inspiratory effort exceeds the flow from the ventilator. However, if the patient's inspiratory demand exceeds the flow provided by the ventilator, inspiratory pressures will drop. When this flow dyssynchrony occurs, a "scooping" effect (pressure rise vertically is slow compared to horizontal progression) appears in the pressure waveform. This flow dyssynchrony usually

occurs during volume control ventilation where flow is set by the clinician. Using an inspiratory flow of at least 60 L/min for most adults may decrease the occurrence of flow dyssynchrony; however, higher flows may be required in some patients. All patients should be periodically assessed for presence of scooping of the pressure waveform and ventilator settings adjusted appropriately. **Figure 14-2** provides an example of flow dyssynchrony during inspiration.

Pressure Control Ventilation and Pressure Support Ventilation

During PCV or PSV the pressure waveform is usually square or rectangular. This square pressure waveform is achieved because the ventilator automatically varies inspiratory flow to maintain the targeted pressure throughout inspiration. In the beginning of the breath,

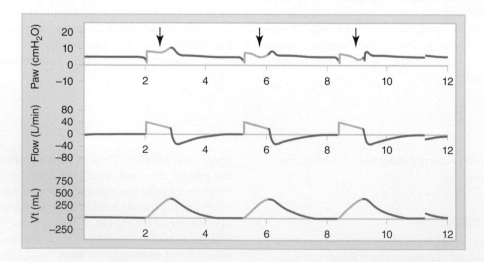

FIGURE 14-2 Pressure, flow, and volume versus time graphics during VCV: decelerating flow pattern. Note: The arrows depict the scooping of the pressure waveform due to the patient's effort exceeding the set inspiratory flow of the ventilator. Note that the flow and volume waveform did not change because these are set parameters.

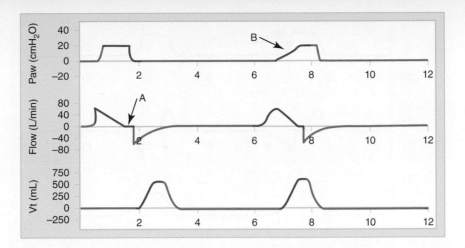

FIGURE 14-3 Pressure, flow, and volume versus time graphics during PCV: slow rise time. Note: Arrow A identifies the point where inspiratory flow has reached zero and the pressure set on the ventilator has equilibrated in the lung. Arrow B identifies the slope or rise to pressure that may be observed when using a pressure limited mode. In the second waveform, the rise time or slope is set too slow and should be set faster.

inspiratory flow is high in order to reach the targeted pressure and then decelerates as pressure in the lung increases. During the inspiratory phase with PCV, once the pressure in the alveoli matches the targeted pressure set on the ventilator, inspiratory gas flow will stop and a plateau will occur (see **Figure 14-3**). At this point, the PIP and plateau pressure will be equal and reflect alveolar pressure. With PCV, the I-time is set by the operator, and when the set I-time is reached the ventilator cycles to the expiratory phase (i.e., time cycled to expiration).

With PSV, the inspiratory phase is terminated when gas flow decreases to a certain predetermined level (i.e., flow cycled to expiration). An inspiratory plateau pressure is never reached during PSV because this mode is primarily flow cycled and inspiratory flow should not reach zero before the expiratory phase begins. During inspiration, the rate of the initial rise in pressure is determined by the *rise time setting*. A rounding of

the pressure waveform can occur when using PSV or PCV due to a slow rise time setting (see Figure 14-3). This is can be corrected by increasing the rise time or slope. If the rise time is set too fast, overshooting will occur, resulting in a "dog ear" on the left side of the pressure waveform (see **Figure 14-4**). This overshoot is corrected by the slowing rise time or decreasing the slope until the artifact disappears from the pressure waveform. Occasionally a dog ear or upward inflection on the right side of the pressure waveform at the end of inspiration may occur (see **Figure 14-5**). This upward inflection on the left side of the pressure–time curve occurs when inspiratory time is too long and the patient is actively exhaling before the ventilator breath ends. This patient–ventilator cycle dyssynchrony increases the patient's WOB. This dyssynchrony can be alleviated by decreasing the set inspiratory time during PCV or increasing the percent flow cycle during PSV.

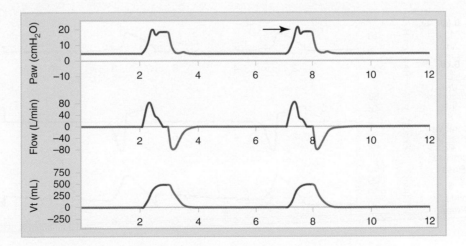

FIGURE 14-4 Pressure, flow, and volume versus time graphics during PCV: rapid rise time. Note: The arrow here is depicting an inspiratory rise that is set to fast resulting in overshoot on the pressure waveform. Rise time or slope should be slowed down until overshoot is eliminated.

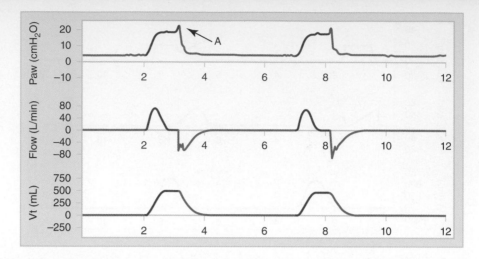

FIGURE 14-5 Pressure, flow, and volume versus time graphics during PCV: dyssynchrony. Note: Arrow A is identifying the patient actively exhaling against the set pressure and results in an upward deflection on the right side. It is generally corrected by shortening the inspiratory time.

Volume Waveforms

Volume waveforms provide a visual representation of inspired and expired tidal volume during mechanical ventilation (see Figure 14-1). When the inspired tidal volume provided by the ventilator exceeds the exhaled volume from the patient, there is either air trapping or a leak in the system (see **Figure 14-6**). The patient–ventilator system must be closed with minimal leaks in order to effectively ventilate patients using standard modes of ventilation. Leaks can occur in the ventilator circuit, artificial airway, or within the patient (e.g., bronchopleural fistula [BPF]). When a leak is suspected, the ventilator circuit must be carefully inspected for the source of the leak. Common sources of leaks include circuit connections, the humidifier, the filter, the temperature probe, and other adaptor connections. If the source of leak is difficult to identify, the volume delivered can be measured at each point along the circuit using a handheld respirometer. If the volume is delivered to the inspiratory side of the patient connection (i.e., "Y") but is not returning on the expiratory side, then the source of the leak is the patient. Leaks around the cuff of an artificial airway are fairly common. Ensuring proper cuff pressure and that the artificial airway is placed at the appropriate depth can resolve this problem. The patient should also be checked for a chest tube and its drainage system observed to see if the water seal is bubbling during inspiration when the patient receives a positive-pressure breath. A pleural air leak (e.g., BPF) is probably present in this case. **Clinical Focus 14-4** describes the evaluation of a patient with a possible air leak.

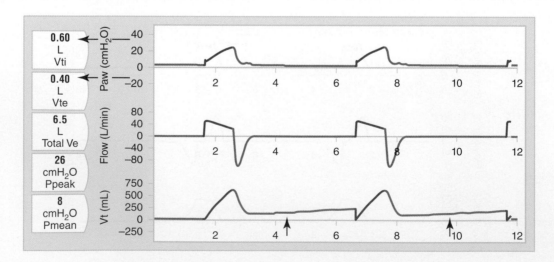

FIGURE 14-6 Pressure, flow, and volume versus time graphics during volume controlled ventilation with a 50% decelerating flow pattern: system leak. Note: The arrows are depicting a leak in the system. Note the difference between inspired and expired tidal volumes.

CLINICAL FOCUS 14-4

Bronchopleural Fistula

A 65-year-old male with a large, right-sided pneumothorax treated with a chest tube was receiving invasive mechanical ventilation in the intensive care unit. There was persistent air bubbling in the chest drainage system 24 hours after chest tube insertion with no re-expansion of the collapsed right lung. Prior to the pneumothorax, the patient was "easy" to ventilate with a tidal volume (V_T) of 500 mL and a rate of 15 breaths/min in the assist-control mode. There was no air leak, and inspired and expired tidal volumes were equal. Following development of the pneumothorax with chest tube insertion, the difference in delivered and exhaled volume was approximately 300 mL on the same ventilator settings with no apparent leak around the endotracheal tube or ventilator circuit. The most recent arterial blood gas results revealed moderate hypercapnia.

Clinical Assessment Questions

1. What is your initial impression of this clinical scenario?
   Continuous air bubbling through the water seal of the drainage system without re-expansion of the collapsed lung indicates that a bronchopleural fistula (BPF) may be present. BPF represents communication between the bronchial tree and pleural space causing air leak from the lungs into pleural cavity. The large difference between inspired and exhaled tidal volume confirms the presence of a large leak in the system.

2. How would you manage this situation?
   In this case, there was a continuous air leak into the pleural space that prevented re-expansion of the collapsed lung. In such cases, it may be necessary to insert a second large-bore chest tube that can facilitate air removal from the pleural space, thus aiding in lung re-expansion. The size of the air leak is sometime calculated as leak rate in liters per minute (L/min). The following equation can be used to calculate the pleural leak (L/min):

   Pleural leak = Respiratory rate × Difference in delivered and exhaled V_T per breath =
   Pleural leak = 15 breaths/min × 300 mL leak per breath = 4.5 L/ min

   Thus, in this case a gas leak of 4.5 L/min was causing inadequate ventilation and moderate hypercapnia in the patient.

   Ventilator strategies should be aimed at minimizing volume loss through the fistula by limiting tidal volume and pressures to reduce alveolar overdistension and allow the fistula to begin healing. Shortening inspiratory times, limiting PEEP, and reducing the respiratory rate may also be tried. Permissive hypercapnia may be required. If hypercapnia becomes unacceptable in patients with BPF, the use of pressure control ventilation (PCV) may result in adequate ventilation even when the air leak is large. PCV will increase flow and inspired volume to compensate for the volume lost to the leak. There are reports of using high-frequency ventilation (HFV), airway pressure release ventilation (APRV), or independent lung ventilation when severe BPF persists, but there is no strong evidence that these measures significantly improve outcomes. BPF requires aggressive management of the underlying cause.

Flow Waveforms

Flow waveforms graphically display the inspiratory and expiratory gas flow rate versus time during mechanical ventilation (see Figure 14-1). In the volume control mode of ventilation, the inspiratory flow rate or inspiratory time is set by the operator, depending on the manufacturer of the ventilator. For ventilators with an adjustable inspiratory flow rate control (e.g., Puritan Bennett 840, Puritan Bennett 980, Covidien), the set tidal volume, inspiratory flow rate, and ventilator flow waveform determine the inspiratory time (I-time). Generally, for adult patients the inspiratory flow rate is set between 40 and 80 L/min, which results in an I-time of about 0.80 to 1.0 second.

Selectable flow pattern options in the volume control mode vary depending on the ventilator manufacturer, but commonly include a square wave and descending ramp. In the volume control mode, increasing the inspiratory flow rate decreases I-time, and decreasing the inspiratory flow rate increases I-time. In this type of ventilator, a change from a square wave to a descending ramp increases I-time, and a change from a descending ramp to a square wave decreases I-time time (volume control mode). It should be noted that as inspiratory flow rate increases, the difference between PIP and plateau pressures also increases due to increased R_{aw}.

The pressure waveform developed is affected by the tidal volume, the inspiratory flow rate, and the inspiratory flow waveform. For example, a square wave flow pattern tends to result in a linear increase in pressure, whereas a decelerating (descending ramp) flow pattern tends to result in a more curvilinear pressure waveform. It should also be noted that when changing from a square wave to a descending ramp flow waveform, the inspiratory flow rate must be increased to maintain the same I-time.

With certain types of adult ventilators, the primary adjustable controls in the volume control mode are tidal volume, inspiratory time, and respiratory rate (e.g., Servo-s, MAQUET; Hamilton S1, Hamilton Medical AG, Dräger Evita, Dräger). These ventilators allow the operator to directly set the inspiratory time in the control mode, and I-time is maintained regardless of the tidal volume or flow waveform settings.

PSV and PCV Flow and Pressure Waveforms

As mentioned earlier, with PSV and PCV the inspiratory flow rate is variable and generally assumes a decelerating (descending) pattern (see Figure 14-3). With both PSV and PCV, inspiratory pressure rapidly increases to a preset value. Unlike volume control ventilation, an increase in R_{aw} or decrease in C_{rs} will not change PIP. With changes in C_{rs} or R_{aw}, inspiratory flow rate and tidal volume may vary in the PCV or PSV modes. For example, with increased R_{aw} more time is required for the pressure set on the ventilator to equilibrate with the lungs in the PCV mode. If the inspiratory flow does not reach zero and pressures between the ventilator and lungs do not equilibrate, than delivered tidal volume will decrease. Airway secretions are common causes of increased R_{aw} that may reduce tidal volume in the PSV or PCV modes. Airway

secretions or water in the circuit can sometimes be seen as small squiggly variations in the flow and/or pressure waveforms, especially upon exhalation (see **Figure 14-7**). Remember, however, that the increased R_{aw} or decreased C_{rs} will increase PIP during volume controlled ventilation.

Flow waveforms can be particularly helpful in determining when the pressure set on the ventilator has equilibrated in the lungs when using a pressure-limited, time-cycled mode (e.g., PCV). Inspection of the waveform can then be used to set I-time during a PCV breath. If inspiratory flow on the flow waveform does not reach zero at the end of the inspiratory phase, I-time can be lengthened until it does. Increasing I-time in the PCV mode, and thus allowing pressures to equilibrate, will usually achieve a larger delivered tidal volume without increasing PIP (see **Figure 14-8**).

Air Trapping and Auto-PEEP

Flow waveforms are also useful in identifying air trapping and the presence of **auto-PEEP**. Auto-PEEP, also known as intrinsic or occult PEEP, is the pressure that results from gas trapped in the lungs when inspiration begins before expiration is complete. Auto-PEEP can be measured by using the ventilator controls to institute an *expiratory hold*. The patient must be passive during the hold, and the hold must last long enough to allow the gas trapped in the lung to equilibrate with the pressure transducer of the ventilator. This expiratory hold allows for measurement of **total-PEEP** (auto-PEEP + set PEEP). Auto-PEEP is calculated by subtracting set PEEP from total-PEEP. It can be seen on the expiratory side of a flow waveform when the expiratory flow of gas does not reach zero before inspiration begins (see **Figure 14-9**).

Air trapping results in auto-PEEP and is more likely to occur when I:E ratios are $\geq 1:1$. High respiratory rates in assisted modes with a set inspiratory time

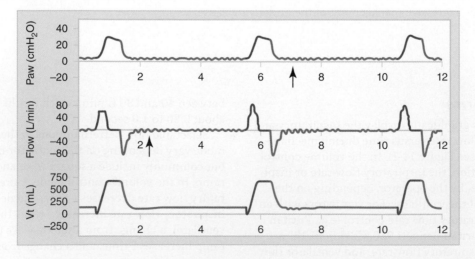

FIGURE 14-7 Pressure, flow, and volume versus time graphics during PCV: secretions. Note: These arrows are pointing to small squiggly variations in flow and/or pressure waveforms, indicating the presence of secretions and/or condensation in the system.

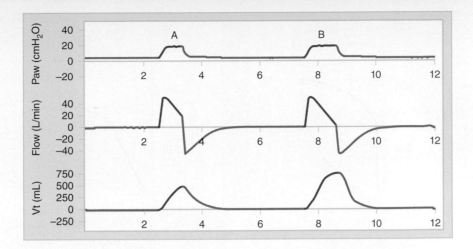

FIGURE 14-8 Pressure, flow, and volume versus time graphics during PCV: short inspiratory time. Note: In breath "A," inspiratory time is too short and flow is not reaching zero. Inspiratory time is longer in breath "B," allowing inspiratory flow to reach zero, resulting in a larger tidal volume.

can result in decreased expiratory time, an inverse I:E ratio, and the development of auto-PEEP. Patients with obstructive lung disease (e.g., COPD) may develop (or worsen) air trapping and auto-PEEP during mechanical ventilation if adequate time for exhalation is not provided. Auto-PEEP increases alveolar pressures and may increase the risk of barotrauma. Increased thoracic pressures due to auto-PEEP may cause hemodynamic compromise (e.g., increased pulmonary vascular resistance and decreased venous return, cardiac output, and blood pressure). Auto-PEEP can also make it more difficult for the patient to trigger a mechanical breath from the ventilator, and this may lead to dyssynchrony and increased WOB.

Auto-PEEP can sometimes be eliminated or reduced by adjusting the ventilator controls to increase E-time. If auto-PEEP cannot be eliminated by increasing E-time, the clinician can increase the set PEEP level to just below the auto-PEEP value in an attempt to improve ease of ventilator triggering and reduce WOB. Besides shortening I-time or adding PEEP, the clinician can attempt to increase total cycle time by changing to SIMV mode and decreasing the set SIMV rate. Another option if the patient is tachypneic due to pain and/or anxiety is to administer analgesics and/or sedation to make the patient more comfortable.

Pressure–Volume Curves

Pressure–volume curves, sometimes referred to as *pressure–volume loops,* can be used to assess several aspects of patient–ventilator interaction. Typically, pressure values are depicted on the *x*-axis and volume values are depicted on the *y*-axis of a pressure–volume curve. The larger the swing to the left (negative) side of the pressure axis before triggering the ventilator, the greater the patient effort and the greater the imposed WOB.

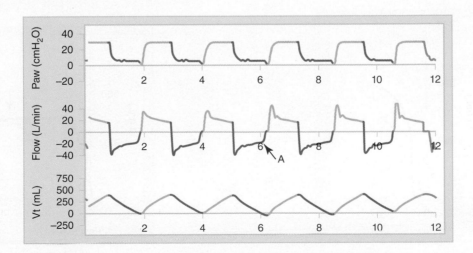

FIGURE 14-9 Pressure, flow, and volume versus time graphics during PCV: air trapping. Note: Arrow A identifies air trapping because inspiration is beginning before expiration is complete. The patient's high respiratory rate on an assisted mode with a set inspiratory time is resulting in the air trapping.

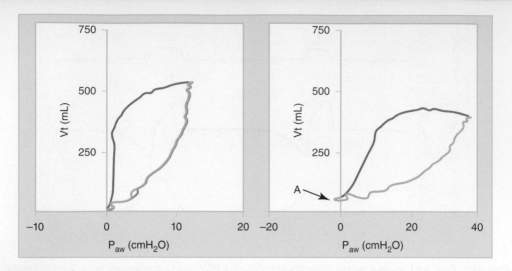

FIGURE 14-10   Pressure-volume loop during an assisted mechanical breath. Note: The left loop depicts flow triggering while the right loop depicts pressure triggering. Arrow A is identifying the additional imposed WOB created by pressure triggering in this patient.

Setting the ventilator's trigger (i.e., sensitivity) such that the patient can trigger the ventilator with minimal effort without autotriggering will lessen the imposed WOB (see **Figure 14-10**). If the graphic pressure tracing stays left of the baseline (i.e., negative) after inspiration has begun, inspiratory flow is probably set too low. If the patient's inspiratory demand exceeds the inspiratory flow provided by the ventilator, WOB will increase. The resulting patient–ventilator dyssynchrony may result in patient discomfort, and the patient may begin "fighting the ventilator." Inadequate inspiratory gas flow provided by the ventilator can be identified using a pressure–volume curve and observing the classic sign of a figure eight (8), as shown in **Figure 14-11**. The "live" breath-by-breath pressure–volume tracing generated during a mechanical breath should move in a counterclockwise fashion with a slight curvilinear shape similar to a football. Inadequate inspiratory flows in the face

of increased patient effort will cause the inspiratory limb of the curve to be deflected to the left (i.e., inward), and WOB will increase. Increased R_{aw} will cause the inspiratory limb of the curve to be deflected to the right (i.e., bowed outward). Changes in C_{rs} will cause changes the slope of the pressure–volume curve. Increased compliance shifts the pressure–volume curve up and to the left (i.e., towards the vertical y-axis), whereas reduced compliance shifts the pressure–volume curve down and to the right (i.e., towards the horizontal x-axis). If the pressure–volume curve flattens horizontally at the end of the inspiratory portion of the breath cycle, then alveolar overdistension is likely (see **Figure 14-12**). A strong patient inspiratory effort can create a similar pattern that should not be confused with overdistension. Alveolar overdistension can result in barotrauma, and ventilator settings should be adjusted to avoid ventilator-associated lung injury (VALI).

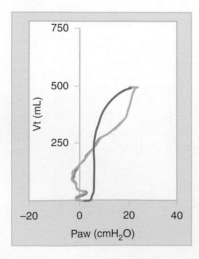

FIGURE 14-11   Pressure-volume loop during VCV: low flow. Note: This loop is a classic "figure eight" sign depicting an inadequately set inspiratory flow.

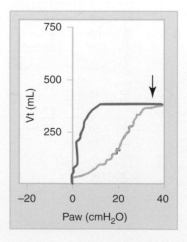

FIGURE 14-12   Pressure-volume loop during VCV: overdistension. Note: The arrow identifies the alveolar overdistension.

Pressure–Volume Curves and PEEP

Static pressure–volume curves have been suggested to determine the best PEEP and tidal volume. The lower inflection point (LIP) is the point where the inspiratory pressure–volume curve stops moving horizontally and starts to move more vertically. Setting PEEP just above the LIP (e.g., LIP pressure +2 cm H_2O) is probably a good place to begin when seeking the best PEEP needed for alveolar stability and highest compliance. The upper inflection point (UIP) of the pressure–volume curve is the point at which the curve begins to flatten, or "beak." The UIP is thought to represent the point at which compliance begins to decrease significantly due to over-distension of the lung. Static pressure volume–curves, however, are difficult and time consuming to obtain and are generally not used in the ICU for those reasons. A slow flow, pressure–volume curve provides an alternative, which may allow identification of the best PEEP and selection of appropriate tidal volume in the ICU. A slow-flow pressure–volume curve (flow < 10 L/min) in the apneic patient can be used to identify the LIP on the pressure–volume curve as a guide to setting PEEP. The UIP can also be identified on a slow-flow pressure-volume curve. Ventilator parameters might then be adjusted to ensure ventilation is between the LIP and UIP in an attempt to avoid ventilator-associated lung injury.

Flow-Volume Loops

Observation of graphically displayed flow-volume loops during mechanical ventilation can be useful to identify obstruction, response to a bronchodilator, and airway leaks. Not unlike a flow-volume loop obtained in the PFT laboratory, flow-volume loops obtained during mechanical ventilation allow the clinician to identify peak inspiratory flow (PIF), peak expiratory flow (PEF), and associated volumes. An obstructive disorder can be identified by observing a reduction in expiratory gas flow rates on the flow-volume loop. In a similar fashion, the response to administration of a bronchodilator can be assessed. If there is an improvement in expiratory gas flow on the flow-volume loop following bronchodilator administration, a positive response is likely. Flow-volume loops can also be useful to identify endotracheal tube or airway leaks. In these cases, the inspiratory volume will be clearly greater than the expiratory volume, as displayed on the flow-volume loop.

Monitoring the Patient Airway

Invasive mechanical ventilation requires the placement of an endotracheal or tracheostomy tube, and an important aspect of monitoring and assessment is related to the artificial airway. Once placed, the respiratory care clinician must ensure that the artificial airway is in proper position and does not move or become dislodged from its confirmed location. Proper placement of an endotracheal tube (ETT) should be confirmed by the clinician performing the intubation. The clinician should directly observe the passage of the ETT through the vocal cords. The position of the ETT within the trachea is then verified by auscultation, capnometry, and observation of condensation in the airway. The right and left side of the chest should be auscultated to ensure that bilateral breath sounds are present. If the ETT has been advanced too far into the airway, right-side bronchial intubation may occur. In this case, breath sounds are typically present on the right side of the chest and absent (or very diminished) on the left. The stomach should also be auscultated while ventilating the patient with a manual resuscitator bag to ensure that esophageal intubation has not occurred; no sounds of air movement should be present over the stomach. The distance from the gingiva or teeth to the carina is approximately 21 cm for an adult female and 23 cm for an adult male, although this will vary greatly in different patients based on their height, size, and neck characteristics.[9,10] Proper depth of an ETT should be confirmed via a chest x-ray. It is important that the tip of the ETT be several centimeters above the carina. If the ETT is too deep, it may extend into the right bronchus, resulting in absent ventilation on the left and development of left-sided atelectasis. Flexion and/or rotation of the neck can cause the ETT to advance as much as 2 cm further into an adult patient's airway.[11,12] Even without bronchial intubation, if the ETT is too close to the carina, left-sided atelectasis may occur due to uneven airflow distribution between right and left lungs caused by the angles of the bronchi. For these reasons it is recommended that the tip of the ETT be placed 3 to 5 cm above the carina.

Visualization of the carina on the chest x-ray can be difficult for a number of reasons (e.g., infiltrates, poor-quality image). When it is difficult to visualize the carina on chest x-ray, it is sometimes helpful to ensure that the tip of the ETT is below the level of the clavicles on x-ray. This assumes a properly positioned patient and x-ray machine (the machine must be perpendicular to the patient's chest when the image is obtained). In the acute care setting patients are often rotated in the bed, causing the clavicles to appear higher or lower than their true position. Another thoracic landmark that may be helpful is the superior aspect of the aortic arch. This landmark is typically located about 3 to 5 cm above the carina, and positioning the tip of the ETT at the same level should be acceptable. The superior aspect of the aortic arch can also be difficult to identify on some x-rays. Endotracheal tubes have centimeter markings along their length, and this allows the depth of the tube at the level of the front teeth or gum line to be noted at the time of the postintubation chest x-ray. The ETT is then monitored for proper position at least every 12-hour shift.

Once proper ETT position is established, it is important to ensure that the ETT is stable and does not move, resulting in accidental extubation or inadvertent bronchial intubation. There are a number of devices on the market that can be used to secure an ETT instead of traditional tape. Ventilator circuits can become heavy due to condensation from humidity or secretions accumulating in the circuit. For this reason it is recommended that the ventilator circuit be positioned and supported in such a way to avoid any traction on the artificial airway, especially if the artificial airway is a new tracheostomy. The patient's skin around a new tracheostomy can be very sensitive and painful. Dislodgement of the tracheostomy tube can be catastrophic if the tube is accidentally pulled out and the stoma closes.

Airway cuff pressures should be checked every shift and maintained between 20 to 25 cm H_2O. This pressure is high enough to seal the airway for most patients and lessen the risk of aspiration of secretions. Maintaining cuff pressures at this pressure is usually part of the hospital's ventilator protocol to prevent ventilator-associated pneumonia (VAP). Maintaining pressures greater than 25 cm H_2O can cause tracheal tissue ischemia. Ischemia occurs if the cuff pressure against the tracheal mucosa exceeds the mucosal capillary blood pressure. Tracheal mucosal ischemia can result in airway-associated complications such as tracheal stenosis, tracheal malacia, and tracheal esophageal fistula. Occasionally, small airways (≤ 7.0 mm ID) are placed in larger adults. This can result in a situation where the artificial airway cuff cannot seal unless the cuff pressure is > 25 cm H_2O. In these cases, the lowest cuff pressure that results in a seal at the end of inspiration from a mechanical breath should be used.

RC Insights

It is recommended that the endotracheal tube tip be positioned 3 to 5 cm above the carina.

Noninvasive Monitoring

Noninvasive monitoring is an integral part of the care and monitoring of patients in the critical care setting. Advancements in technology and software have made it possible to monitor patients' status with less invasive testing. Noninvasive monitoring techniques are now available that allow for automated notification of healthcare professionals via computer tablets or cell phones when monitored parameters stray outside of the desired range. This technology should be used to improve patient outcomes by allowing quicker decision making.

Pulse Oximetry

Use of **pulse oximetry** to measure oxygenation has become a common part of critically ill patients'

assessment. Oximetry equipment allows for the noninvasive measurement of hemoglobin's oxygen saturation in the arterial blood. Many pulse oximeters also display heart rate and pulsatile waveform. Measurement of oxygen saturation using pulse oximetry (SpO_2) is considered an important vital sign in the acute care setting.[13,14] When reviewing SpO_2 values, it is important to remember that other factors affect the patient's overall oxygenation (e.g., hemoglobin level, cardiac output, tissue perfusion). It is important to assess the patient's general appearance, color, heart rate, respiratory rate, mental status, perfusion, and history when making decisions concerning oxygen needs. Hemoglobin has the capacity to bind with other molecules than oxygen (e.g., carbon monoxide [CO]), and many pulse oximeters are inaccurate in certain situations (e.g., carbon monoxide poisoning).

Based on the spectrophotometric principle of light absorption described in the Beer-Lambert law, pulse oximeters emit two different wavelengths of light through blood-filled capillary beds.[15] Red light emitted at 660 nm is highly absorbed by deoxygenated hemoglobin (deoxyhemoglobin) and barely absorbed by oxygenated hemoglobin (oxyhemoglobin). Emitted near-infrared light at 940 nm, in contrast, is highly absorbed by oxyhemoglobin and barely absorbed by deoxyhemoglobin. A photodiode sensor on the opposite side of the capillary bed measures the remaining unabsorbed light. The difference between the transmitted light and remaining unabsorbed light is used to determine the amount of oxygen bound to hemoglobin and is immediately displayed as a percentage to the clinician.[15,16] In addition to oxygen saturation, heart rate, based on the pulsatile differences in the remaining unabsorbed light, is computed and displayed.[17]

In order for this principle to work accurately and efficiently, the pulse oximeter probe must be properly placed. **Table 14-1** lists factors that may cause inaccurate pulse oximetry values.[16] When placed on the fingers or toes, movement or lack of perfusion may cause inaccuracies to occur. In some cases, removal of fingernail polish (especially in the case of black polish) may be necessary to obtain an accurate reading. To combat inaccuracies, pulse oximeter companies have redesigned their probes so they can be placed on different areas of the body. The forehead, ears, nose, and neck are now commonly used as sites for SpO_2 measurement to try to overcome shortcomings involving ambient light, skin/nail pigmentation, and motion artifact.[18]

Once the oximeter probe is correctly in place, proper interpretation of the displayed values is essential. Normal ranges for saturation and heart rate vary depending on the patient population. Although the normal range of SpO_2 tends to differ from patient to patient (based on age and cardiopulmonary status), an SpO_2 reading of 95% to 97% or greater is generally considered normal, though this will vary with the patient's age and

TABLE 14-1
Causes and Mechanisms of Unreliable Spo_2 Readings

1. Causes of intermittent drop-outs or inability to read Spo_2
   a. Poor perfusion due to a number of causes (e.g., hypovolemia, vasoconstriction)
2. Causes of falsely normal or elevated Spo_2
   a. Carbon monoxide poisoning
   b. Sickle cell anemia vaso-occlusive crises (overestimation of FO_2Hb and underestimation of Sao_2)
3. Causes of falsely low Spo_2
   a. Venous pulsations
   b. Excessive movement
   c. Intravenous pigmented dyes
   d. Inherited forms of abnormal hemoglobin
   e. Fingernail polish (some colors)
   f. Severe anemia (with concomitant hypoxemia)
4. Causes of falsely low or high Spo_2
   a. Methemoglobinemia
   b. Sulfhemoglobinemia
   c. Poor probe positioning
   d. Sepsis and septic shock
5. Causes of falsely low FO_2Hb as measured by a co-oximeter
   a. Severe hyperbilirubinemia
   b. Fetal Hb (HbF)

Reprinted from *Respiratory Medicine*, 107(6), Chan ED, Chan MM, Chan MM, Pulse oximetry: Understanding its basic principles facilitates appreciation of its limitations, pages 789–799, Copyright 2013, with permission from Elsevier.

elevation. For example, patients in Denver, Colorado, would be expected to have a lower Spo_2 value due to altitude. We would usually become concerned if Spo_2 dropped below 92% or less than 88% in chronic lung disease patients (e.g., COPD).

Today, some pulse oximeters include co-oximetry capabilities and can measure other types of hemoglobin, such as carboxyhemoglobin (COHb), methemoglobin (metHb), and total hemoglobin (tHb) in the blood.[16] Other newer measurements now available include acoustic respiration rate (RRa), oxygen content (SpOC), pleth variability index (PVI), perfusion index (PI), and patient state index (PSI). Although the efficacy of these alternative types of oximetry are not yet proven, values and percentages can be used to trend, monitor, and analyze disease progression.[19] Chapter 8 provides additional detail regarding pulse oximetry.

RC Insights

An Spo_2 reading of 95% to 97% or greater is considered normal. Become concerned if the Spo_2 drops below 90% to 92% (or < 88% in chronic lung disease patients).

Capnography

End-tidal carbon dioxide ($ETCO_2$ or $PETCO_2$) reflects the CO_2 that is exhaled from the alveolar units, and $PETCO_2$ should approximate alveolar CO_2 tension (i.e.,

$P_ACO_2 = PETCO_2$). $ETCO_2$ is affected by ventilation, physiologic dead space, lung perfusion, and metabolism. Continuous, noninvasive measurement of $ETCO_2$ has become increasingly popular in the intensive care setting. **Capnometry** is defined as detecting the presence or absence of CO_2 exhaled during a normal respiratory cycle. Capnography, on the other hand, refers to a graphical depiction of PCO_2 values plotted against time and allows for the measurement of $ETCO_2$. $ETCO_2$ represents the partial pressure level of CO_2 at the end of expiration (i.e., $PETCO_2$). A normal exhaled CO_2 tracing consists of three parts, or phases: (1) a period of dead space emptying with no CO_2, (2) an abrupt rise in CO_2 as terminal airways and alveoli begin to empty, and (3) an alveolar plateau that ends in an $ETCO_2$ measurement (see **Figure 14-13**). In normal patients, $ETCO_2$ is generally within 2 to 5 mm Hg of the actual $Paco_2$. Thus, in the absence of pathology $Paco_2$ and $ETCO_2$ should be approximately the same. The difference between $ETCO_2$ and $Paco_2$ is sometimes referred to as the $ETCO_2$–$Paco_2$ gradient. This gradient ranges from an average of only about 0.3 mm Hg in patients with low V_D/V_T to an average of 18 mm Hg in patients with high V_D/V_T. Thus, $ETCO_2$ appears to be a useful indicator of $Paco_2$, even in patients with significant lung disease, provided that the expected increase in the $ETCO_2$–$Paco_2$ gradient is taken into consideration. Deviations from the normal capnographic tracing may also be useful to identify airway obstruction (see **Figure 14-14**), rapid shallow breathing, ventilation–perfusion mismatch, inadequacy of cardiopulmonary resuscitation efforts, or a large air leak. Measurement of $ETCO_2$ during cardiopulmonary resuscitation (CPR) may be helpful in assessing chest compressions; $ETCO_2$ of 10 to 20 mm Hg suggests compressions are effective, < 10 mm Hg suggests that compressions need improvement. With the return of spontaneous circulation (ROSC), $ETCO_2$ will increase significantly (e.g. $ETCO_2$

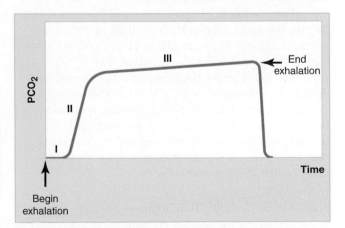

FIGURE 14-13 Capnogram. Phase I, dead space emptying with no CO_2; Phase II, an abrupt rise in CO_2 as anatomic dead space changes and terminal airways and alveoli begin emptying; and Phase III, an alveolar plateau that ends in an $ETCO_2$ measurement.

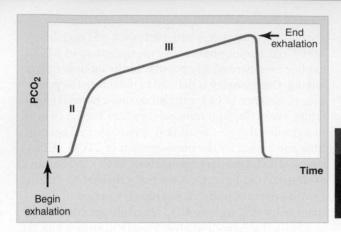

FIGURE 14-14 Capnogram produced with airflow obstruction.

of 35-45 mm Hg) as blood flow to the lungs improves. **Box 14-1** lists some common causes of changes in $ETCO_2$.

As a stand-alone substitute for measuring $Paco_2$, $ETCO_2$ is considered to be inadequate.[20] Nevertheless, with the advent of faster and smaller microprocessors, the use of capnography in conjunction with other respiratory parameters can help to provide an assessment of changes in patients' cardiopulmonary status. Capnography should be used to identify trends and suggest the need for further investigation. Capnography provides a measure of cardiopulmonary status on a breath-by-breath basis. This has led to an increase in usage by paramedics and emergency departments to predict impending respiratory failure, as well as measure the effectiveness of cardiopulmonary resuscitation (CPR) efforts.[21–23]

Use of capnography also allows for calculation of the ratio of dead space to tidal volume (V_D/V_T). It is calculated by subtracting mean exhaled CO_2 ($P\bar{E}co_2$) from $Paco_2$ and dividing the difference by $Paco_2$ ($V_D/V_T = (Paco_2 - P\bar{E}co_2)/Paco_2$). A normal $P\bar{E}co_2$ is about 28 mm Hg, and a normal V_D/V_T is 0.30, or 30%. The normal range for V_D/V_T is 20% to 40%. V_D/V_T is slightly higher during mechanical ventilation. The V_D/V_T ratio multiplied by the tidal volume is the physiologic dead space volume ($V_D = V_T \times V_D/V_T$). This volume is excluded from the calculation of alveolar ventilation because it does not participate in gas exchange. An increase in physiologic dead space and V_D/V_T means that an increase in minute volume will be required in order to maintain a normal $Paco_2$.

Transcutaneous Monitoring

Transcutaneous monitoring (TCM) is another noninvasive assessment that is used in critically ill patients to monitor ventilation and oxygen. TCM is thought to provide an estimate of what is occurring at the tissue level in terms of gas exchange and tissue perfusion.

TCM devices use modified blood gas electrodes for monitoring of oxygenation and ventilation. Compared to pulse oximetry and capnometry, these devices are better correlated with actual $Paco_2$ and Pao_2.[24]

BOX 14-1

End-Tidal Carbon Dioxide Measurement

The partial pressure of end-tidal carbon dioxide ($Petco_2$) generally reflects alveolar carbon dioxide (P_Aco_2) levels.

$Petco_2$ will generally increase with:
- Decreased alveolar ventilation (decreased $\dot{V}_A$) due to:
  - Decreased tidal volume
  - Decreased respiratory rate
  - Decreased minute volume
- Increased CO_2 production (increased $\dot{V}co_2$) due to:
  - Agitation
  - Shivering
  - Pain
  - Anxiety
  - Recovery from sedation
  - Fighting the ventilator

$Petco_2$ will generally decrease with:
- Increased alveolar ventilation due to:
  - Increased tidal volume
  - Increased respiratory rate
  - Increased minute volume
- Very small tidal volumes approaching dead space volumes
- Rapid, shallow breathing
- Decreased CO_2 production (decreased $\dot{V}co_2$)
  - Sleep
  - Cooling
  - Relaxation
- Decreased lung perfusion
  - Decreased cardiac output
  - Pulmonary embolus

$Petco_2$ may be absent with:
- Apnea
- Cardiac arrest
- Complete airway obstruction
- Ventilator disconnect
- Ventilator malfunction

Data from: Wilkins RL, Stroller JK, Kacmarek RM. *Egan's Fundamentals of Respiratory Care.* St. Louis, MO: Mosby; 2009: 1115–1152.

Transcutaneous P_{O_2}

Use of transcutaneous monitoring of oxygen partial pressure (Ptc_{O_2}) was first described in 1971 by Eberhard et al. and Huch et al.[25] Modified blood gas sensors monitor the capillary P_{O_2} through the skin by heating the tissue to a minimum of 41° C, melting the lipid layer, and altering the stratum corneum. This heating causes hyperemia and increases the skin permeability, greatly enhancing the oxygen diffusion speed between the tissues and the sensor at the skin surface. The measured skin P_{O_2} level is then adjusted to account for increased metabolism and oxygen consumption at the sensor site. As the skin temperature is raised, oxygen diffusion from the capillary bed increases, improving correlation between the measured Ptc_{O_2} and arterial Pa_{O_2}.[25]

Today, most transcutaneous O_2 sensors are heated to 42° to 45° C, with a recommended accuracy-based temperature of 44° C. Unfortunately, the increased temperatures may cause thermal injuries such as skin blisters, burns, erythema, or skin tears. Thus, these sensors must be repositioned intermittently based on the patient's skin sensitivity and thickness.[26]

Fluctuations in cardiac output and increased peripheral resistance can significantly affect the accuracy of TCM and may serve as an indicator of poor tissue perfusion. Following trends and taking multiple factors into account is important when using TCM. Tissue edema, for instance, can greatly increase the oxygen diffusion distance, causing Ptc_{O_2} to falsely underrepresent arterial Pa_{O_2}. Thus, TCM does not provide a replacement for the invasive measurement of Pa_{O_2} levels in critically ill patients.[27]

Transcutaneous CO_2

Transcutaneous monitoring of CO_2 pressure (Ptc_{CO_2}) was discovered shortly before its P_{O_2} monitoring counterpart. In 1960, Severinghaus first described the use of a "specially designed temperature-stabilized tissue P_{CO_2} electrode" to detect P_{CO_2} on slightly blanched skin. By 1969, Johns et al. had determined that the P_{CO_2} detected with these specialized electrodes correlated with blood Pa_{CO_2} within the range of 20 to 70 mm Hg. By the late 1970s, Ptc_{CO_2} had become common in many neonatal ICUs for estimating blood Pa_{CO_2}.[25]

Similar to Ptc_{O_2} monitoring, heating of the skin electrodes greatly increases Ptc_{CO_2} correlation with Pa_{CO_2}. Although sensor probe temperatures as low as 37° C have been reported to have good correlation with Pa_{CO_2} levels, a temperature of 42° C is currently recommended by most manufacturers. Similarly, increased temperatures may cause thermal injuries if the electrode sites are not changed every few hours. Today, Ptc_{CO_2} electrodes are combined with Ptc_{O_2} monitors, and their use is growing in popularity in the pediatric and adult acute care setting.[25,28]

Exhaled Nitric Oxide

Nitric oxide (NO) is another exhaled respiratory gas that is measured noninvasively to detect airway inflammation. Since its discovery in 1987, the fraction of **exhaled nitric oxide (FeNO)** has been studied to better understand its correlation with respiratory disease and associated inflammation. Initially named as the endothelium-derived relaxing factor (EDRF), it was quickly discovered to be the smallest and lightest systemic biological messenger in mammals. In lung physiology, epithelium-derived relaxing factor (EpDRF) was similarly confirmed to be NO. It plays an extensive role in cardiovascular, neurologic, immune, and metabolic disease. Today, NO is monitored in the clinical environment to determine disease severity and progression.[29]

Although monitoring of FeNO has become more common, interpretation of the results obtained is not as clearly defined. Because every human body is different in NO production, defining a normal level of exhaled NO is difficult. However, based on large population sampling and expert opinion, the American Thoracic Society (ATS) was able to create a few guidelines with some recommendations and boundaries for FeNO value interpretation. **Table 14-2** lists the causes of low FeNO (values < 25 parts per billion [ppb] for adults and < 20 ppb for children). Although a low FeNO value can be obtained when noneosinophilic airway inflammation is present, this lower limit is generally considered to be consistent with little or no airway inflammation. FeNO values are considered high when they are greater than 50 ppb for adults and greater than 30 ppb for children. They are considered to be acutely rising when they vary more than 40% from a predetermined baseline. These criteria are being reassessed in various patient populations. For example, FeNO values in pregnant asthmatics are higher than healthy, pregnant non-asthmatics. **Table 14-3** lists causes of higher FeNO values. Very high FeNO values are associated with deteriorating or uncontrolled eosinophilic airway inflammation. With these predetermined boundaries of maximal and minimal acceptable levels of FeNO, the general outline proposed in **Table 14-4** can be followed to interpret FeNO levels.[30]

During the expiratory phase of a normal respiratory cycle, extensive NO monitoring has made it possible to determine the predominant site of increased FeNO within the lungs. Chemiluminescence analyzers,

---

RC Insights

FeNO values are considered high when they are > 50 ppb for adults, > 30 ppb for children, or acutely rising (more than 40% from a predetermined baseline). These values imply deteriorating or uncontrolled eosinophilic airway inflammation.

TABLE 14-2
Diagnosis and Monitoring of Low FeNO (FeNO < 25 ppb in adults, FeNO < 20 ppb in children)

Diagnosis

- In a symptomatic patient (chronic cough, wheeze, and/or shortness of breath for 6 weeks) presenting for the first time will be unlikely to benefit from inhaled corticosteroids. Possible etiologies include:
  - Pulmonary/airway causes
    - Rhinosinusitis
    - Noneosinophilic asthma
    - Reactive airways dysfunction syndrome
    - COPD
    - Bronchiectasis
    - Cystic fibrosis, primary ciliary dyskinesia
    - Postviral bronchial hyperresponsiveness syndrome
    - Vocal cord dysfunction
  - Nonpulmonary causes
    - Anxiety, hyperventilation
    - Gastroesophageal reflux disease
    - Cardiac disease/pulmonary hypertension/pulmonary embolism
  - Confounding factors
    - Smoking
    - Obesity

Monitoring

- In a symptomatic patient with an established diagnosis of asthma, possible etiologies include:
  - Asthma
    - Noneosinophilic asthma (probably steroid unresponsive)
  - Additional or alternative diagnosis
    - Vocal cord dysfunction
    - Anxiety, hyperventilation
    - Bronchiectasis
    - Cardiac disease
    - Rhinosinusitis
    - Gastroesophageal reflux disease
- In an asymptomatic patient with an established diagnosis of asthma:
  - Implies adequate dosing and good adherence to anti-inflammatory therapy.
  - Inhaled corticosteroid dose may possibly be reduced (repeat FeNO weeks later to confirm this judgment; if it remains low, then relapse is unlikely).

Reprinted with permission of the American Thoracic Society. Copyright © 2014 American Thoracic Society. Dweik RA, Boggs PB, Erzurum SC, Irvin CG, Leigh MW, Lundberg JO, et al. 2011. An Official ATS Clinical Practice Guideline: Interpretation of Exhaled Nitric Oxide Levels (FeNO) for Clinical Applications. *American Journal of Respiratory and Critical Care Medicine* 184(5):602–615, Table 3. Official Journal of the American Thoracic Society.

TABLE 14-3
Diagnosis and Monitoring of Elevated FeNO (FeNO > 50 ppb in adults, FeNO > 35 ppb in children) or Rising FeNO (FeNO > 40% change from previously stable levels)*

Diagnosis

- In a symptomatic patient (chronic cough and/or wheeze and/or shortness of breath during past 6 weeks) presenting for the first time, possible etiologies include:
  - Atopic asthma
  - Eosinophilic bronchitis
  - COPD with mixed inflammatory phenotype
  - Trial of inhaled corticosteroid treatment may be beneficial

Monitoring

- In a symptomatic patient with asthma, possible etiologies include:
  - High persistent allergen exposure
  - Issues with inhaled corticosteroid delivery
    - Poor medication adherence
    - Incorrect inhaler technique
    - Limited drug deposition
  - Insufficient dose of inhaled corticosteroid:
    - Likely to respond to increased inhaled or oral corticosteroid
  - Rarely, truly steroid-resistant asthma (FeNO will remain high after a trial of systemic steroid)
  - Rarely, Churg-Strauss syndrome, pulmonary eosinophilia
- In an asymptomatic patient:
  - No change in the dose of inhaled corticosteroid dosing (refer to patient's FeNO trend over time)
  - Withdrawing inhaled corticosteroid may result in a relapse
  - An increase in therapy is still indicated in some patients and may be a risk factor for an exacerbation
  - Elevated FeNO may be normal in some patients

* Values are likely to change as additional studies are completed.
Reprinted with permission of the American Thoracic Society. Copyright © 2014 American Thoracic Society. Dweik RA, Boggs PB, Erzurum SC, Irvin CG, Leigh MW, Lundberg JO, et al. 2011. An Official ATS Clinical Practice Guideline: Interpretation of Exhaled Nitric Oxide Levels (FeNO) for Clinical Applications. *American Journal of Respiratory and Critical Care Medicine* 184(5):602–615, Table 4. Official Journal of the American Thoracic Society.

such as Aerocrine's NIOX, measure the levels of NO exhaled at a constant flow rate of about 50 L/m. With a near-constant flow rate, acute changes in measured NO during exhalation can then be correlated with specific regions of the lung, which may contain signs of eosinophilic/noneosinophilic inflammation. Advances in newer, more portable devices, such as Aerocrine's NIOX-MINO and the NOBreath by Bedfont Scientific Ltd., have made the ability to trend and monitor FeNO in the primary care setting a reality.[31–33]

Cardiac Monitoring

Monitoring of the cardiovascular system is another major part of critical care monitoring. The heart plays a vital role in gas exchange, transport of essential elements, and waste removal for all organs within the body; therefore, careful and ongoing monitoring is essential in critically ill patients. Due to its importance, many invasive and noninvasive devices exist to monitor the heart as well as alert healthcare providers when an intervention may be needed.

Electrocardiography Monitoring and Analysis

In the ICU, noninvasive telemetry and pulse oximetry are often used as stand-alone tools to monitor heart rate, cardiac rhythm, and SpO_2. Generally, a continuous two-lead or six-lead ECG rhythm "strip" is graphically displayed on the monitor providing the necessary

TABLE 14-4
General Outline for FeNO Interpretation

Diagnosis
- Symptoms (cough and/or wheeze and/or shortness of breath) present during past 6 or more weeks
  - FeNO < 25 ppb (< 20 ppb in children)
    - Eosinophilic airway inflammation unlikely
    - Alternative diagnoses
    - Unlikely to benefit from inhaled corticosteroids
  - FeNO 25 to 50 ppb (20 to 35 ppb in children)
    - Be cautious
    - Evaluate clinical context
    - Monitor change in FeNO over time
  - FeNO > 50 ppb (> 35 ppb in children)
    - Eosinophilic airway inflammation present
    - Likely to benefit from inhaled corticosteroids

Monitoring (in patients with diagnosed asthma)
- Symptoms present
  - FeNO < 25 ppb (< 20 ppb in children)
    - Possible alternative diagnoses
    - Unlikely to benefit from increase in inhaled corticosteroids
  - FeNO 25 to 50 ppb (20 to 35 ppb in children)
    - Persistent exposure to allergens
    - Inadequate inhaled corticosteroid dose
    - Poor adherence
    - Steroid resistance
  - FeNO > 50 ppb (> 35 ppb in children)
    - Persistent exposure to allergens
    - Poor medication adherence or improper inhaler technique
    - Inadequate inhaled corticosteroid dose
    - Risk for exacerbation
    - Steroid resistance
- Symptoms absent
  - FeNO < 25 ppb (< 20 ppb in children)
    - Adequate inhaled corticosteroid dose
    - Good adherence
    - Inhaled corticosteroid taper
  - FeNO 25 to 50 ppb (20 to 35 ppb in children)
    - Adequate inhaled corticosteroid dosing
    - Good adherence
    - Monitor for change in FeNO
  - FeNO > 50 ppb (> 35 ppb in children)
    - Inhaled corticosteroid withdrawal or dose reduction may result in relapse
    - Poor adherence to inhaler technique

Data from: Dweik RA, Boggs PB, Erzurum SC, et al. An official ATS clinical practice guideline: interpretation of exhaled nitric oxide levels (FeNO) for clinical applications. *Am J Respir Crit Care Med.* 2011;184(5):602–615.

information needed for monitoring critically ill patients. Monitoring lead placement on the chest allows for some patient mobility and comfort. Additionally, automated external defibrillator (AED) analysis can be started earlier during CPR with as few as two leads placed on the chest.[23,34]

For routine monitoring, ECG leads are placed on the upper right arm, upper left arm, and lower chest or abdomen. With this configuration most telemetry systems can provide basic monitoring to the bedside clinician of heart rate and rhythm. In some cases, the detail provided by general telemetry and pulse oximetry may not be enough.[34,35] Six-lead monitoring allows continuous monitoring for the development of ST segment depression, which can be valuable in detecting silent myocardial ischemia in critically ill patients. Although 2-lead or 6-lead telemetry can provide enough information to predict the need for an intervention, a complete 12-lead ECG is often necessary to provide supplemental information regarding the heart's conducting system. The 12-lead ECG provides 12 perspectives of the heart, which can help locate the cause of an irregular heart rate or rhythm. With 12 leads, defects in the heart's electrical conducting system can be identified by specific anatomic location, allowing for advanced, targeted treatment strategies.[34,36]

Once the ECG has been generated, it is vital that the bedside clinician can easily visually recognize an irregular heart rate or rhythm and decide on a course of action.[37] Some patients may have an abnormal rhythm and remain asymptomatic, whereas other patients begin to exhibit symptoms of cardiovascular compromise before it is visualized on the ECG. Thus, the bedside clinician's knowledge of the patient's baseline heart rate and rhythm as well as expertise in these basic abnormal rhythms can greatly improve intervention time, if indicated.[38] Chapter 10 provides additional detail regarding ECG monitoring, to include examples of common irregular rhythm strips.

Hemodynamic Monitoring

Understanding and monitoring hemodynamics are essential to managing patients with cardiopulmonary disorders. Hemodynamics is defined as the study of blood flow through the body.[39] **Figure 14-15** provides a brief overview of blood flow through the body. Assessing hemodynamics should be completed using a systematic approach. The blood moves from the right side of the heart through the lungs to the left side of heart and then out through the systemic system. If something prevents blood from moving forward, it will begin to increase the pressure behind this point. An example would be overdistending the lungs with excessive PEEP. High levels of PEEP increase pulmonary artery and right atrial pressure, which decreases venous return to the heart. Reduction of venous return to the right side of the heart can lead to jugulovenous distension (neck vein distension) and peripheral edema. If blood return to the left heart is significantly reduced, cardiac output may decline, resulting in decreased systemic blood pressure, especially in preload-dependent patients. To detect changes in hemodynamics it is important to compare measured values to normal ranges (see **Table 14-5**).

Arterial blood pressure can be measured noninvasively with a blood pressure cuff and stethoscope by auscultating for Korotkoff sounds as the pressure in the

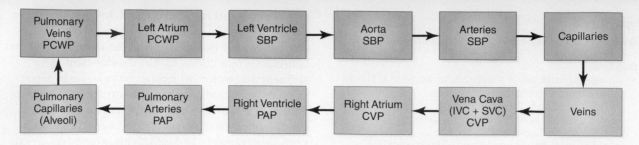

FIGURE 14-15 Hemodynamic cycle. CVP, central venous pressure; IVC, inferior vena cava; SVC, superior vena cava; PAP, pulmonary artery pressure; SBP, systemic blood pressure; PCWP, pulmonary capillary wedge pressure.

cuff is deflated. Limitations and complications of the noninvasive measurement of blood pressure include inaccuracies due to improperly sized cuffs, skin injury, and extremity ischemia.[40] Blood pressure can also be measured invasively with a fluid-filled arterial catheter connected to a pressurized transducer. Arterial lines are generally inserted in patients who are hyper- or

TABLE 14-5
Normal Values for Hemodynamic Measurements[1]

Variable	Units	Normal Range
Systolic blood pressure (SBP)	mm Hg	90–140
Diastolic blood pressure (DBP)	mm Hg	60–90
Mean arterial pressure (MAP)	mm Hg	80–100
Pulmonary artery systolic pressure (PASP)	mm Hg	20–35
Pulmonary artery diastolic pressure (PADP)	mm Hg	5–15
Mean pulmonary artery pressure (MPAP)	mm Hg	10–20
Right ventricular systolic pressure (RVSP)	mm Hg	15–30
Right ventricular end-diastolic pressure (RVEDP)	mm Hg	0–8
Central venous pressure (CVP)	mm Hg	4–8
Pulmonary artery wedge pressure (PAWP)	mm Hg	6–12 (< 18)
Cardiac output (CO)	L/min	4–8 (varies with size of patient)
Cardiac index (CI)	L/min/m²	2.5–4.0

[1.] Normal values are approximate and different sources list different ranges.

Data from: Critical Care Clinics 12 (4), Nelson LD, The new pulmonary artery catheters: right ventricular ejection fraction and continuous cardiac output, page 795, Copyright 1996.

hypotensive and who require frequent titration of vaso-active drugs. Limitations and complications to invasive measurement of blood pressure include inaccuracies when the transducer is not level with the heart, obstruction of the catheter, injury to the radial artery and nerve, bleeding, extremity ischemia, and increased risk of a bloodstream infections.[40] An arterial line produces an arterial pressure waveform with a peak representing systolic pressure followed by a dicrotic notch due to the closure of the aortic valve and ending at diastolic pressure (see **Figure 14-16**). Arterial lines overestimate the systolic pressure and underestimate the diastolic pressure, but are usually very accurate for monitoring the mean arterial pressure. It is important to monitor the appearance of the arterial waveform for damping, because this would indicate that values may be inaccurate. Arterial waveform damping appears as a narrowing and/or flattening of the waveform.

Central venous pressure (CVP) is measured through a line inserted via the external jugular or subclavian vein and advanced until the tip is in the superior vena cava. Besides monitoring CVP, this central venous line allows for venous blood sampling and fluid and medica-tion administration. Complications associated with a central venous line are related to insertion (bleeding, pneumothorax, nerve injury), catheter malposition (arrhythmias, tricuspid valve injury), and bloodstream infections.[40] Connecting the central line to a pressur-ized, fluid-filled transducer at the level of the heart allows CVP to be measured continuously. This setup will display CVP waveforms on the patient's cardiac monitor. A CVP waveform is composed of a, c, and v waves, which represent atrial systole, tricuspid valve closure, and ventricular contraction, respectively (see **Figure 14-17**). A properly placed central line will allow the CVP obtained to reflect right atrial pressures and intravascular volume status. Large "a waves" or "cannon a waves" occur with tricuspid stenosis or atrioventricu-lar dissociation because the atrium contracts against a narrow or closed tricuspid valve.[40] Likewise a large "v wave" may reflect tricuspid regurgitation.

A pulmonary artery catheter is placed when right ventricular; pulmonary artery systolic, diastolic, and

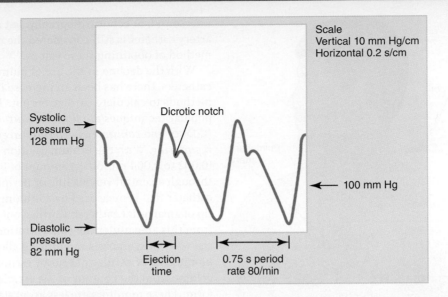

FIGURE 14-16 Arterial pressure waveform.

Courtesy of Hess DR, MacIntyre NR, Mishoe SC, Galvin WF, and Adams AB.

mean; and pulmonary capillary wedge pressures are needed. This catheter can also measure cardiac output via a thermistor located at its distal end. The catheter is placed either through the external jugular or left subclavian vein. The catheter is guided through the heart until it reaches the pulmonary artery and wedges (see **Figure 14-18**). As the pulmonary artery catheter floats through the right atrium, right ventricle, pulmonary artery, and ultimately wedges, it reflects the characteristic waveforms and pressures associated with these locations (see **Figure 14-19**). It is important that this catheter is placed in lung zone 3 where pulmonary artery and venous pressures are greater than the

alveolar pressures (see **Figure 14-20**). This placement will allow for the pulmonary capillary wedge pressure to be reflective of left atrial pressure.

Complications are similar to those associated with a central line and include bleeding, pneumothorax, nerve injury, catheter malposition, arrhythmias, valve injury, ventricular injury, pulmonary infarction, and bloodstream infections. Insertion of a pulmonary artery catheter is indicated to assess the degree of pulmonary hypertension, cardiomyopathy, valvular disease, or vascular volume and determine the type of shock.[40] Hemodynamic parameters can also be measured noninvasively using bioimpedance/bioreactance,

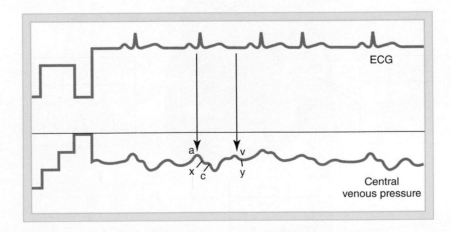

FIGURE 14-17 Central venous pressure waveform. The a wave is associated with atrial contraction. The x descent is the period following artial emptying before the tricuspid valve closes, c wave. The v wave reflects ventricular contraction followed by the y descent as the right ventricle begins to fill during diastole.

Courtesy of Hess DR, MacIntyre NR, Mishoe SC, Galvin WF, and Adams AB.

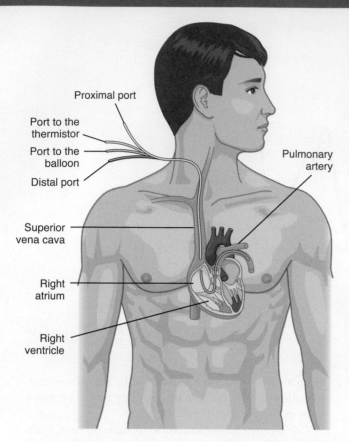

FIGURE 14-18 Pulmonary artery catheter. Pulmonary artery catheter and its associated ports are used to measure various pressures and cardiac output.

ultrasound, or echocardiography, but a pulmonary artery catheter is still considered the most accurate method of obtaining these values.[41,42]

With the decline in the use of pulmonary artery catheters, there has been an increase in less-invasive methods to calculate cardiac output. Two of the more popular techniques are *lithium dilution cardiac output* (LiDco) and *continuous arterial waveform analysis monitoring*. With the lithium dilution method, a small (0.002 to 0.004 mmol/kg) amount of lithium is injected through a central venous line or peripheral intravenous catheter that is measured by a lithium electrode on the tip of an arterial catheter. Cardiac output is calculated from this area under the concentration curve.[43] Arterial waveform analysis monitoring allows continuous monitoring of cardiac output by estimating the stroke volume from the contour of the arterial pressure waveform. These monitors are less accurate if the artery stiffens or arterial compliance decreases. Accuracy may be improved if periodically calibrated against LiDco.[43] Newer third-generation uncalibrated pulse contour analysis monitors have been shown to accurately report cardiac output changes based on changes in preload, but may lose accuracy when a vasoactive drug is used.[44]

Hemodynamic monitoring devices are generally designed to measure the different pressures at particular points within the body. **Table 14-6** provides a listing of currently available hemodynamic monitoring methods and devices. **Box 14-2** lists the properties of an ideal hemodynamic monitoring device. Although

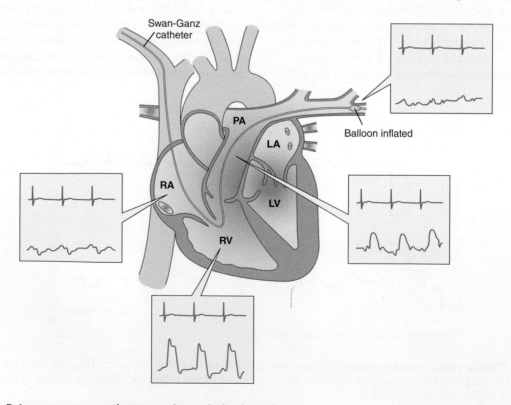

FIGURE 14-19 Pulmonary artery catheter waveforms during insertion.

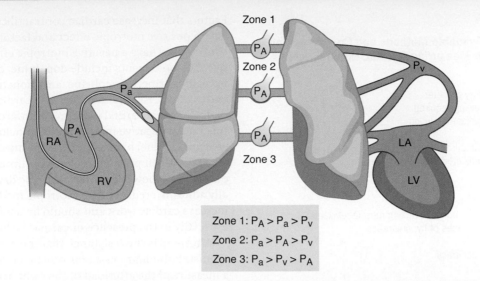

Zone 1: $P_A > P_a > P_v$

Zone 2: $P_a > P_A > P_v$

Zone 3: $P_a > P_v > P_A$

FIGURE 14-20 Pulmonary artery catheter placement. The pulmonary artery catheter should be placed in Zone 3 of the lungs so alveolar pressures are less than pulmonary artery and venous pressures.

Courtesy of Hess DR, MacIntyre NR, Mishoe SC, Galvin WF, and Adams AB.

there are currently no devices that encompass all of these characteristics, an effort should be made to select a device that includes as many as possible.[45]

Hemodynamic measurements are frequently used to manage patients experiencing severe hemodynamic compromise. Remember that blood moves from the right side of the heart through the lungs to the left side of heart and then out through the systemic circulatory system. The global measure of blood flow through the body is cardiac output. Cardiac output is determined by stroke volume and heart rate. The determinants of stroke volume are preload, cardiac contractility, and afterload.

Preload is the filling pressure exerted upon the ventricles during diastole. CVP is a measure of the filling pressure of the right ventricle, and pulmonary artery occlusion or pulmonary capillary wedge pressure (PAOP = PCWP) is a measure of the filling pressure of the left ventricle. Normal CVP is about 4 to 8 mm Hg, and normal PCWP is about 6 to 12 mm Hg. These measures are usually reflective of intravascular volume: the higher the pressure, the higher the intravascular volume, and vice versa. The CVP is also influenced by lung disease (hypoxic vasoconstriction) and mechanical ventilation (positive pressure) and thus the CVP can be elevated even in patients with volume depletion. However, if ventricular volume is low, administering fluids will increase stroke volume, which increases cardiac output. This increase in cardiac output will continue as fluid is administered until the ventricles are maximally stretched. If excessive fluids are administered, fluid overload may occur, and pulmonary edema and/or peripheral edema may develop.

Cardiac output versus the CVP or PCWP pressures can by plotted on a ventricular function curve to determine the filling pressures associated with the highest cardiac output. Besides fluid management, CVP and PCWP are helpful in identifying cardiovascular disorders. When CVP is elevated and PCWP is normal or decreased, a pulmonary embolism or cor pulmonale from high pulmonary artery pressures (PAP) may be present. In cardiogenic shock, both CVP and PCWP are elevated. In septic shock, CVP and PCWP are often normal or reduced. Monitoring and maintaining appropriate filling pressures are important in managing critically ill patients. With the ability of measuring cardiac output and stroke volume (amount of blood ejected from the ventricle with each contraction) by

---

BOX 14-2

Preferred Characteristics of Critical Care Monitoring Devices

- Accurate measurement of clinically relevant variables
- Ease of use
- Rapid response time
- Low maintenance
- Low cost
- Minimally invasive
- Minimal (or no) complications or hazards associated with device

Data from: Vincent JL, Rhodes A, Perel A, et al. Clinical review: Update on hemodynamic monitoring—a consensus of 16. *Crit Care.* 2011;15(4):229.

TABLE 14-6

Examples of Available Methods and Corresponding Limitations for Measuring Cardiac Hemodynamics

Thermodilution
- Pulmonary artery catheter
  - Invasive, training required

Transpulmonary indicator dilution
- PiCCO
  - Decreased accuracy
  - Need for dedicated arterial catheter
- LiDCO
  - Decreased accuracy
  - Need for lithium injection
  - Interference by nondepolarizing muscle relaxants; inaccurate in cases of hyponatremia
- COstatus
  - Decreased accuracy
- VolumeView
  - Decreased accuracy
  - Need for dedicated arterial catheter

Arterial-pressure waveform derived
- PiCCO, LiDCO, Vigileo, MostCare
  - Decreased accuracy
  - Need for optimal arterial pressure tracing

Esophageal Doppler
- CardioQ, WAKle TO
  - Training required
  - Intermittent measurement

Suprasternal Doppler
- USCOM
  - Difficult in some patients

Echocardiography
- Vivid, Sonosite MicroMaxx, Philips CX50
  - Training required
  - Intermittent measurement

Partial CO_2 rebreathing
- NiCO
  - Less reliable in respiratory failure

Bioimpedance
- Lifegard, TEBCO, Hotman, BioZ
  - Less reliable in critically ill patients
  - Not applicable in cardiothoracic surgery

Bioreactance
- NICOM
  - Validated in only one study in critically ill patients

PiCCO, pulse contour cardiac output; LiCo, lithium dilution cardiac output; CO status, a minimally invasive technique incorporating ultrasound signals.

Data from: Vincent JL, Rhodes A, Perel A, et al. Clinical review: Update on hemodynamic monitoring—a consensus of 16. *Crit Care.* 2011;15(4):229.

noninvasive means, reliance on CVP to predict volume status has become less important.

Contractility is the strength with which the heart contracts. If the force of cardiac contraction increases, stroke volume and cardiac output will also increase.

Factors that increase cardiac contractility are said to have a positive inotropic effect and factors that decrease contractility have a negative inotropic effect. Positive inotropic agents include dopamine, dobutamine, norepinephrine, epinephrine, amrinone/milrinone, and digitalis. Factors that decrease cardiac contractility include myocardial ischemia or infarction. Agents that have a negative inotropic effect include β-blockers, calcium channel blockers, and some antiarrhythmic agents.[46] When preload has been optimized and cardiac output is still low, a positive inotropic drug is generally administered. Positive inotropic medications may increase cardiac work and should be used with caution, especially in the presence of cardiac ischemia.

Afterload is the resistance that the heart pumps against. Pulmonary vascular resistance (PVR) provides a measure of the afterload of the right heart. Systemic vascular resistance (SVR) provides a measure of the afterload of the left heart. When PVR or SVR are reduced, cardiac output will generally increase. When PVR or SVR are elevated, cardiac output will generally decrease. When increased afterload decreases cardiac output, it can sometimes be compensated for by an increase in preload. This scenario can become a vicious cycle sometimes seen with systemic hypertension. With systemic hypertension, left ventricular afterload increases. As the body retains fluid, preload and cardiac output increase. This further increases blood pressure and afterload, putting additional stress on the heart.

PVR is calculated by subtracting PCWP from mean PAP and dividing this by cardiac output ($\dot{Q}_T$): [PVR = (MPAP – PCWP)/$\dot{Q}_T$ × 80]. A normal PVR is 110 to 250 dyne/sec/cm^{-5}. SVR is calculated by subtracting CVP from mean arterial pressure (MAP) and dividing this by cardiac output [SVR = (MAP – CVP)/$\dot{Q}_T$ × 80]. A normal SVR is 900 to 1400 dyne/sec/cm^{-5}.[44] PVR is elevated with pulmonary hypertension, severe atelectasis, or lung overdistension. PVR is normally at its lowest when the lung is at functional residual capacity. Acidosis, hypoxemia, and hypercarbia all increase PVR. SVR is elevated with cardiogenic shock, systemic hypertension, volume depletion, and hypothermia. SVR may also be increased with the use of vasoactive drugs such as vasopressin, epinephrine, or high-dose dopamine. SVR is reduced in distributive shock (e.g., sepsis), acidosis, and when vasodilating drugs are administered, such as nitroprusside, clonidine, or hydralazine. **Table 14-7** provides examples of common cardiopulmonary disorders and characteristic hemodynamic variables.

RC Insights

CVP represents the right heart's preload; PCWP represents the left heart's preload. Normal CVP is about 4 to 8 mm Hg; normal PCWP is about 6 to 12 mm Hg. These measures usually reflect intravascular volume.

RC Insights

A normal PVR and SVR are 100 to 250 and 800 to 1200 dyne-sec/cm^{-5}, respectively. PVR or SVR have a direct effect on cardiac output; as they increase, cardiac output will tend to decrease.

TABLE 14-7
Characteristic Hemodynamic Variables for Common Cardiopulmonary Disorders

Condition	CVP	PAP	PCWP	PVR	SVR	CO	BP
Fluid overload	↑	↑	↑	↑ or N	↑ or N	↑ or N	↑ or N
Left ventricular failure	↑	↑	↑	↑	↑ or N	↓	↓
Hypovolemic shock	↓	↓	↓	↑ or N	↑	↓	↓
Septic shock	↓ or N	↓ or N	↓ or N	↓ or N	↓	↑	↓
Cardiogenic shock	↑	↑	↑	↑ or N	↑	↓	↓
Pulmonary embolus	↑	↑	↓ or N	↑	↑	↓ or N	↓ or N
Lung overdistension	↑	↑	↓	↑	↑	↓	↓
ARDS	↓ or N	↑	↓ or N	↑ or N	↑ or N	N	↑ or N

↑, increased; ↓, decreased; N, normal; CVP, central venous pressure; PAP, pulmonary artery pressure; PCWP, pulmonary capillary wedge pressure; PVR, pulmonary vascular resistance; SVR, systemic vascular resistance; CO, cardiac output; BP, blood pressure; ARDS, acute respiratory distress syndrome.

Managing hemodynamics is critical to maintaining oxygen delivery to the organs and tissues. **Oxygen delivery ($\dot{D}o_2$)** is determined by cardiac output ($\dot{Q}_T$) and arterial content of oxygen (Cao_2); $\dot{D}o_2 = \dot{Q}_T \times Cao_2 \times 10$. Cao_2 is calculated using the following formula:

$$Cao_2 = (Hb \times 1.34 \times Sao_2) + (Pao_2 \times 0.003)$$

where Hb is hemoglobin, Sao_2 is arterial oxygen saturation, and Pao_2 is the partial pressure of arterial oxygen. These formulas should make it clear that cardiac output, Hb, and Sao_2 greatly impact oxygen delivery to the tissues. Normal oxygen delivery is about 1000 mL/min. $\dot{D}o_2$ adjusted for body surface area (BSA) is 550 to 650 mL/min/m². Normal oxygen consumption ($\dot{V}o_2$) is about 250 mL/min or 100 to 140 mL/min/m² BSA.[47] Usually $\dot{D}o_2$ greatly exceeds $\bar{V}o_2$; however, a decrease in cardiac output, Hb, or Sao_2 can significantly reduce oxygen delivery. $\dot{V}o_2$ can increase due to tissue injury, sepsis, fever, and increased levels of muscle activity (e.g., shivering, agitation). If $\dot{V}o_2$ exceeds $\dot{D}o_2$ then anaerobic metabolism will begin to produce lactate, and a lactic acidosis may ensue. Monitoring partial pressure of mixed venous oxygen ($P\bar{v}o_2$) and mixed venous oxygen saturation ($S\bar{v}o_2$) can be helpful in identifying if oxygen delivery is adequate. As $\dot{D}o_2$ decreases or $\dot{V}o_2$ increases, $P\bar{v}o_2$ and $S\bar{v}o_2$ will decrease. A normal $P\bar{v}o_2$ is about 35 to 40 mm Hg, and a normal $S\bar{v}o_2$ is 75%. A $P\bar{v}o_2 < 27$ mm Hg and $S\bar{v}o_2 < 50\%$ are associated with lactic acidosis. When managing critically patients, we try to maintain the $S\bar{v}o_2$ at 60% to 75%; sepsis guidelines suggest maintaining $S\bar{v}o_2 \geq 70\%$. An $S\bar{v}o_2$ greater than 77% is associated with sepsis, hypothermia, cyanide poisoning, or high cardiac output.[45] **Box 14-3** provides additional information regarding $S\bar{v}o_2$.

RC Insights

When managing critically patients, try to maintain the $S\bar{v}o_2$ at 60% to 75%; with sepsis, keep $S\bar{v}o_2 > 70\%$.

BOX 14-3

Mixed Venous Oxygen Saturation

Normal values and causes for abnormally increased or decreased mixed venous oxygen saturation are as follows:
- Elevated $S\bar{v}o_2$ ($S\bar{v}o_2 > 77\%$)
  - Sepsis (e.g., peripheral shunt)
  - Left-to-right cardiac shunt (e.g., VSD, PDA, ASD, AVSD)
  - Marked elevation in cardiac output
  - Cyanide poisoning
  - Wedged pulmonary artery catheter when sample drawn

(continues)

- Normal $S\bar{v}o_2$ ($S\bar{v}o_2 \geq 70\%$ but $\leq 77\%$)
  - Normal tissue oxygen delivery and extraction
- Decreased $S\bar{v}o_2$
  - $S\bar{v}o_2 < 70\%$ but $\geq 50\%$
    - Compensatory O_2 extraction due to decreased O_2 delivery (e.g., decreased Cao_2, decreased cardiac output) or increased O_2 demand (e.g., increased metabolic rate)
  - $S\bar{v}o_2 < 50\%$ but $\geq 30\%$
    - Extraction of O_2 is insufficient and O_2 supply (e.g., Do_2) is less than O_2 demand
    - Anaerobic metabolism and lactic acidosis begin
  - $S\bar{v}o_2 < 30\%$ but $\geq 25\%$
    - Anaerobic metabolism results in severe lactic acidosis
  - $S\bar{v}o_2 < 25\%$
    - Cellular hypoxia and death

$S\bar{v}o_2$, mixed venous oxygen saturation; VSD, ventricular septal defect; PDA, patent ductus arteriosus; ASD, arterial septal defect; AVSD, atrioventricular septal defect; Do_2, oxygen delivery ($Do_2 = Cao_2 \times$ Cardiac output); Cao_2, arterial oxygen content ($Cao_2 = 1.34 \times$ Hb $\times$ Sao_2 + 0.003 Pao_2); Hb, hemoglobin; Sao_2, arterial O_2 saturation; Pao_2, arterial O_2 tension.
Data from: Jonas MM, Transer SJ. Lithium dilution measurement of cardiac output and arterial pulse waveform analysis: an indicator dilution, calibrated beat-by-beat system for continuous estimation of cardiac output. *Curr Opin Crit Care*. 2002;8:257–261.

Summary

This chapter highlighted the need to combine assessment fundamentals with the ability to gather information from various monitoring systems to determine appropriate interventions or changes in the care of acutely or critically ill patients. As the level of monitoring and/or assessments increases, so does the cost of care provided. Insufficient monitoring or assessment places patients at additional risk. The cost-benefit relationship of monitoring provided must be considered in today's critical care environment as resources become limited. A number of ventilatory parameters should be assessed when monitoring critically ill patients. Certainly the trending of respiratory rate and tidal volume play a critical role. If the respiratory care clinician visualizes good chest rise, auscultates bilateral breath sounds, and counts a normal respiratory rate in a spontaneously breathing patient, ventilation should be sufficient to maintain adequate oxygenation and carbon dioxide removal. Alternatively, a decreasing tidal volume and increasing respiratory rate are signs of increased WOB and possible impending ventilatory failure. A rapid, shallow breathing pattern often indicates a high WOB, and patients may be unable to maintain their oxygenation and/or ventilation. Serial measures of slow vital capacity that decline below 15 mL/kg (IBW) or 1.0 L are widely accepted as indications of impending ventilatory failure and poor respiratory muscle strength, especially in patients with neuromuscular disease.

If mechanical ventilation is provided, ventilated patients should be assessed for patient–ventilator synchrony and appropriate lung mechanics. Use of ventilator graphics is integral in this process. Common issues that can be identified using ventilator graphics include flow and trigger dyssynchrony, air trapping/auto-PEEP, changes in compliance and resistance, and air leaks.

Noninvasive monitoring is routinely used in managing critically ill patients. This technology should be used to improve patient outcomes by allowing for faster and better decision making. Spo_2 is part of the standard vital sign assessment in today's ICU. An Spo_2 reading of 95% to 97% or greater is considered normal. If Spo_2 decreases to less than 90% to 92% (or less than 88% in chronic lung disease), further assessment is indicated to determine the severity and extent of an oxygenation disturbance. It must also be remembered that pulse oximetry has many limitations, and an adequate Spo_2 does not necessarily mean that the patient is well oxygenated.

Capnography and $ETCO_2$ are affected by the level of ventilation, physiologic dead space, lung perfusion, and metabolic rate. Capnography is commonly used in the intensive care setting for monitoring ventilation and assessing lung perfusion during resuscitation. Transcutaneous monitoring is a noninvasive assessment that may provide information regarding tissue oxygenation and perfusion. Exhaled nitric oxide (NO) is another exhaled respiratory gas that is measured noninvasively to detect airway inflammation.

Critically ill patients frequently require more invasive measurement of hemodynamic parameters. The global measure of blood flow through the body is cardiac output. Cardiac output is determined by heart rate, preload, contractility, and afterload. CVP is a measure of the right heart's preload, and PCWP is a measure of the left heart's preload. A normal CVP is 4 to 8 mm Hg, and a normal PCWP is 6 to 12 mm Hg. PCWP and CVP usually reflect intravascular volume in a direct relationship, and as they increase cardiac output will also increase until fluid overload occurs. If preload is normal but cardiac output is low, there is a contractility and/or afterload problem. Contractility is the strength with which the heart contracts. If an inotropic drug is given (or dose increased), contractility and cardiac output will usually increase. The afterload of the right heart is determined by PVR, and the afterload of the left heart is determined by SVR. When PVR or SVR increase, cardiac output may decrease, or vice versa. Septic patients routinely have low SVRs and require vasoactive drugs to increase SVR. Managing hemodynamics is critical to maintain perfusion and oxygen delivery to the organs and tissues. When managing critically patients, the clinician should try to maintain the $S\bar{v}o_2$ above 60% and most often in the range of 70% to 75%.

Key Points

▶ Tachypnea is often the body's response to hypoxia, hypercarbia, pyrexia, pain, and/or anxiety.

▶ Decreasing tidal volume and increasing respiratory rate (e.g., rapid shallow breathing) are signs of fatiguing respiratory muscles and respiratory distress. Providing inspiratory assist with a positive pressure device may be needed to prevent ventilatory failure in such patients.

▶ If a mechanically ventilated patient becomes tachypneic in the assist-control mode, the delivered minute volume and the I:E ratio will increase. These patients should be monitored for air trapping.

▶ A slow vital capacity (SVC) < 15 mL/kg IBW or 1.0 L is indicative of potential ventilatory problems and poor respiratory muscle strength.

▶ A vital capacity < 20 mL/kg IBW, an MIP > −30 cm H_2O, and an MEP < 40 cm H_2O indicates poor respiratory muscle strength and possible ventilatory failure.

▶ During volume control ventilation, if both PIP and plateau pressure increase there is a compliance problem. If PIP increases but the plateau pressure remains the same, there is an airway resistance problem.

▶ During PCV, decreases in the compliance will cause exhaled tidal volume to decrease and inspiratory flow to reach zero quickly. Increasing R_{aw} will cause peak inspiratory and expiratory flows to decrease and may cause tidal volume to decrease if inspiratory flow no longer reaches zero before inspiration terminates.

▶ When flow dyssynchrony occurs during volume control ventilation, a scooping effect (pressure rise vertically is slow compared to horizontal progression) may appear in the pressure waveform.

▶ Volume waveforms are helpful in identifying air leaks.

▶ When expiratory flow does not return to zero before the next breath begins, air trapping is present, which results in auto-PEEP.

▶ With pressure–volume curves, if the graphic tracing stays negative compared to baseline after inspiration has begun, inspiratory flow is set too low.

▶ Inadequate inspiratory flow rates provided by the ventilator cause patient discomfort and increased WOB. This pattern creates a classic figure eight (8) sign when seen on ventilator graphics.

▶ The endotracheal tube (ETT) tip should be positioned 3 to 5 cm above the carina.

▶ The ETT cuff pressure is maintained between 20 to 25 cm H_2O.

▶ An Spo_2 reading of ≥ 95% to 97% is considered normal. An Spo_2 < 90% to 92% (< 88% with chronic lung disease patients) is a cause for concern.

▶ In normal patients, $ETCO_2$ is generally within 2 to 5 mm Hg of the actual $Paco_2$.

▶ $ETCO_2$ deviations may be due to airway obstruction, rapid shallow breathing, ventilation–perfusion mismatch, inadequacy of cardiopulmonary resuscitation efforts, or a large leak.

▶ Fluctuations in cardiac output and increased PVR can significantly affect the accuracy of transcutaneous monitoring and may serve as an indicator of poor tissue perfusion.

▶ FeNO values are considered high when they are > 50 ppb for adults or > 30 ppb for children. They are considered acutely rising if they are more than 40% from a predetermined baseline. These values imply deteriorating or uncontrolled eosinophilic airway inflammation.

▶ Cardiac output is determined by stroke volume and heart rate. The determinants of stroke volume are preload, contractility, and afterload.

▶ CVP is the right heart's preload, and PCWP is the left heart's preload.

▶ A normal CVP is 4 to 8 mm Hg, and a normal PCWP is 6 to 12 mm Hg. These measures usually reflect intravascular volume.

▶ If cardiac contractility increases, cardiac output will increase. Factors that increase contractility have a positive inotropic effect, and factors that decrease it have a negative inotropic effect.

▶ Afterload is the resistance that the heart pumps against. The afterload of the right heart is pulmonary vascular resistance (PVR). The afterload of the left heart is systemic vascular resistance (SVR).

▶ When PVR or SVR are elevated, cardiac output may decrease.

▶ Managing hemodynamics is critical to maintain perfusion and oxygen delivery to the organs and tissues.

▶ A normal $P\overline{v}o_2$ is 35 to 40 mm Hg, and a normal $S\overline{v}o_2$ is 75%. As oxygen delivery decreases or consumption increases, $P\overline{v}o_2$ and $S\overline{v}o_2$ will decrease.

References

1. Harvey S, Stevens K, Harrison D, et al. An evaluation of the clinical and cost-effectiveness of pulmonary artery catheters in patient management in intensive care: A systematic review and a randomized control trial. *Health Technol Assess.* 2006;10(29):iii–iv, ix–xi, 1–133.

2. Hofer CK, Rex S, Ganter MT. Update on minimally invasive hemodynamic monitoring in thoracic anesthesia. *Curr Opin Anaesthesiology.* 2014;27(1):28–35.

3. O'Donnell DE. Ventilatory limitations in chronic obstructive pulmonary disease. *Med Sci Sports Exerc.* 2001;33(7 Suppl):S647–55.

4. Mehta S. Neuromuscular disease causing acute respiratory failure. *Respir Care.* 2006;51(9):1016–1023.

5. Hutchinson D, Whyte K. Neuromuscular disease and respiratory failure. *Pract Neurol.* 2008;8(4):229–237.

6. Hautmann H, Hefele S, Schotten K, Huber RM. Maximal inspiratory mouth pressures (PIMAX) in healthy subjects—what is the lower limit of normal? *Respir Med.* 2000;94(7):689–693.

7. Thille AW, Rodriguez P, Cabello B, Lellouche F, Brochard L. Patient-ventilator asynchrony during assisted mechanical ventilation. *Intensive Care Med.* 2006;32(10):1515–1522.

8. Barrera R, Melendez J, Ahdoot M, et al. Flow triggering added to pressure support ventilation improves comfort and reduces work of breathing in mechanically ventilated patients. *J Crit Care.* 1999;14(4):172–176.

9. Roberts J, Spadafora M, Cone D. Proper depth placement of oral endotracheal tubes in adults prior to radiographic confirmation. *Acad Emerg Med.* 1995;2(1):20–24.

10. Sitzwohl C, Langheinrick A, Schober A, et al. Endobronchial intubation detected by insertion of endotracheal tube, bilateral auscultation, or observation of chest movements: randomised trial. *BMJ.* 2010;9(341):c5943.

11. Kim JT, Kim HJ, Ahn W, et al. Head rotation, flexion, and extension alter endotracheal tube position in adults and children. *Can J Anaesth.* 2009;56(10):751–756.

12. Yap S, Morris R, Pybus D. Alterations in endotracheal tube position during general anaesthesia. *Anaesth Intensive Care.* 1994;22(5):586–588.

13. Tierney LM Jr., Whooley MA, Saint S. Oxygen saturation: A fifth vital sign? *West J Med.* 1997;166(4):285–286.

14. Neff TA. Routine oximetry. A fifth vital sign? *Chest* 1988;94(2):227.

15. Mendelson Y. Pulse oximetry: Theory and applications for noninvasive monitoring. *Clin Chem.* 1992;38(9):1601–1607.

16. Chan ED, Chan MM, Chan MM. Pulse oximetry: Understanding its basic principles facilitates appreciation of its limitations. *Respir Med.* 2013;107(6):789–799.

17. Kamlin COF, Dawson JA O'Donnell CPF, et al. Accuracy of pulse oximetry measurement of heart rate of newborn infants in the delivery room. *J Pediatr.* 2008;152(6):756–760.

18. DeMeulenaere S. Pulse oximetry: uses and limitations. *J Nurse Pract.* 2007;3(5):312–317.

19. *Taking Noninvasive Monitoring to New Sites and Applications.* Irvine, CA: Masimo Corporation; 2012.

20. Pekdemir M, Cinar O, Yilmaz S, Yaka E, Yuksel M. Disparity between mainstream and sidestream end-tidal carbon dioxide values and arterial carbon dioxide levels. *Respir Care.* 2013;58(7):1152–1156.

21. Manifold CA, Davids N, Villers LC, Wampler DA. Capnography for the nonintubated patient in the emergency setting. *J Emerg Med.* 2013;45(4):626–632.

22. Ortega R, Connor C, Kim S, Djang R, Patel K. Monitoring ventilation with capnography. *N Engl J Med.* 2012;367(19):e27.

23. Neumar RW, Otto CW, Link MS, et al. Part 8: Adult advanced cardiovascular life support: 2010 American Heart Association Guidelines for Cardiopulmonary Resuscitation and Emergency Cardiovascular Care. *Circulation.* 2010;122(18 Suppl 3):S729–S767.

24. Pilbeam SP, Cairo JM. Mechanical ventilation: Physiological and clinical applications. St. Louis, MO: Mosby-Elsevier; 2006.

25. Eberhard P. The design, use, and results of transcutaneous carbon dioxide analysis: Current and future directions. *Anesth Analg.* 2007;105(6 Suppl):S48–S52.

26. Restrepo RD, Hirst KR, Wittnebel L, Wettstein R. AARC clinical practice guideline: Transcutaneous monitoring of carbon dioxide and oxygen: 2012. *Respir Care.* 2012;57(11):1955–1962.

27. Weaver LK. Transcutaneous oxygen and carbon dioxide tensions compared to arterial blood gases in normals. *Respir Care.* 2007;52(11):1490–1496.

28. Tobias JD. Transcutaneous carbon dioxide monitoring in infants and children. *Paediatr Anaesth.* 2009;19(5):434–444.

29. Munakata M. Exhaled nitric oxide (FeNO) as a non-invasive marker of airway inflammation. *Allergol Int.* 2012;61(3):365–372.

30. Dweik RA, Boggs PB, Erzurum SC, et al. An official ATS clinical practice guideline: Interpretation of exhaled nitric oxide levels (FeNO) for clinical applications. *Am J Respir Crit Care Med.* 2011;184(5):602–615.

31. Barnes PJ, Dweik RA, Gelb AF, et al. Exhaled nitric oxide in pulmonary diseases: A comprehensive review. *Chest.* 2010;138(3):682–692.

32. Menzies D, Nair A, Lipworth BJ. Portable exhaled nitric oxide measurement: Comparison with the "gold standard" technique. *Chest.* 2007;131(2):410–414.

33. Kapande KM, McConaghy LA, Douglas I, et al. Comparative repeatability of two handheld fractional exhaled nitric oxide monitors. *Pediatr Pulmonol.* 2012;47(6):546–550.

34. Madias JE. A comparison of 2-lead, 6-lead, and 12-lead ECGs in patients with changing edematous states: Implications for the employment of quantitative electrocardiography in research and clinical applications. *Chest.* 2003;124(6):2057–2063.

35. Fox L, Kirkendall C, Craney M. Continuous ST-segment monitoring in the intensive care unit. *Crit Care Nurse.* 2010;30(5):33–43; quiz 44.

36. Reilly RB, Lee TC. Electrograms (ECG, EEG, EMG, EOG). *Technol Health Care.* 2010;18(6):443–458.

37. Becker DE. Fundamentals of electrocardiography interpretation. *Anesth Prog.* 2006;53(2):53–64.

38. Thavendiranathan P, Bagai A, Khoo C, Dorian P, Choudhry NK. Does this patient with palpitations have a cardiac arrhythmia? *JAMA.* 2009;302(19):2135–2143.

39. Hollenberg SM. Hemodynamic monitoring. *Chest.* 2013;143(5):1480–1488.

40. Govert JA, Hess DR. Hemodynamic monitoring. In: Hess DR, MacIntyre NR, Mishoe SC, et al. (eds.). *Respiratory Care: Principles and Practice,* 2nd ed. Sudbury, MA: Jones & Bartlett Learning; 2012: 87–100.

41. Vincent JL, Rhodes A, Perel A, et al. Clinical review: Update on hemodynamic monitoring—a consensus of 16. *Crit Care.* 2011;15(4):229.

42. Busse L, Davison DL, Junker C, Chawla LS. Hemodynamic monitoring in the critical care environment. *Adv Chron Kid Dis.* 2013;20(1):21–29.

43. Jonas, MM, Tanser SJ. Lithium dilution measurement of cardiac output and arterial pulse waveform analysis: An indicator dilution, calibrated beat-by-beat system for continuous estimation of cardiac output. *Curr Opin Crit Care.* 2002;8:257–261.

44. Meng L, Phuong Tran N, Alexander BS, et al. Impact of phenylephrine, ephedrine, and increased preload on third-generation Vigileo-FloTrac and esophageal Doppler cardiac output measurements. *Anesth Analg.* 2011;113(4):751–757.

45. Bloos F, Reinhart K. Venous oximetry. *Intensive Care Med.* 2005;31(7):911–913.

46. Restrepo RD. Cardiac output measurement. In: Heuer AJ, Scanlan CL (eds.). *Wilkins' Clinical Assessment in Respiratory Care,* 7th ed. Maryland Heights, MO: Elsevier-Mosby: 2014:373–395

47. Vines DL. Respiratory monitoring in critical care. In: Heuer AJ, Scanlan CL (eds.). *Wilkins' Clinical Assessment in Respiratory Care,* 7th ed. Maryland Heights, MO: Elsevier-Mosby: 2014;314–347.

CHAPTER

15

Obstructive Sleep Apnea and Other Sleep-Related Breathing Disorders

Paul Ingmundson, Angela C. Hospenthal, and Maureen Koops

CHAPTER OUTLINE

CHAPTER OBJECTIVES

1. Describe the normal stages of sleep.
2. Explain what is measured during a sleep study.
3. Identify the causes of sleep apnea.
4. Understand the scope of sleep apnea as it relates to the general population.
5. Recognize the individual with a breathing-related sleep disorder in the clinical setting.
6. Distinguish among obstructive sleep apnea, central sleep apnea, and mixed sleep apnea.
7. Appreciate other coexisting disease states in the patient with obstructive sleep apnea.
8. Explain diagnostic strategies for sleep apnea.
9. Outline treatment options for each type of sleep apnea.
10. Describe how a positive pressure device can be used to treat obstructive sleep apnea.
11. Understand the differences among the various positive pressure airway devices used to treat sleep apnea.
12. Discuss the barriers to adherence in treating sleep apnea.

KEY TERMS

bilevel positive airway
  pressure (BiPAP)
central sleep apnea (CSA)
continuous positive airway
  pressure (CPAP)

electroencephalogram
  (EEG)
hypopnea
obstructive sleep apnea
  (OSA)

polysomnography
positive airway pressure
  (PAP)
rapid eye movement (REM)
  sleep

respiratory effort–related
  arousal (RERA)
sleep-disordered breathing
  (SDB)

Overview

Sleep disorders affect millions of individuals in the United States and inadequate sleep may result in motor vehicle and other accidents, as well as contributing to the severity of illness in a number of chronic diseases including diabetes, obesity, hypertension, and cancer. Diagnosis and treatment of sleep-disordered breathing has become an important part of the respiratory care clinician's role.

Introduction to Respiration in Sleep

Hypoventilation occurs during sleep, primarily due to a reduction of tidal volume with a minimal decrease in respiratory rate. This hypoventilation leads to relative hypoxemia (a decrease of 3 to 10 mm Hg in Po_2) and hypercapnia (an increase of 2 to 3 mm Hg in Pco_2) in normal individuals. These changes are slightly more pronounced in **rapid eye movement (REM) sleep** than non-REM (NREM) sleep.[1] Given that the sleep period causes respiratory perturbations in healthy individuals, in susceptible individuals the act of sleeping can cause marked pathologic breathing with significant detrimental effects on overall health and general well-being.

Sleep Stages

The diagnosis of sleep-disordered breathing has evolved since the widespread adoption of overnight sleep recording (nocturnal polysomnography, or NPSG) in the 1970s. Consensus definitions have been promulgated by the American Academy of Sleep Medicine (AASM).[2]

Sleep in adults is defined by changes in three sets of electrophysiologic parameters: the **electroencephalogram (EEG)**, electrooculogram (EOG), and electromyogram (EMG). Sleep in adults is composed of two distinct physiologic states: rapid eye movement (REM, or stage R) sleep and nonrapid eye movement (NREM) sleep. NREM sleep is subdivided into three distinct substages: N1, N2, and N3. Sleep generally begins with a light transitional state, stage N1, characterized by low-voltage, mixed-frequency waves in the EEG. EEG waves increase in amplitude and decrease in a dominant EEG frequency as sleep progresses through stages N2 and N3. Stage N2 sleep is characterized by distinct EEG features known as spindles and K-complexes, and it accounts for 40% to 50% of total sleep time in normal adults. Stage N3, sometimes called "slow-wave" sleep, is characterized by a high-voltage, low-frequency (fewer than four cycles per second) EEG (**Figure 15-1**). In normal sleep, stages N1, N2, and N3 progress over approximately 90 minutes before the first appearance of REM sleep. REM sleep is characterized by a low-voltage, mixed-frequency EEG, similar to what is observed in wakefulness, accompanied by muscle atonia. In REM sleep, an active, wake-like EEG is observed, along with rapid eye movements in the EOG and a loss of muscle tone in the EMG. The combination of intense cerebral activation in the EEG, frequently associated with the vivid hallucinatory experience of dreaming, accompanied by the functional paralysis of the skeletal muscles, has led some investigators to identify REM sleep as "paradoxical" sleep. The loss of upper airway muscle tone makes the REM state particularly vulnerable to upper airway obstruction, although changes in ventilatory control may give rise to increases in the frequency of central apneas in NREM sleep in some clinical syndromes such as complex sleep apnea.[3]

In normal adult sleep, the NREM phase precedes the REM phase, and the two phases repeat in a cycle every 90 minutes, with slow-wave sleep predominating in the two 90-minute cycles and REM sleep predominating later in the night.

Specific pediatric criteria are available for scoring sleep stages and respiratory events in children. These pediatric criteria are used for patients younger than 13 years of age. Either the adult or pediatric criteria can be used for patients between 13 and 17 years of age.

The sleep stages in infants and children differ from those of adults. In adults, the posterior dominant rhythm used to determine sleep onset is the alpha

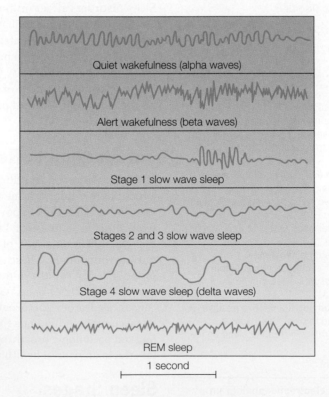

Quiet wakefulness (alpha waves)

Alert wakefulness (beta waves)

Stage 1 slow wave sleep

Stages 2 and 3 slow wave sleep

Stage 4 slow wave sleep (delta waves)

REM sleep

1 second

FIGURE 15-1 EEG waveforms of stages of sleep. Stages: Wake, N1, N2, N3, R (REM).

rhythm. In infants and children, this posterior dominant rhythm is slower and has a higher voltage. Sleep spindles are seen in all normal infants by 9 weeks of age, but K-complexes are usually not present until 5 to 6 months of age. Slow-wave activity has the same frequency in both adults and children, but is usually of a much higher voltage in children.

Sleep-stage organization evolves over the life span. Infants typically spend 16 hours of the 24-hour day asleep, and infant sleep is polyphasic, with multiple periods of sleep and wakefulness occurring throughout the 24-hour day. Polyphasic sleep persists in preschool children, with afternoon naps generally persisting until age 6 or 7.

Sleep stages in infants and children differ from the stages observed in adults. The phase of sleep generally identified as REM sleep in infants is generally labeled *active sleep*, whereas the NREM sleep stages are collectively identified as *quiet sleep*. Sleep-stage scoring in infants will also include epochs labeled as *indeterminate* or *transitional* sleep to describe segments that cannot be categorized as either active (REM) or quiet (NREM) sleep. Sleep-onset REM, or active sleep, is typical in infants. REM and NREM stages alternate every 60 to 70 minutes in early infancy, with the REM/NREM sleep cycle gradually lengthening to 90 minutes over the first year of life. REM sleep constitutes approximately 50% of infant sleep, with the percentage gradually decreasing to 20% to 25% by age 10. Slow-wave (stage N3) sleep, with high-amplitude EEG waves, persists through childhood and decreases dramatically with the onset of puberty. The proportion of stage N3 sleep continues to decrease gradually from adolescence into adulthood and senescence.

Sleep-disordered breathing (SBD) disrupts the orderly progression of sleep stages. Patients with SDB typically have increased amounts of stage N1, or transitional, sleep; an increased number of awakenings; and decreased time spent in REM and slow-wave sleep. SDB results in a loss of sleep continuity, or sleep fragmentation, as well as episodes of hypoxemia; both sleep fragmentation and hypoxemia may have independent contributions to the clinical manifestations and increased cardiovascular risks associated with SDB.

Recording Parameters

The current standard for diagnosing sleep apnea is an overnight sleep study attended by a technician (i.e., NPSG). An overnight recording consists of the continuous monitoring of a set of electrophysiologic signals. Electrophysiologic signals required for defining sleep stages (EEG, EOG, and EMG) are used to identify sleep and wake states. EMG signals derived from the anterior tibia of the lower extremities are used to monitor movements during sleep. Respiratory signals acquired during nocturnal polysomnography typically include at least

two signals to measure airflow. Oronasal thermistors are used to evaluate airflow based on the temperature difference between inspired and expired air and are the primary signal used in the identification of apneas. Nasal pressure transducers are used in the evaluation of airflow changes associated with hypopneas. Respiratory effort is measured by bands placed around the thorax and abdomen using respiratory inductance plethysmography (RIP) or polyvinylidene fluoride (PVDF) sensors. Esophageal manometry is an alternative approach to evaluating respiratory effort. Oxygen saturation is evaluated by means of pulse oximetry. Hypoventilation is monitored with devices measuring either end-tidal or transcutaneous Pco_2 (**Figure 15-2**). Pco_2 monitoring is used in adults where hypoventilation is suspected, and it is required in polysomnographic evaluations in children. A compilation of signals from these various sensors (**Figure 15-3**) are viewed by the polysomnographer remotely in real time and are simultaneously recorded for formal interpretation by a sleep specialist at the conclusion of the study. Other parameters that are typically included in a comprehensive attended polysomnographic evaluation include video monitoring (particularly important in the assessment of parasomnias), audio channels assessing snoring, and position sensors to provide continuous monitoring of body position.

Definitions

Sleep-disordered breathing in adults is characterized by several distinct events, which are summarized in **Table 15-1**.

In adults, apnea is defined as a near-complete (> 90%) cessation of airflow lasting ≥ 10 seconds. Apneas are classified into three subtypes:

- **Obstructive sleep apnea (OSA)**: Cessation of airflow for ≥ 10 seconds, with evidence of sustained inspiratory effort.
- **Central sleep apnea (CSA)**: Cessation of both airflow and inspiratory effort for ≥ 10 seconds.
- *Mixed apnea*: Cessation of both airflow and inspiratory effort in the initial portion of the event, followed by a resumption of effort in the second portion of the event.

Hypopneas are considerably more frequent than apneas in most patients with SDB. A **hypopnea** is defined as a decrease in the signals measuring airflow (nasal thermistors and airflow pressure transducers) of 30% or more for ≥ 10 seconds, accompanied by an O_2 desaturation ≥ 3%. The desaturation criterion for defining hypopneas continues to be a matter of some controversy. The American Academy of Sleep Medicine (AASM) has recommended a definition requiring an oxygen desaturation of ≥ 3%, whereas the Center for Medicare and Medicaid Services (CMS) has maintained

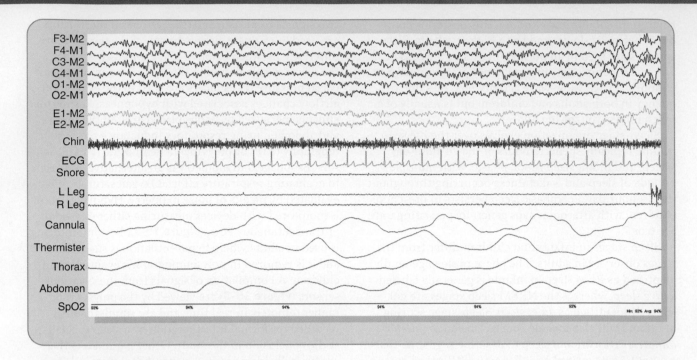

FIGURE 15-2 A typical diagnostic polysomnogram montage.

Courtesy of William Spriggs.

a definition requiring a desaturation ≥ 4%. Hypopneas are further classified into two subtypes:

■ *Obstructive hypopneas*: Hypopneas observed in association with markers of inspiratory effort (snoring, inspiratory flattening in the airflow signal, or thoracoabdominal paradox).

■ *Central hypopneas*: Hypopneas observed in association in the absence of inspiratory effort.

Respiratory effort–related arousals (RERAs) are sleep-disordered breathing events that are not associated with oxygen desaturations of 3% or more. A RERA is a sequence of breaths lasting ≥ 10 seconds associated

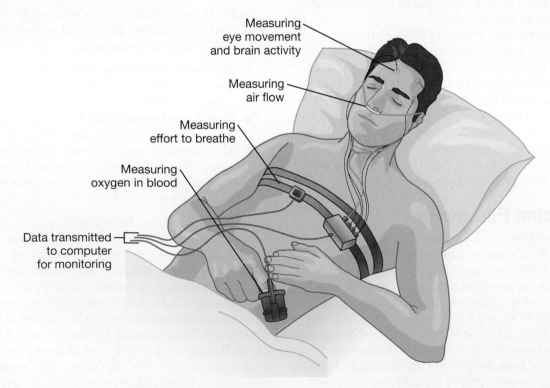

FIGURE 15-3 Compilation of waveforms from multiple sensors.

TABLE 15-1
Sleep-Disordered Breathing Definitions (Adults)

Criteria	Apneas		Hypopneas		Mixed Apneas	RERAs
	Obstructive	Central	Obstructive	Central		
Airflow	No	No	Yes, ≥ 30% reduction	Yes, ≥ 30% reduction	No on initial portion	Decreased but not > 30%
Inspiratory effort	Yes	No	Yes	No	No on initial portion, then effort resumes	Yes
Oxygen desaturation > 3%	Yes	Yes	Yes	Yes	Yes	No

RERA, respiratory effort–related arousal.

with increasing respiratory effort or flattening of the inspiratory portion of the airflow signal that does not meet the criteria for an apnea or hypopnea.

The criteria for scoring obstructive apneas and hypopneas are similar for adults and children except for duration. In adults, an obstructive apnea or hypopnea must last at least 10 seconds, for infants and children the duration is a minimum of two breath cycles. Brief central apneas are normal in infants and children. Therefore, a central apnea is not scored unless it is at least 20 seconds in length or it lasts for two or more breath cycles and is associated with either an oxygen desaturation of ≥ 3% or bradycardia. Finally, monitoring of hypoventilation, typically by means of end-tidal Pco_2 recording, is recommended as a routine part of any pediatric diagnostic study, although it is optional during a positive airway pressure (PAP) titration. The threshold for clinically significant sleep apnea for children is lower than in adults, with an apnea index (AI) of 1.0 or more generally considered abnormal. Consequently, most pediatric sleep specialists regard an apnea index (AI) of more than 1 or an apnea hypopnea index (AHI) of 1.5 as abnormal, and most recommend treatment of any child with an AI greater than 5.

SDB in children is typically associated with evidence of airflow limitation along with periods of hypoventilation associated with elevated Pco_2, oftentimes with minimal changes in oxygen saturation.

Spectrum of Breathing-Related Sleep Disorders

The second edition of the *International Classification of Sleep Disorders* (ICSD-2)[4] lists 14 specific diagnoses that involve abnormal breathing during sleep (Box 15-1). The most clinically relevant disease of the group is obstructive sleep apnea (OSA).

Central Sleep Apnea Syndromes

An intricate communication system between the respiratory centers of the brain and the respiratory anatomy of the chest via chemoreceptors in the bloodstream is required to coordinate each breath. Central sleep apnea (CSA) syndromes include breathing disorders resulting from miscommunication among these entities, usually due to dysfunction in either the cardiovascular or central nervous system (CNS). Thus, cessation of respiratory airflow is due to the centrally mediated cessation of thoracoabdominal inspiratory effort (Figure 15-4).

Cheyne-Stokes breathing (CSB) is the most common form of central sleep apnea, prevailing in 25% to 40% of those with congestive heart failure (CHF) and in nearly 10% of those with stroke.[4] CSB is characterized by recurrent central apneas alternating with a crescendo-decrescendo tidal volume pattern.[5] Heart failure patients who manifest CSB have a worse prognosis than CHF patients with normal breathing.[6]

Central hypoventilation without CSB may be observed in patients with brain tumors, following stroke, or in association with narcotic analgesics. Neuromuscular disorders, including myasthenia gravis, amyotrophic lateral sclerosis (ALS), cerebellar ataxias, myopathies, and chest wall anatomic abnormalities may be associated with ventilatory impairments that are present with central apnea syndromes during sleep. Healthy adults who climb elevations above 5,000 meters, patients with chronic pain who use opioid medications, and premature infants can all suffer from CSA.

CSA syndromes, whether idiopathic, congenital, or due to medical conditions, are characterized by a regular breathing pattern during sleep with periods of hypercapnia and/or hypoxemia. Of these, sleep-related hypoventilation/hypoxemia caused by a medical condition is the most common. Hypoventilation/hypoxemic syndromes due to pulmonary parenchymal diseases include a variety of disorders that result in the inflammation and destruction of the lung interstitium. Vascular disorders resulting in nocturnal blood gas perturbations include pulmonary hypertension and hemoglobinopathies. An essential feature of these conditions is a sustained oxygen desaturation in the absence of airflow limitation or snoring. Hypoventilation/hypoxemic

BOX 15-1

Sleep-Related Breathing Disorders

Central Sleep Apnea Syndromes

    Primary central sleep apnea
    Central sleep apnea due to Cheyne-Stokes breathing pattern
    Central sleep apnea due to high-altitude periodic breathing
    Central sleep apnea due to medical condition not Cheyne-Stokes
    Central sleep apnea due to drug or substance
    Primary sleep apnea of infancy (formerly primary sleep apnea of newborn)

Obstructive Sleep Apnea Syndromes

    Obstructive sleep apnea, adult
    Obstructive sleep apnea, pediatric

Sleep-Related Hypoventilation/Hypoxemic Syndromes

    Sleep-related nonobstructive alveolar hypoventilation, idiopathic
    Congenital central alveolar hypoventilation syndrome

Sleep-Related Hypoventilation/Hypoxemia Due to Medical Condition

    Sleep-related hypoventilation/hypoxemia due to pulmonary parenchymal or vascular pathology
    Sleep-related hypoventilation/hypoxemia due to lower airways obstruction
    Sleep-related hypoventilation/hypoxemia due to neuromuscular and chest wall disorders

Other Sleep-Related Breathing Disorder

    Sleep apnea/sleep-related breathing disorder, unspecified

syndromes due to lower airways obstruction, mainly chronic obstructive pulmonary disease (COPD), are identified by a $Paco_2$ greater than 45 mm Hg during sleep.[4] Neuromuscular diseases and chest wall disorders directly affect the breathing "pump" with resultant hypoventilation, and the subsequent atelectasis contributes to the hypoxemia.

Obstructive Sleep Apnea Syndromes

Whether in the adult or pediatric population, obstructive sleep apnea (OSA) is characterized by repetitive episodes of complete (apnea; **Figure 15-5**) or partial (hypopnea; **Figure 15-6**) upper airway obstruction during sleep. Thus, there is decrement of airflow or complete cessation of airflow in the setting of continued thoracoabdominal inspiratory effort (**Figure 15-7**). The diagnosis of OSA is based on a combination of sleep laboratory criteria and clinical symptoms, which will be discussed in further detail in the following sections.

Clinical Focus 15-1 describes the treatment of a patient with OSA using continuous positive airway pressure (CPAP).

Complex sleep apnea and overlap syndrome are not listed specifically in the current diagnostic manual (*ICSD-2*), although criteria for diagnosis of complex sleep apnea are proposed for inclusion in the third edition (*ICSD-3*) of the manual. Patients who fulfill the diagnostic criteria for OSA but have additional characteristic findings warrant further classification of their disease process into these entities.

Complex Sleep Apnea

A significant number of patients with presentations typical of OSA may demonstrate ventilatory instability, particularly during NREM sleep, that may be aggravated with the application of the most common treatments, which are **continuous positive airway pressure (CPAP)** and **bilevel positive airway pressure (BiPAP)**. 3 Patients with complex sleep apnea may present with "treatment emergent" sleep apnea, where the application of CPAP increases rather than resolves ventilatory instability during NREM sleep, resulting in the emergence of central sleep apnea. The presence of the constellation of sleep-disordered breathing that is worse in

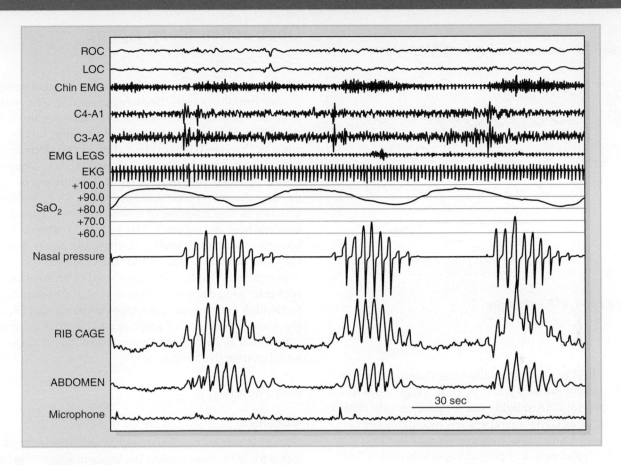

FIGURE 15-4 **CSA waveforms.**

Reprinted with permission of the American Thoracic Society. Copyright © 2014 American Thoracic Society. http://www-archive.thoracic.org/sections/education/sleep-fragments/quiz/waxing-weaning-breathing.html. Official Journal of the American Thoracic Society.

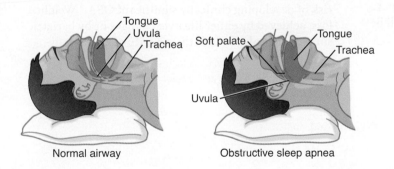

FIGURE 15-5 **Apnea.**

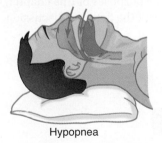

FIGURE 15-6 **Hypopnea.**

NREM sleep rather than REM sleep, the emergence of central apneas with the application of CPAP or BiPAP, and the worsening of sleep-disordered breathing in the supine sleep position, taken together, raises the clinical suspicion for complex sleep apnea. This scenario is particularly common in patients where ventilatory instability may emerge in the context of cardiovascular disease and congestive heart failure. Recent innovations in **positive airway pressure (PAP)** technologies (adaptive servoventilation [ASV] therapy) have been found to

be particularly useful in the treatment of patients with complex sleep apnea syndromes.[3] **Clinical Focus 15-2** describes a patient who may benefit from ASV.

Overlap Syndrome

The coexistence of COPD and OSA in the same patient is overlap syndrome (OS). The upper airway muscles have decreased tone during sleep, and these muscles are further deranged in the presence of OSA and COPD. Patients with OS are older and less obese than those

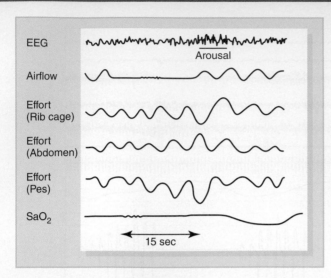

FIGURE 15-7 **OSA waveforms.**

with COPD or OSA alone. Daytime sleepiness may be less apparent in those with OS; thus, a high index of suspicion for OSA should exist for patients with COPD. Autotitrating CPAP therapy is not recommended for those with COPD, thus first-line therapy for OS is CPAP. Hypoxemia may persist, especially during REM sleep, despite relief of obstructive events. Consequently, supplemental oxygen blended in with CPAP therapy is often needed.[1] BiPAP has a role in aiding ventilatory effort during acute exacerbations of COPD. **Clinical Focus 15-3** describes a patient with COPD and OSA.

For the purposes of this chapter, adult OSA will be the focus of the detailed discussion.

Obstructive Sleep Apnea

Epidemiology

Obstructive sleep apnea (OSA) is by far the most prevalent syndrome of sleep-disordered breathing observed in clinical populations. A widely cited study estimated that 4% of men and 2% of women in the labor force younger than age 65 years meet clinical and sleep laboratory criteria for obstructive sleep apnea.[7] Sleep-disordered breathing without clinical symptoms of daytime sleepiness is far more prevalent: 9% of women and 24% of men have five or more apneas and hypopneas per hour during sleep. Many of these patients may not report symptoms such as daytime sleepiness, but they may be at increased risk for the cardiovascular complications that have been reported to be associated with even mild degrees of sleep-disordered breathing.[8] Epidemiologic investigations have estimated that 5% of the adult population in European and North American countries may have clinically significant but undiagnosed obstructive sleep apnea.[1]

Risk Factors

Obesity

Obesity is commonly recognized as an important risk factor for SDB. Even modest increases in weight over the life span may be associated with dramatic increases in the prevalence of sleep apnea. Studies of individuals over time have found that those who experience a 10% increase in weight have a 6- to 10-fold increase in the risk of developing clinically significant OSA.[9] Weight loss, achieved by either lifestyle changes or by bariatric surgery, may also reduce the severity of OSA. Body

---

CLINICAL FOCUS 15-1

Treatment of OSA with Positive Airway Pressure

A 56-year-old man with severe obstructive sleep apnea (OSA) started on continuous positive airway pressure (CPAP) at 15 cm H_2O returns for his 2-week follow-up. He has trouble following asleep with CPAP and finds it difficult to exhale against the pressure.

What adjustments may improve the patient's adherence?

Review the CPAP settings. Determine the ramp time; that is, the time it takes for the pressure to go from an initial low level to the target level. The ramp time can usually be set between 10 and 45 minutes. Increasing the ramp time will delay the time to peak pressure and may allow this patient to fall asleep more easily. Some patients want more pressure, in which case you could reduce or eliminate the ramp time. Most CPAP machines are able to reduce the pressure during exhalation by 1, 2, or 3 cm H_2O pressure. Maximizing the expiratory pressure relief (EPR or C-Flex) may improve this patient's tolerance.

CLINICAL FOCUS 15-2

Adaptive Servoventilation (ASV)

A 67-year-old man with obstructive sleep apnea (OSA) on therapy with continuous positive airway pressure (CPAP) recently hospitalized for congestive heart failure due to severe cardiomyopathy with an ejection fraction less than 30% reports recurrence of excessive daytime sleepiness (EDS). Data downloaded from the CPAP machine indicates excellent adherence, but the periodic breathing index is extremely high.

1. What could explain the patient's recurrent EDS and high periodic breathing index?
    The patient may have developed central sleep apnea due to the Cheyne-Stokes breathing pattern often seen in patients with congestive heart failure. This patient should undergo a repeat positive airway pressure (PAP) titration with adaptive servoventilation (ASV).

mass index (BMI) is the most frequently cited index of obesity associated with increased risk, but other anthropometric measures, in particular neck size, may be better predictors. Neck size greater than 16 inches (40.6 cm) in men and 15 inches (38.1 cm) in women has been found to be correlated with increased risk for clinically significant OSA. The CMS requires documentation of neck circumference as part of the physical examination of patients referred for CPAP treatment for OSA.

Gender

Most studies of the prevalence of sleep-disordered breathing have shown an increased prevalence in males.[8] Patients on testosterone replacement therapy have been found to be at increased risk for the development of SDB, possibly due to decreased respiratory drive associated with increasing testosterone levels with replacement therapy.[10] Postmenopausal women are reported to have increased risk for SDB even after adjusting for the effects of age and weight.[11] Progesterone administration has been found to have modest benefits in treatment of SDB, although application of this therapy has decreased with the widespread adoption of PAP treatment as the first line of therapy.

Age

Abnormalities of breathing during sleep may present from infancy to senescence. OSA is most commonly first diagnosed in middle age, though sleep-disordered

CLINICAL FOCUS 15-3

OSA and COPD

A 63-year-old man with chronic obstructive pulmonary disease (COPD) and obstructive sleep apnea (OSA) on bilevel-therapy inspiratory positive airway pressure (IPAP) 16 cm H_2O and expiratory positive airway pressure (EPAP) 12 cm H_2O presents for follow-up. The patient was hospitalized 3 months ago for pneumonia and COPD exacerbation and required supplemental oxygen during that admission. Since returning home, he has noted an increase in excessive daytime sleepiness (EDS) and new morning headaches. His vital signs are normal, and O_2 saturation per pulse oximetry is 91%. Data from his bilevel machine indicates good adherence and an apnea–hypopnea index (AHI) of < 5 per hour.

1. What could explain this patient's recurrent EDS and morning headaches?
    This patient is likely experiencing nocturnal hypoxemia. This is most likely to occur and to be more profound during REM sleep. Headache is a common symptom in patients with nocturnal hypoxemia, and morning headaches are common due to the increased proportion of REM sleep in the second half of the night, prior to morning awakening. During REM sleep, accessory respiratory muscles are paralyzed.
2. What simple testing could confirm nocturnal hypoxemia?
    An overnight oximetry recording can be used to confirm nocturnal hypoxemia.

breathing in children is increasingly recognized as an important clinical problem.[12] Children with sleep apnea often present with problems with snoring, accompanied by problems with attention, learning, or behavior rather than excessive daytime sleepiness.[13] Prevalence estimates for SDB in children vary widely, ranging from 0% to 5.7%;[14] some of this variation is most likely due to an absence of consensus concerning definitions for SDB in children. The recommended threshold for clinically significant SDP (AI > 1 per hour) is lower than the thresholds applied in adult populations. Surgical treatment (adenotonsillectomy) is generally considered the first line of treatment in children with sleep apnea and adenotonsillar hypertrophy. Rapid maxillary expansion has been proposed as an alternative, although data supporting the efficacy of this treatment are limited.

In adults, SDB appears to increase in prevalence from ages 40 to 60 and level off in later years. Snoring is common in older adults, but the correlation between the diagnosis of SDB and daytime consequences, such as excessive daytime sleepiness, is weaker, as is the correlation with cardiovascular risk, leading some investigators to suggest that SDB in older adults may represent a different clinical syndrome.[15]

Clinical Presentation

Obstructive sleep apnea, sometimes referred to as *obstructive sleep apnea-hypopnea syndrome*, is a common clinical syndrome that has become increasingly recognized over the past 50 years. Initial descriptions of sleep apnea described the syndrome in the context of obesity hypoventilation or "Pickwickian" syndrome, a constellation of symptoms observed in individuals with obesity, hypersomnolence, hypercapnia, erythrocytosis, and cor pulmonale. The advent of clinical investigation of sleep disorders in the 1970s led to a rapid increase in awareness of the prevalence of breathing problems during sleep. It is now recognized that the Pickwickian syndrome is only one subtype of a family of SDB disorders.

Typical presenting symptoms of patients with SDB include habitual snoring, sleep fragmentation with frequent awakenings during sleep, excessive daytime sleepiness, and impairments in concentration, memory, and mood. Loud snoring is a common feature, and probably the most common symptom leading to clinical referral among patients who sleep with bed partners. Nocturia (waking to urinate); decreased libido; and restless, nonrefreshing sleep are other commonly observed clinical correlates. **Table 15-2** details the common history and physical examination findings associated with OSA.[16] **Figure 15-8** describes the Mallampati classification for airway crowding; class 4 suggests increased incidence of OSA and increased difficulty in intubation.

TABLE 15-2
History and Physical Examination Findings Suggestive of Obstructive Sleep Apnea

History	Physical Examination
Daytime symptoms Dry mouth or sore throat upon awakening Headache upon awakening Excessive sleepiness Impaired concentration Irritability Depression **Nighttime symptoms** Snoring/Snorting Choking Gasping Frequent awakenings Restless sleep Nocturia	Elevated blood pressure Elevated body mass index Retrognathia Micrognathia (small lower jaw) Macroglossia (large tongue) Crowded airway appearance (see Figure 15-8): • Low-hanging soft palate • Enlarged tonsils Large neck circumference

Disease Correlates

Obesity is a well-known risk factor for the development of OSA. Studies have suggested that there may be a bidirectional relationship between obesity and OSA: obesity leads to OSA, and OSA may, in turn, lead to further weight gain due to decreased activity levels and increased appetite.[17] A similar pattern of bidirectional causation may be true for diabetes and OSA. Major predisposing or comorbid conditions, such as obesity and diabetes, combined with the pathophysiologic effects of OSA on various organ systems contribute to the development of other significant medical conditions; the most devastating sequelae belong to the spectrum

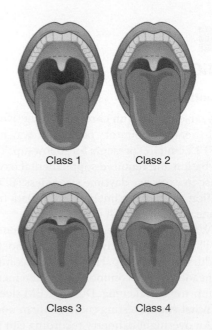

Class 1   Class 2

Class 3   Class 4

FIGURE 15-8 Mallampati classification of airway crowding. Class 1 = normal to Class 4 = severe.

of cardiovascular disease. Hypertension (HTN), coronary heart disease (CHD), congestive heart failure (CHF), arrhythmias, and stroke have all been linked with OSA. Many studies have established an association between HTN, and there is growing evidence in support of a direct causal link of OSA to the development of HTN.[17–19] OSA has been found to have a role in atherogenesis, and thus has been increasingly linked to CHD. In the cohort of patients studied in the Sleep Heart Health Study, an increased likelihood of having CHF was found in those with OSA, independent of other factors.[20] Many types of cardiac arrhythmias have been observed in OSA patients, including atrial fibrillation, atrioventricular blocks, and ventricular tachycardia. Studies have also shown increased risk of stroke in those with OSA.[20] **Box 15-2** lists those disorders that have been linked to sleep apnea.[20]

Polysomnographic Diagnosis and Severity Classification

Diagnosis of OSA is based on a combination of laboratory criteria and clinical symptoms. The severity of SDB is typically characterized by the frequency of sleep-disordered breathing events per hour of sleep. An apnea–hypopnea index (AHI) of five or more events per hour, accompanied by clinical symptoms (excessive daytime sleepiness, impaired cognition, mood disorders, insomnia) or cardiovascular sequelae (hypertension, ischemic heart disease, stroke) meets the threshold for a diagnosis of sleep apnea. An AHI of 15 or more an hour is generally recognized as meeting the criteria for diagnosis in adults regardless of the presence or absence of clinical symptoms. Thresholds for defining apnea severity vary, but an AHI < 15 per hour is generally considered in the mild range, an AHI of ≥ 15 but < 30 per hour is considered moderately severe, and an AHI > 30 per hour is considered severe (**Table 15-3**).

Alternatives to Attended Nocturnal Polysomnography

Increased recognition of OSA has led to rapid growth in referrals for diagnostic evaluations. Attended in-laboratory polysomnography remains the standard for the diagnosis of OSA and the differential diagnosis of other sleep disorders, including movement disorders during sleep and parasomnias. The costs and complexity of attended **polysomnography**, however, coupled with technical innovations in recording technology, has led to increased use of portable monitoring (PM) devices for what is sometimes referred to as home sleep testing (HST) or out-of-center (OOC) testing, as an alternative to attended laboratory-based polysomnography.

The AASM has published clinical guidelines for the use of portable monitors in the diagnosis of sleep apnea.[21] Data acquired from portable monitors can inform the process of arriving at a clinical diagnosis, but it must be utilized within the context of a comprehensive evaluation conducted by a trained sleep medicine specialist. Portable monitors should not be used as "screening tests" for high-risk populations and are most effective in evaluating patients with clinical symptoms of OSA who do not have comorbid medical disorders or symptoms of other comorbid sleep disorders.

Technologies used to assess sleep apnea are generally categorized into four types.[22] Type I devices enable monitoring of seven or more channels by a trained technologist; this corresponds to full nocturnal polysomnography (NPSG), the "gold standard" for clinical sleep assessment. Type II devices provide for the assessment of seven or more channels without the presence of a technologist (unattended polysomnography). Type III devices include a limited set of channels (typically four to seven), usually without EEG; most unattended monitoring is performed with devices corresponding to this category. Type IV devices are monitors with one or two channels using pulse oximetry as one of the signals; data acquired from type IV devices are generally considered insufficient to establish a sleep apnea diagnosis. Unattended portable monitoring with type III portable devices generally includes measures of airflow, oxygenation, and respiratory effort, often with a position sensor, without concurrent measurement of EEG.[23] Because these devices do not measure EEG-defined sleep per se, the indices reported are based on events per hour of recording time, rather than sleep time, and therefore the typical cutoffs used to diagnose sleep apnea (greater than five apneas and hypopneas per hour of recorded sleep) may be underestimated.

BOX 15-2

Disease Sequelae of Obstructive Sleep Apnea

Obesity
Hypertension
Type 2 diabetes
Coronary artery disease
Congestive heart failure
Cardiac arrhythmias
Pulmonary hypertension
Stroke
Metabolic syndrome
Depression
Neurocognitive deficits

TABLE 15-3
Diagnostic Criteria/Severity Levels of Obstructive Sleep Apnea in Adults

	Mild	Moderate	Severe
AHI or RDI*	5 to < 15 events per hour with symptoms	15 to < 30 events per hour	≥ 30 events per hour

AHI, apnea–hypopnea index; RDI, respiratory disturbance index. Note: The RDI is the sum of the AHI and the number of RERAs/per hour. RERA = respiratory effort related arousals (i.e., that are not associated with hypopnea or apnea and occur secondary to respiratory effort trying to overcome obstruction).

It is important to note that the technologies used in portable monitoring are rapidly evolving. Newer devices, such as instrumentation using actigraphy assessment combined with oximetry and the measurement of peripheral arterial tonometry (PAT, Watch-PAT)[24] and devices that use digitized EEG signals in combination with airflow and oximetry[25] show some promise for estimating sleep stages, in addition to respiratory parameters. Devices such as the SleepShirt (Rest Devices, Boston, Mass.) and electrostatic mattresses[26] are examples of technological innovations that seek to provide reliable diagnostic assessment of OSA at low cost with minimally intrusive, or completely nonintrusive, instrumentation.

Treatments

Positional Therapy

Attended nocturnal polysomnograms and unattended home-based sleep studies typically include sensors to monitor sleep position. Positional sleep apnea, conventionally defined as an apnea–hypopnea index in the supine position that is twice or more than the indices derived in other sleep positions, is extremely common. It has been reported that 56% of all patients diagnosed with sleep apnea qualify as having positional sleep apnea.[27] The first therapies proposed for treatment of positional sleep apnea consisted of simple homemade devices, with one to three tennis balls or squash balls placed in a pocket sewn into the midline of the back of the nightshirt. These homemade therapies have been mimicked by low-cost commercial products utilizing shirts or belts with bulky items similar to the tennis ball that act as a positional cue to prevent patients from remaining in a supine posture during sleep.

Positional therapies may be used as a monotherapy for patients who have SDB exclusively in the supine position, or in conjunction with other therapies, such as CPAP or oral appliances. The assessment of sleep position is sometimes overlooked in diagnosis and follow-up, but is oftentimes of critical importance. Some patients treated with CPAP demonstrate radically different pressure requirements in supine versus nonsupine sleep positions, and some patients with severe sleep apnea cannot be treated effectively with CPAP in the supine position but respond well in nonsupine sleep positions. Many patients with position-sensitive

sleep apnea are not aware of the effects of position on the quality of their sleep. It is not unusual for a patient to deny sleeping in the supine position, while objective assessment using either attended or unattended recording demonstrate time asleep in the supine position. The respiratory therapist engaged in follow-up of patients treated with CPAP who remain symptomatic may do well to investigate sleep position in interviewing the patient (in addition to obtaining collateral history from any bed partners) and include a discussion of the role of sleep position and the use of position trainers in treatment planning.

Weight Loss

Approximately 70% of patients with OSA are obese, and the incidence of OSA in obese adults has been estimated at 40%,[28] and subpopulations, such as obese patients with type 2 diabetes, may have prevalence rates as high as 86.6%.[29] The application of intensive lifestyle interventions, emphasizing changes in diet and activity pattern, can be effective in promoting weight loss with concomitant reductions in objective measures of disease severity (AHI) in obese patients with OSA in conjunction with CPAP therapy.[29] Lifestyle counseling is an important component in the comprehensive care of patients with sleep apnea, and addressing lifestyle changes, in conjunction with promoting adherence to CPAP treatment, hold considerable promise for improving long-term outcomes. Bariatric surgery has also been found to be helpful, with one recent review reporting that over 75% of patients undergoing bariatric surgery achieving improvement in indices of OSA severity.[30]

Positive Airway Pressure Devices

Administration of positive airway pressure remains the treatment of choice for patients with OSA. CPAP, autotitrating CPAP, and BiPAP are three ways to mechanically splint the upper airway to prevent its partial or complete collapse during sleep (**Figure 15-9**). Determination of the optimal pressure for PAP therapy is performed in the sleep laboratory.[31] CPAP has been shown to effectively reduce symptoms from sleep fragmentation caused by disordered breathing. The evidence suggests that those with more severe disease show symptom improvement, but a recent study has also shown improved functional outcomes for patients with mild to moderate disease.[32] More important, it

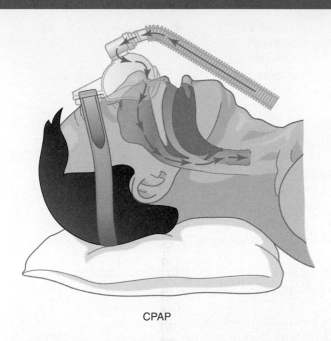

FIGURE 15-9 Continuous positive airway pressure (CPAP).

has demonstrated a positive effect on disease sequelae, such as HTN.[20] Many studies have noted significant impact of CPAP therapy on cardiovascular morbidity and mortality, likely achieved from impacting the diseases that are risk factors for the development and progression of cardiovascular disease. In a recent study, the use of autotitrating CPAP reduced blood pressure, lowered blood lipid levels, and reversed the metabolic syndrome.[33]

Continuous Positive Airway Pressure

Positive airway pressure is most commonly delivered in patients with OSA by CPAP units (Figure 15-10). Pressurized air flows continuously through the upper airway to overcome the critical transmural pressure noted in airway obstruction. Thus, CPAP acts as a pneumatic splint to maintain airway patency throughout the respiratory cycle. It is observed in the sleep lab that the amount of positive pressure needed to overcome partial or full collapse of the airway can vary depending on body position and stage of sleep. For most patients, the optimal pressure for CPAP prescription is based on the pressure required to eliminate apneic and hypopneic episodes during REM stage sleep in the supine position. Box 15-3 lists the recommended practice parameters for the use of CPAP.

Autotitrating Continuous Positive Airway Pressure

A variety of factors ranging from weight changes, nasal congestion, sedative use, sleep stage, and body position can affect CPAP requirements. Self-titrating CPAP units were subsequently developed to attempt to match these changing pressure requirements throughout the night. Sensors allow for continuous airflow and pressure monitoring at the mask level for analysis of breath-related fluctuations. The auto-CPAP unit detects these fluctuations (snoring) based on an algorithm and changes the pressure level accordingly. The pressure is again modified if no further breathing fluctuations are detected. Therapeutic efficacy of autotitrating CPAP administration was found to be equal to constant pressure CPAP.[31] Not all patients, however, are candidates for autotitrating CPAP therapy. Patients with CHF; patients with significant lung disease, such as COPD; patients expected to have nocturnal arterial oxyhemoglobin desaturation due to conditions other than OSA (e.g., obesity hypoventilation syndrome); patients who do not snore (either naturally or as a result of palate surgery); and patients who have central sleep apnea syndromes are not currently candidates for autotitrating CPAP therapy.[34] **Box 15-4** details practice parameters for auto-CPAP use.

Bilevel Positive Airway Pressure (BiPAP)

BiPAP (pronounced "Bi-PAP") therapy allows delivery of two pressure levels, with the expiratory level typically at least 4 cm H_2O lower than the inspiratory level. Patients may theoretically prefer BiPAP to CPAP due to less effort required to breathe against lower expiratory pressures; however, there was no difference found in the average hours of CPAP or BiPAP use over a 12-month observation period of OSA patients.[35] Nevertheless, it is common practice to offer BiPAP therapy to those intolerant of CPAP. BiPAP may have more clinical relevance in OSA patients with concomitant CHF or COPD. Box 15-3 lists the recommended practice parameters for the use of BiPAP.

Adaptive Servoventilators

Certain sleep apnea syndromes, specifically, central sleep apnea and complex sleep apnea, are treated suboptimally with CPAP therapy.[36] Adaptive servoventilation (ASV) uses an automatic, minute ventilation–targeted device that performs breath-to-breath analysis and adjusts its settings accordingly.[37] A constant minute ventilation is maintained as the machine adjusts the airflow per the patient's respiratory effort. There is growing evidence that ASV is more effective than CPAP in relieving abnormal breathing patterns in complex sleep apnea and central sleep apnea syndromes.

Treatment Issues in Positive Airway Pressure Therapy

Although there is no clear definition of adherence, 4 hours of nightly PAP use is typically the acceptable minimum duration to be considered compliant.

BOX 15-3

Practice Parameters for CPAP and BiPAP Use

Recommendations

4.1.1 Treatment with CPAP must be based on a prior diagnosis of OSA established using an acceptable method. (Standard)

4.1.2 CPAP is indicated for the treatment of moderate to severe OSA. (Standard)

4.1.3 CPAP is recommended for the treatment of mild OSA. (Option)

4.1.4 CPAP is indicated for improving self-reported sleepiness in patients with OSA. (Standard)

4.1.5 CPAP is recommended for improving quality of life in patients with OSA. (Option)

4.1.6 CPAP is recommended as an adjunctive therapy to lower blood pressure in hypertensive patients with OSA. (Option)

4.2.1 Full-night, attended polysomnography performed in the laboratory is the preferred approach for titration to determine optimal positive airway pressure; however, split-night, diagnostic-titration studies are usually adequate. (Guideline)

4.3.1 CPAP usage should be objectively monitored to help assure utilization. (Standard)

4.3.2 Close follow-up for PAP usage and problems in patients with OSA by appropriately trained healthcare providers is indicated to establish effective utilization patterns and remediate problems, if needed. This is especially important during the first few weeks of PAP use. (Standard)

4.3.3 The addition of heated humidification is indicated to improve CPAP utilization. (Standard)

4.3.4 The addition of a systematic educational program is indicated to improve PAP utilization. (Standard)

4.4.1 After initial CPAP setup, long-term follow-up for CPAP-treated patients with OSA by appropriately trained health care providers is indicated yearly and as needed to troubleshoot PAP mask, machine, or usage problems. (Option)

4.4.2 CPAP and BiPAP therapy are safe; side effects and adverse events are mainly minor and reversible. (Standard)

4.5.1 While the literature mainly supports CPAP therapy, BiPAP is an optional therapy in some cases where high pressure is needed and the patient experiences difficulty exhaling against a fixed pressure or coexisting central hypoventilation is present. (Guideline)

4.5.2 BiPAP may be useful in treating some forms of restrictive lung disease or hypoventilation syndromes associated with daytime hypercapnia. (Option)

AASM Levels of Recommendations

Standard: This is a generally accepted patient care strategy that reflects a high degree of clinical certainty. The term *standard* generally implies the use of Level I evidence, which directly addresses the clinical issue, or overwhelming Level II evidence.

Guideline: This is a patient care strategy that reflects a moderate degree of clinical certainty. The term *guideline* implies the use of Level II evidence or a consensus of Level III evidence.

Option: This is a patient-care strategy that reflects uncertain clinical use. The term *option* implies inconclusive or conflicting evidence or conflicting expert opinion.

Suggestions vary from 4 hours per night to 6 hours per night to 4 hours per night for 5 nights each week, but it may be best to determine adherence based on the clinical benefits derived by each patient.[38] When 4 hours per night is used as expected adherence to therapy, reports note that 46% to 83% of adults with OSA are nonadherent.[39] Possible barriers to adherence are listed in **Box 15-5**.[40]

Strategies to improve adherence in those with anxiety or depression include pharmacotherapy (e.g., anxiolytics and antidepressants). Use of benzodiazepine anxiolytics at bedtime requires caution, because these agents can further worsen the apneic–hypopneic episodes. In patients with posttraumatic stress disorder (PTSD), daytime sleepiness at baseline was predictive of adherence, whereas nightmares were predictive of

BOX 15-4

Practice Parameters for Auto-CPAP Use

Recommendations

1.1   APAP* is not recommended to diagnose OSA. (Standard)

1.2   Patients with congestive heart failure, significant lung disease such as chronic obstructive pulmonary disease, patients expected to have nocturnal arterial oxyhemoglobin desaturation due to conditions other than OSA (e.g., obesity hypoventilation syndrome), patients who do not snore (either naturally or as a result of palate surgery), and patients who have central sleep apnea syndromes are not currently candidates for APAP titration or treatment. (Standard)

1.3   APAP devices are not currently recommended for split-night titration. (Standard)

1.4   Certain APAP devices may be used during attended titration with polysomnography to identify a single pressure for use with standard CPAP for treatment of moderate to severe OSA. (Guideline)

1.5   Certain APAP devices may be used in an unattended way to determine a fixed CPAP treatment pressure for patients with moderate to severe OSA without significant comorbidities (CHF, COPD, central sleep apnea syndromes, or hypoventilation syndromes). (Option)

1.6   Patients being treated with fixed CPAP on the basis of APAP titration or being treated with APAP must have close clinical follow-up to determine treatment effectiveness and safety. This is especially important during the first few weeks of PAP use. (Standard)

1.7   A reevaluation and, if necessary, a standard attended CPAP titration should be performed if symptoms do not resolve or if the APAP treatment otherwise appears to lack efficacy. (Standard)

AASM Levels of Recommendations

Standard: This is a generally accepted patient care strategy that reflects a high degree of clinical certainty. The term *standard* generally implies the use of Level I evidence, which directly addresses the clinical issue, or overwhelming Level II evidence.

Guideline: This is a patient care strategy that reflects a moderate degree of clinical certainty. The term *guideline* implies the use of Level II evidence or a consensus of Level III evidence.

Option: This is a patient care strategy that reflects uncertain clinical use. The term *option* implies inconclusive or conflicting evidence or conflicting expert opinion.

*APAP, autotitrating positive airway pressure or autotitrating CPAP
Reproduced from: Sharma SK, Agrawal S, Damodaran D, et al. CPAP for the metabolic syndrome in patients with obstructive sleep apnea. *N Engl J Med*. 2011;365:2277–2286.

nonadherence.[40] Medication to mitigate nightmares, such as prazosin, and psychological counseling are important adjunctive therapies for PTSD patients with OSA on CPAP. Patients with dementia may have difficulty remembering when and how to use their equipment; they may be able to adhere better to therapy if social support is available at home. The adherence of patients with poor insight and perception of risks of untreated disease or personality types with negative affectivity can be improved with group cognitive behavioral therapy and standard education.[41]

Patients with physical barriers such as nasal congestion or rhinorrhea may be given a trial of topical nasal corticosteroid sprays or nasal anticholinergic sprays, respectively. Surgical correction of nasal obstruction has also been shown to improve adherence.[42] Mouth or throat dryness is a common complaint. It is important to review medications used by patients, because these may contribute to mouth dryness (e.g., sedating antihistamines, tricyclic antidepressants). Oftentimes, oral mucosal dryness is due to suboptimal use of the humidifier. Retraining and liberal use of a humidifier at home may improve these symptoms.[43] With liberal use of humidification, condensation can occur in the tubing and mask apparatus; some patients may complain of excessive water collection in these areas, which, in turn, adds to their nonadherence. If this occurs, home techniques can be employed to prevent excessive condensation, and heated hoses are available that can be used specifically for that purpose. **Clinical Focus 15-4** describes a patient with nasal congestion associated with the treatment of OSA.

BOX 15-5

Possible Barriers to Adherence of Positive Airway Pressure Therapy

Psychological

Anxiety/claustrophobia
Depression
Posttraumatic stress disorder (PTSD)
Dementia
Personality type
Poor insight to disease
Lack of significant sleepiness

Physical

Nasal congestion or rhinorrhea
Eye irritation from air leaks
Nasal/mouth/throat dryness
Aerophagia (swallowing of air into the gastrointestinal tract)

Device Related

Pressure intolerance
Device type
Ill-fitting mask
Humidification control
Noise

Socioeconomic

Low education level
Low-income status
Lack or loss of health insurance
Lack of social support at home

Healthcare Delivery

Poor equipment support
Poor technical support
Poor follow-up

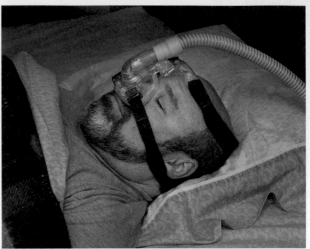

A

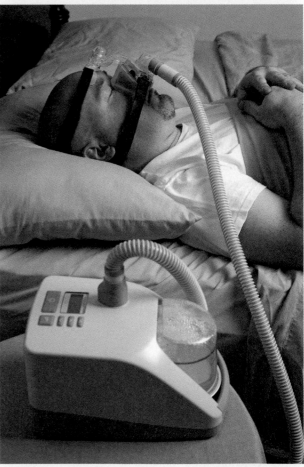

B

FIGURE 15-10 CPAP masks. (A) CPAP mask shown for treatment of obstructive sleep apnea. (B) Patient with CPAP machine for use at night.

(A) © Howard Sandler/ShutterStock, Inc.; (B) © Amy Walters/ShutterStock, Inc.

Device-associated barriers to adherence are challenging to address. Mask issues are best addressed by close follow-up by the clinician and CPAP technician to ensure proper mask type and proper fitting. There are a myriad of brands and types of masks (**Figure 15-10**) that the patient should be allowed to try before giving up on PAP therapy. Strategies to improve tolerance to pressure can include the use of pressure-relief systems. Changing modalities (e.g., switching from CPAP to BiPAP[44]) may improve adherence in some patients, though most of the data suggests that no particular modality is more likely to achieve better adherence.[35] Sometimes, compromising on a lower air pressure with gradual titration (i.e., ramping) to the optimal pressure determined during a formal titration study can be effective in improving adherence.

Initial and continued patient education is important in achieving and maintaining adherence. Regular visits

Improving Adherence to Treatment

A 49-year-old man with obstructive sleep apnea (OSA) started on therapy with continuous positive airway pressure (CPAP) at 14 cm H_2O pressure presents for his 2-week follow-up. Patient complains of increased nasal congestion and occasional awakenings due to water condensation on his face.

1. How can you improve nasal congestion associated with CPAP?

   Nasal congestion is a common complaint among CPAP users. Ensure the use of heated humidification in conjunction with CPAP. The application of nasal saline nightly can provide relief. Additionally, nasal steroids can also be beneficial.

2. How can you reduce the potential for water condensation?

   Heated humidification is routinely used with CPAP. Water condensation within the tubing and/or mask is a common problem. Increasing the heat may help, but often cold tubing is the problem. When the warm air from the humidifier travels through the cold tubing, condensation is likely to occur. Tubing insulators can be purchased or made from socks. Heated tubing is available as an optional feature for most CPAP units and will usually resolve the problem.

with the CPAP clinic to download compliance data will also aid the sleep clinic team in helping the patient become successful with CPAP therapy.

Oral Appliances

Oral appliances (OA) have been used for many years in the management of snoring, and more recently have gained popularity in the treatment of OSA. A number of OAs have been tested and marketed. Most of the devices are fitted by a dentist and inserted by the patient into the oral cavity prior to sleep. The most popular devices are splints designed to advance the position of the mandible relative to the maxillary teeth (**Figure 15-11**). OAs have gained attention and popularity as alternatives to CPAP for patients who have difficulty adapting to CPAP therapy for long-term treatment. Adherence rates for OAs have been reported to be better than CPAP, with patients wearing the devices on 77% of nights in the first year (per self-report) after initiating treatment.[45] Although OA therapy appears to be accepted by many patients who have difficulty tolerating CPAP, it does not appear to be as effective as CPAP in terms of reducing the overall AHI or reducing indices of oxygen desaturation. OAs are currently recommended as therapeutic options for patients with mild to moderately severe OSA, but are generally not considered appropriate for patients with severe OSA, severe daytime sleepiness, or severe nocturnal O_2 desaturations.

Oral appliances have been developed using both fixed-position designs and adjustable positioners. Although data evaluating outcomes with objective measures, including polysomnography, suggest both designs can be effective, reviews of the evidence suggest that adjustable devices may produce greater reductions

in the frequency of sleep-disordered breathing events and be associated with more successful outcomes.[46]

Nasal Valves

Challenges in achieving patient adherence in the use of CPAP therapy continues to motivate the search for alternative approaches to treatment. Provent Nasal Therapy (Theravent, Inc., Belmont, CA.) has been developed as a therapeutic alternative. The device consists of a one-way valve that is inserted into the nares and secured by means of a strip of adhesive material. The device permits the free flow of air on inspiration, while generating expiratory flow resistance on exhalation. The valve thus generates expiratory positive airway pressure (EPAP) without the use of any external power source, hypothetically stabilizing the pharynx

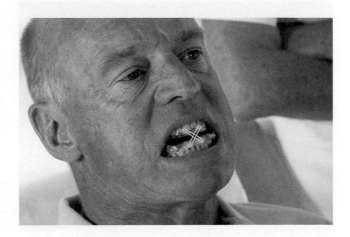

FIGURE 15-11 TAP3©.

© CHASSENET/age fotostock

and preventing upper airway collapse. Data evaluating the efficacy of this treatment are limited, but industry-supported studies have shown reduction in the average AHI from an average of 24.5 events per hour at baseline to 13.5 per hour at the initiation of treatment, and 15.5 per hour following 30 nights of home use, without any significant adverse effects.[47] The reduction in AHI for these patients did not appear to be associated with any normalization in the parameters used to measure sleep continuity or sleep architecture. The evidence to date suggests that this treatment may be considered for patients with mild to moderate OSA who are unable to tolerate CPAP, but data concerning efficacy have not established nasal valves as a first line of treatment (**Figure 15-12**).

Surgical Interventions

Several surgical interventions have been proposed for treatment of OSA. Surgery is not a first-line therapy for the treatment of OSA in adults. All patients with mild to moderately severe OSA should be offered therapy with PAP and oral appliances before considering surgery. If the patient does not tolerate or refuses these therapies, then surgical intervention can be considered.

Tracheostomy, either permanent or temporary, creates a surgical bypass of the upper airway and may provide immediate relief for upper airway obstruction. Tracheostomy may be considered in emergent situations for patients with serious medical complications, including cor pulmonale, uncontrolled hypertension, or life-threatening arrhythmias. However, tracheostomy is rarely considered acceptable by patients as a lifelong treatment.

Uvulopalatopharyngoplasty (UPPP) involves the removal of redundant tonsillar tissue, resection of the uvula, and remodeling of the soft palate. UPPP was first introduced in the United States by Fujita and colleagues in 1981.[48] Initial reports of high rates of success with UPPP proved overly optimistic; subsequent reviews aggregating multiple case series have estimated the overall success rate at approximately 40%.[47–49]

Laser-assisted uvuloplasty (LAUP) is an office-based procedure in which a CO_2 laser is used as an alternative to conventional surgery to remodel the uvula and soft palate. The procedure appears to have limited value in treating OSA, and its application now is primarily restricted to treatment of snoring and mild sleep-disordered breathing.

Radiofrequency tissue ablation (RTA) uses a radiofrequency probe inserted into soft tissue structures in the upper airway. The application of low-frequency radio waves using this procedure can induce fibrotic changes, resulting in a shrinking and stiffening of soft tissue. RTA is currently used primarily to treat snoring or in combination with other surgical approaches.

Palatal implants (Pillar procedure) have been proposed as a minimally invasive alternative to UPPP and LAUP. The procedure involves the surgical insertion of three strips of polyester material into the soft palate to increase its stiffness and reduce upper airway vibration and collapse. A meta-analytic review found that palatal implants are associated with reduced snoring and decreases in AHI scores in patients with mild to moderately severe OSA,[50] although it is unclear if the size of the effects is clinically meaningful. One placebo-controlled investigation found that a clinically meaningful reduction in the AHI was observed in only 26% of patients treated with palatal implants, as compared to10% of patients in the control group.[51]

Surgical treatment procedures aimed at remodeling the soft palate are often thought to fail because patients may experience obstruction at the base of the tongue. Several surgical approaches have been proposed to address this problem. Genioglossus advancement-hyoid myotomy and suspension (GAHMS) places tension on the tongue musculature and can prevent the retroplacement of the tongue during sleep. Mandibular osteotomy, alone or in combination with advancement of the maxilla (maxillomandibular advancement, MMA), addresses the problem of obstruction at the base of the tongue. Although individual surgical approaches to treatment seem to show modest success rates at best, surgical protocols involving phased, multiple procedures have reported higher success rates.[52]

Nasal reconstruction (septoplasty, alar valve or alar rim reconstruction, turbinectomy) is generally not effective as a treatment for OSA, but it may reduce mouth breathing, relieve snoring, and improve acceptability and tolerability of PAP therapy. Adenotonsillectomy is generally considered a first-line treatment for children with adenotonsillar hypertrophy, but it is less likely to be of clinical benefit in adults. An alternative surgical approach for obese patients with OSA is bariatric surgery. OSA is not an indication for bariatric surgery, but bariatric surgery can improve and

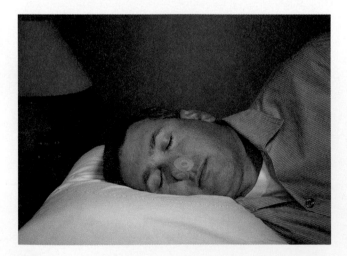

FIGURE 15-12 Provent ©.

even normalize the AHI, especially in morbidly obese patients. It is important to note that OSA can recur several years after surgery even when there has not been significant weight regain.[53]

In conclusion, tracheostomy is very effective in relieving airway obstruction but should only be considered in patients with severe OSA when other treatment options have failed, the patient refuses other therapies, or it is considered clinically urgent.[54] Success rates for other surgical procedures have generally been modest, although surgical protocols involving multiple procedures, addressing multiple possible sites of obstruction, may yield better results. CPAP or other PAP therapies remain the first choice of treatment for most adult patients. Surgical treatment of OSA is generally to be considered only if PAP treatment and other noninvasive therapies (oral appliances) cannot be tolerated. Decisions to undergo surgical treatment require a careful assessment and full discussion of possible risks as well as benefits.

Other Sleep Disorders

Disorders of breathing during sleep share symptoms that overlap with other sleep disorders, and comorbid sleep disorders may complicate the management of sleep-disordered breathing. *Narcolepsy* is a disorder associated with severe excessive daytime sleepiness. It needs to be considered as part of the differential diagnosis in patients presenting with a complaint of hypersomnolence. *Insomnia* is a highly prevalent sleep problem. Many patients with sleep-disordered breathing will present with complaints of difficulties initiating or maintaining sleep. Patients with sleep-disordered breathing and comorbid symptoms of insomnia are often prescribed sedative hypnotics prior to referral for diagnostic evaluation, and the use of benzodiazepines for the treatment of insomnia may aggravate sleep-disordered breathing and complicate the diagnosis and management of OSA. *Restless legs syndrome* (RLS) and *periodic limb movements during sleep disorder* (PLMD) may present with restless sleep and excessive daytime sleepiness. Patients with OSA who experience persistent motor restlessness during sleep despite effective treatment of their sleep-disordered breathing with CPAP need to be evaluated for RLS and possible PLMD. Parasomnias such as sleep terrors and confusional arousals from sleep may be observed in patients with severe sleep apnea who experience repetitive arousals and chronic partial sleep deprivation, and evaluation for possible sleep-disordered breathing is an important consideration in the differential diagnosis of patients presenting with parasomnia complaints.

Key Points

▶ Sleep-disordered breathing requires careful assessment, diagnosis, and treatment.

▶ Sleep in adults is composed of two distinct stages: rapid eye movement (REM) and non-REM (NREM) sleep. NREM sleep is further subdivided into three distinct substages.

▶ In normal adults, NREM sleep precedes REM sleep, and these two stages repeat in a cycle every 90 minutes.

▶ Sleep stages in infants and children differ from the stages observed in adults.

▶ Sleep-disordered breathing disrupts the normal progression of sleep stages.

▶ Sleep apnea may be classified as obstructive, central, or mixed.

▶ OSA is characterized by episodes of apnea or hypopnea to upper airway obstruction during sleep.

▶ Obstructive sleep apnea (OSA) is defined as a cessation of airflow for 10 or more seconds with evidence of a sustained inspiratory effort on the part of the patient.

▶ Central sleep apnea is the cessation of both airflow and inspiratory efforts for at least 10 seconds.

▶ Hypopnea is defined as a decrease in airflow of at least 30% for at least 10 seconds accompanied by arterial oxygen desaturation of at least 3%.

▶ Respiratory effort-related arousals (REFRAs) are a form of sleep-disordered breathing not associated with oxygen desaturation.

▶ The current "gold standard" for diagnosing sleep apnea is an overnight sleep study attended by a trained technologist, although the use of portable technologies for home sleep testing has increased.

▶ Brief apneas are normal in infants and children

▶ Cheyne-Stokes breathing (CSB) is the most common form of central sleep apnea.

▶ Patients with brain tumors, stroke, neuromuscular disorders and those receiving narcotics may exhibit central hypoventilation without CSB.

▶ Complex sleep apnea refers to the development of central apnea or hypopnea during the treatment of OSA using positive airway pressure (e.g., CPAP or BiPAP).

▶ COPD patients with OSA are said to have overlap syndrome; CPAP with supplemental oxygen (as needed) is the first line of therapy.

▶ Typical symptoms of sleep-disordered breathing include snoring, frequent awakenings, excessive daytime sleepiness, and impairments in memory, mood, and concentration.

▶ Risk factors associated with sleep-disordered breathing include age, gender, obesity, upper airway or craniofacial abnormalities, and certain medical conditions (e.g., CHF, COPD, stroke).

▶ Pickwickian syndrome is one subtype of sleep-disordered breathing that combines obesity, hypersomulance, hypercapnea, increased RBCs, and cor pulmonale.

▶ An apnea–hypopnea index (AHI) of five or more events per hour combined with clinical symptoms allows for the diagnosis of sleep apnea.

▶ Patients who have sleep-disordered breathing only in the supine position may be candidates for positional therapy.

▶ Positive airway pressure (e.g., CPAP or BiPAP) remains the treatment of choice for patients with OSA.

▶ OSA in obese patients may improve with weight loss.

▶ Auto-titrating CPAP and adaptive servoventilators provide alternatives to traditional CPAP.

▶ Causes of nonadherence to prescribed positive airway pressure therapy should be investigated and corrected, if possible.

▶ Other possible treatments for OSA include oral appliances, nasal valves, and surgical interventions.

▶ Other sleep disorders include narcolepsy, insomnia, restless legs syndrome (RLS), periodic limb movements during sleep disorder (PLMD), and parasomnias (e.g., sleep terrors).

References

1. Hospenthal MAC, Adams S. Obstructive sleep apnea in chronic obstructive pulmonary disease: The overlap syndrome. *Curr Respir Med Rev.* 2012;8(2):131–136.

2. Berry RB, Brooks R, Gamaldo CE, et al. *The AASM Manual for the Scoring of Sleep and Associated Events: Rules, Terminology, and Technical Specifications*, Version 2.0. Darien, IL: American Academy of Sleep Medicine; 2012.

3. Gilmartin GS, Daly RW, Thomas RJ. Recognition and management of complex sleep-disordered breathing. *Curr Opin Pulm Med.* 2005;11(6):485–493.

4. American Academy of Sleep Medicine. *International Classification of Sleep Disorders, 2nd ed. Diagnostic and Coding Manual.* Westchester, IL: American Academy of Sleep Medicine; 2005.

5. Harrison TR, King CE, Calhoun JA, et al. Congestive heart failure. Cheyne–Stokes respiration as the cause of paroxysmal nocturnal dyspnea at the onset of sleep. *Arch Intern Med.* 1934;53(6):891–910.

6. Hanly PJ, Zuberi-Khokhar NS. Increased mortality associated with Cheyne–Stokes respiration in patients with congestive heart failure. *Am J Respir Crit Care Med.* 1996;153(1):272–276.

7. Young T, Palta M, Leder, R et al. The occurrence of sleep-disordered breathing among middle-aged adults. *N Engl J Med.* 1993;328:1230–1235.

8. Young T, Peppard PE, Gottlieb DJ. Epidemiology of obstructive sleep apnea. *Am J Respir Crit Care Med.* 2001;165(9):1271–1239.

9. Peppard PE, Young T, Palta M, et al. Longitudinal study of moderate weight change and sleep-disordered breathing. *JAMA.* 2000;284(23):3015–3021.

10. Sandblom RE, Matsumoto AM, Schoene RB, et al. Obstructive sleep apnea syndrome induced by testosterone administration. *N Engl J Med.* 1983;308(9):508–510.

11. Young T, Finn L, Austin D, et al. Menopausal status and sleep disordered breathing in the Wisconsin Sleep Cohort Study. *Am J Respir Crit Care Med.* 2003;167(9):1181–1185.

12. Mitchell RB. Sleep-disordered breathing in children: Are we underestimating the problem? *Eur Respir J.* 2007;25(2):216–217.

13. Lal C, Strange C, Bachman D. Neurocognitive impairment in obstructive sleep apnea. *Chest.* 2012;141(6):1601–1610.

14. Marcus CL, Brooks LJ, Draper KA, et al. Diagnosis and management of childhood obstructive sleep apnea syndrome. *Pediatrics.* 2012;130(3):e714–e755.

15. Young T. Sleep-disordered breathing in older adults. Is it a condition distinct from that in middle-aged adults? *Sleep.* 1996;19(7):529–530.

16. Mannarino MR, Di Filippo F, Pirro M. Obstructive sleep apnea syndrome. *Eur J Intern Med.* 2012;23(7):586–593.

17. Romero-Corral A, Caples DO, Lopez-Jimenez F, Somers VK. Interactions between obesity and obstructive sleep apnea: Implications for treatment. *Chest.* 2010;137(3):711–719.

18. Pack AI, Gislason T. Obstructive sleep apnea and cardiovascular disease: A perspective and future directions. *Prog Cardiovasc Dis.* 2009;51(5):434–451.

19. Marin JM, Agusti A, Villar I, et al. Association between treated and untreated obstructive sleep apnea and risk of hypertension. *JAMA.* 2012;307(20):2169–2176.

20. Mannarino MR, Di Filippo FD, Pirro M. Obstructive sleep apnea syndrome. *Eur J Int Med.* 2012;23(7):586–593.

21. Collop NK, Anderson WM, Boehlechke B, et al. Clinical guidelines for the use of unattended portable monitors in the diagnosis of obstructive sleep apnea in adult patients. *J Clin Sleep Medicine.* 2007;3(7):737–747.

22. Standards of Practice Committee of the American Sleep Disorders Association. Practice parameters for the use of portable recording in the assessment of obstructive sleep apnea. *Sleep.* 1994;17(4):372–377.

23. Collop NA, Tracy SL, Kapur V et al. Obstructive sleep apnea devices for out-of-center (OOC) testing: Technology evaluation. *J Clin Sleep Med.* 2011;7(5):531–548.

24. Bar A, Pillar G, Dvir I, et al. Evaluation of a portable device based on peripheral arterial tone for unattended home sleep studies. *Chest.* 2003;123(3):695–703.

25. Westbrook PR, Levendowski DJ, Cvetinovic M, et al. Description and validation of the apnea risk evaluation system: A novel method to diagnose sleep apnea-hypopnea in the home. *Chest.* 2005;128(4):2166–2175.

26. Kirjavainen T, Polo O, McNamara S, et al. Respiratory challenge induces high frequency spiking on the static charge sensitive bed (SCSB). *Eur Respir J.* 1996;9(9):1810–1815.

27. Richard W, Kox D, den Herder C, et al. The role of sleep position in obstructive sleep apnea syndrome. *Eur Arch Otorhinolaryngol.* 2006;263(10):946–950.

28. Vgontzas AN, Tan TL, Bixler EO, et al. Sleep apnea and sleep disruption in obese patients. *Arch Intern Med.* 1994;154(15):1705–1711.

29. Thomasouli M, Brady EM, Davies MJ, et al. The impact of diet and lifestyle management strategies for obstructive sleep apnoea in adults: A systematic review and meta-analysis of randomized controlled trials. *Sleep Breath.* 2013;17(3):925–935.

30. Sarkhosh K, Switzer NJ, El-Hadi M, et al. The impact of bariatric surgery on obstructive sleep apnea: A systematic review. *Obesity Surg.* 2013;23(3):414–423.

31. Ficker JH, Wiest GH, Lehnert G, Wiest B, Hahn EG. Evaluation of an auto-CPAP device for treatment of obstructive sleep apnea. *Thorax.* 1998;53(7):643–648.

32. Weaver TE, Mancini C, Maislin G, et al. Continuous positive airway pressure treatment of sleepy patients with milder obstructive sleep apnea: Results of the CPAP Apnea Trial North American Program (CATNAP) randomized clinical trial. *Am J Respir Crit Care Med.* 2012;186(7):677–683.

33. Sharma SK, Agrawal S, Damodaran D, et al. CPAP for the metabolic syndrome in patients with obstructive sleep apnea. *N Engl J Med.* 2011;365(24):2277–2286.

34. Morgenthaler TI, Aurora RN, Brown T, et al. Practice parameters for the use of autotitrating continuous positive airway pressure devices for titrating pressures and treating adult patients with obstructive sleep apnea syndrome: An update for 2007. An American Academy of Sleep Medicine report. *Sleep.* 2008;31(1):141–147.

35. Reeves-Hoche MK, Hddgel DW, Meck R, et al. Continuous versus bilevel positive airway pressure for obstructive sleep apnea. *Am J Respir Crit Care Med.* 1995;151(2 Pt 1):443–449.

36. Allam JS, Olson EJ, Gay PC, Morgenthaler TI. Efficacy of adaptive servoventilation in treatment of complex and central sleep apnea syndromes. *Chest.* 2007;132(6):1839–1846.

37. Cassina T, Chiolero R, Mauri R, Revelly JP. Clinical experience with adaptive support ventilation for fast-track cardiac surgery. *J Cardiothoracic Vasc Anesth.* 2003;17(5):571–575.

38. Archbold KH, Parthasarathy S. Adherence to positive airway pressure therapy in adults. *Curr Opin Pulm Med.* 2009;15(6):585–590.

39. Weaver TE, Grunstein RR. Adherence to continuous positive airway pressure therapy: The challenge to effective treatment. *Proc Am Thorac Soc.* 2008;5(2):173–178.

40. El-Soh AA, Ayyar L, Akinnusi M, Relia S, Akinnusi O. Positive airway pressure adherence in veterans with posttraumatic stress disorder. *Sleep.* 2010;33(11):1495–1500.

41. Richards D, Bartlett DJ, Wong K, Malouff J, Grunstein RR. Increased adherence to CPAP with a group cognitive behavioral treatment intervention: A randomized trial. *Sleep.* 2007;30(5):635–640.

42. Friedman M, Soans R, Joseph N, Kakodkar S, Friedman J. The effect of multilevel upper airway surgery on continuous positive airway pressure therapy in obstructive sleep apnea/hypopnea syndrome. *Laryngoscope.* 2009;119(1):193–196.

43. Ryan S, Doherty LS, Nolan GM, McNicholas WT. Effects of heated humidification and topical steroids on compliance, nasal symptoms, and quality of life in patients with obstructive sleep apnea syndrome using nasal continuous positive airway pressure. *J Clin Sleep Med.* 2009;5(5):422–427.

44. Ballard RD, Gay PC, Strollo PJ. Intervention to improve compliance in sleep apnea patients previously non-compliant with continuous positive airway pressure. *J Clin Sleep Med.* 2007;3(7):706–712.

45. Ferguson KA, Cartwright R, Rogers R, Schmidt-Nowara W. Oral appliances for snoring and obstructive sleep apnea: A review. *Sleep.* 2006;29(2):244–262.

46. Lettieri CJ, Paolino N, Eliasson AH, Shah AA, Holley AB. Comparison of adjustable and fixed oral appliances for the treatment of obstructive sleep apnea. *J Clin Sleep Med.* 2011;7(5):439–445.

47. Rosenthal L, Massie CA, Dolan DC, et al. A multicenter, prospective study of a novel nasal EPAP device in the treatment of obstructive sleep apnea: Efficacy and 30-day adherence. *J Clin Sleep Med.* 2009;5(6):532–537.

48. Fujita S, Conway W, Zorick F, Roth T. Surgical correction of anatomic abnormalities of sleep apneas syndrome: Uvulopalatopharyngoplasty. *Otolaryngol Head Neck Surg.* 1981;89(6):923–934.

49. Sher A, Schechtman K, Piccirillo JF. The efficacy of surgical modifications of the upper airway in adults with obstructive sleep apnea syndrome. *Sleep.* 1996;19(2):156–177.

50. Choi JH, Kim SN, Cho JH. Efficacy of the Pillar implant in the treatment of snoring and mild-to-moderate obstructive sleep apnea: A meta-analysis. *Laryngoscope.* 2013;123(1):269–276.

51. Steward DL, Huntley TC, Woodson BT, Surdulescu V. Palate implants for obstructive sleep apnea: Multi-institution, randomized, placebo-controlled study. *Otolaryngol Head Neck Surg.* 2008;139(4):506–510.

52. Riley RW, Powell NB, Guilleminault C. Obstructive sleep apnea syndrome: A review of 306 consecutively treated surgical patients. *Otolaryngol Head Neck Surg.* 1993;108(2):117–135.

53. Morgenthaler TI, Kapen S, Lee-Chiong T, et al. Practice parameters for the medical therapy of obstructive sleep apnea. *Sleep.* 2006;29(8):1031–1035.

54. Aurora N, Casey K, Kristo D, et al. Practice parameters for the surgical modifications of the upper airway for obstructive sleep apnea in adults. *Sleep.* 2010;33(10):1408–1413.

© VikaSuh/ShutterStock, Inc.

CHAPTER OUTLINE

CHAPTER OBJECTIVES

1. Describe the significance of each element of the perinatal history.
2. Describe the methods used to estimate the gestational age of the fetus and of the newborn at the time of delivery.
3. Discuss the purpose for each specific fetal diagnostic test and any associated potential procedural risks.
4. Explain methods to measure lung maturity of the fetus.
5. Describe typical fetal heart rate and patterns and the three-tiered system used to determine care.
6. List the tests used to determine fetal well-being.
7. Explain alterations of the amniotic fluid and how it influences the risk assessment of the fetus.
8. Calculate the estimated date of delivery (EDD).
9. Identify the purpose and components of the APGAR score and interpret the results.
10. Summarize maternal, fetal, and neonatal effects of common infections.
11. Describe neonatal physical assessment techniques.
12. Recognize abnormal neonatal assessment findings and list possible causes.
13. Understand the dynamics of the neonatal cardiovascular system.
14. Recognize physical and developmental differences and approaches to children of different ages.
15. Describe the pediatric assessment to include history and physical examination and diagnostic testing.
16. Recognize deviations from age-related pediatric assessment findings and explain possible causes.
17. List the types, purposes, and key values for neonatal and pediatric diagnostic and laboratory tests.

KEY TERMS

amniocentesis	Grey Turner's sign
amniotic fluid volume (AFV)	grunting
APGAR score	guarding
apnea	head bobbing
bradypnea	human chorionic
capillary blood gases	gonadotropin (hCG)
chest wall retractions	last menstrual period (LMP)
contraction stress test (CST)	lecithin/sphingomyelin ratio (L/S ratio)
crackles	Naegele's rule
date of conception	nasal flaring
Doppler ultrasound	new Ballard score (NBS)
Down syndrome	phosphatidylglycerol (PG)
Dubowitz scoring system	skin testing
fetal heart rate (FHR)	spina bifida
fetal movement	startle reflex
fetal nonstress test (NST)	stridor
fetal quickening	surfactant-to-albumin ratio (TDx FLM II)
foam stability index (FSI)	sweat chloride test
functional residual capacity (FRC)	transcutaneous monitoring
gestational age	transillumination
grasp reflex	triple test
gravida	type II alveolar cells

Overview

This chapter provides an introduction to the assessment of neonatal and pediatric patients, with a focus on factors affecting the cardiopulmonary system. Assessment of the fetus is described to include fetal and maternal history, estimates of gestational age, and assessment of fetal well-being and lung maturity. Assessment of the newborn is then reviewed to include vital signs, physical examination, and laboratory assessment. Pediatric patient assessment is then described to include history and physical examination, diagnostic imaging and laboratory testing, and common abnormalities.

Introduction to Neonatal/Pediatric Assessment

The assessment of the newborn or pediatric patient is different from that of an adult. When a child is sick, the child often does not act the same as an adult would with a similar illness; treating pediatric patients as if they were "little adults" can cause unanticipated problems. In addition, many healthcare providers who do not routinely work with infants and children may be intimidated by a perception of their fragile nature. Being sick and in a healthcare environment surrounded by strangers can frighten an already stressed child, which can make the evaluation more difficult.

Infants and children include a broad spectrum of ages. For our purposes, we will consider infants as those 0 to 12 months of age. *Neonates* are infants 0 to 28 days of age; *young infants* are 29 to 90 days old. *Toddlers* are children 1 to 3 years of age. Children 3 to 5 years of age are *preschool age*, and children 6 to 12 years are *school age*. *Adolescents* are those children 13 to 18 years of age though some (e.g., WHO) define adolescence as between ages 10 and 19.

This chapter is designed to help the respiratory care clinician develop the assessment skills needed for the evaluation of neonatal and pediatric patients. Discussion starts with the assessment of the fetus and continues with newborn and pediatric patient evaluation, including physical and diagnostic examinations and interpretation of results.

Assessment of the Fetus

History

The first step in an assessment is obtaining a patient history. The mother's demographic information, past obstetric history, and general medical history should be reviewed. Access to the obstetric and gynecologic (OB/GYN) medical records can also provide valuable historical information. The initial history should include the date of the woman's **last menstrual period (LMP)**; estimated date of confinement (EDC; i.e., when delivery is expected); history of live births (both premature and full term); and history of abortion, if any. The exact **date of conception** may not be known, but can be estimated as 11 to 21 days after the first day of the LMP in women with a regular menstrual cycle. A normal menstrual cycle is 28 days with fertilization most likely on day 14, although many women do not have a regular 28-day cycle.

Typically, the obstetric history is described in terms of whether this is a first pregnancy or one of multiple pregnancies. The term **gravida** refers to the number of pregnancies. For example, gravida one (G1) indicates that it is a woman's first pregnancy, whereas G3 would indicate a woman who has been pregnant three times. The term *para* (P) refers to the number of viable live births; therefore, P2 would refer to a woman who has had two live births. Abortion is noted as *Ab*. Abortion can be further divided into spontaneous abortions (i.e., miscarriages), which are noted as *SAb*, or therapeutic abortions, which are noted as *TAb*. A woman with a pregnancy history listed as G1, P1, Ab0 would have a past obstetric history of one pregnancy resulting in one live birth and no history of abortion. It is also important to note if the fetus or previous children were conceived naturally or by in vitro fertilization. A review of the mother's prenatal care record is important in evaluating the mother and fetus, providing patient education, and identifying risk factors that may lead to problems during pregnancy or following delivery.[1]

The mother's general medical history is also important. It is important to identify prior health issues, such as lung disease (e.g., asthma), cardiovascular disease (e.g., hypertension), or metabolic disease (e.g., obesity [specifically, excess abdominal fat], anorexia, malnutrition, or disorders of lipid metabolism), that may affect the pregnancy. *Metabolic syndrome* refers to obesity, hypertension, high cholesterol, and elevated blood glucose levels. This syndrome can predispose patients to cardiovascular disease, stroke, kidney disease, and diabetes. Diabetic mothers are at increased risk for premature delivery. Infants born prematurely have higher incidents of respiratory distress syndrome (RDS) and other health-related issues. A history of infectious disease and its treatment should be documented, because infections may be passed from the mother to the fetus. All medications should also be recorded, as well as use of alcohol, tobacco (e.g., cigarette smoking), or illicit drugs. A large number of drugs, medications, and chemicals are reproductive toxins.[1] These range from certain antibiotics (e.g., trimethoprim) to antidepressants and anticonvulsants; pregnancy risk tables for medications are available from the Food and Drug Administration (FDA).[1] Environmental factors that may have an adverse effect on the fetus should be recorded to include occupational hazards, lead exposure, exposure to pesticides, or exposure to mercury.[1] Lead is found in some older buildings that have lead-based paint. Consumption of fish known to have high mercury levels (e.g., shark, swordfish, king mackerel) should be avoided.[1]

Previous live births should be noted to include whether births were premature or if there were any problems with the newborn. If a previous child was diagnosed with a genetic disorder or syndrome, it may increase the potential risk of the fetus developing the same condition. The family history is also important because it may reveal genetic disorders (e.g., cystic fibrosis, sickle cell disease, Down syndrome) in family members that may place the fetus at risk. Social factors of concern include domestic abuse, substance abuse, or conditions in the home that may put the mother or child in danger.

Physical examination of the mother should include measurement of vital signs, height, weight, body mass index (BMI), and other routine physical assessment procedures.[1] Laboratory examinations should include a standard panel of tests as well as any additional tests suggested by specific risk factors.[1] Diagnostic screening for specific genetic disorders (e.g., cystic fibrosis) may be performed, as indicated.

Gestational Age

Gestational age should be estimated because it provides valuable information to enable proper preparation to care for the newborn, if born prematurely. Gestational age can also guide decisions regarding possible induction of labor in postterm situations. Obtaining gestational age can be straightforward when women know the date when the fetus was conceived. If they are unsure, other ways to assess gestational age include menstrual cycle history, physical examination, and use of ultrasound imaging. The use of fetal ultrasound imaging is helpful because the length of the fetus correlates with the age of the fetus.[2] Fetal ultrasound examinations are often performed during the first trimester in order to estimate gestational age and provide early diagnosis of fetal congenital malformations.[3]

Most newborns delivered at less than 32 weeks have premature lungs and surfactant deficiency. These newborns are at the highest risk of developing RDS. Newborns delivered between 32 and 39 weeks also may develop RDS or other complications. **Box 16-1** lists common complications associated with preterm birth.

Fetal Lung Maturity

Tests to measure lung maturity are important because proper care can be provided quickly and accurately when this information is known. The following paragraphs describe a variety of tests used to assess fetal lung maturity.

Human chorionic gonadotropin (hCG) is a hormone produced by the mother after conception. It is found in the mother's blood or urine and is measured to confirm pregnancy as well as provide some indication of gestational age. hCG levels increase as the fetus develops (see **Table 16-1**).[4] Levels peak around weeks 8 and 9 and then decrease.[4] Measurement of hCG is sometimes combined with measurement of other blood hormones and alpha-fetoprotein (AFP) in order to detect certain birth defects (e.g., spina bifida, Down syndrome, anencephaly). When these three substances—AFP, hCG, and estriol (uE3)—are measured, it is referred to as a **triple test**. With the addition of a fourth hormone, inhibin A, it is known as a *quad test*.[5] It is important to keep in mind that these tests are used to screen if the mother is at risk of carrying a baby with a genetic disorder; it is not a confirmation of a genetic disorder.

BOX 16-1

Complications of Premature Birth

Full term is birth occurring from 38 to 42 weeks of gestation. Infants born before 37 weeks of gestation are considered to be preterm, or premature. Premature birth has a number of short- and long-term complications.

Short-term complications:

- Respiratory distress syndrome (RDS)
- Retinopathy of prematurity
- Patent ductus arteriosis (PDA)
- Bronchopulmonary dysplasia
- Sepsis
- Intraventricular cerebral hemorrhage
- Gastrointestinal tract infection and inflammation (e.g., necrotizing enterocolitis)

Long-term complications

- Chronic health issues
- Growth impairment
- Frequent hospitalization
- Impaired cognitive skills
- Neurologic problems
- Impaired lung function

Data from: Mandy GT. Long-term complications of the premature infant. In: *UpToDate*, Basow DS (ed.), UpToDate, Waltham, MA, 2013; Mandy GT. Short-term complications of the premature infant. In: *UpToDate*, Basow DS (ed.), UpToDate, Waltham, MA, 2013.

Amniocentesis is an invasive procedure in which the clinician obtains a fluid sample from the amniotic sac for analysis. A long, thin needle is inserted through the mother's abdomen into the uterus and amniotic sac and a small sample of amniotic fluid is withdrawn. The use of ultrasound imaging to guide amniocentesis reduces the risk of damaging the fetus or inducing a miscarriage.[6] Amniocentesis is used to detect birth defects in at-risk patients as well as for estimating lung maturation. The fluid obtained may be tested to include measurement of alpha-fetoprotein (AFP) because AFP increases with certain genetic abnormalities. Amniocentesis for genetic studies is typically performed between weeks 15 and 17 of gestation.[7] Amniocentesis for the purpose of determining fetal lung maturity is typically performed after week 32, but not at week 40 or later.[7] *Full term* is generally considered to be 38 to 42 weeks; babies born before 37 weeks are *premature* (or *preterm*). Infants born at 37 or 38 weeks are sometimes considered *early term,* whereas infants born after 42 weeks are considered *postterm.*[8] In the past,

TABLE 16-1
Pregnancy Status Based on Serum Human Chronic Gonadotropin (hCG) Levels

From Conception	From LMP	mIU/mL or IU/L
7 days	3 weeks	0–5
14 days	28 days	3–426
21 days	35 days	18–7340
28 days	42 days	1080–56,500
35–42 days	49–56 days	7650–229,000
43–64 days	57–78 days	25,700–288,000
57–78 days	79–100 days	13,300–253,000
17–24 weeks	2nd trimester	4060–165,400
25 weeks to term	3rd trimester	3640–117,000
Several days postpartum		Nonpregnant levels (< 5)

LMP, last menstrual period.
Data from: Johnson W. The best hCG diet site. hCG levels by week: A guide for pregnant women. November 23, 2011. Available at http://besthcgdietsite .com/1050/hcg-levels-by-week-%E2%80%93-a-guide-for-pregnant-women.

TABLE 16-2
Lecithin/Sphingomyelin (L/S) Ratio and Phosphatidylglycerol (PG) Level

Lung Maturation	L/S Ratio	PG
Mature	> 1.9	Present
Borderline	1.5–1.9	Absent
Immature	< 1.5	Absent

amniocentesis was suggested as a way to determine if a baby could be delivered early and safely if the mother or child's health was at risk.[9] Current evidence suggests that this is not the case, because lung development does not correlate with the development of other body systems.[9] Some evidence suggests, however, that there may be biomarkers found in amniotic fluid that indicate if a baby may be safely delivered earlier than expected.[10]

As the fetal lung matures, surfactant begins to be secreted that can then be found in the amniotic fluid. Surfactant is secreted by **type II alveolar cells** beginning at about 20 weeks of gestation.[11] Mature surfactant, which contains the phospholipid **phosphatidylglycerol (PG)**, does not appear until about week 35.[11] Lecithin and sphingomyelin are two other phospholipids found in neonatal surfactant. After about week 32 of gestation, the concentration of lecithin in the amniotic fluid increases, while sphingomyelin levels remain constant.[12,13] Thus, an increase in the surfactant **lecithin/sphingomyelin ratio (L/S ratio)** is associated with fetal lung maturation. The L/S ratio can be measured in amniotic fluid along with PG concentration and then be used to determine the maturity of the lung (see **Table 16-2**).[14,15] An L/S ratio ≥ 2.0 indicates lung maturity.[12,16] L/S measurements are affected by both blood and meconium in the amniotic fluid.[12,13] PG measurements, in addition to the L/S ratio, provide a better assessment of lung maturation. Unlike the L/S ratio,

PG levels are not affected by the presence of blood and meconium.[12,13] Measurement of the L/S ratio and PG are technically complex and time consuming.[17]

Another test to determine fetal lung maturity is the **surfactant-to-albumin ratio (TDx FLM II)**.[17–20] Specifically, this test measures the surfactant phospholipid present in amniotic fluid reported as milligrams surfactant present per gram of albumin.[17,19] A surfactant-to-albumin ratio (SAR) > 55 mg/g suggests that the lung is mature, and values < 40 mg/g suggest that the lung is immature.[12,17,19,20] Little data are available to assist the clinician in interpreting intermediate values between 40 and 54 mg/g, though the probability of RDS increases with decreasing SAR and decreasing gestational age.[13,20] For example, a gestational age of ≤ 30 weeks with an SAR ≤ 20 is associated with an incidence of RDS of ≥ 90%.[21] In contrast, a gestational age of 36 weeks with an SAR of 60 is only associated with an incidence of RDS of slightly more than 1%.[20,21] Both blood and meconium may cause inaccurate test results.[12,13,20] Although this test showed positive results as a predictor of RDS, currently the TDx FLM II is not being manufactured and is no longer available for clinical use.[17]

The **foam stability index (FSI)** is a rapid bedside biophysical test used to predict fetal lung maturity. A sample of amniotic fluid is placed in a test tube filled with a known concentration of ethanol and the sample is shaken. When sufficient surfactant is present, a stable foam ring will form; mature surfactant stabilizes the bubbles, and this is known as a positive "shake test." Serial dilutions of ethanol (42% to 58%) are used to calculate the FSI and thus quantify the amount of surfactant present.[17,22] However, blood or meconium in the sample will interfere with test results, and such samples should not be used.[13] The FSI test has fallen out of favor and has largely been replaced by other methods to assess lung maturation.[13,17]

Lamellar body count (LBC) is a direct measurement of the surfactant that is produced by the type II pneumocyte in the fetal lungs. Increased lamellar body production is reflected by an increase in amniotic fluid phospholipids and the L/S ratio.[23] These bodies are large enough to be counted. If there are fewer than 15,000 per microliter, this suggests pulmonary immaturity; counts of 50,000 per microliter or greater suggest pulmonary maturity.[23,24] This count is not significantly affected by meconium or blood.[24] In addition, the LBC can be used in women who develop gestational diabetes.[13,24] The current consensus is that if the LBC is < 15,000 or > 50,000 then no additional testing needs to be done; however, if the count is between 15,000 and 50,000 it is considered indeterminate, and additional phospholipid testing is needed to determine lung maturity.[13] **Table 16-3** provides a summary of current tests used to assess fetal lung maturity.

Amniotic fluid also contains fetal cells that can be analyzed to determine if the fetus has a chromosomal abnormality (e.g., trisomy 21, a form of Down syndrome), enzyme deficiencies (e.g., Tay-Sachs, a rare genetic disorder), or other genetic mutations (e.g., sickle cell disease). Newer noninvasive methods are available that can detect some of these chromosomal abnormalities using a sample of maternal blood, but these tests are currently used for screening purposes only.[25] If any of these tests are positive, an amniocentesis is usually performed to confirm the diagnosis.[26]

Fetal Movement

Fetal movement provides another tool for assessment of the fetus.[27] Fetal movement can be assessed by maternal observation; the mother can usually sense this movement around 17 to 20 weeks. This is called **fetal quickening**. Keeping a diary of fetal movement is encouraged for women who are at high risk. The diary should include timing, strength, and duration of fetal movement over a set period of time. The mother should also record what she was doing at the time (eating, exercising, sleeping, etc.). Several studies have reported a significant correlation between maternal perception of fetal movement and movements confirmed by ultrasound scanning.[28] By about week 28, the mother should feel 10 movements within a 1- to 2-hour period with minimal stimulation to the baby.[28] The movements could be kicks, punches, or jabs. Usually, the number is attained very quickly. A reduction of fetal movement is an indicator of compromised fetal well-being.[29] A lack of vigorous motion may relate to abnormalities of the central nervous system or, less commonly, to muscular dysfunction, skeletal abnormalities, or mechanical restriction of the lower extremities. Inactivity has been documented in fetuses with major malformations such as hydrocephalus, bilateral renal agenesis (failure of the kidneys to develop), and bilateral hip dislocation.[28] Excess activity, defined clinically as an average of more than 40 perceived motions per hour for at least 14 days, may represent a fetal anomaly such as anencephaly.[28]

TABLE 16-3
Fetal Lung Maturity Testing

Quantification of Surfactant Components	Mature	Transitional	Immature
Lecithin/sphingomyelin (L/S) ratio	> 0.20	1.5–2.0	< 1.5
Phosphatidylglycerol	Present	Trace	Absent
Desaturated phosphatidylcholine	> 70	50–70	< 50
Surfactant/albumin ratio (fluorescence polarization)—TDx-FLM II assay (mg surfactant/g albumin)*	> 55	40–54 is indeterminate	< 40
Lamellar body count (per microliter)	≥ 50,000	>30,000 to 40,000 may be mature	< 30,000
Foam stability index (FSI) using amniotic fluid samples	≥ 47	47%	<47%
Shake test (foam stability test) of amniotic fluid to alcohol dilution of 1:2	Foam ring persists for 15 minutes after shaking.		
Tap test using amniotic fluid and HCl/diethyl ether and "tap" tube several times	< 6 bubbles in ether layer at 10 minutes		
Optical density of amniotic fluid (turbidity) at a wavelength of 650 nm.	≥ 0.15		
Visual inspection of amniotic fluid (turbidity)	Cannot read printed material through tube because of turbidity.		

*Test currently not available
Data from: Zanelli SA, Kaufman D. Surfactant replacement therapy. In: Walsh BK, Czervinske MP, DiBlasi RM (eds.). *Perinatal and Pediatric Respiratory Care*, 3rd ed. St. Louis, MO: Saunders-Elsevier; 2010: 252.

Rapid, seizure-like movement has been described among brain-dead fetuses.[28] If prenatal asphyxia or neurologic disease is present, the newborn may require resuscitation at birth. If the mother notices any abnormal movements, she should contact her healthcare provider. Other techniques to assess fetal movement include fetal ultrasound, which can also provide additional useful information, such as heart rate and pattern.

Fetal Heart Rate

Fetal heart rate (FHR) and pattern can vary in response to blood volume changes, acidemia, hypoxemia, and sympathetic or parasympathetic (e.g., vagal) stimulation.[28,30,31] The FHR is usually obtained through a **Doppler ultrasound** device secured to the mother's abdomen. Ultrasound monitoring can be used for a baseline measure or for longer term monitoring during labor. FHR monitoring may detect hypoxemic and acidotic conditions. A normal fetal heart rate ranges from 110 to 160 beats per minute (bpm).[32]

Fetal heart rate patterns can be described as "reassuring" or "nonreassuring." A reassuring pattern indicates that the fetus is in no distress at the time of assessment, though it does not predict future patterns. Stable or reassuring FHR patterns include the following:[33]

- A baseline fetal heart rate of 110 to 160 bpm
- Absence of late or variable FHR decelerations
- Moderate FHR variability (6 to 25 bpm)
- Gestational age–appropriate FHR accelerations

FHR accelerations with stimulation (e.g., uterine contractions) are normal, and clinicians should not be overly concerned about small changes in FHR pattern.[33] For example, compression of the fetus's head as it passes through the birth canal will typically cause vagal stimulation and FHR deceleration.

Nonreassuring FHR patterns are of concern because they suggest fetal comprise or a declining ability for the fetus to handle the stress of labor. These may be associated with fetal hypoxia or metabolic acidosis. Fetal scalp testing is used to assess the fetus for the presence of acidemia. The clinician performs the fetal scalp test by placing a finger on the fetus's head or gently pinching the scalp with the finger or a clamp. Normally, fetal scalp stimulation will result in an increase in FHR ($\geq$ 15 bpm) for > 15 seconds. The absence of FHR acceleration following fetal scalp stimulation is associated with about a 50% chance of acidosis.[21] In the presence of nonreassuring FHR patterns, both the mother and the fetus need urgent assessment. **Table 16-4** lists nonreassuring FHR patterns.[21]

The National Institute of Child Health and Human Development has developed a three-tier system to help clinicians identify certain FHR patterns. They are as follows:[21,33,34]

- *Category I*: Normal. Category I FHR tracings are predictive of normal fetal acid-base status at the time of observation.
- *Category II*: Indeterminate or "atypical" FHR tracings. These tracings require evaluation and continued surveillance.
- *Category III*: Abnormal. FHR patterns are associated with abnormal fetal acid-base status at the time of observation and require prompt evaluation.

Depending on the clinical situation, efforts to treat the abnormal FHR pattern may include provision of maternal oxygen, change in maternal position, discontinuation of labor stimulation, treatment of maternal hypotension, and treatment of frequent uterine contractions (e.g., tachysystole), if present. If a Category III pattern does not resolve with these measures, delivery should be undertaken.[33,34] **Table 16-5** provides further description of the three tiers.

Tests of Fetal Well-Being

Several additional tests can help clinicians assess the well-being of the fetus. The simplest one is fetal movement, which was discussed earlier. As the fetus moves or is subjected to stress, such as a contraction, it requires more blood flow. The normal response is an increase in the fetal heart rate. Therefore, if the placenta is functioning properly, the heart rate should increase with activity or stress. If the placenta is compromised, when the fetus experiences a lack of blood flow when events occur and is stressed, the heart rate may not change.

A common prenatal test is the **fetal nonstress test (NST)**. In this noninvasive test, the fetal heart rate is monitored by attaching a belt on the mother's abdomen. Another belt is placed to measure the contractions. An increase in the fetal heart rate due to fetal movement is expected, and at term most fetal movements should elicit FHR accelerations.[35,36] A normal, healthy fetus will typically show an increase in FHR by at least 15 bpm for at least 15 seconds at least twice within a given 20-minute window.[35,36] An NST that lacks sufficient FHR accelerations over a 40-minute period is considered nonreactive.[35,36] A nonreactive NST is normal early in gestation (e.g., 24 to 28 weeks of gestation), but by weeks 28 to 32 most NSTs should be reactive.[36] Loss of reactivity is associated with the fetal sleep cycle, but may also occur due to central nervous system (CNS) depression, acidosis, immaturity, maternal ingestion of sedatives, and fetal cardiac or neurologic anomalies.[35,36] A fetus with a nonreactive NST near the time of birth may require resuscitation and further monitoring after delivery.[37,38]

Vibroacoustic stimulation is sometimes used during the fetal NST.[27] Vibratory sounds are generated using a special device and transmitted to the fetus across the

TABLE 16-4
Assessment of Fetal Heart Rate

Baseline Rate		
Baseline Rate (bpm)	**Terminology**	**Possible Causes**
< 110	Bradycardia	Prolonged cord compression, cord prolapse, tetanic uterine contractions, paracervical block, epidural or spinal anesthesia, maternal seizures
110–160	Normal	
> 160	Tachycardia	Fetal hypoxia, maternal fever, maternal or fetal anemia, and certain medications (e.g., atropine, hydroxyzine, sympathomimetics)

The baseline rate is the mean FHR over a 10-minute interval (excluding periodic changes, periods of marked variability, and segments that differ by more than 25 bpm). The baseline must be identifiable for 2 minutes during the interval (but not necessarily a contiguous 2 minutes), otherwise it is considered indeterminate.

Baseline Variability	
Baseline Variability	**Description**
Absent	Fluctuations in baseline that are irregular in amplitude and frequency
Minimal	Fluctuations in baseline minimal
Moderate	Fluctuations in baseline moderate
Marked	Fluctuations in baseline marked

Baseline variability is measured in a 10-minute window. The amplitude is measured peak to trough. There is no distinction between short- and long-term variability.
A prolonged acceleration is ≥ 2 minutes but < 10 minutes. An acceleration of 10 minutes or more is considered a change in baseline.

Deceleration	
Type of Deceleration	**Description**
Early deceleration	A gradual decrease and return to baseline of the FHR associated with a uterine contraction. The nadir (lowest point) of the FHR and the peak of the contraction occur at the same time. The deceleration's onset, nadir, and termination are usually coincident with the onset, peak, and termination of the contraction.
Variable deceleration	An abrupt decrease in FHR below the baseline. The decrease is ≥ 15 bpm, lasting ≥ 15 seconds and < 2 minutes from onset to return to baseline. The onset, depth, and duration of variable decelerations commonly vary with successive uterine contractions.
Late deceleration	A gradual decrease and return to baseline of the FHR associated with a uterine contraction. The deceleration is delayed in timing, with the lowest point (the nadir) of the deceleration occurring after the peak of the contraction. The onset, nadir, and recovery usually occur after the onset, peak, and termination of a contraction.
Prolonged deceleration	A decrease in FHR below the baseline of 15 bpm or more, lasting at least 2 minutes but < 10 minutes from onset to return to baseline. A prolonged deceleration of 10 minutes or more is considered a change in baseline.

Gradual changes are defined as those taking ≥ 30 seconds from the onset of the deceleration or acceleration to its peak or nadir. Abrupt changes occur in < 30 seconds.

bpm, beats per minute; FHR, fetal heart rate.
Data from: Macones GA, Hankins GD, Spong CY, et al. The 2008 National Institute of Child Health and Human Development workshop report on electronic fetal heart rate monitoring. *Obstet Gynecol*. 2008;112:661–666; National Institute of Child Health and Human Development Research Planning Workshop. Electronic fetal heart rate monitoring: Research guidelines for interpretation. *Am J Obstet Gynecol*. 1997;17:1385–1390.

TABLE 16-5
Three Categories for Fetal Heart Rate Interpretation

Category I: Normal
- Baseline rate: 110 to 160 bpm
- Baseline FHR variability: Moderate
- Late or variable decelerations: Absent
- Early decelerations: Present or absent
- Accelerations: Present or absent

Category II: Atypical

Category II includes patterns that cannot be categorized as Category I or III.

Examples of atypical patterns include:

Baseline Rate
- Bradycardia not accompanied by absent baseline variability
- Tachycardia

FHR Variability
- Minimal baseline variability
- Absent baseline variability not accompanied by recurrent decelerations
- Marked baseline variability

Accelerations
- Absence of induced accelerations after fetal stimulation

Periodic or Episodic Decelerations
- Recurrent variable decelerations accompanied by minimal or moderate baseline variability
- Prolonged deceleration ≥ 2 minutes but < 10 minutes
- Recurrent late decelerations with moderate baseline variability
- Variable decelerations with other characteristics, such as slow return to baseline "overshoots" or "shoulders"

Category III: Abnormal
- Absent baseline FHR variability and any of the following
  - Recurrent late decelerations
  - Recurrent variable decelerations
  - Bradycardia

  OR
- Sinusoidal pattern

bpm, beats per minute; FHR, fetal heart rate.
Data from: Macones G, Ramin SM, Barss V (eds). Management of intrapartum category I, II, III fetal heart tracings. UptoDate, 2013.

mother's abdomen. The stimulation is directed at the fetus's head at predetermined stimulation levels for several seconds.[27] The goal is to stimulate the startle reflex and induce fetal heart rate acceleration.[27,29] If fetal heart rate acceleration occurs, then fetal acidemia is unlikely. By the third trimester, an increase in the FHR baseline within 10 seconds of at least 10 bpm for at least 180 seconds should occur.[27,35] If there is no FHR acceleration, then fetal acidemia may be present and further assessment should be performed.[27]

Similar to a fetal NST is the **contraction stress test (CST)**, which is also known as an *oxytocin challenge*. Fetal heart rate is monitored while uterine contractions are stimulated. This is usually done by giving the mother dilute intravenous oxytocin. As the uterus contracts, there is a decrease in the partial pressure of oxygen (Po_2) of the blood that the baby receives via the placenta.[35] The fetal heart rate will normally decrease

and then quickly return to normal. A decrease in FHR that does not return to baseline may indicate placental insufficiency.[35] Slowing of the FHR during a contraction is considered a late FHR deceleration. A CST is considered positive when late decelerations occur during at least 50% of the contractions.[34,35] A suspicious CST is one where the decelerations are not consistent (< 50% of the contractions).[34,35] A negative CST obtained 1 week prior to delivery predicts fetal survival (assuming no clinical change in the interim). If the CST is abnormal (positive), further evaluation is needed.[34] A positive CST could result from maternal conditions (e.g., respiratory disorders, hypovolemia, uterine hyperstimulation) or fetal conditions (e.g., placental insufficiency, umbilical cord compression).[35] Variable decelerations should prompt ultrasound evaluation of the amniotic fluid volume and umbilical cord. Equivocal tests are usually repeated within 24 hours unless other indications for emergent delivery are present.[35] Management of preterm pregnancies with positive CST results will vary based on the circumstances.[35] A positive CST is associated with decreased APGAR scores and increased mortality.[35]

Assessment of the amniotic fluid volume is useful to assess the health of the fetus. The amniotic fluid provides the fetus with a source of water, protects the fetus from trauma, and allows for normal movements critical for anatomic development.[39,40] **Amniotic fluid volume (AFV)** abnormalities could indicate premature rupture of membranes, fetal congenital anomalies, chromosomal abnormalities, or fetal growth restriction.[35] Low AFV is also associated with an increased risk of adverse perinatal outcomes. The volume of amniotic fluid varies as the fetus develops. The assessment of amniotic fluid is performed by ultrasound using one of the following techniques:[41,42]

- Single deepest pocket (SDP) measurement
- Amniotic fluid index (AFI) measurement
- Two-diameter amniotic fluid pocket
- 2 × 1 cm or 2 × 2 cm pocket technique

The values derived from assessment of amniotic fluid volume are then compared to expected values based on gestational age. Abnormally high AFV (polyhydramnios) may be caused by birth defects, maternal diabetes, fetal anemia, and incompatible fetal–mother blood type. Abnormally low amniotic fluid values (oligohydramnios) may be caused by premature rupture of the placenta membranes, impaired fetal urine production, insufficient blood flow to the placenta (i.e., placental insufficiency), poor fetal growth, and genetic defects.

Fetal ultrasound testing can be used to derive a biophysical profile (BPS or BPP). The BPS incorporates the following variables: fetal tone, movement, breathing, AFV, and the results of the fetal NST.[29,43,44] **Table 16-6** provides examples of normal and abnormal scores. The

TABLE 16-6
Biophysical Profile

Biophysical Variable	Normal Score (+2 points each)	Abnormal Score (0 points each)
Fetal breathing movements	One of more episodes of > 30 seconds in 30 minutes	No breathing movements or none lasting > 30 seconds in 30 minutes
Fetal body movement	Three or more discrete body/limb movements in 30 minutes	Fewer than three movements of body/limbs in 30 minutes
Fetal tone	At least one episode of extension with return to flexion movements of limb	Absent or incomplete extension with only partial return to flexion movements
Reactive fetal heart rate	Two or more acceleration of > 15 bpm lasting 15 seconds with movement in 20 minutes	Fewer than two such accelerations in 30 minutes or < 15 bpm
Amniotic fluid level	One or more amniotic fluid pockets measuring >10 mm in two perpendicular planes	No amniotic fluid pocket or pockets in < 10 mm in two planes

Normal: 8–10 points; 2 points are awarded for each normal finding.
Modified from: James D. Monitoring the biophysical profile. *Br J Hosp Med.* 1993;49:561–563.

presence of specific biophysical variables (e.g., fetal breathing, body movement, tone, reactive FHR, good AFV) suggests the absence of significant hypoxemia or acidemia at the time of testing. The fetus may be compromised if there is a loss of accelerations of the FHR, decreased movement, decreased muscle tone, and decreased AFV.[43,44] The presence or risk of fetal acidemia is minimal when the BPS score is 8 to 10 and rises as the score decreases. A low BPS score indicates that the fetus is at risk of having fetal acidemia and has an increased risk of fetal compromise and/or death.[36]

Estimating the Delivery Date

The baby's delivery date can be determined in several ways. Most mothers know approximately when the fetus was conceived and can count forward 40 weeks. **Naegele's rule** can be used to determine the estimated date of delivery (EDD). Using this rule, EDD is calculated by adding 1 year and then counting back 3 months from the last menstrual cycle and adding 7 days. For example, if the last menstrual period occurred July 1, 2015, the estimated date of delivery would be calculated as follows:

1. EDD = (Last menstrual period + 1 year) – 3 months + 7 days =
2. (July 1, 2015 + 1 year) – 3 months + 7 days =
3. July 1, 2016 – 3 months + 7 days =
4. April 1, 2016 + 7 days = April 8, 2016

Thus, the estimated date of delivery for this patient would be April 8, 2016.

Another common way to determine the delivery date is based on the size of the uterus. Uterine size correlates to the approximate gestational age and is sometimes described based on the size of specific fruits. At 6 to 8 weeks of gestational age the uterus should be about

the size of a small pear; at 8 to 10 weeks it should be about the size of an orange; at 10 to 12 weeks the uterus should be about the size of a grapefruit.

Ultrasound is often used to estimate gestational age and delivery date and is superior to LMP or physical exam alone.[2,3] Ultrasound may be especially useful in mothers who have irregular menstrual cycles or when the child was conceived using hormone therapy. Ultrasound should be performed during the first trimester to determine fetal biometrics.[48] The ultrasound during the first trimester provides the following biometrics: gestational sac, yolk sac, crown rump length, and cardiac activity.[45] During the second and third trimesters, the following biometrics are measured: biparietal index, cephalic index, head circumference, femur length, and abdominal circumference.[45]

Assessment of the Newborn

History

As discussed in the previous section, obtaining a good maternal and fetal history is essential. The maternal history, pregnancy history, and family history will often help predict if the newborn will have complications, either during the delivery or afterwards. The fetal history is also important in determining if the fetus has been stressed or exposed to acidemia, which may compromise the fetus.

During labor, the fetus is exposed to cyclic decreases in blood flow as well as compression of the body as it passes through the birth canal. It is important to know if there is meconium in the amniotic fluid, because this is an indicator that the fetus has been stressed or may have experienced some fetal asphyxia and alert the clinician to the possibility of meconium aspiration. The duration of labor and any vaginal bleeding should be noted. The fetus may also be at risk for acquiring a maternal infection. Maternal fever and elevated white blood cell count, tender uterus, fetal tachycardia, and prolonged rupture of the membranes for more than 24 hours are associated with fetal infections transferred from the mother. Foul-smelling or colored amniotic fluid may also suggest infection.

The delivery method should be noted: vaginal, cesarean section (C-section), spontaneous, forceps (low, middle, or high), or vacuum extraction. Infants who need help during delivery may be at risk for developing complications postdelivery. Any drugs that the mother received are important to note, because some drugs may pass across the placenta and negatively affect the newborn. Spinal anesthetics may cause the mother to have a lower blood pressure, which may, in turn, compromise oxygen delivery to the fetus.

Assessment Following Delivery

Once the baby is delivered, proper resuscitation is vitally important. Hypoxia and hypoventilation, no matter the cause, can drive a neonate back into fetal circulation, requiring major interventions (including ECMO) to reverse. Upon delivery, the first three questions should be: (1) Is the baby full term? (2) Is the baby breathing and/or crying? (3) Does the baby have good muscle tone? If the question is yes to all of these questions, then the baby should be dried, warmed, and placed in the arms of the mother. If not, then the initial steps for neonatal resuscitation should be taken. Clinicians should calculate an APGAR (appearance, pulse, grimace, activity, respiration) score soon after birth. The **APGAR score** provides a standardized assessment of the newborn infant that is simple, quick, and reliable.[46] The APGAR score is composed of five metrics (heart rate, respiratory effort, muscle tone, reflex irritability, and color) each scored 0 to 2 points.[46] APGAR scores are assigned at 1 and 5 minutes. If the infant is experiencing problems, scores may be repeated. As an infant's condition deteriorates, the APGAR score will decline. Typically, cyanosis will occur first, followed by changes in reflex irritability, muscle tone, respiratory effort, and heart rate. As the infant improves, APGAR scores increase; first the heart rate will improve, followed by improvements in respiratory effort, reflex irritability, color, and muscle tone. **Table 16-7** provides an illustration of the APGAR scoring system. **Figure 16-1** provides an algorithm for neonatal resuscitation.

Gestational Age at Birth

A normal pregnancy results in birth at 38 to 42 weeks of gestation. As discussed in previous sections, gestational age can be determined by maternal report, fetal ultrasound, or other gestational age assessment method. Women who have received prenatal care should have an early fetal ultrasound on record; the gestational age of the fetus is usually determined at that time. However, if the mother is unsure of when the baby was conceived, there was no prenatal assessment, or there is a large difference between the maternal date given and the ultrasound date, then estimation of gestational age at birth should be completed. The newborn is considered to be *full term* when the gestational age is 39 to 40 weeks (i.e., ≥ 39 weeks and < 41 weeks). A newborn is considered to be *late term* is if the gestational age is ≥ 41 weeks and < 42 weeks. A gestational age of ≥ 42 weeks is considered *postterm* or *postmature*. A baby is considered to be *premature* if the gestational age is < 37 weeks or < 259 days; gestational age of 37 to 38 weeks is considered *early term*.

A normal birth weight is about 3.4 kg (about 7.5 lbs), with a range of about 2.7 to 4.6 kg (5.5 to 8.8 lbs).[47] Birth weight increases with gestational age, and low birth weight is associated with prematurity. Premature (preterm) and low-birth-weight infants have higher mortality than term infants and are at risk for development of a number of short- and long-term complications ranging from RDS to chronic health issues.

TABLE 16-7
APGAR Score

Parameter	0 points	1 point	2 points
Heart rate	None	< 100 bpm	> 100 bpm
Respiratory effort	None	Weak, irregular	Strong cry
Color	Body pale or blue, extremities blue	Body pink, extremities blue	Completely pink
Reflex (irritability to suction)	No response	Grimace	Cry, cough, or sneeze
Muscle tone	Limp	Some flexion	Well flexed

Apgar, Virginia M.D., A Proposal for a New Method of Evaluation of the Newborn Infant, *Current Researches in Anesthesia & Analgesia* 32(4), July/August, pp. 260–267, 1953. Used by permission of Wolters Kluwer Health. http://www.anesthesia-analgesia.org/content/32/4/260.full.pdf+html.

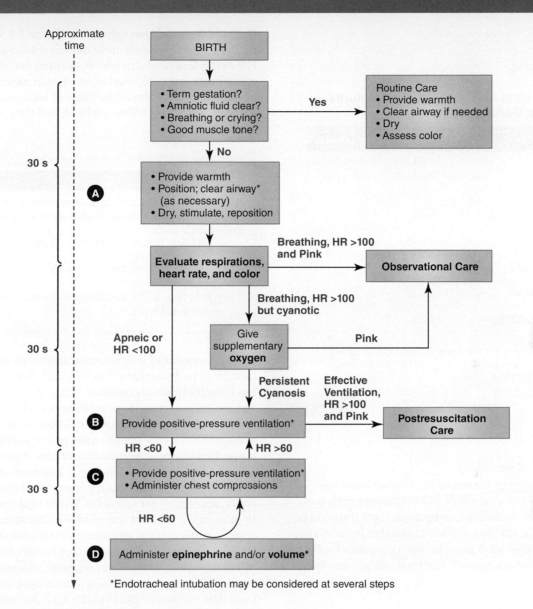

FIGURE 16-1 Algorithm for resuscitation of the neonate.

Reproduced from: Neonatal resuscitation guidelines. *Circulation.* 2005;112(suppl I):IV-188–IV-195. Reprinted with permission of the American Academy of Pediatrics.

Mortality is about 230 per 1000 live births in infants born with a birth weight of < 1500 grams (< 1.5 kg) and about 50% in patients born at < 25 weeks of gestation.[48] **Box 16-2** summarizes the nomenclature used related to gestational age at birth; **Box 16-3** provides examples of normal and low birth weights for newborns.

The **Dubowitz scoring system** provides a method to help determine the gestational age of the newborn at the time of birth. The Dubowitz score incorporates 21 physical and neurologic assessments. Eleven physical criteria are assigned scores of 0 to 4, and 10 neuromuscular criteria are scored from 0 to 5. Higher scores indicate greater maturity. The scores are added and then plotted on a graph to estimate gestational age.[49] A problem with the Dubowitz scoring system is that it

has not been validated for preterm infants. Although considered an acceptable tool for neonates born prematurely, it tends to overestimate their gestational age. Another concern that limits its utility is severity of illness in the critically ill neonate. The Ballard score is a modified form of the Dubowitz assessment that is preferred because it takes into account infant prematurity. The Ballard score is calculated within 30 to 42 hours of birth. The Ballard is fast and can be done on very sick infants.[50] The Ballard method was further refined as the **new Ballard score**, which allows for the assessment of infants born as early as 20 weeks.[51] **Figure 16-2** illustrates the Ballard examination score. **Box 16-4** describes common neonatal cardiopulmonary disorders.

BOX 16-2

Classification of Infant Term and Maturity Based on Gestational Age

Terminology	Gestational Age (weeks)
Postterm	≥ 42
Late term	41
Full term	39–40
Early term	37–38
Late preterm (premature)	33–36
Very premature	26–32
Extremely premature	≤ 25

Data from: Mandy GT. Incidence and mortality of the premature infant. In: *UpToDate*, Basow DS (ed.), UpToDate, Waltham, MA, 2013.

Newborn Vital Signs

An assessment of the major vital signs (heart rate [HR], respiratory rate [RR], blood pressure [BP], body temperature, and oxygen saturation [SpO_2]) should be completed at the first available opportunity following birth.[52,53] **Table 16-8** provides normal ranges for these vital signs for normal and low-birth-weight newborns.

BOX 16-3

Classification of Newborns by Birth Weight

Birth Weight (grams)	Classification
2500–4600	Normal
1500–2499	Low
1000–1499	Very low
< 1000	Extremely low

Data from: Mandy GT. Incidence and mortality of the premature infant. In: *UpToDate*, Basow DS (ed.), UpToDate, Waltham, MA, 2013; Medline Plus. Birth weight. November 6, 2013. Available at http://www.nlm.nih.gov/medlineplus/birthweight.html.

It should be noted that values for HR and RR will normally vary fairly significantly but fall within a range. For example, a newborn who is sleeping may have a lower heart rate compared to one who is agitated or crying. Vital signs should be taken at least once an hour for the first 6 hours following birth and then every 8 to 12 hours.

RC Insights

Under normal conditions, PaO_2 can be estimated using oxygen saturation as a guide. The PaO_2 is normally about 30 mm Hg lower than the SpO_2.

- If the SpO_2 is 90%, then the patient's PaO_2 is approximately 60 mm Hg.
- If the SpO_2 is 80%, then the patient's PaO_2 is approximately 50 mm Hg.
- If the SpO_2 is 70%, then the patient's PaO_2 is approximately 40 mm Hg.

Measurement of infant temperature may be done rectally or in the axillary space. Rectal thermometry has been traditionally considered the "gold standard," and rectal temperature generally reflects core temperature.[53–55] Axillary temperature has been shown to correlate well with core temperature in newborns, though it may be a less reliable indicator of core temperature in infants and pediatric patients.[52–55] Tympanic membrane temperature measurement (i.e., ear probe) should generally be reserved for infants at least 2 months of age.[52] In most cases, the best way to take a newborn's temperature is at the axillary site using an infrared thermometer.[53–55] The infant may be in an open crib, unless the infant requires a warmer or incubator. Normal newborn axillary temperature taken in an open crib ranges from 97.0° to 98.6° F (36.1° to 37° C).[53] Normal rectal temperature values are 99.6° ± 1° F (37.6° ± 1° C).[52–55]

Elevated core body temperature can be caused by an overly warm environment or infection, though newborns may not develop a fever with infection because their thermoregulation system is still immature.[54,55] Fever in the neonate may be viral or bacterial in origin; fever can be a sign of a serious bacterial infection (SBI). Causes of SBI include sepsis, pneumonia, meningitis, gastroenteritis, or urinary tract infection.[54] Special consideration should be made for neonates with a rectal temperature ≥ 38° C (100.4° F). Clinicians should send cultures (e.g., blood, urine, CSF) and potentially start empiric antibiotic therapy, particularly if an SBI is suspected.[55] Newborns with signs of pulmonary disease should also have a chest radiograph.[54]

Hypothermia refers to a reduced core body temperature. Because of their large surface area in proportion to their body mass, newborns are sensitive to environmental temperature and "cold stress." Newborns have a surface area to body mass ratio three times greater than a typical adult and are thus more likely to lose

Neuromuscular Maturity

Score	-1	0	1	2	3	4	5
Posture							
Square window (wrist)	>90°	90°	60°	45°	30°	0°	
Arm recoil		180°	140–180°	110–140°	90–110°	<90°	
Popliteal angle	180°	160°	140°	120°	100°	90°	<90°
Scarf sign							
Heel to ear							

Physical Maturity

Skin	Sticky, friable, transparent	Gelatinous, red, translucent	Smooth, pink; visible veins	Superficial peeling and/or rash; few veins	Cracking, pale areas; rare veins	Parchment, deep cracking; no vessels	Leathery, cracked, wrinkled
Lanugo	None	Sparse	Abundant	Thinning	Bald areas	Mostly bald	
Plantar surface	Heel-toe 40–50 mm: –1 < 40 mm: –2	> 50 mm, no crease	Faint red marks	Anterior transverse crease only	Creases anterior 2/3	Creases over entire sole	
Breast	Imperceptible	Barely perceptible	Flat areola, no bud	Stippled areola, 1–2 mm bud	Raised areola, 3–4 mm bud	Full areola, 5–10 mm bud	
Eye/Ear	Lids fused loosely: –1 tightly: –2	Lids open; pinna flat; stays folded	Slightly curved pinna, soft slow recoil	Well curved pinna, soft but ready recoil	Formed and firm, instant recoil	Thick cartilage, ear stiff	
Genitals (male)	Scrotum flat, smooth	Scrotum empty, faint rugae	Testes in upper canal, rare rugae	Testes descending, few rugae	Testes down, good rugae	Testes pendulous, deep rugae	
Genitals (female)	Clitoris prominent, labia flat	Clitoris prominent, small labia minora	Clitoris prominent, enlarging minora	Majora and minora equally prominent	Majora large, minora small	Majora cover clitoris and minora	

Maturity Rating

Score	Weeks
-10	20
-5	22
0	24
5	26
10	28
15	30
20	32
25	34
30	36
35	38
40	40
45	42
50	44

FIGURE 16-2 Ballard examination score.

Reprinted from Journal of Pediatriacs 119(3), Ballard JL. New Ballard score, expanded to include extremely premature infants, pages 417–423, Copyright 1991, with permission from Elsevier.

heat quickly. Premature infants may have a surface area to body mass ratio that approaches six times that of an adult, which makes them extremely sensitive to low environmental temperatures. Respiratory care clinicians should be aware of room temperature, moisture content, airflow, and the temperature of objects in the room (e.g., examination tables), because these may affect the newborn's ability to maintain a normal body

BOX 16-4

Neonatal Cardiopulmonary Disorders

Respiratory distress syndrome (RDS)
- Pathophysiology: Surfactant deficiency in premature infants; lung inflammation and injury, pulmonary edema, and hypoxemia.
- Clinical manifestations: Tachypnea, nasal flaring, expiratory grunting, retractions, cyanosis.
- Diagnosis: Clinical manifestations, arterial blood gas measurements.
- Treatment: Surfactant therapy, oxygen therapy, CPAP, ventilator support, supportive care.

Transient tachypnea of the newborn (TTN)
- Pathophysiology: Pulmonary edema due to delayed clearance of alveolar fluid following birth.
- Clinical manifestations: Tachypnea, increased work of breathing, similar to RDS; occurs more often in term or late preterm infants.
- Diagnosis: Clinical picture and exclusion of other causes of respiratory distress.
- Treatment: Oxygen therapy, neutral thermal environment, and supportive care.

Neonatal pneumonia
- Pathophysiology: Bacterial, viral, or fungal infection resulting in alveolar lung disease.
- Clinical manifestations: Similar to RDS; tachycardia, apnea, poor perfusion, temperature instability, and acidosis.
- Diagnosis: Clinical findings, cultures (blood, cerebrospinal fluid), chest radiograph.
- Treatment: Empiric antibiotic therapy, supportive care, oxygen therapy and ventilatory support as needed.

Meconium aspiration
- Pathophysiology: Aspiration of intrauterine meconium resulting in obstruction, inflammation, infection, and surfactant disruption; hypoxemia, acidosis, and persistent pulmonary hypertension (PPHN) may also occur.
- Clinical manifestations: Amniotic fluid stained with meconium at birth; neurologic depression, respiratory distress, retractions, tachypnea, accessory muscle use, cyanosis, grunting, nasal flaring, increased anteroposterior chest diameter.
- Diagnosis: Clinical findings, meconium stain, chest x-ray (densities, overinflation), arterial blood gases (hypoxemia, increased $Paco_2$).
- Treatment: Oxygen therapy and ventilatory support, correction of acidosis, empiric antibiotic therapy, supportive care (neutral thermal environment, nutrition), and circulatory support as needed; avoid infant agitation.

Persistent pulmonary hypertension of the neonate (PPHN)
- Pathophysiology: Pulmonary circulatory system abnormalities.
- Clinical manifestations: Tachypnea, respiratory distress, cyanosis, presence of another respiratory problem (e.g., meconium aspiration, pneumonia, RDS).
- Diagnosis: Clinical findings, oximetry, arterial blood gas measurements, chest x-ray, electrocardiogram, and echocardiography.
- Treatment: Supportive care; treatment of underlying lung disease (e.g., RDS, pneumonia); oxygen therapy and ventilatory support, as needed; severe cases may require inhaled nitric oxide therapy (iNO), extracorporal membrane oxygenation (ECMO).

Sepsis in the newborn
- Pathophysiology: Bacterial infection (e.g., Group B streptococcus [GBS], *E. coli*).
- Clinical manifestations: Fever, respiratory distress, low APGAR, anorexia, vomiting, jaundice, lethargy, cyanosis.
- Diagnosis: Clinical picture, complete blood count (CBC), blood cultures, risk factors present (e.g., membrane rupture, preterm birth).
- Treatment: Antibiotic therapy, supportive care, monitoring.

Bronchopulmonary dysplasia (BPD)
- Pathophysiology: Exposure of the immature lung due to oxygen toxicity, barotrauma from mechanical ventilatory support and infections resulting in airway injury, inflammation, and fibrosis.
- Clinical manifestations: Asthma-like symptoms in children, reduced exercise tolerance, sleep disorders (hypoxemia, hypoventilation), repeated respiratory infections.
- Treatment: Improved management of premature infants (e.g., surfactant therapy, corticosteroid therapy); bronchodilators are effective in some patients; treatment/prevention of infection.

TABLE 16-8
Normal Values for Vital Signs in the Neonatal Patient

Birth Weight (g)	Systolic/Diastolic Blood Pressure (mm Hg)	Mean Blood Pressure (mm Hg)
> 600	45/20	25
> 1000	48/25	35
> 2000	50/30	40
> 3000	50/35	45
> 4000	65/40	50
Newborn older than 12 hours	75/50	60
Respiratory rate: 40–60 breaths/min	Respiratory rate varies in pre-term and term infants	
Heart rate: 100–160 bpm	Heart rate varies in pre-term and term infants	

Data from: Versmold HT, Kitterman JA, Phibbs RH, Gregory GA, Tooley WH. Aortic blood pressure ranges during the first 12 hours of life in infants with birth weight 610 to 4,220 grams. *Pediatrics*. 1981;67:607–613.

temperature. Avoidance of cold stress is important, and any procedures that expose the newborn to low environmental temperatures may put the baby at risk. This is especially true of preterm and low-birth-weight infants; care should be taken to maintain a neutral thermal environment for all newborns.

Anatomic shunts that occur in the newborn may take several hours or days to close. To assess for shunting, pulse oximetry should be done in two places: a preductal site and a postductal site. In the neonate, cardiac shunt may occur where blood is shunted right to left, left to right, or bidirectionally. Shunts may also be systemic to pulmonary or pulmonary to systemic. A pulmonary shunt occurs when blood is perfusing the lungs but no ventilation takes place. It has been suggested that all newborns have pre- and postductal oxygen saturations documented between 24 to 48 hours of birth to assess for shunt. The best place to measure preductal oxygen saturation (SpO_2) is the right hand; the best place to obtain a postductal SpO_2 is the left hand or lower extremities.[56] The current threshold for a positive screening relates to both the absolute reading by the pulse oximeter as well as the difference between the two extremities. A pulse oximetry SpO_2 reading of $\geq 95\%$ in either extremity with a $\leq 3\%$ absolute difference between the upper and lower extremity would be considered a normal, or "pass," screening test.[56] If a newborn does not pass this test, then additional screening to rule out either pulmonary or cardiac defects should be carried out, including an echocardiogram. Some shunts may stay open 48 hours, and the patient

may show no sign of cyanosis or heart murmur.[56–58] It is not recommended that a pulse oximeter screen be performed to rule out cardiac defects during the first 24 hours following birth unless the patient is being discharged.[56–58]

RC Insights

The newborn's oxygen saturation should increase by 5% each minute for the first 5 minutes of life:
- 1-minute targeted preductal SpO_2 is 60% to 65%.
- 2-minute targeted preductal SpO_2 is 65% to 70%.
- 3-minute targeted preductal SpO_2 is 70% to 75%.
- 4-minute targeted preductal SpO_2 is 75% to 80%.
- 5-minute targeted preductal SpO_2 is 80% to 85%.

Note that it may take up to 10 minutes or longer for the SpO_2 to reach 85% to 95% in the newborn.

It should be noted that fetal hemoglobin differs from adult hemoglobin. Fetal hemoglobin is present from approximately the last 7 months of gestation until about 6 months of age.[59] Neonates typically have fetal hemoglobin values of 80% to 90%; values may be higher if the baby is born prematurely.[59] An important difference between adult and fetal hemoglobin is the affinity for oxygen; fetal Hb has a much greater affinity for O_2. This allows blood coming from the placenta to have a higher oxygen content even though the partial pressure of O_2 is very low. In other words, because of fetal hemoglobin a lower PaO_2 results in a higher O_2 saturation. However, due to the higher affinity of fetal Hb for O_2, there is less offloading of oxygen from the hemoglobin to the body cells at the tissue level.[59] The P_{50} value for fetal hemoglobin (i.e., the partial pressure of oxygen at which the hemoglobin is 50% saturated; lower values indicate greater affinity) is roughly 19 mm Hg, whereas adult hemoglobin has a value of approximately 27 mm Hg. A recent study of neonates showed that a PaO_2 of 50 to 75 mm Hg resulted in an SpO_2 of 96% to 97%.[59] The same PaO_2 in an adult would result in an SpO_2 of only approximately 85% to 94%.[59] For this reason, a sick child may have a higher pulse oximetry reading than might be expected with a given PaO_2, providing the healthcare provider with a false sense of security.

Cardiovascular Function and Heart Rate

Newborn heart rates are typically 100 to 160 bpm; blood pressure varies with birth weight and is generally $\leq 70/50$ mm Hg.[60,61] The brachial or femoral sites are usually used to assess pulse, and blood pressure is typically measured using a blood pressure cuff and noninvasive blood pressure device. Common causes of newborn tachycardia (HR > 160 bpm) include crying or other distress (e.g., pain, fever). Other causes of tachycardia in the newborn include congenital heart defects, reduced cardiac output or hypotension (e.g., shock), and certain medications. Causes of newborn bradycardia (HR < 100 bpm) include hypothermia, hypoxia, vagal stimulation, certain drugs, grunting (e.g., Valsalva maneuver), and long periods of apnea.[61]

If possible, the pulse and blood pressure should be assessed while the infant is quiet. Initially, both brachial and femoral pulses are often palpated simultaneously; these should feel equal in intensity. If the pulses are weak, it may suggest a decreased cardiac output, such as may occur with a congenital heart defect. Weak pulses in the lower extremities may also occur with a coarctation of the aorta, which can reduce blood flow to the lower extremities. If bounding pulses are detected, then the infant may have a right-to-left shunt due to patent ductus arteriosis (PDA). If the femoral pulse is weak or abnormal, then the radial and pedal pulses should also be evaluated.

In the absence of an indwelling arterial line, the best way to measure blood pressure is by use of an appropriately sized blood pressure cuff and a noninvasive blood pressure monitoring device (e.g., oscillometric method). Neonatal blood pressure increases with gestational age, birth weight, and postnatal age. For example, low-birth-weight and preterm infants are expected to have lower systolic and diastolic blood pressures; pressures should then increase over the first hours and days following birth. If cardiovascular problems are suspected, blood pressures are sometimes measured and compared at all four extremities. Typically, blood pressures in the lower extremities are slightly higher than those measured in the upper extremities. If there is a significant difference in blood pressure between upper and lower extremities or the upper extremity blood pressure is higher than that of the lower extremity, it may be sign of a heart defect. Clinicians should be concerned about hypotension or hypertension in the newborn, because cerebral ischemic injury and intraventricular hemorrhage, along with other injuries, could occur. The normal range for neonatal blood pressure is listed in Table 16-8. The following formula can be used to estimate adequate mean blood pressure for the newborn:

> Adequate mean blood pressure
> = Gestational age (weeks) + 5

The point of maximal impulse (PMI) is the place on the chest where the apical pulse, or apical impulse, is strongest. The apical impulse is located by palpation and is normally felt at the fifth intercostal space at the midclavicular line on the left side.[62] The apical pulse can sometimes be visible as pulsation of the chest wall in the area of the left lower sternal border. The apical impulse can be used to locate the position of the heart. For example, pneumothorax or diaphragmatic hernia may alter heart position. Apical impulse can also be affected by heart size and force of left ventricular contraction.

The best site for cardiac auscultation is also located in the left lower sternal boarder over the PMI. The left lower sternal border can also be palpated for cardiac heave (lifting of the sternum) or thrills (a palpable vibration). Upon auscultation, the first heart sound (S_1) is associated with the concurrent closure of the tricuspid and mitral valves. The second heart sound (S_2) is associated with closure of the pulmonary and aortic valves. S_1 is normally a single sound, whereas S_2 is often a single sound during expiration but split during inspiration. Dextrocardia is a congenital rotation of the heart to the right that may shift heart sounds towards the right side of the chest.

Many infants have benign heart murmurs that resolve in a few hours to days following birth. Causes of heart murmurs at birth include a PDA and a patent foreman ovale. These circulatory pathways are holdovers from the fetal circulation, which usually close shortly after birth as pulmonary vascular resistance decreases and blood flows to the lungs. A cardiology consult should be considered at 48 hours if a murmur does not resolve, because a heart defect may be present. Physical findings associated with congenital heart defects include:[21]

- Loud or moderately loud or harsh heart murmur
- Murmur continues from the beginning of S_1 to the end of S_2 (i.e., "pansystolic" duration)
- Murmur is loudest at upper left sternal border, upper right sternal border, or apex
- Abnormal second heart sound (S_2)
- Absent or diminished femoral pulse

Examples of congenital heart disease are listed in **Box 16-5**.

Respiratory Assessment

The normal newborn respiratory rate is between 40 and 60 breaths per minute and is related to gestational age (i.e., the younger the gestational age, the greater the RR).[60] Shallow and rapid breathing may help to maintain **functional residual capacity (FRC)**, and infants who are in distress may partially close the glottis (grunting) on expiration to help maintain FRC.

RC Insights

Until about 10 years of age, children breathe faster to increase ventilation rather than breathing more deeply because they have fewer and smaller alveoli and less lung volume than adults.

RC Insights

Tidal volume is proportional to weight, at approximately 7 to 10 mL/kg.

BOX 16-5

Congenital Heart Disease

Cyanotic disease
- Anomalous pulmonary venous return
- Coarctation of the aorta (preductal)
- Ebstein's anomaly
- Hypoplastic left heart syndrome (HLHS)
- Pulmonary atresia
- Tetralogy of Fallot (TOF)
- Transposition of the great vessels (TGA)
- Tricuspid atresia
- Truncus arteriosus

Acyanotic disease
- Aortic stenosis
- Atrial septal defect
- Atrioventricular canal
- Coarctation of the aorta (postductal)
- Patent ductus arteriosus (PDA)
- Pulmonic stenosis
- Ventricular septal defect (VSD)

Modified from: Medline Plus. Congenital heart disease. November 5, 2013. Available at http://www.nlm.nih.gov /medlineplus/ency/article/001114.htm.

Respiratory rate may be counted by observation of the motion of the chest or while listening to breath sounds using a stethoscope. Tachypnea (RR > 60 breaths/min) and **bradypnea** (RR < 30 breaths/min) are both sensitive indicators of the newborn's condition. Tachypnea can be due cardiac or lung disease such as a congenital heart defect or untreated RDS. Specifically, tachypnea may be caused by hypoxia, acidosis, fever, anxiety, or pain. Respiratory rate will also increase when the infant is stimulated, crying, or with fever. Bradypnea may be caused by certain medications (e.g., narcotics), hypothermia, or diseases affecting the CNS. Most newborns have an increase in their respiratory rate when stimulated; bradypnea is not a normal response in the neonate. With lung disease, tachypnea followed by abnormally slowed respirations may occur when the work of breathing is high and the infant tires. Thus, bradypnea may signal impending ventilatory failure.

Periods of **apnea** are sometimes seen in the newborn and may be classified as *long apnea* (≥ 20 seconds), *short apnea* (6 to 14 seconds), or as a *respiratory pause* (< 6 seconds).[63–65] Long apnea is a pathologic condition that may be accompanied by cyanosis, bradycardia, pallor, and hypotonia (i.e., decreased muscle tone).[63–65] Brief episodes of short apnea, respiratory pauses, or

"periodic breathing" are normal in preterm and term infants up to 3 months of age.[61] Preterm infants may have very irregular breathing patterns. Any abnormal pattern should be monitored and investigated to make sure it is not an indication of a serious issue.

The chest should be inspected for appearance, symmetry, and chest wall motion during breathing. Chest wall deformities include *pectus excavatum* ("funnel chest") and *pectus caninatum* ("pigeon chest").[66] Chest wall motion in the newborn may be paradoxical (e.g., "see-saw" motion), even in normal infants.

Auscultation of breath sounds should be performed (if possible) while the baby is quiet and in a neutral thermal environment. Similar to listening to the heart sounds, the stethoscope should be warmed and then placed over bare skin. Clear, bronchovesicular breath sounds are normally heard throughout the infant's lungs. Abnormal breath sounds include crackles, wheezes, and absent or diminished breath sounds. **Crackles** are associated with fluid, such as pulmonary edema or pneumonia. Crackles are sometimes heard for a few hours after delivery, especially in newborns born via C-section. Passage through the birth canal normally causes fetal lung fluid to be expelled. Babies born by C-section do not experience this clearing effect and may take several hours following birth to clear fetal lung fluid. Wheezing is associated with narrowed airways, as seen with bronchopulmonary dysplasia.[61] Decreased or absent breath sounds suggest a decrease in airflow, as may occur due to atelectasis, pneumothorax, or infant RDS.[61]

Grunting is a sound made by the closure of the glottis during expiration and is a sign of respiratory distress in the newborn. Grunting may loud or soft and is thought to increase FRC and reduce alveolar collapse. Other signs of respiratory distress include nasal flaring, retractions, and cyanosis. Infants in respiratory distress may have the level of distress quantified by the use of the *Silverman scoring system*. This system grades the infant's appearance based on chest motion, retractions, nasal flaring, and absence or presence of an expiratory grunt (see **Figure 16-3**). The score range is 0 to 10, with 10 indicating severe distress. **Clinical Focus 16-1** and **Clinical Focus 16-2** describe infants with respiratory distress.

Head and Neck Assessment

The infant's head should be assessed for size and shape and the presence of contusions, abrasions, or other abnormalities.[67,68] Head circumference is measured along with other biometric data (e.g., birth weight, abdominal circumference, length). The head is usually the first body part through the birth canal, and as such may initially appear bruised with some molding.[68] The fetal skull is relatively flexible and can change shape under pressure. *Molding* refers to changes in the shape of the baby's head to allow easier passage through the

	Upper chest	Lower chest	Xiphoid retraction	Nares dilation	Expiratory grunt
Grade 0	Synchronized	No retraction	None	None	None
Grade 1	Lag on inspiration	Just visible	Just visible	Minimal	Stethoscope only
Grade 2	See-saw	Marked	Marked	Marked	Naked ear

FIGURE 16-3 Silverman scoring system.

Reproduced with permission from Pediatrics, Vol.17, Page 1-6, © 1956 by the AAP.

CLINICAL FOCUS 16-1

Infant Respiratory Distress

A 28-week premature male was born via vaginal delivery and admitted to the neonatal intensive care unit. At birth, the infant weighed 1200 g and appeared vigorous. APGAR scores at 1 and 5 minutes were 6 and 8, respectively. Over the next hour the infant had worsening distress and was placed on a blended nasal cannula. Deterioration of the patient's respiratory status occurred in the following hours. The respiratory care clinician is called for assessment and support.

1. What actions should the respiratory care clinician take?

   The respiratory care clinician should perform a patient assessment, including general appearance, vital signs, and breath sounds.

   The following information is gathered on this patient.
   - Physical examination: Nasal flaring, expiratory grunting, and moderate to severe retractions.
   - Breath sounds decreased bilaterally.
   - Vital signs:

     Heart rate: 175 bpm

     Blood pressure: 54/40 mm Hg

     Respiratory rate: 80 breaths/min:

     SpO_2: 88%

     Temperature: 37.6° C

2. Based on these findings, what diagnosis should be considered?

   Respiratory distress syndrome (RDS) of the neonate should be considered. The patient was < 1500 g at birth and is in acute distress with an increased work of breathing.

3. What interventions and/or additional diagnostic testing should now be considered?

   The following should now be considered:
   - Place the infant on nasal continuous positive-pressure airway pressure (CPAP) with blended oxygen to maintain adequate saturations.
   - Obtain a chest x-ray.
   - Draw an arterial blood gas 30 minutes after CPAP placement.
   - Provide a neutral thermal environment.

   It is important for the premature infant be placed in a thermoregulated environment to maintain a thermoneutral temperature. Premature infants are prone to high heat loss because of their large skin surface area as compared to their body mass, decreased amount of subcutaneous fat, decreased amount of developed brown fat, and limited ability to increase heat production when they have pulmonary problems (e.g., hypoxia).

An arterial blood gas study and chest x-ray (CXR) is obtained following placement of the patient on CPAP, with the following results:

- Arterial blood gases:
  pH: 7.23
  $Paco_2$: 61 mm Hg
  Pao_2: 40 mm Hg
  Sao_2: 88%.
- Chest x-ray: Opacity and reticulogranular infiltrates with "ground-glass" appearance.

The patient continues to be in acute distress with little apparent improvement in work of breathing.

4. **What is an appropriate assessment of this patient at this time?**

   The blood gas results indicate hypoventilation (acute respiratory distress) with hypoxemia. The chest x-ray results (i.e., increased opacity, ground-glass appearance) and low birth weight are consistent with development of neonatal RDS due to surfactant deficiency.

5. **What steps should now be considered in the management of this patient?**

   The respiratory care clinician should consider placement of an endotracheal tube and institution of mechanical ventilatory support. Surfactant replacement therapy should be administered. Specifically, steps should include:

   - Endotracheal intubation: An infant weighing 1200 g would probably require a 3.0-mm endotracheal tube.
   - Initial mechanical ventilation settings for the patient might include:
     - Mode: Time cycled, pressure limited mode
     - Peak inspiratory pressure (PIP): 20 to 25 cm H_2O
     - Respiratory rate: 30 to 40 breaths/min
     - PEEP: 5 to 8 cm H_2O
     - FIO_2: < 60%

   Surfactant dose and administration should be performed according to manufacturer guidelines.

   The patient stabilizes with some minor ventilator adjustments. If the patient's condition worsens, other possible support measures, such as high-frequency ventilation, should be considered.

CLINICAL FOCUS 16-2

Meconium Aspiration

The respiratory care clinician is asked to be present in the delivery room of a mother with a female baby with a 42-week estimated gestational age. The pregnancy has been uncomplicated, and all the maternal lab values have been normal. Meconium-stained amniotic fluid was present at birth.

1. **What steps and/or interventions should be taken by the clinician to assess the patient?**

   Meconium is fecal material expelled from the fetal intestine into the amniotic fluid. Meconium aspiration occurs as the infant takes the first few breaths following delivery. Meconium aspiration causes airway obstruction, inflammation, and surfactant disruption and may lead to pulmonary infection. Meconium aspiration is more likely in postterm babies (i.e., those born at a gestational age > 41 weeks).

   Because meconium aspiration is likely, the clinician should further assess the infant and prepare to establish and maintain an adequate airway:

   - Assess the baby's initial condition: The baby is limp, apneic, and cyanotic. The meconium is thick and brown.
   - Prepare for immediate oral and tracheal suctioning as per Neonatal Resuscitation Program (NRP) guidelines. Oral and tracheal suctioning are repeated until little meconium was present when suctioning the patient.

(continues)

Following these interventions, the baby continues with poor respiratory effort and remains cyanotic.

2. What additional interventions should the respiratory care clinician consider?

Following establishment of an adequate airway, initial treatment of meconium aspiration may include oxygen therapy and mechanical ventilatory support. Sedation may be required to avoid ventilator–patient dyssynchrony, and surfactant therapy may be useful. Additional diagnostic tests include obtaining a chest radiograph and possibly an echocardiogram to assess cardiac/cardiovascular function.

The infant is intubated and placed on a mechanical ventilator. Upon arrival to the NICU, the ventilator is set to the following:

Mode: Pressure control mode
PIP: 26 cm H_2O
PEEP: 5 cm H_2O
Respiratory rate: 35 breaths/min
F_{IO_2}: 100%

The endotracheal tube is in good position. Initial arterial blood gases (ABG) on these ventilator settings are:
pH: 7.15
Pa_{CO_2}: 70 mm Hg
Pa_{O_2}: 31 mm Hg
HCO_3^-: 13 mEq/L
BE: 16
Sa_{O_2}: 83%

3. What is an appropriate assessment of the patient's initial ventilator settings and resultant arterial blood gases?

The Pa_{O_2} of 31 mm Hg with an Sa_{O_2} of 83% indicates hypoxemia. The patient is acidotic and hypercapnic, even with mechanical ventilatory support.

4. What interventions should the respiratory care clinician suggest at this point?

As noted, the patient is hypoxemic and hypercapnic with a resultant respiratory acidosis. The ventilatory rate should be increased and PEEP may be increased to improve oxygenation:

- Increase the respiratory rate to 40 breaths/min.
- Increase PEEP to 8 cm H_2O.

5. What additional diagnostic studies may be useful at this point in time?

Imaging studies should be ordered. A chest x-ray should be obtained in to assess the degree of lung involvement. An echocardiogram should also be considered to assess the patient's cardiac/cardiovascular status. Meconium aspiration may cause hypoxemia, which, in turn, results in persistent fetal circulation and right-to-left shunt. Additional diagnostic studies may include pre- and postductal oxygen saturations, arterial blood gas studies, chest radiograph, and electrocardiogram.

The chest x-ray for this patient reveals patchy, irregular opacifications and a small right-apical pneumothorax. Pneumothorax is common in patients with meconium aspiration because meconium can plug the airways and cause hyperinflation in local areas. These hyperinflated areas can cause rupture of alveoli into the bronchovesicular bundle (the area of the lung where blood vessels and lymphatics run from the pleura to the mediastinum), resulting in a pneumothorax.

The echocardiogram demonstrates the presence of persistent pulmonary hypertension of the newborn (PPHN). Normally, pulmonary vascular resistance decreases following the first few breaths after birth due to the effects of oxygen, which is a pulmonary vasodilator. Hypoxemia can cause pulmonary vascular resistance to remain abnormally high following birth, resulting in PPHN. Cyanosis, hypoxemia, and respiratory distress are seen with PPHN, due, in part, to the right-to-left shunt that occurs. Echocardiography is the diagnostic test of choice for establishing the presence of PPHN.

6. What additional interventions should be considered?

Pre- and postductal oxygen saturations should be obtained by measuring the Sp_{O_2} in the right thumb (preductal saturation) and the Sp_{O_2} in one of the big toes (right or left; postductal saturation). An Sp_{O_2} difference between the pre- and postductal Sp_{O_2} > 10% is associated with right-to-left shunting. This right-to-left shunt can be caused by a persistent fetal circulation (e.g., patent ductus arteriosis [PDA]). PPHN and PDA often appear together. Inhaled nitric oxide (NO) therapy may be started at 20 ppm to correct this right-to-left shunt. Nitric oxide is a potent pulmonary vasodilator.

Chest tube placement should also be considered to treat the pneumothorax. Surfactant replacement therapy may be useful and should be considered.

Almost immediately after inhaled NO is initiated, the pre- and postductal oxygen saturations increase to $\geq 96\%$. Thirty minutes later, an ABG is obtained with the following results:

pH: 7.24

$Paco_2$: 60 mm Hg

Pao_2: 64 mm Hg

HCO_3^-: 24 mEq/L

BE: −3

Sao_2: 97%

7. What is an appropriate assessment of the patient's condition at this time?

    The pre- and postductal oxygen saturations have improved, suggesting that the inhaled nitric oxide has reduced the right-to-left shunt and lowered pulmonary vascular resistance and pulmonary artery pressure. The arterial blood gases continue to show hypoventilation with a respiratory acidosis, though oxygenation has improved significantly.

8. What additional interventions should be considered at this time?

    The respiratory rate on the ventilator should be increased in order to lower the $Paco_2$. If this fails, high-frequency oscillatory ventilation (HFOV) might be considered. At this point in time, 100% oxygen is no longer necessary. The following actions should be taken:

    • Increase the respiratory rate on the ventilator to 50 breaths/min.

    • Wean the Fio_2, as tolerated, based on SpO_2 and arterial blood gases.

    The decision is made to place the baby on HFOV so that she can stabilize over the next few hours.

    The infant remained on HFOV with inhaled NO days for the next 5 days. The patient was successfully transitioned to conventional ventilation and weaned off inhaled NO. The patient was extubated the following week. Note that if the infant's condition worsened on HFOV, the next escalation in treatment would have been extracorporeal membrane oxygenation (ECMO).

birth canal.[68] Molding typically resolves within a few days following birth.[68] Assessment of the newborn's head will include palpation of the fontanels (the soft spots between cranial bones), skull sutures (lines of articulation between skull bones), and palpation for the presence of craniotabes (abnormal softening of skull bones).[67,68] Edema in the subcutaneous scalp tissues of the scalp and presenting part of the head is common at birth and generally resolves within a few days.[68]

The face should be evaluated for symmetry. If the face is asymmetric, a congenital abnormality may be present. Newborns who were delivered by forceps or had prolonged or difficult labor may be at risk of facial palsy (facial paralysis or loss of movement).[69,70] Facial palsy most commonly affects the muscles around the lips and is most apparent when the baby is crying, though the eyelid and lower face on the affected side may be involved.[69,70] Facial palsy typically resolves in few days to a few weeks.[70]

The eyes should be assessed for spacing, symmetry, and movement. The pupils, sclera (whites of the eye), conjunctiva (membrane covering inner eyelids and sclera), and cornea should be examined. Pupils should be round, regular, and reactive to light in term infants and preterm infants with a gestational age of at least 28 to 32 weeks.[53] The sclera of each eye should be white and clear, though the sclera may have a light blue appearance in preterm infants.[53] The *red reflex*

test refers to a recommended ophthalmic examination to detect cataracts, glaucoma, or other lens or retinal abnormalities. The eyes may be swollen and edematous from the birthing process. To prevent infection, antibiotic ointment or silver nitrate should be applied to the eyes soon after birth. Once the swelling has gone down, one can assess for excessive spacing or slanting of the eyes. For example, infants with **Down syndrome** typically have up-slanting palpebral fissures (the space between the margins of the eyelids) and an epicanthic fold of the inner eyelid.

The ears should be examined for placement, shape, size, and any deformation. If the ears are deformed, abnormally low set, or posteriorly rotated, a genetic abnormality may be present. The ear canals should be present and patent and the tympanic membranes free of infection. As hearing loss at birth is common, the American Academy of Pediatrics recommends a hearing evaluation prior to discharge from the hospital. Undetected hearing loss can hinder the development of speech and language.[71]

Because newborns are obligate nose breathers, special attention should be paid to the shape of the nose, nasal patency, and nasal airflow. Airflow and patency can be assessed by occluding one nare and observing if the infant is able to breathe through the opposing side. The procedure is then repeated for the opposite nare. As an alternative, the clinician can place a piece of string in front of each nare and observe to see if the string moves back and forth as the infant breathes. If the newborn cannot breathe through one nare, then nasal patency should be established by passing a suction catheter to determine if there is a nasal obstruction. If both nares are occluded, then the infant may require intubation because the infant will not be able to breathe adequately through the mouth. A possible diagnosis in an infant that has at least one blocked nare is *choanal atresia,* a congenital disorder in which the nasal passage is blocked. A common presentation for patients with choanal atresia is apnea and cyanosis while at rest; when stimulated, the baby will turn pink.

> **RC Insights**
>
> Infants are obligate nose breathers. The tongue is large and the nasal and oral airway passages are small. Keeping nasal passages patent is essential to care of the infant in distress.

The mouth should be examined next. Many congenital anomalies are linked to oral defects. The mouth should open without any problems. The size of the jaw should be noted. A small jaw might indicate a genetic disorder (e.g., Pierre Robin syndrome). Infants with Down syndrome (i.e., trisomy 21) commonly have a small mouth, small ears, and flattened nose. The lip should be intact, and any clefts should be noted and assessed, because both a small jaw and cleft lip may lead to feeding difficulties. For infants with a small jaw, positioning the baby on his or her belly may provide short-term relief until a surgical repair can be performed.

The neck should be examined for limitations of movement and vertebral anomalies. Neck masses may be visible or palpable and could impair breathing by applying pressure to the trachea. Torticollis (an abnormal asymmetrical neck) may be caused by trauma to the sternocleidomastoid muscle due to a birth injury, intrauterine malposition, or developmental abnormalities of the cervical spine.[53]

Abdominal Assessment

The abdomen should be inspected for size and appearance. The appearance of the umbilical cord should also be assessed. Masses or hernias should be noted. The umbilical cord should be of normal size and free of infection (omphalitis).[53] Abdominal distension may be caused by intestinal obstruction, ascites, or enlarged abdominal organs (e.g., liver).[53] A diaphragmatic hernia, an extremely serious condition, can allow abdominal contents to move into the chest cavity, resulting in a flat or hollow abdominal appearance. The liver and kidneys should be palpable.

Musculoskeletal System Assessment

Congenital anomalies can sometimes be identified by assessing the musculoskeletal system. Joint movement or newborn position may suggest joint contractures. Symmetry of the spine should be assessed. Many infants have a sacral dimple. If the bottom of the dimple can be seen and there are no bony defects, then the dimple may be nothing to be concerned about. However, if the bottom of dimple cannot be seen or there are boney defects, a tuft of hair, and drainage, then the newborn may have the birth defect known as **spina bifida**. A form of spina bifida in which the neural tube forms over the spine is called *myelomeningocele.*

Neurologic Assessment

The neurologic assessment includes determining if the newborn responds normally to the surrounding environment and to stimulation.[68,69] Newborns who are overly irritable, jittery, or lethargic may have a neurologic disorder. A complete neurologic assessment should be done within 24 hours of birth and should include a medical and genetic history of the parents.[68,69]

A number of normal reflexes are present in the newborn. The **grasp reflex** is observed when the newborn grasps a finger that is placed in the palm of its hand. When the soles of the feet are stimulated, the infant's toes should curl down as if the toes are trying to grasp an object (plantar grasp reflex). Other reflexes evaluated in the neonate include the Moro reflex, the stepping reflex, and the **startle reflex**. Most of these reflexes are present around 32 weeks of gestation.[68,69]

> **RC Insights**
>
> Avoiding cold stress is vital to care of the neonate. Newborn infants have a large body surface area compared to their body mass, especially the head, making them very susceptible to hypothermia. Providing adequate heat, wrapping them up, and using hats/caps will help mitigate the effects of cold stress.

Muscle tone is assessed by moving the infant's extremities and noting resistance to the motion.[68,69] Passive tone can be measured by using certain passive maneuvers. For example, the scarf sign assesses the range of shoulder adduction; resistance to this maneuver increases with gestational age.[68,69]

Assessment of the Extremities

The extremities should be assessed and the number, size, and position of the fingers and toes noted. Movement of the arms and legs should be reviewed and color of the hands and feet noted. Acrocyanosis refers to a decrease in oxygen delivery to the extremities, and this may persist for several hours following birth.[62] The skin of the newborn should be assessed for color, rashes, pigmentation, and any unusual markings, edema, or bruising.[62]

Normally, the newborn's skin is pink, though 25% to 50% of term infants develop neonatal jaundice due to high levels of bilirubin in the blood.[62] This condition is even more prevalent in premature infants. Normally, neonatal jaundice does not require treatment, though special blue lights (bili lights) are sometimes used to provide phototherapy that breaks down bilirubin in the skin. One hazard of bili lights is retinal damage, and care should be taken to protect the infant's eyes through use of eye shields.

Laboratory Assessment

If the mother or the newborn show signs of infection or sepsis, laboratory tests may be performed to identify infection. Newborns who are septic may have fever, low APGAR scores, and may be irritable or unresponsive. A sepsis evaluation includes blood cultures, complete blood count (CBC), cerebrospinal fluid (CSF) tap, and urine culture to locate the source of the infection. Blood gas measurement from either a capillary sample or arterial sample may be helpful in determining respiratory status. Newborns tend to have elevated levels of hemoglobin and hematocrit at birth.

Metabolic or endocrine disorders, genetic hemoglobin disorders, and infection are some of the problems that may be detected by the newborn laboratory screen.[72] This testing should be done as close to discharge as possible or before any blood transfusion or dialysis, because it may give false-positives or false-negatives following these procedures. **Table 16-9** lists normal infant laboratory values. **Table 16-10** provides normal cord, neonatal, and pediatric blood gas values.

Assessment of the Pediatric Patient

Pediatric patients encompass a wide range of ages and stages of development. For our discussion we will use the following ranges:

- Newborn/neonate: Birth up to 1 month of age (or up to 28 days of age)
- Infant: 1 month of age to 1 year of age
  - May include newborn/neonatal period as well
- Toddler: 1 to 3 years of age
- Preschool: 3 to 5 years of age
- Primary school age: 5 to 13 years of age
- Secondary school age: 13 to 18 years of age
  - Adolescent: Generally corresponds to teen years; however, may range from between ages 10 and 19.

Children in their late teens (16 to 18 years of age) are sometimes treated as adults.

History

The pediatric medical history may be gathered from the child, the parents, and the healthcare record. Other sources might include people who care for the child, such as guardians, schoolteachers, day care providers, and babysitters. It is also a good idea to be aware of the child's birthing history in order to note if there were any problems that may have led to the current presentation. For the very young child, the history must be obtained from the parents or other caregiver. Older children may provide valuable and relevant information.

When obtaining a medical history, the respiratory care clinician should identify the chief complaint or main concern and then move on to the history of present illness. Next, the past medical history should be obtained. The clinician may then obtain the family history and address any social or environmental issues. Current medications should be reviewed and any nutritional issues addressed. For each medication, the clinician should try and identify the type of medication (prescription, nonprescription, or alternative medicine) and its purpose, dose, and when it was last taken. Before beginning the physical examination, it is a good idea to perform a review of symptoms.

The chief complaint provides the main reason for seeking medical care. This could be something that was observed by the caregiver (e.g., "cough" or "fever") or the child (e.g., "my throat hurts"). Determining the chief complaint is usually the first step in identifying the problem. Questions asked to clarify the problem include symptom timing, location, and triggers or aggravating factors. Medications (if any) taken to treat the symptoms should be noted. It should also be determined if this is a new, seasonal, chronic, or recurring illness. Common respiratory related problems seen in pediatric patients include cough, runny nose, ear pain, sore throat, fever, and sputum production. The child may be short of breath and experience chest pain, wheezing, or chest tightness. The caregiver may note audible stridor or wheezing. The child may be anxious or irritable; lethargy, somnolence, or unresponsiveness can signal severe cardiopulmonary problems.

The family, social, and environmental history may further clarify the problem. For example, genetic problems may "run in the family." Environmental factors may affect specific disease states (e.g., asthma). Where (and with whom) the child lives, the social environment, and daily activities such as day care attendance and school attendance should be noted. The occupation of the primary caregivers, housing conditions, and the presence of secondhand smoke, mold, or pets should be reviewed. The clinician should ask about exposures at school or day care, missed school days due to illness, and the child's grades and/or school performance. Finally, the clinician should inquire about recent travel or if the patient has recently moved from another country or region of the country. Information gathered as part of the patient history may provide the clinician with clues as to why the patient got sick and

TABLE 16-9
Normal Pediatric Laboratory Values

	Age	Normal Values
Chemistry		
Albumin	0–1 year	2.0–4.0 g/dL
	1 year to adult	3.5–5.5 g/dL
Ammonia	Newborns	90–150 mcg/dL
	Children	40–120 mcg/dL
	Adults	18–54 mcg/dL
Amylase	Newborns	0–60 units/L
	Adults	30–110 units/L
Bilirubin, conjugated, direct	Newborns	< 1.5 mg/dL
	1 month to adult	0–0.5 mg/dL
Bilirubin, total	0–3 days	2.0–10.0 mg/dL
	1 month to adult	0–1.5 mg/dL
Bilirubin, unconjugated, indirect		0.6–10.5 mg/dL
Calcium	Newborns	7.0–12.0 mg/dL
	0–2 years	8.8–11.2 mg/dL
	2 years to adult	9.0–11.0 mg/dL
Calcium, ionized, whole blood		4.4–5.4 mg/dL
Carbon dioxide, total		23–33 mEq/L
Chloride		95–105 mEq/L
Creatinine	0–1 year	≤ 0.6 mg/dL
Glucose	1 year to adult	0.5–1.5 mg/dL
	Newborns	30–90 mg/dL
	0–2 years	60–105 mg/dL
	Children to adults	70–110 mg/dL
Iron	Newborns	110–270 mcg/dL
	Infants	30–70 mcg/dL
	Children	55–120 mcg/dL
	Adults	70–180 mcg/dL
Lactic acid, lactate		2–20 mg/dL
Lipase	Children	20–140 units/L
	Adults	0–190 units/L
Magnesium		1.5–2.5 mEq/L

Osmolality, serum		275–296 mOsm/kg
Osmolality, urine		50–1400 mOsm/kg
Phosphorus	Newborns	4.2–9.0 mg/dL
	6 weeks to 19 months	3.8–6.7 mg/dL
	19 months to 3 years	2.9–5.9 mg/dL
	3–15 years	3.6–5.6 mg/dL
	> 15 years	2.5–5.0 mg/dL
Potassium, plasma	Newborns	4.5–7.2 mEq/L
	2 days to 3 months	4.0–6.2 mEq/L
	3 months to 1 year	3.7–5.6 mEq/L
	1–16 years	3.5–5.0 mEq/L
Protein, total	0–2 years	4.2–7.4 g/dL
	> 2 years	6.0–8.0 g/dL
Sodium		136–145 mEq/L
Urea nitrogen, blood	Adults	30–200 mg/dL
	0–2 years	4–15 mg/dL
	2 years to adult	5–20 mg/dL
Uric acid		Male: 3.0–7.0 mg/dL Female: 2.0–6.0 mg/dL
Enzymes		
Alanine aminotransferase (ALT; also referred to as SGPT)	0–2 months	8–78 units/L
Alkaline phosphatase (ALKP)	> 2 months	8–36 units/L
	Newborns	60–130 units/L
	0–16 years	85–400 units/L
Aspartate aminotransferase (AST)	> 16 years	30–115 units/L
	Infants	18–74 units/L
Serum glutamic oxaloacetic transaminase (SGOT)	Children	15–46 units/L
	Adults	5–35 units/L
Creatine kinase (CK)	Infants	20–200 units/L
	Children	10–90 units/L
	Adult male	0–206 units/L
	Adult female	0–175 units/L
Lactate dehydrogenase (LDH)	Newborns	290–501 units/L
	1 month to 2 years	110–144 units/L
	> 16 years	60–170 units/L

(continues)

Blood Gases

	Arterial	Capillary	Venous
pH	7.35–7.45	7.35–7.45	7.32–7.42
PCO_2 (mm Hg)	35–45	35–45	38–52
PO_2 (mm Hg)	70–100	60–80	24–48
HCO_3^- (mEq/L)	19–25	19–25	19–25
TCO_2 (mEq/L)	19–29	19–29	23–33
O_2 saturation (%)	90–95	90–95	40–70
Base excess (mEq/L)	5 to +5	5 to +5	5 to +5

Hematology Values

Age	Hb (g/dL)	Hct (%)	RBC (mill/mm³)	RDW	MCV (fL)	MCH (pg)	MCHC (%)	PLTS (× 10³/mm³)
0–3 days	15.0–20.0	45–61	4.0–5.9	< 18	95–115	31–37	29–37	250–450
1–2 weeks	12.5–18.5	39–57	3.6–5.5	< 17	86–110	28–36	28–38	250–450
1–6 months	10.0–13.0	29–42	3.1–4.3	< 16.5	74–96	25–35	30–36	300–700
7 months to 2 years	10.5–13.0	33–38	3.7–4.9	< 16	70–84	23–30	31–37	250–600
2–5 years	11.5–13.0	34–39	3.9–5.0	< 15	75–87	24–30	31–37	250–550
5–8 years	11.5–14.5	35–42	4.0–4.9	< 15	77–95	25–33	31–37	250–550
13–18 y	12.0–15.2	36–47	4.5–5.1	< 14.5	78–96	25–35	31–37	150–450
Adult male	13.5–16.5	41–50	4.5–5.5	< 14.5	80–100	26–34	31–37	150–450
Adult female	12.0–15.0	36–44	4.0–4.9	< 14.5	80–100	26–34	31–37	150–450

White Blood Cell and Differential

Age	WBC (× 10³/mm³)	Segs	Bands	Lymphs	Monos	Eosinophils	Basophils	Atypical Lymphs	No. of NRBCs
0–3 days	9.0–35.0	32–62	10–18	19–29	5–7	0–2	0–1	0–8	0–2
1–2 weeks	5.0–20.0	14–34	6–14	36–45	6–10	0–2	0–1	0–8	0
1–6 months	6.0–17.5	13–33	4–12	41–71	4–7	0–3	0–1	0–8	0
7 months to 2 years	6.0–17.0	15–35	5–11	45–76	3–6	0–3	0–1	0–8	0
2–5 years	5.5–15.5	23–45	5–11	35–65	3–6	0–3	0–1	0–8	0
5–8 years	5.0–14.5	32–54	5–11	28–48	3–6	0–3	0–1	0–8	0
13–18 years	4.5–13.0	34–64	5–11	25–45	3–6	0–3	0–1	0–8	0
Adults	4.5–11.0	35–66	5–11	24–44	3–6	0–3	0–1	0–8	0

Hb, hemoglobin; Hct, hematocrit; RBC, red blood cell count; RDW, red cell distribution width; MCV, mean corpuscular volume; MCHC, mean corpuscular hemoglobin concentration; PLT, platelets; WBC, white blood cell; segs, segmented neutrophils; bands, band neutrophils; lymphs, lymphocytes; monos, monocytes; NRBC, nucleated red blood cells.
Data from: Pediatric Care Online. Reference Values for Children. October 23, 2013. Available at https://www.pediatriccareonline.org/

TABLE 16-10
Normal Cord, Neonatal, and Pediatric Blood Gas Values

Parameter	Umbilical Artery	Umbilical Vein	Newborn	Infant to Toddler	Child to Adult
pH	7.24	7.32	7.3–7.4	7.3–7.4	7.35–7.45
$PaCO_2$ (mm Hg)	49	38	30–40	30–40	35–45
PO_2 (mm Hg)	16	27	60–90	80–100	80–100
HCO_3^- (mmol/L)	19	20	20–22	20–22	22–24

Courtesy of Hess DR, MacIntyre NR, Mishoe SC, Galvin WF, and Adams AB. *Respiratory Care: Principles And Practice*. 2nd ed. Burlington, MA: Jones and Bartlett Learning; 2011.

what things may be exacerbating the symptoms. For example, a detailed family, social, and environmental history of a 4-year-old child with frequent upper respiratory tract infections may reveal parents that smoke, a grandmother living in a damp, moldy apartment, and attendance at a day care center where there are lots of sick children.

Physical Examination

The physical examination should be conducted in a professional, respectful, warm, and reassuring manner. Ideally, the pediatric patient will be calm and cooperative, but for younger patients this may not be the case. Children are often frightened by a medical setting and may be crying, agitated, or uncooperative. A parent or guardian should be present during the examination, and this may help in securing the child's cooperation. The clinician may use a toy, pictures, or games to further distract the child or set him or her at ease.

Vital Signs

The first set of parameters collected on a pediatric patient is a set of vital signs. These are standard parameters that provide the baseline data for determining the health of the pediatric patient. Normal values for heart rate, respiratory rate, and blood pressure vary with age, with the values for children older than 12 years of age approaching adult normal values. Heart rate, respiratory rate, and blood pressure may also vary if the child is upset or anxious. For example, pulse and blood pressure may be elevated if the child is screaming and moving vigorously; otherwise, values should be normal for the child's age. **Table 16-11** lists the baseline normal values for heart rate and blood pressure for children of different ages. It should be noted that accurate blood pressure measurement in very young children can be difficult; routine measurement in children < 3 years of age may not be typically performed.[73]

A child's temperature will vary depending on the time of the day and the severity of the illness. Although the ideal normal value for body temperature is 98.6° F (37.0° C), some children may tend to have a "normal"

that is slightly warmer or cooler. The most accurate method of assessing a child's temperature is rectally, though forehead, ear, and axillary measurements are acceptable. Normal temperatures for oral, axillary, rectal, and ear measurements are listed in **Table 16-12**.

Oxygen saturation (Spo_2) via pulse oximeter is often assessed as a part of routine vital sign measurement in children. A normal Spo_2 is 95% to 99% while breathing room air; children with lung or heart disease will often have a lower Spo_2.

General Examination

The general physical examination should include assessment of general appearance, vital signs, measurement of growth parameters (e.g., weight, height, head and chest circumference) and examination of the head and neck, chest, abdomen, and extremities. The neurologic examination and assessment of mental status should include level of consciousness, orientation, and reflexes. A complete physical examination will also

TABLE 16-11
Pediatric Vital Signs

Age	Heart Rate (bpm)	Blood Pressure (mm Hg)
0–6 months	90–160	55–90/45–65
6–12 months	80–120	70–100/50–65
1–3 years	70–110	80–105/55–70
3–6 years	65–110	90–110/55–70
6–10 years	70–110	95–110/60–75
> 10 years	55–95	100–125/60–80

General estimate of blood pressure: Systolic BP = 90 mm Hg + (2 × Age in years)
Rough approximation of pulses:
Infant: 160 bpm
Preschool: 120 bpm
Adolescent: 100 bpm

TABLE 16-12
Normal Pediatric Temperature Range (Fahrenheit)

Age	Oral	Rectal	Axillary	Ear	Forehead
0–2 years	—	97.9–100.4	94.5–99.1	97.5–100.4	
3–10 years	95.9–99.5	97.9–100.4	96.6–98.0	97.0–100.0	
> 11 years	97.6–99.6	98.6–100.6	95.3–98.4	96.6–99.7	87.8–96.1

Conversion from degrees Fahrenheit (F) to Celsius (C)					
Degrees Fahrenheit	Degrees Celsius°	Degrees Fahrenheit	Degrees Celsius°	Degrees Fahrenheit	Degrees Celsius°
94.5	34.7	97.9	36.6	99.6	37.6
95.3	35.2	98.0	36.7	99.7	37.6
95.9	35.5	98.4	36.9	100.0	37.8
96.6	35.9	99.1	37.3	100.4	38.0
97.0	36.1	99.5	37.5	100.6	38.1
97.5	36.4				
97.6	36.4				

Modified from: Agrawal S. Normal vital signs in children: heart rate, respirations, temperature, and blood pressure. *Complex Child E-Magazine.* 2008. Available at http://www.articles.complexchild.com/march2009/00114.pdf.

include attention to the skin, lymph nodes, spine, pelvis, and urinary system.

The patient's general appearance provides important assessment information. The clinician should observe the patient carefully and address the following questions:[73]

- Is the patient awake, alert, and oriented?
- Is the patient calm, shy, or anxious?
- Does the patient "look" normal, or does he or she appear to be ill, uncomfortable, or in distress?
- Is the patient irritable, upset, and/or combative?
- If the patient is crying, is the sound weak, loud, or high in pitch?
- Is the patient's weight normal, overweight, or underweight?
- What is the patient's position?

For example, a patient who is seriously ill may appear to be listless with weak crying.[73] Rapid, shallow breathing may suggest a respiratory problem. A child in distress due to an asthma attack may sit forward and brace himself to ease the work of breathing.[73] A child with a sore throat, upper respiratory tract infection, or epiglottitis may be leaning forward and drooling.

The general physical examination should include measurement of height and weight. Values should be compared to expected normal values for children of the same age and gender, and charts and calculators are available for this purpose.[74] If height and/or weight

are less than expected, further investigation should be conducted to determine what maybe causing the slow growth or poor weight gain.[74] Causes of poor weight gain include inadequate caloric intake, problems with food absorption, and excess metabolic demand.

Achievement of *developmental milestones* refers to a child reaching certain motor (e.g., crawling, standing, walking), communication (e.g., speech and language), cognitive, social, and emotional milestones appropriate to the child's age. Children should reach their developmental milestones within a few months of the average for normal children of that age. For example, a 1-year-old is typically shy or nervous around strangers, responds to simple spoken requests, and is able to copy gestures. A 1-year-old child with a developmental delay may not demonstrate these behaviors. Children who have neuromuscular disease (e.g., cerebral palsy, muscular dystrophy) may have difficulty hitting their milestones and be at greater risk of developing respiratory infections, especially if they have a hard time coughing and clearing secretions.

Pulmonary Examination

The pulmonary assessment should include inspection, palpation, percussion, and auscultation and should be done with the child's upper torso exposed. Signs of respiratory distress such as tachycardia, tachypnea, fever, and decreased SpO_2 should be noted.

The respiratory rate is a sensitive indicator of cardiopulmonary status. Typically, children with respiratory distress are tachypneic. Common causes of rapid, shallow breathing in children include pulmonary infection, cardiac disease, and compensation for a metabolic acidosis.[75] Be aware that a fever may cause tachypnea in children; the higher the fever, the higher the respiratory rate. As lung disease worsens, typically work of breathing increases. As respiratory failure ensues, the patient's respiratory rate may decrease as the patient becomes fatigued. An abnormally decreased respiratory rate can also be due to CNS problems, drugs and medications (e.g., narcotics, sedatives), and metabolic disease.[75] Infants may also have variable respiratory rates interspersed with periods of apnea.[75] **Table 16-13** describes normal respiratory rates in awake children.

Breathlessness can sometimes be evaluated by assessing the child's ability to speak without pausing or becoming short of breath. For example, the clinician may count the number of words the child is able to say before the child needs to pause and take a breath. Generally, a short interval between breaths and decreased number of words spoken suggest increased respiratory distress and breathlessness. For a child who does not communicate, note his or her energy level. Observing an infant while feeding may also provide clues to the level of respiratory distress. For example, an infant in distress may only be able to take one or two gulps of milk before a long pause to catch his or her breath.

Head bobbing is another sign of respiratory distress sometimes seen in infants and young children. In infants, head bobbing is caused when the scalene and sternocleidomastoid muscles contract to assist ventilation; the contraction of these muscles during inspiration and relaxation during expiration causes the head to "bob." Specifically, during inspiration, the head is pulled down while the rib cage and clavicles are pulled up; thus the head bobs forward during inspiration.

Other signs of respiratory distress in infants and small children include grunting and **nasal flaring**. As noted earlier, grunting is the sound generated by exhaling against a partially closed glottis. Grunting increases the end-expiratory pressure in the lungs, increases FRC, and may help prevent small airway and alveolar collapse. Typically, grunting is seen in newborns with RSV/bronchiolitis, RDS, pulmonary edema, or atelectasis. Nasal flaring is also an important sign of respiratory distress. Children up to the age of 2 years are obligate nose breathers. When in distress, the nostrils will flare during inspiration as the child tries to increase air movement into the lungs. **Clinical Focus 16-3** provides an example of an infant with bronchiolitis.

Chest Inspection

Inspection of the chest wall should include anterior, posterior, and lateral aspects. Patients who have obstructive lung diseases such as chronic asthma, bronchopulmonary dysplasia (BPD), and cystic fibrosis (CF) may have an increased anteroposterior (AP) thoracic diameter due to air trapping (i.e., a barrel-shaped chest).[75] Inspection of the thorax may also reveal certain congenital deformities. *Pectus excavatum* refers to a chest wall deformity in which the chest appears to be sunken in, and may be referred to as "sunken chest" or "funnel chest." Pectus excavatum is often apparent at birth or shortly thereafter, though it may not become obvious until the early teenage years.[34] *Pectus carinatum* ("pigeon chest") is a less common congenital chest wall deformity in which the sternum bulges out. Pectus carinatum is often identified at birth, though it may not become apparent until early adolescence.[34] *Spinal scoliosis* is a lateral (i.e., sideways) curvature of the spine, whereas *kyphosis* is an anteroposterior curvature of the spine. Scoliosis can be due to a congenital defect, or it may appear later in life and be caused by another disease state or condition (e.g., neuromuscular disease), or it may be due to unknown causes (e.g., idiopathic scoliosis). Kyphoscoliosis is a musculoskeletal disease that combines the two deformities and causes a more significant restrictive pulmonary disease pattern. Causes of kyphoscoliosis in children include neuromuscular disease (e.g., polio, muscular dystrophy, cerebral palsy), rickets (from vitamin D deficiency), and connective tissue disorders (e.g., Marfan syndrome). Kyphoscoliosis may cause chronic hypoventilation, hypoxemia, and pulmonary hypertension (due to chronic hypoxemia).

Observing chest wall motion as the child breathes may also provide clues regarding the patient's respiratory status. **Chest wall retractions** are a sign of respiratory distress. Retractions can be classified as suprasternal, intercostal, subcostal, and substernal. Suprasternal retractions are seen above the clavicle and sternum. Intercostal retractions occur between the ribs. Subcostal retractions may be seen below the lower costal margin of the rib cage. Substernal retractions may be seen below the xiphoid process. Retractions are seen in infants with respiratory distress and older pediatric patients with significant upper airway obstruction.

TABLE 16-13
Normal Respiratory Rates in Awake Children

Age	Respiratory Rate (breaths/min)	Heart Rate (bpm)
Infant (birth – 1 year)	30–60	100–160
1–3 years	24–40	90–150
3–6 years	22–34	80–140
6–12 years	12–30	70–120
> 12 years	12–16	60–100

CLINICAL FOCUS 16-3

Bronchiolitis/RSV

A previously healthy 4-month-old girl presents to the emergency department in January with a 2-day history rhinorrhea and cough. The patient has tachypnea, chest congestion, fever, and an apparent increase in the work of breathing. The patient has not been eating or drinking well for the past 2 days.

1. In order to assess this patient, what steps should the respiratory care clinician take?

    The respiratory care clinician should perform a physical assessment to include general appearance, vital signs, and breath sounds.

    On assessment, the following vital signs are obtained:

    Temperature (axillary): 38.5° C

    Heart rate: 152 bpm

    Respiratory rate: 72 breaths/min

    Blood pressure: 74/46 mm Hg

    SpO_2: 90% on room air

    Breath sounds were bilateral and coarse with fair aeration and wheezing.

2. Based on the examination findings what steps should the respiratory care clinician now consider?

    The patient is in acute distress with an elevated respiratory rate and heart rate. The presence of fever, cough, chest congestion, and decreased oxygen saturation (SpO_2) suggest respiratory tract infection. One of the most common causes of lower respiratory infection in infants is respiratory syncytial virus (RSV). RSV is more common in winter. Wheezing is a common clinical manifestation of RSV in infants. Bronchiolitis or pneumonia may be caused by RSV, which can lead to respiratory failure.

    With bronchiolitis, upper respiratory tract infection may be followed by inflammation of the lower respiratory tract (i.e., the bronchioles). Upper respiratory symptoms may include nasal congestion and rhinorrhea, whereas lower respiratory tract infection may result in crackles and/or wheezing. Infants with bronchiolitis may have difficulty feeding and become dehydrated. Moderate to severe respiratory distress may occur, and some infants experience periods of apnea. Blood gases generally show hypoxemia, which may or may not be accompanied by hypoventilation and acidemia.

3. What interventions and/or additional testing should the respiratory care clinician now consider?

    Based on the assessment findings, the clinician should consider a diagnosis of RSV. Laboratory testing of respiratory secretions (e.g., rapid antigen testing) should be performed to confirm the diagnosis. The treatment of RSV is largely supportive. Oxygen therapy and bronchodilator therapy should be provided. The nasal passages of the infant should be suctioned to make sure that they are clear. Fluids may be administered to treat dehydration. Aerosolized hypertonic saline (3% NaCl) may be delivered to reduce airway edema and mucus plugging in infants.

    The clinician takes the following steps:

    - Suction the nasal passages. The secretions are copious, thick, and yellow. Minimal change in respiratory status is noted following suctioning.
    - Provide oxygen therapy. A nasal cannula is started at 1 L/min to treat the desaturation.
    - Administer a bronchodilator. Albuterol (5 mg) is administered via nebulizer for the wheezing. The recommended dosage of albuterol is 2.5 to 5 mg (diluted in 2.5 to 3 mL of normal saline). Following administration of the bronchodilator, there is minimal change to breaths sounds and slight improvement in work of breathing. Oxygen saturation improves to 94%.

    A peripheral intravenous catheter is placed followed by a fluid bolus for dehydration. The patient is admitted to the hospital because of respiratory distress, increased work of breathing, oxygen requirements, and dehydration.

4. Upon admission to the hospital floor, what interventions should the respiratory care clinician suggest for the patient's continued wheezing, respiratory distress, and increased work of breathing?

    As noted, treatment of RSV is largely supportive and may include oxygen therapy (if oxygen saturations are ≤ 90%), bronchodilator therapy, and fluid support, if indicated.

    The following interventions are ordered:

    - Racemic epinephrine (2.25%) 0.25 to 0.5 mL via nebulizer
    - Hypertonic saline 3% delivered via nebulizer
    - Suctioning of nasal passageways as needed.

All three interventions are completed and result in mild improvements to breath sounds and work of breathing. The bronchodilator therapy is discontinued, because there was minimal evidence of improvement following therapy. The hypertonic saline therapy is continued along with suctioning to maintain clear nasal passages. The patient is stabilized with oxygen therapy, hypertonic saline administration, and frequent nasal suctioning over the next 24 hours. The following day the patient was weaned off the oxygen and was feeding without difficulty. The patient was discharged to home.

Escalation interventions for critically ill patients with bronchiolitis commonly include the use of a high-flow nasal cannula and/or continuous positive airway pressure (CPAP). Less often the use of heliox and/or mechanical ventilation is required.

Retractions are a serious matter and may be a sign of respiratory failure. *Paradoxical breathing*, or asynchronous breathing, is present when the chest wall and abdomen move in opposite positions during breathing. During normal ventilation, the chest wall rises and the diaphragm descends (abdomen rises) on inspiration; the chest falls during exhalation as the diaphragm relaxes. During paradoxical breathing ("see-saw" breathing pattern) the chest wall movement is out of synch with the motion of the diaphragm. This may occur unilaterally with a unilateral pneumonia, pneumothorax, atelectasis, or foreign body obstruction on one side or bilaterally with neuromuscular disease.[75]

In infants, *transillumination* of the chest may help identify pneumothorax. Transillumination of the chest is performed by placing a bright light (typically a bilirubin light) behind the area of the chest where the pneumothorax is suspected. A pneumothorax will be seen as an area of hyperlucency due to the air in the thorax on the affected side.

Palpation

Palpation of the thorax is helpful to assess chest wall movement and to identify abnormal vibrations of the chest wall. For example, tactile rhonchi are vibrations felt over the chest wall caused by secretions vibrating as air flows across the secretions. Vocal fremitus refers to vibrations caused by the patient speaking. Consolidation or atelectasis can sometimes cause an increase in vocal fremitus. Chest wall excursion can be assessed in older children by placing the hands on both sides of the thorax and having the patient breathe; the symmetry of the movement and distance moved can thus be assessed.

Pneumothorax or pneumomediastinum may cause subcutaneous emphysema (subcutaneous air). Subcutaneous emphysema can often be detected by palpating the surface tissue of the chest and neck. It has been described as a crackling sensation under the examiner's fingers, not unlike the snap-crackle-pop of Rice Krispies cereal. Palpating the neck and trachea may also allow clinicians to determine if the trachea has shifted due to air pneumothorax or masses.

Percussion

Percussion of the chest is typically performed on older pediatric patients. Chest percussion is performed by tapping the finger of one hand with the finger with the other hand over areas of the chest with the patient sitting in an upright position. A normal percussion note is resonant. Hyperresonance suggests air trapping or pneumothorax. A dull percussion note suggests atelectasis, consolidation, or pleural effusion.

Auscultation

Normal breath sounds upon auscultation are quiet and clear.[75] Abnormal breath sounds include crackles (formally called rales), gurgles (rhonchi), and wheezes. Crackles may be heard with bronchiolitis, pulmonary edema, and atelectasis (if there is some airflow present). Rhonchi or gurgles are associated with secretions in a larger airway that may clear following cough. Wheezes are high-pitched sounds produced by narrowed or constricted airways. Wheezing may be heard in asthmatics, those with central airway obstruction, or patients with pulmonary edema. With acute, severe asthma exacerbation, it is not uncommon to hear audible wheezes without a stethoscope. Absent or decreased breath sounds can be caused by pleural effusion, atelectasis, or alveolar filling (e.g., pneumonia). Decreased breath sounds in a patient with a severe asthma exacerbation can be an ominous sign. E-A egophany is an "A" sound heard during chest auscultation when the patient says "E" and is associated with pleural effusion or occasionally associated with segmental or lobar consolidation.[75] Loud, course "bronchial" breath sounds heard over the periphery of the chest are also suggestive of parenchymal consolidation (e.g., pneumonia) or microatelectasis.

Stridor is a high-pitcheds monophonic sound that is typically caused by upper airway obstruction due to viral infection (e.g., laryngotracheobronchitis).[79] Other possible causes of stridor include bacterial infection (e.g., epiglottitis), trauma, anaphylaxis, foreign body obstruction, tumors, congenital airway abnormalities (e.g., laryngomalacia), and vocal cord problems.[76] *Stertor* is a low-pitched, wet sound that may sound like snoring and is also suggestive of upper airway obstruction.

Cardiac Examination

The patient's chest should be exposed to allow for inspection, palpation, and auscultation of the precordium. The precordium should be inspected for any pulsations generated by the heart and great vessels. The precordium may be palpated to assess the apical impulse (i.e., the point of maximum impulse [PMI]) or any vibrations or motion (e.g., cardiac thrill, lift, or heave). With enlargement of the heart, the apical impulse may be displaced. A cardiac thrill is a palpable vibration or murmur that may be caused by pulmonary valve stenosis, aortic stenosis, ventricular septal defect, or other cardiac anomalies (e.g., patent ductus arteriosis, coarctation of the aorta).[75]

Auscultation of the Heart

Normal heart sounds correlate with the beating of the heart and closure of the heart valves as the myocardium contracts. The normal heart sounds are S_1 and S_2, which correspond to the "lub-dub" heard when listening to the heart. S_1 is best heard at the apex of the heart and is associated with the closure of atrioventricular valves (mitral, tricuspid).[75] The intensity of S_1 may be increased or decreased. For example, S_1 intensity is increased (i.e., louder) with mitral stenosis and decreased (i.e., softer) with mitral regurgitation. The second heart sound (S_2) signifies the closure of the aortic valve (A_2) and the pulmonary valve (P_2) and is best heard over the upper left sternal border.[75] Normally, the closure of the mitral and tricuspid valves is nearly simultaneous, and S_1 is a single sound.[75] S_2 is normally "split," especially during inspiration. The two components of S_2 (i.e., A_2 and P_2) may be decreased in intensity. For example, an increase in A_2 may be due to systemic hypertension, whereas an increase in P_2 may be due to pulmonary arterial hypertension.[77] A decrease in A_2 may be caused by aortic regurgitation or decreased diastolic arterial pressure; a decrease in P_2 may be caused by decreased pulmonary arterial pressure.[77]

A third (S_3) or fourth heart (S_4) sound is sometimes heard and is occasionally referred to as a *gallop*. If present, S_3 is heard over the apex or lower border of the heart and is louder on expiration. Together, the gallop rhythm of S_1, S_2, and S_3 is sometimes described as

similar to the pronunciation of the word "*Ken*-tucky."[77] S_3 may be "normal" for certain patients or it may be due to cardiac disease (e.g., a failing left ventricle). When an S_4 is heard (i.e., S_1, S_2, and S_4), it may mimic the rhythm of the word "Tennes-*see*."[77] Causes of a S_4 gallop include chronic hypertension resulting in heart disease (e.g., left ventricular stiffness or hypertrophy).[77] When both an S_3 and S_4 occur, it is called a *summation gallop*.

When auscultating the heart, the following sequence is suggested for stethoscope placement:

1. Second right intercostal space: Over the aortic valve.
2. Second left intercostal space: Over the pulmonary valve.
3. Lower left sternal border at the fourth intercostal space: Over the tricuspid valve.
4. Fifth left intercostal space, 1 cm medial to midclavicular line: Over the mitral valve.

Heart murmurs are "whooshing" sounds caused by turbulent blood flow. Vavular heart disease is the most common cause of a heart murmur. Examples include valve regurgitation (mitral, tricuspid, pulmonary, or aortic), valve stenosis (mitral, tricuspid, pulmonary, aortic), and prolapse (mitral, tricuspid). An abnormal opening between the left and right heart (e.g., ventricular septal defect [VSD], atrial septal defect [ASD]) or between the aorta or pulmonary arteries and a heart chamber (e.g., patent ductus arteriosis) may also cause a heart murmur. Murmurs may be systolic, diastolic, or continuous. Cardiac ultrasound imaging (i.e., echocardiography) is the preferred method for determining the cause of a heart murmur.

Abdominal Examination

The abdominal examination should include inspection, auscultation, palpation, and percussion. The patient should be placed on an examining table or bed and positioned for comfort and to relax the abdominal wall muscles. The abdominal area should be exposed, keeping in mind the patient's privacy. The abdomen should be inspected for shape, skin markings, color, and any distension, bulging, protrusion, or abdominal masses. A bluish discoloration with edema and bruising of the umbilicus is called the *Cullen's sign*, which may be associated with a number of disorders, including acute pancreatitis. **Grey Turner's sign** is a similar bluish discoloration (bruising) of the flanks, also associated with acute pancreatitis. The skin should be inspected for surgical scars that should be correlated with the patient history. The abdomen should be inspected for masses. The clinician should determine if masses are abdominal wall masses or intra-abdominal masses. Abdominal wall masses become more prominent with tensing of the abdominal musculature, whereas an intra-abdominal mass may become less prominent.[55] Abdominal wall masses are most commonly due to hernias, neoplasms (benign and malignant), infections, and hematomas. Intra-abdominal masses may be due to abdominal organ disease (e.g., liver, gallbladder, pancreatic, aortic, renal, intestinal, bladder, or uterine disease). Finally, the abdominal wall should be observed for motion with respiration. Normally, the abdominal wall moves concurrently with inspiration. As discussed earlier, asynchrony is a sign of respiratory distress. Rigidity of the abdominal wall as seen with peritonitis may cause this motion to be absent.[55]

Auscultation

The clinician should identify the presence of bowel sounds by listening over the abdomen. The clinician should listen for at least 3 minutes before concluding that bowel sounds are absent. Decreased or absent bowel sounds may be caused by bowel obstruction or appendicitis.[75] Abdominal bruits are "swishing" sounds heard over major arteries that can be caused by arterial stenosis.[75] Rubs can sometimes be heard over the liver, spleen, or an abdominal mass.[78]

Palpation and Percussion

Palpation and percussion of the abdomen is useful for assessment of organ size (e.g., liver, kidney, spleen) and detection and evaluation of an abdominal tumor or mass.[75] With inflammation or abdominal pain, the abdomen may be tense or rigid due to voluntary (e.g., pain) or involuntary (e.g., inflammation) contraction of the abdominal muscles.[75] Abdominal spasm is involuntary and can occur due to peritoneal inflammation, whereas **guarding** is voluntary abdominal muscle contraction in an attempt to avoid or diminish pain.[81] Upon percussion, abdominal areas filled with air (e.g., an air-filled bowel) will be resonant or tympanic, whereas areas filled with liquid will be dull (e.g., the bladder).[75] Ascites (fluid in the peritoneal cavity) may sometimes be detected as dullness in the flank or side.[75] Abdominal pain may worsen with palpation or percussion. Causes of acute abdominal pain in children include constipation, GI tract infection, colic, abscess, and other GI conditions.[79] Appendicitis, trauma, intestinal invagination, inguinal hernia with incarceration, abdominal adhesions (e.g., postop adhesions), and peptic ulcer disease can also cause abdominal pain; these conditions can be life threatening and should be evaluated accordingly.[79]

Skin and Extremities

Skin color and the presence of scars, redness, edema, or sweating should be noted. The nail beds of the fingers and toes and the gums should be pink. Cyanosis is associated with hypoxemia, though it is a variable finding (see also Chapter 5). A pale appearance with cold, clammy skin is associated with shock. Other conditions that may affect skin color and appearance include rash, fever, jaundice, carbon monoxide poisoning, methemoglobinemia, cyanide poisoning, increased P_{CO_2}, burns, and trauma.

Capillary refill should be good, and the skin and extremities should be well perfused. Peripheral edema may be caused by fluid overload, heart failure, sepsis, or decreased plasma albumin. Angioedema (swelling of the face, upper airway, extremities) may be caused by an allergic reaction to a bee sting or insect bite, drug reaction, or food allergy. Excessive sweating may be a sign of respiratory distress, pain, anxiety, fever, or infection. Trauma or surgery may leave surface scars. Children with chronic lung disease (e.g., cystic fibrosis) and those with heart defects may have chronic hypoxemia and digital clubbing.

Eczema (atopic dermatitis) may cause skin rash, redness, swelling, and lesions. Eczema is often seen in patients with asthma or seasonal allergy (e.g., hay fever) and may be seen in children younger than 2 years of age, older children, and in adults. Allergy to pollen, mold, dust mites, soaps, lotions, or cosmetics may cause or worsen eczema. Triad asthma consists of skin rash, mucosal edema, nasal polyps, and aspirin intolerance.

Diagnostic Imaging and Laboratory Testing

Following the history and physical examination, additional imaging and laboratory testing may be required. These diagnostic tests can often clarify or confirm the diagnosis, quantify disease severity, or assess response to therapy. Generally, simple, less expensive and less invasive tests are preferred; however, advanced imaging and invasive diagnostic procedures may be required in some circumstances.

Imaging

Diagnostic imaging is discussed in Chapter 11. Imaging techniques used in children include chest radiography (CXR), computed tomography (CT), ultrasonography, magnetic resonance imaging (MRI), and various nuclear medicine techniques (e.g., PET [positron emission tomography] and PET/CT). Imaging techniques in children can be used for diagnosis, to guide interventional procedures, and for placement of catheters, lines, and tubes. Examples where the chest radiograph may be especially useful include assessment of infants and children with severe respiratory distress, pneumonia, trauma, atelectasis, or pleural effusion and in evaluation of children with chronic cough. The chest radiograph is not generally useful in patients with acute asthma or uncomplicated bronchiolitis. High-resolution CT (HRCT) of the chest may be useful for evaluation of patients with diffuse lung disease. HRCT is also useful to evaluate patients with bronchiectasis, which sometimes occurs with cystic fibrosis (CF).

Imaging studies are also important in evaluation of pediatric patients with cardiac disease. The chest radiograph may identify an enlarged heart and pulmonary congestion due to congestive heart failure. Echocardiography (a form of ultrasonography) can evaluate cardiac structure and function in the evaluation of congenital cardiac defects. A lateral neck radiograph is useful in patients with upper airway obstruction (e.g., croup or epiglottitis). Croup will often show a "steeple sign" on a frontal view of the neck. A neck film of a patient with epiglottitis will show supraglottic narrowing and a thumb-shaped epiglottis (i.e., the "thumb sign"; see also Chapter 11). **Clinical Focus 16-4** provides an example of a patient with epiglottitis.

Pulmonary Function Testing and Blood Gases

Pulmonary function testing is performed to assess lung function and monitor the progression of disease. Specifically, pulmonary function tests (PFTs) in children are useful to evaluate obstructive and restrictive disease, diffusion, and respiratory muscle strength.[80] PFTs sometimes performed on children include:

- Spirometry
  - Forced vital capacity (FVC)
  - Forced expiratory volume in 1 second (FEV_1)
  - FEV_1/FVC (FEV1%)
  - Forced expiratory flow (FEF)
  - Peak expiratory flow rate (PEFR)
- Bronchial challenge tests
- Lung volume measurement
  - Residual volume (RV)
  - Total lung capacity (TLC)
  - RV/TLC ratio
  - Thoracic gas volume (TGV)
- Diffusion capacity
- Exhaled nitric oxide
- Maximal inspiratory and expiratory pressures (i.e., MIP and MEP)

Spirometry is especially useful in the assessment of patients with asthma, cystic fibrosis and BPD. Measures of flow (e.g., FEV_1, FEV_1/FVC, PEFR) are used to measure the degree of obstruction and monitor the effectiveness of therapy. **Clinical Focus 16-5** provides an example of a patient with asthma.

CLINICAL FOCUS 16-4

Epiglottitis

A 3-year-old male presents to the emergency department with inspiratory stridor, labored breathing, hoarse voice, high fever, and drooling.

1. What actions should the respiratory care clinician take at this time?

   The respiratory care clinician should perform an assessment of the patient, including vital signs, physical assessment, and appropriate diagnostic testing. Signs and symptoms are suggestive of upper airway inflammation (e.g., croup or epiglottitis). Epiglottitis represents a medical emergency requiring prompt recognition and treatment.

   The clinician takes the following steps:

   - *Examine the patient.* On examination, the patient's vital signs are:

   Heart rate: 170 bpm

   Blood pressure: 110/86 mm Hg

   Respiratory rate: 65 breaths/min

   SpO_2: 85%.

   Breath sounds are decreased bilaterally, and the patient is having difficulty swallowing.

   - *Determine respiratory status and possible interventions.* The patient is in severe respiratory distress with documented hypoxemia. Fever is associated with infection. Stridor and substernal and intercostal retractions are suggestive of partial upper airway obstruction. Drooling is associated with difficulty in swallowing, as may occur with sore throat, croup, or epiglottitis.

     The patient should be maintained in an upright position, allowing him to lean forward in the sniffing position. Try to keep the patient calm, because agitation can precipitate complete airway obstruction. Do *not* suggest placing the patient in the supine position. Recommend a lateral neck x-ray and consider laryngoscopy (often performed under general anesthesia in the operating room or endoscopy suite). Aerosolized therapies are *not* recommended. Avoid any procedure that may cause additional anxiety, including laboratory studies, until the airway is secured.

   - *Confirm the differential diagnosis.* Epiglottitis is confirmed by lateral neck x-ray or direct visualization of the epiglottis during laryngoscopy performed under general anesthesia. The lateral neck x-ray on this patient reveals an enlarged epiglottis, known as the "thumb sign," thickened aryepiglottic folds, and obliteration of the vallecula.

Securing an airway is the superseding priority for the patient. The patient is taken to the operating room and is given general anesthesia by mask immediately followed by laryngoscopy (which confirmed an enlarged epiglottis) and airway placement by a skilled anesthesiologist. Airway placement is successful, and the patient is moved to the pediatric intensive care unit (PICU). Antibiotics are initiated to treat bacterial infection, which is the most common cause of epiglottitis.

2. Following placement of an endotracheal tube in the operating room and transfer of the patient to the PICU, what steps should the respiratory care clinician now take?

   The clinician should determine the patient's respiratory status and consider possible interventions based on the findings. The patient should receive humidified supplemental oxygen via the endotracheal tube. Mechanical ventilatory support may be needed initially as the patient recovers from anesthesia and sedation. The clinician should assess the patient's breath sounds, respiratory rate, heart rate, and need for mechanical ventilatory support.

Forty-eight hours following insertion of the endotracheal tube, the patient is awake and alert, breathing spontaneously via the endotracheal tube. The upper airway swelling has decreased, as verified by inspection via laryngoscopy. The airway cuff is then deflated and a leak was heard around the endotracheal tube when the patient was "bagged" using a manual resuscitator.

3. What should the respiratory care clinician now do?

   The clinician should confirm the patient's airway stability by measuring the leak around the endotracheal tube with the cuff deflated while providing positive pressure ventilation. If a sufficient leak is present and laryngoscopy reveals reduced inflammation of epiglottis, the artificial airway can be removed.

The presence of a large leak is verified with the endotracheal tube cuff deflated, and the patient is extubated. The clinician recommends observation for another 24 to 36 hours before discharge.

CLINICAL FOCUS 16-5

Pediatric Asthma

A 12-year-old girl presents to the emergency department in September with a 2-day history of cough and wheezing. Over the past 18 months, the child has experienced three hospital admissions for asthma exacerbation. The patient is now in acute distress despite using her inhaler every 3 to 4 hours. The patient is 53 inches tall and weighs 70 lbs (31.8 kg).

1. In order to assess this patient, what steps should the respiratory care clinician take?

   The respiratory care clinician should perform a brief history and physical assessment to include general appearance, vital signs, breath sounds, accessory muscle use, and measurement of peak expiratory flow rate (PEFR) or FEV_1 (if practical).

   On assessment, the following vital signs are obtained:

Temperature (axillary): 37.5° C

Heart rate: 125 bpm

Respiratory rate: 30 breaths/min

Blood pressure: 110/60 mm Hg

SpO_2: 90% on room air

PEFR: 106 L/min (38% of predicted)

   Her breath sounds are bilateral with inspiratory and expiratory wheezing and a prolonged expiratory phase. Note that initial measurement of PEFR in patients with severe or very severe asthma exacerbation may be omitted in order to avoid worsening bronchospasm until after a bronchodilator is given.

2. Based on the examination findings, what steps should the respiratory care clinician now consider?

   The patient is in acute distress with an elevated respiratory rate and heart rate. The presence of distress, tachypnea, accessory muscle use, wheezing, prolonged expiratory phase, cough, and decreased SpO_2 suggest an asthma exacerbation. Common causes of an asthma flare include infection, allergies, irritants, and changes in season or weather. Wheezing and cough are common clinical manifestations of asthma.

(continues)

With asthma exacerbation, the lower airways become inflamed, resulting in bronchospasm, mucosal edema, and increased secretions. The combination of swelling, bronchospasm, and excess mucus causes the airways to become obstructed, making it difficult to breath. Moderate to severe respiratory distress may occur in these patients. The PEFR of 38% predicted suggests severe exacerbation (see also below).

3. What interventions and/or additional testing should the respiratory care clinician now consider?

Based on the assessment findings, the clinician should take steps for evaluation and treatment of severe asthma exacerbation. The treatment of severe asthma exacerbation includes bronchodilator therapy as well as oral corticosteroids (assuming the patient is tolerating oral medications without difficulty). A chest radiograph may be obtained to rule out other causes of respiratory distress.

The treatment of asthma exacerbation in the emergency department setting includes short-acting β-agonist bronchodilator (SABA) therapy (e.g., albuterol) every 20 to 30 minutes by nebulizer or metered dose inhaler (MDI) with holding chamber. As an alternative, continuous nebulization may be performed. If there is slight improvement, therapy should be continued and the patient reevaluated in the emergency department. If there is no improvement, the patient should be admitted.

Oxygen therapy is indicated if the SpO_2 is < 92%, and O_2 is administered to keep the SpO_2 > 92%. Oral steroids should be given, depending on the patient's severity of illness and response to SABA therapy. Asthma exacerbation severity can be assessed based on PEFR or FEV_1 where:

- Mild: FEV_1 or PEF > 70% predicted or personal best
- Moderate: FEV_1 or PEF > 40% but < 70% predicted or personal best
- Severe: FEV_1 or PEF < 40% but > 25% predicted or personal best
- Very severe: FEV_1 or PEF ≤ 25% predicted or personal best

With severe exacerbation, SABA may be combined with ipratropium by small volume nebulizer (or given via MDI with holding chamber) and oral systemic corticosteroids begun. In very severe cases (e.g., impending or actual respiratory arrest) intubation, mechanical ventilation, and 100% oxygen may be required.

Initial albuterol dose in children is weight based and is usually 0.15 mg/kg per dose, with a minimum dose of 2.5 mg and a maximum of 5 mg. Initial therapy is one dose (2.5 to 5 mg) by nebulizer. This is repeated every 20 to 30 minutes for three doses. As an alternative, albuterol may be given continuously by nebulizer. Continuous nebulization dose is 0.5 mg/kg per hour with a maximum dose of 20 mg per hour. MDI dose is one-quarter to one-third puffs per kg or four to eight puffs every 20 to 30 minutes for three doses.

As noted, ipratropium may be given by small volume nebulizer or MDI with spacer. For children weighing less than 20 kg, the ipratropium nebulizer dose is 250 mcg/dose (0.25mg/dose) every 20 to 30 minutes for three doses. For children weighing at least 20 kg, the ipratropium nebulizer dose is 500 mcg/dose every 20 to 30 minutes for three doses. MDI dose is four to eight puffs every 20 minutes for up to 3 hours, as needed. Initially, oral prednisone is given (1 to 2 mg/kg) for a maximum of 60 mg/day.

The clinician takes the following steps:

- Administer bronchodilator. Albuterol (5 mg) is administered via small volume nebulizer every 20 minutes for three doses for wheezing while in the emergency department. Following administration of the bronchodilator, aeration increases, though persistent wheezing is noted, and there is a slight improvement in the work of breathing. SpO_2 improves to 91%.
- Administer oral corticosteroid. The patient tolerates the initial dose of prednisone by mouth.
- Provide oxygen therapy. The patient is placed on a nasal cannula at 2 L/min. SpO_2 improves to 94%.

The patient is admitted to the hospital for acute asthma exacerbation, respiratory distress, persistent wheezing, increased work of breathing, and the need for supplemental oxygen.

4. Upon admission to the hospital floor, what interventions should the respiratory care clinician suggest for this patient?

The clinician should suggest the following:

- Albuterol 5.0 mg via small volume nebulizer every 1 to 3 hours *or* albuterol eight puffs via MDI and holding chamber every 1 to 3 hours.
- Continue oxygen therapy to maintain oxygen saturations > 92%.
- Perform peak flow monitoring before and after bronchodilator therapy.
- Oral corticosteroids twice a day starting the next day (following the initial dose of 1 to 2 mg/kg on day 1). Following the initial dose of prednisone, the dose is 0.5 to 1 mg/kg twice a day for a 3- to 10-day course or until PEFR returns to 70% of predicted or personal best. For children ages 5 to 11 years, the dose is always twice a

day; however, a 12-year-old could receive a single dose once a day or a divided dose twice a day (e.g., 32 mg once a day or 16 mg twice a day). The maximum does of prednisone is 60 mg/day.

- Fluid support, as needed.

The following interventions are ordered:

- Albuterol 1 mg in 3 mL normal saline via nebulizer every 2 hours.
- Oxygen therapy via nasal cannula at 2 L/min, maintaining the SpO2 > 92%.
- Oral steroids twice a day to begin the next day.

All three interventions are continued. Progressive improvement in breath sounds and work of breathing continues over the next 24 hours. Oxygen is then "weaned" to room air (Spo_2 94%). The bronchodilator therapy frequency is reduced to every 4 hours or as needed. The patient is started on an inhaled steroid via MDI to be taken every day for asthma management. The following day the patient and parents receive an asthma education session to review her medications, MDI use and technique, and environmental control measures (i.e., environmental triggers). She is provided an asthma action plan. The patient is then discharged to home with the following:

- Continue SABA via MDI.
- Continue course of oral corticosteroids until complete.
- Continue inhaled steroids via MDI.
- Follow up with primary care provider in 1 week.

* Note that many studies supporting the use of spacers were done with chlorofluorocarbon-based MDIs. Data suggest that HFA do not have increased deposition with holding chambers.
Data from: National Heart, Blood, and Lung Institute Expert Panel Report 3 (EPR 3): Guidelines for the diagnosis and management of asthma. August 28, 2007. Available at https://www.nhlbi.nih.gov/guidelines/asthma/asthgdln.pdf; Sawicki G, Haver K. Acute asthma exacerbation in children: Inpatient management. In: *UpToDate*, Basow DS (ed.), UpToDate, Waltham, MA, 2013.

Vital capacity and lung volumes are used to assess restrictive lung disease (e.g., chest wall deformity, neuromuscular disease, interstitial lung disease [ILD]). Lung volume measurement can be also helpful in assessment of air trapping (e.g., asthma, CF) or restrictive disease.

Measurement of MIP and MEP can help evaluate respiratory muscle strength in patients with neuromuscular disease.[80] Bronchial challenge tests are useful for verifying the presence of hyperactive airways (e.g., suspected asthma). Diffusion testing is sometimes of value in assessing patients with ILD. Exhaled nitric oxide concentration measurement is sometimes used to assess airway inflammation in asthma patients.

Pulmonary function testing requires a degree of patient cooperation for most tests. Obtaining PFTs may be difficult in younger children, though some technologists are able to perform good tests in children as young as 3 years of age.[80] Specialized techniques are sometimes used in younger children. For example, in infants and small children measurement of airway resistance via plethysmography or respiratory system forced conductance oscillation can be performed.[80] Pulmonary function testing is described in more detail in Chapter 12.

Arterial blood gas studies provide for assessment of the pediatric patient's oxygenation, ventilation, and acid-base balance. Blood gas sampling and analysis are discussed in Chapter 8. Sampling techniques used in infants include arterial puncture, arterial line sampling (e.g., umbilical arterial line, radial arterial line), capillary sampling, and the use of venous blood gases.[81] Each

technique has advantages and disadvantages. For neonates and infants younger than 1 year, "heel sticks" are used to obtain capillary blood gas samples. **Capillary blood gases** are useful to assess acid-base status and, to a lesser extent, oxygenation and CO_2 levels. Capillary sampling does not provide a good estimate of arterial oxygen levels in the newborn.[82]

Because arterial blood samples may be difficult to obtain in smaller children and infants, venous blood gases are sometimes used as an alternative.[81] It should also be noted that the pain of an arterial "stick" will often cause a child to cry, altering the blood gas values obtained; many clinical sites avoid performing arterial punctures on small children.

Transcutaneous monitoring of Po_2 and Pco_2 has largely been replaced by pulse oximetry.[82,83] Pulse oximetry (Spo_2) provides a good alternative for assessment of arterial oxygenation; however, the drawbacks and limitations of Spo_2 measurement must also be considered. Table 16-10 provides normal newborn and pediatric blood gas values.

Laboratory Testing

Laboratory testing in infants and children can be of a great value in providing diagnostic information and in assessing disease progression. Pediatric laboratory exams include various tests to assess hematology and coagulation, clinical chemistry and immunology, toxicology and therapeutic drug monitoring, and microbiology. In addition, laboratory exams can be performed on blood, sputum, cerebral spinal fluid, urine, bone marrow, and stool. For routine evaluation of the pediatric patient, common blood tests include the complete blood count (CBC), clinical chemistry, blood cultures, lead test (recommended for all toddlers), and liver function tests. A basic metabolic panel (BMP) is sometimes ordered, which includes measurement of glucose, calcium, sodium, potassium, chloride, carbon dioxide, BUN, and creatinine. In addition, toxicology (for suspected poisoning) and therapeutic drug monitoring can be performed. The **sweat chloride test** is performed in patients to diagnose cystic fibrosis (CF), though molecular techniques to test for CF are now available. Stool samples are sometimes analyzed to test for allergy (e.g., milk protein allergy), infection (e.g., bacteria, parasites), nutrient malabsorption problems, or bleeding. Testing for HIV, pregnancy, or sexually transmitted disease (STD) is sometimes indicated in teens. Normal values for most laboratory tests in children are similar to those found in adults.

Throat cultures (e.g., strep screen) are often done in children with sore throat. Cultures can also be performed on sputum samples, blood, urine, or wounds. Laboratory tests performed on sputum cultures include the Gram stain, culture and sensitivity, and acid-fast bacillus (AFB). Blood cultures may be performed to evaluate possible sepsis. Lumbar puncture with spinal fluid cultures may be performed if a CNS infection is suspected (e.g., meningitis). Chapter 9 provides additional information about laboratory testing.

Skin Testing

The tuberculin skin test is useful in diagnosis of tuberculosis (TB) in children, although a negative test does not rule out TB. Interferon gamma release assays (IGRA) of immune response may also be used to diagnose TB in children, though neither test can discriminate between active and inactive (latent) disease.[84] Allergy **skin testing** may also be performed in children to identify specific allergens.

Other Diagnostic Testing

Polysomnography, more commonly referred to as a sleep study, is sometimes used to determine if a pediatric patient has sleep apnea. Obstructive sleep apnea (OSA) is present when there are episodes of active diaphragmatic movement but no airflow due to airway obstruction. OSA is not uncommon in children and may occur at any age, though it is most common in children between 2 and 6 years old. Central sleep apnea occurs when there are no diaphragmatic movements and no airflow. The brain signals have either stopped or are not reaching the diaphragm. Central sleep apnea in children may be caused by brainstem dysfunction or

tumor. Chapter 15 describes sleep disorders, including sleep apnea.

Bronchoscopy is sometimes performed in children in order to visualize the airways and to obtain tissue or secretion samples, to suction secretions, or to remove foreign bodies. Children are especially susceptible to inhaling small objects, such as small toys or toy parts, hard candy, or peanuts, and bronchoscopy may be required to remove these objects. Chapter 13 describes bronchoscopy.

Summary

The assessment of a fetus, newborn, or child is different than that of an adult patient. Assessment of the fetus will include gestational age, fetal movement, fetal heart rate, and other tests of fetal well-being. Newborn assessment will include gestational age at birth, vital signs (to include the APGAR score), respiratory assessment, and cardiac/cardiovascular assessment. Physical examination of the newborn should include assessment of the head and neck, chest, abdomen, musculoskeletal system, neurologic system, and extremities. Laboratory screens of the newborn should be performed before the baby leaves the hospital. Assessment of the pediatric patient will include history and physical and diagnostic testing. Imaging tests and pulmonary function tests may also be indicated.

Key Points

▶ Obtaining an accurate and thorough medical history provides specific knowledge regarding the patient's past and present status, assists in determining plans of care, and guides future decisions concerning care.

▶ Determination of gestational age provides valuable information regarding expected or potential problems and directly affects the treatment plan for the neonate.

▶ The primary aim of prenatal diagnostic testing is to provide an accurate diagnosis that will allow informed choices to parents of patients at increased risk.

▶ Fetal lung maturity (FLM) tests predict lung maturity (and the likelihood of developing respiratory distress syndrome [RDS]) by measurement of surfactant phospholipids secreted by the lungs into amniotic fluid.

▶ Assessment of heart rate variability is an important part of interpreting a fetal heart rate (FHR) pattern.

▶ New standardized guidelines divide all FHR patterns into one of three differentiating categories.

▶ Fetal well-being tests (e.g., nonstress test, contraction stimulation test, biophysical profile) are designed to evaluate the status of the placenta and

- whether oxygen and nutrition transferred to the fetus are being affected.
- ▶ APGAR scores provide a standardized assessment of the newborn that is quick, simple, and reliable.
- ▶ APGAR scoring is completed at 1 and 5 minutes, and sometimes longer when the condition warrants: 0 to 3 points indicate severe distress, 4 to 6 points indicate moderate distress, and 7 to 10 points indicate no distress.
- ▶ Vital signs must be assessed at the first available opportunity following birth, typically in the following sequence: respirations, heart rate, blood pressure, and temperature.
- ▶ A full head-to-toe examination of the newborn should be completed within 24 hours following birth.
- ▶ The normal pulse rate of a newborn is 100 to 160 bpm. A persistent heart rate < 100 or > 160 bpm is a cause for concern.
- ▶ Transient heart murmurs are often heard after birth, but the presence of a loud murmur, significant differences in blood pressure in the upper and lower extremities, or central cyanosis suggests a cardiac abnormality.
- ▶ Pediatric patients include a wide range of ages and stages of development including: infant, toddler, preschool, school-aged (primary school), and adolescent (secondary school).
- ▶ General appearance of the pediatric patient provides important clinical information in terms of acuity of illness.
- ▶ Respiratory rate is a good indicator of pediatric pulmonary status.
- ▶ A thorough pediatric pulmonary assessment includes inspection, palpation, percussion, and auscultation.
- ▶ Normal heart sounds correspond to the "lub-dub" sound heard when listening to the chest.
- ▶ Heart murmurs are described in a variety of ways, each indicating different types of cardiac abnormality.
- ▶ Pediatric diagnostic tests used to clarify or confirm diagnosis, severity of illness, or responses to therapy and may include laboratory studies of blood and body fluids.
- ▶ Pediatric imaging techniques include radiography, computed tomography, ultrasonography, magnetic resonance imaging, and various nuclear medicine techniques.
- ▶ Pulmonary function tests in pediatric patients provide specific lung capacity, volume, and flow-related information, but require a degree of cooperation and performance from the patient in order to be accurate.
- ▶ Other pulmonary tests used for differential diagnosis in pediatric patients include arterial blood gases, polysomnography, and bronchoscopy.

References

1. Lockwood CJ, Magriples U. Initial prenatal assessment and first trimester prenatal care. In: *UpToDate*, Basow DS (ed.), UpToDate Waltham, MA, 2013.
2. Mongelli M, Wilcox M, Gardosi J. Estimating the date of confinement: Ultrasonographic biometry versus certain menstrual dates. *Am J Obstet Gynecol.* 1996;174(1):278–281.
3. Whitworth M, Bricker L, Neilson JP, Dowswell T. Ultrasound for fetal assessment in early pregnancy. *Cochrane Database Syst Rev.* 2010(4):CD007058.
4. Braunstein GD, Rasor J, Danzer H, Adler D, Wade ME. Serum human chorionic gonadotropin levels throughout normal pregnancy. *Am J Obstet Gynecol.* 1976;126(6):678–681.
5. Healthwise. WebMD. Human chorionic gonadotropin (hCG). May 6, 2010. Available at http://www.webmd.com/baby/human-chorionic-gonadotropin-hcg.
6. Eddleman KM, Sullivan F, Dukes L, et al. Pregnancy loss rates after midtrimester amniocentesis. *Am J Obstet Gynecol.* 2006;108(5):1067–1072.
7. Ghidini A. Diagnostic amniocentesis. In: *UpToDate*, Basow DS (ed.), UpToDate, Waltham, MA, 2013.
8. Medline Plus. Appropriate for gestational age. Accessed December 6, 2013. Available at http://www.nlm.nih.gov/medlineplus/ency/article/002225.htm.
9. ACOG committee opinion no. 560: Medically indicated late-preterm and early-term deliveries. *Obstet Gynecol.* 2013;121(4):908–910.
10. Kim A, Lee ES, Shin JC, Kim HY. Identification of biomarkers for preterm delivery in mid-trimester amniotic fluid. *Placenta.* 2013;34(10):873–878.
11. Beachy W. *Respiratory Care Anatomy and Physiology: Foundations for Clinical Practice*, 2nd ed. St. Louis, MO: Mosby Elsevier; 2007.
12. Leung Pineda V, Gronowski AM. Biomarker tests for fetal lung maturity. *Biomark Med.* 2010;4(6):849–857.
13. Ventolini G, Neiger R, Hood D, Belcastro C. Update on assessment of fetal lung maturity. *J Obstet Gynaecol.* 2005;25(6):535–538.
14. Gluck L, Kulovich MV, Borer RC Jr., Brenner PH, Anderson GG, Spellacy WN. Diagnosis of the respiratory distress syndrome by amniocentesis. *Am J Obstet Gynecol.* 1971;109(3):440–445.
15. Hallman M, Kulovich M, Kirkpatrick E, Sugarman RG, Gluck L. Phosphatidylinositol and phosphatidylglycerol in amniotic fluid: Indices of lung maturity. *Am J Obstet Gynecol.* 1976;125(5):613–617.
16. Hallman MT, Teramo K. Measurement of the lecithin/sphingomyelin ratio and phosphatidylglycerol in amniotic fluid: An accurate method for the assessment of fetal lung maturity. *Br J Obstet Gynaecol.* 1981;88(8):806–813.
17. Gillen-Goldstein J, MacKenzie AP, Funfai EF. Assessment of fetal lung maturity. In: *UpToDate*, Basow DS (ed.), UpToDate, Waltham, MA, 2013.
18. Kesselman EJ, Figueroa R, Garry D, Maulik D. The usefulness of the TDx/TDxFLx fetal lung maturity II assay in the initial evaluation of fetal lung maturity. *Am J Obstet Gynecol.* 2003;188(5):1220–1222.
19. Winn-McMillan TK, Karon BS. Comparison of the TDx-FLM II and lecithin to sphingomyelin ratio assays in predicting fetal lung maturity. *Am J Obstet Gynecol.* 2005;193(3):778–782.
20. Hagen E, Link JC, Arias F. A comparison of the accuracy of the TDx-FLM assay, lecithin-sphingomyelin ratio, and

phosphatidylglycerol in the prediction of neonatal respiratory distress syndrome. *Obstet Gynecol.* 1993;82(6):1004–1008.

21. Willacy H. Heart murmurs in children. 2012. Available at http://www.patient.co.uk/doctor/Heart-Murmurs-in-Children.htm.

22. Sher G, Statland BE, Freer DE, Kraybill EN. Assessing fetal lung maturation by the foam stability index test. *Obstet Gynecol.* 1978;52(6):673–677.

23. Khazardoost S, Yahyazadeh H, Borna S, Sohrabvand F, Yahyazadeh N, Amini E. Amniotic fluid lamellar body count and its sensitivity and specificity in evaluating of fetal lung maturity. *J Obstet Gynaecol.* 2005;25(3):257–259.

24. Neerhof MG, Dohnal JC, Ashwood ER, Lee IS, Anceschi MM. Lamellar body counts: A consensus on protocol. *Obstet Gynecol.* 2001;97(2):318–320.

25. Morain S, Greene MF, Mello MM. A new era in noninvasive prenatal testing. *N Engl J Med.* 2013;369(6):499–501.

26. Bianchi DW, Oepkes D, Ghidini A. Current controversies in prenatal diagnosis 1: Should noninvasive DNA testing be the standard screening test for Down syndrome in all pregnant women? *Prenat Diagn.* 2014;34(1):6–11.

27. Tan KH, Smyth RM. Fetal vibroacoustic stimulation for facilitation of tests of fetal wellbeing. *Cochrane Database Syst Rev.* 2001;(1):CD002963.

28. Velazquez MD, Rayburn WF. Antenatal evaluation of the fetus using fetal movement monitoring. *Clin Obstet Gynecol.* 2002;45(4):993–1004.

29. Lalor J, Devane D. Using the biophysical profile to assess fetal wellbeing. *Pract Midwife.* 2010;13(6):16–17.

30. Renou P, Newman W, Wood C. Autonomic control of fetal heart rate. *Am J Obstet Gynecol.* 1969;105(6):949–953.

31. Gagnon R, Campbell K, Hunse C, Patrick J. Patterns of human fetal heart rate accelerations from 26 weeks to term. *Obstet Gynecol.* 1987;157(3):743–748.

32. Pildner von Steinburg S, Boulesteix AL, Lederer C, et al. What is the "normal" fetal heart rate? *PeerJ.* 2013;1:e82–e82.

33. Macones GA, Hankins GD, Spong CY, Hauth J, Thomas T. The 2008 National Institute of Child Health and Human Development workshop report on electronic fetal monitoring: Update on definitions, interpretation, and research guidelines. *J Obstet Gynecol Neonatal Nurs.* 2008;37(5):510–515.

34. ACOG Practice Bulletin No. 106: Intrapartum fetal heart rate monitoring: Nomenclature, interpretation, and general management principles. *Obstet Gynecol.* 2009;114(1):192–202.

35. Devoe LD. Antenatal fetal assessment: Contraction stress test, nonstress test, vibroacoustic stimulation, amniotic fluid volume, biophysical profile, and modified biophysical profile—an overview. *Semin Perinatol.* 2008;32(4):247–252.

36. ACOG Practice Bulletin. Antepartum fetal surveillance. Number 9, October 1999 (replaces Technical Bulletin Number 188, January 1994). Clinical management guidelines for obstetrician-gynecologists. *Int J Gynaecol Obstet.* 2000;68(2):175–185.

37. Evertson LR, Gauthier RJ, Schifrin BS, Paul RH. Antepartum fetal heart rate testing. I. evolution of the nonstress test. *Am J Obstet Gynecol.* 1979;133(1):29–33.

38. Electronic fetal heart rate monitoring: Research guidelines for interpretation. National Institute of Child Health and Human Development Research Planning Workshop. *Am J Obstet Gynecol.* 1997;177(6):1385–1390.

39. Magann EF, Sandlin AT, Ounpraseuth ST. Amniotic fluid and the clinical relevance of the sonographically estimated amniotic fluid volume: Oligohydramnios. *J Ultrasound Med.* 2011;30(11):1573–1585.

40. Nabhan AF, Abdelmoula YA. Amniotic fluid index versus single deepest vertical pocket as a screening test for preventing adverse pregnancy outcome. *Cochrane Database Syst Rev.* 2008(3):CD006593.

41. Chamberlain PF, Manning FA, Morrison I, Harman CR, Lange IR. Ultrasound evaluation of amniotic fluid volume. I. The relationship of marginal and decreased amniotic fluid volumes to perinatal outcome. *Am J Obstet Gynecol.* 1984;150(3):245–249.

42. Magann EF, Isler CM, Chauhan SP, Martin JN. Amniotic fluid volume estimation and the biophysical profile: A confusion of criteria. *Obstet Gynecol.* 2000;96(4):640–642.

43. Manning FA, Platt LD, Sipos L. Antepartum fetal evaluation: Development of a fetal biophysical profile. *Am J Obstet Gynecol.* 1980;136(6):787–795.

44. Manning FA, Morrison I, Lange IR, Harman CR, Chamberlain PF. Fetal biophysical profile scoring: Selective use of the nonstress test. *Obstet Gynecol.* 1987;156(3):709–712.

45. Laing F, Frates M, Benson C. Ultrasound evaluation during the first trimester of pregnancy. In: *Ultrasonography in Obstetrics and Gynecology.* Philadelphia: WB Saunders; 2000.

46. APGAR V. A proposal for a new method of evaluation of the newborn infant. *Curr Res Anesth Analg.* 1953;32(4):260–267.

47. Medline Plus. Birthweight. Accessed December 6, 2013. Available at http://www.nlm.nih.gov/medlineplus/birthweight.html.

48. Mandy GT, Weisman LE, Kim MS. Incidence and mortality of the premature infant. In: *UpToDate,* Basow DS (ed.), UpToDate, Waltham, MA 2013.

49. Dubowitz LM, Dubowitz V, Goldberg C. Clinical assessment of gestational age in the newborn infant. *J Pediatr.* 1970;77(1):1–10.

50. Ballard JL, Novak KK, Driver M. A simplified score for assessment of fetal maturation of newly born infants. *J Pediatr.* 1979;95(5):769–774.

51. Ballard JL, Khoury JC, Wedig K, Wang L, Eilers-Walsman BL, Lipp R. New Ballard score, expanded to include extremely premature infants. *J Pediatr.* 1991;119(3):417–423.

52. Siedel HM, Ball JW, Dains JE, Flynn JF, Solomon BS, Stewart RW. Examination techniques and equipment. In: Siedel HM, Ball JW, Dains JE, Flynn JF, Solomon BS, Stewart RW (eds.). *Mosby's Guide to Physical Examination,* 7th ed. St. Louis, MO: Mosby Elsevier; 2011: 46–74.

53. McKee-Garrett TM. Assessment of the newborn infant. In: *UpToDate,* Basow DS (ed.), UpToDate, Waltham MA, 2013.

54. Smitherman HF, Macias CG. Evaluation and management of fever in the neonate and young infant. In: *UpToDate,* Basow DS (ed.), UpToDate, Waltham, MA, 2013.

55. Smitherman HF, Macias CG. Definition and etiology of fever in neonates and infants. In: *UpToDate,* Basow DS (ed.), UpToDate, Waltham, MA, 2013.

56. Kemper AR, Mahle WT, Martin GR, et al. Strategies for implementing screening for critical congenital heart disease. *Pediatrics.* 2011;128(5):e1259–e1267.

57. Mahle WT, Newburger JW, Matherne GP, et al. Role of pulse oximetry in examining newborns for congenital heart disease: A scientific statement from the American Heart Association and American Academy of Pediatrics. *Circulation.* 2009;120(5):447–458.

58. Mahle WT, Martin GR, Beekman RH 3rd, Morrow WR; Section on Cardiology and Cardiac Surgery Executive Committee. Endorsement of Health and Human Services recommendation for pulse oximetry screening for critical congenital heart disease. *Pediatrics.* 2012;129(1):190–192.

59. Shiao SY. Effects of fetal hemoglobin on accurate measurements of oxygen saturation in neonates. *J Perinat Neonatal Nurs.* 2005;19(4):348–361.

60. Iliff A, Lee VA. Pulse rate, respiratory rate, and body temperature of children between two months and eighteen years of age. *Child Dev.* 1952;23(4):237–245.

61. Deming DD. Assessment of neonatal and pediatric patients. In: Wilkins RL, Dexter JR, Heuer AJ (eds.). *Clinical Assessment in Respiratory Care,* 6th ed. St. Louis, MO: Elsevier-Mosby; 2010: 68–94.

62. Aloan CA, Hill TV. Physical examination of the newborn. In: Aloan CA, Hill TV (eds.). *Respiratory Care of the Newborn and Child,* 2nd ed. Philadelphia: Lippincott; 1997: 42–56.

63. American Academy of Pediatrics. Task Force on Prolonged Apnea. Prolonged apnea. *Pediatrics.* 1978;61(4):651–652.

64. Hoppenbrouwers T, Hodgman JE, Harper RM, Hofmann E, Sterman MB, McGinty DJ. Polygraphic studies of normal infants during the first six months of life: III. Incidence of apnea and periodic breathing. *Pediatrics.* 1977;60(4):418–425.

65. American Academy of Pediatrics. Task Force on Prolonged Infantile Apnea. Prolonged infantile apnea: 1985. *Pediatrics.* 1985;76(1):129–131.

66. Hoppin AG, Kim MS, TePas E, Torchia MM. What's new in pediatrics. In: *UpToDate*, Basow DS (ed.), UpToDate, Waltham, MA, 2013.

67. Pedroso FS, Rotta N, Quintal A, Giordani G. Evolution of anterior fontanel size in normal infants in the first year of life. *J Child Neurol.* 2008;23(12):1419–1423.

68. McKee-Garrett TM. Assessment of the newborn infant. In: *UpToDate*, Weismen L, Duryea T, Kim M (eds.), UpToDate, Waltham, MA, 2013.

69. Amiel-Tison C. Neurological evaluation of the maturity of newborn infants. *Arch Dis Child.* 1968;43(227):89–93.

70. Medline Plus. Facial nerve palsy due to birth trauma. Accessed December 6, 2013. Available at http://www.nlm.nih.gov/medlineplus/ency/article/001425.htm.

71. Erenberg A, Lemons J, Sia C, Trunkel D, Ziring P. Newborn and infant hearing loss: Detection and intervention. American Academy of Pediatrics. Task Force on Newborn and Infant Hearing, 1998–1999. *Pediatrics.* 1999;103(2):527–530.

72. Kemper AR. Newborn screening. In: *UpToDate*, Basow DS (ed.), UpToDate, Waltham, MA, 2013.

73. Drutz JE. The pediatric physical exam: General principles and standard measurements. In: *UpToDate*, Basow DS (ed.), UpToDate, Waltham, MA, 2013.

74. Kirkland RT. Patient information: Poor weight gain in infants and children. In: *UpToDate*, Basow DS (ed.), UpToDate, Waltham, MA, 2013.

75. Drutz JE. The pediatric physical examination: Chest and abdomen. In: *UpToDate*, Basow DS (ed.), UpToDate, Waltham, MA, 2013.

76. Quintero DR, Fakhoury K. Assessment of stridor in children. In: *UpToDate*, Basow DS (ed.), UpToDate, Waltham, MA, 2013.

77. Chatterjee K. Auscultation of heart sounds. In: *UpToDate*, Basow DS (ed.), UpToDate, Waltham, MA, 2013.

78. Ferguson CM. Inspection, auscultation, palpation, and percussion of the abdomen. In: Walker HK, Hall WD, Hurst JW (eds.). *Clinical Methods: The History, Physical, and Laboratory Examinations*, 3rd ed. Philadelphia: Butterworth; 1990: chapter 93.

79. Ferry GD. Causes of acute abdominal pain in children and adolescents. In: *UpToDate*, Basow DS (ed.), UpToDate, Waltham, MA, 2013.

80. Rosen DM, Colin AA. Overview of pulmonary function testing in children. In: *UpToDate*, Basow DS (ed.), UpToDate, Waltham, MA, 2013.

81. Theodore AC. Venous blood gases and other alternatives to arterial blood gases. In: *UpToDate*, Manaker S, Finlay G (eds.), UpToDate, Waltham, MA, 2013.

82. Adams JM. Oxygen monitoring and therapy in the newborns. In: *UpToDate*, Basow DS (ed.), UpToDate, Waltham, MA, 2013.

83. Restrepo RD, Hirst KR, Wittnebel L, Wettstein R. AARC clinical practice guideline: Transcutaneous monitoring of carbon dioxide and oxygen: 2012. *Respir Care.* 2012;57(11):1955–1962.

84. Adams LV, Starke JR. Tuberculosis disease in children. In: *UpToDate*, Basow DS (ed.), UpToDate, Waltham, MA, 2013.

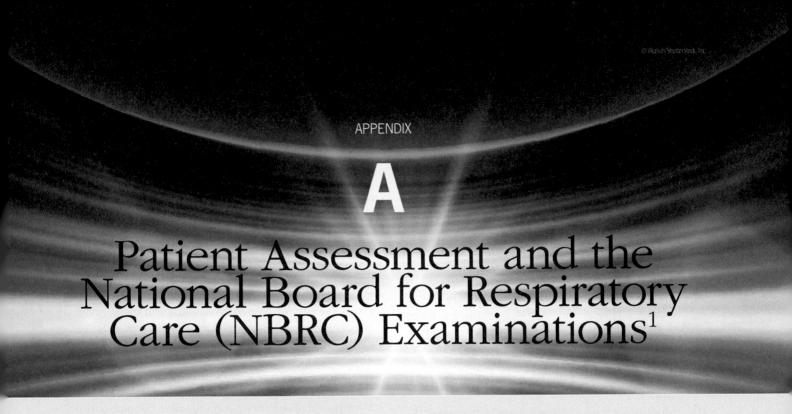

Patient Assessment and the National Board for Respiratory Care (NBRC) Examinations[1]

The National Board for Respiratory Care (NBRC) currently administers a number of different examinations for the certification of respiratory care practitioners. These include the certification examination for entry-level respiratory therapists (CRT), the registry examinations for advanced respiratory therapists (RRT), and the neonatal/pediatric specialty examination. In 2015, the name of the CRT examination changed to the "Therapist Multiple-Choice Examination" which combines the content formerly found on the CRT and RRT written examinations. The minimum passing score for RRT eligibility on this new combined examination is higher than the passing score required for award of the CRT credential. Those passing the Therapist Multiple-Choice Examination with a high enough score will be eligible to take the Clinical Simulation Examination (CSE) for the RRT credential. In addition, the NBRC administers specialty examinations in the areas of pulmonary function technology (i.e., certification examination for entry-level pulmonary function technologist [CPFT] and registry examination for advanced pulmonary function technologist [RPFT]) and a sleep disorders specialty examination. The admission policies for each of these examinations can be found at the NBRC website (see http://www.NBRC.org).

The combined CRT and written RRT examination (i.e., the Therapist Multiple-Choice Examination) is broken down into three major areas: (1) patient data evaluation and recommendations; (2) troubleshooting and quality control of equipment and infection control; and (3) initiation and modification of interventions. Patient data evaluation and recommendations represent about 39% of the questions, while initiation and modification of interventions are about 46% of the combined examination content. What follows is a brief summary

of the content areas of the CRT and RRT examinations directly related to patient assessment and care plan development, with the corresponding book chapters for this text listed.

I. Patient Data Evaluation and Recommendations

A. Evaluate Data in the Patient Record (see Chapter 3)

The review of the patient's medical record should include noting the admitting diagnosis, patient problem list, physician's orders, results of history and physical examinations, laboratory and imaging reports, reports of procedures and progress notes, and patient education. Chapter 3 of the text describes the review of the patient medical record. Specific information found in the patient record and tested on the NBRC CRT and RRT exams includes each of the following areas:[1-3]

1. Patient history to include diagnosis, admission data, history of the present illness, orders, medications, progress notes, DNR status/advance directives, and social history (see Chapters 3 and 4).

2. Physical examination, with an emphasis on the cardiopulmonary system, to include vital signs and physical findings (see Chapters 3 and 5).

3. Artificial airways, chest tubes or other drainage or access devices should be noted (see Chapters 3 and 14).

4. Laboratory data found in the medical record to include CBC, electrolytes, coagulation studies, culture and sensitivities, and sputum Gram stain

(see Chapters 3 and 9). Cardiac enzymes should also be noted (see Chapters 3 and 10).

5. Blood gas analysis results (see Chapters 3 and 8).

6. Pulmonary function and other cardiopulmonary testing results. This should include the results of PFT testing, 6-minute walk tests, metabolic testing (O_2 consumption, CO_2 production, respiratory quotient, energy expenditure) or cardiopulmonary stress testing performed (see Chapters 3 and 12).

7. The results of imaging studies to include chest radiographs, CT scans, MRI, ultrasound, and PET and ventilation–perfusion scans (see Chapters 3 and 11).

8. Maternal, perinatal, and neonatal history and related data to include APGAR scores, gestational age, L/S ratio, and social history (see Chapters 3 and 16).

9. The results of sleep studies related to diagnosis and treatment of sleep disorders (see Chapters 3 and 15).

10. Monitoring data to include trends in vital signs (see Chapter 5); fluid balance; intracranial pressure; weaning parameters (see Chapters 7 and 14); measures of compliance, airway resistance, and work of breathing (WOB) (see Chapters 7 and 14); and noninvasive measures of cardiopulmonary function (e.g., pulse oximetry, capnography, and transcutaneous O_2 and CO_2 measurement (see Chapters 8 and 14).

11. Cardiac monitoring trends to include ECG and other hemodynamic monitoring, cardiac catheterization (see Chapters 10 and 14), and echocardiography (see Chapters 3 and 11).

B. Gather Clinical Information

Following review of the data found in the patient's medical record (see Chapter 3), the respiratory therapist will collect and evaluate additional clinical information needed to develop an appropriate respiratory care plan. This will include completion of the patient history and physical examination (see Chapters 4 and 5); assessment of the patient's oxygenation and ventilation (see Chapters 6 and 7); and ordering and evaluation of additional cardiac, laboratory, and imaging studies (see Chapters 8–11). Additional pulmonary function testing and the use of diagnostic bronchoscopy and related diagnostic testing may be required (see Chapters 12 and 13). In the critical care environment, especially in patients receiving mechanical ventilatory support, additional critical care monitoring and the assessment of monitored results may be needed (see Chapter 14). In addition, certain patients may require sleep studies in order to confirm the presence of sleep-disordered

breathing (see Chapter 15). Specific information covered on the NBRC CRT and RRT examinations/Therapist Multiple-Choice examination includes each of the following areas:[1-3]

Patient Interview (see Chapter 4)

The NBRC examination content outlines[1-3] list clinical information gathered during the patient interview. The patient interview should be completed to determine level of consciousness, orientation, emotional state, and the ability to cooperate. The patient history should also determine the patient's level of pain (if any), the presence of dyspnea, sputum production, and the ability to tolerate exercise. Interview questions should also assess the patient's nutritional status and social history (e.g., smoking, substance abuse). The patient or family should also be questioned regarding any advance directives such as DNR status. In addition, an attempt should be made to determine any patient education or learning needs. Specific items listed on the Therapist Multiple-Choice Examination detailed content outline include:

1. Interviewing the patient for level of consciousness, orientation, emotional state, level of pain (if present), and ability to cooperate.

2. Assessment of dyspnea, sputum production, exercise tolerance, and activities of daily living (ADLs).

3. Tobacco use and smoking history.

4. Environmental exposures, if any.

5. Learning and patient education needs to include assessment of the patient's preferred learning style, culture, and literacy.

Physical Assessment (see Chapter 5)

1. Inspection to assess the patient's overall cardiopulmonary status. This will include general appearance, cyanosis, diaphoresis, breathing pattern, accessory muscle use, chest wall movement, clubbing, edema, and venous distention. Airway assessment should include airway patency, neck range of motion, and assessment for the presence of macroglossia (unusually large tongue). Assessment of cough and any sputum production should be included, noting the amount and character of sputum produced. For neonates, APGAR score and gestational age must be determined, and transillumination of the chest may be performed (see also Chapter 16).

2. Palpation to assess the patient's overall cardiopulmonary status. This should include assessment of pulse, rhythm and force, accessory

muscle use, the presence of asymmetrical chest movements, tactile fremitus, crepitus, airway secretions, any tenderness, and the presence of tracheal deviation.
3. Percussion to assess the patient's cardiopulmonary status.
4. Auscultation to assess the patient's cardiopulmonary status. This should include listening to breath sounds, heart sounds and rhythm, and assessment of blood pressure.

Imaging Studies (see Chapter 11)

A review of the imaging studies should be conducted to assess the patient's cardiopulmonary status and assess for the presence of, or any change in, specific cardiopulmonary abnormalities. According to the NBRC examination content outlines,[1-3] the respiratory therapist should be able to:

1. Identify and evaluate the quality of the chest radiograph to include the exposure of the image (i.e., penetration) and patient positioning.
2. Determine the position of an endotracheal or tracheostomy tube or indwelling tubes or catheters (if present).
3. Evaluate imaging studies for the presence of foreign bodies, heart size and position, pneumothorax, consolidation, pleural effusion, and pulmonary edema, and evaluate the position of and any change in the trachea, mediastinum, or hemidiaphragms.
4. Evaluate lateral neck radiographs in children and be able to identify the presence of epiglottitis, croup, or foreign bodies.

C and D. Perform Procedures to Gather Clinical Information and Evaluate Procedure Results

ECG (see Chapter 10)

According to the NBRC examination content outlines,[1-3] the respiratory therapist should be able to perform and interpret the results of a 12-lead ECG to include evaluation of heart rate, irregular rhythm (if present), and any artifacts.

Noninvasive Monitoring (see Chapters 8 and 14)

According to the NBRC examination content outlines,[1-3] the respiratory therapist should be able to perform and interpret the results of noninvasive monitoring to include pulse oximetry, capnography, and transcutaneous monitoring.

Bedside and Screening Measures of Pulmonary Function (see Chapters 7, 12, and 14)

According to the NBRC examination content outlines,[1-3] the respiratory therapist should be able to perform and interpret the results of measurement of peak flow, tidal volume, minute volume, vital capacity, and screening spirometry—see also below.

Arterial Blood Gases and Acid-Base Balance (see Chapter 8)

According to NBRC exam content outlines,[1-3] the respiratory therapist should be able to perform and interpret the results of arterial sampling (percutaneous and arterial line sampling), arterialized capillary blood sampling, and blood gas and hemoximetry analysis. In addition, the respiratory therapist should be able to perform arterial line insertion and pulse oximetry to include overnight oximetry.

Assessment of Oxygenation (see Chapter 6)

The respiratory therapist must recognize the physical findings associated with hypoxemia and be well-versed in the various measures of oxygenation. According to the NBRC examination content matrixes,[1-3] this should include interpreting the results of pulse oximetry, oxygen titration with exercise, and calculations of $P(A - a)O_2$, P/F ratio, and oxygenation index.

Assessment of Ventilation (see Chapter 7)

The respiratory therapist should be well prepared to assess the cardiopulmonary patient's ventilatory status. This should include an understanding of the relationships among tidal volume, respiratory rate, minute volume, physiologic dead space, and alveolar ventilation. Factors associated with normal ventilation and ventilatory failure should be clearly understood to include recognition of acute or impending ventilatory failure and the need to provide mechanical ventilatory support. According to the NBRC examination content outlines,[1-3] the respiratory therapist should be able to perform and evaluate the results of:

1. Measurement and interpretation of tidal volume, minute volume, vital capacity, peak expiratory flow (PEF), and other measures of lung function obtained via bedside spirometry (i.e., FVC, FEV_1).
2. Measurement and interpretation of lung mechanics to include maximal inspiratory pressure (MIP), maximal expiratory pressure (MEP), compliance, and airway resistance.
3. Measurement of V_D/V_T must also be performed and the results interpreted.

Acute and Critical Care Monitoring and Assessment (see Chapter 14)

The respiratory therapist must be able to assess patient's cardiopulmonary status in the acute and critical care setting. This includes ventilatory parameters, the use of noninvasive monitoring, cardiac and hemodynamic monitoring, and monitoring of the patient airway. According to the NBRC examination content matrixes,[1-3] this should include measurement and evaluation of:

1. Ventilatory volumes and flows (e.g., tidal volume, minute volume, respiratory rate, vital capacity, peak expiratory flow [PEF], FVC, FEV_1 – see Chapters 7 and 12).
2. Lung mechanics including MIP, MEP, and plateau pressure (see Chapters 7 and 14).
3. Pulmonary compliance and airway resistance (see Chapter 7).
4. Ventilator graphics should be reviewed and the results of observation of pressure–volume loops should be interpreted. Auto-PEEP must also be detected, if present (see Chapter 14).
5. Oximetry, transcutaneous monitoring, and capnography should be performed when appropriate, and results interpreted (see Chapters 8 and 14).
6. Spontaneous breathing trials in mechanically ventilated patients (see Chapters 7 and 14).
7. Tracheal tube cuff pressures and/or volumes must also be measured, and the results properly interpreted (see Chapter 14).
8. Hemodynamic monitoring must be performed, and the results properly interpreted. This includes the measurement of blood pressure and CVP (see Chapter 14).
9. ECG monitoring is used in most critically ill patients, and the respiratory therapist must be able to recognize abnormalities (see Chapter 10). The therapist should also be able to perform exhaled nitric oxide measurement and interpret the results (see Chapter 14).

Pulmonary Function Testing (see Chapter 12)

The respiratory therapist must understand the purpose of pulmonary function testing, indications for specific pulmonary function tests, predicted values, the equipment used, and the interpretation of the results of pulmonary function testing. According to the NBRC examination content matrixes,[1-3] this should include

1. Bedside spirometry (PEF, FEV_1, and VC/FVC measurement).
2. 6-minute walk test; oxygen titration with exercise.

3. Stress testing (ECG, SpO_2).
4. Pulmonary function laboratory studies.

Miscellaneous Tests and Examinations

In addition to the tests and related assessment techniques listed above, the NBRC CRT and RRT examination content matrixes[1,2] suggest that the respiratory therapist be able to collect and evaluate the following additional clinical information:

1. Results of various blood tests (e.g., hemoglobin, potassium; see Chapter 9).
2. Obtain diagnostic bronchoscopy and/or bronchoalveolar lavage (BAL) to evaluate atelectasis or hemoptysis and thoracentesis to evaluate pleural effusion (see Chapter 13).
3. Results of sleep studies, continuous positive airway pressure (CPAP)/bilevel positive airway pressure (BiPAP) titration during sleep and overnight pulse oximetry (see Chapter 15), and apnea monitoring (see Chapter 16).

E. Recommend Diagnostic Procedures

The respiratory therapist must understand the indications for specific diagnostic procedures, be able to recommend these procedures when needed and interpret the results. According to the NBRC examination content matrixes,[1-3] this should include:

1. Laboratory blood tests such as measurement of electrolytes and CBC; sputum Gram stain, culture, and sensitivity (see Chapter 9).
2. Skin testing for allergy or tuberculosis (see Chapter 9).
3. Blood gas analysis (see Chapter 8).
4. Noninvasive monitoring such as pulse oximetry, capnography, and transcutaneous monitoring (see Chapters 8 and 14).
5. Exhaled gas monitoring to include measurement of exhaled CO_2, carbon monoxide (CO), and nitric oxide (NO and FeNO – see Chapter 14).
6. ECG (see Chapter 10).
7. Pulmonary function testing (see Chapter 12).
8. Bronchoscopy, bronchoalveloar lavage (BAL), and thoracentesis (see Chapter 13).
9. Hemodynamic monitoring (see Chapter 14).
10. Sleep studies (see Chapter 15).

Respiratory Care Plans (see Chapters 1 and 2)

In addition to reviewing data in the patient medical record, collecting and evaluating additional clinical information, and recommending procedures to obtain additional data, the NBRC examination content outline suggests that as much as 46% of the examination content will be based on the ability to initiate and modify therapeutic and other interventions.[3]

III. Initiation and Modification of Interventions

The respiratory therapist must be able to develop, administer, and modify the respiratory care plan based on the patient's response. This includes airway care, lung expansion therapy, support of oxygenation and ventilation, administration of medications and specialty gases, use of evidence-based practice, emergency care, and patient transport. The therapist must also be able to assist the physician (or other provider) with specific procedures and be able to initiate and conduct patient and family education.

A. Maintain a Patent Airway Including the Care of Artificial Airways (see Chapters 7 and 14)

According to the NBRC detailed content outline for the Therapist Multiple-Choice Examination,[3] this includes properly positioning the patient, recognition of a difficult airway, and establishing and maintaining a patient's airway:

1. The use of specific types of airways and related equipment (e.g., nasopharyngeal airway, oropharyngeal airway, laryngeal mask airway, esophageal-tracheal tubes, supraglottic airways (Combitube, King), and speaking tubes.
2. The use of endotracheal, tracheostomy, and laryngectomy tubes, including providing adequate humidification, performing tracheostomy care, and exchanging artificial airways.
3. Endotracheal intubation, and maintaining appropriate cuff inflation are also listed on the CRT and written RRT summary content outline,[2] but are not specifically listed in the content outline for the Therapist Multiple-Choice Examination.[3] Extubation is listed on both content outlines.[2,3]
4. Applying techniques to prevent ventilator associated pneumonia using protocols.

B. Perform Airway Clearance and Lung Expansion Techniques (see Chapter 2)

According to the NBRC summary content outlines,[1-3] this includes:

1. Suctioning (nasotracheal and orotracheal) and airway care.
2. Postural drainage, percussion, and vibration; high-frequency chest wall oscillation; positive expiratory pressure (vibratory PEP); and intrapulmonary percussive ventilation.
3. Assisted cough, including the "huff cough" and "quad" cough.
4. Lung expansion therapy, including IPPB and incentive spirometry.
5. Providing inspiratory muscle training.

C. Support Oxygenation and Ventilation (see Chapters 2, 6, 7, and 14)

According to the NBRC summary content outlines,[1-3] this includes initiating and adjusting low-flow and high-flow oxygen therapy; minimizing hypoxemia via patient positioning and suctioning; and initiating and adjusting CPAP by mask or nasal appliance (see Chapters 2 and 6). In support of ventilation, the respiratory therapist will initiate and adjust mechanical ventilatory support (e.g., continuous mechanical ventilation, noninvasive ventilation, high-frequency ventilation) and set ventilator alarms (see Chapters 7 and 14). The therapist will use ventilator graphics (i.e., waveforms, scales) to monitor and adjust care, including correction of patient-ventilator dyssynchrony (see Chapter 14). The therapist will also evaluate patients for ventilator discontinuation and apply techniques (e.g., weaning) for liberation from the ventilator (see Chapters 7 and 14). The therapist will also perform lung recruitment techniques, as indicated (see Chapter 14).

D. Administer Medications and Specialty Gases (see Chapters 2 and 14)

According to the NBRC summary content outlines,[1-3] this includes administration of aerosol therapy with specific medications via metered dose inhalers (MDI), small volume nebulizers (SVN), and dry powder inhalers and endotracheal instillation of medications. Specialty gas administration includes heliox and nitric oxide (NO).

E. Ensure Modifications Are Made to the Respiratory Care Plan (see Chapter 2)

According to the NBRC examinations summary content outlines,[1-3] this includes recommendations for:

1. Institution of treatment based on patient's response, treatment of pneumothorax, adjustment of fluid balance, adjustment of electrolyte therapy, insertion or change of an artificial airway, liberation from mechanical ventilation, and extubation and discontinuing treatment based on the patient's response (to include termination of treatment due to an adverse, life-threatening event).
2. Changes in patient position, O_2 therapy, airway clearance techniques, and lung hyperinflation therapy (see Chapter 2).
3. Changes in mechanical ventilation to improve patient synchrony, enhance oxygenation, improve alveolar ventilation, adjust the I:E ratio, and

adjust ventilator settings. Based on ventilator graphics, the therapist should be able to change the type of ventilator, alter mechanical dead space, reduce auto-PEEP, and decrease plateau pressure (see Chapters 6, 7, and 14).

4. Pharmacologic interventions, including administration of bronchodilators, anti-inflammatory drugs, mucolytics and proteolytics; cardiovascular drugs and diuretics; sedatives, hypnotics, analgesics and neuromuscular blocking agents; pulmonary vasodilators (e.g. sildenafil, prostacyclin, inhaled NO); surfactants and vaccines; and changes to drug dosage or concentration (see Chapters 2, 10, 14, and 16).

F. Utilize Evidence-Based Medicine Principles (see Chapters 1 and 2)

According to the NBRC summary content outlines,[1-3] this should include the ability to analyze all of the available information to determine the patient's pathophysiologic state. This review should include any planned therapy, the ability to establish the therapeutic plan and recommend changes in the plan when indicated. Clinical practice guidelines and the application of evidence-based methods include use of the ARDSNet protocols and National Asthma Education and Prevention Program (NAEPP) recommendations.

G. Provide Respiratory Care Techniques in High-Risk Situations

According to the NBRC summary content outlines,[1-3] this includes treatment of cardiopulmonary emergencies (e.g., cardiac arrest, tension pneumothorax, obstructed or lost airway), participation in patient transport (both within and between hospitals), disaster management, and participation in medical emergency teams (MET), such as the rapid response team.

H. Assist a Physician/Provider Performing Procedures (see Chapters 8, 13, and 14)

According to the NBRC summary content outlines,[1-3] this includes intubation, bronchoscopy, thorocentesis, tracheostomy, chest tube insertion, insertion of venous or arterial catheters, moderate (conscious sedation) cardioversion, cardiopulmonary exercise testing, and withdrawal of life support.

I. Initiate and Conduct Patient and Family Education (Chapters 1 and 2)

The therapist should conduct patient and family education with respect to safety and infection control; home care and home care equipment; smoking cessation; pulmonary rehabilitation and disease management to include asthma and COPD; and sleep disorders.[3] According to the NBRC CRT and RRT summary content outline,[1,2] this includes initiating and adjusting apnea monitors, starting treatment for sleep disorders, and modifying respiratory care procedures for use in the home.[1,2] Explaining planned therapy goals to the patient to optimize outcomes, educating the patient and family, and performing health management to include counseling the patient and family concerning smoking cessation are listed.[1,2] Instructing the patient and family to ensure patient safety and infection control and interacting with case managers are also suggested.[1,2]

J. Maintain Records and Communicate Information (see Chapters 3 and 4)

According to the NBRC CRT and RRT summary content outline,[1,2] this should include recording therapy delivered to include interpreting the patient's response to therapy and communicating information regarding the patient's clinical status. This includes information relevant to coordinating patient care and preparing for discharge. Verification of orders, use of computer technology, and maintaining patient safety are included. Communication with the patient and providing patient and family education are also incorporated to include provision of information related to health management and smoking cessation. The new Therapist Multiple-Choice Examination Detailed Content Outline does not include this category.[3]

References

1. National Board for Respiratory Care. *NBRC: Candidate Handbook and Application.* Olathe, KS: Author; 2014.
2. National Board for Respiratory Care. *NBRC: Summary Content Outline for CRT and Written RRT Examinations.* Olathe, KS: Author; 2014.
3. National Board for Respiratory Care. *NBRC: Therapist Multiple-Choice Examination Detailed Content Outline.* Olathe, KS: Author; 2014.

Glossary

2,3-diphosphoglycerate (2,3-DPG) A substance found within the red blood cell that alters the affinity of hemoglobin and oxygen.

A-a gradient [P(A – a)o₂] The calculated difference between the alveolar P_{O_2} and the arterial P_{O_2}.

a-A oxygen ratio (Pao₂/Pao₂) The calculated ratio of the arterial P_{O_2} divided by the alveolar P_{O_2}.

acid Compound that donates or yields a hydrogen ion (H^+) in an aqueous solution; a substance that donates a proton in a proton-transfer reaction.

acid-base status The overall acid-base status reflects both the metabolic and respiratory components of acid-base balance; generally assessed by measurement of arterial blood pH.

acidemia A decrease in arterial blood pH below normal.

acidosis Describes the condition of a pH of less than normal (< 7.35).

activated partial thromboplastin time (aPTT) A test used to determine whether abnormalities of blood clotting are present and to evaluate the effects of anticoagulants when used for treatment.

activities of daily living (ADL) A person's ability to perform daily self-care tasks such as bathing, dressing, preparing meals, walking, housekeeping, shopping, and other tasks that are part of normal daily life. Occupational therapists and other professionals use a number of different assessment tools to evaluate a patient's ability to perform ADLs.

acute alveolar hyperventilation superimposed on chronic ventilatory failure Occurs when patients with chronic ventilatory failure acutely develop respiratory distress and begin to hyperventilate relative to their normal state of chronic alveolar hypoventilation.

acute alveolar hyperventilation A sudden decrease in arterial P_{CO_2} with a corresponding increase in pH.

acute lung injury (ALI) A condition characterized by bilateral infiltrates on chest x-ray, hypoxemia (Pao₂/Fio₂ ratio < 300 mm Hg), and noncardiogenic pulmonary edema. The Berlin definition of acute respiratory distress syndrome (ARDS) redefines ALI as a mild form of ARDS.

acute mountain sickness A condition usually caused by ascent to a mountainous area and the corresponding decrease in barometric pressure and inspired oxygen levels.

acute myocardial infarction Damage of the myocardium due to a lack of adequate blood flow (and oxygen); most commonly caused by a blood clot.

acute respiratory distress syndrome (ARDS) Respiratory disorder characterized by the abrupt onset of respiratory distress; associated with severe hypoxemia and diffuse pulmonary opacities on chest radiograph that are not caused by congestive heart failure or volume overload. Severity is based on the Pao₂/Fio₂ ratio: mild ($200 < $ Pao₂/Fio₂ ≤ 300), moderate ($100 < $ Pao₂/Fio₂ ≤ 200), and severe (Pao₂/Fio₂ < 100). In addition to Pao₂/Fio₂ < 100, severe ARDS criteria include $C_{rs} \leq 40$ mL/cm H_2O, PEEP ≥ 10 cm H_2O, $\dot{V}_F \geq 10$ L/min, and radiographic severity.

acute respiratory failure A general term referring to an inability of the heart and lungs to maintain adequate oxygenation and/or carbon dioxide removal. Acute respiratory failure generally refers to a sudden fall in arterial oxygen levels, with or without CO_2 retention.

[1] Adapted from: Hess DR, MacIntyre Nr, Mishoe SC, Galvin WF, Adams AB. *Respiratory Care: Principles and Practice*. 2nd ed. Sudbury, MA: Jones & Bartlett Learning; 2012.

acute ventilatory failure (AVF) A sudden increase in arterial P_{CO_2} with a corresponding decrease in pH.

acute ventilatory failure superimposed on chronic ventilatory failure Occurs when patients in chronic ventilatory failure begin to acutely hypoventilate, often due to an acute insult (e.g., acute exacerbation of COPD).

admitting diagnosis The provisional diagnosis based on the initial assessment of the patient.

adventitious breath sounds Abnormal breath sounds.

afterload Resistance against which the ventricle must eject blood during contraction; the load that opposes myocardial shortening.

air bronchogram Radiographic abnormality in the image of the bronchi occurring when the alveolar airspaces become filled with fluid, causing increased contrast between the air-filled bronchi and adjacent fluid-filled lung parenchyma, rendering the bronchi lucent and projecting them as branching tubular air-filled structures.

air trapping Condition in the lung in which air is not exhaled because of decreased lung elasticity and/or increased expiratory airway resistance; accompanied by hyperinflation.

airway hyperresponsiveness Condition associated with asthma that is responsive to both specific and nonspecific factors (such as environment, exercise, allergens, and viral infections), whereby the airways constrict too easily and frequently.

airway inflammation Condition that exacerbates asthmatic reactions by the release of mediators, including mast cells, eosinophils, macrophages, epithelial cells, and T lymphocytes, resulting in recurrent exacerbations that manifest as wheezing, progressive shortness of breath, chest tightness, and coughing; may be classified as acute, subacute, or chronic.

airway resistance (R_{aw}) Pressure difference developed per unit flow as gas flows into or out of the lungs.

airway stent An endobronchial device designed to maintain patency of the airway in the presence of central airways obstruction due to benign or malignant causes.

albumin A type of protein found in the blood (i.e., serum albumin) that affects the blood's colloidal osmotic pressure.

alkalemia An abnormal increase in arterial blood pH.

alkalosis An abnormal systemic pH >7.45.

allergen Common triggering mechanism for asthmatic reactions; can be indoor factors (e.g., mold, animal dander, cleaning chemicals, cockroach antigen, dust mites) or outdoor factors (e.g., noxious fumes, gas, tree pollens).

α_1-antitrypsin (AAT) deficiency α_1-antitrypsin is a plasma protein produced in the liver that inhibits trypsin and other proteolytic enzymes; deficiency is associated with the development of emphysema.

altitude hypoxia Low oxygen levels caused by the decrease in barometric pressure associated with increasing altitude.

alveolar dead space (V_D alveolar) Refers to alveoli that are ventilated but not perfused.

alveolar oxygen tension (P_{AO_2}) The partial pressure of oxygen in the alveoli, usually calculated using the alveolar air equation.

alveolar ventilation ($\dot{V}_A$) The volume of gas entering the gas exchange units in the lung (i.e., alveoli) per minute; usually calculated by subtracting physiologic dead space from tidal volume and multiplying the result by the number of breaths per minute.

ambient hypoxia Hypoxia caused by low oxygen levels in a room or confined space.

America Thoracic Society (ATS) A national/international society dedicated to improving global health through research, patient care, and public health. The ATS focuses on pulmonary disease, critical illness, and sleep disorders.

amniocentesis A procedure in which amniotic fluid is withdrawn for analysis.

amniotic fluid volume (AFV) The volume of fluid surrounding the fetus.

anatomic dead space (V_D anatomic) The volume of gas in the conducting airways that extends from the external nares down to and including the terminal bronchioles.

anatomic shunt Blood that moves from the right side of the heart to the left side of the heart via anatomic structures (e.g., a patent ductus arteriosus) without participating in gas exchange.

anemia A decrease in the number of red blood cells or hemoglobin level.

angina Choking, crushing, painful feeling most often associated with cardiac pain caused by hypoxia of the myocardium.

angiography Medical imaging that involves contrast media to visualize blood vessels and organs.

anion gap Difference between the concentrations of serum cations and anions such that the anion gap $= ([Na^+] + [K^+]) - ([HCO_3^-] + Cl^-])$. If the anion gap exceeds 12 mmol/L, excessive unmeasured anions are likely present. Because its concentration is normally low, $[K^+]$ is often omitted from this calculation.

anteroposterior (AP) projection A chest radiographic view in which the x-ray beam passes through the chest from the front to the back.

antiasthmatic medications Medications designed to prevent acute asthma exacerbations, such as the leukotriene antagonists (e.g., zafirlukast) and mast cell stabilizers (e.g., cromolyn or nedocromil).

anti-inflammatory agents Agents that reduce inflammation, such as corticosteroids and nonsteroidal anti-inflammatory drugs (NSAIDs; e.g., ibuprofen).

APGAR score A calculated index used in the assessment of the newborn comprised of the newborn's heart rate, respiratory effort, muscle tone, reflex irritability, and color.

apnea Absence or cessation of breathing.

apnea of prematurity Category or type of cessation of airflow in a premature infant's breathing.

apneustic breathing Abnormal ventilatory pattern in which the patient experiences gasping breaths with an end-inspiratory pause.

arrhythmia/dysrhythmia An abnormal cardiac rhythm; electrical activity of the heart is irregular or abnormally fast (tachycardia) or slow (bradycardia).

arterial blood gases Blood analysis whose primary measurements (P_{O_2}, P_{CO_2}, and pH) provide important information about oxygenation, ventilation, and acid-base status.

arterial blood gas study Laboratory study in which arterial blood is analyzed to determine the P_{O_2}, P_{CO_2}, pH, and Sa_{O_2} of the arterial blood.

arterial oxygen content (Ca_{O_2}) The volume of oxygen carried in the arterial blood, usually expressed as milliliters of oxygen per hundred milliliters of arterial blood or volumes percent.

arterial oxygen saturation (Sa_{O_2}) The percent oxygen saturation of the hemoglobin in the arterial blood.

arterial oxygen tension (Pa_{O_2}) The partial pressure of oxygen in the arterial blood, usually expressed as mm Hg or torr.

arterialized capillary blood gas study A technique sometimes used in infants in which venous blood is obtained following warming of the site from which the blood is taken in order to increase perfusion and "arterialize" the blood. The infant heal stick is an example.

ascites Accumulation of fluid in the peritoneal cavity.

aspiration The accidental entry of foreign materials (e.g., food or liquids) into the lower respiratory tract.

asthma Chronic, inflammatory disorder of the airways in which many cells and cellular elements play a role, in particular, mast cells, eosinophils, T lymphocytes, macrophages, neutrophils, and epithelial cells; causes recurrent episodes of wheezing, breathlessness, chest tightness, and coughing, particularly at night or in the early morning.

asthma trigger Any mechanism that can cause asthmatic reactions, including allergens, pollution, food and drug additives, and viral agents.

atelectasis Incomplete expansion of the lung or the collapse of previously expanded lung tissue, a common noninfectious pulmonary complication after surgery; may be due to many factors, including small, monotonous tidal volumes and inadequate lung distending forces, airway obstruction with gas absorption, and reduction in surfactant levels.

atrial flutter An abnormal atrial cardiac rhythm.

atrioventricular (AV) block A problem in conduction between the atria and ventricles of the heart.

atrioventricular (AV) junction That part of the cardiac conduction system that carries electrical activity from the atria to the ventricles.

atrioventricular (AV) node Located in the septal wall of the right atrium, the AV node receives impulses from the SA node and transmits them to the AV bundle for eventual symmetric distribution throughout the ventricles.

atypical pneumonia Pneumonia caused by any strain of unusual type and characterized by a flulike disease with prodromal symptoms, dry cough, myalgia, malaise, rhinorrhea, and moderate fever; usual pathogens in atypical pneumonia include *Mycoplasma pneumonia*, *Chlamydia psittaci*, *Chlamydophila pneumoniae*, and *Coxielle burnetii*, and respiratory viruses.

auscultation Most commonly used physical assessment technique; involves listening to sounds produced by the body with the aid of a stethoscope placed on bare skin.

auto-PEEP End-expiratory alveolar pressure that is greater than the pressure at the proximal airway, which results from high airways resistance and/or a short expiratory time.

axis deviation Alterations in the electrical axis of the heart.

Bachmann's bundle Part of the electrical conduction system of the heart; the intra-atrial conduction tract.

base Solution that yields a hydroxide ion ($OH-$) in an aqueous solution; species accepting the proton in a proton-transfer reaction.

base excess/deficit (BE/BD) The amount of bicarbonate that would be needed to adjust the pH to normal with a normal partial pressure of arterial CO_2.

basophils A type of white blood cell that tends to increase with certain inflammatory reactions, such as allergies.

bilevel positive airway pressure (BiPAP) Technique in which two levels of pressure are applied during spontaneous breathing.

bilirubin A yellow breakdown product of heme (as in hemoglobin) that is excreted in bile and urine; causes the yellowish color seen with bruises and the yellow color of the skin (i.e., jaundice) seen with liver failure.

Biot's breathing Pattern of breathing symptomatic of elevated intracranial pressure and meningitis; characterized by a short burst of uniform, deep respirations followed by a period of apnea lasting 10 to 30 seconds.

blebs Thin-walled, blister-like tissues on the surface of the lung.

blood urea nitrogen (BUN) Most common nonprotein nitrogenous compound in the blood; measurement used to assess renal function in the adult. Normal values for BUN are between 7 and 21 mg/dL.

body mass index (BMI) A measure to assess whether a person's weight is normal (i.e., healthy weight) or if he or she is overweight or obese based on measurement of height and weight.

body plethysmograph Diagnostic tool that is used to achieve measurements of airway resistance (R_{aw}), airway conductance (G_{aw}), and static lung volumes based on Boyle's law (e.g., FRC, TGV).

body temperature, pressure, and saturated (BTPS) Gas at body temperature, barometric pressure of 760 mm Hg, fully saturated with water vapor.

Bohr effect The effect of P_{CO_2} on the HbO_2 dissociation curve, in which the binding affinity of the hemoglobin to oxygen is inversely related to blood acidity and carbon dioxide concentration.

Borg scale A subjective method of rating a patient's dyspnea using a 0–10 scale.

Boyle's law A physical property of gases stating that the pressure and volume of a gas vary inversely if the temperature remains constant.

brachytherapy Radiotherapy treatment that involves applying an ionizing radiation source near the body area being treated; in respiratory treatment, this usually entails the endobronchial placement of encapsulated radionuclide in close proximity to an endobronchial malignancy.

bradycardia Abnormally slow heart rate (usually < 60 bpm).

bradypnea Slow respiratory rate.

bronchial challenge Use of either methacholine or mannitol to measure responsiveness to general stimuli; usually administered in a pulmonary function lab and followed (usually within 15 minutes) with a short-acting β-agonist that results in a 12% to 15% increase in a patient's forced expiratory volume in 1 second (FEV_1).

bronchial hygiene Respiratory care procedures and techniques used to maintain the mucosal blanket (e.g., humidity therapy) and remove excess secretions (e.g., chest physical therapy).

bronchiectasis Permanent dilatation of the small airways often resulting in sputum retention, excess sputum production, chronic cough, and repeated infection.

bronchiectasis Permanent small airway dilatation and damage that may be congenital or acquired.

bronchitis Inflammation of the bronchi that may be acute or chronic.

bronchoalveolar lavage (BAL) Procedure for collecting an alveolar specimen by use of a bronchoscope or other hollow tube through which saline is instilled into distal bronchi and then withdrawn; also used to describe the specimen thus obtained.

bronchodilator therapy Procedures in which bronchodilator medications are administered, most commonly by inhaled aerosols.

bronchogenic carcinoma A malignant lung tumor that originates in the bronchi.

bronchopulmonary dysplasia Chronic iatrogenic lung disease caused by oxygen toxicity and barotrauma resulting from positive pressure ventilation; incidence is greater in premature infants, perhaps related to the increased requirement for oxygen therapy and mechanical ventilation in this patient population.

bronchoscopy Examination using a bronchoscope that enables inspection of the tracheobronchial tree and related diagnostic and therapeutic maneuvers, including taking specimens for culture, biopsy, and removal of foreign bodies.

bronchospasm Spasm or contraction of the smooth muscle surrounding the small airways.

bullae Airspace enlargements greater than 1 cm; can progressively enlarge and compress adjacent lung tissue, impairing respiratory function.

bundle of His The portion of the electrical conduction system of the heart between the AV junction and the right and left bundle branches.

cachexia A significant loss of appetite or unintended weight loss.

calcification Accumulation of calcium salts; may occur in soft tissue (e.g., lung).

capillary blood gases A term used to refer to the analysis of arterialized blood as an alternative to drawing an arterial blood sample.

capnography Noninvasive technique that measures carbon dioxide levels in inspired and expired gas and displays a capnogram.

capnometry Numeric display of CO_2 measurements taken from the proximal airway.

carbon dioxide production ($\dot{V}CO_2$) The amount of CO_2 produced by the tissues and excreted by the lungs each minute; normally about 200 mL/min in adults.

carbonic acid (H_2CO_3) Product of the hydration of carbon dioxide (CO_2) that ionizes to H^+ and bicarbonate; carbonic acid then forms bicarbonate.

carboxyhemoglobin (COHb) Compound produced by exposing hemoglobin to carbon monoxide; usually inhaled into the lungs and subsequently bound to hemoglobin in the blood, blocking the sites for oxygen transport.

cardiac enzymes Group of enzymes that are released from myocardial tissue and appear in the serum during myocardial injury (usually ischemia).

cardiomegaly Enlarged heart.

cardiopulmonary exercise testing A relatively noninvasive test that measures respiratory gas exchange (oxygen uptake and carbon dioxide output, minute ventilation, and anaerobic threshold), electrocardiography, blood pressure, and pulse oximetry during maximal exercise tolerance.

carina The point at which the trachea bifurcates into the main bronchi.

case control An observational research design in which individuals with a disease are compared to similar individuals without the disease in order to determine if certain factors are associated with disease development.

Centers for Medicare and Medicaid Services (CMS) The federal agency responsible for administration of Medicare, Medicaid, and child health insurance programs. CMS was initially named the Healthcare Financing Administration.

central sleep apnea (CSA) Loss of diaphragmatic and other respiratory muscle function, resulting in the cessation of respiratory effort; apnea stemming from the central nervous system.

central venous pressure (CVP) Pressure measured in the superior vena cava or right atrium and used to estimate intravascular volume status.

charting Term used for recording information in the medical record following a patient interaction,

monitoring procedure, or the administration of medications or other therapy.

chest physiotherapy (CPT) Bronchial hygiene techniques that include postural drainage, percussion, and vibration to mobilize or remove secretions.

chest wall retractions Inward motion of the tissue between the ribs, below the sternum, or above the sternum during inspiration. Retractions are a sign of acute respiratory distress.

chest x-ray An image produced by x-ray beams passing through the thorax.

Cheyne–Stokes breathing Breathing consisting of a repeating pattern in which the rate and depth of breathing increases to a peak, followed by a decrease in the rate and depth of breathing, followed by a period of apnea.

chief complaint In most cases, the reason the patient has sought medical care. Examples of chief complaints include cough, shortness of breath, chest pain, headache, and sputum production.

cholesterol Sterol lipid that combines with phospholipids in the cell membrane to help stabilize its bilayer structure; also used by the body as a starting point in making steroid hormones such as estrogen, testosterone, and cortisol.

chronic alveolar hyperventilation characterized by a low arterial PCO_2 and a normal or near normal pH due to renal compensation.

chronic bronchitis Type of chronic obstructive pulmonary disease (COPD) defined by the presence of cough and sputum production for 3 or more months in 2 successive years in patients who do not have other causes of cough.

chronic obstructive pulmonary disease (COPD) Progressive, irreversible condition characterized by dyspnea and difficulty exhaling, and sometimes including chronic cough.

chronic ventilatory failure A chronic elevation in arterial CO_2 levels with a normal or near normal pH as a result of metabolic compensation.

coagulation The process by which the blood clots.

cohort studies A research design in which a group of subjects is followed over time to determine if certain risk factors are associated with the development of disease.

community acquired pneumonia (CAP) Pneumonia acquired outside the hospital.

complete blood count (CBC) A routine blood test that includes measurement of red blood cells, white blood cells, and platelets.

computed tomography (CT) A radiographic technique that produces an image representing detailed cross sections of tissue using an array of detectors in a variety of angles and a collimated beam of x-rays that rotates in a continuous 360-degree motion around the patient to create cross-sectional images.

congestive heart failure (CHF) Inability of the heart to adequately pump blood; may be right-sided (i.e., right ventricle) or left-sided failure (i.e., left ventricle).

consolidation A condition in which alveoli become filled with fluid, infection, and inflammatory exudate, as with pneumonia.

continuous mandatory ventilation (CMV) System for delivering a set tidal volume (or pressure) and a minimum respiratory rate in which the patient can trigger additional breaths above the minimal rate, but the set volume or pressure is constant at the preset level.

continuous positive airway pressure (CPAP) A ventilation method by which a constant pressure greater than atmospheric pressure is applied to the airway throughout the respiratory cycle.

contractility Feature of muscle tissue, especially cardiac muscle, that allows it to contract by shortening the sarcomeres.

contraction stress test (CST) A test performed on the fetus following administration of oxytocin, which causes uterine contractions. The fetal heart rate is monitored to determine if the fetus may have difficulty during labor contractions.

contrast agent Substance used to outline vessels or organs as part of an imaging study.

co-oximetry Means for measuring carboxyhemoglobin levels, hemoglobin oxygen saturation and methemoglobin.

cor pulmonale Hypertrophy and dilatation of the right ventricle.

coronary angiography Direct imaging of the coronary arteries using cardiac catheterization and subsequent injection of contrast dye; can identify atherosclerotic lesions as well as coronary anomalies, areas of spasm, and acute thrombi.

crackles Fine, high-pitched, discontinuous sounds heard during auscultation of the lungs.

C-reactive protein (CRP) A protein found in the blood, the levels of which rise in response to inflammation.

creatinine Substance formed from creatine metabolism and measured in blood and urine as an indicator of kidney function; creatinine levels are a function of skeletal muscle breakdown, and most creatinine is filtered in the glomeruli with little reabsorption.

creatinine clearance (CrCl) A measure of kidney function; an approximation of glomerular filtration rate as assessed by the volume of blood cleared of creatinine.

critical care monitoring Techniques used to ensure patient safety and adjust care based on the patient's condition. Critical care monitoring techniques include ECG monitoring, vital sign monitoring, hemodynamic monitoring, and monitoring of ventilatory volumes, flows, and pressures during mechanical ventilatory support.

critical illness polyneuromyopathy Disease affecting several areas of the peripheral nervous system at once; diagnosis is confirmed by electromyographic studies.

critical thinking A style of thinking that employs analysis, synthesis, evaluation, and application of information gathered through observation, experience, and other sources of evidence employed to solve problems and guide practice.

cuff-leak test Test to assess for swelling around the endotracheal tube in preparation for possible extubation of the patient.

cyanosis a blue or purple tint to the skin, nail beds, or mucosa associated with low oxygen saturation of the hemoglobin.

cystic fibrosis Disorder that is inherited in an autosomal recessive pattern and affects the exocrine glands, resulting in abnormally thick secretions of mucus.

date of conception The approximate date on which a pregnancy began, usually calculated by estimating 11–21 days from the woman's last menstrual period.

dead space The part of the tidal volume that does not participate in gas exchange; ventilation without perfusion.

dead space to tidal volume ratio (V_D/V_T) The ratio of the physiologic dead space to tidal volume, which is normally in the range of 0.20 to 0.40 (i.e., 20% to 40%).

deep vein thrombosis (DVT) Blood clotting in the legs and pelvis, which usually occurs as a result of venostasis; common in surgical patients and with other causes of immobility, damage to the endothelial wall of the blood vessels, and hypercoagulability states.

delayed-type hypersensitivity (DTH) A cell-mediated response that takes 2 to 3 days to develop.

depolarization The shift in cardiac cell membrane potential that accompanies cardiac muscle contraction.

diabetes mellitus A chronic metabolic disease associated with high blood glucose levels.

diabetic ketoacidosis Buildup of ketones in the blood due to the breakdown of stored fats for energy; a potentially life-threatening complication in patients with diabetes mellitus.

diaphoresis Profuse sweating.

diffusing capacity (D_{LCO}) Number of milliliters of gas that transfer from the lungs across the alveolar–capillary membrane into the bloodstream each minute for each 1 mm Hg difference in the pressure across the membrane.

diffusion defect A deficiency in the ability of gases to cross the alveolocapillary membrane.

diffusion limited Gas transfer in the lung can be perfusion limited or diffusion limited. Carbon monoxide is diffusion limited, whereas nitrous oxide is perfusion limited.

DNR status An advanced directive order that states that if the patient's heart stops beating or he or she stops breathing, he or she should not receive cardiopulmonary resuscitation, no effort to institute an airway, no assisted breathing, and no chest compressions.

Doppler ultrasound Test used to evaluate blood flow through arteries and veins; may be used to evaluate umbilical or cardiac blood flow in the fetus.

Down syndrome A congenital disorder associated with mental retardation, a characteristic physical appearance, and trisomy of chromosome 21.

Dubowitz scoring system A scoring system that provides an assessment of gestational age of the newborn.

dynamic compliance ($C_{dynamic}$) A measure of compliance calculated by dividing the delivered volume by the difference between the peak airway pressure and the baseline pressure; reflects both compliance and airway resistance.

dyspnea Shortness of breath or breathlessness; distressing feeling of inability to breathe or great effort required to breathe.

edema Fluid accumulation in the tissues; in the lungs edema can collect in the interstitial (interstitial edema) or alveolar spaces.

egophony Auscultation sound typical in consolidation of lung tissue, meaning that the normally aerated tissue has been filled with fluid, mucus, pus, or cellular debris; in egophony, *e* sounds like *a*.

Einthoven's triangle The triangle formed from the three limb leads of the ECG.

electrocardiogram (ECG) A test for the evaluation of the electrical activity of the heart.

electroencephalogram (EEG) Recording through the scalp of electrical potentials (activity) from the brain and the changes in these potentials.

electrolytes Any substance containing free ions that make the substance electrically conductive.

electronic health record (EHR) An individual patient's medical record in digital format. Electronic health record systems coordinate the storage and retrieval of individual records with the aid of computers.

electronic medical record (EMR) A medical record in digital format. In health informatics, an EMR is considered by some to be one of several types of electronic health records (EHR), but in general usage EMR and EHR are synonymous.

emphysema Type of chronic obstructive pulmonary disease occurring in patients who experience damage to the lung parenchyma; results in histopathologic evidence of alveolar wall destruction and physiologic evidence of decreased lung elastic recoil, resulting in bullae that eventually enlarge and compress adjacent lung tissue, impairing respiratory function.

endobronchial Within the bronchi.

endobronchial ultrasound (EBUS) The use of ultrasonic probe as part of flexible bronchoscopy for the assessment of endobronchial lesions and lymph nodes.

endocardium The inner layer of the heart that lines the cardiac chambers.

end-tidal P_{CO_2} P_{CO_2} at end-exhaustion (P_{ETCO_2}).

endotracheal tube (ETT) A tube inserted into the trachea via either the nose or mouth to maintain airway patency for delivery of oxygen to the lungs.

enteral nutrition Provision of nutrients through the gastrointestinal tract when the patient is unable to chew or swallow.

eosinophils A type of white blood cell that may be elevated in the presence of multicellular parasites and certain other infections.

epicardium The outer layer of the heart.

epiglottitis Rapidly progressing inflammation of the epiglottis and surrounding tissue that can result in severe airway obstruction.

erythrocytes Red blood cells.

eupnea Normal breathing.

European Respiratory Society (ERS) An international society that seeks to alleviate suffering from respiratory disease and promote lung health.

exacerbation Sudden worsening of respiratory symptoms accompanied by deteriorating lung function; most often, patients will present with increased dyspnea, cough, and changes in the quality or quantity of sputum.

exhaled nitric oxide (FeNO) Marker of airway inflammation, particularly useful in both acute and chronic asthma in both children and adults.

expiratory reserve volume (ERV) The volume of gas that can be exhaled forcefully following a passive exhalation.

false-negative　A test result that suggests that a condition is not present, even though it is present.

false-positive　A test result that suggests that a condition is present when in fact it is not.

family history　The portion of the patient's medical history in which the health of family members is described to include illnesses and causes of death (if applicable). The family history may be especially useful in helping identify diseases that may have a genetic component.

fetal heart rate (FHR)　Heart rate of the fetus as assessed by various types of monitoring equipment.

fetal hemoglobin　Hemoglobin F; has higher affinity to O_2 than adult hemoglobin (hemoglobin A), which can be attributed to the replacement of β-chains in hemoglobin A by γ-chains.

fetal movement　Flutters, kicks, or other movement of the fetus felt by the mother; provides a gross assessment of fetal development.

fetal nonstress test (NST)　A noninvasive test that measures fetal heart rate, contractions, and fetal reactivity.

fetal quickening　Point during pregnancy in which the mother begins to sense fetal movements.

fever　Elevated body temperature above the normal range.

fissures　A cleft or division that separates body tissues; in the lung fissures divide the lung lobes.

flail chest　Multiple rib fractures on one side or two or more adjacent rib fractures in two or more places. The term *flail* refers to the paradoxic motion of the chest resulting from loss of chest wall stability.

flexible bronchoscopy　The type of bronchoscopy that utilizes a flexible fiber-optic scope.

fluoroscopy　A radiologic imaging technique that allows for real-time visualization of internal body structures.

foam stability index (FSI)　A test of the amniotic fluid used to assess lung maturation of the fetus.

forced expiratory volume in 1 second (FEV$_1$)　The volume of gas that can the forcefully exhaled in 1 second following a maximal inspiration.

forced oscillation technique (FOT)　A noninvasive pulmonary function technique used to measure respiratory mechanics.

forced vital capacity (FVC)　Test of pulmonary function that measures the maximal volume of gas that can be expelled forcibly after full inspiration.

foreign body aspiration　Aspiration (inhaling) of foreign material into the lung.

fremitus　Vibrations transmitted through the body; commonly assessed by palpation.

fully compensated　Refers to an acid-base disorder in which a respiratory or metabolic abnormality is compensated by a corresponding adjustment in Pco_2 or bicarbonate levels; the result is a normal or near normal pH.

functional residual capacity (FRC)　The volume of gas remaining in the lungs following a normal, passive expiration.

gestational age　A measure of the age the fetus.

gestational diabetes mellitus　A condition in which pregnant women exhibit abnormally high blood glucose levels.

glomerular filtration rate (eGFR)　The rate of flow of filtered plasma through the kidney.

gram-negative bacteria　Bacteria that have a cell wall composed of a thin layer of peptidoglycan covered by an outer membrane of lipoprotein and lipopolysaccharide and which lose the stain or are decolorized by alcohol in Gram staining; examples include *Haemophilus influenzae, Moraxella catarrhalis, Pseudomonas aeruginosa, Klebsiella* species, *Escherichia coli, Enterobacter* species, *Serratia* species, *Acinetobacter* species, and *Proteus mirabilis*.

gram-positive bacteria　Bacteria whose cell walls are composed of a thick layer of peptidoglycan with attached teichoic acids and which retain the stain or resist decolorization by alcohol in Gram staining; examples include *Streptococcus pneumoniae, Staphylococcus aureus,* and *Enterococcus* species.

grasp reflex　Normal reflex present at birth in which the infant grasps an object placed in the palm of the infant's hand.

gravida　Refers to a pregnant woman.

Grey Turner's sign　Bruising of the sides associated with a retroperitoneal hemorrhage.

ground-glass opacification　A hazy increased attenuation of the lungs, with preservation of bronchial and vascular margins.

grunting　A sound heard in newborns with respiratory distress. It occurs when the glottis is closed in an attempt to maintain lung volume.

guarding　When the patient protects or tries to protect a specific area of the body, usually due to pain.

Guillain-Barré syndrome (GBS)　Acute idiopathic polyneuritis usually presenting as an ascending symmetric paralysis associated with absent tendon reflexes.

HbO$_2$ dissociation curve A graphical representation of the effect of increasing partial pressure of oxygen (x-axis) on the saturation of the hemoglobin with oxygen (y-axis). The resultant curve is sigmoid in shape.

head bobbing A phenomenon most commonly seen in infants that is associated with respiratory distress.

health A state of complete physical, mental, and social well-being, not merely absence of disease or infirmity.

health-related quality of life (HRQOL) The well-being of people and societies as affected by health.

heart murmur An abnormal heart sound caused by blood flow across the heart valve.

heat exhaustion A condition caused by failure of the body to adequately cool itself, often due to exercise under hot, humid conditions.

hematocrit Proportion of whole blood that is red blood cells (the hemoglobin-carrying cells).

hemoglobin (Hb) Iron-containing globular protein consisting of two pairs of polypeptides; primary function is the transport of oxygen from the lungs to the tissues.

hemoglobin A$_{1c}$ A type of hemoglobin that is sometimes measured as part of the assessment of blood glucose levels and in the detection of possible diabetes.

hemolysis Destruction of red blood cells.

hemoptysis Coughing up of blood or blood-containing secretions.

hemostasis The mechanisms by which bleeding stops.

hemothorax Blood trapped in the pleural space, causing a space-occupying lesion; source of blood is typically from fractured ribs lacerating the intercostal blood vessels or lacerating the lung.

hemoximetry The measurement of the oxygen saturation of the hemoglobin.

Henderson-Hasselbalch equation Assertion that the pH of a buffer is determined by the ratio of the concentration of base to the concentration of weak acid.

hilum Depression in the lung where the vessels and nerves enter.

history and physical examination The core components of a patient assessment are the medical history and performance of a physical examination.

history of the present illness (HPI) A history of the present illness that generally includes onset, severity, course over time, any factors that improve or worsen symptoms, and any treatment that has been undertaken.

history The portion of the patient assessment performed by interviewing patients and family members in order to gather the medical history. Includes the chief complaint, history of the current illness, medications, past medical history, family history, and social history.

Holter monitoring A technique for measuring cardiac electrical activity (i.e., ECG) as the patient goes about normal activities.

honeycombing The presence of cystic airspaces with thick, fibrous walls lined by bronchiolar epithelium.

hospital-acquired pneumonia Pneumonia that develops after hospital admission, excluding any infection that is incubating at the time of admission.

human chorionic gonadotropin (hCG) A hormone that is sometimes used as a marker of pregnancy.

hypercapnic respiratory failure Respiratory failure in which there is an elevation in arterial Pco_2; sometimes referred to as "pump failure."

hyperresonant The quality of a sound often produced in percussion technique, that is loud, low pitched, and long; often heard over an emphysematous lung.

hypersomnolence A condition characterized by excessive sleepiness.

hypertension An abnormally elevated blood pressure, usually defined as a diastolic pressure > 90 mm Hg or a systolic pressure > 140 mm Hg.

hyperventilation Rapid, deep, labored breathing resulting in a lowered Pco_2.

hypopnea Abnormally slow, shallow respiration.

hypotension An abnormally low blood pressure, usually < 90/60 mm Hg.

hypothermia A core temperature of 95° F (35° C) or less.

hypoventilation A decrease in ventilation as assessed by an elevation in arterial Pco_2; may be acute, or chronic.

hypovolemic shock Hypotension with end organ dysfunction caused by intravascular volume loss; most commonly due to hemorrhage in a traumatically injured patient.

hypoxemia Deficiency in blood oxygenation; may be caused by inadequate ventilation relative to perfusion (i.e., low $\dot{V}_A/\dot{Q}$ and shunt), which has a greater effect on oxygen uptake by the lung; hypoxemia in adults is usually defined as a Pao_2 of less than 80 mm Hg at sea level.

hypoxemic drive A second ventilatory drive that triggers increased minute ventilation when the Pao_2 is less than 60 mm Hg.

hypoxemic respiratory failure Respiratory failure in which hypoxemia is the predominant feature; sometimes referred to as "lung failure."

hypoxia Decreased tissue oxygenation below adequate levels.

hypoxic hypoxia Also known as alveolar hypoxia, refers to low oxygen levels in the alveoli.

hypoxic pulmonary vasoconstriction Narrowing of the lumen in a pulmonary blood vessel because of low oxygen level.

hysteresis The phenomena in which the manifestation of a physical force lags behind its application; commonly seen in pressure volume curves performed on air-filled lungs.

idiopathic pulmonary fibrosis (IPF) Interstital lung disease that affects predominantly males in the fifth to seventh decade of life; of unknown pathogensis but likely to affect an aberrant host response to injury of the alveolar epithelium and endothelium or a protracted response to the same; a history of a gradual onset of dyspnea with exercise is typical.

imaging studies Various studies that allow for visualization of internal structures or function. Common imaging studies include radiography (e.g., x-rays), CT, MRI, and diagnostic medical sonography (e.g., ultrasonography).

immediate hypersensitivity An allergic reaction that occurs rapidly following re-exposure to an allergen.

immunocompromised Refers to patients who have a compromised immune response.

immunohistochemistry Laboratory tests used to detect antigens in cells of tissue samples.

infarction Tissue death caused by a lack of blood supply and/or oxygen.

inferior vena cava (IVC) filter A type of vascular filter that is implanted into the inferior vena cava to prevent fatal pulmonary emboli.

infiltrate Abnormal fluid accumulation in the lung.

inspection An examination technique that ranges from casual observation to visual scrutiny of the patient.

inspiratory capacity (IC) The maximal amount of gas that can be inhaled following a passive exhalation.

inspiratory time Time interval from the start of inspiratory flow to the start of expiratory flow, including the inspiratory hold (or pause) time.

inspiratory-to-expiratory ratio (I:E) The ratio of inspiratory time to expiratory time.

inspired oxygen tension (P_{IO_2}) The partial pressure of oxygen in inspired gas, which is determined by the fractional concentration of oxygen (F_{IO_2}) and barometric pressure (PB).

insulin A hormone produced in the pancreas that regulates aspects of metabolism to include the conversion of glucose to glycogen.

interferon-gamma-release assays (IGRA) A laboratory test sometimes used for detection of infectious disease, such as tuberculosis.

intermittent positive pressure breathing (IPPB) A form of mechanical ventilatory support usually provided for brief periods of time (10 to 15 minutes) as a form of lung expansion therapy. The positive pressure provided during inspiration is adjusted to achieve an inspiratory volume sufficient to treat or prevent atelectasis, although evidence of the effectiveness of IPPB is limited.

interstital lung disease (ILD) Term used to delineate approximately 200 distinct diseases in which the interstitium is altered by inflammation or fibrosis or both; may affect any of the following structures: the alveolar walls (and lumens), pulmonary microvasculature, interstitial macrophages, fibroblasts, myofibroblasts, and matrix components of the lung.

intervals On an ECG tracing, areas that denote time passage between one specific electrical event and another within a specific cycle (e.g., PR interval, QT interval).

intrapulmonary shunt Blood moves from the right side of the heart through the lungs to the left side of the heart without participation in gas exchange.

junctional premature complex (JPC) An abnormal heart rhythm originating within the AV junction.

Kerley B lines Short lines that appear perpendicular to the pleural surface on a chest radiograph; associated with congestive heart failure.

Kussmaul breathing Hyperventilation as a compensatory mechanism for metabolic acidosis.

kyphosis Forward curvature of the spine.

laboratory studies A broad range of studies, often performed in a clinical laboratory, that include hematology, clinical chemistry, microbiology, and other studies of blood and body secretions.

lactate threshold The point where lactate (lactic acid) begins to accumulate in the bloodstream; also known as the anaerobic threshold.

laminar flow Gas flow in the lung that is smooth, with little turbulence. It is largely present in the distal small airways of the lung.

last menstrual period (LMP) The time from which gestational age is usually calculated.

lateral decubitus A chest radiographic view in which the patient is lying on the side.

lecithin/sphingomyelin (L/S) ratio A test performed on amniotic fluid to determine lung maturity; with an LS ratio of more than 2:1, the lungs are considered mature.

leukemia A type of cancer that causes a proliferation of abnormal white blood cells.

leukocytes White blood cells.

leukocytosis Elevated white cell count; often a sign of significant infection but also can be associated with elevated glucocorticoids (e.g., stress reaction, steroid administration) and a number of hematologic malignancies.

leukopenia Decreased white cell count; often indicates overwhelming infection.

lower airway obstruction Obstruction in the lower airways that is usually considered to begin below the larynx, although some authors consider the lower airways as those below the glottis.

lung compliance (C_L) The stretchability of the lung tissue.

lung expansion therapy Therapy designed to treat or prevent atelectasis by providing deep breaths via positive pressure (i.e., IPPB) or coaching (i.e., incentive spirometry).

lymphadenopathy Abnormal lymph nodes, often enlarged; may be due to infection, malignancy or auto immune disease.

lymphocytes A type of white blood cell involved in immune response; includes T cells, B cells, and natural killer (NK) cells.

macrocytic Larger than normal red blood cells with insufficient hemoglobin.

magnetic resonance imaging (MRI) Imaging that takes advantage of nuclear magnetic resonance.

mass An abnormal "spot" on the lungs at least 3 cm in diameter; may be benign or cancerous.

maximal compensation The maximal adjustment normally possible in compensation for a metabolic or respiratory acid-base disorder. Estimates of expected maximal compensation may be calculated using various formulas.

maximal expiratory pressure (MEP) After a full inhalation, the pressure generated by forced exhalation against an occluded airway.

maximal inspiratory pressure (MIP) After a full exhalation, the pressure generated by forced inhalation against an occluded airway.

maximal voluntary ventilation (MVV) The maximal amount of air that can be moved per minute; the test is usually conducted for 10 to 15 seconds and the volume is reported in liters per minute.

mean airway pressure Average pressure, relative to atmospheric pressure, within the airway during one complete respiratory cycle; directly related to the inspiratory time, respiratory rate, peak inspiratory pressure, and positive end-expiratory pressure.

mean cell (or corpuscular) hemoglobin (MCH) the average mass of hemoglobin per red blood cell.

mean cell (or corpuscular) hemoglobin content (MCHC) The average concentration of hemoglobin in a given volume of blood.

mean cell (or corpuscular) volume (MCV) The average volume of a red blood cell.

mean exhaled carbon dioxide tension ($\overline{PE}co_2$) The average partial pressure of carbon dioxide in exhaled gas; normally about 28 mm Hg.

mean platelet volume (MPV) Average blood platelet size.

mechanical dead space The volume of rebreathed gas due to a mechanical device.

mechanical ventilation A form of respiratory support that typically uses a positive pressure ventilator.

meconium aspiration syndrome Condition that develops when the fetus or newborn inhales meconium; can block the air passages and cause failure of the lungs to expand or other pulmonary dysfunction such as pneumonia or emphysema.

mediastinoscopy Examination of the mediastinum using an endoscope with light and lenses inserted through an incision in the suprasternum.

medical record The medical record in the acute care setting refers to the patient's "chart," which includes the admitting diagnosis, patient data (i.e., name, gender, age, primary physician), physicians' orders, history and physical examination, results of laboratory and imaging studies, monitoring flow sheets, progress notes, and reports of operations or procedures.

meta-analysis A statistical analysis in which the results of multiple randomized controlled trials are combined.

metabolic acidosis Decrease in pH associated with a decrease in buffer (HCO_3^-).

metabolic alkalosis Increase in pH associated with an increase in buffer (HCO_3^-).

metabolic rate Rate at which metabolism occurs, commonly assessed by measuring oxygen consumption and CO_2 production.

metastasis Process by which tumor cells spread to distant parts of the body.

methemoglobin Form of hemoglobin that is produced when the iron in heme is oxidized from Fe^{+2} to Fe^{+3}.

methemoglobinenemia An abnormal condition in the blood in which the concentration of methemoglobin is elevated, resulting in a decrease in the oxygen carrying capacity of hemoglobin.

microalbumin Laboratory test that measures albumin in the urine as a test for kidney damage in people with diabetes or renal disease.

microcytic Abnormally small red blood cells.

minute volume ($\dot{V}_E$) Volume of gas exhaled per minute; respiratory rate times tidal volume.

misallocation Refers to care provided that is not indicated or the failure to provide care that is indicated.

mixed venous blood gas study Refers to the measurement of P_{O_2}, P_{CO_2}, and pH in blood aspirated from a catheter in which the tip lies in the pulmonary artery.

modified Allen test A test performed on the wrist and hand to assess for collateral blood flow prior to a radial artery puncture or radial arterial line insertion.

monocytes A type of white blood cell.

mucosal edema Swelling of the bronchial mucosa, usually due to inflammation or infection.

multiple sclerosis (MS) Demyelinating disease of the central nervous system characterized clinically by repeated remissions and exacerbations of symptoms, including paresthesias, motor weakness, diplopia, blurred vision, bladder incontinence, and ataxia.

muscular dystrophy Heterogeneous group of progressive, hereditary degenerative skeletal muscle diseases in which the respiratory muscles, like any skeletal muscle, become progressively weaker, eventually culminating in respiratory failure and death (respiratory complications are the most common cause of death in these diseases).

musculoskeletal chest pain Pain centered in the chest muscles, ligaments, tendons, joints, or bones. Rib fractures and chest trauma are two examples of possible causes of musculoskeletal chest pain.

myasthenia gravis Autoimmune disorder characterized by impaired transmission of neural impulses across the neuromuscular junction resulting from the destruction of the postsynaptic acetylcholine receptors.

mycobacterial pneumonia Any of a group of pneumonias caused by tuberculous and nontuberculous mycobacteria (NTM) and diagnosed by acid-fast bacilli (AFB) smears and mycobacterial cultures, using nucleic acid probes to detect *Mycobacterium tuberculosis*, *Mycobacterium avium complex*, *Mycobacterium gordonae*, or *Mycobacterium kansasii*.

myocardial infarction (MI) More commonly known as a heart attack, an MI is caused when there is inadequate blood flow (and oxygen delivery) to the heart muscle, resulting in tissue injury. A common cause of an MI is a blockage of one of the coronary arteries.

myocardial ischemia Condition of inadequate blood flow in the coronary arteries that supply the heart muscle; often results in angina.

myocardium The cardiac muscle itself.

Naegele's rule A method for estimating the due date for a pregnancy.

nasal flaring Flaring of the nostrils during inspiration associated with respiratory distress.

negative inspiratory force (NIF) The maximum subatmospheric pressure generated during inspiration against a closed valve; also known as maximum inspiratory pressure (MIP).

new Ballard score (NBS) A scoring method for assessment of gestational age that may be completed shortly after birth.

NIH ARDS Network A clinical research network that was established by the National Institutes of Health (NIH) to accelerate the development of successful management strategies for acute lung injury and the acute respiratory distress syndrome (ARDS).

nitric oxide Colorless gas that is naturally synthesized in human tissue and plays an important role in vascular smooth muscle relaxation, inhibition of platelet aggregation, neurotransmission, and immune regulation.

nodular pattern Multiple round opacifications on the chest radiograph.

non-small-cell lung cancer (NSCLC) Major category of histologic types of lung carcinomas, including adenocarcinoma of the lung, large cell carcinoma, and squamous cell carcinoma.

nosocomial An infection that is acquired in a hospital or nursing home.

non-ST segment elevation MI (NSTEMI) A category of myocardial infarction based on ECG findings.

normochromic A type of anemia in which the hemoglobin levels in the red blood cell are normal but there are insufficient numbers of red blood cells.

normocytic A type of anemia in which red blood cells are of normal size and have normal hemoglobin levels.

nuclear medicine (NM) The medical specialty that incorporates radioactive materials for the diagnosis and treatment of disease.

obesity Having a body mass index (BMI) of greater than 30.

obstructive lung disease Disease characterized by a reduced lumen of the airways within the lungs.

obstructive sleep apnea (OSA) Reduction in airflow to less than 90% of baseline despite persistent respiratory effort.

opacifications (opacity) Areas on a chest radiograph that block the passage of x-ray energy and thus appear white.

open lung biopsy (OLBx) A surgical procedure used to remove a small piece of tissue from the lung; generally performed under anesthesia in the operating room.

opiate Natural or synthetic derivative of morphine, derived from the opium poppy, stimulating opiate receptors in the brain and spinal cord to decrease the sensation of pain; also acts as a potent sedative or cough suppressant.

oral glucose tolerance test (OGTT) A method of testing for diabetes by testing blood glucose levels after a patient drinks a standardize glucose solution.

orthopnea Breathlessness, especially when recumbent.

oximetry Determination of the hemoglobin oxygen saturation of arterial blood using an oximeter.

oxygen consumption ($\dot{V}o_2$) Rate of O_2 uptake by the body, measured by analyzing inspired and expired O_2 in a ventilator circuit; approximately 250 mL/min in the adult under resting conditions.

oxygen delivery ($\dot{D}o_2$) Rate of O_2 transport to the peripheral tissues, expressed as $\dot{D}o_2$; determined by the cardiac output and arterial O_2 content; also referred to as O_2 availability or O_2 transport.

oxygen extraction The difference between the amount of oxygen delivered to the tissues and the amount of oxygen remaining when the blood leaves the tissues.

oxygen extraction ratio (O_2ER) The ratio of the arterial oxygen content minus the venous oxygen content divided by the arterial oxygen content.

oxygen saturation by pulse oximetry (Spo_2) The oxygen saturation of the hemoglobin as measured via pulse oximetry.

oxygen therapy Therapy in which an oxygen delivery appliance (e.g., oxygen mask, nasal cannula) is used to provide an increased Fio_2.

oxygen toxicity Pathologic response of the body and its tissues from long-term exposure to high partial pressures of oxygen.

oxygen-induced hypoventilation Reduced ventilation that results from the administration of high concentrations of oxygen to patients with chronic hypercapnea.

oxygenation status An assessment of the patient's overall oxygenation status requires review of all of the factors that may affect oxygen delivery, uptake, and utilization by the tissues. This may include assessment of inspired oxygen levels, assessment of alveolar ventilation, assessment of gas transfer across the lung, assessment of oxygen loading to include hemoglobin and oxygen saturation, assessment of oxygen delivery, and assessment of tissue uptake and utilization.

P wave The electrical activity of the heart associated with the depolarization of the atria.

P_{50} The partial pressure of oxygen resulting in 50% saturation of the hemoglobin.

pacemaker cells Cells that set the cardiac rhythm and rate.

pack years Measure of patient's smoking exposure; one pack a day for 1 year equals 1 pack year.

palpation Examiner's use of his or her hands to feel for body movement, lumps, masses, and skin characteristics.

Pao_2/Fio_2 ratio A number calculated by dividing Pao_2 by Fio_2 that is used to estimate the severity of hypoxemic respiratory failure.

paradoxical respiration Flail chest movement, characterized by chest wall movement outward on expiration and inward on inspiration.

parenchyma Functional organ tissue; does not include connective and supporting tissue of the organ. Term often used to refer to functional lung tissue.

parenteral nutrition Administration of nutrients by a route other than the alimentary canal.

paroxysmal nocturnal dyspnea Sudden shortness of breath that occurs several hours after a patient lies down; suggests cardiac dysfunction.

partial thromboplastin time (PTT) Clotting time in anticoagulation therapy, best if 2 to 2.5 times the control.

partially compensated When a metabolic or respiratory acid-base disorder is partially compensated by a change in Pco_2 or bicarbonate.

patient outcomes Outcomes of illness and care provided ranging from subjective (e.g., symptoms, such as pain) to physiologic (e.g., blood pressure), to length of illness and recovery, and to health-related quality of life. Other outcomes of interest include patients' knowledge of their disease state or condition, ability to provide self-care, cost, healthcare utilization, and ability to return to school or work.

patient profile A written or oral brief description of the patient to include a statement of the problem, supporting information, and planned care.

patient-ventilator asynchrony A condition in which there is a mismatch between how the patient is breathing and the ventilator is delivering breaths.

peak expiratory flow (PEFR or PEF) The peak flow that can be maximally generated during a forced expiratory maneuver.

peak inspiratory pressure (PIP) The highest pressure measured at the proximal airway during positive pressure ventilation.

pectus carinatum Condition in which the chest bows out at the sternum similar to that of a pigeon.

pectus excavatum Condition in which the sternum is depressed and deviated somewhat like a funnel.

percussion Examination technique in which the examiner places a finger firmly against a body part and then strikes that finger with a fingertip from the other hand, producing sounds that may suggest normal or abnormal tissue.

perfusion without ventilation (shunt) Commonly refers to capillary shunting in which alveoli are not ventilated (e.g., atelectasis, fluid filling) but perfused.

pericardium The sac that contains and covers the heart.

pH Indicates the hydrogen ion concentration [H^+] in a solution; mathematically defined as the negative logarithm of the hydrogen ion concentration.

phenotype The observable physical or biochemical characteristics of an organism, as determined by both genetic makeup and environmental influences.

phosphatidylglycerol (PG) A substance found in pulmonary surfactant that is sometimes measured to determine lung maturity.

physical examination Techniques to gather patient information via inspection, auscultation, palpation, and percussion.

physician's orders Orders by physicians and certain other healthcare providers (e.g., nurse practitioners, physician assistants) for medications, procedures, monitoring and follow-up, and other patient care interventions.

physiologic dead space (V_D physiologic) The volume of gas in the conducting airways (i.e., anatomic dead space) plus the volume of gas in any alveoli that are ventilated but not perfused (i.e., alveolar dead space).

pitting edema Accumulation of excess fluid in the interstitial space beneath the skin, sometimes assessed by pressing on the skin and observing the resultant depression.

plasma bicarbonate (HCO_3^-) The primary base compound in blood that regulates acid-base balance. Bicarbonate is excreted in the kidneys in response to elevation in pH.

plateau pressure ($P_{plateau}$) End-inspiratory alveolar pressure attained during mechanical ventilation (which should, ideally, be kept below 30 cm H_2O) in conjunction with an overall lung protective ventilation strategy.

platelets Blood cells critical to clot formation after vascular injury; produced in the bone marrow.

pleural friction rub Continuous grating sound heard in auscultation of the lungs, resembling two pieces of leather or two hands being rubbed together; occurs when pleurae are inflamed or when fluid accumulates in the pleural cavity.

pleural Term used to refer to the pulmonary pleura.

pleuritic chest pain Chest pain that originates in the pleural space and is often associated with inflammation of the pleura.

pneumocystis pneumonia (PCP) Pneumonia caused by a yeast-like fungus (*Pneumocystis jiroveci*) that may occur in patients with weak immune systems.

pneumomediastinum Air in the mediastinum.

pneumonia Any of several subgroups of respiratory infections; characterized by the inflammation and consolidation of lung tissue caused by infectious agents.

pneumothorax Air in the pleural space that can cause collapse of the lung.

polycythemia An abnormal increase in red blood cells or hemoglobin levels.

polymerase chain reaction (PCR) A method by which microorganisms may be identified by amplification of nucleic acids.

polymorphonuclear neutrophil (PMN, segmented neutrophil, Seg) A type of white blood cell that may be elevated with infection.

polysomnography A sleep study that produces a polysomnogram.

ponopnea Painful breathing.

positive airway pressure (PAP) A general term used to refer to the application of positive pressure during the respiratory cycle.

positive end-expiratory pressure (PEEP) Positive airway pressure during the exhalation phase.

positron emission tomography (PET) Imaging modality used for assessing thoracic pathology, in particular for tumor imaging, providing physiologic and metabolic information, and focusing on the biochemical properties of cells.

posteroanterior (PA) projection A chest radiographic view in which the x-ray beam passes through the chest from the back to the front.

PR segment The portion of the ECG that connects the P wave to the QRS complex.

preload Distending pressure within the ventricle during diastole.

premature atrial contraction (PAC) An abnormal heart rhythm in which there is premature contraction of the atria.

premature junctional complexes (PJCs) Premature beats that originate in the AV node, the area around the AV node, or the bundle of His.

premature ventricular contraction (PVC) An abnormal cardiac rhythm associated with premature contraction of the ventricles.

pressure control ventilation (PCV) Mode of ventilation in which airway pressure is set and remains constant with changes in resistance and compliance.

pressure support ventilation (PSV) A breathing mode in which patient effort is augmented by a clinician determined level of pressure during inspiration.

prevalence How many persons have a given disease or condition in a location at a given time.

problem-oriented medical record (POMR) A problem-based approach to medical record keeping that focuses on a problem list and often includes the use of SOAP notes.

prone position Position in which the patient is lying face-downward.

prothrombin time (PT) Test for coagulation defects, used to evaluate the extrinsic pathway, depending on the levels of factors V, VII, X, and eventually I and II.

protocol A detailed, written description of care to be provided, often including steps to adjust care depending on the patient's response and/or algorithms to guide the healthcare provider in the provision of care.

pulmonary angiography Radiographic examination of the blood vessels of the lungs after injection of an opaque contrast medium into the pulmonary circulation.

pulmonary artery catheter Swan-Ganz catheter, which is inserted into the pulmonary artery, providing pressure measurements, cardiac output determination, and mixed venous blood analysis.

pulmonary capillary oxygen tension ($P_c o_2$) The partial pressure of oxygen in the capillaries adjacent to the alveoli.

pulmonary capillary wedge pressure (PCWP) Measure that provides an estimate of left atrial (LA) and left ventricular end-diastolic or filling pressure (LVDEP).

pulmonary edema Accumulation of excess fluid in the interstitial and alveolar spaces in the lung.

pulmonary embolism Blockage of a pulmonary artery by foreign matter, such as fat, air, tumor tissue, or a thrombus; characterized by dyspnea, sudden chest pain, shock, and cyanosis.

pulmonary function testing (PFT) A collection of studies used to help clinicians identify abnormalities by direct or indirect measurement of lung function.

pulmonary hypertension Abnormally high pressure within the pulmonary circulation.

pulmonary vascular resistance (PVR) Resistance in the pulmonary vascular bed against which the right ventricle must eject blood.

pulse oximetry Technique that measures oxyhemoglobin saturation noninvasively in arterial blood; rapidly detects changes in arterial oxygen saturation.

pulsus paradoxus Abnormal decrease in systolic pressure and pulse wave amplitude during inspiration.

pupillary reflex or response Response of the pupils to light.

Purkinje fibers Those fibers that carry the electrical impulse across the ventricles.

QRS complex That portion of the ECG associated with ventricular contraction.

radiodensity The ability of an object to block x-ray energy, determined by its composition and thickness.

radiolucent Body tissues that are penetrated by x-rays; produces black areas on the chest radiograph.

radiopaque Body tissues that are impenetrable or poorly penetrable to x-rays; produces white or gray areas on the chest radiograph, depending on the extent to which the tissue blocks x-ray penetration.

randomized controlled trial (RCT) The primary study method for testing effectiveness of a medical treatment. Patients are randomized to receive either a treatment or usual care, with a comparison of outcomes to evaluate the effect of treatment.

rapid eye movement (REM) sleep Phase of the sleep cycle marked by the presence of rapid eye movements on electrooculography.

RBC count The number of red blood cells present in the blood; part of a routine complete blood count (CBC).

red blood cell distribution width (RDW) A red blood cell parameter measured as part of a CBC that is particularly sensitive to recent transfusion or maintenance of blood volume through supportive therapies.

refractory hypoxemia Low oxygen levels in the arterial blood that do not respond to conventional oxygen therapy.

repolarization The change in myocardial cell membrane potential in preparation for the next wave of depolarization.

residual volume (RV) The volume of gas remaining in the lung after a forced expiration.

resonant Quality of sound produced upon percussion that is loud, low, and long, such as may be heard over normal lung tissue.

respiratory acidosis Decrease in pH associated with an elevated $Paco_2$.

respiratory alkalosis Increase in pH associated with a decreased $Paco_2$.

respiratory care plan A written plan of the respiratory care to be provided to the patient.

respiratory distress syndrome (RDS) Condition of a newborn characterized by dyspnea with cyanosis; the most common cause for hypoxemic respiratory failure in premature neonates.

respiratory drive Those factors that stimulate breathing.

respiratory effort–related arousal (RERA) Arousals from sleep associated with breathing difficulties that do not meet the criteria for apnea or hypopnea.

respiratory failure A general term referring to an inability of the heart and lungs to provide adequate oxygenation and/or carbon dioxide removal.

respiratory rate (f) The respiratory frequency or number of breaths taken per minute.

restrictive lung disease An abnormality detected by spirometry characterized by reduced lung volumes.

retained secretions Respiratory secretions that are not being properly expelled via the mucociliary escalator and/or cough mechanism.

reticular pattern A linear pattern of all opacification observed on chest x-ray or CT scan of the lung.

reticulonodular pattern An opacification pattern seen on chest x-ray or CT scan of the lung that combines aspects of nodular and reticular patterns.

retinopathy of prematurity Formation of fibrous tissue behind the lens of the eye caused by excessive oxygen administration to premature infants; produces blindness in its worst form; also called retrolental fibroplasia.

retractions Abnormal "sinking in" of the tissue seen on inspiration during marked inspiratory efforts. Most commonly seen between the ribs (i.e., intercostal retractions) and just above (suprasternal) or below the sternum (substernal); may be caused by partial airway obstruction.

rhonchus Deep, rumbling respiratory sound that is more pronounced in auscultation on expiration and is usually continuous, caused by air passing through a partially obstructed airway.

rigid bronchoscopy Introduction of a metal tube into the central airways for diagnostic and therapeutic purposes.

RV/TLC ratio The ratio of the residual volume to the total lung capacity; sometimes used as a measure of pulmonary overinflation.

Sanz electrode Modern pH electrode, which has a small sampling chamber, allowing the use of aliquots of blood volume as small as 25 μL.

sarcoidosis Interstitial lung disease (ILD) in which multiple organ systems usually have noncaseating granulomas; most prevalent ILD of unknown etiology.

Severinghaus electrode Modern Pco_2 electrode, a modification of the PH electrode developed by Stowe in the early 1950s.

shunt Any cardiac or pulmonary condition in which blood passes from the right side of the heart to the left side of the heart without participating in gas exchange.

sickle cell disease A hereditary disorder in which the red blood cells assume a sickle-like shape.

signs The manifestations of a disease state or condition that can be observed by the healthcare provider (e.g., accessory muscle use or intercostal retractions).

silhouette sign Radiologic sign, usually an obliterated border, that helps to localize a radiographic opacity.

sinoatrial (SA) node The heart's natural pacemaker, located in the upper part of the right atrium.

skin testing Testing by injection of the substance subcutaneously; may be used in tuberculosis screening or assessment of allergies.

sleep apnea Sleep disorder in which a person temporarily does not maintain airflow through the nose and mouth, resulting in periodic absence of breathing.

sleep-disordered breathing (SDB) A general term used to refer to a number of different breathing disorders associated with sleep; sleep apnea is one form of sleep disordered breathing.

sleep stages The phases of sleep that are based on the frequencies recorded during an electroencephalogram (EEG).

slow vital capacity (SVC) The maximal amount of air that can be exhaled following a maximal inspiration; gases exhaled slowly to avoid air trapping.

small cell lung cancer (SCLC) Type of lung cancer characterized histologically by the presence of small blue cells on hematoxylin and eosin staining; believed to arise from bronchial neuniendocrine cells.

smoking history The history of the patient's tobacco use, usually recorded as the amount of cigarettes (i.e. packs) or number or cigars consumed per day and the number of years this consumption has continued (i.e., pack years).

SOAP notes A method of charting in the medical record that includes notation of the patient's subjective response (S), objective observations by the healthcare provider (O), assessment of the subjective and objective findings (A), and the plan of action (P) based on these findings.

SOAPIER A form of medical record notation that includes SOAP, the intervention (I), the planned follow-up evaluation (E), and (R) revision of the care plan based on the evaluation findings.

solitary pulmonary nodule (SPN) Lesion, seen on a chest radiograph, that is completely surrounded by lung parenchyma, without other radiographic abnormalities such as pleural effusion or adenopathy.

spectrophotometry Method that identifies substances by their absorption (also called extinction) of specific wavelengths in the electromagnetic spectrum.

spina bifida A congenital disorder associated with incomplete closure of the embryonic neural tube.

spirometer Apparatus for measuring a patient's tidal volume and minute ventilation.

spontaneous breathing trial (SBT) A technique in which the patient is removed from ventilatory support and allowed to breath spontaneously to identify extubation readiness.

sputum Mucus and secretions coughed up from the lower airways.

squamous cell carcinoma Slow-growing malignant tumor of scaly or platelike epithelium.

ST segment elevation MI (STEMI) A classification of myocardial infarction based on ECG appearance of the ST segment.

ST segment Connects the end of the QRS complex to the beginning of the T wave on ECG.

stagnant or circulatory hypoxia Hypoxia due to inadequate cardiac output and/or blood pressure.

startle reflex Normal infant reflex produced by a sudden stimulus.

static total compliance (CST) A measure of the ability of the lung and thorax to stretch together during breathing. It is normally about 60 to 100 mL/cm H_2O.

stress testing A form of cardiac testing in which the goal is to increase the heart rate through the use of physical exertion or the administration of medication. During a stress test, an ECG is recorded, as well as any symptoms the patient may have.

stridor Crowing inspiratory sound, commonly caused by inflammation and edema of the larynx, such as postextubation or croup.

stroke volume Absolute volume of blood ejected during a single contraction of a ventricle.

stroke Cerebrovascular accident; sudden brain abnormality characterized by occlusion by an embolus, thrombus, or cerebrovascular hemorrhage, resulting in ischemia of the brain tissues normally perfused by the damaged vessels.

subcutaneous emphysema Air accumulation in the tissues; associated with alveolar rupture.

submaximal and maximal compensation A respiratory or metabolic acid-base disorder may be uncompensated, submaximally compensated, or maximally compensated. If the disorder is very acute, there is no compensation. If the disorder has been present long enough for maximal compensation, the pH will trend towards normal, but often will not completely normalize. Various formulas are available for predicting maximal compensation.

substernal chest pain Pain centered below the sternum, sometimes associated with cardiac ischemia and myocardial infarction (MI).

surface tension Property of liquid tending to reduce the surface of a liquid to a minimum.

surfactant Surface-active agent, such as soap or detergent, dissolved in water to decrease its surface tension or the tension between the water and another liquid.

surfactant-to-albumin ratio (TDx FLM II) A test of amniotic fluid used to assess lung maturation.

surgical lung biopsy (SLB) Lung tissue sample obtained by surgical procedure, usually performed in the operating room under general anesthesia.

sweat chloride test Method of assessing sodium and chloride excretion from the sweat glands; often the first test done in the diagnosis of cystic fibrosis.

symptoms The manifestations of the disease state or condition experienced by the patient (e.g., shortness of breath or chest pain).

synchronized intermittent mandatory ventilation (SIMV) Mode of breath delivery or ventilation in which a mandatory breath rate is set and the patient determines the tidal volume and rate of the spontaneous breaths between the mandatory breaths, which are synchronized with the patient's spontaneous efforts.

systemic vascular resistance (SVR) The resistance against which the left ventricle must force its stroke volume with each beat.

T wave That portion of the ECG associated with repolarization of the ventricles.

tachycardia Elevated heart rate, usually > 100 bpm.

tachypnea Increased respiratory rate.

tactile fremitus Palpation of vibrations of the chest wall as a patient speaks.

tension pneumothorax Gas under pressure in the pleural space.

The Joint Commission (TJC) A nonprofit accreditation agency that provides accreditation of hospitals, nursing homes, and other healthcare provider institutions and groups.

thoracentesis Removal of pleural fluid from the chest cavity using a needle or small catheter.

thoracic compliance (chest wall compliance, C_C) The stretchability of the thorax or chest wall.

thoracotomy Surgical opening into the thorax or pleural space.

thrombocytes A type of blood cell (i.e., platelet) involved in blood clotting and tissue repair following injury.

thrombocytopenia A relative decrease in the number platelets in the blood.

thrombocytosis An elevated blood platelet count.

thrombolytic therapy Use of drugs such as tissue plasminogen activator, urokinase, or streptokinase to dissolve an arterial clot.

tidal volume (V_T) The volume of gas passively exhaled after a normal inspiration.

tissue plasminogen activator (TPA) Common thrombolytic agent used to help dissolve clots.

total compliance (C_T) The stretchability of the lungs within the thorax; comprises lung compliance and thoracic (or chest wall) compliance in a reciprocal relationship.

total lung capacity (TLC) The maximal amount of air the lungs can hold following a maximal inspiration.

total parenteral nutrition (TPN) Administration of a nutritionally adequate solution that can meet the needs of a patient who cannot eat by mouth.

total-PEEP The total positive expiratory pressure being applied during mechanical ventilatory support or during spontaneous breathing using a PEEP valve.

transbronchial biopsy (TBBx) Primary bronchoscopic technique for evaluating the alveolar compartment, particularly useful for sampling peripheral parenchymal masses, diagnosing a select number of specific interstitial lung diseases, and obtaining tissue specimens for culture or documentation of tissue invasion or microorganism pathogenicity.

transcutaneous monitoring (TCM) A means of respiratory monitoring of blood gases through electrodes applied to the skin.

transient tachypnea of the newborn (TTNB) A self-limiting disorder that presents in term or near-term infants shortly after birth and is characterized by rapid respirations that usually resolve within 24 to 48 hours.

transillumination Technique in which light is shined through the thorax to assess for the presence of air (e.g., pneumothorax).

transitional flow Flow that is neither laminar nor turbulent; occurs where airways divide.

treatment menu A list of the respiratory therapy treatment options available to the respiratory care practitioner. The basic care treatment menu includes oxygen therapy, bronchial hygiene therapy, lung expansion therapy, and techniques for providing ventilatory support.

trepopnea Shortness of breath experienced while lying on one side.

triple test Maternal blood screening test to assess for the likelihood of fetal genetic defects.

tuberculosis Infection that arises by inhalation of *Mycobacterium tuberculi* from infected, coughing individuals and manifesting with malaise, fever, or no symptoms.

turbulent flow Gas flow that is rough and chaotic with a great deal of eddy formation. Turbulence usually occurs in the upper airways, larynx, trachea, and major bronchi.

tympanic Quality of the loud, drumlike, high-pitched sound typically heard over a gastric bubble during percussion examination or over the chest wall with pneumothorax.

type 1 diabetes A metabolic disorder characterized by low or absent insulin levels resulting from autoimmune destruction of the pancreas.

type 2 diabetes An increase in circulating glucose levels because of insulin resistance.

type I alveolar cells Alveolar epithelial cells that form part of the alveolar–capillary complex and cover a large portion (90%) of the alveolar surface, facilitating the movement of gases across this surface.

type II alveolar cells Alveolar cells that produce surfactant and surfactant-associated proteins.

U wave A wave sometimes seen following the T wave on ECG.

ultrasonography Medical imaging that incorporates the use of ultrasound (i.e., diagnostic medical sonography).

uncompensated An acute respiratory or metabolic acidosis or alkalosis in which there is no compensation.

unstable angina A form of angina pectoris that is irregular and may signal the development of a myocardial infarction.

upper airway obstruction Obstruction of the upper airways, which are usually defined as those above the trachea or larynx.

urinalysis Laboratory tests performed on urine.

valvular heart disease Any valvular lesion or abnormality that can be differentiated hemodynamically into two types, although a combination of both may exist: stenotic lesions due to a decreased valve orifice size or impaired valve opening, or regurgitive lesions due to impairment of valve closure.

valvular stenosis Narrowing of a heart valve.

vasopressor Agent used to increase blood pressure through vasoconstriction.

venous admixture The phenomena in which venous blood moves from the right side of the heart to the left side of the circulatory system (i.e., left heart or aorta) and does not participate in gas exchange.

ventilation–perfusion ($\dot{V}/\dot{Q}$) ratio Measure of effective gas exchange in the lung, or $\dot{V}/\dot{Q}$ ratio; ideally, this ratio should be 1.0 for the most effective gas exchange to occur.

ventilation without perfusion Refers to alveoli that are ventilated but not perfused by adjacent capillaries.

ventilator discontinuation The process by which mechanical ventilatory support is withdrawn; may be abrupt or gradual (i.e., weaning).

ventilator weaning A gradual and systematic reduction in ventilatory support.

ventilator-associated pneumonia (VAP) Pneumonia in a mechanically ventilated patient developing after at least 48 hours of mechanical ventilation.

ventilator-induced lung injury Damage to the lungs sustained during mechanical ventilation and caused by any of several factors, including alveolar overdistention and/or cyclical opening of an alveolus during inhalation and closure during exhalation.

ventilatory failure An abnormal elevation in arterial P_{CO_2}; may be acute, subacute, or chronic.

ventricular fibrillation Completely irregular electrical activity of the ventricles associated with an absence of cardiac output.

ventricular flutter An abnormal cardiac rhythm of the ventricles.

video-assisted thorascopic surgery (VATS) Minimally invasive surgical procedure that incorporates a tiny camera and surgical instruments inserted into the thorax to diagnose and treat certain diseases.

viral load The amount of virus present as a measure of the severity of a viral infection.

vital capacity (VC) The maximum volume of gas that can be exhaled from the lungs after a maximal inspiration or inhaled from a point of maximal exhalation.

volume control ventilation Mode of ventilation in which the ventilator controls the inspiratory flow, time, and tidal volume; the tidal volume in this mode is delivered regardless of resistance or compliance.

WBC count The number of white blood cells present in the blood.

WBC differential The percentage or actual number of each type of white blood cell present in the blood.

weaning Removing a patient gradually from dependency on mechanical ventilation while maintaining an appropriate balance between the load placed on the respiratory muscles and the ability of the muscles to meet that load.

weaning parameters Measurements made to determine when liberation from the ventilator might be possible.

wheeze, wheezing Breath sound characterized by either a high- or low-pitched musical quality; caused by high-velocity airflow through a narrowed airway.

whispered pectoriloquy Voice sound heard during auscultation of the lungs, typically heard with lung consolidation.

white blood cells (WBCs) Blood cells that function as part of the immune response in defending against infection or foreign substances; WBCs include polymorphonuclear neutrophils, lymphocytes, monocytes, eosinophils, and basophils.

work of breathing (WOB) Pressure needed to move a volume of gas into the lungs; sometimes assessed using pressure–volume curves.

Index

Note: Page numbers followed by *b, f,* or *t* indicate material in boxes, figures, or tables, respectively.

Equations

Minute ventilation:
$$\dot{V}_E = V_T \times f$$

Physiologic Dead Space:
$$V_D/V_T = (Paco_2 - P\bar{E}co_2)/Paco_2$$
$$V_D = V_D/V_T \times V_T$$

Alveolar Po$_2$ (abridged alveolar gas equation):
$$P_Ao_2 = Fio_2 \times (P_B - 47) - 1.25 \times Paco_2$$

Oxygenation Index:
$$OI = [(\bar{P}_{aw} \times Fio_2)/Pao_2] \times 100$$

Shunt:
$$\dot{Q}_s/\dot{Q}_t = (Cc'o_2 - Cao_2)/(Cc'o_2 - C\bar{v}o_2)$$

Arterial Oxygen Content:
$$Cao_2 = (Hb \times 1.34 \times Sao_2) + (0.003 \times Pao_2)$$

Henderson-Hasselbalch Equation:
$$pH = 6.1 + \log[HCO_3^-/(0.03 \times Paco_2)]$$

Anion Gap:
$$AG = ([Na^+] + [K^+]) - ([Cl^+] + [HCO_3^-])$$
(Because its concentration is small, $[K^+]$ is often omitted from this calculation)

Respiratory System Compliance on Ventilator (aka Total Compliance):
$$C_{rs} = V_T/(P_{plat} - PEEP)$$

Airway resistance (on ventilator):
$$R_{aw} = (PIP - P_{plat})/\dot{V}$$

Ideal Body Weight (aka predicted body weight [PBW]):
Males: $IBW = 50 + 2.3 \times [Height (inches) - 60]$
Females: $IBW = 45.5 + 2.3 \times [Height (inches) - 60]$

Mean Arterial Blood Pressure (estimate):
$$MAP = [systolic + (2 \times diastolic)]/3$$

Cardiac Output:
$$\dot{Q}_T = HR \times SV$$

Fick Equation:
$$\dot{Q}_T = \dot{V}o_2/C(a - \bar{v})o_2$$

Cardiac Index:
$$CI = \dot{Q}_T/BSA$$

Systemic Vascular Resistance:
$$SVR = [(MAP - CVP) \times 80]/\dot{Q}$$

Pulmonary Vascular Resistance:
$$PVR = [(MPAP - PCWP) \times 80]/\dot{Q}$$

Cerebral Perfusion Pressure:
$$CPP = MAP - ICP$$

Work of Breathing:
$$WOB = \Delta P \times \Delta V$$
(1 joule = 10 cm $H_2O \times L$)

Alveolar to Arterial Oxygen Difference:
$$P(A - a)o_2 = P_Ao_2 - Pao_2$$

Oxygen Delivery:
$$\dot{D}o_2 = Cao_2 \text{ (mL } O_2/100 \text{ mL blood)} \times \dot{Q}_T \text{ (mL/min)}$$